Oxford Handbook of
General Practice

Fourth Edition

Chantal Simon
General Practitioner and Executive Editor, InnovAiT

Hazel Everitt
General Practitioner and Clinical Lecturer,
University of Southampton

Françoise van Dorp
General Practitioner

Guest author
Matt Burkes
General Practitioner

OXFORD
UNIVERSITY PRESS

OXFORD
UNIVERSITY PRESS

Great Clarendon Street, Oxford, OX2 6DP,
United Kingdom

Oxford University Press is a department of the University of Oxford.
It furthers the University's objective of excellence in research, scholarship,
and education by publishing worldwide. Oxford is a registered trade mark of
Oxford University Press in the UK and in certain other countries

© Oxford University Press 2014

The moral rights of the authors have been asserted

First Edition published in 2002

Second Edition published in 2005

Third Edition published in 2010

Fourth Edition published in 2014

Impression: 1

Published in the United States of America by Oxford University Press
198 Madison Avenue, New York, NY 10016, United States of America

British Library Cataloguing in Publication Data

Data available

Library of Congress Control Number: 2013945300

ISBN 978–0–19–967103–8

Printed in Italy by
L.E.G.O S.p.A.—Lavis TN

Contents

Luteinizing hormone (LH)	P	0.8–12u/L
Follicle-stimulating hormone (FSH)	P/S	0.8–11.5u/L
		>30u/L post menopause
Prolactin	P	♂ <450u/L
		♀ <600u/L
Prostate-specific antigen (PSA)	P	<50y 0–2.5 micrograms/L 📖 p. 459
		50–59y 0–3.5 micrograms/L
		60–69y 0–4.5 micrograms/L
		>70y 0–6.5 micrograms/L
Thyroxine (free T$_4$)	P	8–22pmol/L
TSH	P	0.35–5.5mLu/L

P = plasma (e.g. heparin bottle); S = serum (clotted—no anticoagulant).

Haematology	**Reference interval**
Haemoglobin	♂ 13.0–17.0g/L
	♀ 12.0–15.0g/L
Red cell count (RCC)	♂ 4.5–5.5 × 10^{12}/L
Erythrocytes	♀ 3.8–4.8 × 10^{12}/L
Packed cell volume (PCV) or haematocrit	♂ 0.40–0.50
	♀ 0.36–0.46
Mean cell volume (MCV)	80–100fL
Mean cell haemoglobin (MCHC)	32.0–36.0g/dL
White cell count (WCC)	4.0–11.0 × 10^9/L
Neutrophils	2.0–7.5 × 10^9/L *40–75% WCC*
Lymphocytes	1.5–4.0 × 10^9/L *20–45% WCC*
Eosinophils	0.04–0.50 × 10^9/L *1–6% WCC*
Basophils	0.02–0.10 × 10^9/L *0–1% WCC*
Monocytes	0.2–1.0 × 10^9/L *2–10% WCC*
Platelet count	150–400 × 10^9/L
Reticulocyte count	♂ 25–135 × 10^9/L
	♂ 20–120 × 10^9/L
	*0.5–2.5%**
Erythrocyte sedimentation rate (ESR)	📖 p. 665
	<50y ♂ 10mm, ♀ 19mm
	51–60y ♂ 12mm, ♀ 19mm
	61–70y ♂ 4mm, ♀ 20mm
	>70y ♂ 30mm, ♀ 35mm
International normalized ratio (INR)	Therapeutic ranges 📖 p. 676

* Only use % if red cell count is normal. Otherwise, use absolute value.

Foreword

pace of change in general practice seems to be accelerating, and there
been a lot of change for the fourth edition of the *Oxford Handbook*
General Practice. For this new edition, we welcome Dr Matt Burkes as
est Editor. He has recently finished GP training and has been responsi-
for the chapters on mental health and skin problems.

ince the last edition of the OHGP, clinical general practice has moved
apace with new treatments, guidelines, and care pathways, changing the
in which we work. There has been a continued move of work from
ondary care to primary care to enable patients to be cared for closer
ome, and our ageing population means that many of our patients have
tiple morbidities that must be managed simultaneously. Furthermore,
must continue to provide high-quality care within an environment of
easing public expectation and decreasing financial resources.

he administration of general practice in the UK is also changing, as the
olved nations' healthcare systems move further apart. GP practices
he UK now need to meet standards imposed by the Care Quality
mmission, and perhaps the biggest change is the abolition of Primary
e Trusts (just in England) and their replacement with GP-led commis-
ing through Clinical Commissioning Groups.

evalidation has also become a reality. All GPs in the UK registered with
General Medical Council must demonstrate their fitness to practise
ry five years. Perhaps unsurprisingly, GP training is changing too. General
ctice has traditionally had the shortest training of all specialties in the
The need for a widening clinical skills and knowledge base, improved
eralist skills to promote health, prevent disease and manage people with
nplex problems in a variety of different settings, and improved public
lth and leadership skills have led to a successful bid by the RCGP to
ance and lengthen GP training to prepare GPs fit for the future.

o address all these factors, within the non-clinical sections of this new
tion of the OHGP, we have included new sections on revalidation,
anced and extended GP training, commissioning, changes to benefits
low income, sickness and disability, and Care Quality Commission
stration. In addition, as well as updating all the clinical information
ne with current guidance within the clinical sections of this edition,
have included photographs within the text for the first time. Due to
ce limitations, we have used these initially just within the dermatology
ophthalmology chapters, and we hope that you will find them useful.

s always, we welcome any feedback from our readers. We would also
to thank the many of you who have contacted us to point out errors,
issions, and ways to improve the OHGP in the past. It is thanks to you
the feedback that you provide that the OHGP continues to develop
neet your day-to-day needs.

CS
HE
FvD

Acknowledgements

s book would not have come into being without input from a large
nber of individuals.

irst, we would like to thank our very select and helpful editorial team at
ford University Press: Helen Liepman, Liz Reeves, and Michael Hawkes.
en was brave enough to commission us to write the first edition of the
ord Handbook of General Practice (OHGP) in 1999 and then moved to
er projects. Liz left us midway through preparation of the third edition
the OHGP to go on maternity leave. Therefore, it has been lovely to
e both back on the team for this fourth edition.

Next, we would like to thank our long-suffering families. Writing and
ting a book like the OHGP is very time-consuming, and we all have
er 'day jobs'. Without the support of our families, a project like the
IGP would not be possible. In alphabetical order, we would like to
e special thanks to our spouses: David Gough, Ruth Searle, Ian Wright,
I Peter Wynn—and children: Adam, Ben, Charlie, Emma, Emily, Flint,
nnah, Helena, Kate, Leif, River, and Sophie.

he OHGP has always had a 'hands-on' feel. That is because it is writ-
by practising GPs who learn new things every day from their patients
I colleagues. We would like to thank all those that we work with for
ir help and support. In particular, we would like to thank the authors,
iwers, and entire Editorial Board of InnovAiT (the RCGP Journal for
s in training), the staff of the Department of Primary Medical Care at
University of Southampton and the GPs, patients, and staff of the fol-
ring practices:

he Banks and Bearwood Medical Centres, Bournemouth, Dorset
)r Godfrey and Partners, Totton, Hampshire
Wilton Health Centre, Wilton, Wiltshire
he Orchard Partnership, Wiltshire
Langley House Surgery, Chichester, West Sussex
Maywood Surgery, Bognor Regis, West Sussex

ally, we would like to give special thanks to all the other many individu-
who contributed, either directly or indirectly, to this edition of the
IGP. We do not always know who you are, as much of the OHGP is
er-reviewed anonymously, but your expert input has been extremely
uable. In particular, we would like to thank:

Mr Richard Newsom (Consultant Ophthalmologist, Southampton
University Hospitals Trust) for his expert help co-authoring Chapter
6 (Ophthalmology).

Dr Helen Dignum (Consultant Haematologist, Portsmouth
Hospitals Trust) for her help providing expert review of Chapter 19
Haematology and immunology) and answering the tricky questions
hat came up when that chapter was sent for anonymous peer review.

Dr Alice Shiner (GP) and **Mr Nikolaos Burbos** (Consultant
Gynaecologist, Norfolk and Norwich University Hospitals Trust) for
heir expert review of Chapter 21 (Gynaecology).

- **Dr Max Watson** (Consultant in Palliative Medicine, Northern Ireland Hospice) for his help with contributions to and review of Chapter 28 (Cancer and palliative care).
- **Dr Roger Gadsby** (GP and Associate Clinical Professor, Univers of Warwick) for his review and expert feedback on Chapter 12 (Endocrinology).
- **Dr Ben Riley** (GP and Medical Director Curriculum, RCGP) for his help providing information about GP training and the RCGP Curriculum for Chapter 4 (Education, monitoring, and research).
- **Dr Waseem Aslam** for his helpful input for the section on multicultural medicine in Chapter 5.
- **RCGP 'Supporting Carers in General Practice' project** (Clinical Leads, Dr Elizabeth Muir, Dr Chantal Simon and Mrs Judith Cameron, the RCGP Professional Programmes Team, and Dr Moir Fraser of the Carers Trust) for providing the information for the pa about carers in Chapter 9.
- **The Cornwall Partnership CASC Team** (Dr Rohit Shankar Dr Giles Richards, Dr Richard Laugharne, and Dr Karl Rathbone) fc allowing us to ask as many questions as we liked about mental heal for Chapter 27.
- **Previous authors and editors of the OHGP** Dr Brian Stevenson, Dr Jon Birtwistle, Dr Knut Schroeder, and Professor To Kendrick.

If there any omissions from this list, we apologize. Please tell us, and v will add your name to the list at the first opportunity.

Abbreviations used in the text

Evidence-based superscripts

NICE guideline

Guideline from a major guideline-producing body

Cochrane review

Clinical evidence

Systematic review or meta-analysis published in a major peer-reviewed journal

Randomized controlled trial published in a major peer-reviewed journal

Referral times

Emergency admission

Urgent referral

Soon referral

Routine referral

Handbook symbols

Note

Warning

OHGP cross reference

Weblink

Telephone number

Female

Male

Controversy

Primary

Secondary

Increased/increasing

Decreased/decreasing

Leading to/resulting in

Approximately

Approximately equal

With or without

Standard abbreviations

AA	Attendance Allowance
AAA	abdominal aortic aneurysm
ABPI	ankle-brachial pressure index
ABPM	ambulatory blood pressure monitoring
ACE	angiotensin-converting enzyme
ACS	acute coronary syndrome
ACTH	adrenocortocotrophic hormone
ADH	antidiuretic hormone
ADHD	attention deficit hyperactivity disorder
AED	automated external defibrillator
AF	atrial fibrillation
AFP/αFP	alpha fetoprotein
AIDS	acquired immune deficiency syndrome
Alk phos	alkaline phosphatase
ALT	alanine aminotransferase
ANF	antinuclear factor
APH	antepartum haemorrhage
ARB	angiotensin receptor blocker
ASD	atrial septal defect
ASO	antistreptolysin O
AST	aspartate aminotransferase
AV	arterio-venous
AXR	abdominal X-ray
BASHH	British Association for Sexual Health and HIV
BCG	Bacille Calmette–Guérin
bd	twice daily
βHCG	beta-human chorionic gonadotrophin
BMA	British Medical Association
BMJ	British Medical Journal
BNF	British National Formulary
BP	blood pressure
bpm	beats per minute

$^{2+}$	calcium
BG	coronary artery bypass graft
F	congestive cardiac failure
G	Clinical Commissioning Group
IC	combined hormonal contraception
ID	coronary heart disease
IS	central nervous system
OC	combined oral contraceptive
PD	chronic obstructive airways disease
	creatinine
P	C-reactive protein
	computerized tomography
A	cerebrovascular accident
D	cardiovascular disease
S	cardiovascular system
KR	chest X-ray
	days
OH	developmental dysplasia of the hip
S	Directed Enhanced Service
H	Department of Health
PJ	distal interphalangeal joint
A	Disability Living Allowance
M	diabetes mellitus
N	district nurse
E	digital rectal examination
VLA	Driving and Vehicle Licensing Authority
T	deep vein thrombosis
V	Epstein–Barr virus
G	electrocardiogram
no	echocardiogram
G	electroencephalogram
T	ear, nose, and throat
AU	early pregnancy assessment unit

ESA	Employment and Support Allowance
ESR	erythrocyte sedimentation rate
ESRD	end-stage renal disease
FBC	full blood count
FBG	fasting blood glucose
FEV$_1$	forced expiratory volume in 1 second
FH	family history
FSH	follicle-stimulating hormone
FSRH	Faculty of Sexual and Reproductive Healthcare
FVC	forced vital capacity
g	grams
GA	general anaesthetic
GI	routine referral
GGT	gamma glutamyl transferase
GMC	General Medical Council
GMS	General Medical Services
GP	general practitioner
GPC	General Practitioner Committee
GTN	glyceryl trinitrate
GTT	glucose tolerance test
GU	genito-urinary
GUM	genito-urinary medicine
h	hours
Hb	haemoglobin
HbA1c	glycosylated haemoglobin
HBPM	home blood pressure monitoring
HBsAg	hepatitis B surface antigen
HDL	high density lipoprotein
Hib	*Haemophilus influenzae* type b
HIV	human immunodeficiency virus
HOCM	hypertrophic obstructive cardiomyopathy
HRT	hormone replacement therapy

V	herpes simplex virus
	health visitor
S	high vaginal swab
	intracranial pressure
	immunoglobulin
)	ischaemic heart disease
	intramuscular
R	international normalized ratio
	information technology
	international units
CD	copper intrauterine device
)	intrauterine device
	progestogen-containing intrauterine system
	intravenous
	intravenous pyelogram
	Jobseeker's Allowance
	jugular venous pressure
	potassium
	kilograms
B	kidney, ureters, and bladder X-ray
	litres
	local anaesthetic
BB	left bundle branch block
	Local Enhanced Service(s)
	liver function tests
	luteinizing hormone
	left iliac fossa
P	last menstrual period
WH	low molecular weight heparin
TI	lower respiratory tract infection
OT	long-term oxygen therapy
Q	left upper quadrant
F	left ventricular failure

LVH	left ventricular hypertrophy
m	metres
mane	in the morning
MAOI	monoamine oxidase inhibitor
M,C&S	microscopy, culture, and sensitivity
MCP	metacarpophalangeal
MCV	mean cell volume
MDI	metered dose inhaler
mg	milligrams
MHRA	Medicines and Healthcare products Regulatory Agency
MI	myocardial infarction
min	minutes
mL	millilitres
MMR	measles, mumps, and rubella
MND	motor neurone disease
mmHg	millimetres of mercury
mo	months
MRI	magnetic resonance imaging
MS	multiple sclerosis
MSU	midstream urine
Na^+	sodium
NAAT	nucleic acid amplification test
NES	National Enhanced Service
NHS	National Health Service
NI	National Insurance
NICE	National Institute for Health and Care Excellence
nocte	at night
NSAID	non-steroidal anti-inflammatory drug
NSTEMI	non-ST elevation myocardial infarction
O_2	oxygen
OA	osteoarthritis
OCD	obsessive–compulsive disorder
od	once daily
OOH	out-of-hours

'C	over-the-counter
N	polyarteritis nodosa
	percutaneous coronary intervention
O	primary care organization
	Parkinson's disease
	pulmonary embolus
FR	peak expiratory flow rate
T	pre-eclamptic toxaemia
CT	primary healthcare team
	Personal Independence Payment
J	proximal interphalangeal joint
H	past medical history
S	Personal Medical Services
	practice nurse
	oral
$_4^{3-}$	phosphate
P	progesterone-only pill
H	post-partum haemorrhage
	per rectum
	as needed
s	four times daily
)F	Quality and Outcomes Framework
	rheumatoid arthritis
BB	right bundle branch block
GP	Royal College of General Practitioners
OG	Royal College of Obstetricians and Gynaecologists
)	rhesus factor
	right iliac fossa
A	road traffic accident
Q	right upper quadrant
	seconds
	subcutaneous
	systemic lupus erythematosus
L	space-occupying lesion

SNRI	serotonin and noradrenaline reuptake inhibitor
SSRI	selective serotonin reuptake inhibitor
stat	immediately
SpO_2	peripheral oxygen saturation
STEMI	ST elevation myocardial infarction
STI	sexually transmitted infection
SVC	superior vena cava
TB	tuberculosis
TCA	tricyclic antidepressant
tds	three times daily
TFT	thyroid function tests
TIA	transient ischaemic attack
u	units
U&E	urea and electrolytes
UC	ulcerative colitis
URTI	upper respiratory tract infection
US(S)	ultrasound scan
UTI	urinary tract infection
VF	ventricular fibrillation
VSD	ventriculoseptal defect
VT	ventricular tachycardia
WCC	white cell count
wk	weeks
y	years

❶ *All other abbreviations are defined in the text on the page in which the appear.*

Elderly care and child health flags: conditions peculiar to children elderly people, or in which management varies for these groups, are flag as follows:

Child health

Elderly care

What is general practice?

What is general practice?

*'Generalism describes a philosophy of practice which is person, not dise
centred; continuous, not episodic; integrates biotechnical and biographical ,
spectives; and views health as a resource for living and not an end in itsel,*

In the early 19th century, when apothecaries, physicians, and surgeons provi
medical care, the term 'general practitioner' became applied to apothecaries
ing the Membership Examination of the Royal College of Surgeons of Engla

Over the past 60y, general practice has established itself as the corr
stone of most national healthcare systems. In so doing, general pra
tioners (GPs or family physicians) have shown the intellectual framew
within which they operate is different from, complementary to, but no
demanding than that of specialists.

What is medical generalism? The RCGP defines medical general
as: 'An approach to the delivery of healthcare that routinely applie
broad and holistic perspective to the patient's problems.' It invol
- Seeing the person as a whole and in the context of his/her family an
  wider social environment
- Using this perspective as part of the clinical method and therapeutic
  approach to all clinical encounters
- Being able to deal with undifferentiated illness and the widest range
  patients and conditions
- In the context of general practice, taking continuity of responsibility
  people's care across many disease episodes and over time
- Also in general practice, coordinating care as needed across
  organizations within and between health and social care

The role of the GP In the UK, >90% of the population is registe
with a GP. GPs diagnose illness, treat minor illness within the commur
promote better health, prevent disease, certify disease, monitor chrc
disease, and refer patients requiring specialist services. General practic
the primary point of access to healthcare services.

Although patients have an average of 5.5 consultations with their GP ev
year in the UK, only 1 in 20 consultations results in a secondary care refe
Everything else is dealt with in the primary care setting. To do this, GPs m
- Have a working knowledge of the whole breadth of medicine
- Maintain ongoing relationships with their patients—they are the onl
  doctors to remain with their patients through sickness and health
- Focus on patients' response to illness rather than the illness itself,
  taking into account personality, family patterns, and the effect of the
  on the presentation of symptoms
- Be interested in the ecology of health and illness within communitie
  and in the cultural determinants of health beliefs, and
- Be able to draw on a far wider range of resources than are taught
  in medical school, including intuition, knowledge of medicine,
  communication skills, business skills, and humanity

---

[1] Reeve J (2010) Protecting generalism—moving on from evidence-based medicine? *BJGP* **60**:

ddition to day-to-day medical care of their patients, GPs in the UK
e a number of additional roles:

atekeeping GPs control access to hospital-based services, enabling
st-effective care

avigating GPs work with patients/carers to guide them effectively
d safely through the healthcare system

ervice redesign and improvement GPs manage service provision
ithin their own practices, and beyond their practice boundaries

esearch GPs need critical appraisal skills to understand and apply
levant evidence to inform clinical decision making. They need to be
mpetent in collecting and analysing data for service improvement,
d must collaborate effectively in primary care-based research

ducation GPs can be effective teachers in a wide range of contexts,
ducating patients, practice staff, medical students and junior doctors,
llow GPs, and the general public

eadership Many GPs have leadership roles—in their own practices,
ithin their localities, or nationally

at is the difference between GPs and specialists? Marshall
inker contrasted the role of generalists and specialists as shown in
e 1.1

ble 1.1 Differences between GPs and specialists

s	Specialists
lude the presence of serious disease	Confirm the presence of serious disease
erate uncertainty—managing ients with undifferentiated symptoms	Reduce uncertainty—investigating until a diagnosis is reached
lore probability seeing patients n a population with a relatively low dence of serious disease	Explore possibility seeing a preselected population of patients with a relatively high incidence of serious disease
rginalize danger—recognizing and ng on danger signs even when gnosis is not certain	Marginalize error—ensuring accurate diagnosis and treatment

perform their roles well, GPs must show empathy for their patients;
agement and commitment to involve themselves in every aspect of
ent care; appreciation of the limits of their skills and expertise; and
fessionalism in their dealings with both patients and colleagues.

ther information

ependent Commission on Generalism Guiding patients through com-
ity: modern medical generalism (2011) ℘ www.rcgp.org.uk

GP Medical Generalism: Why expertise in whole person medicine
ters (2012) ℘ www.rcgp.org.uk

on C (2009) From generalism to specialty: a short history of general
tice. *InnovAiT* **2**:2–9.

inker M (2009) General practice and the new contract. In: Bevan G,
inker M (eds) *Greening the White Paper*. London: Social Marketing
ndation.

General practice in the UK

Today, along with opticians, dentists, and pharmacists, GPs form the 'f line' of the NHS in the UK, providing primary medical care and actin 'gatekeepers' to the secondary care system.

Workload ~97% of the British population are registered with a Patients register with a practice of their choice in their area—wl families are often registered with the same practice. Once registe patients stay with that practice for an average of 12y. GPs carry ~300 million consultations/y in England alone—82% at the surgery 4% at the patient's home. 70% of the GP's total workload is spent wi patient, while >20% is currently spent on administration.

Working hours Standard working hours are 8 a.m. to 6.30 p.m normal working weekdays for GMS and most PMS practices althc this is currently under review with a proposed change to 8 a.m.–8 cover 7 days a week. Practices may provide 'extended hours' as a (📖 p. 21); to qualify, the practice must provide 30min of additional o ing time/1,000 registered patients at times agreed with the PCO acc ing to local needs. Some practices also provide OOH care (📖 p. How workload is distributed between individual doctors and PHCT is a matter for each practice to decide.

Primary care provider Term used to designate any organization viding NHS primary care services.

Primary care contracts The provider contract with the local F defines services primary care providers will provide, standards to ach and payments they will receive. Currently, there are 4 contract types:
- General Medical Services (GMS) (📖 p. 20)
- Personal Medical Services (PMS) (📖 p. 28)
- Alternative Provider Medical Services (APMS) (📖 p. 29)
- Primary Care Led Medical Services (PCLMS) (📖 p. 29)

Primary care performer list List of all doctors deemed compe to provide primary medical care held by the PCO.

Partnership Group of self-employed contractors working togethe. mutual benefit. A partnership can become a primary care provider as as ≥1 partner is a GP. Although traditionally partnerships are made u GPs only, practice managers, nurses, allied health professionals, and p macists can be included within partnerships.

Independent contractor status Around half of all GPs in the work as independent contractors, providing core primary healthcare vices and additional services as negotiated within their contract. As s these GPs are self-employed, running small businesses or practices. have management responsibilities for staff, premises, and equipment. S most GPs receive a profit share, the amount each GP is paid depends only on income to the practice, but also expenditure:

Income

- **Private work** Includes: private appointments (e.g. clinical assistant, industrial appointments); insurance examinations/reports; private medical examinations and certificates (e.g. HGV licence application
- **Income from the NHS** GMS, PMS, or APMS contract work

penditure

Running costs of the practice Staff salaries; premises (rent, rates, repairs, maintenance, insurance); service costs (heating, water, electricity, gas and telephone bills, stationery and postage); training costs, etc.

Capital expenses Purchase of new medical and office equipment

Salaried GP A GP employed by a PCO, practice, or alternative provider medical services (APMS). PCOs and GMS practices are bound by a tionally agreed model contract, with a salary within a range set by the view Body. PMS practices can make their own arrangements. Salaried sts have advantages for those who do not want to commit to long-term orking within one practice or become involved with managerial tasks. y tends to be less than that of independent contractors.

GP retainer Provides an opportunity for doctors with other commitents to maintain medical skills before returning to full- or part-time nployment at a later date (usually within 5y). Practices approved for the tainer scheme must provide adequate education, supervision, and support. Members of the scheme must:
Have 'licence to practise' (📖 p. 69) and maintain their GMC registration
Work ≥12, but ≤208 paid service sessions a year (one session = 3.5h); most work 2–4 sessions/wk
Do ≥28h of educational sessions/y and take a professional journal

Freelance GP or locum Works for practices or PCOs by a regular or ermittent arrangement or by providing medical cover on a one-off basis. nds to be self-employed and charge on a sessional basis. Long-term cums should make their own pension provision or apply to join the NHS heme. Some freelance GPs work from 'locum chambers' with administtive support to help with bookings and payments.

GP with special interest (GPwSI) 📖 p. 70

GP registrar GP in 3rd/4th year of specialty training 📖 p. 64

Practice boundaries Practices set geographical boundaries around eir practices agreed with their PCOs. Currently, practices only accept w patients onto the practice list who live within that boundary. In gland, practice boundaries for patient registrations will be abolished er October 2014. However GPs will not be required to do home visits patients living outside their practice boundaries; these will become the sponsibility of NHS England Local Area Teams.

Practice lists All patients registered with a particular primary care prorder. Lists may be *open* (accepting new patients) or, by agreement with e PCO for a set period of time, *closed* to new patients 📖 p. 46.

Polyclinics Also referred to as 'Darzi centres' are found in urban cenes throughout the UK. They may be owned and run by the NHS, large P practices, private companies, or Foundation Trusts. *Key features:*
Large premises serving up to 50,000 patients and housing up to 25 GPs
GP services alongside other health services, e.g. dentists, pharmacists
Extended services—consultant outpatient appointments, physiotherapy, routine diagnostic services, e.g. ECG, X-ray
Extended opening—urgent care 18–24h/d and routine
GP appointments in the evenings and at weekends

Good medical practice for GPs

GMC duties of a doctor[1]
- Make the care of your patient your first concern
- Protect and promote the health of patients and the public
- Provide a good standard of practice and care
  - Keep your professional knowledge and skills up to date
  - Recognize and work within the limits of your competence
  - Work with colleagues in the ways that best serve patients' interes
- Treat patients as individuals and respect their dignity
  - Treat patients politely and considerately
  - Respect patients' right to confidentiality
- Work in partnership with patients
- Listen to patients and respond to their concerns and preferences
  - Give patients the information they want or need in a way they can understand
  - Respect patients' right to reach decisions with you about their treatment and care
  - Support patients in caring for themselves to improve and maint their health
- Be honest and open and act with integrity
  - Act without delay if you have good reason to believe that you c a colleague may be putting patients at risk
  - Never discriminate unfairly against patients or colleagues
  - Never abuse your patients' trust in you or the public's trust in t profession

You are personally accountable for your professional practice and m always be prepared to justify your decisions and actions.

Good medical practice for GPs[2]
- **Good clinical care** Provide best possible clinical care for patients
- **Maintaining good medical practice** Monitor, review, and continuou strive to improve performance of yourself and your practice
- **Teaching and training, appraising and assessing** 📖 p. 60
- **Relationships with patients** Communicate with and listen to views opinions of your patients; use terms/information they can understan respect their privacy and dignity at all times
- **Working with colleagues** Ensure effective communication channels within/outside the practice; ensure an environment for personal/ professional development for everyone working within the practice
- **Probity** Behave in a proper fashion, ensuring honesty and openness all matters. Avoid conflicts between personal and professional roles Research 📖 p. 82
- **Health** GPs must be able to perform their roles to an adequate standard and be safe to practise. Concerns about performance 📖 p. 69

[1] Reproduced with permission of the GMC
[2] Summarized from Good medical practice for GPs (2008) 🔗 www.rcgp.org.uk

ntinuity of care A patient seeing the same healthcare worker over
e. In the UK, this has been the norm, but continuity of care is becoming
available.

sons for continuity of care A practitioner's sense of responsibility
ard his/her patients ↑ with duration of relationship and number of
tacts. Continuity builds trust, creates a context for healing, and ↑ prac-
ner's and patient's knowledge of each other. *Evidence:*
  patient and doctor satisfaction
  compliance
  uptake of preventive care, and
etter use of resources (time spent in the consultation, discriminatory
se of laboratory tests, and admission to hospitals)

ents' desire for personal care depends on the reason for the encoun-
Most find it important to see their own GP for serious medical condi-
s and emotional problems.

sons why continuity of care is becoming less available Problems bal-
ng accessibility, flexibility, and continuity of care:
octor factors Flexible careers, special interests, and managerial
esponsibilities all limit the availability of GPs to their patients
atient factors 24h society, in which patients want to be seen at
eir convenience rather than when their GP is available, makes it
npossible to maintain continuous care. For minor problems and
mergencies, patients do not mind who they see—as long as they see
omeone who can deal with their problem quickly
ystem factors Changing roles—nurse practitioners and other
ealthcare professionals commonly take on tasks which used to be
one by GPs; clinical governance structures mean that patients with
articular conditions are managed in clinics specifically for those
onditions within the practice; other primary healthcare providers,
.g. NHS 111, walk-in clinics, and separate out-of-hours cover
rrangements, further fragment care

tioning A full discussion on rationing healthcare is beyond the
pe of this handbook, but, with continued innovation, rising demand,
limited resources, it will become an increasingly important factor
medicine worldwide. To some extent, there is already rationing by
ault—medicines and certain treatments are not provided on the
S or have very long waiting lists. Government bodies, such as NICE,
luate services and develop guidelines for healthcare professionals
ut medicines and services which are both clinically and cost-effective.
vitably, this will mean that some groups will feel they are being deprived
he treatment they require. It will remain a contentious issue.

rther information
praisal and revalidation 📖 p. 68
C/RCGP Good medical practice for GPs (2008) ℬ www.rcgp.org.uk
C Duties of a doctor ℬ www.gmc-uk.org

Stress in general practice

Increasing stress is a feature of society as a whole. GPs score twice national average on stress test scores. Similar figures are seen if anxi scores are used, and 1 in 4 GPs are classed as suffering from depressi depression screening tools are used. Burnout describes the syndrom emotional exhaustion, depersonalization, low productivity, and feelin low achievement. Studies of British GPs consistently find significant bers of GPs in all age groups are affected.

Causes of stress in general practice Insecurity about w (particularly changes in NHS structure and complaints), isolation, relationships with other doctors, disillusionment with the role of changing demands, work–home interface, demands of the job (particu time pressure, problem patients, and emergencies during surgery ho patients' expectations, and practice administration.

Roots of stress Many of the main stressors for GPs appear to created or perpetuated by doctors' own policies: overbooking pati starting surgeries late, accepting commitments too soon after surgerie due to finish, making insufficient allowances for extra emergency pati and allowing inappropriate telephone or other interruptions. Higher average pressure scores occur in doctors with fast consultation compared to those with slower rates.

General characteristics of a stressed person at work are La concentration, poor timekeeping, poor productivity, difficulty in co rehending new procedures, lack of cooperation, irritability, aggres withdrawal behaviour, resentment, ↑ tendency to make mistakes, resistance to change.

Effects of stress
- **Effects on clinical work** One study showed frustrated doctors are more willing to take undesirable short cuts in treating patients; and that those doctors with negative feelings of tension, lack of time, and frustration have poor clinical performance (measured by an ↑ prescription rate and lack of explanation to patients)
- **Effects on practices** Stress has effects on the practice too, resultin in mistakes, arguments or angry outbursts, poor relationships with patients and staff, increased staff sickness and turnover, and accide
- **Effects at home** Stressed GPs may develop problems in their relationships with their partners and family at home, becoming uncommunicative at home or work, and more withdrawn and isola

Experience of stress does not necessarily result in damage. The exte stress necessary to ↓ performance or satisfaction levels will depen the doctor's personality, biographical factors, and coping methods, concurrent illness or coexisting life event may have additive effects can ↑ vulnerability to stress or ↓ ability to cope.

Alcohol Doctors commonly use alcohol as a coping method for st The BMA estimates 7% of doctors are addicted to alcohol and/or c chemical substances, with half of those addicted to alcohol alone.

Interventions and solutions

Improve your working conditions, e.g. longer booking intervals for patient consultations; develop a specialist clinical or academic interest within or outside the practice; learn to decline extra commitments. GPs with high stress levels do not necessarily have low morale, but there is a close correlation between levels of job satisfaction and morale—job satisfaction seems to protect against stress

Look at your own behaviour and attitudes Stop being a perfectionist; resist the desire to control everything; don't judge your mistakes too harshly

Look after your own health and fitness Set aside time for rest and relaxation; make time for regular meals and exercise

Allow time for yourself and your family Do not allow work to invade family time. Consider changes in working arrangements to allow more time for leisure and family

Don't be too proud to ask for help As well as formal channels for seeking help, there are several informal doctor self-help organizations and counselling services (see Useful contacts)

Chronic stress 📖 p. 1002

Useful contacts

Occupational Health Services Available to GPs whose health is causing performance concern.

BMA Doctors for Doctors Service and BMA Counselling Service. Provides members and their families (normally resident with them) with help, counselling, and personal support. Also produces a 'doctors' health and well-being' webpage ☎ 0845 9 200 169 🖰 www.bma.org.uk

British Doctors and Dentists Group Support group of recovering medical and dental drug and alcohol users. Students are also welcomed. Gives confidential help and advice through a local recovering doctor or dentist. ☎ 0779 2819 966

Cameron Fund Provides help and support solely to GPs and their dependants. It can meet needs that vary from those of the elderly in nursing homes to young, chronically sick doctors and their families, and those suffering from relationship breakdown or financial difficulties following the actions of professional regulatory bodies. ☎ 020 7388 0796

Sick Doctors Trust A confidential intervention and advisory service for alcohol- and drug-addicted doctors, run by doctors for doctors. *24h helpline:* ☎ 0370 444 5163 🖰 www.sick-doctors-trust.co.uk

Doctors' Support Network (DSN) Aims to raise awareness of mental health concerns, encourage, doctors to look after their mental health and to seek help early. Confidential, anonymous support service, allowing doctors to talk about issues affecting them, whether mental health, work problems, or anything else ☎ 0844 395 3010

Royal Medical Benevolent Fund Provides specialist information and advice, and necessary financial assistance due to age, ill health, disability, or bereavement. ☎ 020 8540 9194

General practice within the wider NHS

In 1948, the National Health Service (NHS) was formed, giving free hea care for the entire population of the UK paid for by the taxpayer. NHS is now the largest organization in Europe. The structure of the N varies from country to country within the UK.

England (See Figure 1.1)

- **Secretary of State for Health** Head of the NHS responsible to Parliament
- **Department of Health (DH)** Sets overall health policy in England, is headquarters for the NHS, and is responsible for developing and putting policy into practice
- **Monitor** Independent regulator of healthcare in England
- **NHS Commissioning Board** Key link between the DH and NHS. Advises Clinical Commissioning Groups (CCGs) and holds them to account. Manages the budget allocated to the NHS, distributing it to CCGs, and also directly commissions primary care and national servi
- **Healthwatch England** Part of the Care Quality Commission. Provides feedback from service users through a network of Local Healthwatch organizations to the Secretary of State for Health, NH Commissioning Board, Monitor, and local authorities
- **Clinical Commissioning Groups (CCGs)** Cornerstone of the NHS responsible at a local level for planning, providing, and commissioni health services from service providers, and improving the health/ well-being of the local population
- **Health and Wellbeing Boards** Work with patients, CCGs, and loc authorities to develop a *Joint Strategic Needs Assessment* (JSNA) in order to improve health/well-being of the local population. The JSN then influences commissioning decisions across health, public, healt and social care, thus promoting integrated health/social care
- **NHS Trusts** Provide hospital and specialist community services

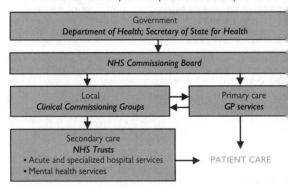

Figure 1.1 Structure of the NHS in England

Northern Ireland The *Department of Health, Social Services and Public Safety* (DHSSPS) is responsible for:

Health and Social Care Board Agent of the DHSSPS in planning, commissioning and purchasing services for the residents of Northern Ireland, including primary care services

6 Health and Social Care Trusts Cover the whole of Northern Ireland (Belfast, Northern, Southern, Western, South Eastern, and Northern Ireland Ambulance Service) and directly provide services to people in their areas

19 Health Agencies Provide national services, e.g. Public Health Agency; Blood Transfusion; Northern Ireland Cancer Screening

Patient and Client Council Provides patient/client feedback to shape services

Further information ☞ http://www.n-i.nhs.uk

Scotland

Scottish Government Health Directorate Responsible both for NHS Scotland and for the development and implementation of health and community care policy

NHS Boards Health services are delivered through 14 regional NHS Boards. These Boards provide strategic leadership and performance management for the entire local NHS system in their areas and ensure that services are delivered effectively and efficiently. NHS Boards are responsible for the provision and management of the whole range of health services in an area, including hospitals and general practice

Special Boards and Public Health Body Scotland has seven Special Boards delivering services across the whole of Scotland e.g. Scottish Ambulance Service; NHS24. In addition, there is one Public Health Body

Further information ☞ www.show.scot.nhs.uk

Wales The NHS is Wales' largest employer (7% workforce).

National Advisory Board Responsible for providing independent advice to the Welsh Minister for Health and Social Services

National Delivery Group The Chief Executive, NHS Wales, is responsible for providing the Welsh Minister for Health and Social Services with policy advice and for exercising strategic leadership and management of the NHS. To support this role, the Chief Executive chairs a National Delivery Group, forming part of the Department for Health and Social Services (DHSS). This group is responsible for overseeing the development and delivery of NHS services across Wales

Local Health Boards (LHBs) 7 boards secure/deliver healthcare services in their areas. LHBs are responsible for commissioning GP services from practices, and community and secondary care services

NHS Trusts 3 Trusts deliver services that operate throughout Wales. These are: Public Health Wales, Welsh Ambulance Services NHS Trust, Velindre NHS Trust offering cancer care services, and the Welsh Blood Service

Community Health Councils 7 statutory lay bodies (one for each LHB) that represent the interests of the public

Further information ☞ http://www.wales.nhs.uk

Organizations important to general practice

British Medical Association (BMA) Voluntary professio association and independent trade union of doctors. >80% of UK doct are members. Also runs a publishing house, producing books and journ (including the BMJ); negotiates doctors' pay and terms of service; prov advice about matters related to work practice; provides educational research facilities, accommodation, dining facilities, and financial servi The General Practitioners Committee (GPC) is a subgroup.

Further information ☎ 020 7387 4499 ✍ www.bma.org.uk

Care Quality Commission (CQC) A independent public body. functions are to:
- Assess management, provision and quality of health and social care i England (including GP practices)
- Regulate the independent healthcare sector through registration, annual inspection, monitoring complaints, and enforcement
- Publish information about the state of health and social care
- Consider complaints about NHS organizations that the organizatior themselves have not resolved
- Coordinate reviews and assessments of health and social care and carry out investigations of serious failures in the provision of care

Further information ✍ www.cqc.org.uk

General Medical Council (GMC) Licenses doctors to prac medicine in the UK. It investigates complaints against doctors and the authority to revoke a doctor's licence, if appropriate. It also monit standards of undergraduate, postgraduate, and continuing med education and provides information about good medical practice.

Further information ✍ www.gmc.org.uk

General Practitioners Committee (GPC) BMA commit with authority to deal with all matters affecting NHS GPs, represen all doctors in general practice, whether or not they are a member of BMA. The committee is recognized as the sole negotiating body for gen practice by the DH.

Further information ✍ www.bma.org.uk

Independent Complaints Advocacy Service (ICAS) Supp patients and their carers wishing to pursue a complaint about their N treatment or care.

Local Medical Committee (LMC) Committee of GPs represer tive of GPs in their area. All GPs (including locums and salaried doct are represented by LMCs. *Functions:*
- **Statutory** Consultation regarding administration of the GMS and PN contracts; involvement with disciplinary and professional conduct committees; representation of GPs as a whole
- **Non-statutory** Advice on all matters concerning GPs; communicati between GPs; links with other bodies; helping individual GPs

National Association of Sessional GPs (NASGP) Acts as a voice and resource for all NHS GPs who work independently of the traditional 'GP principal' model. This includes GP locums, retainers, salaried GPs, and GP assistants.

Further information ℘ www.nasgp.org.uk

National Institute for Health and Care Excellence (NICE) Special authority which aims to provide patients, health and social care professionals, and the public with authoritative guidance on 'best practice' and thus improve the quality/consistency of health and social care services. It evaluates health technologies and reviews management of specific conditions.

Further information ℘ www.nice.org.uk

NHS Business Services Authority (NHSBSA) 📖 p. 141

Patient Advice and Liaison Service (PALS) Provided by all healthcare organizations running hospitals, GP or community health services. Equivalent service in Scotland is the Patient Advice and Support Service (PASS). Aims to:

- Advise and support patients, their families, and carers
- Provide information on NHS services
- Listen to and record concerns, suggestions, or queries. PALS can liaise directly with NHS staff and managers regarding patients' concerns
- Help to sort out problems quickly
- Direct NHS users to sources of independent advice and support, e.g. Independent Complaints Advocacy Services (ICAS)

Royal College of General Practitioners (RCGP) Founded to 'encourage, foster and maintain high standards within general practice and to act as the voice of GPs on issues concerned with education, training, research and standards'. Services include:

- Publishing—books and journals including *British Journal of General Practice* and *InnovAiT*
- Education—online learning, courses, conferences
- Revalidation support, including e-portfolio
- Representation of GPs at national and international levels
- International collaboration, including international membership section
- Support for specific groups, e.g. First5 (for GPs within 5y of their Certificate of Completion of Training); AiT Committee for GPs in training

Statutory responsibilities include:

- Developing and updating the GP training curriculum
- Setting and managing the UK licensing examination for general practice
- Managing certification and recertification

3 grades of membership:

- **Members** are entitled to speak and vote at meetings, and to use the designation MRCGP (📖 p. 66)
- **Fellows** Highest grade of membership; holders use the designation FRCGP (📖 p. 66)
- **Associates** For doctors still in training. Associates can participate in College activities but cannot vote or use the designation MRCGP

Further information ℘ www.rcgp.org.uk

Practice in other countries

It is beyond the scope of this book to discuss different systems of health care and practice regulations outside the UK; however, in most countries there is a registration body (usually termed the 'Medical Council') which ensures doctors are qualified and fit to practise; an organization representing the interests of the medical profession generally (often termed the 'Medical Association'); and separate specialist bodies representing the interests of family practitioners. Details can be obtained from the following websites:

International Directory of Medical Regulatory Authorities Lists worldwide medical regulatory bodies and contact details. ✆ www.iamra.com

World Organization of Family Doctors (WONCA) Includes list of member organizations and contact details.
✆ www.globalfamilydoctor.com

European Union of General Practitioners/Family Physicians Gives overview of different healthcare systems in member states and contacts for member organizations. ✆ www.uemo.eu

Medical Association of South East Asian Nations (MASEAN) Contains contact details for Medical Associations in Brunei, Cambodia, Indonesia, Laos, Malaysia, Myanmar (Burma), Philippines, Singapore, Thailand, and Vietnam. ✆ www.masean.org

Country-specific information

Australia
- Australian Medical Council ✆ www.amc.org.au
- Australian Medical Association ✆ www.ama.com.au
- Royal Australian College of General Practitioners ✆ www.racgp.org.au

Canada
- Medical Council of Canada ✆ www.mcc.ca
- Canadian Medical Association ✆ www.cma.ca
- College of Family Physicians of Canada ✆ www.cfpc.ca

China
- Chinese Medical Association ✆ www.cma.org.cn

Hong Kong
- Medical Council of Hong Kong ✆ www.mchk.org.hk
- Hong Kong Medical Association ✆ www.hkma.org
- Hong Kong College of Family Physicians ✆ www.hkcfp.org.hk

India
- Medical Council of India ✆ mciindia.org
- Indian Medical Association ✆ www.ima-india.org

Ireland (Eire)
- Irish Medical Council ✆ www.medicalcouncil.ie
- Irish Medical Organization ✆ www.health.ie
- The Irish College of General Practitioners ✆ www.icgp.ie

Japan
- Japan Medical Association ✍ www.med.or.jp
- Japan Primary Care Association ✍ www.primary-care.or.jp

New Zealand
- Medical Council of New Zealand ✍ www.mcnz.org.nz
- New Zealand Medical Association ✍ www.nzma.org.nz
- Royal New Zealand College of General Practitioners
  ✍ www.rnzcgp.org.nz

Pakistan
- Pakistan Medical and Dental Council ✍ www.pmdc.org.pk

Singapore
- Singapore Medical Council ✍ www.smc.gov.sg
- Singapore Medical Association ✍ www.sma.org.sg
- College of Family Physicians Singapore ✍ www.cfps.org.sg

South Africa
- Health Professions Council of South Africa ✍ www.hpcsa.co.za
- South African Medical Association ✍ www.samedical.org
- South African College of Family Physicians ✍ www.collegemedsa.ac.za

USA
- Educational Commission for Foreign Medical Graduates (ECFMG)
  ✍ www.ecfmg.org
- American Medical Association (AMA) ✍ www.ama-assn.org
- Federation of State Medical Boards ✍ www.fsmb.org
- American Board of Family Practice ✍ www.abfp.org
- American Academy of Family Physicians ✍ www.aafp.org

Contracts

Partnership agreements

Partnership disputes are common. A properly drafted partnership agreement may prevent disputes and, if they do occur, may lessen their impact

Partnership at will A partnership without an up-to-date written agreement is a 'partnership at will', governed by the 1890 Partnership Act. A 'partnership at will' is a very unstable situation as:

- All partners are deemed to have equal profit shares, unless there is clear evidence to the contrary
- Decisions are made by simple majority
- Notice may be served by any partner on the others without their prior knowledge or consent
- Dissolution of the partnership may take immediate effect, and no reason needs be given to justify it
- Dissolution may result in the forced sale of all partnership assets (including the surgery premises) and redundancy of all staff
- There is nothing to prevent any partner, or group of partners, from immediately forming a new practice/partnership to the exclusion of the other partner(s) once the practice is dissolved

Partnership agreements Should be drawn up every time a new partner joins or leaves a practice. Employed doctors and retainers also require contracts of employment. An agreement checklist is included in Box 2.1. Detailed guidance is produced by the BMA, and further guidance can be obtained from local BMA offices and LMCs.

Partnership disputes However good a partnership agreement is, disputes still occur. Advice on partnership and employment matters is available from the BMA and LMC, and the BMA also provides conciliation services (contact local office). Legal battles are expensive, and the BMA will not fund partnership disputes. Try to resolve matters amicably.

Discrimination It is unlawful for any partnership to discriminate on grounds of age, gender, marital status, colour, race, nationality (including citizenship), ethnic or national origins when appointing a new partner or in the way they treat an existing partner. The BMA will consider backing GPs to take such matters to industrial tribunals—contact the local office. Applications should be made on forms available via local Job Centres and must be made within 3mo of the last act of discrimination.

Contracts of employment for salaried GPs Model terms and conditions of service for a salaried GP and a model offer letter of employment are available from the BMA or DH websites. Nationally agreed salary scales apply and are compulsory for GMS, but not PMS, practices.

Responsibilities towards employed GPs 📖 p. 36

Box 2.1 Partnership agreement checklist

- **Business detail** Purpose of the business; premises and basis of occupation. If premises are owned by the partners, state procedure for valuation, payment of the retiring partner, and investment of the incoming partner
- **Assets** Specify assets, their ownership, arrangements for valuation and interest payments. It is illegal to sell goodwill in NHS practices
- **Income and allowances** Definition of practice income; allowable expenses
- **Profit sharing** Distribution of practice NHS income and other NHS allowances; distribution of income from non-NHS work
- **Accounting** Accounting and banking arrangements; cheque signing; access to accounts and bank statements
- **Taxation** Arrangements for paying tax; obligations of each partner
- **Pension arrangements**
- **Retirement/suspension/expulsion** Reasons for suspension/expulsion; process of suspension/expulsion; mechanisms of voluntary leaving/ retirement; division of assets in the event of retirement. May include a restrictive clause preventing the outgoing doctor working in the practice area for a period of time after leaving—seek legal advice
- **Leave** Holiday entitlement; basis of deciding who has holiday when; study leave; sabbatical leave; sick leave; maternity, paternity, and adoption leave; compassionate leave
- **Obligation** NHS obligations; non-NHS work within the practice; other work outside the practice; educational activities; obligations to each other; hours of work
- **Decisions and disputes** Decision-making process; process to manage disputes; process to dissolve partnership. Ensure that who pays legal fees for who in the event of a dispute is included
- **Correct procedure** Ensure each partner has signed and dated the agreement and that their signature has been witnessed. It is recommended that each partner should take independent legal advice and not rely on the 'practice solicitor' for sole advice

Further information

DH ✎ www.dh.gov.uk
BMA ✎ www.bma.org.uk
Equality and Human Rights Commission ☎ 0845 604 6610 (England); 0845 604 8810 (Wales); 0845 604 5510 (Scotland)
✎ www.equalityhumanrights.com

General Medical Services Contract

Although there may be some differences in process in each of the four countries of the UK, the principles of the General Medical Services (GMS) Contract apply to all.

Primary Care Organization (PCO) PCOs vary across the nations of the NHS but, for the purposes of GP Contracts, are the:
- NHS Commissioning Board in England (NHS England)
- NHS Boards in Scotland
- Local Health Boards in Wales, and
- Health and Social Care Trusts in Northern Ireland

The Contract The GMS Contract is a contract made between an individual practice and a PCO. All the partners of the practice, at least one of whom must be a GP, have to sign the contract. It includes:
- National terms applicable to all practices (the 'Practice Contract')
- A description of which services will be provided by that practice, i.e.
  - Essential services
  - Additional services if not opted out
  - Out-of-hours cover if not opted out
  - Enhanced services if opted in
- A level of quality of essential and additional services that the practice 'aspires' to
- Support arrangements, e.g. for IT and premises
- A summary of the total financial resources

Essential services Services that all practices *must* undertake. These include:
- **Day-to-day medical care of the practice population** Health promotion, management of minor and self-limiting illness, and referral to secondary care services and other agencies as appropriate,
- **General management of patients who are terminally ill**, and
- **Chronic disease management**

Additional services Services that the practice will *usually* undertake but may 'opt out' of. If the practice opts out, the PCO takes responsibility for providing the service instead. The practice then receives a ↓ global sum payment. The services included are:
- **Cervical screening** Opting out results in a 1.1% ↓ in global sum
- **Contraceptive services** Opting out → 2.4% ↓ in global sum
- **Vaccinations and immunizations** Opting out of vaccinations and immunizations altogether results in a 2% ↓ in global sum; opting out of childhood immunizations leads to a 1% ↓ in global sum
- **Child health surveillance** (excluding the neonatal check). Opting out leads to a 0.7% ↓ in global sum
- **Maternity services, excluding intrapartum care** (which is an enhanced service). Opting out causes a 2.1% ↓ in global sum
- **Certain minor surgery procedures** Curettage, cautery, cryocautery of warts/verrucae and other skin lesions—opting out results in a 0.6% ↓ in global sum

Out of hours (OOH) care Practices can 'opt out' of providing an OOH service. The decision must be made for the whole practice—individual doctors within a practice cannot 'opt out' alone. The cost of opting out for a practice is 7% of the global sum. Practices that have opted out of OOH can offer surgeries or consultations within the OOH period as an extended opening hours Directed Enhanced Service by agreement with their local PCO.

Enhanced services Are commissioned by the PCO and paid for in addition to the global sum payment. There are 3 types:

- **Directed Enhanced Services (DES)** Services under national direction with national specifications and benchmark pricing that all PCOs *must* commission to cover their population. These services change from year to year and include payment targets for childhood immunizations, influenza vaccinations, and more complex minor surgery, e.g. joint injections, incisions/excisions
- **National Enhanced Services (NES)** These services have national minimum standards and benchmark pricing but are not directed (i.e. PCOs do *not* have to provide these services). Examples include: anticoagulation monitoring; treatment of drug/alcohol misuse; minor injury services
- **Local Enhanced Services (LES)** Services developed locally to meet local needs. In England, these may be commissioned by CCGs, e.g. special services for refugees

Further detail

Other parts of the GMS Contract covered in greater detail in this book include:

- Carr-Hill Formula 📖 p. 24
- Dispensing 📖 p. 23
- GP pay 📖 p. 22
- Minimum Practice Income Guarantee 📖 p. 23
- IT 📖 p. 22
- Premises 📖 p. 22
- Quality payments 📖 p. 22
- Seniority 📖 p. 23

Further information

DH The GMS Contract ℘ www.dh.gov.uk
BMA The GMS Contract and supporting documents ℘ www.bma.org.uk
NHS Employers ℘ www.nhsemployers.org

GP pay under the GMS Contract

A total sum for GMS services is given to each primary care organization (PCO) as part of a bigger unified budget allocation. PCOs vary across the four nations of the NHS, but, for the purposes of GP payments, they are the NHS Commissioning Board in England, NHS Boards in Scotland, Local Health Boards in Wales, and Health and Social Care Trusts in Northern Ireland.

Payment to practices comprises the following components
- The global sum +
- Quality payments +
- Enhanced services payments +
- Payment for premises +
- IT payments +
- Dispensing payments (if applicable)

The Global Sum Major part of the money paid to practices. It is paid monthly and intended to cover practice running costs. It includes provision for delivery of essential services and additional/OOH services (if not opted out); staff costs; career development; and locum reimbursement (e.g. for appraisal, career development, and protected time).

Quality payments Payment for quality is made in 2 ways:
- **Aspiration payments** Advance payments to allow practices to develop services to achieve higher quality standards. Practices agree their aspirations for quality points the following year with their PCO. Aspiration payments are made monthly alongside global sum payments and amount to roughly 70% of the points achieved in the previous year (for 2012/13, this was equivalent to 2011/12 points achieved × £133.76/point × 70% × adjustment for list size and composition)
- **Achievement payments** Payments made for the practice's actual achieved number of points in the Quality and Outcomes Framework (📖 p. 26) as measured at the start of the following year. Aspiration payments that have already been received are deducted from the total (i.e. actual payment = achievement payment − aspiration pay already received)

Payment for extra 'enhanced' services Paid to practices that provide Directed Enhanced Services, National Enhanced Services, and/or Local Enhanced Services.

Payment for premises and information technology GP premises are funded in many different ways. The GP contract has provision to reimburse practices that rent their premises the cost of the rent, or pay practices that own their premises for the use of those premises. The PCO also reimburses all the IT costs of the practice.

Dispensing GPs Any GP, in an area classified as rural, may apply to dispense to any of his/her patients living >1 mile from the local pharmacy, as long as this would not render the pharmacy's business unviable. A series of fees are paid for providing this service in a similar way to that in which community pharmacists are funded and in addition to the GMS global sum.

Carr-Hill Allocation Formula GMS resource allocation formula for allocating funds for the Global Sum and quality payments. The formula takes the practice population and then makes a series of adjustments based on the profile of the local community, taking account of determinants of relative practice workload and costs. The resulting 'allocation factor' is then applied to the global sum and quality payments made to the practice—📖 p. 24.

Minimum Practice Income Guarantee (MPIG) Designed to protect those practices that lost out when the GP Contract changed in 2004. It is the difference between the Global Sum allocation (GSA) under the new GMS Contract and the Global Sum equivalent (GSE)—the amount the practice would have earned providing the same service under the old Contract. If GSA < GSE, a correction factor (CF) is applied so that GSA + CF = GSE. MPIG is now being slowly phased out.

Seniority payments Payment system based on years of NHS service. Superannuable income is used as a measure of that service. From 2014 this scheme has not been open to new GPs and it will end for all GPs in 2020.

Carr-Hill Allocation Formula

Geographical and social factors result in differing workload for GPs (see Table 2.2). The Carr-Hill Formula allocates payment to practices on the basis of the practice population, weighted for factors that influence relative needs and costs in order to reflect the differences in workload these factors generate.

Age-sex adjustments Older people and children <5y require the most GP care. The Carr-Hill formula uses an age-sex curve to adjust payments to practices based on the age and gender of their registered populations (see Table 2.1).

Table 2.1   Age-sex workload index (using males aged 5–14 = 1)

Age	0–4	5–14	15–44	45–64	65–74	75–84	85+
Male	3.97	1.00	1.02	2.15	4.19	5.18	6.27
Female	3.64	1.04	2.19	3.36	4.90	6.56	6.72

❶ A different age-sex curve is used for Scotland.

Nursing and residential homes Patients in nursing and residential homes generate more workload through ↑ travelling time. The workload factor applied is 1.43.

List turnover Areas with high list turnovers often have higher workload, as patients tend to have more consultations in their first year of registration in a practice. A factor of 1.46 is applied to all new registrations.

Additional needs In the UK (apart from Scotland) Standardized Limited Long-Standing Illness (SLLI) and the Standardized Mortality Rate for those <65y (SMR <65) are best at explaining variations in workload over and above age and sex. They are related to workload by a complex formula used to make the payment adjustment.

Scotland SMR <65 together with unemployment rate, elderly people (>65y) on income support, and households with ≥2 indicators of deprivation are used in the adjustment formula.

Staff Market Forces Factor (MFF) Reflects geographical variation in staff costs practices incur.

Rurality Rural practices have ↑ practice costs (see Table 2.2). Adjustment is made to payments based on a complex formula using average distance patients live from the practice and population density. An additional adjustment is made for a few small practices in Scotland to allow for economies of scale (small practices incur disproportionately high costs as many expenses—particularly relating to premises—must be met regardless of practice size).

Table 2.2 Comparison of inner city and rural practice

	Inner city practice	Rural practice
Deprivation	Above average unemployment; workers on low pay; ↑ single parents; ↑ sick and disabled	1 in 4 rural households live in poverty. Deprivation is more covert
Access to care	Highly mobile populations → fragmented care Non-English speakers (e.g. refugees) have limited access to care Cultural issues can restrict care	Public transport is often poor. Costs of private transport are increasing, making it impossible for some patients to attend the surgery or hospital. Home visiting rates are ↑, and visiting is arranged by geography rather than urgency
Patterns of illness	Social class gradients are found for many different causes of morbidity and mortality	Certain conditions are rarely seen in the town, e.g. poisoning with organophosphate insecticides
Workload	Social deprivation →↑ consultation rates, ↓ consultation times, multiple problems, and heavy workload. ↑ land costs, elderly buildings, and ↑ crime rates → poor premises and ↓ patient, GP, and staff morale	GPs in rural areas take longer to do home visits and may need to travel further to attend meetings or educational events
Recruitment	Potential recruits are dissuaded from applying due to heavy workload, environment, and high property costs	Difficulty recruiting due to ↑ working hours, ↓ income, lack of out-of-hours cover (still the case in some rural Scottish practices) and difficulties covering time off for educational activities

Further information

DH The GMS Contract—Annex D ℘ www.dh.gov.uk

Quality and Outcomes Framework

The Quality and Outcomes Framework (QOF) was developed for the GMS Contract, but there are similar arrangements for those working with other contracts. Financial incentives encourage high quality care.

The domains The QOF is divided into 2 domains (see Table 2.3):
- Clinical indicators, and
- Public health

Indicators Every domain has a set of 'indicators' relating to quality standards that can be achieved within that domain. The indicators are developed by expert groups based on best available evidence and are updated regularly. All data should be available from practice clinical systems. Indicators are split into 3 different types:
- **Structure,** e.g. is a disease register in place?
- **Process,** e.g. is a particular measure being recorded? Is action being taken where appropriate?
- **Outcome,** e.g. how well is the condition being controlled?

Quality points All achievement against quality indicators converts to points. Each point has a monetary value.
- **Yes/no indicators** Points are awarded only if the result is +ve
- **Range of attainment** For most clinical indicators, it is not possible to attain 100% results, so a range of satisfactory attainment is specified. Minimum standard is usually 40–50%. Points are allocated in linear fashion by comparison of attainment against the maximum standard, e.g. if the maximum is 90%, the minimum 40% and the practice achieves 65%, the practice receives 25/50 (i.e. ½) of the available points
- **Minimum standard** All points are awarded if the criterion is met in more than a certain % of cases

Exception reporting Prevents practices being penalized when unable to meet targets due to factors beyond their control, e.g. patients fail to attend for review or medication is contraindicated. It applies to indicators where level of achievement is determined by % of patients reaching the designated level. Practices report number of exceptions for each indicator set and individual indicator. Ensure the reason why a patient has been 'excepted' from the QOF is identifiable in the clinical record.

Reporting on quality Since April 2013, most data for calculating QOF payments have been obtained through the General Practice Extraction Service (GPES) which takes information directly from GP IT systems. Summarized data are then used by the Calculating Quality Report Service (CQRS) to enable calculation of payments for QOF. There is also an annual quality review visit by the PCO. Based on achievement, the PCO confirms level of achievement funding attained and discusses points the practice will 'aspire' to the following year. The process is confirmed in writing and signed off by both parties.

❶ The GPES and CQRS system are also used for calculating payments for National, Directed, and Local Enhanced Services.

Table 2.3 Calculation of points for QOF payments

Components of total points score	Points	Way in which points are calculated
Clinical indicators	425	Achieving preset standards in management of:
		• Asthma • Epilepsy
		• Atrial fibrillation • Heart failure
		• Cancer • Hypertension
		• Chronic kidney disease • Learning disability
		• Mental health
		• COPD • Osteoporosis
		• Coronary heart disease (2° prevention) • Stroke and TIA
		• Palliative care
		• Dementia • Peripheral arterial disease
		• Depression
		• DM • Rheumatoid arthritis
Public health	124	Achieving preset standards in:
		• Blood pressure
		• Obesity
		• Primary prevention of CVD
		• Smoking
		• Additional services
		• Cervical screening
		• Contraception
Total possible	549	

! The QOF changes from year to year. The domains listed here are correct for 2013/14. In 2012/13, the average value of 1 point was:
- England £133.76
- Scotland £133.47
- Wales £133.69
- Northern Ireland £129.88

Further information

BMA The Quality and Outcomes Framework and supporting documents
℡ www.bma.org.uk
NHS Employers ℡ www.nhsemployers.org
GPES ℡ www.hscic.gov.uk/gpes
CQRS ℡ www.systems.hscic.gov.uk/cqrs

Other provider contracts

Personal Medical Services (PMS) Contract The option to become or stay a PMS practice remains an alternative contracting arrangement in the UK. At present, ~40% of GP practices in England work under PMS contracts. *Features*:

- The GMS Contract is a nationally agreed, locally managed contract; the PMS Contract is a locally agreed, locally managed contract
- The PMS contract alters the way the primary care provider, not individual doctor, is paid
- As decision making is closer to the patient, theoretically, PMS Contracts give better flexibility to meet local needs and solve problems
- Practices are paid to provide a package of services, but PMS Contracts do not necessarily contain all the elements of the GMS Contract and may contain others, in addition, by local negotiation. How the practice provides those services is up to the practice
- As for GMS practices, payments to PMS practices are adjusted for practice factors that ↑ workload using the Carr-Hill Formula
- Practices can opt out of additional and OOH services

Budget Most PMS budgets consist of:

- **Practice costs** Staffing, equipment, IT, and premises costs
- **Core services** Services patients would expect to receive from any GP. This is equivalent to the GMS Contract's 'essential' services
- **Additional services** Both those usually expected from a GP (maternity, minor surgery, contraception) and those usually provided by other community/secondary care services, e.g. community nursing or community-based specialist services (e.g. endoscopy, ultrasound). Extra services not usually provided by the GP are known as 'PMS plus'. These services are roughly equivalent to both the additional and enhanced services under the GMS Contract
- **Prescribing budget** (optional)
- **Dispensing budget** (for dispensing practices only)

Quality payments PMS practices can apply for aspiration and achievement payments in the same way as GMS practices. In order to reflect the local nature of the contract, quality standards do not have to be the same as those contained in the QOF. Nevertheless, all standards must be rigorous, evidence-based, monitored fairly, assessed against criteria agreed between PCOs/provider, and paid at appropriate rates.

Specialist PMS Provide medical services to meet the needs of special groups. Patients do not need to be registered for all 'core' primary care services. This enables practices to develop innovative, bespoke models of service delivery tailored to specific needs of groups poorly served in the established primary care system. Some examples are:

- Primary care services for vulnerable groups, e.g. the homeless, refugees
- Specialist services, e.g. outpatient elderly care, home-based palliative care, dermatology, ultrasound, community rehabilitation for stroke
- Specific service provision, e.g. services for violent patients, OOH care, teenage contraceptive services, sexual health clinics

Alternative Provider Medical Services (APMS) PCOs may commission APMS to provide:
   Essential services,
   Additional services (including where GMS/PMS practices opt out),
   Enhanced services, and
   OOH services

APMS contracts for the provision of primary medical services can be made with anyone, for example:
   Existing GMS/PMS practices—through a separate contract
   Groups of other healthcare professionals, e.g. community nurses
   Individuals
   Private companies—including those from overseas
   Secondary care trusts
   Voluntary sector organizations

APMS may be used where specific needs arise, e.g. through practice vacancies or in areas with rapidly expanding populations where extra capacity is needed.

Primary Care Led Medical Services (PCLMS) Under PCLMS, primary medical services are delivered directly by employees of the PCO.

Further information
DH ℘ www.dh.gov.uk

Commissioning

In the Health and Social Care Bill (2011), the UK government laid the foundation for groups of GPs and other clinical professionals to group together in Clinical Commissioning Groups to take on formal responsibility for commissioning the majority of NHS services in England, working in partnership with other health professionals, local communities, and local authorities.

Aims of commissioning

- To design improved patient pathways
- To enable more efficient use of funds so that savings can be used to provide better patient services
- To enable improved community and hospital services that better meet the needs of patients

Clinical Commissioning Groups (CCGs) Every GP practice in England must be part of a CCG. CCGs do not cross local authority boundaries unless there is a clear benefit to patients from doing so.

Governing body Every CCG must have a governing body/board that has decision-making powers. It must meet in public and publish minutes of meetings. The governing body must include

- ≥2 lay members—one with a lead role in championing patient and public involvement and the other with a lead role in overseeing key elements of governance; one of the lay members will either be the chair or the deputy chair of the governing body
- One registered nurse (not employed by a local provider), and
- One doctor from secondary care (not employed by a local provider)

The commissioning cycle See Figure 2.1

Planning Assessment is made of the needs of the local population and resources available. Information is provided by advisory groups set up local to enable CCGs to do this, national clinical networks (providing expert clinical advice), and clinical senates providing a regional overview of service provision. Where identified needs do not have matching resources, the CCG identifies or develops the necessary resource or capacity to meet that need.

❶ CCGs must develop plans in line with the local Joint Strategic Needs Assessment formed in collaboration with patients and the local authority. Health and Wellbeing Boards can refer commissioning plans back to the NHS Commissioning Board if they feel CCGs are not doing this.

Contracting Once resource and need are matched, the CCG commissions services for local patients. CCGs must offer contracts out to tender to 'any qualified provider'. A qualified provider may be an existing NHS organization, or any other organization (including private sector) able to provide the service required. Contracts should cover quality standards, access targets, volumes, prices, and other issues identified.

Monitoring Once a provider is selected and a contract is made, the CCG is responsible for monitoring delivery and ensuring that delivery is kept on track. Funding passes from the CCG to the provider under the terms of the contract.

Revision If delivery is not on track or the needs of the CCG change with time, agreements should be reviewed and revised.

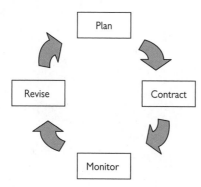

Figure 2.1 The commissioning cycle

A detailed discussion of how each of these stages actually works is beyond the scope of this text.

Although primary care commissioning has only been implemented in England at present, the principles of commissioning are the same whichever organization is commissioning services. Therefore, GPs all over the UK can become involved and influence commissioning decisions by Primary Care Organizations.

Practice management

GPs as managers

'If you have time to do something wrong; you have time to do it right'
W. Edwards Deming

GP partners in a practice have dual roles as both clinicians and managers of small businesses. As such, they must co-operate with their partners and practice manager to run the business side of the practice and with primary health care team members to cover all aspects of the clinical work.

Definition Management is the process of designing and maintaining an environment in which individuals, working together, efficiently accomplish selected aims. The manager coordinates individual effort towards the group goal. To do this, he/she needs technical skill (knowledge specific to the business of the organization); human skill (ability to work with people); conceptual skill (ability to see the 'big picture'); and design skill (ability to solve problems). There are 5 managerial functions:

- **Planning** Involves selecting missions and objectives and the actions to achieve them—requires decision making
- **Organizing** Defining roles—ensuring all tasks necessary to accomplish goals are assigned to those people who can do them best
- **Staffing** Ensuring all positions in the organizational structure are filled with people able to fulfil those roles
- **Leading** Influencing people so that they will contribute to organization and group goals
- **Controlling** Measuring and correcting individual and organizational performance to ensure events conform to plans

Management and teamwork Key features which contribute to successful teamwork are:

- **Communication** Information sharing, feedback, and grievance airing
- **Clear team rules** Especially with regard to responsibility and accountability. Make sure these are understood by everyone
- **Sympathetic leadership** Any team needs a co-coordinator to direct its efforts. A weak leader may allow the team to drift, but an autocratic leader may be too directive and diminish the status of other team members and thus ↓ the effectiveness of the team
- **Clear decision-making process** Especially if differences of opinion
- **Pooling** Knowledge, experience, skills, resources, and responsibility for outcome
- **Specialization of function** Team members must understand and respect the role and importance of other team members
- **Delegation** Work of the team is split between its members. Each member leaves the others to carry out functions delegated to them
- **Group support** Team members share and are committed to a common, agreed purpose or goal which directs their actions

Practice meetings Essential to ensure necessary decisions are made; review policies and agree standards of care; review the financial position of the practice; educate and inform practice members; aid communication; and improve morale of practice members.

Risk management Primary care is about risk and uncertainty, but sometimes unnecessary risks cause ourselves and our patients unnecessary harm. Defence organization records suggest ~½ all successful negligence claims reflect poor clinical judgement on the doctor's part; the other ½ represent avoidable mishaps which would be susceptible to risk management approaches—often failures in simple administrative systems, communication failures, inadequate records, or lack of training.

Risk management means taking steps to minimize risk and keep ourselves and others as safe as possible. All the major defence organizations run risk management programmes for their members. There are 4 stages:

1. Identify the risk—through analysis of complaints and comments from GPs, other practice staff, or patients; through significant event audit (📖 p. 81); or by using material provided by the defence organizations to identify common pitfalls
2. Assess frequency and severity of the risk
3. Take steps to reduce or eliminate the risk
4. Check the risk has been eliminated

Categories of risk relevant to general practice
- Clinical care, e.g. prescribing errors
- Non-clinical risks to patient safety, e.g. security and fire hazards
- Risks to the health of the workforce, e.g. hepatitis B
- Organizational risks, e.g. failure to safeguard confidential information and unlicensed use of computer software
- Financial risks, e.g. employment of a new staff member

Key safety issues for primary care
- **Diagnosis** 28% of reported errors
- **Prescribing** 1 in 5 prescriptions contains a prescribing error; one in 550 prescriptions contains a serious error; 9% hospital admissions are due to potentially avoidable problems with prescribed drugs. 4% of drugs are incorrectly dispensed each year
- **Communication** Poor communication is a major cause of complaints; 28% of patients have discrepancies between the drugs prescribed at hospital discharge and those they receive in the community
- **Organizational change** In industry, better teamwork, communication, and leadership ↓ adverse incidents

In each case, consider
- **Organizational and management factors** Financial resources/ constraints; practice policies; and organization
- **Work environment factors** Staffing levels; skill mix; work load; equipment
- **Team factors** Team structure; communication; supervision
- **Individual (staff) factors** Knowledge and skills; competence; physical and mental health
- **Task factors** Availability and use of protocols/guidelines; availability and accuracy of test results
- **Patient factors** Condition (complexity and seriousness); language and communication; personality and social factors

Practice staff

Practices employ an array of staff. Staff costs are included in the Global Sum (📖 p. 22) paid to a practice.

Recruiting staff

- Review the post—does the post need to be filled or the duties changed?
- Prepare a job description stipulating duties and hours of work
- Prepare a profile of the person required
- Decide on a salary range; the BMA can give advice
- Advertise the post
- Set a closing date for applications
- Shortlist candidates
- Interview—decide who will interview, what points must be covered, and who will ask questions; ask similar questions to all candidates, and score the responses at the time
- Make a decision on the preferred candidate—if in doubt, defer the appointment or re-interview preferred candidates
- Confirm the job offer by letter asking for a formal letter of acceptance in return
- Plan an induction course for the new employee; a probationary period can be helpful for both employer and employee
- Produce a contract of employment

Employment law Very complex field which changes rapidly. If in doubt, contact your local BMA office for advice. *Major points:*

Contract of employment Sample contracts are available from the BMA. Employees have a contract of employment from the day they accept their job—even if it is not written. All employees must be provided with a written statement of the main particulars of their employment <2mo after their start date. This must include: pay, hours, holidays, notice period, disciplinary and grievance procedures.

Pay Workers must be paid ≥ the national minimum wage for every hour worked. Deductions can only be made if authorized by legislation, contract of employment, or in advance in writing by the employee. All employees must receive an itemized pay statement at, or before, the time they are paid, including all deductions.

Notice After 1mo employment, an employee must give ≥1wk notice. An employer must give an employee ≥1wk notice after 1mo, 2wk after 2y, 3wk after 3y, and so on up to 12wk after ≥12y, unless other notice periods are specified in the contract of employment.

Redundancy pay After 2y continuous employment, employers must make 'redundancy payments' related to employee's age, length of continuous service with the employer (to a maximum of 20y), and weekly pay.

Pensions All employees must belong to a pension scheme. The NHS pension scheme is available to practice employees.

Working time Parents of children <6y or disabled children <18y and carers may request flexible working patterns; employers have a duty to consider their requests. Working Time Regulations (1998) apply to agency workers and freelancers as well as employees and include:

- Average working week ≤48h (although individuals can opt to work longer)
- 1d off each week
- Minimum 5.6wk paid annual leave
- 20min in-work rest break if the working day is ≥6h
- 11 consecutive hours' rest in any 24h period (night workers must work ≤8h/d)

Time off Employees are entitled to time off for illness; antenatal care; emergencies involving a dependant; certain public duties (e.g. jury service); to look for another job; and approved trade union activities.

Maternity leave All pregnant employees are entitled to 52wk maternity leave (26wk ordinary maternity leave + 26wk additional maternity leave) regardless of length of service. Women are entitled to return to their own or an equivalent job after their leave. Similar arrangements exist for adoptive mothers.

Paternity leave Employees who have worked for their employer for ≥26wk by the 15th wk before the baby is due and up to the birth of the child are entitled to 1–2wk paternity leave which must be completed within 56d of the birth. Fathers may also claim additional paternity leave for up to 26wk from 20wk to 1y after birth/adoption to look after their child if the mother returns to work.

Parental leave After 1y employment, employees are entitled to 13wk unpaid parental leave for each child born or adopted up to the child's 5th birthday (or 5y after adopted). Parents of disabled children can take 18wk up to the child's 18th birthday.

Health and safety of staff 📖 p. 38

Discrimination Employers must not, either directly or indirectly, discriminate against their staff on the basis of age, race, gender, or disability.

Unfair dismissal Employees of >1y standing (or on maternity, paternity, or adoption leave) are entitled to a written statement of reasons for dismissal. Employers must not dismiss an employee unfairly.

Further information

ACAS Provides advice for employers and employees 📞 0845 747 4747 🖱 www.acas.org.uk

HM Government Information about 'Employing people' 🖱 www.gov.uk

Equality and Human Rights Commission 📞 0800 444 205 Textphone: 0800 444 206 🖱 www.equalityhumanrights.com

GP premises

Funding of premises GPs may either own or rent the property in which they practice:

- **GPs who own surgeries** GPs may own surgeries by themselves or in partnership. They receive a payment ('notional rent') for allowing their private buildings to be used for NHS purposes. Payment is based on the current market rental (CMR) value of the property as assessed by the district valuer. When a new GP partner joins a practiced he/she may be expected to buy into the practice to contribute a share of previous investment in the practice premises and equipment
- **GPs who rent surgeries** Can claim reimbursement from their PCO for the rent they pay as long as it is 'reasonable' as assessed by the district valuer
- **Cost rent scheme** This scheme is no longer available, but many surgeries remain on it. Finance for building, refurbishment, or modification of GP premises was originally raised by the partners. The PCO reimburses the interest payments on the loans taken out to do this
- **Improvement grants** Available via PCOs in some circumstances

❶ New premises/refurbishments must meet national minimum standards.

Disabled access The Equality Act (2010) gives disabled people rights of access to goods, facilities, and services. A disabled person is defined as 'someone who has a physical or mental impairment that has a substantial and long-term adverse effect on his or her ability to carry out normal day-to-day activities'. Practices must:

- Not refuse to take disabled people onto a practice list or provide a lower standard of service due to their disability
- Make reasonable adjustments to their premises and the way they deliver their services so that disabled people can use them

Building regulations and access for disabled patients The building regulations exist to ensure the health and safety of people in and around all types of buildings. Part M deals with access/facilities for disabled people. All new buildings/alterations to existing buildings must be accessible to and useable by anyone, including those with disabilities.

Health and safety The basis of British health and safety law is the Health and Safety at Work Act 1974. The Act sets out the general duties employers have towards employees and members of the public, and employees have to themselves and to each other.

Responsibilities of GPs as employers The Management of Health and Safety at Work Regulations 1999 (the Management Regulations) give clear guidance about employers' duties towards their staff.

1. Employers with ≥5 employees must carry out a risk assessment and record the significant findings. HSE leaflet '5 Steps to Risk Assessment' gives more information
2. Make arrangements for implementing the health and safety measures identified as necessary by the risk assessment
3. Appoint competent people (usually the practice manager) to help implement the arrangements

4. Set up emergency procedures (e.g. fire drills)
5. Provide clear information and training to employees
6. Work together with other employers sharing the same workplace

Other important pieces of health and safety legislation

- **Employers' Liability (Compulsory Insurance) Regulations 1969**
  Require employers to take out insurance against accidents and ill health to their employees and display the insurance certificate
- **Health and Safety Information for Employees Regulations 1989**
  Require employers to display a poster, telling employees what they need to know about health and safety
- **Workplace (Health, Safety and Welfare) Regulations 1992** Cover a wide range of basic health, safety, and welfare issues, such as ventilation, heating, lighting, and seating
- **Reporting of Injuries, Diseases and Dangerous Occurrences Regulations 1995 (RIDDOR)** Require employers to notify certain occupational injuries, diseases, and dangerous events
- **Health and Safety (Display Screen Equipment) Regulations 1992** Set out requirements for work with visual display units (VDUs)
- **Personal Protective Equipment (PPE) Regulations 1992** Require employers to provide appropriate protective clothing and equipment
- **Provision and Use of Work Equipment Regulations (PUWER) 1998** Require that equipment provided, including machinery, is safe
- **Manual Handling Operations Regulations 1992** Cover moving of objects by hand or bodily force
- **Health and Safety (First Aid) Regulations 1981** Cover requirements for first aid
- **Control of Substances Hazardous to Health Regulations 2002 (COSHH)** Require employers to assess the risks from hazardous substances and take appropriate precautions
- **Gas Safety (Installation and Use) Regulations 1998** Cover safe installation, maintenance and use of gas systems and appliances in domestic and commercial premises

Further information

Health and Safety Executive ℘ www.hse.gov.uk

Computers and classification

Computers in practices Under the GMS Contract, PCOs directly fund 100% of IT costs. PMS practices are similarly reimbursed.

Almost all practices now use computers on a daily basis. All specialist GP systems must be approved by the DH (termed 'Systems of Choice'—see Table 3.1). The software covers all aspects of practice from appointment systems, through clinical care, to audit and reporting.

Table 3.1 GP Systems of Choice (GPSoC) suppliers

Supplier	Systems	Web address for information
TPP	SystmOne	℘ www.tpp-uk.com
EMIS	LV	℘ www.emis-online.com
	PCS	
	Web	
Advanced Health and Care	Crosscare	℘ www.advancedcomputersoftware.com
InPractice	Vision 3	℘ www.inps.co.uk
iSOFT	Premiere	℘ www.isofthealth.com
	Synergy	
Microtest	Evolution	℘ www.microtest.co.uk
	Practice	
	Manager II	

Electronic GP records Most GPs maintain all records on computer, i.e. they are 'paperless'.

Read codes Code all aspects of patient care in general practice in the UK. They code in a hierarchical way, e.g. all operations are quantified by 7...; all appendix operations as 770; all emergency excisions of abnormal appendix as 77001. Characters in the code can be numerical or alphabetical. The huge number (58^5) of possible combinations ensures there are enough unused Read codes to accommodate changes.

SNOMED Clinical terms (CT) New coding system that will eventually replace Read coding. The aim is that all healthcare systems in the UK will use the same coding system, allowing a single unified patient record

Summary Care Record (SCR) Electronic summary of patient medication list and drug allergies. Extracted from GP IT systems and can be viewed by healthcare staff in other settings.

NHSnet Intranet connecting NHS organizations which are protected from the Internet by a firewall. This enables NHS users to access the internet but outside users cannot access protected NHSWeb sites. All GP practices in the UK are connected to the NHSnet enabling e-mail, internet access, electronic exchange of information (e.g. laboratory/X-ray results, discharge summaries, out-patient clinic letters), shared information portals, and many other benefits.

Choose and book (C&B) National service that combines electronic booking and choice of place, date and time for first outpatient appointments. *Features:*

- A list of available services and indicative waiting list times for the first outpatient appointment is displayed to the GP
- Appointments can be booked by the GP in the surgery (if the secondary care provider is linked to the C&B system and there is no PCO referrals management system in operation) or patients may receive booking forms at home to book appointments themselves later via the internet or by telephone. This ensures that appointments are made at dates and times convenient for the patient
- Patients and/or clinicians can opt to use any appropriate service paid for by the NHS, whether hospital or community based
- Patients may cancel or alter their appointments at a later date by the same mechanism without going back to the GP
- Each referral is allocated a unique number (UBRN), enabling referral letters to be submitted and retrieved electronically
- The 'advice and guidance' facility enables GPs to contact consultants for advice via C&B

Use of e-mail in the GP surgery 📖 p. 96

On-line patient access In England, all GPs must offer the facility for on-line appointment booking by patients and on-line prescription requests. Proposals to allow patients access to their own summary care record are underway.

Electronic transmission of prescriptions Practices using this service can generate and transmit electronic prescriptions. The electronic prescription is transmitted to the Electronic Prescription Service (EPS). Patients 'nominate' a dispenser to receive their prescriptions who downloads the prescription to issue it. No paper prescription is required.

Care.data Under the Health and Social Care Act 2012, the Health and Social Care Information Centre (HSCIC) can extract personal confidential data (PCD) about patients from GP practice IT systems for planning services or secondary uses (e.g. commissioning, research). This can be done without seeking patient consent. If patients wish to opt out they must actively refuse; otherwise it is assumed that consent has been given.

Electronic sickness certification 📖 p. 125

Further information

NHS Connecting for Health 🖰 www.connectingforhealth.nhs.uk
- GP Systems of Choice
- Electronic prescribing
- Choose and book
- SNOMED CT

DH Good practice guidelines for general practice electronic patient records (v. 4–2011) 🖰 www.dh.gov.uk
British Computer Society Primary health care specialist group 🖰 www.phcsg.org.uk

Useful websites for GPs

Website	Description
Organizations	
www.nhs.uk	NHS
www.dh.gov.uk	Department of Health
www.gmc-uk.org	GMC
www.bma.org.uk	BMA
www.rcgp.org.uk	Royal College of GPs
www.the-mdu.com	UK medical defence organizations
www.mps.org.uk	
www.mddus.com	
Guidelines/books/journals/evidence-based medicine	
www.mapofmedicine.com	Map of Medicine®
www.nice.org.uk	NICE
www.sign.ac.uk	SIGN
www.gpnotebook.co.uk	GP Notebook—online textbook
www.bnf.org	BNF and BNF for Children
www.medicine.ox.ac.uk/bandolier	Bandolier
www.ncbi.nlm.nih.gov/pubmed	PubMed Central
www.bmj.com	BMJ and other BMJ Group journals
www.bmjjournals.com	
www.rcgp.org.uk/Publications/BJGP.aspx	British Journal of General Practice
http://ino.sagepub.com/	InnovAiT—journal for GPs in training
www.elearning.rcgp.org.uk	RCGP Online Learning Environment
www.freemedicaljournals.com	Portal to free medical journals online
www.freebooks4doctors.com	Portal to free medical books online
Other useful medical sites	
www.patient.co.uk	Patient information leaflets
www.rcgp.org.uk	RCGP
www.rcgp-curriculum.org.uk	GP curriculum
www.bma.org.uk	BMA
www.doctors.net.uk	Doctors net
www.adviceguide.org.uk	Citizens Advice Bureau
www.direct.gov.uk	Government guide to services

Website	Description
www.nhs.uk	NHS Choices
www.nhsemployers.org	NHS Employers
Useful non-medical sites	
www.google.co.uk	Search tool
www.bt.com	Telephone directories
www.yell.com	
www.royalmail.com	Postcode finder
www.hmrc.gov.uk	Online self-assessment tax form
www.rac.co.uk	Online travel information—roads
www.thetrainline.com	Train—tickets and timetables
www.streetmap.co.uk	Maps
www.amazon.co.uk	Online book shop
www.bbc.co.uk	General information; news
www.lastminute.com	Travel, gifts, and leisure

Eligibility for free healthcare

Eligibility to receive free hospital care in the UK Is determine by whether a person is resident in the UK and not related to nationality payment of National Insurance or taxes.

Patients from abroad

- Anyone coming to the UK intending to stay for <3mo does not fulfill the qualifying criteria for free non-emergency NHS care
- For patients coming to the UK intending to stay for 'settled purpose', entitlement to free treatment begins on arrival in the UK—there is n qualifying period of residency before free treatment starts

British nationals returning to the UK

- A British resident on extended holiday or a business trip still counts a ordinarily resident and is entitled to free healthcare on return
- Someone who has emigrated, but returns from time to time to take advantage of free NHS care, does not qualify; treat UK nationals permanently resident abroad like any other overseas visitor (unless embassy staff, merchant seamen, in the armed forces, or pensioners)
- Persons (with the exception of pensioners) leaving the UK for >3mo should *not* continue to be registered with a GP; the onus is on patien to inform the authorities and surrender their medical cards
- UK state pensioners who live in the UK for 6mo and the European Economic Area for 6mo every year are entitled to free NHS care; those who have lived in the UK for >10y continuously in the past wh return to the UK under any other circumstances are also entitled to free treatment 'the need for which arises during a visit to the UK'

UK residents going abroad

- Doctors should *not* provide NHS scripts for conditions that might ari whilst the patient is away, e.g. traveller's diarrhoea
- Prescribing interval for any repeat medication should be related to the next time that medication would normally be reviewed. Generall this should not be >13wk; the prescribing doctor retains medicolegal responsibility for the duration of the prescription
- If the doctor does decide to prescribe for the patient's stay abroad (e.g. if repeat supplies cannot be obtained at the destination or the drug prescribed has a narrow therapeutic index), it is essential to inform the patient of the need to consult a doctor for any regular monitoring as well as the need to consult a doctor in the event of an unforeseen complications or symptoms

General rules for treatment of overseas visitors to the UK

- **Emergency or immediately necessary treatment** (including worsening of pre-existing conditions, oxygen, and renal dialysis) must be offered to overseas visitors free of charge for a period of ≤14d. There is no obligation to provide non-emergency treatment. It is the decision of the GP whether care is deemed necessary
- **Non-emergency care** Provided on a private, paying basis

- **Reciprocal healthcare arrangements and refugees** (whether or not awarded leave to stay) are regarded as ordinarily resident. Treat in the same way as NHS patients
- **Hospital admission** A&E services are free as are compulsory psychiatric treatment and treatment for certain communicable diseases
- **NHS prescriptions** can be issued to overseas residents, but quantities supplied should be no more than necessary for immediate purposes; overseas visitors are charged normal NHS prescription fees

❶ GPs can register any patient as an NHS patient, but the patient may not be eligible for specialist/hospital care. If registration is refused, the practice must provide a non-discriminatory reason in writing (e.g. the practice only registers patients residing in the area for settled purpose).

General rules for British patients travelling abroad <60 countries worldwide have any sort of healthcare agreements with the UK. When travelling abroad, always have comprehensive medical insurance.

The European Health Insurance Card (EHIC) The EHIC entitles holders to reduced cost, or sometimes free, medical treatment that becomes necessary whilst in another European Economic Area (EEA) country or Switzerland. The EHIC can be obtained online from ℘ www.ehic.org.uk or at any Post Office. Countries this applies to are listed in Table 3.2. Each country has its own rules—details for individual countries are available on the DH travel advice website. British citizens moving to another EEA country are not entitled to use an EHIC to obtain medical treatment.

Other reciprocal agreements The UK has reciprocal agreements with certain other countries for the provision of urgently needed medical treatment at ↓ cost or free. Countries and the services available are listed on the DH travel advice website. Only urgently needed treatment is provided on the same terms as for residents of that country. Proof of British nationality or UK residence is required.

Table 3.2 Countries in which an EHIC can be used

• Austria	• Greece	• Netherlands
• Belgium	• Hungary	• Norway
• Bulgaria	• Iceland	• Poland
• Cyprus (but not Northern Cyprus)	• Ireland	• Portugal
	• Italy	• Romania
• Czech Republic	• Latvia	• Slovakia
• Denmark	• Liechtenstein	• Slovenia
• Estonia	• Lithuania	• Spain
• Finland	• Luxembourg	• Sweden
• France	• Malta	• Switzerland
• Germany		

Further information

NHS Choices Travel advice website
℘ www.nhs.uk/nhsengland/Healthcareabroad/pages/Healthcareabroad.aspx

JET LIBRARY

Registration and practice leaflets

Registration process Patients can apply to join a practice list b handing in their medical card at the practice or completing an applicatio form. For children, a parent or a guardian can make the application.

- **Open lists** Practices with open lists must consider all applications to join their list They can only refuse if they have reasonable grounds for doing so, which do not relate to the applicant's race, gender, social class, age, religion, sexual orientation, appearance, disability, or medica condition. Reasonable grounds include living outside the practice area When an application is refused, the practice must inform the applican in writing of the reasons for refusal
- **Closed lists** Practices with closed lists can only consider applications from immediate family members of patients already registered

Once the practice has accepted the application, it must then inform th PCO. The PCO confirms the application has been accepted to the prac tice and patient.

List closure Practices wishing to close their lists to new registration must inform the PCO in writing. The PCO must then enter into discussio with the practice to provide support to keep the list open. If that is no possible, the list will be closed for a specified period of time. Ofte closure is requested due to high list size. In that instance, a list size can b set so that the list re-opens when it falls below that limit.

Practice boundary 📖 p. 5

Newly registered patients When a patient has been accepted ont a practice list, or assigned to a practice list by a PCO, the practice mus offer the patient a consultation for a routine health check (the 'ne patient check') within 6mo of registration.

Routine health checks for other groups Practices must offer consultation for a routine health check to all:

- Patients aged 16–75y who have not been seen by a healthcare professional within the practice in the past 3y
- Patients aged >75y who have not been seen by a healthcare professional within the past year

❶ In England, patients aged 40–74y are eligible for a free NHS healt check and personalized assessment of risk under a scheme launched i 2009. Mechanisms for delivery of the check vary across England, but G surgeries may provide checks as a Local Enhanced Service.

Temporary residents Patients may register with a practice on short-term basis for treatment or advice if they are living temporarily (fo >24h but <3mo) in the practice area.

Emergency and immediately necessary treatment A practic must provide services required in core hours for the immediate necessary treatment of:

- Anyone injured or acutely unwell as a result of an accident or medical emergency at any place in its practice area

Anyone whose application for inclusion in the practice list (as a permanent or temporary resident) has been refused and who is not registered with another provider in the area

Anyone who is in the practice area for <24h

Removing patients from the practice list 📖 p. 56

Assignments PCOs may assign patients to any open practice list if the patient has problems registering with a practice. PCOs can only assign patients to closed lists if all other local practice lists are also closed and an assessment panel has approved the placement.

Practice leaflets Each practice is required to produce a practice leaflet to distribute to patients. In Wales, the practice leaflet must be in Welsh and English. The practice leaflet aims to inform patients about the practice, the services provided, and how to access them. In addition it informs patients of their rights and responsibilities. Most practices also take the opportunity to include general health information and information about self-management of minor illness.

Content of the practice leaflet Practice leaflets *must* be updated annually and include details of:

The name of the practice (and if the contract is with a partnership, names of partners and their status within the partnership; if the contract is with a company, names of directors, company secretary, shareholders, and the address of the company's registered office)

Names and professional qualifications of those providing medical care

Whether the practice teaches or trains healthcare professionals

Practice area, including reference to a map, plan, or postcode

Addresses of all practice premises, telephone and fax numbers, and website address (if any)

Services available, including details of routine health checks for patients aged >75y not seen in the past year or aged 16–75y and not seen in the previous 3y

Access for disabled patients and, if not, alternative arrangements for providing them with services

Registration process

Opening hours and methods of accessing services (including home visits) within those hours

Out-of-hours arrangements (including who is responsible for their provision) and how to access them

Arrangements for dispensing drugs (if applicable) and repeat prescriptions

Name and address of any local walk-in centre, telephone number of NHS 111 service (or equivalent) and details of online NHS health information

Complaints procedure

Rights and responsibilities, including the right of patients to express a preference of practitioner (and the way that they can express that); responsibility to keep appointments

Action that will be taken if a patient is aggressive or abusive

Access to patient information and the patient's rights of confidentiality

Name, address, and telephone number of the responsible PCO

The primary healthcare team

The GP does not function alone. Doctors within general practice are a integral part of a team of professionals that care for patients in the community—the primary healthcare team (PHCT). Precise composition PHCTs depends on the overall aims of the team, needs of the practic population, and practice characteristics. *Team members include GPs and:*

Practice manager General manager of the practice in liaison wit the partners. *Roles include:* staff appointments, supervision, trainin and dismissals; duty rotas; liaison with outside organizations (e.g. PCC and other primary healthcare team members (e.g. community nurses ar health visitors); maintenance of premises and equipment and financi planning. Most practice managers have management qualifications.

Practice nurse Duties can vary but include 'traditional' nursing task health promotion; immunizations; new registration checks; speciali clinics (e.g. asthma, DM, etc.); administration and audit.

Nurse practitioner Specially trained nurse who takes on clinic responsibility for specific aspects of care she has been trained for eith within the GP surgery or in patients' own homes, e.g. filtering out-of-hou calls or managing heart failure. Seen as a way to alleviate pressure on GP Nurse practitioners are at least as effective as GPs in the roles they perforr

District nurse Qualified nurse who has a community nursin qualification recognized by the Nursing and Midwifery Council. Most wo is conducted in patients' homes, particularly in looking after the chronical ill or those recently discharged from hospital. District nurses are usual employed by local community trusts or PCOs and coordinate their ow team of community nurses.

Community matron Highly experienced, senior nurse who wor closely with a limited number of patients who are high-intensity users health and social services (usually with serious, long-term conditions a complex range of conditions). The community matron acts as a 'cas manager' and single point of access to provide, plan, and organize care.

Health visitor Works with individuals, families, and groups in preventiv medicine, health promotion, and education. Health visitors visit all babi after the midwife ceases to attend, carry out developmental assessme checks, and advise on general care and immunization. Some health visito have a role exclusively for the elderly. Health visitors must be trained nurs and registered as health visitors with the Nursing and Midwifery Council.

Midwife Important link between hospitals, GPs, and other members the primary healthcare team in obstetric care. May practise independen when dealing with uncomplicated pregnancies but are obliged to refer a doctor in the event of complications. Midwives must be registered wi the Nursing and Midwifery Council.

Administrative and clerical staff Perform all the non-clinical task necessary to keep the practice running. Training varies.

Receptionists Perform an essential role as the interface between the general public and the GPs and nursing staff. Good interpersonal skills are essential. Training varies.

Community pharmacist Increasing role within practices—managing repeat prescribing, monitoring prescribing practices, and advising on prescribing policy.

Social worker Helps people live more successfully within the local community by helping them find solutions to their problems. Social workers tend to specialize in either adult or children's services:

Adult services Roles include working with people with mental health problems or learning difficulties in residential care; working with offenders by supervising them in the community and supporting them to find work; working with older people or disabled people at home, helping to sort out problems with their health, housing, or benefits

Children/young people services Roles include providing assistance and advice to keep families together; working in children's homes; managing adoption and foster care processes; providing support to younger people leaving care or who are at risk or in trouble with the law; or helping children who have problems at school or are facing difficulties brought on by illness in the family

Other team members Might include dieticians, occupational therapists, physiotherapists, and/or complementary therapists (such as psychological therapists).

Intermediate care Community-based service working closely with the PHCT. Provided by multidisciplinary teams. Provision and team composition varies across the UK but may include specialist doctors and/or GPs, nurses, physiotherapists and occupational therapists, home carers, and social workers. Usually provided in patients' own homes but can also involve community hospitals and/or short-term nursing/residential care placements. Common service features:

Time-limited (usually <6wk)

Targeted at people who would otherwise face prolonged hospital stays or inappropriate admission to hospital

Aims to maximize independence and enable people to remain living in their own homes

Further information

Association of Medical Secretaries, Practice Administrators & Receptionists (AMSPAR) ☎ 020 7387 6005 ⌕ www.amspar.co.uk
Nursing and Midwifery Council (NMC) ☎ 020 7637 7181 (registrations: ☎ 020 7333 9333) ⌕ www.nmc-uk.org
Royal College of Nursing ⌕ www.rcn.org.uk
Royal College of Midwives ⌕ www.rcm.org.uk
Community Practitioners' and Health Visitors' Association
⌕ www.unitetheunion.org/cphva
British Association of Social Workers ⌕ www.basw.co.uk

Confidentiality

Respect for confidentiality is also an essential requirement for the preservation of trust between patient and doctor. Failure to comply with standards can lead to disciplinary proceedings and even restriction/cessation of practice.

Caldicott Principles for disclosure of patient information

- **Justify the purpose** Patients may agree to identifiable information about themselves being released to specific individuals for known purposes. Implied consent applies when patients are aware that personal information may be shared and of their right to refuse but make no objection. Patients must have a realistic opportunity to refuse—and if they do refuse, clearly document that and respect their decision
- **Do not use patient identifiable information unless it is absolutely necessary** It is not necessary to seek consent to use anonymous information. If in doubt, seek advice from the BMA or your defence organization. Health information used for secondary purposes, e.g. planning, teaching, audit, should—when possible—be anonymous
- **Use the minimum patient identifiable information**
- **Access to patient identifiable information should be on a strict 'need to know basis'**
- **Everyone should be aware of their responsibilities**
- **Understand and comply with the law**

Special circumstances

Children (<16y) Disclosure can be authorized by a person with parental responsibility. Young people, mature enough to understand the implications, can make their own decisions and have a right to refuse parental access to their health record.

Mentally incapacitated adults Assessment of capacity to consent to information disclosure is time- and decision-specific. A mentally incapacitated adult can consent to information disclosure if the person is able to:
- Understand the concept of authorizing/prohibiting sharing of information
- Retain that information long enough to make a decision
- Weigh up the implications of disclosure or non-disclosure, and
- Communicate a decision

Otherwise, decisions must be based on an evaluation of the person's best interests, taking into account the views of the patient's representative(s) and reflecting the individual's expressed wishes and values.

❶ Except in Scotland, parents are able to consent for mentally incapacitated 16–17y olds.

The deceased Legislation covering records made since 1st November 1991 permits limited disclosure in order to satisfy a claim arising from death. Where there is no claim, there is no legal right of access to information.

Breaching confidentiality Only breach confidentiality in exceptional cases and with appropriate justification. This includes discussing a patient with another health professional not involved currently with that patient's care. Wider disclosure to people loosely associated with care (e.g. support staff in residential care settings) requires patient consent.

Situations where breach of confidentiality may be justified
- **Emergencies** Where necessary, to prevent or lessen a serious and imminent threat to the life or health of the individual concerned or another person (unless previously forbidden by the patient)
- **Statutory requirement** Ask under which legislation it is sought—check the legislation before disclosing if unsure
- **The public interest** What is in the public interest is not defined. The BMA has produced guidance
- **Public health** Reporting notifiable diseases (statutory duty)
- **Required by court or tribunal**
- **Adverse drug reactions** Routine reporting to the Medicines and Healthcare Products Regulatory Agency (□ p. 146)
- **Complaints** As part of GMC performance procedures involving doctors

Legal considerations
- **Human Rights Act (1998)** Establishes a right to 'respect for private and family life' and creates a general requirement to protect the privacy of individuals and preserve confidentiality of their health records. Compliance with the Data Protection Act and common law of confidentiality should satisfy requirements
- **Common law of confidentiality** Built up from case law where practice has been established by individual judgements. The key principle is that information confided should not be used or disclosed further, except as originally understood by the confider, or with their subsequent permission, except in exceptional circumstances (see Breaching confidentiality)
- **Data Protection Act (1998)** Imposes constraints on processing of personal information. Also requires personal data to be protected against unauthorized/unlawful processing and accidental loss, destruction, or damage. Also applies to personnel records
- **Administrative law** The extent the NHS can access confidential information to perform its functions is set down in statutes
- **Health and Social Care Act (2001)** Allows for certain exceptions to confidentiality laws to be made, e.g. for use in cancer registries
- **Freedom of information Act (2000)** Applies to all NHS bodies, including GP practices. Practices are required to produce a publication scheme detailing all information routinely published by the practice. In addition, members of the public can make written requests to see any information recorded by the practice in any format. These rights are restricted by certain exemptions, e.g. personal data

Further information
GMC Guidance on good practice—confidentiality ℘ www.gmc-uk.org
BMA Confidentiality and people under 16 ℘ www.bma.org.uk
Information Commissioner's Office Data Protection ℘ www.ico.gov.uk

Consent

Consent Implies willingness of a patient to undergo examinatio investigation, or treatment (collectively termed 'procedure' on this page It may be expressed (i.e. specifically says yes or no/signs a consent form or implied (i.e. complies with the procedure without ever specifical agreeing to it—use with care). For consent to be valid, patients:
- Must be competent to make the decision,
- Have received sufficient information to take it, and
- Not be acting under duress

⚠ Under 'common law', touching a patient without valid consent may constitute the civil or criminal offence of battery, and if the patient suf fers harm as a result of treatment, lack of consent may be a factor in any negligence claim. Never exceed the scope of the authority given by a patient, except in an emergency.

If you are the doctor carrying out a procedure, it is *your responsibility* t discuss it with the patient and seek consent. The task may be delegate but the responsibility *remains* yours.

Information to include
- Reasons why you want to perform the procedure
- Nature, purpose, and side effects (common and serious) of proposed procedure
- Name of the doctor with overall responsibility
- Whether students or other 'trainees' will be involved
- Whether part of a research programme or outside usual procedure
- Reminder that patients have a right to seek a 2nd opinion and/or can change their minds about a decision at any time

And for therapeutic procedures/treatments
- Details of diagnosis and prognosis (including uncertainties)
- Management options—including the option not to treat and other options that you cannot offer—and, for each option, an estimation of likely risks, benefits, and probability of success
- Details of follow-up in order to monitor progress or side effects

❶ Document if a patient does not want to be fully informed befor consenting.

Written consent It is good practice to seek written consent if:
- The procedure is complex or involves significant risks ('risk' means ar adverse outcome, including complications and side effects)
- The procedure involves general/regional anaesthesia or sedation
- Providing clinical care is not the primary purpose of the procedure
- It has consequences for employment, social, or personal life of the patient
- The procedure is part of a project or programme of approved research

Establishing capacity to make decisions 📖 p. 122

Mentally incapacitated adults The Mental Capacity Act (2005), and equivalents in Scotland and NI, enables patients' advocates (usually friends, relatives, or carers) or suitable professionals (e.g. doctors, social workers) to act in patients' best interests on their behalf. This includes provision of medical care. Before acting:

Take all factors affecting the decision into consideration

Involve the patient with the decision making as far as possible

Take the patient's previous known wishes into consideration, and

Consult everyone else involved with the patient's care/welfare

In situations in which there is disagreement about the patient's best interests, the decision can be referred to the Court of Protection.

Advance statements 📖 p. 123

Children (<16y) A competent child is able to understand the nature, purpose, and possible consequences of a proposed procedure as well as the consequences of not undergoing that procedure. This is termed '*Gillick competence*' after the court case in which the principle was established (Gillick v West Norfolk and Wisbech AHA [1986] AC 122).

A competent child may consent to treatment. However, if treatment is refused, a parent or court may authorize procedures in the child's best interests*. Where a child is not judged competent, *only* a person with parental responsibility may authorize/refuse investigations or treatment. If in doubt, seek legal advice.

Emergencies When consent cannot be obtained, you may provide medical treatment, provided it is limited to what is immediately necessary to save life or avoid significant deterioration in the patient's health. Respect the terms of any advance statement/living will you are aware of.

Further information

GMC 🕸 www.gmc-uk.org
Consent: patients and doctors making decisions together (2008)
0–18 years: guidance for all doctors (2007)

Office of the Public Guardian Making decisions: a guide for people who work in health and social care (2007) 🕸 www.publicguardian.gov.uk

---

Note: In Scotland, parents do not have this power to overrule a competent child's decision.

Complaints

Sadly, complaints are a fact of life for most GPs (see Figure 3.1). The mo constructive and least stressful approach is to view them as a learnin experience and a chance to improve practice risk management strateg Always contact your local LMC ± defence organization if you are direct implicated in a complaint. Patients who complain generally want:

- Their complaint to be heard and investigated promptly
- Their complaint to be handled efficiently and sympathetically
- To receive a genuine apology if mistakes have occurred
- To be assured that steps will be taken to prevent a recurrence

Time limits for complaints NHS complaints can only be accepted

- <1y after the incident which is the subject of the complaint, or
- <1y after the date at which the complainant became aware of the matter

After that time, complaints can only be accepted if there is good reaso for delay and it is possible to effectively investigate.

A 3y time limit after the incident (or after the date upon which the clai ant became aware that the incident might have caused harm) is placed o civil clinical negligence cases, except for children who may claim until the 21st birthday.

Conciliation Is a way of dealing with complaints that helps to avo adversarial situations. Either party can ask the local PCO for conciliatio but both parties must agree to it taking place. By bringing the two sid together with a neutral conciliator, it aims to:

- Explain and clarify matters for both parties
- Ensure both parties are really listening to each other
- Ensure the process is unthreatening and helpful

Records of complaints A file on the complaint, including a copy all correspondence, should be kept separate from clinical records of t patient and, if the patient leaves the practice, should not be sent on wi the clinical notes.

Private sector Most private sector healthcare providers have the own complaints resolution procedures. Patients should contact t organization concerned for details.

Disciplinary procedures There is no direct connection betwee complaints procedures and disciplinary action. If a complaints procedu reveals information indicating the need for disciplinary action, it is th responsibility of the PCO to act. If they decide there has been a breach the terms of service, the PCO can fix a penalty, if appropriate.

Further information

Risk management 📖 p. 35
BMA 🖰 www.bma.org.uk
Medical defence organizations

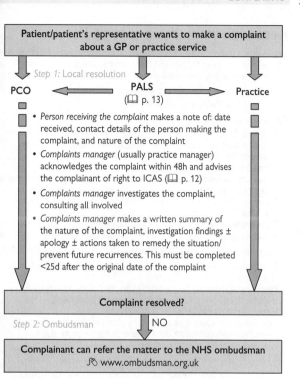

Patient/patient's representative wants to make a complaint about a GP or practice service

Step 1: Local resolution

PCO   **PALS** (📖 p. 13)   **Practice**

- *Person receiving the complaint* makes a note of: date received, contact details of the person making the complaint, and nature of the complaint
- *Complaints manager* (usually practice manager) acknowledges the complaint within 48h and advises the complainant of right to ICAS (📖 p. 12)
- *Complaints manager* investigates the complaint, consulting all involved
- *Complaints manager* makes a written summary of the nature of the complaint, investigation findings ± apology ± actions taken to remedy the situation/ prevent future recurrences. This must be completed <25d after the original date of the complaint

Complaint resolved?

Step 2: Ombudsman | NO

Complainant can refer the matter to the NHS ombudsman 🖰 www.ombudsman.org.uk

Figure 3.1 The NHS complaints procedure for general practice

Removal from the practice list

Removal of a patient from a practice list can be distressing for both patient and GP. In England and Wales ~53,000 patients/y are transferred by PCO at the request of the GP; ~1,000/y because of an act or threat of violence

❶ Practice policies for removing patients and dealing with threats/violence should be stated in practice leaflets.

Situations that justify removal

- **Violence** Physical violence or verbal abuse towards doctors, practice staff, premises, or other patients. Includes violence or threatening behaviour by other household members not registered with the practice and/or pets (e.g. dogs)
- **Crime and deception** Deliberate deceit to obtain a service or benefit; obtaining drugs under false pretences for non-medical reasons; use of the doctor to conceal or aid criminal activity; stealing from practice premises
- **Distance** New residence outside the designated outer boundary of the practice area, with failure to register with another GP

Situations that never justify removal

- **Costly treatment** GPs can apply for an ↑ in their prescribing budget to allow for this
- **Particular conditions** If a particular condition demands costly treatment, out-of-area referrals, or expensive equipment, accommodation can be made at PCO level
- **Age** General practice is about looking after patients from cradle to grave. Although patients >75y do result in higher costs, this is reflected in allocation of funds to the practice

Situations that do not normally justify removal

- **Disagreement with the patient's views** Patients must have freedom to choose whether to accept a GP's advice. The GP can try to influence the view but should not remove a patient if he or she fails to concur
- **Critical questioning and/or complaints** Complaints to the practice via normal in-house channels can be constructive and help improve services; they do not usually justify removal of the patient from the practice list. However, personal attacks on a doctor or allegations that are clearly unfounded indicate a serious breakdown in doctor–patient relationship and could justify removal

Patients' rights to change doctor Patients also have a right to change their doctor. They are not required to give reasons or any period of notice, and there is no requirement for the GP to be notified.

Other family members Removal of other family members should not automatically follow removal of a patient from a practice list unless removal of that patient makes ongoing care of the rest of the household impossible.

retrievable breakdown of the doctor–patient relationship he most contentious reason for removal from a practice list. Causes the ost problems. As a good doctor–patient relationship is fundamental to uccessful care, it is in the interest of both patient and GP that the patient oves to another practice list if that relationship breaks down. Difficulty ises when the patient sees matters differently.

Inform appropriate members of the practice Discuss reasons for breakdown in relationship (e.g. chronic stress, mental illness, cultural differences) and factors that contribute to the situation; consider solutions/alterations in procedures that might help

Inform the patient Consider arranging a meeting to discuss matters (can be done through the in-house complaints framework). Explain the nature of the problem and elicit the patient's perspective; be prepared to give ground and compromise

If discussion fails to resolve the problem Suggest the patient sees another GP within the practice (although discuss the patient's feelings about the possibility of being treated by the ex-GP in an emergency). Consider giving advice about alternative practices in the area. If the situation continues, then consider removal from the practice list

emoving patients from the practice list

Warn the patient A practice can only request removal of a patient from a practice list if, within 12mo prior to the date of its request to the PCO for removal, it has warned the patient that he/she is at risk of removal and explained the reasons for that. Exceptions to this are violent patients, patients who have moved outside the practice area, and those for whom it would be unsafe or impractical to issue a warning

Inform the PCO in writing of your decision. Give full patient details. Except in the case of violent patients, removal will not take effect until the 8th day after the request is received by the PCO unless the patient is accepted by, allocated, or assigned to another GP sooner than this. The patient is always notified by the PCO

Write to the patient about the decision and reason for removal (take advice from your medical defence organization, if needed). Include information on how to register with another practice and reassurance that the patient will not be left without a GP. Take care to ensure reasons given are factual and the tone of the letter is polite and informative

nmediate removal of any patient who has committed an act f violence Includes actual or threatened physical violence or verbal buse leading to fear for a person's safety.

Notify the police (or, in Scotland, either the police or the procurator fiscal) about the violent behaviour

Notify both the PCO and the patient of the removal in writing. The PCO has a duty to provide alternative primary medical care services by commissioning specialized directed enhanced services, e.g. GPs with secure facilities for consulting

urther information

MA ⌖ www.bma.org.uk

Education, monitoring, and research

Education in primary care

Teaching and training in primary care at every level should:
- Be based on evidence
- Train the doctor to be part of an integrated and comprehensive healthcare system
- Have a balanced agenda across clinical topics (prevention, diagnosis, cure, care, and palliation), practice organization and management, team working, audit, and research

Teaching in general practice Most GPs are involved in teaching to some extent. This may involve:
- Teaching medical students, foundation doctors, or GP registrars within the practice
- Helping to train new practice staff
- Arranging your own and/or your colleagues' continuing education programme

Teaching can be very rewarding but also brings stresses (e.g. preparation of material). Payments are available to GPs who take medical students, foundation doctors, and/or GPs in training into their surgeries for teaching and there are a few teaching posts within UK universities for GPs.

As a teacher, it is your responsibility to ensure you are competent to fulfil the task. Take steps to acquire proficiency in teaching skills. Local medical schools often run courses for prospective teachers.

Learning styles Different people have different learning styles. Depending on a person's preferred learning style, the starting point for an educational initiative will be different:
- **'Why'** (concrete, reflective) Learners learn best when they know why something is relevant and how it will apply to their work
- **'What'** (abstract, reflective) Learners learn best when given plenty of time to think about things and link different concepts in their mind
- **'How'** (abstract, active) Learners like to work actively on well-defined tasks and learn by trial and error
- **'What if'** (concrete, active) Learners learn best by applying course material in new situations and solving problems they create for themselves
- **Serialist** Learners like to see the 'big picture' first
- **Holist learners** Like to take learning bit by bit in small chunks
- **Individual learners** Prefer to learn on their own
- **Group learners** Prefer to learn with others

Principles of self-directed and adult learning The learner takes responsibility for defining learning needs; setting goals; identifying resources; implementing appropriate activities; and evaluating outcomes. Adults are motivated by education that:
- Is based on mutual trust and respect
- Allows them to take responsibility for their own learning
- Actively involves them
- Is perceived as relevant
- Is based on, and builds on, previous experience

Is focused on problems
Can be immediately applied in practice
Involves cycles of action and reflection

Personal development plans (PDPs) Outline areas of knowledge in need of update and ways in which these needs can be met. PDPs are an integral part of junior doctor training, GP training, and the appraisal process. Ask:

What you need to learn—specific, measurable objectives
Why you need to learn it
How you plan to learn it
How you will know *whether* you have learnt it
How your intentions link to *past* and *future* learning
The *timescale* for your learning

'SMART' criteria—learning objectives should be:
Specific
Measurable
Achievable
Realistic
Timed (i.e. there should be a deadline for achieving them)

Methods of identifying learning needs Numerous—include:
Gap analysis
Significant event analysis (📖 p. 81)
Objective tests of knowledge and skill
Self-assessment through diary, log book, or weekly review
Video assessment of performance
Criterion-based audit (📖 p. 80)
Patient satisfaction surveys (📖 p. 84)
Risk assessment (📖 p. 35)
Peer assessment/multisource feedback

Medical students Are taught in general practice as:
Early patient contact is helpful to enable students to relate theoretical concepts to the reality of medical practice. General practice settings are especially good for teaching concepts of health and illness behaviour and the effect of family and social settings on illness
Clinical skills can be taught successfully in general practice, and the one-to-one teaching that can be undertaken within GP surgeries is an excellent teaching resource

Foundation doctors 📖 p. 62

GP training 📖 p. 64

Continuing professional development (CPD) The aim of CPD is to sustain professional development of doctors and help them to provide high-quality patient care throughout their careers. Doctors need to demonstrate that they have up-to-date knowledge across the spectrum of general practice to become a registered GP and then need to show they are continuing to update and expand their knowledge to meet the requirements of appraisal and revalidation (📖 p. 68).

Foundation doctors in primary care

Newly qualified doctors spend their first working year (F1) doing three hospital placements before obtaining full registration. In the second year (F2), 42% have a 4mo attachment to primary care.

Who employs foundation doctors? Foundation programmes are hosted by acute hospital trusts. The trust recruits the doctors, arranges placements, employs them through their 2y programme, provides indemnity, appoints educational supervisors, and is responsible for assessment.

F2 placements in general practice
- Made by employing trusts; practices have no say about who they take
- Educational deaneries are responsible for appointing practices for F2 placements, and interested practices should contact their local deanery
- Practices must be of adequate standard and have an approved supervisor for their F2s; the standard required of the practice is similar to that required of training practices (📖 p. 65)—practices are inspected by their deanery to check that they meet the criteria
- GP F2 supervisors need not be GP trainers. To attain approval, potential supervisors undergo a short training course organized by the deanery; they are paid at a rate related to the trainer rate

Expectations of F2 doctors F2 doctors:
- Are expected to do 7 clinical sessions/wk, 1 session of supervised study, 1 session of project work, and attend a half day group session at their host trust. No OOH work is expected. Part-time working is allowed, but training must be undertaken on a $\geq\frac{1}{2}$-time basis
- Are entitled to study leave (up to 1wk) and annual leave
- Can sign prescriptions; practical procedures must be supervised
- Need an initial induction period, working with practice staff and the wider primary healthcare team and sitting in with a trained GP
- Are likely to need longer consultation times than standard 10min slots
- Need to have a fully trained GP available whenever they are seeing patients to provide advice and support, monitor their performance, and debrief at the end of the session

ePortfolio Compulsory record of training. The doctor must prove that he/she has attained all the competences required (see Box 4.1) before progression to specialist training. *Includes:*

- Core procedures
- Clinical supervisor-end-of placement report
- Placement supervision group report
- Team assessment of behaviour (TAB)
- Educational supervisor end-of-year report

Supervised learning events (SLE) Three types are commonly used:
- **Direct observation of doctor/patient encounters** An experienced colleague watches the F2. Tools available: direct observation of procedural skills (DOPS)—for practice procedures; mini clinical evaluation exercise (Mini-CEX)—for clinical consultations
- **Case-based discussion (CBD)** Structured case review with a senior clinician
- **Developing the clinical teacher**

Further information
The Foundation Programme ℘ www.foundationprogramme.nhs.uk

Box 4.1 Foundation level syllabus

1: Professionalism
- Behaviour in the work place
- Continuity of care
- Leadership
- Teamworking
- Time management

2: Relationship and communication with patients
- Communication in difficult circumstances
- Communication with patients
- Treats the patient as the centre of care within a consultation
- Complaints
- Consent

3: Safety and clinical governance
- Risks of fatigue, ill health, and stress
- Quality and safety improvement

4: Ethical and legal issues
- Medical ethical principles/ confidentiality
- Legal framework of medical practice
- Comprehension of relevance of outside bodies to professional life

5: Teaching and training

6: Maintaining good medical practice
- Life-long learning
- Evidence, guidelines, care protocols, and research

7: Good clinical care
- Makes patient safety a priority in clinical practice
- Undertakes regular patient review
- Medical record-keeping and correspondence
- History and examination
- Safe prescribing
- Infection control and hygiene
- Diagnosis and clinical decision-making
- Safe use of medical devices
- Interface with different specialties and with other professionals

8: Recognition and management of the acutely ill patient
- Promptly assesses the acutely ill, collapsed, or unconscious patient
- Manages patients with impaired consciousness, including seizures
- Responds to acutely abnormal physiology
- Manages pain
- Manages sepsis
- Manages acute mental disorder and self-harm

9: Resuscitation and end-of-life care
- Resuscitation
- End-of-life care and appropriate use of Do Not Attempt Resuscitation (DNAR) orders/advanced decisions

10: Patients with long-term conditions
- Manages patients with long-term conditions
- Supporting patient decision-making
- Patient education and public health
- Nutrition
- Discharge planning
- Health promotion

11: Investigations

12: Procedures

Becoming a GP in the UK

GP vocational training in 2014 Involves 3y full-time (or the equivalent part-time) specialty training after the Foundation years: 18mo in selected hospital specialty posts and 18mo as a GP registrar in general practice under the supervision of a GP trainer.

Broad-based training (BBT) In place of the usual first year of specialist training (ST1), a 2y BBT scheme is currently being piloted in 7 deaneries. Junior doctors do 6mo of each of paediatrics, general medicine, general practice, and mental health before going into the ST2 year of their chosen specialty.

GP training in the future Approval was gained in 2012 to enhance & extend GP training to better prepare future GPs for independent practice. If implemented as planned, the new 4y programme will focus on:
- Enhancing clinical skills
- Enhancing generalist skills
- Enhancing leadership skills

The vision includes
- Experience of working in general practice early in training
- Spending ≥24mo in primary care to learn how to manage complex patients with multiple morbidities
- Specialist-led training in child and mental health
- More scope to tailor training to individual trainee needs
- More innovative and integrated placements in a range of settings
- A 'Quality Improvement Project' in the local community

Distribution of training Enhanced GP training will include:
- 12mo in relevant specialist posts approved by the GMC
- 12mo used flexibly by deaneries to create GP training placements in a range of hospital, community, and general practice settings
- 24mo in general practice placements

Recruitment and selection Applications for GP training must be made online to the National Recruitment Office for General Practice Training (NRO):
- All applicants meeting GP training entry criteria are invited to attend a national shortlisting assessment consisting of a machine-markable test
- Candidates are sorted in rank order; highest scoring applicants are invited to attend a selection centre at their highest preferred location. Selections centres in England are the regional deaneries. Scotland, Wales, and NI each have a single selection centre
- The selection centre assessment comprises 3 workplace-based assessments, which include a patient simulation exercise. Following assessment, highest ranked applicants are offered training places in that area
- Appointable candidates without training places are placed on a reserve list for the deanery. Any reserve candidates not offered local places are entered into national clearing

Criteria for training practices Each region sets its own criteria for selection of practices to train prospective GPs. These relate to:
- The trainer as a doctor
- The trainer as a teacher, and
- The training practice

Practices must demonstrate high-quality clinical care and administration, and a commitment and capability to educate a GP registrar. Details of local requirements can be obtained from regional deanery offices.

RCGP Curriculum (updated 2012—see Figure 4.1, 🕮 p. 67). Access at 🕾 www.rcgp-curriculum.org.uk. Describes the core knowledge, skills, and attitudes required to be a competent GP.

InnovAiT RCGP journal for GPs in training. Provided free to all GPs in training and available at subsidized rate to other RCGP members, medical students, and Foundation doctors. Acts like a rolling textbook, covering GP curriculum every 3y.

The RCGP Certification Unit evaluates general practice training and makes recommendations for Certificates of Completion of Training (CCT) to the GMC. Anyone undertaking a training programme, leading to a CCT, should register with the Certification Unit.

Certification of Completion of Training
- During training, on completion of each placement, the clinical supervisor completes an assessment of the trainee's performance
- The GP educational supervisor signs this assessment off as confirmation that there has been satisfactory progress in acquiring the relevant curriculum competences
- The portfolio of assessments is reviewed and endorsed by the deanery, at least annually (Annual Panel Review)
- Submission of this portfolio, together with successful completion of the MRCGP, enables a GP in training to apply for the CCT via the RCGP Certification Unit

Certification of Eligibility for GP Registration (CEGPR) CEGPR (previously called Article 11) is an alternative route for doctors who are not eligible for a CCT but believe that their training, qualifications, and experience are equivalent (e.g. all, or part, of their training outside the UK or in a non-approved training post). Trainees who begin a 3y planned programme for a CCT and decide to shorten it, by including posts not in their GP programme, must also apply for a CEGPR. This type of application is more complex and time-consuming than the CCT route. Application is online to the GMC, with submission of a portfolio of evidence.

Further information
🕾 www.rcgp.org.uk/gp-training-and-exams/gp-certification-overview.aspx

Further information

Gerada C, Riley B and Simon C Preparing the future GP : the case for enhanced GP training (2012) 🕾 www.rcgp.org.uk
RCGP ☎ 020 3188 7400 🕾 www.rcgp.org.uk
National Recruitment Office for General Practice Training (NRO) 🕾 www.gprecruitment.org.uk

Membership of the Royal College of GPs

Membership of the RCGP (MRCGP) The MRCGP is an examination of professional competency based on modern educational theory and an evidence-based approach to assessment designed to test GPs in training across the spectrum of knowledge, skills, behaviours, and attitudes defined by the RCGP Curriculum (see Figure 4.1).

Passing the 3 different components of the MRCGP is compulsory for all doctors wishing to become GPs in the UK:

Applied Knowledge Test (AKT) 200 multiple-choice questions test whether the candidate can apply knowledge in the context of general practice. Computer-based assessment held at Pearson VUE computer centres across the country. Questions are distributed as follows: clinical medicine (80%); administration and informatics (10%); research, appraisal evidence-based medicine, and statistics (10%).

Clinical Skills Assessment (CSA) Assesses behaviour in a mock surgery in which patients are played by actors. The candidate performs 13 consultations, each of 10min duration. The CSA is currently only available at the RCGP in Euston and takes place 3 times a year in February, May and November.

Workplace-Based Assessment (WPBA) Continuous qualitative assessment of performance in training based on the ePortfolio and trainer's report. The evidence collected in the Trainee ePortfolio is reviewed at least 1×/12mo by the deanery Annual Review of Competence Progression (ARCP) panel to ensure the trainee is ready to move into the next year of training.

First5® On gaining their CCT, newly qualified GPs can receive additional support through the RCGP to the first point of revalidation at 5y through the RCGP First5® programme.

Fellowship of the RCGP Is awarded in recognition of a significant contribution to medicine in general, and general practice in particular. It recognizes a significant contribution to: the health and welfare of the community; the science or practice of medicine; the aims of RCGP; or any organization which benefits general practice. The candidate (nominee), nominator, and two seconders must each complete a form and a supporting statement. The achievement categories are:

- Clinical practice
- Patient-centred practice
- Leadership
- Teaching and education
- Innovation and creativity
- Academic and research

The nominator emails the completed paperwork to the candidate's local RCGP Faculty for consideration by the Faculty's fellowship committee which considers the application, then makes a recommendation to RCGP Council. Approved candidates are formally elected as Fellows at the RCGP Annual General Meeting or Spring Meeting.

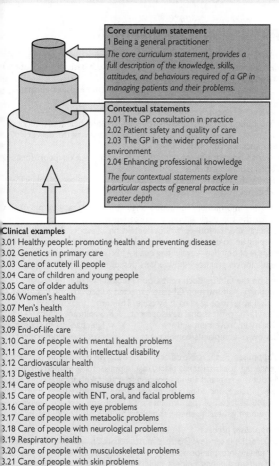

Core curriculum statement
1 Being a general practitioner
The core curriculum statement, provides a full description of the knowledge, skills, attitudes, and behaviours required of a GP in managing patients and their problems.

Contextual statements
2.01 The GP consultation in practice
2.02 Patient safety and quality of care
2.03 The GP in the wider professional environment
2.04 Enhancing professional knowledge

The four contextual statements explore particular aspects of general practice in greater depth

Clinical examples
3.01 Healthy people: promoting health and preventing disease
3.02 Genetics in primary care
3.03 Care of acutely ill people
3.04 Care of children and young people
3.05 Care of older adults
3.06 Women's health
3.07 Men's health
3.08 Sexual health
3.09 End-of-life care
3.10 Care of people with mental health problems
3.11 Care of people with intellectual disability
3.12 Cardiovascular health
3.13 Digestive health
3.14 Care of people who misuse drugs and alcohol
3.15 Care of people with ENT, oral, and facial problems
3.16 Care of people with eye problems
3.17 Care of people with metabolic problems
3.18 Care of people with neurological problems
3.19 Respiratory health
3.20 Care of people with musculoskeletal problems
3.21 Care of people with skin problems

The clinical examples apply the competences in the core statement 'Being a general practitioner' to population groups or to organ-based conditions.

Figure 4.1 The RCGP Curriculum (2012)

Further information
RCGP ☎ 020 3188 7766 🖥 www.rcgp.org.uk

Appraisal and revalidation

Appraisal Requires all doctors wishing to practise medicine in the UK to undergo a formal review on a yearly basis. It is the basis of revalidation to maintain a licence to practise and aims to:
- Set out personal and professional development needs, career paths and goals, and agree plans for them to be met
- Review the doctor's performance, and consider the doctor's contribution to quality and improvement of local healthcare services
- Optimize the use of skills and resources in achieving the delivery of high-quality care
- Offer an opportunity for doctors to discuss and seek support for their participation in activities
- Identify the need for adequate resources to enable service objectives to be met

Supporting information The supporting information that doctors need to bring for the appraisal falls under 4 broad headings:
- General information—provides context on all aspects of work
- Keeping up to date—maintaining/enhancing quality of work
- Review of practice—evaluating quality of current practice
- Feedback on practice—how others perceive your work

Based on the GMC's document Good Medical Practice, there are 6 types of supporting information GPs are expected to provide and discuss at their appraisal at least once in each 5y cycle. They are:
- Continuing professional development
- Quality improvement activity
- Review of complaints/compliments
- Significant events
- Feedback from colleagues
- Feedback from patients

The appraiser Responsible officers of the designated bodies are accountable for ensuring appraisal takes place, that appraisers are properly trained to carry out this role and are in a position to undertake appraisal of a doctor's whole practice, including clinical performance, and where appropriate specialist aspects of performance, e.g. research, service delivery, or management issues. In general, appraisers for GPs will be other GPs.

The appraisal process
- **Before the interview** Doctors must prepare an appraisal document containing evidence and supporting evidence about their practice and personal needs. Folders should be submitted to the appraiser ≥2wk prior to appraisal interviews to allow adequate time for preparation. Various electronic toolkits and portfolios are available
- **At the interview** Doctor and appraiser agree a summary of achievement in the past year, objectives for the next year, key elements of a personal development plan, and actions expected of the organization
- **After the interview** A summary document is produced (usually by the doctor being appraised) and a joint declaration signed that the appraisal has been carried out properly

Licence to Practise The GMC introduced licences to practise in November 2009. All registered doctors were able to request a licence to practise; all doctors eligible for registration with the GMC since November 2009 have also been licensed. The GMC licence (rather than GMC registration) signifies to patients that a doctor has the legal authority to write prescriptions and sign death certificates. GPs working in the NHS, either on a permanent or locum basis, need to be:
- Licensed by the GMC
- Listed on the GMC's General Practice Register
- Included on an NHS Performers List

Revalidation Was formally introduced in December 2012. All licensed doctors need to be relicensed every 5y.

Process of revalidation Doctors need to provide supporting information that shows that they keep up to date and remain fit to practise. GPs are accountable to their local 'designated body' and 'responsible officer'. In order for Responsible Officers to recommend maintenance of a GP's Licence to Practise, they need to be satisfied that:
- The GP has participated in an annual appraisal process that covers all of their medical practice, and
- There are no unresolved concerns about the doctor's performance

Responsible officer's recommendations to the GMC
- **Positive recommendation** The doctor should be revalidated and his/her Licence to Practise continued
- **Deferral: insufficient information** Revalidation cannot be recommended because the doctor has not provided enough information; the doctor will be asked to provide additional information
- **Notification of failure to engage** The doctor has failed to engage with local systems and processes that support revalidation

The GMC will withdraw a Licence to Practise if:
- The doctor tells them that it is no longer required
- The doctor does not pay the appropriate fee
- The doctor does not take part in the revalidation process when asked
- A Fitness to Practise panel directs that the doctor's registration should be suspended or erased

❶ Doctors have a right of appeal against any decision to withdraw, or refuse to restore, their Licence to Practise or Specialist Certificate.

⚠ **Concerns about performance** Any GP with concerns about their own, or a colleague's, performance should discuss the matter confidentially with the secretary of their LMC, the clinical governance lead/performance information manager of their PCO, or the GMC.

Further information
RCGP 🔗 www.rcgp.org.uk
- Principles of GP appraisal (2008)
- Guide to revalidation for GPs (2013)
GMC 🔗 www.gmc-uk.org/doctors/revalidation.asp
NHS Revalidation Support 🔗 www.revalidationsupport.nhs.uk/index.php

Career options for GPs

Times are changing in general practice. Doctors considering a life as a G
want a more flexible and varied career than in the past.

Career options within the NHS

Clinical assistant or hospital practitioner The GP works within a hospit
setting on the wards or in outpatients, providing a specialist service
under direct supervision of a hospital consultant. Posts are usually
advertised in the medical/GP press ± locally. Generally poorly paid.

GP with special clinical interest (GPwSI) GPs who, in addition to their
normal GP duties, provide a specialist service to meet the needs of their
local community. They might deliver a specialist clinical service beyond
the scope of normal general practice, undertake advanced procedures,
or develop services. The main difference between a GPwSI and clinical
assistant is that the GPwSI receives referrals from other GPs and will
decide on the appropriate treatment independently and not under direc
supervision of a consultant, but with the support of secondary care.
Posts are usually advertised to local GPs. In order to be classed as havin
a special interest, GPs must:
- Have undertaken particular training in the specialty or have a proven
  track record of expertise in the specialty
- Regularly update knowledge through attendance at courses,
  conferences, or meetings and through reading
- Look after a specific group of patients with the condition
- Audit practice in the specialty area, demonstrating quality of care

Medical adviser or consultant in primary care Medical advisers c
directors in ambulance trusts, NHS Direct sites, etc. Some national NH
agencies have GP advisers or directors too, e.g. National Commissionir
Board. Posts are either advertised or obtained by direct approach.

Providing GMS/PMS ± enhanced medical services 📖 p. 4

Providing postgraduate medical education e.g. GP tutor, GP trainer (1 i
8 GPs are GP trainers), course organizer. Approach local director or dea
of postgraduate medical education.

Working for local PCO/CCG/Deanery e.g. serving on a committee, clinic
tutor, GP appraiser, etc. Contact local PCO.

Opportunities outside the NHS

Academic posts A GP may be employed solely by a university or jointly b
a university and the NHS. Posts include undergraduate teachers, lecturer
and research posts. Contact local university departments of gener
practice or look for posts advertised in the medical/GP press.

Clinical sessions for commercial companies and charities, e.g. scho
doctor for a private school.

Complementary medicine Seek specialist training. Contact representative bodies of the specialty chosen.

Forensic work, e.g. police surgeon, coroner (☏ 020 8979 6805), expert witness (🖰 www.ewi.org.uk).

Media work/medical author Some sort of professional journalism qualification is useful. The BMJ offers a 1y registrar post for doctors with 3–5y experience. Courses are also available through the BMA and Medical Journalists Association 🖰 www.mja-uk.org. If you have an idea for a book, contact the medical commissioning editor of a reputable publisher to discuss your ideas.

Medical adviser posts within GP and other medical organizations, e.g. RCGP, MDU, GMC. Posts may be advertised or appointments made through election or direct approach. Contact the relevant organization.

Medicals for benefits Examining Medical Practitioners (EMPs) carrying out fitness to work and disability assessments on behalf of the Department for Work and Pensions (DWP).

Medical politics GPs serve on local medical committees (LMCs) on an elected basis. Contact the local LMC and ask about standing for election.

Work for government agencies, e.g. armed forces as a civilian medical practitioner or the territorial army. Usually civilian posts are advertised in the medical/GP press. For commissioned posts, contact service recruitment offices.

Occupational medicine Contact: Faculty for Occupational Medicine 🖰 www.facoccmed.ac.uk

Prison doctor Posts are usually advertised in the medical/GP press.

Sports medicine, e.g. for professional sportsmen; in private clinics. Doctors are required to have a knowledge of sports injuries, their treatment, rehabilitation, and prevention. They also need to know about other aspects of sport, e.g. drugs in sport, nutrition, travel problems. Contact: British Association of Sport and Exercise Medicine 🖰 www.basem.co.uk

Work abroad Contact: RCGP International Department E-mail: international@rcgp.org.uk; RedR UK 🖰 www.redr.org.uk; Voluntary Service Overseas 🖰 www.vso.org.uk. Overseas posts are also advertised in the medical press.

Clinical governance and CQC

Clinical governance is defined as '*a framework through which organization are accountable for continuously improving the quality of their services ar safeguarding high standards of care by creating an environment in whic excellence in clinical care will flourish.*'

Essential elements of clinical governance See Figure 4.2

What does clinical governance entail?
- Within practices, individual doctors must consider their own professional development and educational needs, and regular assessment must be made of performance and development of other health professionals engaged by practices
- Within practices, there must be continuous review and appraisal of procedures and standards—RAID:
  - Review—gather all stakeholders together to look at a topic
  - Agree—strategy to take forward
  - Intervene—make changes decided upon
  - Demonstrate—the effect of changes through audit (🕮 p. 80), patient satisfaction questionnaires, prescribing data, etc.
- Deficiencies in knowledge, skills, or experience must be acted upon through appropriate education and professional development
- Resources should be provided to help develop clinical governance, e.g time out for audit, funding for courses and educational activities

Concerns about GP performance 🕮 p. 69

Care Quality Commission (CQC) The Health and Social Car Act 2008 required any individual, partnership, or organization providir healthcare services in the UK to register with the CQC as a service provide Registration had to be completed by April 2013 for general practice.

Regulated activities Practices must register for any of the 'regulated activities' that they perform. The CQC lists 15 different regulated activitie Those usually applicable to general practice are:
- Treatment of disease, disorder or injury—all practices
- Diagnostic and screening procedures—all practices
- Surgical procedures—minor surgery (does not include cryotherapy or nail surgery)
- Maternity and midwifery services—ante- or postnatal care
- Family planning services—only practices that insert IUDs

Essential standards There are currently 28 essential standards althoug this may change in the near future. Practices must provide evidence tha they meet 16 to be registered with CQC (the remaining 12 relate ongoing provision of the service):
- Outcome 1: Respecting and involving people who use services
- Outcome 2: Consent to care and treatment
- Outcome 4: Care and welfare of people who use services
- Outcome 5: Meeting nutritional needs
- Outcome 6: Cooperating with other providers
- Outcome 7: Safeguarding people who use services from abuse

Outcome 8: Cleanliness and infection control
Outcome 9: Management of medicines
Outcome 10: Safety and suitability of premises
Outcome 11: Safety, availability, and suitability of equipment
Outcome 12: Requirements relating to workers—staff properly
qualified and able to do their jobs
Outcome 13: Staffing—enough staff to provide the service
Outcome 14: Supporting workers—proper training and supervision,
chances to develop/improve skills
Outcome 16: Assessing and monitoring the quality of service
provision—quality checking systems to manage risks
Outcome 17: Complaints
Outcome 21: Records—accuracy, safe keeping, and confidentiality

If practices do not comply, they may still be registered but must ensure
that they take steps to manage any risks posed by non-compliance and
must submit an action plan to explain the steps that will be taken to meet
compliance with a target date for achievement.

Monitoring After registration, the CQC inspects practices on a regular
basis to ensure that they continue to meet essential standards.

Figure 4.2 How does clinical governance fit with other quality initiatives?

Further information
Care Quality Commission ℘ www.cqc.org.uk

Evidence-based medicine

Definition Conscientious, explicit, and judicious use of current be[st] evidence in making decisions about the care of individual patients.

The 5 steps of evidence-based medicine (EBM) are

1. Convert clinical information needs into answerable questions
2. Track down the best evidence with which to answer them (see Table 4.2 for useful web resources)
3. Critically appraise that evidence for its validity and usefulness (Table 4.1 explains grading of evidence)
4. Apply the results of this appraisal in clinical practice
5. Evaluate your clinical performance e.g. through audit ([ ] p. 80)

Practising EBM involves integrating individual clinical expertise wit[h] the best available external clinical evidence from systematic researc[h.] The problem for the clinician on the ground is finding and interpreting th[e] appropriate evidence for the clinical situation. If good-quality evidence [is] out there (and there are many under-researched areas in medicine)—ho[w] do you access it? When do you find the time to search for it? How do yo[u] assess its quality and relevance?

Critical appraisal The process of assessing and interpreting eviden[ce] by systematically considering its validity, results, and relevance. Essenti[al] to avoid misinterpretation and misuse of evidence in practice. In all case[s] before integrating evidence into practice, consider:

- Are the results of the study valid?
- What are the results?
- Will they help me in caring for my patients?

Critical Appraisal Skills Programme (CASP) appraisal tools are availab[le] from ♫ www.casp-uk.net

Table 4.1 Classification and grading of evidence: most → least reliable

Grade	Evidence level	Definition: *evidence obtained from...*
A	Ia	Meta-analysis of randomized controlled trials
	Ib	At least one randomized controlled trial
B	IIa	At least one well-designed controlled study without randomization, e.g. case–control study, cohort study
	IIb	At least one other type of well-designed quasi-experimental study
	III	Well-designed non-experimental descriptive studies, such as comparative studies, correlation studies, and case studies
C	IV	Expert committee reports or opinions and/or clinical experience of respected authorities

Table 4.2 Useful web resources

	Website: ℘ http:// + suffix
General information	
NHS Evidence	www.evidence.nhs.uk (has guidelines index and numerous links to EBM websites)
Bandolier	www.medicine.ox.ac.uk/bandolier/
Evidence Based Medicine	ebm.bmjjournals.com
ScHARR	www.shef.ac.uk/scharr/about
Guidelines	
NICE	www.nice.org.uk
Scottish Intercollegiate Guidelines Network (SIGN)	www.sign.ac.uk
eGuidelines	www.eguidelines.co.uk (registration needed)
National Guidelines Clearing House (US)	www.guideline.gov
Systematic reviews	
Cochrane library	Access via: www.thecochranelibrary.com
Clinical Evidence (BMJ Publishing)	www.clinicalevidence.com
Health Technology Assessment (HTA)	www.hta.ac.uk
Drugs and Therapeutics Bulletin (DTB)	dtb.bmj.com (subscription required)
NICE—Medicine and Prescribing support evidence summaries	www.nice.org.uk/mpc/
PubMed'	Access via BMJ website (www.bmj.com) or NHS Evidence (www.nhs.evidence.nhs.uk)

When searching, aim to retrieve all the most relevant citations with a minimum of junk.
A useful tip is to use the 'Clinical Queries' or 'Systematic Reviews' filter to restrict the amount
of information retrieved.

Further information

Sackett DL, Straus SE, Richardson WS, *et al.* (2000) *Evidence-based Medicine: How to Practice and Teach EBM* (2nd ed). Edinburgh: Churchill Livingstone. ISBN: 0443062404

Winloch I. (1996) *The Pocket Guide to Critical Appraisal*. London: BMJ Books. ISBN: 072791099X

Greenhalgh T. (2000) *How to read a paper* (2nd ed). London: BMJ Books. ISBN: 0727915789

Jones R. (2013) *Critical reading for primary care: The BJGP/RCGP toolkit* ℘ www.rcgp.org.uk

Glossary of terms used in evidence-based medicine

Absolute risk reduction/increase The absolute arithmetic differen in rates of bad outcomes between experimental and control participan in a trial, calculated as the difference in experimental event rate (EER) a control event rate (CER).

Bias Systematic disposition of certain trial designs to produce resul consistently better or worse than other trial designs. Always consid whether a study is biased before accepting its conclusions.

Further information ℘ www.medicine.ox.ac.uk/bandolier/Extraforband Bias.pdf

Case–control study Involves identifying patients who have the outcom of interest (cases) and control patients without the same outcome, a looking back to see if they had the exposure of interest.

Cohort study Involves identification of two groups (cohorts) patients: one that received the exposure of interest, and one that did n and following these cohorts forward for the outcome of interest.

Confidence interval (CI) Quantifies uncertainty in measuremen Usually reported as 95% CI, which is the range of values within which can be 95% sure that the true value for the whole population lies.

Control event rate (CER) The rate at which events occur a control group. It may be represented by a percentage (e.g. 10%) proportion (e.g. 0.1).

Cost–benefit analysis Assesses whether the cost of an intervention worth the benefit by measuring both in the same (usually monetary) uni

Further information ℘ www.medicine.ox.ac.uk/bandolier/painre download/whatis/Cost-effect.pdf

Cross-sectional study Observation of a defined population at a sing point in time or time interval.

Experimental event rate (EER) Rate at which events occur in experimental group, expressed as a percentage or proportion (see CER

False negative/positive 🕮 p. 171

Likelihood ratio (LR) Likelihood that a given test result would expected in a patient with the target disorder compared with t likelihood that the same result would be expected in a patient witho the target disorder. Gives an indication of accuracy of a clinical test. T higher the likelihood ratio, the better the test at detecting the disorder.

Meta-analysis Systematic review that uses quantitative methods summarize the results.

Further information
℘ www.medicine.ox.ac.uk/bandolier/painres/download/whatis/Meta-An.pc

Number needed to treat (NNT) A measure of the difference between active treatment and control treatment. An NNT of 1 describes a situation where an event occurs in every patient given the active treatment but no patient in the comparison group. There are few circumstances in which a treatment is 100% effective and placebo completely ineffective, so NNTs of 2–3 indicate an effective intervention.

Calculating NNT

A = Number who had successful outcome with the intervention
    ÷ total number who had the intervention
B = Number who had successful outcome with control ÷ total
    number who had the control

$$NNT = \frac{1}{A - B}$$

Further information

◊ www.medicine.ox.ac.uk/bandolier/painres/download/whatis/NNT.pdf *and*
◊ www.medicine.ox.ac.uk/bandolier/Extraforbando/NNTextra.pdf

Number needed to harm (NNH) Compares the number having a side effect in the intervention group against the number having that side effect in the comparison group. If no one in the control group and no one in the comparison group has an unwanted effect the NNH will be infinity. Therefore, the NNH should be as large as possible.

Odds ratio (OR) Odds of an event are calculated as the number of events divided by the number of non-events. The odds ratio is the ratio of the odds in the experimental group compared to the control group. For epidemiological studies looking for factors causing harm, an odds ratio >1 indicates the factor the experimental group was exposed to caused harm. For experimental studies looking for a decrease in events through treatment, an odds ratio <1 indicates a positive result. Often expressed as a percentage.

Positive predictive value 📖 p. 171

Relative risk or risk ratio (RR) Ratio of risk in the treated group (EER) to risk in the control group (CER). RR = ERR/CER. It is used in randomized trials and cohort studies. If the RR = 1, there is no difference between the two groups for that measure.

Relative risk reduction (RRR) Difference between the EER and CER (EER – CER) divided by the CER. Usually expressed as a percentage.

Sensitivity 📖 p. 171

Specificity 📖 p. 171

Systematic review Summary of the medical literature that uses explicit methods to perform a thorough literature search and critical appraisal of individual studies and uses appropriate statistical techniques to combine results of studies of acceptable quality.

Clinical guidelines, protocols, and integrated care pathways

Clinical guidelines Defined as 'user-friendly statements that bri together the best external evidence and other knowledge necessary ; decision making about a specific health problem'. Over recent years, the has been a dramatic ↑ in publication of guidelines and protocols. They a to ↓ harmful or expensive variations in clinical practice, improve hea care outcomes, and encourage rapid dissemination of useful innovatio Good clinical guidelines have 3 properties—they:

- Define practice questions and identify all their decision options and outcomes
- Identify, appraise, and summarize best evidence about prevention, diagnosis, prognosis, therapy, harm, and cost effectiveness
- Identify the decision points at which the evidence needs to be integrated with individual clinical experience and clinical circumstance in deciding a course of action

Advantages and disadvantages of guidelines

Advantages

- Provide guidance for busy clinicians—a consistent basis for decision-making
- Practical framework for common problems and chronic disease
- Summaries the available research evidence
- Can be used as a basis for continuing medical education
- Justification for expenditure—can aid cost-effective use of limited resources
- Facilitate the audit cycle

Disadvantages

- Poor-quality guidelines can reinforce poor practice
- Lack of relevance of the guidelines to the clinical setting—much of the 'evidence' used to develop guidelines comes from secondary care and may not reflect the situation in primary care
- Tendency to uniformity—can stifle innovation
- Resistance to change—new methods may not be considered until a new guideline is produced
- Increased risk of litigation
- Cost—guidelines are time-consuming to develop and update
- Lack of ownership—guidelines developed by others may not feel relevant
- Difficulties in implementation—guidelines that are not user-friendly and well disseminated will not be used

efore starting to use a guideline Always ask:
s this guideline valid, important, and applicable in my practice?'

the answer is yes, then consider
What barriers exist to implementation?
Can they be overcome?
Can you enlist collaboration of key colleagues?
Can you meet the educational and administrative conditions that are
likely to determine the success or failure of implementing the strategy?

rotocol Is the term reserved for guidelines at the more rigid end of
e spectrum. These are very specific guidelines which are expected to
e followed in detail, with little scope for variation, e.g. resuscitation
rotocols.

ntegrated care pathway (ICP) ICPs amalgamate all the anticipated
ements of care and treatment of the multidisciplinary team for a
articular patient group in order to achieve agreed outcomes. Any
eviation from the plan is documented as variance—the analysis of which
rovides information for the review of current practice. ICPs aim to:
Facilitate introduction of guidelines and systemic audit into clinical
practice
Improve multidisciplinary communication and care planning
Reach or exceed existing standards
Decrease unwanted practice variation
Improve clinician–patient communication and patient satisfaction
Identify research and development questions
Cross the interface between primary, secondary, and social care

rading/classification of evidence 📖 p. 74

urther information
HS Evidence—guidelines database, integrated care pathways database,
d useful information on development of guidelines.
ⓢ www.evidence.nhs.uk
ICE ℘ www.nice.org.uk
cottish Intercollegiate Guidelines Network ℘ www.sign.ac.uk
Guidelines ℘ www.eguidelines.co.uk (free registration required)
ational Guidelines Clearing House (US) ℘ www.guideline.gov

Audit

Audit is defined as the systematic critical analysis of quality of health care. Its purpose is to appraise current practice (*What is happening?*) by measuring it against preselected standards (*What should be happening?*) to identify and implement areas for change (*What changes are needed?*) and then improve performance.

Audit differs from research, as research aims to establish what best practice is globally; audit aims to discover how close practice is to best practice on a local level and identify ways of improving care. Audit is a continuous process and an integral part of clinical governance ([] p. 72). All practices in the UK are involved in audit in some way.

Aims of audit
- Improved care of patients
- Enhanced professionalism of staff
- Efficient use of resources
- Aid to continuing education
- Aid to administration
- Accountability to those outside the profession

Criterion-based audit—the audit cycle The process of identifying areas of care to be audited, implementing necessary changes, and periodically reviewing the same issues is known as the audit cycle—see Figure 4.3.

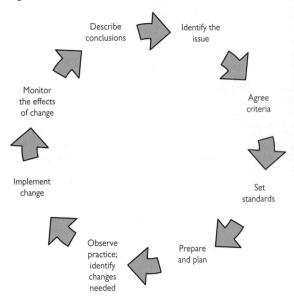

Describe conclusions

Identify the issue

Monitor the effects of change

Agree criteria

Implement change

Set standards

Observe practice; identify changes needed

Prepare and plan

Figure 4.3 The audit cycle

Choosing a topic Any practice matter—clinical or administrative. Make sure the topic is important, manageable, clearly defined, and data are available to assess the criteria chosen. Good starting points are significant events, QOF targets, complaints, National Service Framework or clinical guideline topics, and personal observations.

Choosing criteria Criteria are specific statements of what should be happening. Criteria might be those laid down for quality payments, 'gold standard' care as defined in guidelines, or generated within the practice. Use evidence-based criteria wherever possible. All criteria have to be measurable—ideally with data already collected.

Setting standards Standards are minimum levels of acceptable performance for a criterion. 100% achievement of standards is unusual, so set realistic standards based on quality framework levels and standards achieved by other practices (e.g. comparative practice data, audits from other practices) or previous audits within the practice.

Observing practice You can collect information from: computer registers; medical records; questionnaires—patients, staff, or GPs; data collection sheets (e.g. drugs in doctor's bag are all in date).

Comparing results with standards Consider why standards have not been met. What should be done? Who's going to do it? When? How?

Repeating the audit cycle To ensure action taken is effective.

Significant event audit Process in which individual episodes (when there has been a significant occurrence, either beneficial or deleterious) are analysed in a systematic and detailed way to ascertain what can be learnt about the overall quality of care and to indicate changes that might lead to future improvements. Methods of reporting—see Table 4.3.

Table 4.3 Methods of reporting significant event audits

Reporting method 1	Reporting method 2
Description of event This should be brief and can be in note form	*What happened?*
Learning outcome This should describe the aspects which were of high standard and those that could be improved. Where appropriate, it should include why the event occurred	*Why did it happen?* *Was insight demonstrated?* *Was change implemented?*
Action plan The decision(s) taken need to be contained in the report. The reasons for these decisions should be described together with any other lessons learned from the discussion	

Further information

NICE Best practice in clinical audit
☞ www.nice.org.uk/niceMedia/pdf/BestPracticeClinicalAudit.pdf
RCGP Occasional Paper 70: significant event audit (1995)
☞ www.rcgp.org.uk

Research in general practice

Discovery of new knowledge (*research*) and spreading that knowledg (*dissemination*) is essential for provision of high-quality care. GPs may b involved in research at many levels—as part of an academic department, i a research general practice, or just taking part in a project. Drug compan research—💷 p. 148.

The research process See Figure 4.4

National Institute for Health Research (NIHR) Commissions an funds NHS and social care research in England and provides infrastructur to support both studies and researchers within the NHS. 🕾 www.nihr.ac.u

Primary Care Research Network (PCRN) One of a numbe of research networks that operate under the umbrella of the NIHP Focusses on areas of research for which primary care has particula responsibility: disease prevention, health promotion, screenin early diagnosis, and the clinical management of long-term condition Studies may be accepted onto its portfolio if the topic of the researc falls within the remit of the PCRN and funding has been obtaine through a recognized funding body as a result of open competition an peer review. The PCRN keeps a list of all the studies in its portfoli 🕾 www.crncc.nihr.ac.uk/about_us/pcrn

Within the PCRN, there are eight local research networks. These pr vide support to researchers developing proposals and studies within th portfolio through network-funded staff. This can be anything from hel with formulation of a study proposal, through identification of subjects an recruitment, to help with data management.

❶ A separate Primary Care Research Network operates in Scotland.

University departments of general practice Most UK medic schools have a department of primary care. There are few GP academ posts, but these departments are invaluable sources of advice and suppo if you contemplate doing any original research of your own.

RCGP Supports research by giving advice to GPs, providing researc training fellowships and research funding through the Scientific Foundatic Board, sponsoring research units and research practices, and administerir a quality assessment scheme for research practices. 🕾 www.rcgp.org.uk

Ethics An ethics committee must pass all medical research involvir human participants. Information, contacts, and application forms ar available from the National Research Ethics Service 🕾 www.nres.nhs.uk

Funding Numerous sources of funding for primary care researc are available (including NIHR, RCGP, Medical Research Council, an Wellcome Trust), but all are keenly fought for. Take time preparing you protocol. Ask for advice. It helps to have an experienced researcher a co-applicant on the application form or as project supervisor.

Turn your idea into a specific research question
- What is your aim/hypothesis?
- Review the literature (p. 74)
- Is your idea novel?
- Why does it matter?

Design the study and develop your methods
- Involve participants/other researchers
- Qualitative or quantitative methodology?
- Survey design/sample size
- How are you going to choose/randomize participants?
- Who is going to do the work?

Obtain permissions, funding, and PCRN acceptance
- Ask the healthcare Trust in which the research will be performed
- Ensure that you contact the research governance officer of the organization within which your research will be carried out, and comply with local and national requirements
- Obtain ethics permission
- Obtain funding to cover the costs of the study and staff required
- Gain acceptance onto the PCRN (or another research network) portfolio

Collect and collate data Remember the importance of data protection (p. 51).

Analyse and interpret data
- Consider involving a professional statistician for quantitative data
- Think about the implications of the study findings
- Identify how findings can be put into practice

Write up and disseminate findings
- Journal articles
- Conference presentations
- Press releases
- Submission for higher degrees

Figure 4.4 The research process

Outcomes in general practice

Within the NHS, there are ↑ demands for accountability/improvement in quality of care. To measure this requires use of appropriate outcomes

Patient satisfaction Implies meeting both the wants and needs of the patient. Satisfaction measures are increasingly being used to judge the effectiveness of the NHS. Surveys of satisfaction show ~80% of patients are overall satisfied with GP care, but, if questioned more specifically about different components of care (e.g. information provided, communication etc.), fewer than half are completely satisfied.

Revalidation Measuring patient satisfaction of ≥34 patients using validated tool approved by the GMC is a requirement for GPs once in every 5y revalidation cycle. Approved surveys include:
- **GMC Patient Questionnaire** ℘ www.gmc-uk.org
- **Consultation and Relational Empathy (CARE) measure** ℘ www. gla.ac.uk/researchinstitutes/healthwellbeing/research/generalpractice/ caremeasure/use/
- **Improving Patient Questionnaire (IPQ)** ❶ Charge payable. ℘ www.cfepsurveys.co.uk
- **Doctors' Interpersonal Skills Questionnaire (DISQ)** ❶ Charge payable. ℘ www.cfepsurveys.co.uk
- **Consultation Satisfaction Questionnaire (CSQ)** ❶ Charge payable. ℘ www.patientdynamics.co.uk

GPs must reflect on results and address any development needs.

Peer feedback Is a tool widely used in business to assess worker performance. It may take many forms—from team meetings during which colleague feedback is encouraged, through annual appraisal by a practice manager, to 360° or multi-source feedback forms.

Revalidation Feedback from ≥12 professional colleagues representing the range of your professional activities, using a validated *multi-source feedback* (MSF) tool approved by the GMC, is a compulsory element of revalidation and must be performed once in every 5y cycle. Approved MSF tool include:
- **GMC Colleague Questionnaire** ℘ www.gmc-uk.org
- **2Q MSF** ℘ www.tipportfolio.co.uk/example2q.aspx
- **Colleague Multi-Source Feedback tool for Revalidation** ❶ Charge payable. ℘ www.mylmc.com
- **Sheffield Peer Review Assessment Tool Version 2 (GP-SPRAT)** ❶ Charge payable. ℘ www.waspsoftware.co.uk
- **Colleague Feedback Evaluation Tool Version 2 (CFET)** ❶ Charge payable. ℘ www.cfepsurveys.co.uk
- **Edgecumbe Doctor 360°** ❶ Charge payable. ℘ www.doctor360.co.uk

GPs must reflect on results and address any development needs.

Comparative practice data The government's '*transparency agenda*' has resulted in publication of data held by government departments on the performance of public services, including general practice. Data now in the public domain are listed in Box 4.2.

Box 4.2 GP practice data available in the public domain

Demographic

- GP practice location
- Patient registrations
- Deprivation
- Expected and actual prevalence of disease

Impact on NHS resources

- A&E attendances
- Length of stay
- Admissions (elective and unplanned)
- Referral/outpatient appointments

Infrastructure

- IT services
- Number of GPs

Patient experience

QOF performance

Referrals There are wide variations in referral rates (~3–12/100 consultations) not accounted for by population characteristics. Experience in a specialty ↑ referrals, implying high referrers are not always inadequate.

Referral management schemes Attempts have been made to judge appropriateness of referrals either at practice or at locality level through referral management schemes. All referrals are scrutinized to judge whether the referral is needed at all and (if referral is warranted) whether referral is being made to the most cost-effective service.

Prescribing rates There are wide variations in prescribing rates, e.g. variation in the rate of statin prescription cannot be accounted for by population characteristics; prescription rates for antibiotics for minor illness vary widely between GPs. Whether and how these reflect quality of care is controversial, but comparison of practice prescribing data within localities and prescribing quality targets are driving down prescribing costs.

Procedures Comparisons of procedure outcome (e.g. inadequate smear rates, diabetic outcome measures, immunization rates) between practices can be a way to identify individuals or practices clearly performing less well than others. The reasons must then be investigated.

Doctors' ability to detect illness There are wide variations between GPs in their ability to detect certain illnesses, e.g. mental illness. GPs adept at identifying mental health problems have empathy, early eye contact; use directive rather than closed questioning; clarify the complaint at an early stage. Whether this is a marker of quality of care or just the diversity of general practice is debatable.

Compliance/concordance 📖 p. 142

Further information

RCGP Review of colleague and patient survey instruments (2012) ℗ www.rcgp.org.uk

NHS Choices Patient information and practice scorecards available to compare practices ℗ www.nhs.uk

NHS Information Centre Practice comparative data ℗ https://indicators.ic.nhs.uk

Consulting and certification

The consultation

Over the past 15y, there has been a 40% ↑ in demand for GP appointments in the UK. Each patient now has an average of 5.5 appointments/y. Older people have the highest consultation rate (those >80y have 13.5 appointments/y), and consultation rate is set to ↑ as the population ages.

Potential barriers to effective communication Lack of time, language problems, differing gender, age, ethnic or social background of doctor and patient, 'sensitive' issues to address, 'hidden' or differing agendas, prior difficult meetings, lack of trust between doctor/patient.

The consultation Good communication is essential for all aspects of a GP's work. The consultation is the cornerstone of general practice and focusses on successful information exchange. Various consultation models exist (📖 p. 90) to help GPs evaluate their consultations and make optimum use of the time available. There is no 'correct' way to perform a consultation. Approach will vary according to situation and participants.

Patient centredness Means that the patient's viewpoint is considered and integrated into the diagnosis and decision-making process (see Figure 5.1). It improves patient satisfaction and may improve health outcomes. It consists of 6 interactive components:
- Exploring the disease and illness experience
- Understanding the whole person in context
- Finding common ground regarding management
- Incorporating prevention and health promotion
- Enhancing the doctor–patient relationship
- Being realistic

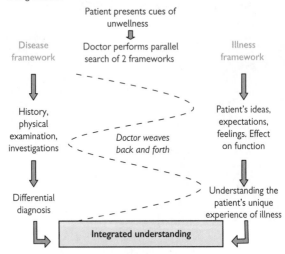

Figure 5.1 The patient-centred process

Patient recall Many studies suggest that >50% (some estimate up to 90%) of information has been forgotten within a few minutes of leaving the surgery. Characteristics of memorable information:
* The patient perceives it as important
* The patient understands it (avoid the use of jargon and medical terms, keep language brief and simple, support with sketches/diagrams ± patient information sheets)
* The information is given early in the consultation
* The information is given in small chunks (not too much at once)

Consultation length Although consultations are usually booked at 10min intervals in the UK, average consultation length is now 11.7min. Instead of managing acute illness, GPs now focus on management of long-term conditions, resulting in ↑ complexity of consultations. Despite this, UK consultations are still a third shorter than those in other parts of the world, e.g. the USA, Switzerland, New Zealand, Belgium, or Australia.

Timekeeping Running late is stressful and frustrating for patients. General practice does not fit conveniently into 10min (or any other size) slots. Even the best time keepers occasionally run late. *Tips:*
* **Endeavour to run to time** Start on time; make appointments long enough (e.g. book double appointments for difficult problems, schedule catch-up slots in the middle of surgeries, change to longer appointments); break difficult problems or multiple problems up into chunks
* **If you are running late** Ask reception staff to apologize to patients as they check in, and tell them the expected delay

Benefits of longer consultation times Include:
* ↑ patient and doctor satisfaction
* ↑ identification of psychosocial problems
* Improved doctor–patient communication
* ↑ health promotion
* ↓ reconsultation rates
* ↓ minor illness prescribing

Heartsink patients Characterized by:
* Frequent presentation—the top 1% of attenders at GP surgeries generate 6% of GP workload
* Highly complex and often multiple problems—some real, others not
* Exasperation generated between patient and doctor

❶ It is a two-way process. Some GPs report more heartsink patients than others. The problem relates to the GP's perception of patients as well as the patients themselves. *GP risk factors*: perception of high workload; low job satisfaction; lack of training in counselling or communication; lack of postgraduate skills.

Management strategy Do a detailed review of notes ± chart of life.
* Agree contacts (e.g. limit to one GP, agree appointment frequency)
* Agree an agenda within consultations, e.g. problem list—1 problem/visit
* Employ reattribution techniques—see Somatization disorder, 🔲 p. 997
* Avoid unnecessary investigation and referral
* Be aware of your own reaction to the patient
* Acknowledge that such patients can be genuinely ill
* Consider psychiatric diagnoses—especially chronic anxiety, depression, somatization disorder. Screening questionnaires can be useful
* Consider referral for CBT and/or specialist mental health support

Consultation models

The consultation process has been extensively studied—each mode views it from a slightly different perspective. A brief overview of each presented here—for more information, consult the original texts:

The medical model Traditional model. History taking → examination → investigation → diagnosis → treatment → follow-up. Does not recognize the complexity and diversity of the consultation in general practice.

Balint, 1957 *The Doctor, His Patient and The Illness*—a philosophy rather than a consultation model:
- Psychological problems are often manifested physically
- Doctors have feelings. Those feelings have a role in the consultation
- Doctors need to be trained to be more sensitive to what is going on in the patient's mind during a consultation
Reference: Churchill Livingstone; ISBN: 0443064601

Berne, 1964 *Games People Play*—describes how to recognize behaviours ('games') patients might use and roles patient and doctor might adopt—'Parent, Adult and Child'.
Reference: Penguin Books; ISBN: 0140027688

RCGP, 1972 *The triaxial approach*—physical, psychological and social aspects of the consultation.
Reference: Working party of the RCGP, 1972

Becker and Maiman, 1975 *Health Belief Model*—Involves exploration of concerns, beliefs, and expectations of the patient. 5 elements:
- Health motivation
- Perceived vulnerability
- Perceived seriousness
- Perceived costs/benefits of an action
- Cues to action—stimuli/triggers for beliefs
Reference: Med Care 1975 **13** 10–24

Heron, 1975 *Six Category Intervention Analysis*—6 types of intervention a doctor could use with a patient:
1. Prescriptive
2. Informative
3. Confronting
4. Cathartic
5. Catalytic
6. Supportive
Reference: University of Surrey, 1975

Byrne and Long, 1976 *Doctors talking to patients*—6 aspects:
1. Doctor establishes a relationship with the patient
2. Doctor attempts to/actually discovers the reason for attendance
3. Doctor conducts verbal ± physical examination
4. Doctor or doctor + patient or the patient consider the condition
5. Doctor (occasionally the patient) details treatment and investigation
6. Consultation is terminated—usually by the doctor
Reference: RCGP; ISBN: 0850840929

Stott and Davis, 1979 *Exceptional potential of the consultation.* 4 tasks:
1. Management of presenting problems
2. Management of continuing problems
3. Modification of help-seeking behaviour
4. Opportunistic health promotion
Reference: JRCGP 1979 **29** 201–5

Helman's folk model, 1981 *Disease vs. illness in general practice:*
- What has happened?
- Why to me?
- Why has it happened?
- Why now?
- What would happen if nothing were done about it?
- What should I do and who should I consult for further help?
Reference: JRCGP 1981 **31** 548–52

Pendleton et al., 1984 *The doctor's tasks:*
- Define the reason for patient's attendance
- Consider other problems (continuing problems and at-risk factors)
- Choose an appropriate action for each problem (involves negotiation between doctor and patient)
- Achieve a shared understanding of the problem (doctor and patient)
- Involve the patient in the management and encourage the patient to accept appropriate responsibility
- Use time and resources appropriately
- Establish and maintain a relationship (between doctor and patient)
Reference: Oxford University Press; ISBN: 0192632884

Neighbour ('The Inner Consultation'), 1987 *Checkpoints:*
- Connecting (doctor establishes rapport with the patient)
- Summarizing (doctor clarifies the patient's reason for consulting)
- Handing over (doctor/patient negotiate and agree a management plan)
- Safety netting (doctor/patient plan for the unexpected—managing uncertainty)
- Housekeeping (doctor is aware of his/her own emotions)
Reference: Petroc Press; ISBN: 1900603675

Fraser, 1992 & 1999 *Areas of competence:*
1. Interviewing and history taking
2. Physical examination
3. Diagnosis and problem-solving
4. Patient management
5. Relating to patients
6. Anticipatory care
7. Record-keeping
Reference: Butterworth Heinemann; ISBN: 0750640057

Kurtz and Silverman, 1996 & update 2002 *Calgary—Cambridge Observation Guide*—5 tasks:
1. Initiating the session
2. Gathering information
3. Building the relationship
4. Giving information—explaining and planning
5. Closing the session
Reference: Medical Education 1996 **30** 83–9 & Academic Medicine 2003 **78** (8) 802–9

Warren 2002 *4 avenues of analysis (BARD):*
- Behaviour—non-verbal and verbal—needs of patient/personality of GP
- Aims—purpose of the consultation and priorities
- Room—setting for the consultation
- Dialogue—tone of voice, what is said, etc.
Reference: Update 5.9.2002 152–4

Launer 2002 *Narrative-based approach.* 6 key concepts:
- Conversations
- Curiosity
- Circularity
- Contexts
- Co-creation
- Caution
Reference: Radcliffe Publishing; ISBN: 1857755391

Patient records

General principles

Be factual, consistent, and accurate Write records in an indelible fashion as soon as possible after an event/encounter has occurred. Ensure logical sequence; be clear, unambiguous, legible, and concise. Use standard coding techniques if using an electronic record. Wherever possible, write notes openly whilst patients/carers are present in terms they can understand. Date, time, and sign (or otherwise identify yourself) on all entries.

Be relevant and useful Record:
- **Information you have on which to base your decisions** Problems presented to you by the patient; relevant aspects of past and family history; examination findings and test results you already have
- **Your impression of the situation** How you see the problem—may include diagnosis, differential diagnosis, prognosis
- **Plan of action** Negotiated between patient and doctor—may include tests requested, prescriptions given, referrals made
- **Information shared and advice given** Relevant worries or concerns voiced by the patient; information provided to the patient; advice given—especially contingency plans if things do not go to plan and review/follow-up arrangements
- **Other essential information** e.g. correspondence to/from other agencies; whether a sickness certificate was issued, for how long and the reason stated on the certificate; if consent for disclosure of information (🕮 p. 50) or treatment/examination (🕮 p. 52) was given

Do not include Abbreviations (especially unconventional ones); jargon; personal views about behaviour or temperament unless they have a bearing on the management of the patient.

Electronic patient records 🕮 p. 40
Summary Care Record (SCR) 🕮 p. 40
Confidentiality 🕮 p. 50

Amending records Rectify errors of fact or judgement. Any alterations or additions should be dated, timed, and signed in such a way that the original entry can still be seen. Patients may request correction of information they believe is incorrect—you must record the patient's view. Highlight amendments and reasons for them.

Access to records Under the Data Protection Act 1998, patients have a right of access to health records which:
- Are about them and from which they can be identified
- Consist of information relating to their health or condition, and
- Have been made in connection with their care

❶ Most records doctors make are included whenever they were made.

Who can seek access?

• Any competent person may seek access to their own health records, including competent children (📖 p. 50)
• Any person with parental responsibility may apply for access to records of a child (<18y or <16y in Scotland). Where >1 person has parental responsibility, each may apply independently without consent of the other parent
• A third party authorized by a competent person may seek access to that person's records (e.g. a solicitor or insurance company), but proof of permission from the patient must be provided. If there is doubt, contact the patient to verify consent has been given (📖 p. 50)

Mentally incapacitated adults Where access is sought and the individual to whom the patient records pertain lacks capacity to give permission, decisions must be based on an evaluation of the person's best interests, taking into account the views of the person's representative(s) and reflecting the individual's expressed wishes and values—📖 p. 50.

Access to dead patients' records 📖 p. 50

Requests for access Nothing prevents doctors from giving patients access to their records on an informal basis, provided there is no reason preventing disclosure. Information must *not* be disclosed if it:
• is likely to cause serious physical or mental harm; *or*
• relates to a third party who has not given consent for disclosure (when not a health professional who has cared for the patient)

❶ If unsure, take advice from the BMA or your defence organization.

Formal applications for access must be in writing and accompanied by the appropriate fee. Patients are entitled to a permanent copy of information (e.g. photocopy, printout), which must be accompanied by an explanation of any unintelligible terms. Access must be given within 40d of receipt of the fee and request. Contact BMA for current fees.

Security of records Do not leave records (electronic or manual) unattended in easily accessible areas. When not in use, ideally store all files and portable equipment under lock and key. Query the status of strangers. Highlight any concerns to the practice/security manager. Do not reveal how security systems operate.
• **Manual records** Store files closed and in logical order. Use a tracking system to monitor the whereabouts of files, and return files taken away as soon as they are no longer required
• **Electronic records** Do not leave a terminal unattended and logged in. Do not share logins or reveal your password to others. Change passwords regularly, and avoid using short or obvious ones. Always clear the screen of a previous patient's information before seeing another. Use a password-protected screen saver to prevent casual viewing of patient information by others

Further information

Access to health records by patients. BMA 🖰 www.bma.org.uk
GMC Guidance on good practice—confidentiality 🖰 www.gmc-uk.org

Telephone consulting and home visits

To cope with ↑ demand for GP appointments, the past 20y have seen the proportion of GP consultations that take place over the telephone rise from 3% to 12%; simultaneously, the proportion of consultations taking place in patients' own homes has fallen from 9% to 3.5%.

Emergency telephone consultations Nearly all requests for emergency care are made by telephone. *General rules:*

- Train surgery staff to handle distressed callers, recognize serious problems, and act appropriately when such calls are received
- Where possible, use a single number for patients to access help. If using an answering machine, ensure the message is easily heard and contains clear instructions
- Appear helpful from the outset. Keep calm and friendly—even if provoked; worried callers often appear abrupt or demanding
- Record the time of the call, date, patient's name, the address the patient is at and a contact telephone number, brief details of the problem, and action taken (even if calls are being recorded)
- Collect only information you need to decide whether a visit or urgent surgery appointment is necessary. If a visit is necessary, collect enough information to decide how quickly the patient should be seen and whether extra equipment or help is needed. If a visit is not necessary, decide whether other actions, such as an urgent surgery appointment, would be more appropriate
- If giving advice, make it simple and in a language the patient can understand. Repeat to make sure it has been understood. Consider asking the patient/carer to repeat what you have told them. Always tell callers to ring back if symptoms change or they have further worries
- If a visit is indicated, ensure the address is right and ask for directions if you are not sure where to go. Try to give a rough arrival time
- In some cases (e.g. major trauma, large GI bleeds, MI, stroke, burns, overdoses), call for an emergency ambulance at once
- If a call seems inappropriate, consider the reason for it, e.g. depression might provoke recurrent calls for minor ailments

⚠ If in doubt—see the patient.

Routine telephone consultations Occur in different ways:

- Telephone triage systems to filter requests for surgery appointments
- Telephone clinics where patients are free to ring with their problems
- Telephone message books, and/or
- Bookable telephone slots in surgery time

The telephone is a useful way to answer simple queries without wasting surgery time. Examples include:

- Consultations for minor, self-limiting conditions or conditions that do not require an examination
- Follow-up of surgery consultations, e.g. to give results, or to offer management advice/prescription following investigations

The biggest drawbacks of telephone consultations are:
- Inability to examine the patient, and
- Lack of visual cues to aid communication

Be alert for verbal cues (e.g. lowering of the voice, hesitations, signs of distress). Ask about ideas/concerns, and invite the patient to ask questions. Before giving advice, ensure you have sufficient information upon which to base your judgement. If examination is needed, see the patient.

Home visiting Home visits may be routine checks for housebound patients or emergency visits for patients temporarily unable to get to the surgery. Home visits done in working hours are usually done by practices under their GMS/PMS contract, but, in some areas, home-visiting services are provided by the PCO and practices are able to 'opt out'.

Routine visits Conducted like ordinary surgery consultations. Seeing patients in their own home may give valuable extra information.

Emergency visits
- Try to stick to the problem you have been called about
- Take a concise history and examine as appropriate
- Make a decision on management, and explain it to the patient and any carers in clear and concise terms they can understand. Repeat advice several times ± write it down
- Record history, examination, management suggested, and advice given for the patient's notes
- Always invite the patient and carers to ring you again should symptoms change, the situation deteriorate, or further worries appear
- For inappropriate calls, take time to educate the patient and/or carers about self-management and use of emergency GP visiting services
- Always consider hidden reasons for seemingly unnecessary visits

Being prepared
- Ensure you have a reliable car with a full tank of fuel
- Have a good street map and in-car electronic navigation system
- Carry a mobile phone and large, strong torch in the car
- Check your drug box is fully stocked and all items are in date
- Check all equipment carried is operational and carry spare batteries
- Carry a list of emergency telephone numbers and know which chemists have extended opening hours and/or carry the chemist's rota

Safety and security
- In all cases, ensure someone else knows where you are going, when to expect you back, and what to do if you do not return on time
- If going to a call you are worried about, either take someone with you to sit in the car or call the police to meet you there before going in
- If you are uncomfortable, make sure you can get out. Note the layout of the property, and make sure you have a clear route to the door
- Set up your mobile phone to call the police or your base at a single touch of a button. Consider carrying an attack alarm
- If possible, have separate bags for drugs and consultation equipment; leave the drug box locked out of sight in the boot of the car when visiting

Referral letters and electronic media

Referral letters Good communication is essential when referring patients to other doctors and agencies. Electronic pre-filled word processing templates may fill in some information automatically, but ensure that all referral letters include:

- Address of the referrer (including telephone number, if possible), name and address of registered GP if not the referrer, and date of referral
- Name, address, telephone number, and date of birth of the patient (and any other identifiers available, e.g. hospital or NHS number)
- Name of the person to whom the patient is being referred (or department if not a named individual)
- Presenting condition—history, examination, investigations already performed with results, treatments already tried with outcomes
- Relevant past medical history and family history
- Current medication, and any intolerances/allergies known
- Reason for referral (what you want the recipient of the letter to do), e.g. to investigate symptoms, to reassure parents
- Any other relevant information, e.g. social circumstances
- Signature (and name in legible format) of referrer ± GMC number
- Ensure that a copy of the referral letter is stored on the patient's electronic record

Use of e-mail in the GP surgery

Dissemination of information E-mail is widely used in the UK to disseminate (cascade) information to GPs, e.g. NICE, DH, MHRA, PCOs

Communication with doctors/other healthcare providers Many communications between doctors occur by e-mail both within practice and also between practices/other healthcare providers (e.g. consultant advice by email). ❶ E-mail transfer between non-NHS e-mail accounts should never be considered secure or confidential.

Communication with patients ~80% of the UK population now have access to e-mail. Cyber-savvy patients increasingly want to be able to communicate with healthcare professionals by e-mail, but e-mail has been used relatively little to date due to concerns over quality of e-mail content, time lag, confidentiality, and liability. Its use is likely to develop further. Successful use of e-mails depends on both the doctor and patient having a clear understanding of its role, advantages, and limitations.

Guidelines for e-mail consultations with patients

- Establish turnaround time; do not use e-mail for urgent matters
- Warn users that e-mail is not secure and that they cannot assume confidentiality just because they are communicating with a doctor
- Advise patients not to use a work or multi-user e-mail
- Retain copies of e-mail communications with patients
- Instruct patients to put the category of transaction in the subject line of the message for filtering: prescription, appointment, medical advice
- Request that patients put their name and date of birth in the message for identification purposes

- Configure an automatic reply to acknowledge receipt of messages
- Send a new message to inform the patient of completion of the request; ensure that others are not copied into the reply
- Avoid giving person-specific information or confirming information given by the patient—it may not be the patient
- Never write anything that you would not be happy to see printed on a newspaper front page
- Request that patients use reply to acknowledge reading your message
- Append a standard block of text to the end of e-mail messages to patients which contains the GP's full name, contact information, and reminders about security and the importance of alternative forms of communication for emergencies
- Explain to patients that their messages should be concise
- Remind patients when they do not adhere to the guidelines

Social media Internet-based websites/tools allowing users to create/share content between networks of people, e.g. Facebook, LinkedIn, Twitter, YouTube. Social media are used successfully by doctors to:
- Establish wider/more diverse social and professional networks
- Engage the public and colleagues in debates
- Facilitate public access to accurate health information, and
- Improve patient access to services

Risks of social media use
- Loss of personal privacy
- Potential breaches of confidentiality
- Online behaviour that might be perceived as unprofessional, offensive, or inappropriate by others
- Risks of posts being reported by the media or sent to employers

Guidance on social media use The BMA, GMC, and RCGP have all produced guidelines for doctors on the use of social media. *Key points:*
- Social media blurs boundaries between public/professional lives
- Adopt conservative privacy settings where available, but be aware that not all information can be protected on the web
- Ethical and legal duties to protect patient confidentiality apply equally on the internet as to other media
- It is inappropriate to post informal, personal, or derogatory comments about patients or colleagues on public internet forums
- Doctors who post online should declare any conflicts of interest
- Do not accept Facebook friend requests from current/former patients
- Defamation law can apply to any comments posted on the web made in either a personal or professional capacity
- Be conscious of online image and its impact on professional standing

Further information
Car J, Sheikh A (2004) Email consultations in healthcare. *BMJ* **329**:435–42.
BMA Using social media: practical and ethical guidance for doctors and medical students (2012) ℰ www.bma.org.uk
GMC Doctor's use of social media: a draft for consultation (2012) ℰ www.gmc-uk.org
RCGP Draft social media highway code (2012) ℰ www.rcgp.org.uk

Organization of out-of-hours services

What is urgent care? Urgent care refers to the range of responses that the health and care services provide to people who need, or perceive that they need, urgent advice, care treatment or diagnosis. Urgent 'same day' appointments currently account for 1 in 3 daytime consultations in general practice, so all GPs must have the skills/knowledge to manage patients with a perceived urgent care need. Effective GPs can manage patients with urgent care needs so that 'dangerous diagnoses' are not missed and A&E and acute hospital services are used efficiently.

What are OOH services? Urgent primary medical care is provided by out-of-hours (OOH) services from 6.30 p.m. to 8 a.m. on weekdays and throughout weekends and public holidays—a total of at least 70% of every week. In England alone, every year primary care OOH services:
- Receive 8.6 million calls, and
- Complete 6.8 million assessments—3 million in out-of-hours primary care centres (44%), 2.9 million by telephone (43%), and 0.9 million through home visits (13%)

1.5% of the calls dealt with are considered 'life-threatening' emergencies and 15% are classified as 'urgent'.

'Opting out' of OOH Both PMS and GMS practices can 'opt out' of providing an OOH service. The decision must be made for the whole practice; individual doctors within a practice cannot 'opt out' alone. The cost of opting out is 7% of the global sum (or PMS equivalent).

OOH work by 'opted out' practices There is nothing to stop practices that have opted out from offering surgeries or consultations within the time periods specified as OOH. These services can be paid for through the practice global sum or under the 'extended opening' DES.

Choice of OOH provider PCOs can consider a range of alternative OOH care providers as long as accreditation standards are met. Only where a practice is exceptionally remote, will the PCO be able to require a practice to continue providing OOH care. Special arrangements for payment then exist. *Several schemes currently operate side by side:*
- **In-practice rota** Traditional model of cover that is now increasingly rare; usually organized in a rota between practice GPs and largely based on home visiting
- **Extended rota** GPs on-call in rotation for a small group of practices
- **GP co-operative** GPs within an area grouped together (often >100 practices in a co-op) to cover the OOH period either between themselves or by employing other GPs; often several GPs are on call at any time, e.g. one doing visits; one taking calls; one seeing patients in a clinic
- **Hospital-based OOH cover** GPs and primary care nurses in A&E departments
- **Commercial OOH service** OOH provided by a commercial profit-making organization employing GPs and specialist nurses
- **NHS 111 and NHS24** 24h nurse-led telephone advice service available throughout England (NHS 111), Wales (NHS 111 Wales)

and Scotland (NHS 24) designed as first-line services aiming to have links to local primary care and OOH services; the telephone services are supported by websites providing healthcare information

- **NHS walk-in centre** Walk-in clinics tend to offer nurse consultation and use NHS diagnosis and management algorithms; most are sited in urban areas and aim to provide easier access to medical care
- **Enhanced paramedic service** Providing initial assessment of patients who are unable to get to OOH centres and/or patient transport to OOH centres
- **Enhanced community nursing team** Providing care to patients terminally ill and initial assessment of patients who do not feel able to get to an OOH centre for other reasons

Challenges for GPs when providing OOH care

- Higher proportion of very ill patients; GPs may need to commence resuscitation or critical illness management protocols more frequently
- Often no information about patients apart from the information that the patient/carer provides
- Much bigger team—GPs often do not know other team members and may be unfamiliar with their working environment
- OOH GPs may work alone for a high proportion of their time doing home visits or manning an out-of-hours clinic
- Access to drugs and some services may be limited
- First contact is almost always over the telephone and good communication skills are needed to provide accurate assessment, triage to appropriate care, and ensure safety netting

The future of NHS OOH care Over recent years, the NHS OOH service has been criticized for variability in coverage and care provided, access difficulties because of the variety of different out-of-hours providers operating across the UK, and being poor value for money.

The government has made a commitment to provide a coherent 24h urgent care service. In some parts of the UK, the NHS 111 service is being used to route all urgent but non-emergency calls in the out-of-hours period through a single triage system—giving advice or directing callers to the appropriate service (e.g. A&E, ambulance call, GP home visit, or GP appointment). Since 2014, GP practices have a responsibility for monitoring the quality of OOH services for their registered patients.

Pre-hospital emergency care To meet calls for increasing sophistication of pre-hospital emergency care, a new sub-specialty has been developed. For GPs, particularly those working in urgent care settings or with populations that are geographically remote from acute specialist services, expertise in this sub-specialty would clearly be beneficial. However, currently GP training does not allow GPs to meet the basic entry requirement for this sub-specialty. Changes in GP training should remedy this.

Further information

NHS 111 ☎ 111 🖰 www.nhsdirect.nhs.uk
NHS Direct Wales ☎ 0845 4647 🖰 www.nhsdirect.wales.nhs.uk
NHS 24 ☎ 08454 242424 🖰 www.nhs24.com

The doctor's bag

⚠ The GP's bag must be lockable and not be left unattended during home visits. If left in the car keep the bag locked and out of sight—preferably in the boot. Consider having a separate bag for drugs and consultation equipment and only get the drug bag out of the boot of the car if it is needed. Keep the bag away from extremes of temperature.

Consider including the following (exact contents will vary according to location and circumstances):

Diagnostic equipment
- Stethoscope
- Sphygmomanometer
- Thermometer
- Gloves, jelly, and tissues
- Torch
- Otoscope
- Ophthalmoscope
- Tongue depressors
- Peak flow meter
- Pulse oximeter
- Fluorescein sticks
- Urine dipsticks
- Capillary blood glucose tester and appropriate test strips
- Tourniquet, vacutainer (or syringe), and needles
- Patella hammer
- Swabs
- Specimen containers
- Vaginal speculum ± sponge forceps
- Fetal stethoscope/Doppler

Administrative equipment
- Mobile telephone ± charger
- Controlled drugs record book
- Envelopes
- Headed notepaper
- Local map
- Pathology/X-ray forms
- Prescription pad
- List of useful telephone numbers
- BNF/MIMS
- Obstetric calculator
- Peak flow chart/wheel
- Book for keeping a record of patient encounters
- Temporary resident records
- List of local chemists and out-of-hours opening times
- Small amount of change for parking, etc.
- Quick reference text, e.g. *Oxford Handbook of General Practice*

Other equipment
- Airway ± Laerdal mask
- Oxygen cylinder and mask with reservoir bag
- Automated external defibrillator
- Nebulizer
- Spacer device
- IV cannula
- IV giving set and fluids
- Needles/syringes
- Bandages
- Gauze swabs
- Adhesive plasters
- Scissors
- Skin closure strips
- Suturing equipment/skin glue
- Urinary catheter and bag
- Antiseptic sachets
- Dressing pack
- Sharps box

Drugs for the doctor's bag *Consider:*

Injectables
- Adrenaline (epinephrine)
- Naloxone
- Benzylpenicillin injection
- Cefotaxime injection
- Lorazepam/diazepam
- NSAID, e.g. diclofenac
- Local anaesthetic, e.g. lidocaine
- Opioid analgesic, e.g. morphine, diamorphine
- Thrombolytic therapy (if >½h from nearest acute hospital and have training)

- Antiemetic, e.g. domperidone, prochlorperazine
- Antihistamine, e.g. chlorphenamine
- Hydrocortisone injection
- Diuretic, e.g. furosemide
- Syntometrine
- Glucagon ± IV glucose
- Major tranquillizer, e.g. haloperidol, chlorpromazine

Oral drugs
- Antacid
- Antibiotics (adult tablets and paediatric sachets), e.g. amoxicillin + erythromycin/clarithromycin + trimethoprim
- Antihistamine

- Rehydration tablets/sachets
- Aspirin
- Lorazepam
- Paracetamol tablets + suspension
- Prednisolone tablets (soluble)
- NSAID, e.g. ibuprofen

Other drugs
- GTN spray
- Bronchodilator for nebulizer
- Salbutamol inhaler + spacer
- GlucoGel® glucose gel

- Glycerin suppositories
- Rectal diazepam
- Diclofenac suppositories
- Domperidone suppositories

⚠ Check drugs at least 2x/y to see they are still in date and usable; commercial databases (e.g. 🖱 www.doctorsbaguk.com) that store data about drugs in the GP's bag can be useful to alert you when drugs go out of date. Record origin, batch number, and expiry date of *all* drugs administered to patients or dispensed to them to take themselves.

Drugs given to patients from the doctor's bag should be
in a suitable container and properly labelled with:
- Patient's name
- Drug name
- Drug dosage
- Quantity of tablets
- Instructions on use
- Relevant warnings
- Name and address of the doctor
- Date
- Warning 'Keep out of reach of children'

Further information

Drugs and Therapeutics Bulletin Drugs for the doctor's bag 1—adults (September 2005), and Drugs for the doctor's bag 2—children (November 2005)

Social factors in general practice

> 'The task of medicine is to promote health, to prevent disease and to treat the sick … These are highly social functions'
>
> H.E. Sigerist, *Civilization and Disease* (1943

Inverse care law Julian Tudor Hart's inverse care law states that 'the availability of good medical care tends to vary inversely with the need of the population served'. This paradox is true across different diseases and healthcare systems. Health inequalities are not inevitable and addressing social factors can contribute significantly in reducing them; 60% of health improvement in the past century is not attributable to advances in medical care but instead to changes in social factors, such as better housing.

Deprivation Social deprivation is linearly associated with death from all causes, with no threshold and no upper limit. Most pronounced effect are in relation to infant mortality, morbidity/mortality from chronic illness (particularly musculoskeletal, CVD, and respiratory conditions), and teenage pregnancy. This is not a new problem nor one unique to the UK Disparity in health is closely related to income. In the UK an ↑ proportion of the population is now living on <50% of average income than 20y ago— the mortality gap has grown proportionately.

Impact on general practice Higher incidence of illness →↑ requirement for primary care team services and ↑ use of OOH and A&E service amongst deprived communities. This is recognized in the UK in the Carr Hill Index which allocates funds to practices (📖 p. 24).

Benefits for people with low income 📖 p. 104

Homelessness

Temporary accommodation Adverse effects of living in temporary accommodation are well documented:
- Adults have an ↑ incidence of depression than people of similar social standing in their own homes
- Homeless women are 2x as likely to have problems in pregnancy and 3x as likely to require admission in pregnancy
- ¼ of babies born to women living in bed and breakfast accommodation are of low birthweight (national average <1 in 10)
- Children from these families are less likely to receive their immunizations, more likely to have childhood accidents and have higher incidence of minor respiratory tract and diarrhoeal diseases

Sleeping rough Poor diet, poor accommodation, and lack of access to medical services are universal problems in this group. Less than 70% are registered with a GP. Many homeless people will suffer from a triad of poor physical health, mental health, and substance misuse; the average age of death is 40–44y. Homeless people have a higher than average use of emergency and hospital inpatient services as a result. Evidence shows that if primary care services are provided, homeless people will use them

Divorce Divorcees of all ages are at greater risk of premature death (2x ↑ for men aged 35–42y) than married people—mainly from cardio- and cerebrovascular disease, cancer, suicide, and accidental death. There is also a similar ↑ in morbidity. Children of divorced parents have ↑ risk of il ealth from the time of separation until adult life—with children <5y old when their parents separate being particularly vulnerable. These children re also more prone to psychiatric illness later in life and are more likely o become divorced themselves.

Employment and unemployment

> *'Without work all life goes rotten'* Albert Camus

ffects of work have been compared to effects of vitamins—we need a ertain amount to be healthy, then there is a plateau where extra does not elp—and too much is harmful. There is good evidence that unemploy- ent causes both ↑ mortality (from CVD, cancers, suicide, violence, ccidents) and ↑ morbidity (depression, CVD). Threat of unemployment one can cause morbidity—in one study, GP consultation rates rose by 0% and referral rates by 60% after it was announced a factory would lose. Increases were found in other family members too.

Refugees and asylum seekers The Geneva Convention defines refugee as any person who, 'owing to well-founded fear of being ersecuted for reasons of race, religion, nationality, membership of a articular social group or political opinion, is outside the country of his ationality and is unable or, owing to such fear, is unwilling to return it.' Refugees are entitled to free healthcare in the UK. *Consider:*

Language, cultural, and religious issues (📖 p. 106)

Physical needs Health needs are diverse depending on country of origin and previous level of healthcare. Always consider infectious diseases, e.g. hepatitis B, HIV, TB, and malaria. Ensure refugees claim all health-related benefits available to them (e.g. free prescriptions)

Psychological needs Depression, anxiety, panic attacks, agoraphobia, and poor sleep are common. Symptoms are often reactions to past experiences and current situation. Social isolation, unemployment, deprivation, hostility, and racism compound them. Use medication if appropriate but also address other issues. ⚠ Although telling their story is helpful for some refugees, 'active forgetting' is the way some people cope with their difficulties

Victims of torture May present with many non-specific health problems. Some are the result of physical trauma—most are of mixed physical and psychological origin. Considerable time and patience is needed to manage them but it is worth it. Advice and support is available from Freedom from Torture (🖰 www.freedomfromtorture.org)

Family Many will have left other family members behind. They may not know their whereabouts or even if they are alive or dead. The Red Cross or Red Crescent can help with tracing (🖰 www.redcross.org.uk)

Useful contacts

Shelter For homeless people ☎ 0808 800 4444 🖰 www.shelter.org.uk
RELATE Relationship counselling ☎ 0300 100 1234 (telephone counselling ost £40/h in 2013) 🖰 www.relate.org.uk
Relationships Scotland ☎ 0845 119 2020
🖰 www.relationships-scotland.org.uk
Refugee Council 🖰 www.refugeecouncil.org.uk
Asylum Aid ☎ 0207 354 9264 🖰 www.asylumaid.org.uk

Benefits for people on low income

Universal Credit Benefit introduced in October 2013 to replace:

- Income Support
- Child Tax Credit
- Working Tax Credit
- Income-based Jobseeker's Allowance
- Housing Benefit
- Budgeting Loans/Advances
- Income-related Employment and Support Allowance
- Social Fund—Sure Start Maternity Grants, Funeral Payment, and Cold Weather Payments

❶ Starts in Northern Ireland from April 2014; existing claimants of ol benefits should be transferred to Universal Credit by the end of 2017.

Low income benefits not replaced by Universal Credit

- **Contributions-based Jobseeker's Allowance** Is a non-income assesse benefit paid for ≤26wk to people ≥19y and under state pension age who are unemployed or working <16h/wk, capable of and available fo work; and have paid sufficient National Insurance in one of the two complete tax years before the start of the year the claim is made
- **Local authority payments** Council Tax Benefit, Community Care Grants, and Crisis Loans for general living expenses have been replaced with payments from local authorities. Local schemes vary
- **Short-term advances** Provided by the Department for Work and Pensions if financial hardship because of issues with benefit payments
- **Automatic health benefits** People claiming low income benefits can claim free NHS prescriptions, dentistry, eye tests/glasses, wigs and fabric supports, travel to hospital, and milk/vitamins for pregnant and breastfeeding women and children <5y. This system continues, but 'passported' benefits gradually ↓ as income ↑

Who can claim Universal Credit? Adults resident in the UK:

- ≥18y and under state pension age
- Not in full-time education, and
- Who have accepted a Claimant Commitment

16–17y olds and students may be able to claim under limited circun stances. Claim via the Benefits Line ☎ 0800 055 6688 or download clai forms from ℛ www.gov.uk

Capital rules People with savings/capital of ≥£16,000 cannot clai Universal Credit. For those with savings/capital of £6,000–£16,00 payments are ↓ by £1/wk for each £250 of savings >£6,000.

Amount paid Payments are paid monthly. Amount depends on:

- **Age** Whether >25y and is single/has a partner
- **Children** One rate for first child; lower rate for additional children; supplement if a child is disabled
- **Childcare costs** Up to 70% of childcare costs if lone parent, both partners are at work or partner able to look after children is working
- **Inability to work** Higher rates are paid for those in the support grou than the work-related activity group (📖 p. 124)
- **Carer status** If caring for a severely disabled person for >35h/wk
- **Housing** If pay rent or a mortgage; also covers service charges

Benefits cap Amount of benefit usually cannot exceed £500/wk if a lone parent or part of a couple, or £350 if single. Certain benefits are excluded when calculating the cap. These include:

- Bereavement payments
- Funeral payments
- Cold weather payments
- Free school meals
- Sure Start Maternity Grants
- Statutory sick pay
- Statutory maternity, paternity, or adoption pay
- Local authority council tax, housing, or discretionary payments

The cap does not apply:

- If the household gross monthly earnings are equivalent to >16h/wk at the national minimum wage
- For 39wk if someone in the household was working for >1y prior to claiming and combined gross earnings were >£430
- If anyone in the household is claiming Attendance Allowance, Disability Living Allowance, Personal Independence Payments, Industrial Injuries Benefits, War Widow/Widower's Pension, or War Disablement Pension/Armed Forces Compensation Scheme Payments
- If either partner is unfit for work after Work Capability Assessment

Working and Universal Credit Both unemployed and working people can claim Universal Credit to supplement low income.

Claimant Commitment Claimants may be placed into one of four groups:

No work-related requirements No need to seek work if: earning > individual threshold (national minimum wage if working 35h/wk); deemed not capable of work under the Work Capability Assessment (📖 p. 124); responsible for a child <1y; over state pension age; carer; pregnant and <11wk prior to EDD; <15wk postnatal; age 16–21y with no parental support in full-time, non-advanced education

Work-focussed interview requirement (but no obligation to seek work) If responsible for a child aged 1–5y or lone/nominated foster carer for a foster child aged <16y (18y if care needs)

Work preparation requirement If assessed by the Work Capability Assessment as having limited capability for work (📖 p. 124)

All work-related requirements Apply to everyone else—individuals must seek and be available for work

Volunteering People claiming Universal Credit can do voluntary work for maximum of half the hours they are expected to seek work for (i.e. if seeking full time work, can do ≤17.5h of voluntary work).

Earnings disregards and tapers When people move back into work, some income can be kept before the amount of Universal Credit ↓. The amount that can be kept (*Earnings disregard*) varies according to whether single, lone parent, partner but no children, partner and children and/or previously in the work-related activity group after Work Capability Assessment. Once disregarded earnings have been taken into account, as earnings ↑, Universal Credit ↓ at a rate of 65p for every £1 of net earnings (the *taper*).

Further information

Jobcentre Plus ☎ 0800 055 6688 🖰 www.gov.uk

Multicultural medicine

Britain is a multicultural and multifaith society. It is important that providers of care take into account cultural and spiritual needs.

⚠ Table 5.1 is a rough guide to religious differences which affect health care. It is forcibly brief and cannot address all the many variations. Everyone is an individual, and there is a real danger of 'pigeonholing' patients by religion or ethnic background and making incorrect assumptions as a result. Always ask patients/family about their own preferences.

Communication Effective communication is essential. Do not assume English proficiency; it is important to ascertain that you understand the patient and that the patient understands you.
- Ask the patient to let you know if he/she does not understand; consider using an interpreter
- Speak clearly and slowly and repeat important information; avoid jargon, confusing phrases, double negatives, and rhetorical questions
- Ask patients to tell you what you have said to check comprehension
- Be wary of sounding condescending—English skills are not a reflection of a hearing disorder or level of intelligence

Respect beliefs and attitudes People have different reaction towards illness, life, and death. Ask patients to provide you with information about their own ideas, e.g for newly arrived immigrants, ask: 'Could you tell me what would happen to you if you were in your country?'

Using interpreters Interpreters are an important resource in providing a voice for patients whose proficiency in English is poor or insufficient for the situation. In general, anyone who has been in an English-speaking country for <2y will need an interpreter. Sometimes a friend or another family member can be used but if sensitive issues have to be discussed or it is essential that the information is translated accurately, use a professional.
General tips:
- Anticipate an interpreter will be needed where possible, and pre-book someone of the same gender who speaks the same language/dialect and will be ethnically acceptable to the patient
- Explain that the interpreter is bound to maintain confidentiality
- Face and speak in the first person directly to the patient, not the interpreter; interpreters are solely there to convey information in a language both patient and doctor can understand—not to analyse information or decide what should or should not be conveyed

Useful contacts

Ethnologue Language guide ℘ www.ethnologue.com/country_index.asp
Interpreter services (fees payable) *Language line* ☎ 0800 169 287℘
℘ www.languageline.co.uk
NHS Direct Multilingual health information and advice. ☎ 0845 464℘
℘ www.nhsdirect.nhs.uk

Table 5.1 Religious differences important in healthcare

Religion	Dietary restrictions	Fasting	Transfusion/transplant	Family planning	Death
Buddhist	Mainly vegetarian	N/A	No objections	No objections—abortion not allowed	Cremation preferred—no objections to post-mortem
Christian	None	N/A	No objections	Some approve of natural methods only	Burial or cremation—no objections to post-mortem
Hindu	Most do not eat beef. Some are strict vegetarian	Fasting involves limiting type of foods	No objections	No objections	Strong preference to die at home. The body should not be touched by non-Hindus. All adults are cremated—no post-mortems unless legally required
Muslim	No pork. Other meat must have been killed in a special manner (halal). Alcohol is prohibited	Fasting sunrise → sunset during Ramadan	Variable—some Muslims may not consent to transplant	Variable—some Muslims do not approve	All Muslims are buried. No post-mortems unless legally required
Jehovah's witness	No foods containing blood or blood products. No alcohol	N/A	No blood transfusion or organ transplant. Dialysis is usually permitted	No objections	Burial or cremation—no objections to post-mortem
Jewish	No pork, rabbit, or shellfish. Meat prepared in kosher fashion. Liberal Jews may not adhere to dietary restrictions	Orthodox Jews may fast for Yom Kippur	No objections	Some orthodox Jews prohibit contraception. Most Jewish boys are circumcised 8d after birth	Burial is preferred. No post-mortems unless legally required
Sikh	No beef. Most are vegetarian. Alcohol is forbidden	N/A	No objections	Allowed but not openly discussed	Children and adults are cremated

Breaking bad news

It is never easy to break bad news. GPs do it frequently, but police officer are rated as showing more sympathy than doctors.

Why is breaking bad news hard?

- **Admission of failure** When we tell patients bad news, it is often an admission that we have failed. When we fail we naturally question what we have done and when looking at our practice in retrospect, it is easy to find fault. Feelings of guilt are common
- **Fear of the reaction of the patient** We all have a desire to avoid unpleasantness but sharing information with patients may be a positive way forwards. Even if news is bad it gives patients control of the situation

Guidelines for sharing bad news with a patient

DO	DON'T
• Plan the consultation as far as possible. Check the facts first, and ensure you have all the information. Ensure privacy and freedom from interruption	• Lie or fudge the issue
• Set aside enough time	• Get your facts wrong
• Ask if the patient would like a relative or friend with them. Make sure you introduce yourself and find out their name and relationship to the patient	• Break bad news in public
• Make eye contact—watch for non-verbal messages. Sit at the same level as the patient	• Give the impression of being rushed or distant
• Use simple and straightforward language	• Give too much information. It is better to be concise—the finer points can be filled in later
• Allow silence, tears, or anger	• Interrupt or argue
• Be prepared to go over facts again	• Say that 'nothing can be done'—there is always something that can be done
• Answer questions	• Meet anger with anger
• Reflect on what the patient or relative have said to allow you to modify your understanding of their feelings	• Say you 'know how they feel'—you don't
• Take into account the patient's current health, e.g. if in pain, then sort out the pain and schedule a further discussion when the patient is more comfortable	• Be frightened to admit you don't know something
• Offer ongoing support	• Use medical jargon
	• Leave the patient with no follow-on contact
	• Agree to withhold information from the patient

Common problems

What if the relatives do not want you to tell the patient? With adults of sound mind, information is confidential to the patient and can only be released, even to close relatives, with the patient's permission. Relatives who say they do not want the patient to know often do so to protect their relative. It is important to recognize they know your patient best. First, explore their worries and point out the difficulties of the patient not knowing. Often once a relative realizes that the patient knows things are not right and needs help and support to face the situation, they come round to the patient being told. Stress that you will not lie to a patient if asked a direct question

How do you know if the patient wants to know? Most people (80–90%) *do* want to know. Assume this is the case and then feel your way carefully. Give the patient ample opportunity to say that they do not want to know

How do you respond to questions you cannot answer? The best way to deal with this is to say that you do not have all the answers but will answer when you can, find out what you can, and say when you do not know

Confirmation and certification of death

⚠ The death certification process in England and Wales is currently under review and likely to change in the near future.

English law *does not* require a doctor:
- To confirm death has occurred or that 'life is extinct'. A doctor is only required to certify what, in their opinion, was the cause
- To view the body of a deceased person. There is no obligation to see/ examine a body before issuing a death certificate
- To report the fact that death has occurred

English law *does* require the doctor who attended the deceased during the last illness to issue a certificate detailing the cause of death. Certificates are provided by the local Registrar of births, marriages, and deaths. A special certificate is needed for infants of <28d old.

Death in the community 1 in 4 deaths occur at home.

Expected deaths In all cases, advise to contact the undertakers and ensure the patient's own GP is notified.
- **Patient's home** Visit as soon as is practicable
- **Residential/nursing home** If possible the GP who attended during the patient's last illness should visit and issue a death certificate. The 'on-call' GP is often requested to visit. There is no statutory duty to do this but it is reassuring for the staff at the home and often necessary before staff are allowed to ask for the body to be removed

Unexpected and/or 'sudden' death If called, advise the attendant to call the emergency services. Visit and take a rapid history from any attendants. Then:
- **Resuscitate if appropriate** Drowning and hypothermia can protect against hypoxic neurological damage; brains of children <5y old are more resistant to damage
- **Report the death to the coroner** If any suspicious circumstances or circumstances of death are unknown/unclear—call the police

Alternatively, if police or ambulance service is already in attendance and death has been confirmed, suggest the police surgeon is contacted.

Cremation Cremation Regulations (2008) require two doctors to complete a certificate to establish identity and that the cause of death is not suspicious before a person can be cremated. The person arranging the funeral may see the forms and pays a fee to each doctor. Two parts:
- **Cremation 4** Completed by the patient's usual medical attendant— usually his/her GP
- **Cremation 5** Completed by another doctor who must have held full GMC registration (or equivalent) for ≥5y and is not connected with the patient in any way nor directly connected with the doctor who issued cremation form 4—usually a GP from another practice

⚠ Pacemakers and radioactive implants must be removed from the deceased before cremation can take place.

Notification of death to the coroner The coroner can be contacted via the local police. Reporting to the coroner does not automatically entail post-mortem. The coroner, once circumstances of death are clear, may advise the GP to tick and initial box A on the back of the certificate, which advises the registrar that no inquest is necessary. Deaths that *MUST* be reported to the coroner are listed in Box 5.1.

❶ In Scotland deaths are reported to a procurator fiscal. The list of reportable deaths is the same with the addition of deaths of foster children and the newborn.

Recording deaths at the practice Death registers are useful. Routine communication of deaths to all members of the primary healthcare team and other agencies involved with the care of that patient (e.g. hospital consultants, social services) avoids the embarrassing and distressing situation of ongoing appointments and contacts being made for that patient. Record the death in the notes of any relatives/partner registered with the practice.

Benefits available after a death
- For widows/widowers 📖 p. 114
- Funeral payment 📖 p. 115

Box 5.1 Deaths that must be reported to the coroner
- Sudden or unexpected deaths
- Accidents and injuries
- Industrial diseases, e.g. mesothelioma
- Service disability pensioners
- Deaths where the doctor has not attended within the past 14d
- Deaths arising from ill treatment, e.g. abuse, neglect, starvation, hypothermia
- Cause of death unknown
- Deaths <24h after hospital admission
- Poisoning (chronic alcoholism and its sequelae are no longer notifiable per se)
- Medical mishaps (including anaesthetic complications, short- or long-term complications of operations, drugs—whether therapeutic or addictive)
- Abortions
- Prisoners
- Stillbirths (when there is doubt about whether the baby was born alive)

Patient advice and support
Department of Work and Pensions (DWP)
- What to do after a death in England and Wales (2009)
  🖰 www.dwp.gov.uk/docs/dwp1027.pdf
- Funeral payment: information and online application form
  🖰 www.gov.uk

Scottish Executive What to do after a death in Scotland (2006)
🖰 www.scotland.gov.uk/Publications/2006/04/12094440/0

Organ donation

Over 10,500 people in the UK are waiting for an organ transplant that could save or dramatically improve their life, but ~3,700 transplants are carried out each year. There is a desperate need for more donors. In 2011 1,000 people died while waiting for a transplant.

Absolute contraindications to any organ donation There are only 2 absolute contraindications to organ donation: HIV disease and Creutzfeldt–Jakob disease (or other neurodegenerative diseases associated with infectious agents).

Donor cards and the NHS Organ Donor Register Potential donors should always discuss their wishes with their relatives. They can register their desire to donate their organs after death by adding their names to the NHS Organ Donor Register and obtaining an Organ Donor Card. Contact the NHS Organ Donor Line ☎ 0300 123 2323 or sign up online at ✆ www.organdonation.nhs.uk

Blood donation New donors age, 17–65y are accepted. Donors may donate whole blood or platelets. Different blood transfusion services operate in the devolved nations of the UK. *Contacts:*
- England ☎ 0300 123 2323 ✆ www.blood.co.uk
- Northern Ireland ☎ 028 9032 1414 ✆ www.nibts.org
- Scotland ☎ 0845 90 90 999 ✆ www.scotblood.co.uk
- Wales ☎ 0800 25 22 66 ✆ www.welsh-blood.org.uk

Bone marrow donation Bone marrow donation is open to people aged 18–49y who are blood donors (although may register at the time of first donation). Volunteers are HLA tissue-typed using DNA from white blood cells. Tissue type is recorded in the British Bone Marrow Registry. Donation involves a small operation in which bone marrow is harvested—usually from iliac crests.

Stem cell donation Peripheral stem cell donation is open to people aged 18–49y who are blood donors (although may register at the time of first donation). As for bone marrow donation, volunteers are HLA tissue-typed using DNA from white blood cells. Their tissue type is recorded within the British Bone Marrow Registry.

Donating stem cells involves daily injection of a growth factor (filgastrim) for 4d; this releases stem cells into the peripheral blood. Stem cells are harvested on day 5 using a cell separator from venous blood collected from one arm; the blood is returned through a vein in the other arm.

Cord blood stem cell donation When delivering their babies in certain hospitals in England, women can opt to donate cord blood for stem cell harvesting. ☎ 020 8437 1740 ✆ www.nhsbt.nhs.uk/cordblood

Surgical organ donation from living donors Two main types:
Donation at the time of routine operation Femoral heads can be donated at the time of hip replacement; skin can be donated at the time of cosmetic surgery (e.g. apronectomy)
Surgery to remove living organs 1 kidney, part of lung, liver or small intestine. Usually close relatives. Removal of the organ/part-organ involves a major operation for the donor. Risks to donor must be weighed against benefits to recipient

Heart-beating donation after death Donors must be maintained on life-support machine at the time of death and until the organs are removed. The role of the GP in these situations is pre-emptive (information about Organ Donor Register) and to support families to make the decision whether to donate. Organs that can be donated: kidneys, hearts, liver, lungs, pancreas, corneas, heart valves, bone, and skin.

Non-heart beating donation after death Most important group for GPs as donation can occur up to 24h after death (sometimes up to 48h) even if the patient dies in the community. Contact NHS Blood and Transplant ☎ 0300 123 2323. Tissues that can be donated:

No upper age limit	*<60y*
Corneas	• Heart valves
Skin	• Tendons
Bone	

Donation of whole body for medical education The donor *must* give authorization for donation prior to death. Relatives should contact the medical school with which the donor has made arrangements after the donor's death. Medical schools arrange collection of the body and a simple funeral. Not all bodies are accepted.

Tissue donation after death for research purposes Can be done in addition to donation for transplantation—organs for transplant are taken first.

Contact Human Tissue Authority ☎ 020 7269 1900 🖰 www.hta.gov.uk

Approach to relatives Many families find the act of donation a source of comfort. Even when the person who has died is on the Organ Donor Register, donation will be discussed with family members. However, if person has agreed to donation prior to death and this is recorded on the Organ Donor Register, the family has no legal right to overrule that decision.

The coroner For any patient normally referred to the coroner, the coroner's permission must be gained before tissues are removed.

Further information
NHS Blood and Transplant ☎ 0300 123 2323 🖰 www.organdonation.nhs.uk

Bereavement, grief, and coping with loss

Models of grief In the traditional model, the bereaved person moves through phases until 'recovery':
- **Initial shock** Sense of unreality, detachment, disbelief, or 'numbness'. Lasts from hours to days
- **Yearning** Pangs of grief, episodes of intense pining, and a desire to search interspersed with anxiety, guilt, and self-reproach
- **Despair** The permanence of the loss is realised. Despair and apathy, social withdrawal, poor concentration, pessimism about the future
- **Recovery** Rebuilding of an identity and purpose in life

Recent models Grief represents an oscillation between loss- and restoration-focussed behaviour, demonstrated by swings in mood, thoughts, and behaviour between memories of the dead person and 'getting on with life'. Avoidance or denial of the loss is common and part of the process.

Health consequences of bereavement
- ↑ mortality (↑ deaths from CVD, cirrhosis, suicide, accidents) particularly in first 6mo. *Risk factors:* ♂ > ♀, age <65y, lower social class
- **Mental health problems** Depression, anxiety, ↑ risk of suicide, substance abuse, identification reaction (hypochondriacal disorder—symptoms mimic those of deceased, e.g. chest pain if died from MI), insomnia, self-neglect
- **Physical problems** Fatigue, aches and pains (e.g. headaches, musculoskeletal pain), appetite change, GI symptoms, ↓ immune response (↑ minor infection)
- **Others** Interference with family life, education and employment, social isolation/loneliness, ↓ income

Role of the primary care team Develop a practice policy for bereaved patients. Flag notes. Consider staff training and active follow-up of bereaved patients. If the person who has died is registered with the practice, ensure all medical referrals/appointments are cancelled.

Bereaved children Children understand what death is by 8y, and even children of 2–3y have some understanding of death. Exclusion makes children isolated and often makes the death of someone they know more, not less, painful. Prepare children for a death if possible and give them a chance to have their questions answered. If a child has problems seek specialist help.

Bereavement benefits Payable to men and women whose spouses have died—including civil partnership, but cohabitation does not qualify except in Scotland. Claims can be made on forms available from the bereavement services helpline ☎ 0845 606 0265 or online via 🖰 www.gov.uk Current benefits available:
- **Bereavement payment** Claim <12 mo after death. Lump sum payable if spouse has paid enough National Insurance contributions or death was caused by employment and the recipient is below state pension age at the time of the death

Bereavement allowance Paid for 52wk from the date of bereavement to spouses >45y and < retirement age, not bringing up children

Widowed parent's allowance Paid to widows/widowers with children or if pregnant

Funeral payment One-off payment for people on low income to help with funeral costs

• **War widows/widowers** ☎ 0800 169 2277 🖰 www.veterans-uk.info

❶ Bereavement payment, bereavement allowance, and widowed parent's allowance will be merged into a single payment 'Bereavement Support Allowance' consisting of a single lump sum payment and monthly allowance (higher for people with dependent children) payable to widows/widowers for 1y after death of a spouse.

Abnormal grief reactions Whether a grief reaction is normal or abnormal depends on individual circumstances—personality, situation surrounding death, and cultural expectations. Recognized patterns of abnormal grief are:

• Inhibited grief—grief is absent or minimal
• Delayed grief—late onset, *and*
• Prolonged or chronic grief—inability to rebuild life in any way

If abnormal grief is suspected Monitor carefully. Consider referral for bereavement counselling, e.g. to CRUSE. Consider clinical depression (📖 p. 1000) or post-traumatic stress disorder (📖 p. 998). If symptoms are persistent or worsening despite treatment or if there is suicidal risk, refer to the mental health team for specialist advice.

Risk factors for poor outcome after bereavement

Predisposing factors

• Multiple prior bereavements
• Poor social or family support
• Low self-esteem
• Being male
• History of mental illness, e.g. depression, anxiety, suicidal attempts/ threats
• Ambivalent or dependent relationship with the deceased

Situations where the circumstances of death may cause particular problems for the bereaved

• Sudden or unexpected death
• Death due to AIDS or suicide
• Multiple deaths (e.g. disasters)
• Death of parent when child or adolescent
• Miscarriage; death of baby, child, or sibling
• Cohabiting partners, same sex partners, extramarital relationship
• Deaths where those bereaved may be responsible
• Deaths from murder, high media profile, or involving legal proceedings
• Where a post-mortem and/or inquest is required

Further information

CRUSE ☎ 0844 477 9400 🖰 www.crusebereavementcare.org.uk

National Association of Widows ☎ 024 7663 4848 🖰 www.widows.uk.net

Occupational illness

If a patient develops an occupational disease, a doctor is obliged to notify the employer in writing, with the patient's consent. The doctor does not need to make a judgement about whether the disease is, in that particular case, caused by the occupation.

Employers must then inform the Reporting of Injuries, Diseases and Dangerous Occurrences Regulations (RIDDOR) incident contact centre (☎ 0845 300 9923 ⌖ www.hse.gov.uk/riddor). Self-employed patients must contact RIDDOR themselves.

Patients who do not give consent for the doctor to notify their employer may allow the doctor to inform the employer's occupational health department or RIDDOR directly instead.

Notifiable industrial diseases   ❶ This is not a complete list:

- Poisoning by industrial agents, e.g. lead, arsenic, mercury
- Repetitive strain injury
- Vibration white finger
- Bursitis, e.g. housemaid's knee
- Occupational asthma
- Folliculitis and acne (associated with work with tar, pitch, or oils)
- Occupational infection, e.g. hepatitis B in healthcare workers, anthrax in farmers
- Chrome ulceration
- Irritant dermatitis, e.g. hairdressers' dermatitis
- Tenosynovitis, e.g. as a result of repeated movements of the hand/wrist
- Pneumoconiosis
- Extrinsic allergic alveolitis
- Occupational deafness
- Occupational cancers, e.g. nasopharyngeal cancer in woodworkers, bladder cancer in plastic workers, cancers as a result of ionizing radiation, mesothelioma due to asbestos exposure

Industrial injury   Injured employees should always report details of any accident to their employer and record them in the accident book as soon as possible—however trivial the injury. Employers must inform RIDDOR of:
- Dangerous incidents—even if no one was hurt
- Incidents where death or serious injury occurs
- Incidents resulting in injury requiring >3d absence from work
- Incidents involving gas

Prescribed industrial disease   Disease for which benefit is paid if the applicant worked in a job for which that disease is 'prescribed' and it is likely the employment caused the disease. Claims may be made at any time with the exceptions of occupational deafness (claim <5y after leaving employment) and occupational asthma (claim <10y after leaving employment). The list of prescribed diseases is similar to, but not the same as, the list of notifiable diseases.

Benefits that may be payable

Industrial injuries disablement benefit Available to employed earners for injuries resulting from accidents or certain (prescribed) illness arising as a result of employment, even if the employee was either part or wholly to blame. 'Industrial' covers virtually all forms of work. For accidents, claims can be made at any time after the event but benefit is paid only if there are still effects of the injury after the 91st day.

Payable if the person was a paid employee at the time of the accident or when he/she contracted the disease; *and* disability is assessed at ≥14% (exceptions: occupational deafness >20%; dust-related lung disease—no level). If a patient claims benefit for >1 industrial accident or disease, assessments may be added together and benefit awarded on the total.

Reduced earnings allowance Accident occurred/disease was contracted prior to 1st October 1990, disablement assessment of ≥1%, *and*
• Unable to work, *or*
• Unable to work at normal job, *or*
• Working less hours at normal job

Retirement allowance Reduced earnings allowance becomes retirement allowance at age 60y (♀) or 65y (♂). It is paid at 25% the rate of reduced earnings allowance when a claimant stopped work.

Constant attendance allowance For people so disabled that they need constant care and attention and who are getting disablement benefit for disability assessed at 100%. Four rates of benefit.

Exceptionally severe disablement allowance For people who get constant attendance allowance at high rate and where need for attendance is likely to be permanent.

❶ People who suffer from industrial diseases or have suffered disability as a result of an industrial accident are also eligible to apply for benefits available for any disabled individuals (📖 p. 222–8).

Making claims Through local Industrial Injuries Disablement Benefits offices. A full list of prescribed industrial diseases is also available from these offices. Some claims can be made online. For further information contact ☎ 0845 603 1358 🖰 www.gov.uk

Further information

RIDDOR Incident contact centre ☎ 0845 300 9923
🖰 www.hse.gov.uk/riddor
Citizens Advice Bureau 🖰 www.adviceguide.org.uk
Trade Unions

Victims of crime

Victims of crime need treatment of injuries and emotional support.
- Note the date, time, and place of the event
- Record injuries in detail (physical and psychological)—including measuring the size of lacerations and bruises. Record all information carefully as it may be needed for legal cases
- Arrange for photographs to be taken, if appropriate (police may arrange this)
- Encourage reporting of the incident to the police—the patient will not be eligible for criminal injury compensation if it is not reported
- Give patient details of local victim support groups
- If the patient's safety is an issue, contact the duty social worker for a place of safety

Rape and indecent assault If a patient reports rape or indecent assault and is willing to report the matter to the police, do not examine her/him. The case against the assailant could be won or lost on the basis of evidence gained by examination of an alleged victim so it is best done by a doctor trained and experienced in such work.

If the patient will not report the matter to the police
- Take a full history of the event. Note LMP, contraception, and sexual history
- Suggest that the patient attends a Sexual Assault Referral Centre (SARC) if available locally for forensic/medical examination and specialist advice and support

If there is no SARC or the patient is unwilling to attend
- Make a note of any injuries and take photographs if possible and appropriate. Do not insist on examination if the patient is unwilling. Ensure a chaperone is present if any examination is attempted
- Discuss the need for emergency contraception, prophylactic antibiotics (e.g. azithromycin 1g po stat), blood tests at 3mo to exclude transmission of syphilis and at 3–6mo for exclusion of seroconversion for HIV
- If at high risk for HIV transmission, refer to A&E for consideration of prophylaxis (📖 p. 744)
- Discuss the need for counselling, and inform the patient about the victim support scheme and Sexual Assault Referral Centres
- Arrange follow-up in 2–3wk

Criminal injuries compensation For victims of violent crimes—even if the attacker is not identified. Compensation is paid for the injury, loss of earnings, and expenses. Claim online or by telephone 📞 0300 00 3601 🖥 www.cica.gov.uk

Post-traumatic stress disorder (PTSD) 23% assault victims and 80% rape victims develop PTSD. ♀:♂ ≈ 2:1. Defined as significant symptoms 1mo after the event—i.e. flashbacks, nightmares, survivor guilt, mood changes, detachment, poor concentration, insomnia, anxiety, and depression. Alcohol abuse, work, and relationship problems are common. Symptoms may last years. See 📖 p. 998.

Domestic violence 📖 p. 120

Non-accidental injury in children 📖 p. 924

Elder abuse 📖 p. 121

Patient information and support
Victim support ☎ 0845 3030 900 🖰 www.victimsupport.org
Victim Support Scotland ☎ 0845 603 9213
🖰 www.victimsupportsco.org.uk
Rape Crisis England and Wales ☎ 0808 802 9999 🖰 www.rapecrisis.org.uk
(a list of SARCs and local Rape Crisis Centres can be obtained from this
website)
Rape Crisis Scotland ☎ 08088 01 03 02 🖰 www.rapecrisisscotland.org.uk
Survivors UK Provides resources for men who have experienced any
form of sexual violence ☎ 0845 122 1201 🖰 www.survivorsuk.org

Domestic violence: the GP's role

Domestic violence Is defined as any incident or pattern of incident of controlling, coercive or threatening behaviour, violence, or abus between those aged ≥16y who are/have been intimate partners or famil members regardless of gender or sexuality. This can encompass, but is n limited to, the following types of abuse:

- Psychological
- Sexual
- Financial
- Physical
- Emotional

Controlling behaviour Acts designed to make people subordinate dependent by isolating them from sources of support, exploiting the resources/capacities for personal gain, depriving them of means needed fc independence, resistance ± escape, and regulating their everyday behaviou

Coercive behaviour Act/pattern of acts of assault, threats, humiliatic and intimidation or other abuse used to harm, punish, or frighten victims

Prevalence Although men may be the victims of domestic violenc ~80% of reported domestic violence is against women by male partner Domestic violence affects ~1 in 4 women and is the most common forn of interpersonal crime: 60%—current partner; 21%—former partner; ha suffer >1 attack; 1 in 3 have been attacked repeatedly.

Effects High incidence of psychiatric disorders, particularly depressio and self-damaging behaviours, e.g. drug/alcohol abuse, suicide/parasuicid

Factors preventing the victim leaving the abusive situation
- Loss of self-esteem makes victims think they are to blame
- Disruption of the family and children's relationship with partner
- Loss of intimate relationship with partner
- Fear of partner
- Risk of homelessness
- Fall in income
- Fear of the unknown

Presentation General practice is often the first place in which victim seek formal help, but only 1 in 4 actually reveals the true nature of th problem. Without appropriate intervention, violence continues and ofte ↑ in frequency and severity. By the time injuries are visible, violence ma be a long-established pattern. On average, victims will be assaulted 3 times before reporting it to police.

Guidelines for care
- Consider the possibility of domestic violence—ask directly
- Emphasize confidentiality
- Document—accurate, clear documentation, over time at successive consultations may provide cumulative evidence of abuse and is essential for use as evidence in court, should the need arise
- Assess the present situation—gather as much information as possible
- Provide information; offer help to make contact with other agencies
- Devise a safety plan, e.g. give the phone number of local women's refuge; advise to keep some money and important financial and legal documents hidden in a safe place in case of emergency; help plan an escape route in case of emergency

❶ Do not pressurize the victim into any course of action. If the patient decides to return to the violent situation, she or he will not forget the information and support given. In time this might give her/him the confidence and back-up needed to break out of the situation.

⚠ If children are likely to be at risk, you have a duty to inform social services or the police, preferably with the patient's consent.

Assault 🕮 p. 118

Non-accidental injury in children 🕮 p. 924

Elder abuse Single or repeated act or lack of appropriate action, occurring within any relationship where there is an expectation of trust, which causes harm or distress to an older person. Prevalence is 4% (↑ with age; ♀:♂ ≈ 2:1)—neglect 1.2%; financial 1%; interpersonal 1.8%. Older people may report abuse but often do not. Different forms may coexist:
» **Physical**, e.g. cuts, bruises, unexplained fractures, burns
» **Psychological**, e.g. unusual behaviour, unexplained fear, appears helpless or withdrawn
» **Financial**, e.g. removal of funds by carers, new will in favour of carer
» **Sexual**, e.g. vaginal or anal bleeding, genital infections
» **Neglect**, e.g. malnourished, dehydrated, poor personal hygiene, late requests for medical attention

Signs Inconsistent story from patient and carer; inconsistencies on examination; fear in presence of carer; frequent attendance at A&E; frequent requests for GP visits; carer avoiding GP.

Management Talk through the situation with the patient, carer, and other services involved in care. Assess the level of risk. Consider admission to a place of safety—contact social services and/or police as necessary; seek advice from Action on Elder Abuse.

Adult safeguarding An adult (>18y) at risk of harm:
» May be in receipt of community care services by reason of mental/ other disability, age, or illness, and
» May be unable to take care of him/herself, or
» Is unable to protect him/herself from serious harm/exploitation

If suspected, contact the local social services adult safeguarding lead (with consent of the individual being harmed if able to give consent).

Further information

Department of Health Responding to domestic abuse: a handbook for health professionals (2005) Available from ℘ www.dh.gov.uk
Home Office Domestic violence ℘ www.homeoffice.gov.uk
BMA Safeguarding vulnerable adults—a toolkit for GPs (2011) ℘ www.bma.org.uk

Useful contacts

Womens' Aid ☎ 0808 2000 247 ℘ www.womensaid.org.uk
Men's Advice Line ☎ 0808 801 0327 ℘ www.mensadviceline.org.uk
Action on Elder Abuse ☎ 0808 808 8141 ℘ www.elderabuse.org.uk
Police domestic violence units
Local authority social services departments
Local authority housing departments

Fitness to make decisions

Definition Mental capacity is the ability to take actions affecting daily life (e.g. when to get up, what to wear, what to eat) and/or make more major decisions (e.g. where to live, how to manage money).

Mental Capacity Act (2005) Came into force in 2007 in England and Wales. Similar legislation applies elsewhere in the UK. It specifies who can take decisions on behalf of other people and allows people to plan ahead for a time when they may lack capacity. Five key principles:

- Every adult has the right to make decisions and must be assumed to have capacity to make them unless proved otherwise
- Every adult must be given all possible help and support to make decisions, and to communicate those decisions where necessary, before he/she can be assumed to have lost capacity
- Making an unwise decision does not mean that a person lacks capacity to make that decision
- Anything done or any decision made on behalf of someone who lacks capacity must be done in his/her best interests
- Anything done or any decision made on behalf of someone who lacks capacity should be the least restrictive of his/her basic rights/freedoms

Assessing capacity A GP asked to give an opinion on a patient's mental capacity should:

- Have access to the patient's records and ideally know the patient
- Seek information from friends, relatives, carers, and/or the patient's independent mental capacity advocate, if one has been appointed
- Examine the patient and assess the type and degree of deficit
- Decide if there is an impairment of, or disturbance in, the functioning of the patient's brain or mind
- If there is a disturbance, decide if the patient is able to make the particular decision in question—in particular:
  - Can the patient understand the relevant information, including the likely consequences of making/not making that decision?
  - Can the patient retain that information?
  - Can the patient use or weigh that information as part of the process of making the decision?
  - Can the patient communicate that decision by any means?
- Decide if assessment should be postponed while measures are taken to improve capacity
- Record all the above information

❶ Even if you think a proposed action is in the patient's best interests you must not judge the patient capable if that is not clearly the case. If in doubt, seek a second opinion.

Capacity to consent to medical treatment 📖 p. 53

Lasting Power of Attorney (LPA) Replaced *Enduring Power of Attorney* (EPA) in October 2007. Patients with EPAs can still use them. An LPA is a legal document that lets individuals appoint someone they trust to make decisions for them. It can be drawn up at any time whilst the person

s capacity but has no legal standing until it is registered with the Office
the Public Guardian. Two types:

Property and affairs LPA Allows the 'attorney' to make decisions
about the management of money, property, and affairs. Unless specified
otherwise, can be used even when the individual retains capacity

Personal welfare LPA Allows the 'attorney' to make decisions about
healthcare and welfare, including decisions to refuse or consent to
treatment, and decide on place of residence. Only active when the
LPA is registered and the individual lacks capacity to make decisions.
The attorney can make decisions about life-sustaining treatment only if
the LPA specifies that

ourt of Protection If a person, by reason of mental disorder,
comes incapable of managing his or her affairs but has not previously
ned an LPA, it may be necessary for someone, usually the nearest
ative, to apply to the Court of Protection for the appointment of a
ceiver' to do so. The medical practitioner will be asked to complete
m CP3. Alternatively, if the patient's affairs are simple (e.g. state
nsion), direct arrangements can be made with relevant authorities.

estamentary capacity The capacity to make a will. Anyone can
ke a will provided that they understand the nature and effect of making
vill, extent of property being disposed of and claims others may have
that property, and the decision is not the result of their condition (e.g.
e to a delusion).

Decisions do not have to seem rational to others, especially if consist-
t with pre-morbid personality.

dvance decision Statement about wishes regarding medical
atment in case the individual becomes incapable of making that decision
er. Advance decisions are legally binding.

Respect any refusal of treatment as long as the decision is clearly
applicable to circumstances, there is no reason to believe the individual
has altered that decision, and the decision was not made under duress

Advance decisions do not have to be written, except those refusing
ife-sustaining treatment which must be: specific to a particular
treatment (e.g. refusal to have CPR); written; signed by the person
making the decision (or a representative if unable to sign) and a witness

Advance decisions cannot include decisions about treatment the
person would like, only treatment the person refuses, and cannot
nclude directions to end the person's life prematurely

Doctors may not be willing to carry through an advance directive. In
uch cases they should refer the patient to another doctor who is

The BMA recommends doctors should *not* withhold 'basic care' (e.g.
ymptom control), even in the face of a directive which specifies that
he patient should receive no treatment

Where a formal advance statement is not available, take patients'
nown wishes into consideration

rther information

fice of the Public Guardian ✆ www.publicguardian.gov.uk
dical defence organizations

Certifying fitness to work

Individuals must self-certify for the first 7d of incapacity, then sickne
certification from a GP is needed until the WCA is carried out.

Own occupation test Applies to those claiming Statutory Sick P
(SSP) for the first 28wk of illness. The GP assesses if the patient is fit
do his/her *own* job.

Work Capability Assessment (WCA) Is carried out
employment advisers contracted to the Department for Work a
Pensions (DWP). It is not diagnosis-dependent and assesses a varie
of different mental/physical health dimensions for ability to work. It
performed within the first 13wk of any claim for Employment Suppo
Allowance (ESA) or Universal Credit and applies to:
● Everyone after 28wk incapacity
● Those who do not qualify for the own occupation test from the start
of their incapacity (i.e. do not qualify for SSP)

Initial information All applicants are asked to fill in the 'Limited capabili
for work' questionnaire which explores how the individual's medic
problem affects ability to work. Sometimes medical reports from GPs m
be sought by the Department of Work and Pensions at this stage. G
have a contractual obligation to complete and return these reports.

Medical examination In the majority of cases, more information will
needed to be able to assess the claim, and the claimant is then invited f
a face-to-face medical examination assessing mental and physical abili
to work. Groups considered unfit to work without medical examinatio
include pregnant women, people with severe physical or learning disabili
and those who are terminally ill.

Classification Based on these assessments people may be placed into o
of 3 groups:
● Fit to work
● Work-related activity group, or
● Support group

Those placed in the *work-related activity group* take part in work-focusse
interviews with personal advisers and are provided with a range of suppo
to help them prepare for a return to work.

Those placed in the *support group* have an illness/disability that has
severe effect on ability to work. They are not expected to take part in a
work-related activity but can choose to do so if they wish.

Appeals Once a decision has been made about ESA/Universal Credit, th
individual's GP is informed and no further sickness certification is neede
If the claimant disagrees with the decision, he/she can ask for it to b
reconsidered, and if that fails to alter the decision, can appeal. GPs mu
continue sickness certification pending the appeal decision.

Equality Act 2010 An employer has to make 'reasonable adjustment
to avoid an employee with an ongoing health problem/disability being p
at a disadvantage (e.g. adjusting working hours or providing equipment'

Forms for certifying incapacity to work

SC1 Self-certification form for people not eligible to claim SSP who wish to claim ESA/Universal Credit. Certifies first 7d of illness. Available from local benefits offices and GP surgeries.

SC2 As SC1 but for people who can claim SSP. Available from employers, local benefits offices, and GP surgeries.

Med 3: Statement of Fitness for Work Filled in by a GP or hospital doctor who knows the patient for periods of incapacity likely to be >7d. Traditionally handwritten but most practices now have the facility to issue computer generated Med3 forms.

During the first 6mo of incapacity can only be issued for a maximum period of 3mo. Gives the doctor two options:
* The patient is unfit for work
* The patient may be fit for work—this allows the GP to recommend circumstances under which the patient may be able to return to work, e.g with restricted duties or reduced hours

The form gives space for the GP to record the patient's functional limitations. This is designed to allow the employer to make adjustments to facilitate the employee's return to work.

The Statement of Fitness for work may be issued:
* On the day of your assessment of the patient (telephone consultations are acceptable)
* On a date after your assessment of the patient if you think that it would have been reasonable to issue a Statement on the day of your assessment of the patient
* After consideration of a report about the patient from another doctor or registered healthcare professional

Only one Statement of Fitness for Work can be issued per patient per period of sickness. If mislaid, reissue, and mark 'duplicate'.

⚫ Employers may not request certification that employees 'need not refrain from work'—if required, this should be requested as a private service from an occupational health physician or GP

Mat B1 Signed by doctor or midwife. Provided to pregnant women once within 20wk of EDD. Enables her to claim statutory maternity pay and other benefits (📖 p. 785).

Private certificates Some employers request a private certificate in the first week of sickness absence. They should request it in writing. If the GP chooses to provide the service, he or she may charge, both for a private consultation and the provision of a private certificate. The company should accept full responsibility for all fees incurred by the patient.

Further information

Department for Work and Pensions. Getting the most out of the fit note: GP guidance (2013) � www.gov.uk/government/uploads/system/uploads/attachment_data/file/183249/fitnote-gps-guidance.pdf
Disability rights: employment ℒ www.gov.uk

Time off work

131 million working days were lost to sickness in the UK in 2011 costing
>£100 billion. The most common reasons for sickness absence were:
- Musculoskeletal problems (35 million days lost)
- Minor illnesses (27.4 million days lost)
- Stress, depression, and/or anxiety (13.3 million days lost)

Facts and figures
- Sickness absence ↑ with age; ♀ have higher rates than ♂
- There has been a ↓ in amount of sick leave over the past 20y
- 16% of sick leave is for >20d, but this accounts for 32% of lost time
- The longer someone is not working, the less likely that person is to
  return to work; someone who has been off sick for ≥6mo has an 80%
  chance of being off work for 5y

Benefits of returning to work Going back to work promotes
recovery, ↑ physical/mental health and well-being, and ↓ social exclusion
poverty. In contrast, long periods out of work can cause/contribute to:
- ↑ consultation, medication consumption, and hospital admission rates
- 2–3x ↑ risk of poor general health and mental health problems, and
- 20% excess mortality

The role of the GP When someone of working age presents with a
problem that affects ability to work, record a brief occupational history:
- Address the underlying health problem and any personal, psychological,
  organizational, or social factors preventing return to work
- Wherever possible, suggest work adjustments where appropriate to
  enable a patient to return to work (e.g. graduated work or transitional
  arrangements) or instead of signing the patient off work; do this
  through the 'remarks' section of the Med3 (📖 p. 125)
- Involve occupational health professionals

Certification of time off work 📖 p. 124

Post-operative time off work See Table 5.2

Time off work for emergencies In many cases, patients have the
legal right to take time off work to deal with an emergency involving
someone who depends on them, but they may only be absent for as long
as it takes to deal with the immediate emergency; employers do not have
to pay for time taken off.

Dependants Include spouse or partner, children, parents, or anyone living
with the patient as part of their family. Others who rely wholly on the
patient for help in an emergency may also qualify.

Emergencies include situations in which a dependant:
- Is ill and needs help
- Goes into labour
- Is involved in an accident or assaulted
- Needs the patient to arrange their longer term care
- Needs the patient to deal with an unexpected disruption or
  breakdown in care, such as a childminder or nurse failing to turn up
- Dies and the patient must make arrangements/attend the funeral

Table 5.2 List of expected time off work for uncomplicated procedures

Operation	Minimum expected (wk)	Maximum expected if no complications (wk)
Angiography/angioplasty	<1	4
Appendectomy	1	3
Arthroscopy (knee)	1	4
Cataract surgery	<1	2
Cholecystectomy	2	12
Colposcopy ± cautery	<1	<1
CABG or valve surgery	6	12
Cystoscopy	<1	<1
D&C, ERPC, or TOP	<1	<1
Femoropopliteal grafts	4	12
Haemorrhoid banding	<1	<1
Haemorrhoidectomy	2	4
Hysterectomy	2	8
Inguinal or femoral hernia	1	6
Laparoscopy ± sterilization	<1	<1
Laparotomy	6	12
Mastectomy	2	12
Pacemaker insertion*	<1	<1
Pilonidal sinus**	2	8
Retinal detachment	<1	Avoid heavy work life-long
Total hip/knee replacement	6	26
TURP	2	8
Vasectomy	<1	2

* Driving—see 🕮 p. 130.

** If time off for dressings is allowed.

These are not hard and fast rules—alter them to fit individual circumstances (e.g. laparoscopic procedures often entail less time off than open procedures; patients performing hard manual jobs may require more time off work).

Fitness to drive

⚠ Driving licence holders/applicants have a legal duty to inform the DVLA of any disability likely to cause danger to the public if they drove

Driving licence types

- **Group 1** Ordinary licence for driving a car/motorcycle. Minimum age 17y (16y if disabled). Old licences expire at 70th birthday and then must be renewed 3-yearly. Applicants are asked to confirm they have no medical disability. If so, no medical examination is necessary. New photocard licences are automatically renewed 10-yearly until age 70y
- **Group 2** Enable holders to drive lorries and buses. Minimum age 21y. Initially valid until 45th birthday then renewable by medical examination every 5y until 65th birthday. >65y renewable annually. Applicants must bring form D4 (available from post offices) with them. Examinations take ~½h. A fee may be charged by the GP

Determining fitness to drive Patients with any disorder which may cause danger to others if they drove should be advised not to drive and to contact the DVLA. The DVLA gives advice on when they can restart

Breaking confidentiality When a patient continues to drive despite advice by a doctor to stop, a doctor has an *obligation* to break confidentiality and inform the DVLA.

If the patient does not understand the advice to stop driving Inform the DVLA immediately.

If the patient does understand but continues to drive
- Explain your legal duty to inform the DVLA if the patient does not stop driving
- If he/she still refuses to stop driving, offer to refer to a colleague for a second medical opinion—on the understanding that the patient stops driving in the interim
- If the patient still continues driving—consider action, such as recruiting the next of kin to the cause (but beware of breach of confidentiality)
- If all else fails, inform the DVLA in confidence. Before doing this, write to the patient to inform him/her of your intended actions and consider contacting your medical defence organization for advice. Once the DVLA has been informed, you should also write to the patient to confirm that a disclosure has been made

Conditions affecting fitness to drive 📖 p. 130

Multiple medical conditions Combination of multiple medical conditions, each insufficient itself to disqualify from driving, may together render a person unfit/unsafe to drive. If this is the case, advise the patient not to drive and seek clarification from the DVLA.

Driving after surgery Drivers do not need to notify the DVLA unless a condition likely to affect safe driving persists >3mo (certain exceptions

ly for neurological and cardiovascular disorders). It is the responsibility
ᵉe driver to ensure that he/she is in control of the vehicle at all times. It
ⁿt also be advisable for the driver to check with his/her insurer before
ᵣrning to drive after surgery. *Consider:*

ᵉcovery from anaesthesia (sedation and cognitive impairment)
ⁿpairment due to analgesia (sedation and cognitive impairment)
ⁿysical restrictions due to the surgery or the underlying condition

abled drivers Who want to learn to drive or return to driving
ᵒwing onset of their disability should have an assessment of their
ⁱng ability and/or advice on controls and adaptations needed. Licences
ʸ be limited to adapted vehicles. A list of driving assessment centres
ˢ be obtained from the Forum of Mobility Centres ☎ 0800 559 3636
ʷww.mobility-centres.org.uk

Impairment due to medication
ˢ an offence to drive/attempt to drive whilst unfit through drugs; the
ʷ does not distinguish between illegal/prescribed drugs. GPs prescrib-
ᵍ/dispensing medication that may affect ability to drive safely should
ᵥise their patients of that risk.

ual acuity Drivers must be able to read in good light (with glasses
ᵒntact lenses) a number plate containing figures 79mm high and 57mm
ᵉ at a distance of 20.5m (20m where the characters are 50 mm wide).
ᵈdition, Group 2 drivers must have corrected vision of ≥6/9 (best eye)
≥6/12 (other eye); they should stop driving if uncorrected acuity in
ᵉr eye is <3/60.

al field defects and diplopia If drivers develop diplopia or are found
ᵃve a visual field defect, they should stop driving and inform the DVLA.
ᵘp 1 licence holders may be able to drive if patching or lenses control
ᵖpia or are able to meet DVLA criteria for field defects.

t belt exemption GPs can sign a form to exempt patients (e.g. those
colostomies) from having to wear a seat belt. Consider very carefully the
ᵒns for exemption in view of the weight of evidence in favour of seat belts.

ther information

A *At a glance guide to the current medical standards of fitness to drive*
ᵐedical practitioners available from 🖰 www.dft.gov.uk/dvla
ⁱcal advisers from the DVLA can advise on difficult issues—contact:
Medical Adviser, Drivers Medical Group, DVLA, Swansea SA99 1TU
☎ 01792 782337 or E-mail: medadviser@dvla.gsi.gov.uk (medical pro-
ᵒnals only)
Forum of Mobility Centres ☎ 0800 559 3636
ʷww.mobility-centres.org.uk
tificates of Exemption from Compulsory Seatbelt Wearing Can be
ᵃined from ☎ 0300 123 1002 or online at 🖰 www.orderline.dh.gov.uk

ient information

ing with a disability or health condition 🖰 www.gov.uk
A Customer enquiries ☎ 0300 790 6806 (for car or motorcycle drivers)
☎ 790 6807 (bus, coach, or lorry drivers) 🖰 www.dft.gov.uk/dvla

Brief guide to DVLA fitness to drive

For UK drivers, the DVLA provides detailed condition-specific g[u]ance about fitness to drive. This is regularly updated. Always check most recent version of the DVLA *At a glance guide to the current m[e]cal standards of fitness to drive for medical practitioners* available fr[om] ♒ www.dft.gov.uk/dvla

Loss of consciousness/altered awareness

Reflex vasovagal syncope Definite prevocational factors, typical prodro[me] and occurs only when standing, No driving restrictions.

Likely cardiovascular cause Abnormal ECG, clinical evidence of struct[ural] heart disease, >1 episode in 6mo, or syncope causing injury when sitt[ing] lying. Inform the DVLA. Stop driving.
- **If no cause found/treated** Group 1—6mo; Group 2—12mo
- **If cause is treated** Group 1—4wk after the event; Group 2—3mo after the event

Likely first fit Seizure markers: no reliable prodrome; tongue bit[e] incontinence; unconsciousness/amnesia >5min; headache after the att[ack]
- **Group 1** 6mo off driving unless clinical factors/investigation results [that] suggest seizure risk ≥20%/y
- **Group 2** 5y off driving. Licence restored if on no anti-epilepsy medication for 5y, recent neurologist assessment, and no clinical fact[ors/] investigations (e.g. EEG, brain scan) that indicate seizure risk is >2%/y

Epilepsy Inform the DVLA; licence revoked.
- **Group 1** Until 1y after last attack (special rules apply if fits only occ[ur] in sleep). If withdrawing medication, stop driving during period of withdrawal and 6mo afterwards
- **Group 2** Until 10y fit-free off all medication

Chronic neurological disease e.g. Parkinson's disease, deme[ntia] MND. Inform the DVLA. Licensing depends on clinical condition.

Significant head injury Inform the DVLA.
- **Group 1** Inform DVLA; usually 6–12mo off driving
- **Group 2** Stop driving; may restart if seizure risk is <2%/y and no ot[her] impairment likely to affect safe driving

Sleep apnoea Stop driving. Restart if symptoms adequately contro[lled]

CVA/TIA/amaurosis fugax
- **Group 1** Do not inform DVLA. 1mo off driving. Resume if clinically[...]
- **Group 2** Inform the DVLA. 1y off driving

Arrhythmia Stop driving and inform DVLA if has caused/is likely t[o] cause incapacity. Otherwise may continue driving. If symptomatic:
- **Group 1** Licence restored when attacks controlled for ≥4wk
- **Group 2** Licence restored when attacks controlled for ≥3mo and i[f] left ventricular ejection fraction is >0.4

Pacemaker insertion Includes box change.
- **Group 1** Stop for 1wk   • **Group 2** Stop for 6wk
- Other implantable defibrillator devices—see DVLA guidance

Hypertension Group 1—continue driving unless symptomatic. **Group 2**—stop if systolic ≥180 or diastolic ≥100mmHg until controlled.

Acute coronary syndromes

Group 1 If successful treatment with angioplasty—stop driving for 1wk. Otherwise, stop driving for 1mo

Group 2 Licence revoked. Reviewed after 6wk with medical examination and exercise ECG

Stable angina

Group 1 Stop driving until symptoms controlled if attack whilst at the wheel, at rest, or with emotion

Group 2 Inform DVLA. Licence revoked until symptom-free >6wk— renewal requires medical examination and exercise ECG or equivalent

Coronary revascularization

Group 1 Do not inform DVLA. Angioplasty/stenting—stop driving for 1wk; restart when clinically fit thereafter. CABG—stop driving for 1mo

Group 2 Inform DVLA. Licence revoked for 6wk after angioplasty or 3mo after CABG. Reviewed with medical examination and exercise ECG or equivalent prior to relicensing

Diabetes mellitus Do not notify DVLA unless:

Insulin-controlled Inform DVLA.

Group 1 Licence issued (1, 2, or 3y) if hypoglycaemia awareness, <2 episodes of hypoglycaemia requiring assistance of another in 12mo, and appropriate blood glucose monitoring

Group 2 1y licence issued if no episodes of hypoglycaemia requiring assistance of person in the past 12mo, hypoglycaemia awareness, monitors blood glucose ≥2x/d using a glucose meter with a memory function, and annual specialist review when ≥3mo of blood glucose readings must be available

Tablets causing hypoglycaemia (e.g. sulfonylurea, glinide)

Group 1 If regular review of DM and <2 episodes of hypoglycaemia requiring assistance from another in 12mo, may drive; no need to inform the DVLA. Otherwise, inform the DVLA and stop driving

Group 2 Inform the DVLA. 1, 2, or 3y licence is issued if: hypoglycaemia awareness, <2 episodes of hypoglycaemia requiring assistance of another in 12mo, and monitors blood glucose ≥2x/d

Psychosis Inform DVLA. Licence revoked.

Group 1 Restored if well and stable for ≥3mo, compliant with treatment, and free from adverse drug effects which would impair driving. Specialist report required

Group 2 Restored after 3y if stable and off antipsychotic medication which might affect ability to drive. Specialist report required

Drug or alcohol misuse or dependency DVLA arranges assessment prior to licence restoration.

Group 1 6mo off driving—1y after detoxification for alcohol, opioid, cocaine, or benzodiazepine dependence, or alcohol/drug-related seizure

Group 2 Licence revoked 1y; 3y if alcohol dependence or misuse of opiates, cocaine, or benzodiazepines; 5y if alcohol/drug-related seizure

Fitness for other activities

Fitness to fly Passengers are required to tell the airline at the time of booking about any conditions that might compromise their fitness to fly. The airline's medical officer must then decide whether to carry them

Hazards of flying
- Cabin pressure—oxygen levels are lower than at ground level and gas in the body cavities expands 30% in flight
- Inactivity and dehydration
- Disruption of routine
- Alcohol consumption
- Stress and excitement

Contraindications to flying
- **Respiratory disease**
  - Suspected pneumothorax/pneumomediastinum—patients should not fly for 14d after complete resolution of pneumothorax
  - Chronic lung disease—if a patient can walk >50m or climb a single flight of stairs without significant breathlessness, he/she should be fit to fly. Supplementary oxygen can be provided in flight for patients unable to walk this far but the patient must pre-book this with the airline and there is usually a fee
- **Heart disease** Patients should not fly if they have unstable angina, poorly controlled heart failure, or an uncontrolled arrhythmia, Patients should also refrain from travelling <10d after uncomplicated MI (3–4wk if complicated recovery) and for 3–5d after angioplasty
- **Thrombo-embolic disease** Patients should not travel with a DVT before established on anticoagulants
- **Neurological disease** Patients should not travel for 3d after stroke, or if epileptic, <24h after a grand mal fit
- **Infectious disease** Patients must not travel with untreated infectious disease
- **Psychiatric illness** Patients should not travel if they have disturbed or unpredictable behaviour that could disrupt the flight
- **Fractures** Flying is restricted for 24–48h (depending on the length of the flight) after the plaster cast has been fitted
- **Haematological disease** Anaemia (<7.5g/dL) and recent sickling crisis may restrict flying
- **Pregnancy** Most airlines will not carry women >36wk pregnant (third trimester if multiple pregnancy) or with history of premature delivery, cervical incompetence, bleeding, or ↑ uterine activity
- **Ear problems** Flying with otitis media or sinusitis can result in pain ± perforation of the ear drum. Patients are advised not to fly until symptoms resolve
- **Babies** <2d old should not fly (preferably <7d old)
- **Surgery** Patients should not travel <10d after surgery to the chest, abdomen, or middle ear. Any other procedure where gas is introduced into the body also needs careful consideration

Precautions
- Carry all regular medication especially relief medications (e.g. salbutamol, GTN spray) in the cabin
- For people who have to time their medication carefully keep to the times that medication was taken at home for duration of flight, e.g. for patients with DM—take snacks to eat and take insulin at normal times
- Drink plenty of liquid (non-alcoholic) to prevent dehydration
- Do calf exercises/get up and walk up and down at intervals to prevent venous stasis in the legs—those at risk of venous thrombo-embolism should wear compression stockings for the flight
- Pre-warn airlines of special needs so that they can accommodate them, e.g. extra leg room, special diet, oxygen in-flight, transport to and from the aeroplane

Further information
Civil Aviation Authority (CAA) *Am I fit to fly?* ℘ www.caa.co.uk

Fitness to perform sporting activities 📖 p. 500

Pre-employment certification It is becoming increasingly common for GPs to be asked about the 'medical' suitability of candidates to perform a job. This is not part of the GP's terms of service and therefore a GP can refuse to give an opinion. In all cases where an opinion is given, a fee can be claimed. Common examples are:
- Forms for childminders
- Care home staff—proof of 'physical and mental fitness'
- Food handlers—certificates of fitness

⚠ Remember—signing a form may result in legal action against you should the patient NOT be fit to undertake an activity.

Where possible, include a caveat, e.g. 'based on information available in the medical notes, the patient appears to be fit to…, although it is impossible to guarantee this.'

If unsure, consult your local LMC or medical defence organization for advice.

Medicines and prescribing

NHS prescriptions

'A doctor is a man who writes prescriptions till the patient either dies or is cured by nature'

John Taylor (1694–1761)

At any one time, 70% of the UK population is taking medicines. Three quarters of people >75y are taking prescribed medicines, and 36% of older people take ≥4 different medications on a regular basis. 1.7 million prescriptions are dispensed daily within the NHS to prevent illness, cure existing illness, and give symptomatic relief, costing >£8.2 billion/y (>10% NHS costs).

Prescribing forms a major part of any GP's workload. Bad prescribing wastes resources, deprives patients from a chance to benefit, and may cause illness. Medicines should be prescribed only when necessary, and, in all cases, benefits of prescribing should be weighed against risks.

❶ Currently, only patients in England pay prescription charges. There are no prescription charges in Wales, Northern Ireland, or Scotland.

Prescription pre-payment certificate (PPC) If not entitled to free prescriptions (see Table 6.1) but needing a lot of medication (>3 prescriptions/3mo or >13/y), it is cheaper for a patient to purchase a 'pre-payment certificate'.

There are 3 ways to purchase a PPC:
* Internet ℘ www.nhsbsa.nhs.uk/HealthCosts
* Telephone ☎ 0300 330 1341
* From a pharmacy registered to sell PPCs. List available at ℘ www.nhsbsa.nhs.uk/HealthCosts

Refunds Send the NHS Business Services Authority a letter explaining the reason for refund to: NHS Business Services Authority, PPC Issue Office, 152 Pilgrim Street, Newcastle-upon-Tyne, NE1 6SN.
* **Full refund** May be claimed if; <1mo after purchase the holder becomes entitled to free prescriptions or dies
* **Partial refund** May be claimed if the holder dies >1mo after issue or if the holder becomes entitled to free prescriptions 1–4mo after issue

Reclaiming money spent whilst awaiting an exemption certificate or PPC Ask for an official receipt at the pharmacy when the drug is paid for (FP57 England). Claim money back within 3mo.

Drugs cheaper over-the-counter (OTC) Many drugs commonly prescribed in primary care (e.g. paracetamol, topical steroid nasal sprays, oral antihistamines, ibuprofen) are cheaper than a prescription charge to buy OTC. Before prescribing for patients who pay prescription charges always consider:
* Is this medication available to purchase OTC?
* Would it be cheaper to buy OTC in the quantities required?

Table 6.1 Free prescription entitlement in England

Free prescription entitlement	Action needed
• Prescription for contraception • >60 or <16y of age or 16–18y of age in full-time education • Patient or family receiving Universal or Pension Credit	Tick the box on reverse of prescription form
Pregnant women and women who have had a baby <12mo ago (MatEx)	Fill in form FW8 as soon as pregnancy is confirmed. Exemption certificates last 1y from EDD. If FW8 is completed after the baby is born, the MatEx certificate lasts 12mo after the date of birth. Includes dentists' charges
Certain conditions (MedEx): • DM (unless diet-controlled only) • Myxoedema/need for thyroxine • Hypoparathyroidism • Epilepsy requiring continuous anticonvulsants • Permanent fistula (e.g. colostomy) needing stoma dressing/appliance • Hypoadrenalism (including Addison's disease) needing replacement therapy • Hypopituitarism, including diabetes, insipidus • Myaesthenia gravis • Cancer • Unable to go out without the help of another person due to a continuing physical disability	Fill in form FP92A (available from doctors' surgeries). Requires a doctor's signature to confirm the condition when applying for exemption. Certificate lasts 5y or until 60th birthday, if sooner
War pensioners—prescriptions related to pensionable condition only	Apply through Veterans-UK ☎ 0800 169 22 77
Low income and <£16,000 savings (higher if in residential care) or pending application for any benefit listed above	Students may be eligible. Includes opticians' and dentists' charges. Apply through the NHS Low Income Scheme (LIS) on form HC1 ☎ 0845 850 1166 *or* ⬥ www.nhsbsa.nhs.uk/HealthCosts

❶ Leaflet HC11 (*Help with Health Costs*) is available from Post Offices, some pharmacies and GP surgeries, or from ⬥ www.nhsbsa.nhs.uk/ HealthCosts/792.aspx

Writing prescriptions

⚠ Legal responsibility for prescribing lies with the person who signs the prescription form.

British National Formulary (BNF) Contains a list of all drugs that a registered medical practitioner can prescribe on NHS prescription. It does not include homeopathic drugs which can be prescribed on NHS prescription, nor aids and appliances. There is a separate but linked BNF concerned with prescribing for children. Dentists and nurses have their own limited formulary.

Further information
BNF ℘ www.bnf.org

Claiming for items dispensed by a non-dispensing GP All GPs may claim payment for dispensing certain items that are supplied and personally administered by the GP or practice staff on behalf of the GP. Claims are made on form FP10 (GP10) to the PPA and must state the name of the patient, item dispensed, and manufacturer of the item. Claimable items are:

- Vaccines
- Anaesthetics
- Injections
- Sutures
- Skin closing strips
- IUCDs
- Contraceptive caps/diaphragms
- Diagnostic reagents
- Pessaries that are appliances (e.g. ring pessary)

❶ Different arrangements apply for high volume vaccines, e.g. influenza.

Prescription writing NHS prescriptions are written on form FP10 (GP10 in Scotland). They should be legible and in indelible ink. They are valid for 13wk from the date written on them. *Include:*
- Patient details—full name, address, and age/date of birth if <12y
- Date
- Full name of the drug (not abbreviated), with quantity to be supplied and dose interval (avoid the use of decimal points, e.g. for quantities <1g, write in mg). If you want a description of the drug included on the label, then write it on the prescription (e.g. 'for asthma')
- Deletion of any unused space (e.g. by striking through)
- Signature of the prescriber in ink
- Name and address of the prescriber

❶ Special rules apply for controlled drugs—🕮 p. 151.

Computer-issued prescriptions (form FP10(C)) Should contain the same information as their handwritten equivalents. They must still be signed in ink by the responsible clinician.

Guidelines are available from the Joint Computing Group of the GPC and RCGP (a summary is available in the BNF ℘ www.bnf.org).

Non-NHS prescriptions The same rules apply to the writing of private prescriptions as NHS prescriptions but private prescriptions should not be written on FP10 forms (normally headed notepaper is used). There are no restrictions upon which drugs can be prescribed.

Private prescriptions for controlled drugs Controlled drugs in Schedules 2 and 3 (including temazepam) presented for dispensing in the community (but not in hospitals) must be written on specially designated forms available from local PCOs. These forms must include the prescriber's unique 6-digit identification number issued specifically for their private prescribing activity.

Nurse prescribers (*BNF*—Appendix NPF) There is a list of preparations approved by the Secretary of State which may be prescribed on form FP10P (form HS21(N) in Northern Ireland, form GP10(N) in Scotland, forms FP10(CN) and FP10(PN) in Wales) by nurses for NHS patients. Nurses who have undergone additional training can prescribe from the nurse prescribers' extended formulary list.

Dentists (*BNF*—Appendix DPF) Can prescribe medication for dental conditions to their NHS patients on form FP10(D) (GP14 in Scotland).

Emergency supply of medicines by pharmacists In emergency situations pharmacists can dispense prescription-only medicines (POM). In general ≤5d supply can be dispensed.

Patient information Since 1994, all newly licensed/relicensed medicines dispensed in an original pack must be accompanied by a patient information leaflet (PiL). Despite the fact most drugs are now supplied with PiLs, doctors should make patients aware of 'substantial or special risks when offering treatment'. How much information to give is unclear. Information regarded as important by patients is: name of the drug; what to do if a dose is missed; purpose of treatment; precautions (e.g. effect on driving); when and how to take the medicine; problems with alcohol and other drugs; unwanted effects and what to do about them.

Security of prescriptions Prescription theft and fraud are common and wastes valuable NHS resources. *Basic precautions:*
- **Prescriptions** Should not be left unattended at reception desks; should not be left in a car where they might be visible; and when not in use should be kept in a locked drawer both at the surgery and at home
- **Writing prescriptions** Draw a diagonal line over the blank part of the form under the prescription; write the quantity in words and figures for drugs prone to abuse (even if not controlled drugs); make alterations clear and unambiguous and add your initials against any altered items

If prescription fraud is suspected ☎ 0800 028 40 60.

Further information
NHS Protect ✆ www.nhsbsa.nhs.uk/protect

Cost-effective prescribing

Generic prescribing Use of generic names when prescribing is one of the simplest ways to ↓ cost of drugs to the NHS but only 63% drugs prescribed by GPs in the UK are prescribed generically.

Every marketed drug has a chemical name, generic name, and a proprietary or brand name. For as long as the drug's patent is valid, the company that developed the drug will derive income from prescription whatever the name on the prescription. Once the patent has expired, competitors can manufacture the drug and market it under its generic or an alternative brand name. If the drug is prescribed generically, the pharmacist decides which brand to supply and market forces drive price ↓.

Advantages of generic prescribing Cost ↓, professional convenience (there are often several brand names for one drug—using generic names everyone knows they are talking about the same thing), ↑ convenience to the patient (pharmacists do not stock each brand of a given drug and, if prescribed by brand name, may have to order a supply—usually generic preparations of all commonly used drugs are available).

Reasons not to prescribe generically
- **Drugs with a low therapeutic index**, e.g. lithium, carbamazepine, phenytoin, ciclosporin—dosage is carefully titrated against plasma concentration or response. Small differences in plasma concentrations can be clinically significant
- **Modified-release formulations**, e.g. diltiazem, nifedipine, aminophylline, or theophylline products. Composition and pharmacokinetic properties are very difficult to standardize
- **Formulations containing ≥2 drugs** Some do have generic names (e.g. co-amilofruse 5/40)—others do not. Do not make up a generic name if the combination drug does not have one

Evidence-based prescribing Decisions on what to prescribe when, were, in the past, largely based on guesswork or faith. With the advent of information from randomized controlled trials and their evaluation using systematic reviews and other techniques, such decisions can now be based (at least in part) on scientific evidence. Failure to do this may cause patients to suffer unnecessary side effects of ineffective drugs, deprive patients the chance to benefit from effective treatments and waste valuable resources. *Sources of information:* 📖 p. 74.

NICE 📖 p. 13

Rationing 📖 p. 7

Practice formularies An agreed practice formulary is an effective way to limit prescribing and costs of prescribing. Compiling a formulary from scratch is a daunting prospect but there are many formularies available, which can then be modified according to evidence that emerges and reviewed within a practice (contact PCO prescribing lead). When compiling or reviewing a formulary consider: evidence of efficacy; safety; cost effectiveness; and local policy.

NHS Business Services Authority (NHSBSA) Special Health Authority which provides a wide range of services to the NHS including:
- Payments to pharmacists for prescriptions dispensed in primary care
- Provision of information on costs and trends in prescribing
- Payments to dentists for work undertaken on NHS contracts and provision of information on costs of dental care
- Management of the NHS Pension Scheme
- A range of health benefits schemes (Low Income Scheme, Exemption schemes, pre-payment certificates)
- Administration of the European Health Insurance Card (EHIC) scheme
- Management of the NHS Injury Benefits Scheme
- Provision of the NHS Protect service

Prescribing information The NHSBSA provides practices with information on their prescribing via the ePFIP (Electronic Prescribing and Financial Information for Practices) system. This is available by registration at ℘ www.nhsbsa.nhs.uk/963.aspx. Information can be used to improve prescribing habits, manage prescribing costs, and produce formularies and prescribing policies. Four types of report are available.

Practice detailed prescribing information (PDPI) Shows prescribing amounts and costs broken down, according to the BNF, for each prescriber in a practice. A new report is created online each time a report is requested. A data selector allows the user to choose the parameters of the report, e.g. prescribers, time periods (1–24mo), BNF groups.

Prescribing analysis report Analysis of the practice prescribing during the reporting period. Produced at both a monthly and quarterly level. The report shows total level of prescribing trends in prescribing, a breakdown of prescribing in the 6 highest cost BNF therapeutic groups, the top 20 leading cost drugs in the practice and the top 40 BNF sections by cost in the practice. Practice prescribing is also compared with last year's level and with the PCO and national levels.

Prescribing monitoring document (PMD) Shows the cost of prescribing to enable management of the drugs element of unified budgets. 2-page report—the first page is a practice statement (or annual return in March); the second is an annual profile of cumulative expenditure.

Local comparative practice data The prescribing team from the PCO can provide comparative prescribing data for practices within its area. This takes the form of overall data (number of items dispensed, costs) or can be broken down into specific drug areas. Looking at comparative data can identify areas in which the practice is over- or under-prescribing and can highlight expensive drugs being used for which there are cheaper, equally effective alternatives.

Further Information
NHSBSA ℘ www.nhsbsa.nhs.uk
UK Medicines Information ℘ www.ukmi.nhs.uk
Electronic Medicines Compendium ℘ www.medicines.org.uk

Medicines management and concordance

Medicines management Defined as 'facilitating the maximum benefit and minimum risk for medicines for individual patients'. Encompasses the way medicines are selected, procured, delivered, prescribed, administered, and reviewed to optimize use. *Components are:*
- Optimizing a medication regime (right drug at the right time)
- Facilitating adherence to medication, addressing beliefs and fears as well as physical problems as a result of drugs
- Organizing supply and administration support, such as repeat dispensing systems
- Providing monitoring and feedback systems

Concordance Is a process of prescribing and medicine taking based on partnership. Patient concordance (or rather lack of it) is a major challenge in general practice. For drugs to be optimally effective they should be taken as directed by the prescriber. Concordance sufficient to attain therapeutic objectives occurs about 50% of the time—1:6 patients take medication exactly as directed; 1:3 take medication as directed 80–90% of the time; 1:3 take medication 40–80% of the time; the remaining 16–17% take medication as directed <40% of the time. 20% of prescriptions are never 'cashed'.

'White-coat concordance' Phenomenon in which 90% of patients take regular medication as directed for a period before a check-up—may mask effects of non-concordance.

Consequences of non-concordance
- Failure to attain therapeutic targets, e.g. failure to take antihypertensive medication reduces the possible benefit in terms of stroke reduction by 30–50%
- Wastage of precious resources (~£250 million worth of medicines are returned to pharmacies each year for disposal—the true quantity wasted is many times that)

Causes of non-concordance
- **Patient beliefs** Strongest predictor of concordance—how natural a medicine is seen to be, the dangers of addiction and dependence, the belief that constant use may lead to ↓ efficacy have all been shown to influence concordance
- **Lifestyle choices**
  - Unpleasant side effects (especially if not pre-warned)
  - Inconvenience (e.g. multiple daily dosage regimes—though little difference between od and bd dosage)
  - No perceived benefit
- **Information** Instructions not understood or poor understanding of the condition/treatment
- **Practical** Forgetfulness; inability to open containers

- **Professional**
  - Doctor–patient relationship (there is a link between patient satisfaction with the consultation and subsequent concordance)
  - Inappropriate prescribing; mistakes in administration/dispensing

Improving concordance ~70% patients want to be more involved in decisions about treatment. Doctors underestimate the degree to which they instruct and overestimate the degree to which they consult and elicit their patients' views. The doctor's task is, by negotiation, to help patients choose the best way to manage their problem. Patients are more likely to be motivated to take medicines as prescribed when they:

- Understand and accept the diagnosis
- Agree with the treatment proposed
- Have had their concerns about the medicines specifically and seriously addressed

Ways to improve concordance

- Use simple language and avoid medical terms
- Discuss reasons for treatment and consequences of not treating the condition, ensuring information is tailored, clear, accurate, accessible, and sufficiently detailed
- Seek the patient's views on their condition
- Agree course of action before prescribing
- Explain what the drug is, its function, and (if known and not too complex) its mechanism of action
- Keep the drug regime as simple as possible—od or bd dosing preferable, especially long term
- Seek the patients' views on how they will manage the regime within their daily schedule and try to tie in with daily routine (e.g. take one in the morning when you get up)
- Discuss possible side effects (especially common or unpleasant side effects)
- Give clear verbal instructions and reinforce with written instructions if complex regime, elderly, or understanding of patient is in doubt
- Deal with any questions the patient has
- Repeat information yourself and also ask patients to repeat information back to you to reinforce information
- If necessary arrange review within short time of starting medicine to discuss progress or queries, or arrange follow-up by another member of the primary healthcare team (e.g. asthma nurse to check inhaler technique 2–3wk after starting inhaler)
- Address further patient questions and practical difficulties at follow-up
- Monitor repeat prescriptions

Further information

NICE Medicines adherence (2009) ℜ www.nice.org.uk
GMC Good practice in prescribing and managing medicines and devices (2013) ℜ www.gmc-uk.org

Repeat prescribing

80% of NHS prescriptions are for repeat medication. Good practice is essential to ensure wastage (>10% of total prescribing costs) is kept to a minimum. *Essential elements are:*

- **Written explanation** of the repeat prescribing process for patients and carers
- **Practice personnel with dedicated responsibility** ensure patient recall and regular medication review
- **Agreed practice policies** for repeat prescriptions, e.g. duration of supply; procedure if someone 'runs out' but is not authorized to have more
- **Authorization check** each time a prescription is signed
- **Compliance check** for under or over use (prescription frequency)
- **Equivalence check** all regular prescriptions are for the same duration of treatment so that prescription requests can be synchronized
- **Regular housekeeping** keeps records of medication up to date (including dosage instructions)—particular care is needed after hospital discharge when medication could have been substantially changed
- **Training of practice staff**

Review process Invite the patient ± carer. *Areas to cover:*

- **Explain** what you want to do in the review and the reasons for it
- **Compile a list** of all medicines being taken/used including: prescribed medication; OTC drugs; herbal/homeopathic medicines; illicit drugs; and medicines borrowed from others. *Compare* the list of drugs generated with the prescription record
- **Concordance.** Find out whether and how medication is taken
- **Explore** understanding of the purpose of the medication and consequences of not taking it and how much, how often, when
- **Discuss** misconceptions/queries
- **Ask about side effects**
- **Review relevant monitoring tests**, e.g. TFTs; INR; HbA1c
- **Review practical aspects.** Problems ordering/receiving repeat prescriptions; using medicines, e.g. problems opening containers; with formulations, e.g. difficulty swallowing tablets; reading labels—can request large print; remembering to take medication—consider reminder chart, multi-compartment compliance aid, altering times of doses to fit in better with daily schedule
- **Check** necessity and appropriateness of all prescriptions (see Figure 6.1)

Further information

BNF ✍ www.bnf.org
UK Medicines Information ✍ www.ukmi.nhs.uk
Electronic Medicines Compendium ✍ www.medicines.org.uk

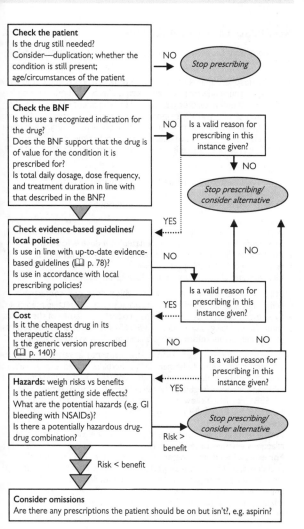

Figure 6.1 Deciding whether a prescribed drug is appropriate

Adverse drug reactions

'I don't want two diseases - one nature-made and one doctor-made'

Napoleon Bonaparte, St Helena (1820)

In 5–17% hospital admissions, an adverse drug reaction is implicated. Any drug may produce unwanted or unexpected effects. Common side effects are listed in the BNF or drug data sheet but any patient can have an allergic reaction or idiosyncratic response to any drug. The possibility of rare (<1:5,000) or delayed reactions means that safety of new medicines cannot be established until they have been used for some time in a large population. A 24h Freefone service is available for information ☎ 0800 100 3352.

Classification
- **Type A**—Common and relate to the pharmacology of the drug (e.g. constipation with opioids)
- **Type B**—Rare, unpredictable, and often serious

Within this classification, reactions may be:
- **Allergy** Anaphylaxis, allergic rash
- **Toxic effect**, e.g. ataxia with carbamazepine if dose is too high
- **Predictable** Well-recognized side effect, e.g. dry mouth with amitriptyline, GI bleeding with aspirin
- **Idiosyncratic** Unpredictable and unique to the individual

Defective medicines A medicine which does not conform to its specification is deemed defective. Report suspected defective medicines, with as much detail as possible on the product and nature of the defect, to: dmrc@mhra.gsi.gov.uk or ☎ 020 3080 6574. There is an online reporting form and further information available at: ᛰ www.mhra.gov.uk.

Suspected adverse reactions Any suspected adverse reaction to any therapeutic agent, whether OTC, herbal/alternative medication, or prescribed by a doctor, should be reported to the Medicines and Healthcare Products Regulatory Agency (MHRA, CHM Freepost, London SW8 5BR). Forms ('Yellow cards') are available from that address or in the back of the BNF. Alternatively, report online at ᛰ yellowcard.mhra.gov.uk.
- **For new drugs** (marked ◆ in BNF). Doctors are asked to report all reactions whether or not causality is clear
- **For established drugs** Doctors are asked to report all reactions in children; and all serious suspected reactions even if the effect is well documented (e.g. anaphylaxis, blood disorders, renal or liver impairment, drug interactions). Well-known, relatively minor side effects (e.g. constipation with opioids, insomnia with SSRIs) should *not* be reported

Prevention of adverse reactions

- Never use a drug unless there is a good indication
- Always ask patients if they have had reactions previously to a drug before prescribing
- Ask about other drugs patients are taking (including self-medication); consider interactions
- Consider the effects of age and hepatic or renal impairment
- Prescribe as few drugs as possible—the more drugs, the more likelihood of interactions
- Give clear instructions about how to take the drug
- Wherever possible use drugs you are familiar with; if using a new drug be alert to side effects
- Warn patients about potentially serious side effects (e.g. risk of GI ulceration with NSAIDs)

Consumer Protection Act (1987) If a patient is damaged by a defective product, liability falls on the producer unless outside the EC when it falls on the importer. If the importer cannot be identified, liability falls on the supplier. This is important for GPs. Those who dispense are at greatest risk but all GPs occasionally supply drugs in an emergency or for procedures within the surgery (vaccinations, minor surgery, contraception). Always record manufacturer, batch number, and expiry date when using such drugs and keep records of storage of drugs and maintenance of equipment.

Poisoning 📖 p. 1116

Poisons information

TOXBASE Poisons database ℔ www.toxbase.org
UK National Poisons Information Service ☎ 0844 892 0111
℔ www.npis.org

Licensing

In the UK, the Medicines Act (1968) makes it essential for anyone who manufactures or markets a drug for which therapeutic claims are made to hold a licence. The Licensing Authority, working through the Medicines and Healthcare Products Regulatory Agency (MHRA), can grant both Manufacturer's Licence and Marketing Authorization (which allows a company to market and supply a product for specified indications). Although doctors usually prescribe according to the licensed indications, they are not obliged to.

Prescribing outside licence There may be occasions when a doctor feels it is necessary to prescribe outside a drug's licence.

- **Generic formulations** for which indications are not described. The prescriber has to assume the indications are the same as for branded formulations
- **Use of well-established drugs for proven but not licensed indications**, e.g. amitriptyline for neuropathic pain
- **Use of drugs for conditions where there are no other treatments** (even if the evidence of their effectiveness is not well proven) This often occurs in secondary care when new treatments become accepted. GPs may become involved if a patient is discharged to the community and the GP asked to continue prescribing. ❶ The person signing the prescription is legally responsible
- **Use of drugs for individuals not covered by their licensed indications** Frequently occurs in paediatrics

⚠ Before prescribing any medication (whether within or outside the licence) weigh risks against benefits. The more dangerous the medicine and the flimsier the evidence base for treatment, the more difficult it is to justify the decision to prescribe.

When prescribing licensed drugs for unlicensed indications, it is important to inform patients and carers of what you are doing and why. Explain that the patient information leaflet (PiL) will not have information about the use of the drug in these circumstances. Record in the patients notes your reasons for prescribing outside the licensed indications for the drug.

Clinical trials Drug discovery and development is a protracted process (>10y) costing huge sums of money (≈£100 million). Clinical testing is conventionally divided into five stages:

- **Phase I trials** clinical pharmacology in normal volunteers
- **Phase II trials** preliminary small-scale studies
- **Phase III trials** large-scale trials (several thousands of patients often). Once complete application is made for a licence to sell the drug
- **Phase IV trials** post-marketing surveillance—large-scale follow-up of patients using the drug to establish evidence long-term efficacy and safety
- **Phase V trials** further trials to compare efficacy and safety with other marketed compounds and explore new indications

GPs are unlikely to be involved before phase III. Taking part in trials can benefit both patients and the practice but consider proposals carefully before embarking on a project.

Research in general practice 📖 p. 82

Questions to ask before agreeing to take part in a clinical trial

- Are the aims and objectives of the study defined?
- What is the design?
- Which drug is to be tested?
- What are the end points?
- Are the criteria for identifying patients clear and explicit?
- Are the numbers to be recruited specified and feasible?
- Are the observations to be made clearly and vigorously defined?
- Are the arrangements for providing information to patients and for obtaining informed consent satisfactory?
- Has ethical approval of the study been obtained?
- Are the financial arrangements clearly set out (minimum— reimbursement of patients' expenses and reimbursement of practice expenses)
- Has adequate provision been made for compensation in the event of injury to patients in the course of the study?

Controlled drugs

Misuse of Drugs Act (1971) Controls manufacture, supply, and possession of controlled drugs. Penalties for offences are graded according to perceived harmfulness of the drug into three classes:
- **Class A**, e.g. cocaine, diamorphine (heroin), methadone, LSD, ecstasy
- **Class B**, e.g. oral amphetamines, barbiturates, cannabis, codeine
- **Class C**, e.g. most benzodiazepines, androgenic and anabolic steroids

Misuse of Drugs Regulations (2001) Defines persons authorized to supply and possess CDs while carrying out their professions and describes the way this is to be done. Five schedules of drug are defined:
- **Schedule 1** Drugs not used for medicinal purposes, e.g. LSD. Possession and supply are prohibited except with special licence
- **Schedule 2** Drugs subject to full CD controls (written dispensing record, kept in locked container, CD prescription regulations), e.g. diamorphine, cocaine, pethidine
- **Schedule 3** Partial CD controls (as Schedule 2, but no need to keep a register—some drugs subject to safe custody regulations), e.g. barbiturates, temazepam, meprobamate, buprenorphine
- **Schedules 4 and 5** Most benzodiazepines, anabolic and androgenic steroids, HCG, growth hormone, codeine. Controlled drug prescription requirements do not apply nor do safe custody requirements

❶ Preparations in Schedules 2 and 3 are identified throughout the British National Formulary (BNF) by the symbol **CD** (controlled drug).

Controlled drugs register All healthcare professionals who hold personal stock of any Schedule 2 drugs must keep their own controlled drugs register, and they are personally responsible for keeping this accurate and up to date. Out-of-date drugs should be recorded and destroyed in the presence of an authorized witness (police, PCO official).

Prescriber's responsibilities If prescribing controlled drugs for medicinal purposes, you have a responsibility:
- To avoid creating dependence by unnecessarily introducing controlled drugs to patients
- For careful monitoring to ensure the patient does not gradually ↑ the dose of drug to a point where dependence becomes more likely
- To avoid being an unwitting source of supply for addicts. If you suspect an addict is going round surgeries with intent to obtain supplies, contact your PCO so that they can issue a warning to other practices

Prescribing for drug misusers 📖 p. 189
Notification of drug misusers 📖 p. 188

Writing prescriptions for CDs Any prescription for Schedules 2 and 3 controlled drugs (with the exception of temazepam) must contain the following details written so as to be indelible:

- The patient's full name, address, and age—if the patient is homeless, 'no fixed abode' is an acceptable address
- The patient's NHS (in Scotland, Community Health Index) number
- Name and form of the drug, even if only one form exists
- Strength of the preparation and dose to be taken
- The total quantity of the preparation, or the number of dose units, to be supplied in both words and figures, e.g. 'Morphine sulfate 10mg (ten milligram) tablets, one to be taken twice daily. Supply 60 (sixty) tablets, total 600 (six hundred) milligrams'
- Signature of the prescriber (must be handwritten) and date. It is good practice to include the GMC number of the prescriber as well
- The address of the prescriber

❗ Apart from in exceptional circumstances, prescriptions for CDs in Schedules 2, 3, and 4 should be limited to a supply of ≤30d treatment. The validity period of NHS and private prescriptions for Schedules 1, 2, 3, and 4 controlled drugs is restricted to 28d. Schedules 2 and 3 drugs should not be prescribed on repeat prescriptions or under repeat dispensing schemes.

Travelling abroad with controlled drugs For patients or doctors travelling abroad with Schedules 2 or 3 drugs, an export licence may be required. Further details are available from 🔊 www.gov.uk/travelling-controlled-drugs. Patient applications to the Home Office for an import/export licence for a CD must be accompanied by a supporting letter from the prescribing doctor stating:

- The patient's name and address
- The quantities of drugs to be carried
- The strength and form in which the drugs will be dispensed
- The country of destination
- The dates of travel to and from the UK

For clearance to import the drug into the country of destination, it is advisable to contact the Embassy or High Commission of that country prior to departure

Further information

National Prescribing Centre (NPC) *A guide to good practice in the management of controlled drugs in primary care* (England) (2009) 🔊 www.npc.co.uk
British National Formulary 🔊 www.bnf.org
Advisory Council on the Misuse of Drugs 🔊 www.gov.uk/government/organisations/advisory-council-on-the-misuse-of-drugs

Prescribing for special groups

Borderline substances (*BNF* Appendix 2 🕸 www.bnf.org) For certain conditions, foods and toilet products can be regarded as drugs and prescribed on NHS prescription (e.g. gluten-free foods for coeliac disease, nutritional supplements for disease-related malnutrition). The Advisory Committee on Borderline Substances advises on which products are available for certain specified conditions. Products should not be prescribed for any other condition. Use form FP10 (GP10 in Scotland) and endorse with the letters 'ACBS'.

Renal impairment Renal function ↓ with age but may not be reflected by raised creatinine due to ↓ muscle mass. Always assume mild to moderate renal failure if prescribing for the elderly. Renal impairment can change the effects of drugs by:

- **Inability to excrete the drug** May cause toxicity. Dose reduction or increase in interval between doses may be necessary
- **Increased sensitivity to drugs** (even if elimination is unimpaired)
- **Poor tolerance of side effects** Nephrotoxic drugs may have more serious side effects
- **Lack of effectiveness** When renal function is reduced

Degree of renal impairment Estimated glomerular filtration rate (eGFR), based on serum creatinine, age, gender, and ethnic origin, is now provided to GPs when renal function tests are done.

- **Mild renal impairment** eGFR 60–89mL/min/1.73m^2
- **Moderate renal impairment** eGFR 30–59mL/min/1.73m^2
- **Severe renal impairment** eGFR <30mL/min/1.73m^2

Further information BNF Guidance on prescribing: prescribing in renal impairment 🕸 www.bnf.org; patients on dialysis—consult local renal unit.

Hepatic impairment Problems do not tend to arise until late stages of liver failure when there is jaundice, ascites, or evidence of encephalopathy. Problems are due to:

- **Impaired drug metabolism** Many drugs are metabolized by the liver. In severe liver failure dose may need to be ↓ ± dosage interval ↑. A few drugs are excreted in the bile unchanged and may accumulate in patients with obstructive jaundice (e.g. rifampicin, fusidic acid)
- **Hypoproteinaemia** Liver disease is associated with ↓ plasma protein. This affects binding of drugs. Highly protein-bound drugs (e.g. phenytoin, prednisolone) can become toxic in normal dosage
- **Hepatotoxicity** Liver toxicity will have ↑ effect if hepatic reserve is already ↓
- **Clotting** Blood clotting factors are made in the liver. In liver disease effects of oral anticoagulants are ↑
- **Encephalopathy** Drugs that depress cerebral function (e.g benzodiazepines, opioids) can precipitate encephalopathy if severe liver failure
- **Fluid retention** Drugs causing fluid retention (e.g. NSAIDs) make oedema and ascites worse

Further information BNF Guidance on prescribing: prescribing in hepatic impairment 🕸 www.bnf.org.

Palliative care 📖 pp. 1028–47

Prescribing for the elderly 📖 p. 206

Pregnancy 📖 p. 784. Drugs taken by the mother can harm the fetus at any stage in pregnancy. *Mechanisms:*

- **1st trimester** Teratogenesis causing congenital malformations. Greatest risk—wks 3–12
- **2nd/3rd trimesters** Toxic effects; effects on growth/development
- **Around labour** May affect labour or have adverse effects on the newborn baby

Only prescribe if essential, especially in the 1st trimester. Stick to tried and tested drugs when possible (see *BNF* Guidance on prescribing: prescribing in pregnancy ℬ www.bnf.org); use smallest effective dose; avoid new drugs. ❶ Lack of information does not imply safety.

Further information UK Teratology Information Service ☎ 0844 892 0909 ℬ www.uktis.org

Breastfeeding Drugs taken by a mother breastfeeding can affect the child by inhibiting lactation or entering the milk and causing toxicity to the infant. Therapeutic doses in the mother can cause toxicity in the infant if the drug is concentrated in milk (e.g. iodides). Avoid prescribing, wherever possible. Stick to tried and tested drugs (see *BNF* Guidance on prescribing: prescribing in breast feeding ℬ www.bnf.org).

Prescribing for children

⚠ Keep all medicines out of the reach of children (and, preferably, in a locked cupboard). Dispose of unwanted medicines by returning them to a pharmacy for destruction.

- Children differ from adults in their response to drugs. Consult the BNF for Children or Paediatric Vade Mecum before prescribing unfamiliar drugs. Always check doses carefully. Many drugs are not licensed for use with children
- Paediatric suspensions often contain sugar. For long-term use or children having frequent prescriptions, consider sugar-free versions
- Do not advise adding medicines to infant feeding bottles—they may interact with milk and the dose will be ↓ if not all the contents are drunk
- Information on drugs used to treat rare paediatric conditions: Alder Hey Children's Hospital (☎ 0151 252 5381) or Great Ormond Street Hospital (☎ 020 7405 9200)
- Report *all* adverse reactions on Yellow Cards 📖 p. 146

Driving whilst taking drugs 📖 p. 129 or ℬ www.dvla.gov.uk/medical/ataglance.aspx

Drugs and sport 📖 p. 501

Further information

British National Formulary ℬ www.bnf.org
UK Medicines Information ℬ www.ukmi.nhs.uk
Electronic Medicines Compendium ℬ www.medicines.org.uk

Complementary medicine

In the UK, ~90% of the population have tried complementary or alternative medicine (CAM) at some time (see Table 6.2). But, although CAM undoubtedly helps many individuals, its use remains controversial.

Reasons for caution Lack of:
- **Evidence of effectiveness** There are many anecdotal reports and small-scale observational studies of +ve effects of complementary therapies, but large-scale, high-quality studies tend to be –ve
- **Regulation of practitioners** At present, anyone can set up as a practitioner of alternative medicine. Regulation has been proposed and is likely to come into force over the next few years. Until then, it is important to find a reputable practitioner with accredited training who is a member of a recognized professional body. It is also important to ensure any practitioner used carries professional indemnity insurance
- **Regulation of products** At present, most complementary 'medicines' are sold as foods rather than medicines and do not hold a product licence. No licensing authority has assessed efficacy, safety, or quality and interactions with conventional medicines are unknown. Complementary medicines can, and do, cause adverse effects—just because they are natural does not mean they are safe

Legal position of GPs

Practising complementary medicine Conventionally trained doctors can administer alternative treatments. The *'Bolam test'* applies—in other words, if a doctor has undergone additional training in a complementary discipline and practises in a way that is reasonable and would be considered acceptable by a number of other medically qualified complementary practitioners, his or her actions are defensible.

Referring to complementary medicine practitioners
- **Delegation to non-medically qualified practitioner** Ask:
  - *Is my decision to delegate to this complementary therapy appropriate?* Evidence-based decisions are most persuasive; commonly accepted but unproven indications are also acceptable
  - *Have I taken reasonable steps to ensure that the practitioner is qualified and insured?* Usually sufficient to ensure he/she is a member of the main professional regulatory body responsible for that discipline. Main bodies require members to be fully indemnified
  - *Has my medical follow-up been adequate?* Continue following up chronic conditions as usual. Do not issue repeat prescriptions without having sufficient information to ensure safe prescribing
- **Referral to a medically qualified practitioner/state registered osteopath or chiropractor** Same legal situation as when referring to another conventional healthcare practitioner. As long as the decision to make the referral is appropriate (see Delegation to non-medically qualified practitioner above), all further responsibility is taken over by the practitioner providing the service

Further information
Bandolier ॐ www.medicine.ox.ac.uk/bandolier/booth/booths/altmed.html

Table 6.2 Commonly used complementary therapies

Therapy	Features
Acupuncture	Needles are used to alleviate symptoms or cure disease Mechanism of action remains unclear. Two broad forms: • *Traditional acupuncture* Based on Chinese medicine where health is a balance between ying and yang. Illness is imbalance, and treatment aims to restore balance • *Modern acupuncture* Uses modern anatomy and physiology **Evidence:** mixed—good evidence that effective for back pain, idiopathic headache, and migraine; knee pain; and post-operative nausea/vomiting **Variants:** auriculotherapy; transcutaneous electrical nerve stimulation (TENS); reflexology
Homeopathy	From the Greek, meaning 'treatment of similars'. Works on the principle that like cures like. A remedy is chosen that mimics the symptoms displayed by the patient. Most remedies are serially diluted in steps of 1:10 (decimal x) or 1:100 (centesimal c). Manufacture is controlled by the Medicines Act **Evidence:** with higher dilutions (>12c), a theoretical problem arises as the solution may not contain any molecules of the mother substance. However, meta-analysis suggests that overall effective
Herbal medicine	Use of plants for medicinal purposes. Although traditional medicine uses many plant extracts (e.g. digoxin, morphine), herbal medicine uses plant extracts and not isolated constituents. All herbal medicines must be registered in order to be sold in the UK **Evidence:** there is evidence of effectiveness of many herbal remedies, including: saw palmetto (benign prostatic hyperplasia); echinacea (common cold); St John's wort (depression); feverfew (migraine) **Variants:** aromatherapy is the use of concentrated aromatic plant oils. No good evidence of effectiveness. Oils commonly used include, lavender oil (insomnia, burns, blisters); tea tree oil (skin infection; head lice); peppermint oil (indigestion); valerian oil (anxiety, insomnia)
Dietary manipulation	*Healing foods* Are commonly used, e.g. cranberry juice for UTI; soya to ↓ menopausal symptoms; ginger to ↓ nausea *Nutritional medicine* Involves giving supplements of vitamins, minerals, amino acids, or essential fatty acids. There is some evidence of effectiveness, e.g. glucosamine for OA; calcium and vitamin D supplements for ↓ osteoporosis; vitamin B_6 for premenstrual tension *Probiotics* Orally administered microbial cell preparations. Some evidence of effectiveness for treatment of gastrointestinal conditions *Environmental medicine* Based on the premise that individuals develop intolerances to environmental substances—most commonly foods. Exclusion diets improve symptoms. The most common culprits are caffeine, milk, gluten, and citrus fruit
Osteopathy & chiropractic	Physical treatments aimed at restoring the alignment of the joints and improving functioning of the body. Already under statutory regulation. Good evidence of effectiveness, particularly for back pain
Hypno- therapy	Hypnotherapy consists of training the patient to relax very deeply—often with a focus, a scene, smell, touch sensation, or colour to aid this process. May be helpful for pain relief

Minor surgery

'A minor operation: one performed on someone else'
Unaccredited
Penguin Dictionary of Humorous Quotations, 2001

Providing minor surgery

Minor surgery in GMS practices Under the GMS contract, minor surgery can be provided as an additional service or directed enhanced service.

Minor surgery as an additional service
- Includes curettage and cautery and, in relation to warts, verrucae, and other skin lesions, cryocautery
- In all cases a record of consent of the patient to treatment and a record of the procedure itself should be kept
- Payment is included within the global sum payment. If a practice does not want to provide this service, it must 'opt out' and global sum payment is ↓ by 0.6%

Minor surgery as a directed enhanced service Extends the range of procedures beyond those practices are expected to do as an additional service. For the purpose of payment, procedures have been divided into 3 groups:
- Injections—muscles, tendons, and joints
- Invasive procedures—including incisions and excisions
- Injections of varicose veins and piles

Payment Treatments are priced according to the complexity of the procedure, involvement of other staff, and use of specialized equipment. Terms for this must be negotiated locally. Typical figures are £40 for a joint injection or £80 for a simple excision.

Minor surgery in PMS practices PMS contracts are negotiated on an individual basis with the local PCO/CCG. In most cases however, the contract provides for similar arrangements and payments to those in place for GMS practices.

Qualification to provide minor surgery Practices can provide minor surgery as a directed enhanced service if they can demonstrate they have the necessary facilities and personnel (partner, employee, or subcontractor) with the necessary skills. This includes:
- Adequate equipment
- Premises compliant with national guidelines as contained in Health Building Note 46: General Medical Practice Premises (DH)
- Nursing support
- Compliance with national infection control policies—sterile packs from the local CSSD, disposable sterile instruments, using approved sterilization procedures, etc.
- Ongoing training in minor surgery, related skills, and resuscitation techniques
- Regular audit and peer review to monitor clinical outcomes, rates of infection, and procedure

Location and equipment A suitable room, adequate lighting, the appropriate equipment, and sufficient uninterrupted time is needed for successful minor surgery. An experienced assistant is also a great help. Sterile instruments and gloves and aseptic technique are essential.

- **Basic minor surgery sets** Usually contain a scalpel; several sizes of blade (e.g. size 11 and 15); toothed forceps; needle holder; fine scissors; artery forceps; skin hook; curette
- **Additional equipment required** Skin preparation liquid (e.g. chlorhexidine); local anaesthetic (e.g. lidocaine 1%); suitable sized needles and syringes; sterile towels; swabs; sterile specimen pots; suture materials and dressings for the wound. For joint injection, ensure that you have steroid and local anaesthetic drawn up and suitably sized needles available before starting

⚠ Always make sure you know how many blades, sutures, needles, and swabs you have, and ensure that you have accounted for and safely disposed of them at the end of the procedure.

Consent Patient consent for the procedure must be sought and recorded in the notes. This involves giving enough information about the procedure and other possible treatment options to allow the patient to make an informed decision about whether to proceed; the patient and consenting doctor should then both sign the consent form and the form should be filed in the patient's medical records.

Histological examination All tissue removed by minor surgery should be sent for histological examination unless there are exceptional or acceptable reasons for not doing so.

Documentation Maintain full, legible, accurate records. Include:
- History of the complaint
- Examination findings
- Diagnosis
- Full details of the procedure undertaken—include dose, batch number, expiry date and quantities of drugs, size and number of sutures, and
- Follow-up arrangements

If the patient is not registered with the practice undertaking the minor surgery, then a complete record of the procedure must be sent to the patient's registered practice for inclusion in the GP notes.

Follow-up and outcome Should be recorded in the patient's notes. Advise the patient:
- What to expect after the procedure
- Precautions to take after the procedure
- When to return for suture removal
- Signs that would indicate the need for reconsultation
- About the expected recovery/healing time

Arrange a follow-up appointment for all but the most straightforward procedures.

Basic techniques

⚠ Never attempt a procedure if you are unsure about it—know the boundaries of your experience and abilities.

Local anaesthesia

- 0.5–2% lidocaine, Xylocaine®, and procaine are the most commonly used preparations
- Epinephrine (1:200,000) added to local anaesthetic ↓ bleeding and prolongs anaesthesia, but do not use epinephrine in areas supplied by end arteries (i.e. fingers, toes, penis, ear, nose)
- The safe maximum dose of local anaesthetic in adults is 20mL of 1% solution (less in elderly and children)—overdose causes fits or cardiac arrhythmias

Administering local anaesthetic

- Pre-warn patients local anaesthetic stings before numbing and that they will still be able to feel pressure—but not pain. If pain is felt more anaesthetic is needed
- Clean the skin, insert a small needle intradermally, and raise a small bleb before infusing more deeply
- Always pull back on the syringe plunger before injecting to check that you are not in a blood vessel
- Anaesthetic must be infused all around the excision site. This may require several needle insertions—try to do this through an already numb area to ↓ discomfort for the patient
- Allow time for anaesthetic to take effect (2–5min) before proceeding

Suturing Suture and needle types—📖 p. 163

- Various techniques for suturing and knot tying can be used (e.g. interrupted, continuous, subcuticular)
- Always make a careful record of the number of stitches and when they should be removed
- Usually, stitches need removal after 3–5d on the face, 7–14d on the back and legs, and 5–7d elsewhere
- Skin closure strips can be used instead of or in addition to stitches in some circumstances

Cautery Chemical (silver nitrate) or electrocautery are used alone, or in combination with other methods (e.g. curettage), to secure haemostasis or destroy tissue. *Suitable conditions:* nose bleeds, spider naevi, telangiectasia.

⚠ *Do not* use electrical cautery for patients with a cardiac pacemaker.

Implants Subcutaneous implants are prescribed for several conditions (e.g. prostate cancer). Most implants come pre-packaged with an insertion cannula and information leaflet—always read and follow the instructions if administering a new product and ensure position of implant and timing of administration is correct.

Contraceptive implants 📖 p. 760

Joint and soft tissue injection Steroids can have a potent local anti-inflammatory effect and dramatically improve certain musculoskeletal problems. Most joint injections are straightforward and can be undertaken within a general practice setting.

General rules
- Always use aseptic technique
- Do not inject if there is local sepsis (e.g. cellulitis) or any possibility of joint infection
- Never inject into the substance of a tendon—this may cause rupture (in tenosynovitis steroid is injected into the tendon sheath)
- Injections should not require pressure on the syringe plunger—if so the needle is probably not correctly located (tennis elbow is an exception)
- Undertake as few injections as possible to settle the problem—often one is sufficient. If no improvement after 2–3 then reconsider the diagnosis
- Do no more than 3–4 injections/patient/appointment and no more than 3–4 in any single joint—more than this ↑ risk of systemic absorption and joint damage

Preparation for the procedure
- Take a history, make a careful examination and have a clear diagnosis before considering injecting steroids
- Gather the needles, syringes, a sterile container (for sending aspirated fluid), steroid, local anaesthetic, skin preparation fluid (e.g. chlorhexidine or surgical spirit), cotton wool, and adhesive spot plaster beforehand
- The injected joint should be rested for 2–3d afterwards, if possible—certainly avoid heavy activity. Make sure the patient is comfortable, has given informed consent, and knows what to expect

Steroid preparations (↑ order of potency) Hydrocortisone acetate, methylprednisolone acetate, triamcinolone hexacetonide.

Local anaesthetic (LA) (e.g. lidocaine 1%) can be mixed with the steroid for some injections—LA effect occurs immediately and lasts 2–4h. The patient may then experience some return of symptoms (pain) before the steroid takes effect—warn the patient.

Follow-up
- Some injections are painful at administration—this is normal for tennis elbow and plantar fasciitis
- Steroid injection may cause temporary flushing and worsening of blood sugar control in patients with DM
- Severe or increasing pain ~48h after injection may indicate sepsis—advise the patient to return urgently if this occurs
- If steroid is injected close to the skin surface (as in tennis elbow), skin dimpling and pigment loss can occur—warn the patient

Most hospital rheumatology departments have a joint injection clinic and are happy to allow GPs to watch to gain experience

Further information
Silver T (2011) *Joint and Soft Tissue Injection: Injecting with Confidence* (5th edn). Radcliffe Publishing. ISBN 1846195004.

Removal of skin lesions

Ensure that you have had training in the techniques—learning by experience is much better than from a book. There are many courses available.

Excision of skin lesions

- Gain written consent—ensure you have warned the patient about the likely size of the scar and the possibility of keloid (especially if the lesion is on a risk area, e.g. upper back and chest)
- Work out the direction of the skin contour lines, clean and anaesthetise the area ($\square$ p. 160)
- An elliptical incision—~3x as long as it is wide—is suitable for most lesions. Place the incision in the skin contour lines if possible (marking the incision line can be helpful)
- Cut through the skin at right angles to the surface with a smooth sweep of the blade
- Use a skin hook to lift the skin from one end of the ellipse
- Use the scalpel blade to remove the skin from the subcutaneous fat
- Save the excised specimen for histology
- Close the wound by carefully apposing the edges (slightly everted) using interrupted non-absorbable sutures. Avoid tension in the sutures and knot securely. Large wounds may benefit from the use of deep absorbable sutures to reduce skin tension

Curettage

- Useful for seborrhoeic warts, pyogenic granuloma, keratoacanthoma, or single viral warts. Not suitable for naevi
- Use only if the diagnosis is certain—scrapings can be sent for histology but the architecture of the lesion is lost
- Numb the area with local anaesthetic and remove the lesion with gentle scooping movements using a curette spoon
- Finally cauterize the base of the lesion

Cryotherapy

- Liquid nitrogen can be used to treat viral and seborrhoeic warts, skin tags, and solar keratoses
- Local arrangements for delivery of liquid nitrogen differ—often a clinic session to treat all suitable lesions at the same time is helpful
- If diagnosis is uncertain excise the lesion, or take a biopsy prior to freezing
- A cotton wool bud or nitrogen spray gun can be used to apply liquid nitrogen for approximately 10s until a thin frozen halo appears at the base of the lesion
- A blister forms <24h after treatment—the lesion then falls off with the blister
- Repeat treatment may be needed after 4wk

Side effects Pain, failure to remove the lesion, skin hypopigmentation, ulceration of lower leg lesions (especially in elderly patients).

⚠ **Rules for removing skin lesions**

- **Only** remove benign lesions (unless you have specific training to excise low-risk BCCs)—refer suspicious lesions to a specialist for expert management
- **Only** remove lesions that you are confident you can cope with. Take special care with lesions on the face or lip margin—the scar may be very noticeable
- **Send all** excised lesions for histology—place in formalin and carefully label with the site and side

Suture types

- **Absorbable** e.g. catgut, Dexon, Vicryl—used to stitch deep layers to help ↓ tension
- **Non-absorbable** e.g. silk, prolene, nylon—used for closure of skin wounds after minor surgery

Needle types Straight, curved, cutting, or round-bodied. Surgical site and personal preference dictate which to use—a cutting needle is usually used for skin.

Suture thickness (gauge) Indicated by a number (10/0 is fine and 2/0 thick). For skin closure: 6/0 or 5/0 is usually used for the face, 3/0 on legs and back, and 4/0 elsewhere.

Lower and upper limb injections

The knee Joint effusions are common (e.g. trauma, ligament strains, OA, RA, gout). Aspirated fluid should be clear/slightly yellow and not purulent. Send any fluid aspirated for analysis. Aspiration of fluid can:

- Help make a diagnosis, e.g. gout
- Be a therapeutic procedure—draining a tense effusion can relieve pain
- Precede administration of steroids, e.g. RA flare

⚠ Any sign of infection within the joint prohibits steroid use.

Technique for aspiration and joint injection

- Lie the patient on couch with knee slightly bent—place a pillow under the knee as this relaxes the muscles
- Palpate the joint space under the lateral or medial edge of the patella and inject/aspirate just below the superior border of the patella with the needle horizontal—see Figure 7.1
- Use a green (21 gauge) needle
- If aspirating and then injecting steroids maintain the needle in position and swap the syringe
- Normal doses of steroid are triamcinolone 20mg or methylprednisolone 40mg
- In prepatella bursitis aspiration and injection of hydrocortisone 25mg into the bursa can help settle inflammation

Plantar fasciitis Painful area in the middle of the heel pad. Steroid injection (e.g. triamcinolone 10–20mg) into the most tender spot can help. Injection hurts, so advise analgesia. Mixing lidocaine 1% with the steroid can help.

Technique
Two methods are commonly used (see Figure 7.2):
- Injection through the tough skin of the sole (more accurate), or
- Lateral approach (less painful)

Rest the foot for several days afterwards and use an in-shoe heel pad. Rupture of the plantar fascia is a rare complication.

Tenosynovitis Causes pain and stiffness in the line of the tendon and crepitus over the affected tendon. The most common site is the base of the thumb (de Quervain's tenosynovitis). Injecting steroid and LA (e.g. hydrocortisone 25mg + 1mL 1% lidocaine) into the space between tendon and sheath can help.

Technique

- Insert the needle along the line of the tendon just distal to the point of maximum tenderness
- Advance the needle proximally into the tendon (felt as a resistance) and then slowly withdraw until the resistance disappears. The tip of the needle is then in the tendon sheath
- It is now safe to inject—the tendon sheath may swell
- Advise the patient to rest the affected area for several days and avoid the precipitating activity

Figure 7.1 Knee joint injection or aspiration

Plantar fascia

Alternative injection point

Figure 7.2 Injection of plantar fasciitis

Patient information

Arthritis Research UK Patient information 'Local steroid injections' ☏ 0870 850 5000 🖰 www.arthritisresearchuk.org

Carpal tunnel syndrome *Technique*:
- Sit the patient with hand resting on a firm surface, palm up. Palmaris longus tendon can be seen by wrist flexion against resistance
- Insert the needle at the distal skin crease, at 45° to the horizontal, pointing towards the fingers, just ulnar (little finger) side of the palmaris tendon (see Figure 7.3). If palmaris longus is absent (10%), inject between flexor digitorum superficialis and flexor carpi radialis tendons
- Use a green (21 gauge) needle. Advance it to half its length. If sudden pain in the fingers, you have hit the median nerve—withdraw the needle and reposition it
- Inject steroid e.g. 10mg triamcinolone—if there is resistance the needle is not in the right place. Do not use LA as it causes finger numbness
- Rest the hand for several days afterwards

Elbow *Technique for tennis/golfer's elbow injection:*
- Sit the patient with the elbow flexed to 90°
- Palpate the most tender spot and insert the needle into that spot
- Inject 0.1–0.2mL of steroid (e.g. hydrocortisone 25mg/mL). There will be resistance. Without taking the needle out, move the needle in a fan shape injecting small amounts of steroid—try to inject all the tender area. Warn about the possibility of skin dimpling or pigment loss
- Pain of injection may last 48h—warn the patient in advance, advise resting the arm and analgesia

❶ For tennis elbow, steroid injection has significantly better effects in the short term (~6wk) but poorer outcome long term compared to physiotherapy[R].

Shoulder Injection may help rotator cuff problems, frozen shoulder, subacromial bursitis, and RA. Use an anterior or posterior approach for shoulder joint injection and lateral approach for the subacromial space.

Technique: Anterior approach
- Sit patient with the arm relaxed at the side, slightly externally rotate.
- Insert the needle (green, 21 gauge) horizontally into the gap between the head of humerus and the coracoid process, ensuring the needle is lateral to the coracoid process—see Figure 7.4(a). Insert the needle for most of its length to reach the joint space
- Inject 1mL steroid e.g. triamcinolone 20mg + 1mL 1% lidocaine. There should be no/little resistance to injection—if there is, the needle is wrongly positioned

Technique: Lateral approach to subacromial space Sit the patient with arm hanging down to the side. Palpate the posterolateral corner of the acromion. Insert the needle horizontally into the space under the acromion—see Figure 7.4(b). Inject 5mL 0.5% bupivacaine + triamcinolone 20mg.

AC joint injection Can help the pain of OA. *Technique*:
- Palpate the joint space—insert the needle anteriorly or superiorly—if you go too far, you may enter the shoulder joint—see Figure 7.4(c)
- Only 0.2–0.5mL can be injected as small joint space. Use a blue (23 gauge) needle and do not add LA

Palmaris longus tendon
Flexor carpi radialis
Flexor retinaculum

Flexor digitorum superficialis

Flexor tendon sheath

Figure 7.3 Injection of the carpal tunnel

⚠ Warn patients that pain may worsen for up to 48h after injection before it improves.

(c)

Acromion

Subacromial bursa

(b)

Long head of biceps synovial sheath

Medial border of deltoid

Lateral end of clavicle

Coracoid process

(a)

Figure 7.4 Shoulder joint injection
Reproduced from Collier J, Longmore M, Amarakone K (2013) *Oxford Handbook of Clinical Specialties*, with permission from Oxford University Press.

Patient information

Arthritis Research UK Patient information 'Local steroid injections'
☎ 0870 850 5000 🖰 www.arthritisresearchuk.org

Healthy living

Prevention and screening

In all disease, the goal is prevention.

Definitions
- **Primary prevention** Prevention of disease occurrence
- **Secondary prevention** Controlling disease in early form (e.g. carcinoma in situ)
- **Tertiary prevention** Prevention of complications once the disease is present (e.g. DM)

Barriers to prevention
- **Patient** Blinkering ('It'll never happen to me'); rebellion ('I know it's bad—but it's cool'); poor motivation (path of least resistance)
- **Doctor** Time; money—health promotion takes time and personnel; motivation—health promotion is repetitive and boring
- **Society** Pressure from big business (e.g. cigarette advertising); other priorities; ethics (e.g. public uproar at threats not to offer cardiac surgery to smokers)

Prevention of coronary heart disease 📖 p. 242

Screening The idea of screening is attractive—the ability to diagnose and treat a potentially serious condition at an early stage when it is still treatable. An ideal screening test must pick up all those who have the disease (have high sensitivity) and must exclude those who do not (high specificity). It must detect *only* those who have a disease (high positive predictive value) and should exclude *only* those who do not have the disease (high negative predictive value). See Table 8.1.

The Wilson–Jungner criteria All screening tests should meet the following criteria before they are introduced to the target population:
- The condition being screened for is an important health problem
- Natural history of the condition is well understood
- There is a detectable early stage
- Treatment at early stage is of more benefit than at late stage
- There is a suitable test to detect early stage disease
- The test is acceptable to the target population
- Intervals for repeating the test have been determined
- Adequate health service provision has been made for the extra clinical workload resulting from screening
- Risks, both physical and psychological, are < benefits (see Table 8.2)
- Costs are worthwhile in relation to benefits gained

UK screening programmes
- >40y health checks—📖p. 242
- Cervical cancer—📖 p. 728
- Breast cancer—📖 p. 694
- Colon cancer—📖 p. 392
- Chlamydia—📖 p. 740
- Antenatal—📖 p. 796
- Neonatal bloodspot—📖 p. 850
- Neonatal hearing—📖 p. 856
- Child health surveillance—📖 p. 846
- Diabetic retinopathy—📖 p. 357
- Abdominal aortic aneurysm—📖 p. 284

Table 8.1 Performance of screening tests

		Disease	
		Present	Absent
Test	*Positive*	True positive (a)	False positive (b)
	Negative	False negative (c)	True negative (d)
Sensitivity = a/(a+c)		Negative predictive value = d/(c+d)	
Specificity = d/(b+d)		Positive predictive value = a/(a+b)	

Performance of screening tests See Table 8.1. For a screening programme to be effective and ↓ morbidity and mortality there must be:
- Adequate participation of the target population
- Few false-negative or false-positive results
- Screening intervals shorter than the time taken for the disease to develop to an untreatable stage
- Adequate follow-up of all abnormal results
- Effective treatment at the stage detected by screening

⚠ There is no ideal screening test. Always explain:
- Purpose of screening
- Likelihood of positive/negative findings and possibility of false-positive/negative results
- Uncertainties and risks attached to the screening process
- Significant medical, social, or financial implications of screening for the particular condition or predisposition
- Follow-up plans, including availability of counselling and support services

Table 8.2 Benefits and disadvantages of screening

Benefits	Disadvantages
• Improved prognosis for some cases detected by screening	• Longer morbidity in cases where prognosis is unaltered
• Less radical treatment for some early cases	• Overtreatment of questionable abnormalities
• Reassurance for those with negative test results	• False reassurance for those with false-negative results
• Increased information on natural history of disease and benefits of treatment at early stage	• Anxiety and sometimes morbidity for those with false-positive results
	• Unnecessary intervention for those with false-positive results
	• Hazard of screening test
	• Diversion of resouces to the screening programme

Further information

Wilson JMG, Jungner G (1968) *Principles and Practice of Screening for Disease.* Public Health Paper No. 34. Geneva: World Health Organization.

Prevention of travel-related illness

Pre-travel assessment 8wk pre-departure where possible. *Check:*
- Age
- General health
- Where and when intending to travel (including areas within a country and stopovers elsewhere)
- Type of accommodation
- Purpose of travel
- Previous experience (including experience with antimalarials)
- Current vaccination status

Health risks

- **Environmental hazards (e.g. changes in altitude/climate)** Avoid rapid changes of altitude—take time to readjust; avoid sunburn. Advise women taking combined hormonal contraception and trekking to altitudes of >4500m for >1wk to consider an alternative method of contraception
- **Accidents** Avoid potentially dangerous tasks under the influence of alcohol, e.g. swimming, driving. Avoid motorbikes—especially without helmets and protective clothing
- **Illness abroad** MI causes 61% deaths related to international travel. Do not travel if unwell. Ensure adequate insurance including repatriation costs. Take enough supplies of regular medication when travelling to last the entire trip, and take preventative steps to avoid infection
- **Transport related problems**
  - Fitness to fly: 📖 p. 132
  - Motion sickness (take OTC medication if afflicted)
  - Jet lag
  - DVT—on flights >3h: drink plenty of water, avoid alcohol, regularly get up and walk around, consider prophylactic support stockings
- **Psychological effects of travel**

Prevention of travellers' diarrhoea 50% travellers experience some diarrhoea. Most cases last 4–5d. 1–2% last >1mo.
- Take care to eat and drink uncontaminated food and water
- Food should be freshly cooked and hot
- Avoid salads and cold meats/fish
- Eat fruit that can be peeled
- Stick to drinks made with boiling water or bottled drinks and water with an intact seal; avoid ice in drinks
- Use water purification tablets if necessary

Action If diarrhoea occurs when abroad advise patients to use oral rehydration fluids. Only take antidiarrhoeals if impossible to get to a toilet. Seek medical advice if blood in stool, fever, or not resolving in 72h (24h for the elderly or infants).

⚠ Do not use antidiarrhoeals if blood in stool, fever, or <10y old.

Prevention of malaria[ND]

- **Awareness of risk** High-risk areas are Central and South America; South East Asia; Pacific islands; sub-Saharan Africa—however brief the time there. Pregnant and asplenic patients are at particular risk

- **↓ mosquito bites** Mosquitoes bite at night
  - *Accommodation*—sleep in screened accommodation spraying screens with insecticide each evening and use a pyrethroid vaporizer. If screens are not available use a permethrin-impregnated bed net (kits are available)
  - *Person*—in the evenings wear long-sleeved shirts and trousers; protect limbs with diethyl toluamide-containing repellant
- **Chemoprophylactic drugs** See Table 8.3. Regimes vary with location and time of year. Information is available via the Travax website (℘ www. travax.nhs.uk—registration needed) and travel information clinics
- **Awareness of residual risk** Chemoprophylaxis is not 100% effective. Advise all travellers to malaria regions to seek medical advice if unwell for up to 6mo after return. Malaria is a great mimic. Have a high level of suspicion

Prevention of HIV and hepatitis B and C

- Avoid casual sexual contacts. If these occur use barrier methods of contraception (Femidom®, condoms)
- Avoid shared needles (e.g. tattooing/ear piercing/drugs)
- Medical kits—if travelling to high-risk areas, take a clearly labelled medical kit containing sutures, syringes, and needles for use in emergencies
- Avoid blood transfusion. Two-thirds blood donations in the developing world are unscreened. Know your blood group. Have good travel insurance, including repatriation costs. In an emergency the Blood Care Foundation can arrange screened blood to be provided anywhere in the world (☎ 01403 262652; ℘ www.bloodcare.org.uk)
- Vaccination for hepatitis B prior to travelling

Vaccination 4% deaths related to travel are due to infectious disease—ensure fully vaccinated for areas intending to visit. Information is available from the Travax website (℘ www.travax.nhs.uk)—registration is needed.

Table 8.3 Antimalarial chemoprophylactic drugs

Drug	Dose	Start	Stop
Chloroquine	310mg weekly	1wk before entering malaria area	4wk after leaving malaria area
Mefloquine	250mg weekly	2.5wk before entering malaria area	4wk after leaving malaria area
Proguanil	200mg daily	1wk before entering malaria area	4wk after leaving malaria area
Malarone® (proguanil + atovaquone)	1 tablet daily	1–2d before entering malaria area	1wk after leaving malaria area
Doxycycline	100mg daily	1–2d before entering malaria area	4wk after leaving malaria area

Useful information

Health Protection Agency (HPA) Guidelines for malaria prevention in travellers from the UK (2007) ℘ www.hpa.org.uk
Fit for Travel Information for people travelling abroad from the UK. Includes a list of yellow fever vaccination centres ℘ www.fitfortravel.nhs.uk

Diet

The role of the GP and primary care team
- **Screening** Identification of obese patients and patients in need of dietary advice for other reasons
- **Assessment** Current diet, motivation, and barriers to change
- **Discussion and negotiation** Exploration of knowledge about diet; negotiation of goals
- **Goal setting** Provide information and 2–3 food-specific goals on each occasion—set a series of mini-targets that appear realistic and achievable; tailor them to existing diet and usual schedule
- **Monitoring progress**

Barriers to a good diet
- Ignorance—posters in surgeries/leaflets may help
- Cultural differences—modify information to be relevant
- Enjoyment—perception of healthy diet is not enjoyable
- Poverty—fresh fruit/vegetables and lean meat/fish are expensive—some elements are cheap, e.g. potatoes, pasta, rice
- Lifestyle—convenience foods contain a lot of salt, sugar, and fat
- Peer pressure—children are under pressure to eat sweets, crisps, etc.
- Habits of a lifetime—we like the foods we have grown up with
- Confusion about what is good—packaging may be misleading, e.g. breakfast cereals claiming health messages but containing high sugar
- Mixed messages—one minute the press says something is good for you, the next it causes some horrible disease and should be avoided
- Fatalism/apathy

The ideal diet See Figure 8.1, 📖 p. 176. Adjust composition/portion size of each meal to maintain a healthy weight. Include a variety of foods:
- **Use starchy foods** (e.g. bread, rice, pasta, potatoes) As the main energy source
- **Eat plenty of fruit and vegetables** (>5 portions of fruit and/ vegetables/d) Do not overcook vegetables; steaming is preferable to boiling, and keep the delay between cutting and eating fruit/vegetables to a minimum
- **Eat plenty of fibre** Good sources are: high-fibre breakfast cereals, beans, pulses, wholemeal bread, potatoes (with skins), pasta, rice, oats, fruit/vegetables
- **Eat fish** At least 2x/wk. including one portion (max. two portions if pregnant) of oily fish (e.g. mackerel, herring, pilchards, salmon). ↓ cooked red or processed meat; consider substituting meat with vegetable protein (e.g. pulses, soya)
- **Choose lean meat** Remove excess fat/poultry skin and pour off fat after cooking; avoid fatty meat products (e.g. sausages, salami, meat pies); boil, steam, or bake foods in preference to frying; when cooking with fat use unsaturated oil (e.g. olive, sunflower oil) and use cornflour rather than butter and flour to make sauces
- **Use skimmed milks** And low-fat yoghurts/spreads/cheese (e.g. Edam or cottage cheese)

- **Avoid adding salt** to foods. Aim for <6g of salt/d. Avoid processed foods, crisps, and salted nuts
- **Avoid adding sugar** and cut down on sweets, biscuits, and desserts
- **Drink at least 4–6 pints (2–3L) of fluid daily** Preferably not tea, coffee, or alcohol. Drinking a large glass of water with meals and instead of snacks can reduce the urge to overeat
- **Avoid excessive alcohol intake** <21u/wk for men and <14u/wk for women—📖 p. 184

Obesity 📖 p. 178

Weight loss Non-specific symptom. Treat the cause. *Consider*:
- **GI causes** Malabsorption, malnutrition, dieting
- **Chronic disease** Hyperthyroidism, DM, heart failure, renal disease, severe COPD, degenerative neurological/muscle disease, chronic infection (e.g. TB, HIV) or infestation
- **Malignancy**
- **Psychiatric causes** Depression, dementia, anorexia

Malnutrition 50% of women and 25% of men aged >85y are unable to cook a meal alone. Malnutrition is common amongst the elderly.

Poor nutritional status Slows rate of wound healing, ↑ risk of infection, ↓ muscle strength, is detrimental to mental well-being, and ↓ the ability of elderly people to remain independent.

Risk factors
- Low income
- Living alone
- Mental health problems (e.g. depression)
- Dementia
- Recent bereavement
- Gastric surgery
- Malabsorption
- ↑ metabolism
- Difficulty eating and/or swallowing (stroke, neurological disorder, MND)
- Presence of chronic disease (e.g. Crohn's disease, UC, IBS, cancer, COPD, CCF)

Management
- **General advice** Encourage to eat more and ↑ consumption of fruit and vegetables; consider using nutritional, vitamin (e.g. vitamin D for the housebound and institutionalized), and mineral supplements
- **Inability to prepare meals/shop** Consider referral to social services, meals on wheels, community dietician; community day centre; local voluntary support organization
- **Difficulty with utensils** Consider aids/equipment, e.g. special cutlery, non-slip mats—consider OT referral
- **Nausea** Consider antiemetics
- **Swallowing difficulty** Investigate cause. If none found or unable to resolve the problem, consider pureed food and/or thickened fluids

Further information

Scientific Advisory Committee on Nutrition (SACN) ⅌ www.sacn.gov.uk
British Nutrition Foundation ⅌ www.nutrition.org.uk
Malnutrition Universal Screening Tool (MUST) ⅌ www.bapen.org.uk/screening-for-malnutrition/must/introducing-must
NICE Nutrition support in adults (2006) ⅌ www.nice.org.uk

Fruits and vegetables

Bread, other cereals, and potatoes

Meat, fish, and alternatives

Foods containing fat
Foods containing sugar

Milk and dairy foods

Figure 8.1 The plate model. Developed nationally to communicate current recommendations for healthy eating. It shows rough proportions of the various food groups that should make up each meal.

What is a portion of vegetables or fruit?

One portion of vegetables or fruit is roughly equivalent to:
- 1 normal portion (2 tablespoons) of any vegetable
- 1 dessert bowl of salad
- 1 large fruit, e.g. apple, banana, orange, pear, peach, large tomato, or a large slice of pineapple or melon
- 2 smaller fruits, e.g. satsumas, plums, kiwi fruits, apricots
- 1 cup of small fruits, e.g. strawberries, raspberries, blackcurrants, cherries, grapes
- 1 tablespoon of dried fruit
- 2 large tablespoons of fruit salad, stewed or canned fruit in natural juices
- 1 glass (150mL) of fresh fruit juice

Avoiding snacking Discourage uncontrolled snacking of junk food between meals. Advise patients to ask themselves the following questions when they feel like eating between meals:
- **Am I hungry?** If unsure, wait 20min, and then ask the same question again
- **When was the last time I ate?** If <3h ago, it may not be real hunger
- **Could a small snack tide me over until the next meal?** Have ready-to-eat fruits or vegetables on hand for this

Height in metres

Weight in kilograms	1.36	1.40	1.44	1.48	1.52	1.56	1.60	1.64	1.68	1.72	1.76	1.80	1.84	1.88	1.92	1.96	2.00
125	68	64	60	57	54	51	49	46	44	42	40	39	37	35	34	33	31
123	67	63	59	56	53	51	48	46	44	42	40	38	36	35	33	32	31
121	65	62	58	55	52	50	47	45	43	41	39	37	36	34	33	31	30
119	64	61	57	54	52	49	46	44	42	40	38	35	35	34	32	31	30
117	63	60	56	53	51	48	46	44	41	40	38	36	35	33	32	30	29
115	62	59	55	53	50	47	45	43	41	39	37	35	34	33	31	30	29
113	61	58	54	52	49	46	44	42	40	38	36	35	33	32	31	29	28
111	60	57	51	51	48	46	43	41	39	38	36	34	33	31	30	29	28
109	59	56	50	50	47	45	43	41	39	38	35	34	32	31	30	28	27
107	58	55	52	49	45	44	42	40	38	36	35	33	32	30	29	28	27
105	57	54	51	48	45	43	41	39	37	35	34	32	31	30	28	27	26
103	56	53	50	47	45	42	40	38	36	35	33	32	30	29	28	27	26
101	55	52	49	46	44	42	39	38	36	34	33	31	30	29	27	26	25
99	54	51	48	45	43	41	39	37	35	33	32	31	29	28	27	26	25
97	52	49	47	44	42	40	38	36	34	33	31	30	28	27	26	25	24
95	51	48	46	43	41	39	37	35	34	32	31	29	28	27	26	25	24
93	50	47	45	42	40	38	36	34	33	31	30	29	27	26	25	24	23
91	49	46	44	42	39	37	36	34	32	31	29	28	27	26	25	24	23
89	48	45	43	41	39	37	35	33	32	30	29	27	26	25	24	23	22
87	47	44	42	40	38	36	34	32	31	29	28	27	26	25	24	23	22
85	46	43	41	39	37	35	33	32	30	29	27	26	25	24	23	22	21
83	45	42	40	38	36	34	32	31	29	28	27	26	25	23	23	22	21
81	44	41	39	37	35	33	32	30	29	27	26	25	24	23	22	21	20
79	43	40	38	36	34	32	31	29	28	27	26	24	23	22	21	21	20
77	42	39	37	35	33	32	30	29	27	26	25	24	23	22	21	20	19
75	41	38	36	34	32	31	29	28	27	25	24	23	22	21	20	19	19
73	39	37	35	33	32	30	29	27	26	25	23	23	22	21	20	19	18
71	38	36	34	32	31	29	28	26	25	24	23	22	21	20	19	18	18
69	37	35	33	32	30	28	27	26	24	23	22	21	20	19	18	18	17
67	36	34	32	31	29	28	26	24	23	22	21	20	19	18	17	17	17
65	35	33	31	30	28	27	25	24	23	22	21	19	19	18	18	17	16
63	34	32	30	29	27	26	25	23	22	21	20	19	19	18	17	16	16
61	33	31	29	28	26	25	24	23	22	21	20	19	18	17	17	16	15
59	32	30	28	27	26	24	23	22	21	20	19	18	17	17	16	15	15
57	31	26	27	26	25	23	22	21	20	19	18	17	16	16	15	15	14
55	30	30	27	25	24	23	21	20	19	19	18	17	16	16	15	14	14
53	29	29	26	24	23	22	21	20	19	18	17	16	16	15	14	14	13
51	28	26	25	23	22	21	20	19	18	17	16	16	15	14	14	13	13
49	26	25	24	22	21	20	19	18	17	17	16	15	14	14	13	13	12
47	25	24	23	21	20	19	18	17	17	16	15	15	14	13	13	12	12
45	24	23	22	21	19	18	18	17	16	15	15	14	13	13	12	12	11
43	23	22	21	20	19	18	17	16	15	15	14	13	13	12	12	11	11

- BMI <18.5—underweight
- BMI 18.5–24.9—acceptable weight
- BMI 25–29.9—overweight
- BMI 30–39.9—obese
- BMI ≥40—morbid obesity

Figure 8.2 Body mass index (BMI) ready reckoner for adults.

For children, BMI child reference tables must be used (available from ✎ www.health forallchildren.co.uk). Overweight is defined as weight ≥ 91st centile; obese as weight ≥ 98th centile.

Obesity

Obesity is one of the most important preventable diseases in the UK (se
Table 8.4). The best measure of obesity is body mass index (BMI).

Classification BMI (weight in kg ÷ (height in m)^2) (see Figure 8.2):
- 18.5–24.9 Healthy weight
- 25–29.9 Overweight
- >40 Obesity III (Morbid obesity)
- 30–34.9 Obesity I
- 35–39.9 Obesity II

} Obesit

Waist circumference See Table 8.5. Alternative measure of bod
fat correlated with CHD risk, DM, hyperlipidaemia, and ↑ BP. Measure
halfway between the superior iliac crest and the rib cage. Use in additio
to BMI to aid assessment of health risks.

Causes
- Physical inactivity
- Smoking cessation—mean weight ↑ 3–4kg
- Polygenic genetic predisposition—~1 in 3 obese people—more prone
  to obesity again after successful dieting
- Childbirth—especially if not breastfeeding
- Drugs—steroids, antipsychotics (e.g. olanzapine), contraceptives
  (especially depo-injections), sulfonylureas, insulin
- Endocrine causes (rare)—hypothyroidism, Cushing's syndrome, PCOS–
  only investigate if there are other symptoms/signs of endocrine disease
- Ongoing binge eating disorder (📖 p. 1015)
- Cultural factors
- Low education

Prevention Begins in childhood with healthy patterns of exercise/diet

Management When the body's intake > output over a period of tim
obesity results. Management aims to reverse this trend on a long-ter
basis through healthy diet, adjustment of calorie intake, physical exercis
and psychological support.

Initial assessment Assess willingness to change, eating behaviour ar
diet, physical activity, psychological distress, and social and family facto
affecting diet. Check a baseline BMI and waist circumference. Check B
blood glucose, and fasting lipid profile.

Advice Whether willing to change or not, provide advice on risks
obesity, and benefits of **healthy eating** (📖 p. 174) and **physical exercis
** (📖 p. 180). Tailor your advice to the individual. If unwilling to chang
reinforce this information at each encounter with the patient.

Diet Advise a weight loss diet for any patient who is overweight/obes
and willing to change:
- ↓ **calorie diets** All obese people lose weight on a low-energy intake.
  Aim for weight loss of 1–2lb (0.5–1kg)/wk using a ↓ in calorie intake
  ~600kcal/d with a target BMI of 25, in steps of 5–10% of original weigh
  There is no health benefit of weight ↓ below this. If simple diet sheet
  are not effective, refer to a dietician
- **Very low calorie diets** (<1,000kcal/d). Only limited place in
  management—use for a maximum of 12wk for obese patients when
  weight loss has plateaued

Table 8.4 Health risks of obesity

Greatly increased risk (RR >3)	Slightly increased risk (RR 1–2)
Mortality (BMI >30)	Cancer (breast in post-menopausal women, endometrial, oesophageal, colon)—14–20% of cancer deaths are due to obesity
Type 2 DM (BMI of 35 confers a 92x ↑ risk of DM)	
Gall bladder disease	
Dyslipidaemia	Reproductive hormone abnormalities
Insulin resistance	PCOS
Breathlessness	Impaired fertility
Sleep apnoea	Low back pain
	Stress incontinence
Moderately increased risk (RR 2–3)	Anaesthetic and post-operative risk
CHD (5–6% deaths are due to obesity)	Fetal defects associated with maternal obesity
↑ BP	Suicide
OA (knees)	School/workplace prejudice
Hyperuricaemia/gout	

Table 8.5 Waist circumference with excess risk (RR ≥3) of CHD and DM

Waist circumference	White Caucasians	Asians
Male	≥102cm (40 inches)	≥90cm (36 inches)
Female	≥88cm (35 inches)	≥80cm (32 inches)

🛈 For every 1cm ↑ in waist circumference, the RR of a CVD event ↑ by ~72%.

Drug therapy BNF 4.5.1. Orlistat (120mg tds with food) is the only drug licensed for treatment of obesity in the UK. It acts by ↓ fat absorption. Consider if a 3mo trial of supervised diet/exercise has failed and BMI ≥30kg/m² *or* ≥27kg/m² + co-morbidity (e.g. DM, ↑ BP). Continue treatment >3mo only if weight ↓ is ≥5% of initial body weight.

Surgery Consider if BMI >40kg/m² and non-surgical measures have failed. Adjustable gastric banding is the most common procedure. *Complications:* band slippage/damage; gastric erosion, pouch dilatation; infection; malabsorption.

Group and behavioural therapy Group activities, e.g. Weight Watchers, have a higher success rates in producing/maintaining weight ↓. Behavioural therapy together with low calorie diets is also effective.

Maintenance of weight loss Once a patient has lost weight, continue to monitor diet. Ongoing follow-up helps to sustain weight loss. Weight fluctuation (yo-yo dieting) may be harmful.

Further information

SIGN Management of obesity (2010) ℘ www.sign.ac.uk
NICE Obesity: the prevention, identification, assessment and management of overweight and obesity in adults and children (2006) ℘ www.nice.org.uk
National Obesity Forum ℘ www.nationalobesityforum.org.uk

Exercise

In the UK, 60% of adults are not active enough to benefit their health.

Recommended amounts of activity
- **Adults** ≥30min/d moderate intensity exercise on ≥5d/wk
- **Children** ≥1h/d moderate intensity exercise every day

Assessing levels of physical activity
See Table 8.6. Use a validated tool to assess levels of physical activity, e.g. General Practitioner Physical Activity Questionnaire (GPPAQ).

Health benefits of exercise Regular physical activity:

↓ risk of
- DM—through ↑ insulin sensitivity[S]   • Obesity[S]—📖 p. 178
- Cardiovascular disease—physically inactive people have ~2x ↑ risk of CHD and ~3x ↑ risk of stroke[S]
- Osteoporosis—exercise ↓ risk of hip fractures by ½[S]
- Cancer—↓ risk of colon cancer ~40%. There is also evidence of a link between exercise and ↓ risk of breast and prostate cancers[S]

Is a useful treatment for
- ↑ BP—can result in 10mmHg drop of systolic and diastolic BP; can also delay onset of hypertension[S]
- Hypercholesterolaemia—↑ high-density lipoprotein (HDL), ↓ low-density lipoprotein (LDL)[C]
- MI (📖 p. 260) and COPD (📖 p. 316)
- DM—improves insulin sensitivity and favourably affects other risk factors for DM, including obesity, HDL/LDL ratio, and ↑BP
- HIV—↑ cardiopulmonary fitness and psychological well-being[C]
- Arthritis and back pain—maintains function[C]
- Mental health problems—↓ intensity of depression; ↓ anxiety[S]

Benefits the elderly
- Maintains functional capacity   • ↓ risk of falls and hip fracture
- ↓ levels of disability   • Improves quality of sleep[C]

Negotiating change See Figure 8.3.

Table 8.6 Physical activity index (PAI) derived from the GPPAQ

Physical exercise and/or cycling (h/wk)	Occupation			
	Sedentary	Standing	Physical	Heavy manual
0	Inactive	Moderately inactive	Moderately active	Active
Some but <1	Moderately inactive	Moderately active	Active	Active
1–2.9	Moderately active	Active	Active	Active
≥3	Active	Active	Active	Active

Figure 8.3 Management plan for increasing activity levels

Effective interventions

- **Healthcare** Counselling is as effective as more structured exercise sessions. Specialist rehabilitation schemes are available for patients with specific conditions (e.g. post-MI, COPD); exercise schemes operate in some areas, offering low cost, supervised exercise for patients who might otherwise find it unacceptable to visit a gym and are accessed via GP 'prescription'; many sports facilities offer special sessions for pregnant women, the over-50s, and people with disability
- **Workplace** Interventions to ↑ rates of walking to work are effective
- **Schools** Appropriately designed and delivered physical education curricula can enhance physical activity levels. A whole-school approach to physical activity promotion is effective
- **Transport** Well-designed interventions ↑ walking/cycling to work
- **Communities** Community-wide approaches ↑ activity

Further information

NICE Physical activity guidance (2006) ☏ www.nice.org.uk
DH The General Practice Physical Activity Questionnaire (2006)
☏ www.dh.gov.uk

Smoking

Facts and figures In England, 21% of adults (σ 21%; φ 20%) smoke. Prevalence is highest amongst those aged 20–24 (32%) and lowest aged >60y (12%). 6% school children aged 11–15y are regular smokers (φ 10% σ 8%). Surveys of smokers show 73% want to stop and 30% intend to give up in <1y—but only ~2%/y successfully give up permanently.

Risks of smoking Smoking is the greatest single cause of illness and premature death in the UK. Half of all regular smokers will die as a result of smoking—106,000 people/y. Smoking is associated with ↑ risk of:

- **Cancers** ~29% all cancer deaths. Common cancers include: lung (>90% are smokers); lip; mouth; stomach; colon; bladder
- **Cardiovascular disease** CHD, CVA, peripheral vascular disease
- **Chronic lung disease** COPD, recurrent chest infection, exacerbation of asthma (29% of respiratory deaths result from smoking)
- **Problems in pregnancy** PET, IUGR, preterm delivery, neonatal and late fetal death
- **DM**
- **Osteoporosis**
- **Thrombosis**
- **Dyspepsia and/or gastric ulcers**

Passive smoking is associated with
- ↑ risk of coronary heart disease and lung cancer (↑ by 25%)
- ↑ risk of cot death, bronchitis, and otitis media in children

Helping people to stop smoking Advice from a GP results in 2% of smokers stopping—5% if advice is repeated[CE]. See Figure 8.4.

Aids to smoking cessation *BNF 4.10*

Nicotine replacement therapy (NRT) ↑ the chance of stopping ~ 1½x[N]. All preparations are equally effective[C]. Start with higher doses for patients highly dependent. Continue treatment for 3mo, tailing off dose gradually over 2wk before stopping (except gum which can be stopped abruptly). Contraindicated immediately post-MI, stroke, or TIA, and for patients with arrhythmia.

Bupropion (Zyban®) Smokers (>18y) start taking the tablets 1–2wk before intended quit day (150mg od for 3d, then 150mg bd for 7–9wk) ↑ cessation rate >2x[N]. *Contraindications:* epilepsy or ↑ risk of seizures, eating disorder, bipolar disorder.

Varenicline (Champix®) Smokers (>18y) start taking the tablets 1wk before intended quit day (0.5mg od for 3d, 0.5mg bd for 4d then 1mg bd for 11wk). ↓ dose to 1mg od if renal impairment/elderly. ↑ cessation rate >2x. If the patient has stopped smoking after 12wk, consider prescribing a further 12wk treatment to ↓ chance of relapse. *Contraindications:* caution in psychiatric illness.

Alternative therapies Hypnotherapy may be helpful in some cases[C].

Support In many areas, 'stop smoking' services are provided by PCOs. These programmes vary but generally consist of a combination of group education, counselling and support ± individual support in combination with nicotine replacement, bupropion, or varenicline.

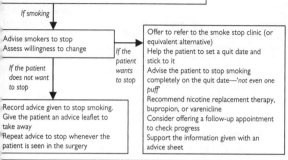

Remind smokers of the importance of stopping smoking with
leaflets and posters around the surgery
Assess smoking status of all patients at least 1×/y if possible

If smoking

Advise smokers to stop
Assess willingness to change

If the patient wants to stop

If the patient does not want to stop

Offer to refer to the smoke stop clinic (or
equivalent alternative)
Help the patient to set a quit date and
stick to it
Advise the patient to stop smoking
completely on the quit date—'*not even one
puff*'
Recommend nicotine replacement therapy,
bupropion, or varenicline
Consider offering a follow-up appointment
to check progress
Support the information given with an
advice sheet

Record advice given to stop smoking.
Give the patient an advice leaflet to
take away
Repeat advice to stop whenever the
patient is seen in the surgery

Nicotine withdrawal symptoms
• Urges to smoke (70%)
• ↑ appetite (70%—mean 3–4kg weight ↑)
• Depression (60%)
• Restlessness (60%)
• Poor concentration (60%)
• Irritability/aggression (50%)
• Night-time awakenings (25%)
• Light headedness (usually first few days
after quitting—10%)

igure 8.4 Management plan for smokers in the surgery

⚠ **Smoking cessation medication** Prescibe *only* for smokers who
commit to a target stop date. Initially, prescribe only enough to last 2wk
after the target stop date, i.e 2wk nicotine replacement therapy, 3–4wk
bupropion, or 3wk varenicline. Only offer a second prescription if the
smoker demonstrates continuing commitment to stop smoking.

❶ If unsuccessful, the NHS will not fund another attempt for ≥6mo.

mokeless tobacco Misri India tobacco, qimam, naswar, gul, khaini,
utkha, zarda, mawa, Manipuri, or bethel quid with tobacco. Particularly
sed in South Asian communities. Carries risk of nicotine addiction, CVD,
ental disease, and mouth/throat cancer. Provide brief advice and consider
RT to help with stopping.

urther information
ICE ℘ www.nice.org.uk
  NRT and bupropion for smoking cessation (2002)
  Brief interventions and referral for smoking cessation in primary care
  and other settings (2006)
  Varencline for smoking cessation (2007)
  Smokeless tobacco cessation: South Asian communities (2012)

seful contacts
HS Smokefree ☏ 0800 022 4332 ℘ http://smokefree.nhs.uk
ction on smoking and health (ASH) ☏ 020 7739 5902
℘ www.ash.org.uk
uit ☏ 0800 00 22 00 ℘ www.quit.org.uk

Alcohol

'An alcoholic is someone you don't like who drinks as much as you do'

Dylan Thomas (1914–1953)

Alcohol misuse is a major public health and social concern. Alcohol-related problems cost the NHS ~£1.7 billion/y. Most harm is caused by non-dependent drinkers. Screening and brief interventions in primary care can identify drinkers in this group and ↓ consumption and harm.

Recommended limits for alcohol consumption See Table 8.7.

Prevalence of excess alcohol use

- Hazardous/harmful drinking—excess drinking causing potential or actual harm but without dependence—affects 32% ♂; 15% ♀
- Binge drinking (>8u for ♂ or >6u for ♀ in 1d)—affects 21% ♂; 9% ♀
- Alcohol dependence—affects 6% ♂; 2% ♀

Health risk Continuum—individual risk depends on other factors too (e.g. smoking, heart disease). *Alcohol-associated problems:*

Death 15–22,000 deaths/y in the UK are associated with alcohol misuse (most related to stroke, cancer, liver disease, accidental injury/suicide).

Social

- Marriage breakdown
- Absence from work
- Loss of work
- Social isolation
- Poverty
- Loss of shelter/home

Mental health Anxiety, depression, and/or suicidal ideas; dementia and/or Korsakoff's ± Wernicke's encephalopathy (🕮 p. 581).

Physical

- ↑ BP
- CVA
- Sexual dysfunction
- Brain damage
- Neuropathy
- Myopathy
- Cardiomyopathy
- Infertility
- Gastritis
- Pancreatitis
- DM
- Obesity

- Fetal damage
- Haemopoietic toxicity
- Interactions with other drugs
- Fatty liver
- Hepatitis
- Cirrhosis
- Oesophageal varices ± haemorrhage
- Liver cancer

- Cancer of the mouth, larynx, and oesophagus
- Breast cancer
- Nutritional deficiencies
- Back pain
- Poor sleep
- Tiredness
- Injuries due to alcohol-related activity (e.g. fights)

Beneficial effects of alcohol Moderate consumption (1–3u/d) ↓ risk of non-haemorrhagic stroke, angina pectoris, and MI.

Table 8.7 Recommended levels of alcohol consumption

Recommended limits (units)	Men	Women	As a rough guide:
			1 unit = 8g of alcohol
Weekly	<21	<14	½ pint of beer (strong beer >1.5u)
Daily	<8	<6	A small glass of wine/sherry or A spirit measure of spirits (in Scotland 1.2u)

Box 8.1 The alcohol use disorders identification test (AUDIT)

Questions assessing hazardous alcohol use	Questions assessing dependence symptoms		Questions assessing harmful alcohol use		
Question	Score: 0	1	2	3	4
1. How often do you have a drink containing alcohol?	Never	<1x /mo	2–4x /mo	2–3x /wk	≥4x /wk
2. How many drinks containing alcohol do you have on a typical day when you are drinking?	1/2	3/4	5/6	7–9	≥10
3. How often do you have 6 or more drinks on one occasion?	Never	<1x /mo	Monthly	Weekly	Daily/ almost daily
4. How often during the last year have you found that you were not able to stop drinking once you started?	Never	<1x /mo	Monthly	Weekly	Daily/ almost daily
5. How often during the last year have you failed to do what was normally expected of you because of drinking?	Never	<1x /mo	Monthly	Weekly	Daily/ almost daily
6. How often during the last year have you needed a first drink in the morning to get yourself going after a heavy drinking session?	Never	<1x /mo	Monthly	Weekly	Daily/ almost daily
7. How often during the last year have you had a feeling of guilt or remorse after drinking?	Never	<1x /mo	Monthly	Weekly	Daily/ almost daily
8. How often during the last year have you been unable to remember what happened the night before because of your drinking?	Never	<1x /mo	Monthly	Weekly	Daily/ almost daily
9. Have you or someone else been injured because of your drinking?	No		Yes—not in the last year		Yes—in the last year
10. Has a relative, friend, doctor or other health care worker been concerned about your drinking or suggested that you cut it down?	No		Yes—not in the last year		Yes—in the last year
					Total:

Action*:

Audit score 0–7	Alcohol education
Audit score 8–15	Simple advice
Audit score 16–19	Simple advice + brief counselling + continued monitoring
Audit score 20–40	Referral to specialist for evaluation and treatment

* Provide the next highest level of intervention to patients who score ≥2 on Questions 4, 5 and 6, or 4 on Questions 9 or 10.

Reproduced with permission from the World Health Organization.

Management of alcohol misuse

Assessing drinking

Suspicious signs/symptoms ↑ and uncontrolled BP; excess weight; recurrent injuries/accidents; non-specific GI complaints; back pain; poor sleep; tired all the time.

Ask Use standardized questionnaires to identify patients with harmful and hazardous patterns of alcohol consumption, e.g. AUDIT (see Box 8.1).

Risk factors
- Previous history
- Family history
- Poor social support
- Work absenteeism
- Emotional and/or family problems
- Financial and legal problems
- Drug problems
- Alcohol associated with work, e.g. publican

Examination Smell of alcohol, tremor, sweating, slurring of speech, ↑ BP; signs of liver damage.

Investigations FBC (↑ MCV); LFTs (↑ GGT identifies ~25% of heavy drinkers in general practice; ↑ AST; ↑ bilirubin). USS—fatty liver/cirrhosis. Often incidental findings.

Alcohol management strategies   See Figure 8.5.

Patients drinking within acceptable limits Reaffirm limits.

Non-dependent drinkers Brief GP intervention → ~24% ↓ drinking. Present results of screening interventions, e.g. AUDIT (📖 p. 185) and identify risks. Provide information about safe amounts of alcohol and harmful effects of exceeding these. Assess whether the patient is receptive to change. If so, agree targets to ↓ consumption, give encouragement, and negotiate follow-up.

Alcohol-dependent drinkers Suffer withdrawal symptoms if they ↓ alcohol consumption (e.g. anxiety, fits, delirium tremens—📖 p. 1070).
- If wanting to stop drinking—refer to the community alcohol team; suggest self-help organizations, e.g. Alcoholics Anonymous; involve family and friends in support
- Detoxification in the community usually uses a reducing regimen of chlordiazepoxide over a 1wk period (20–30mg qds on days 1 and 2; 15mg qds on days 3 and 4; 10mg qds on day 5; 10mg bd on day 6; 10mg od on day 7 then stop)
- Community detoxification is contraindicated for patients with:
  - Confusion or hallucinations
  - History of previously complicated withdrawal (e.g. withdrawal seizures or delirium tremens)
  - Epilepsy or fits
  - Malnourishment
  - Severe vomiting/diarrhoea
  - ↑ risk of suicide
  - Poor co-operation
  - Failed detoxification at home
  - Uncontrollable withdrawal symptoms
  - Acute physical or psychiatric illness
  - Multiple substance misuse
  - Poor home environment

If ambivalent/unwilling to change Provide information; reassess and re-inform on each subsequent meeting; support the family.

Assess the amount of alcohol patients are drinking on a regular basis when they
are seen in the surgery for other reasons

and

Ask any patients presenting with symptoms/signs which could be associated with
excessive alcohol consumption about the amount of alcohol they drink

Drinking within acceptable limits
(♂ <21u/wk; ♀ <14u/wk)
Reaffirm safe drinking limits

Drinking excessively
(♂ >21u/wk; ♀ >14u/wk)

Record advice given to ↓ alcohol
Give the patient an advice leaflet
Repeat advice to cut down whenever
the patient is seen in the surgery

NO

Willing to change?

YES

Non-dependent drinker
Provide advice
Keep a diary of alcohol consumption
Agree targets
Follow-up

Dependent drinker
Provide advice
Refer to the community
alcohol team
Consider detoxification

Figure 8.5 Alcohol management strategy

Vitamin B supplements People with chronic alcohol dependence
are frequently deficient in vitamins, especially thiamine—give oral thiamine
indefinitely (if severe, 200–300mg/d; if mild, 10–25mg/d)^G. During detoxification in the community—give thiamine 200mg od for 5–7d.

Relapse Common. Warn patients; encourage to re-attend. Be supportive. Maintain contact (↓ frequency and severity of relapses^G). Consider
drugs to prevent relapse, e.g. acamprosate, disulfiram (specialist initiation).

Delirium tremens 📖 p. 1070   **Alcohol and driving** 📖 p. 131

Further information
WHO Alcohol Use Disorders Identification Test (AUDIT): guidelines for
use in primary care 🖰 www.who.int
NICE 🖰 www.nice.org.uk
  Alcohol dependence and harmful alcohol use (2011)
  Alcohol use disorders—preventing the development of hazardous and
  harmful drinking (2010)
  Alcohol use disorders—physical complications (2010)

Patient advice and support
Drinkline (government-sponsored helpline) ☎ 0800 917 8282
Alcoholics Anonymous ☎ 0845 769 7555
🖰 www.alcoholics-anonymous.org.uk
ADFAM Support for families ☎ 020 7553 7640 🖰 www.adfam.org.uk

Assessment of drugs misuse

14% of men and 8% of women aged 16–59 report taking illicit drugs in the past year. The majority of patients on treatment programmes report opioid misuse (heroin—54%; methadone—13%) but the most frequently abused drugs are cannabis, amphetamine, ecstasy, and cocaine. Three factors appear important: availability of drugs; vulnerable personality; and social pressures—particularly from peers.

Detection Warning signs suggesting drug misuse:

Use of services Suspicious requests for drugs of abuse (e.g. no clear medical indication, prescription requests are too frequent).

Signs and symptoms
- Inappropriate behaviour
- Lack of self-care
- Unexplained nasal discharge
- Unusually constricted/dilated pupils
- Evidence of injecting (e.g. marked veins)
- Hepatitis or HIV infection

Social factors Family disruption, criminal history.

Assessment Assess on >1 occasion before deciding how to proceed. Exceptions are severe withdrawal symptoms and/or evidence of an established regime requiring continuation. Points to cover:

General information
- Check identification (ask to see an official document)
- Contact with other agencies (including last GP)—check accuracy
- Current residence; family—partner, children
- Employment/finances
- Current legal problems
- Criminal behaviour—past and present

History of drug use/risk taking behaviour
- Reason for consulting now and willingness to change
- Current and past usage
- Knowledge of risks
- Unsafe sexual practices

Medical and psychiatric history
- Complications of drug abuse, e.g. HIV, hepatitis, accidents
- General medical and psychiatric history and examination
- Alcohol abuse
- Overdose—accidental/deliberate

Investigations
- Consider urine toxicology to confirm drug misuse
- Consider blood for FBC, LFTs, hepatitis B, C and HIV serology (with consent and counselling—🕮 p. 744), and other tests according to medical history/examination

Specific drugs See Table 8.9, 🕮 p. 190. ❶ Gabapentin/pregabalin are increasingly being used as drugs of abuse, particularly in prisons.

Notification of drug misusers Report patients who start treatment for drug abuse to the relevant authorities (see Table 8.8). All types of problem drug misuse should be reported. Databases cannot be used as a check on multiple prescribing as data are anonymized.

Table 8.8 National drug misuse databases/centres

England	National Drug Treatment Monitoring System (NDTMS) ☎ (020) 7972 1964 🖰 www.nta.nhs.uk/ndtms.aspx
Scotland	Substance Misuse Programme (SMP) ☎ (0131) 275 6348
Wales	Welsh National Database for Substance Misuse substance.misuse-queries@wales.nhs.uk
Northern Ireland	Northern Ireland Drug Misuse Database (NIDMD) ☎ (028) 9052 2520

Driving and drugs misuse 📖 p. 131 **Overdose** 📖 p. 1116

Controlled drugs regulations 📖 p. 150

Prescribing for drug misusers Approach with special caution. Some controlled drugs can be dispensed to substance misusers in instalments providing they are prescribed on special NHS prescription forms (FP10 MDA—England; WP10 MDA—Wales; GP10—Scotland; HS21—NI). As a general principle, prescribe substitute opioid medicines in daily instalments. *Specify*: number of instalments; intervals to be observed between instalments, and if necessary instructions for supplies at weekends or bank holidays; total quantity of CD providing treatment for a period ≤14d; quantity to be supplied in each instalment.

❶ The prescription must be dispensed on the date on which it is due.

Other equipment for drug misusers Doctors, pharmacists, and drug workers may provide supplies of alcohol swabs, sterile water (≤10 ampoules of 2mL or less), mixing utensils, filters, and citric acid to drug misusers for the purposes of harm reduction.

Travelling abroad with controlled drugs 📖 p. 151

Advice and support for patients and their families
'Talk to FRANK' (England and Wales) Government-run information, advice, and referral service ☎ (24 hour) 0800 77 66 00
🖰 www.talktofrank.com
'Know the Score' (Scotland) ☎ 0800 587 5879 🖰 www.knowthescore.info
Drugscope Information about drug misuse and how to get treatment 🖰 www.drugscope.org.uk
Drugs-info Information about substance abuse for families of addicts 🖰 www.drugs-info.co.uk
ADFAM Support for families of addicts ☎ 020 7553 7640
🖰 www.adfam.org.uk
Benzodiazepines 🖰 www.benzo.org.uk
Solvent abuse ☎ 01785 810762 🖰 www.re-solv.org

❶ The RCGP Substance Misuse Unit provides certificate courses in management of drug abuse 🖰 www.rcgp.org.uk

Table 8.9 Commonly misused substances in the UK

Name (street/ trade names include)	How usually taken	Effects sought	Harmful effects
Heroin (smack, horse, gear, H, junk, brown, stag, scag, jack)	Injected, snorted, or smoked	Drowsiness, sense of warmth and well-being	Physical dependence, tolerance Overdose can lead to coma and death Sharing injecting equipment brings risk of HIV or hepatitis infection
Cocaine (coke, charlie, snow, C)	Snorted in powder form, injected	Sense of well-being, alertness and confidence	Dependence, restlessness, paranoia Damage to nasal membranes
Crack (freebase, rock, wash, stone)	Smokable form of cocaine	Similar to those of snorted cocaine but initial feelings are much more intense	As for cocaine but, because of the intensity of its effects, crack use can be extremely hard to control May additionally cause lung damage ('crack lung')
Ecstasy (E, XTC, doves, disco bisuits, echoes, scooby doos) Chemical name: MDMA	Swallowed, usually in tablet form	Alert and energetic, but with a calmness and a sense of well-being towards others. Heightened sense of sound and colour	Possible nausea and panic Overheating and dehydration if dancing that can be fatal Use has been linked to liver and kidney problems Long-term effects are not clear but may include mental illness and depression
LSD (acid, trips, tabs, dots, blotters, microdots)	Swallowed on a tiny square of paper	Hallucinations, including distorted or mixed-up sense of vision, hearing, and time. An LSD trip can last as long as 8–12h	There is no way of stopping a bad trip which may be a very frightening experience Increased risk of accidents Can trigger long-term mental problems
Magic mushrooms (shrooms, mushies)	Eaten raw or dried, cooked in food, or brewed in a tea	Similar effects to those of LSD, but the trip is often milder and shorter	As for LSD, with the additional risk of sickness and poisoning
Amphetamines (speed, whizz, uppers, billy, sulph, amp)	In powder form, dissolved in drinks, injected, sniffed/ snorted	Stimulates the nervous system, wakefulness, feeling of energy and confidence	Insomnia, mood swings, irritability, panic The comedown (hangover) can be severe and last for several days

(Continued)

Table 8.9 (Cont.)

Name (street/trade names include)	How usually taken	Effects sought	Harmful effects
Khat (quat, chat)	Chewed as leaves	Stimulant, ↓ sleep, calm	Insomnia, irritability, panic
Barbiturates (barbs, downers)	Swallowed as tablets or capsules, injected—ampoules	Calm and relaxed state, larger doses produce a drunken effect	Dependency and tolerance Overdose can lead to coma or death Severe withdrawal symptoms
Cannabis (hash, dope, grass, blow, ganja, weed, shit, puff, marijuana)	Rolled with tobacco into a spliff, joint, or reefer and smoked, smoked in a pipe, or eaten	Relaxed, talkative state, heightened sense of sound and colour	Impaired coordination and increased risk of accidents Poor concentration, anxiety, depression Increased risk of respiratory diseases, including lung cancer
Tranquillizers (brand names include: Valium, Ativan, Mogadon (moggies), temazepam (wobblies, mazzies, jellies)	Swallowed as tablets or capsules, injected	Prescribed for the relief of anxiety and to treat insomnia, high doses cause drowsiness	Dependency and tolerance Increased risk of accidents Overdose can be fatal Severe withdrawal symptoms
Anabolic steroids (many trade names)	Injected or swallowed as tablets	With exercise, can help to build up muscle. However, there is some debate about whether drug improves muscle power and athletic performance	*For men:* erection problems, risk of myocardial infarction or liver disease *For women:* development of male characteristics Injecting equipment brings risk of HIV or hepatitis infection
Poppers (alkyl nitrates, including amyl nitrate with trade names such as Ram, TNT, Thrust)	Vapours from small bottle of liquid are breathed in through mouth or nose	Brief and intense head-rush caused by a sudden surge of blood through the brain	Nausea and headaches, fainting, loss of balance, skin problems around the mouth and nose Particularly dangerous for those with glaucoma, anaemia, breathing, or heart problems
Solvents (including lighter gas refills, aerosols, glues). Some painter thinners and correcting fluids	Sniffed or breathed into the lungs	Short-lived effects similar to being drunk, thick-headed, dizziness, possible hallucinations	Nausea, blackouts, increased risk of accidents Fatal arrhythmias can cause instant death

Management of drugs misuse

Aims to ↓ risk of infectious diseases; ↓ drug-related deaths; and ↓ criminal activity used to finance drug habits.

Avoid working in isolation. Anyone involved in substitute prescribing should wherever possible be doing so through their local shared care arrangements. The GP and primary healthcare team have a vital role in:

- Identifying drug misusers
- Assessing health/willingness to modify drug behaviour (see Figure 8.6)
- Referring for specialist assessment and treatment of drug abuse, and
- Routine screening/prevention (e.g. cervical screening, contraception)

General measures If ongoing care, at each meeting consider:

Education

- Safer routes of drug administration, e.g. smoking/rectal administration for heroin abusers. Discourage IM/subcutaneous administration
- Specific risks of drugs (e.g. psychosis with amphetamines; local risks, such as contaminated street drugs)
- Safe injecting advice and overdose prevention
- Safe sexual practices/condom use
- Driving and drug misuse (📖 p. 131)   • Other local services

Medical care

- Treatment of/advice about complications of drug misuse
- Testing/treatment for blood-borne disease, e.g. hepatitis B or C, HIV

Hepatitis B immunization For injecting drug misusers not already infected immune and close contacts of those already infected. Use accelerated regime—immunization at 0, 7, and 21d, and a booster after 12mo.

Treatment of dependence

- Set realistic goals—aim to help the patient remain healthy, until, with appropriate care and support, he/she can achieve a drug-free life. Consider ↓ in illicit drug use, ↓ duration of periods of drug use, ↓ risk of relapse, ↓ need for criminal activity to finance drug misuse, improving personal and social functioning. These aims are often best met by maintenance substitute prescribing, e.g. with methadone/ buprenorphine for heroin abuse
- Set conditions for acceptable behaviour/treatment withdrawal. Agree on the pharmacy to be used and involve the pharmacist
- Review regularly and include the whole team
- Give contact numbers for community support organizations (📖 p. 189)
- Send notification to national authority (📖 p. 188), if not already done
- Seek advice/refer to a community substance misuse team as needed

Further information

DH Drug misuse and dependence—guidelines on clinical management (2007) 🕾 www.nta.nhs.uk/guidance
NICE Substance misuse interventions (2007) 🕾 www.nice.org.uk
National Treatment Agency for Substance abuse 🕾 www.nta.nhs.uk
Substance Misuse Management in General Practice (SMMGP)
🕾 www.smmgp.org.uk

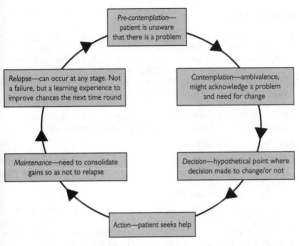

Figure 8.6 Stages of change in addiction

Safe injecting advice
- Never inject alone
- Always inject with the blood flow and rotate sites—avoid neck, groin, penis, axilla, foot and hand veins, and any infected areas/ swollen limbs—even if veins are distended
- Use sterile, new injecting equipment with the smallest bore needle possible and dispose of all equipment safely after use
- Avoid unsuitable preparations e.g. crushed tablets and/or injecting cocktails of drugs (injection of heroin and cocaine together is known as 'speedballing' or 'snowballing')
- Learn basic principles of first aid and CPR (provide information on courses available). Encourage calling for an ambulance
- Poor veins indicate poor technique—find out what the patient is doing

Preventing overdose Be aware of risk factors:
- Injecting heroin
- Longer injecting career
- Recent non-fatal overdose
- High levels of use/intoxication
- High levels of alcohol use
- Lowered tolerance through detoxification/imprisonment
- Depression, suicidal thoughts
- Multiple drug use—particularly CNS depressants
- Sharing equipment/other high risk injecting behaviour—may indicate low concern about personal risk
- Not being on a treatment programme or premature exit from a methadone programme

Insomnia

From the Latin meaning 'no sleep': describes a perception of disturbed or inadequate sleep. ~1:4 of the UK population (♀ > ♂) are thought to suffer in varying degrees. *Prevalence:* ↑ with age, rising to 1 in 2 amongst the over 65s. Causes are numerous—common examples include:

- **Minor, self-limiting** Travel, stress, shift work, small children, arousal
- **Psychological** ~½ have mental health problems: depression, anxiety, mania, grief, alcoholism
- **Physical** Drugs (e.g. steroids), pain, pruritus, tinnitus, sweats (e.g. menopause), nocturia, asthma, obstructive sleep apnoea

Definition of 'a good night's sleep'

- <30min to fall asleep
- Maintenance of sleep for 6–8h
- <3 brief awakenings/night
- Feels well rested and refreshed on awakening

Management Careful evaluation. Many do not have a sleep problem themselves but a relative feels there is a problem, e.g. the retired milkman continuing to wake at 4 a.m. Others have unrealistic expectations, e.g. they need 12h sleep/d. Reassurance alone may be all that is required.

For genuine problems

- **Eliminate physical problems preventing sleep,** e.g. treat asthma or eczema; give long-acting painkillers to last the whole night; consider HRT or fluoxetine for sweats; refer if obstructive sleep apnoea is suspected (📖 p. 338)
- **Treat psychiatric problems**, e.g. depression, anxiety
- **Sleep hygiene**—see Box 8.2
- **Relaxation techniques**—compact discs (borrow from libraries or buy from pharmacies); relaxation classes (often offered by local recreation centres/adult education centres); many physiotherapists can teach relaxation techniques
- **Consider drug treatment** Last resort. Benzodiazepines may be prescribed for insomnia 'only when it is severe, disabling, or subjecting the individual to extreme distress'.

Drug treatment Benzodiazepines (e.g. temazepam), zolpidem, zopiclone, and low-dose TCA (e.g. amitriptyline 10–75mg) nocte are all commonly prescribed for patients with insomnia.

- *Side effects:* amnesia and daytime somnolence. Most hypnotics do affect daytime performance and may cause falls in the elderly. Warn patients about their effect on driving and operating machinery
- Only prescribe a few weeks' supply at a time due to potential for dependence and abuse

⚠ Beware the temporary resident who has 'forgotten' his/her night sedation.

Box 8.2 Principles of 'sleep hygiene'

- Don't go to bed until you feel sleepy
- Don't stay in bed if you're not asleep
- Avoid daytime naps
- Establish a regular bedtime routine
- Reserve a room for sleep only (if possible). Do not eat, read, work, or watch TV in it
- Make sure the bedroom and bed are comfortable, and avoid extremes of noise and temperature
- Avoid caffeine, alcohol, and nicotine
- Have a warm bath and warm milky drink at bedtime
- Take regular exercise, but avoid late night hard exercise (sex is OK)
- Monitor your sleep with a sleep diary (record both the times you sleep and its quality)
- Rise at the same time every morning regardless of how long you've slept

Complications of insomnia ↓ quality of life; ↓ concentration and memory, affecting performance of daytime tasks; relationship problems; risk of accidents. 10% motor accidents are related to tiredness.

Patient information and support
Royal College of Psychiatrists Patient information sheets
℘ www.rcpsych.ac.uk

Chronic disease and elderly care

❶ In other sections of this book, where management differs from the norm for elderly patients, the text is highlighted in a box marked with this symbol.

Chronic disease management

The predominant disease pattern in the developed world is one of chronic or long-term illness. In the UK, 41% of adult ♂ and 43% of adult ♀ report a long-term illness. This figure is increasing as our population ages. People with long-term conditions are very intensive users of services; they account for 52% of GP appointments, 65% of outpatient appointments, and 77% of hospital bed days.

Although details of chronic illness management depend on the illness, people with chronic diseases of all types have much in common with each other. They all have similar concerns/problems and must deal not only with their disease(s) but also its impact on their lives/emotions.

Common patient concerns

- Finding and using health services and other community resources
- Knowing how to recognize/respond to changes in a chronic disease
- Dealing with problems and emergencies
- Making decisions about when to seek medical help
- Using medicines and treatments effectively
- Knowing how to manage stress/depression that go with chronic illness
- Coping with fatigue, pain, and sleep problems
- Getting enough exercise
- Maintaining good nutrition
- Working with your doctor(s) and other care providers
- Talking about your illness with family and friends
- Managing work, family, and social activities

Personal Health Budgets Being introduced in 2014 for all those receiving NHS Continuing Care and will also be available to others with chronic disease who would benefit from increased flexibility of services. Sum of money allocated to enable tailored care to meet individual health/well-being needs. Based on a care plan developed between patient and lead healthcare professional; signed off by the PCO.

Common elements of effective chronic illness management

- **Involvement of the whole family** Chronic diseases do not only affect the patient but everyone in a family
- **Collaboration** Between service providers, patients and carers. Negotiate and agree a definition of the problem; agree targets and goals for management; develop an individualized self management plan
- **Personalized written care plan** Take into account patient/carers' views and experience and the current evidence base
- **Tailored education in self-management** A patient with diabetes spends ~3h/y with a health professional—the other 8757h he or she manages his/her own condition. Helping patients with chronic disease understand and take responsibility for their conditions is vital
- **Planned follow-up** Pro-active follow-up according to the care plan—use of disease registers and call-recall systems is important

- **Monitoring of outcome and adherence to treatment** Use of disease/treatment markers; monitoring of concordance, e.g. checking prescription frequency; medicine management programmes—📖 p. 142
- **Tools and protocols for stepped care** Provide a framework for using limited resources to greatest effect; step professional care in intensity—start with limited professional input and systematic monitoring, then augment care for patients not achieving an acceptable outcome; initial and subsequent treatments are selected according to evidence-based guidelines in light of a patient's progress
- **Targeted use of specialist services** For those patients who cannot be managed in primary care alone
- **Monitoring of process** Continually monitor management through clinical governance mechanisms (📖 p. 72)

Risk profiling In recent years computer software has been produced that can identify 'high-risk' patients from information on GP IT systems and through service usage data. This helps to target resources towards those patients and improve outcomes.

Depression and chronic disease[N] Depression affects 30–50% of those with epilepsy, CVD, dementia, cancer, type 2 DM, and arthritis. It adversely affects prognosis in those patients, but treatment of depression can improve prognosis. Depression is associated with:
- ↑ mortality, ↑ morbidity, ↑ disability, and poorer quality of life
- ↑ prevalence of smoking and sedentary lifestyles
- Poorer chronic disease outcomes measures, e.g. higher HbA1c levels
- ↑ use of services and ↑ healthcare costs
- Poor concordance with medication and management plans

Detection of depression Use NICE depression screening questions:
- During the last month, have you often been bothered by feeling down, depressed, or hopeless?
- During the last month, have you often been bothered by having little interest or pleasure in doing things?

A positive response to either of these questions should prompt further assessment with the following three questions: *During the last month have you often been bothered by*:
- Feelings of worthlessness?   • Thoughts of death?
- Poor concentration?

Further assessment and management 📖 p. 1000

Residential care homes 220,000 people live in residential care in England; 77% are elderly with long-term health conditions. Of younger residents, 61% have learning disabilities; 21% have mental illness; 17% have physical disability, and 2% have substance misuse problems. Chronic disease management for residents of care homes is frequently neglected. Ensure that chronic disease management checks take place, including routine blood monitoring, physical health checks, and medication review.

Further information

NICE Depression in adults with a chronic physical health problem (2009) ✍ www.nice.org.uk

Medically unexplained symptoms

Medically unexplained symptoms (MUS) are physical symptoms for which no organic cause can be demonstrated. GPs deal with MUS in about 25% of consultations, and MUS cost the NHS £3.1 billion/y. MUS cause disability as severe as that originating from organic pathology.

Epidemiology MUS are common throughout the world in all ages. Risk factors for development of MUS include:
- ♀ > ♂
- Stressful life events, e.g. illness or death of a close relative, domestic violence, history of child abuse
- Media campaigns that highlight specific diseases
- Physical illness/trauma

Classification MUS can be divided into 3 types of complaint:
- Pain of a specific location, e.g. back pain, headache, fibromyalgia
- Functional disturbance in a particular organ, e.g. IBS, palpitations
- Fatigue/exhaustion e.g. chronic fatigue syndrome

Many patients have >1 MUS. There are also common overlaps of symptoms, e.g. patients with IBS often meet diagnostic criteria for chronic pelvic pain and vice versa.

Concurrent psychological illness 30% of patients with MUS have an underlying psychiatric problem—usually anxiety or depression.

Underlying mechanism Two mechanisms seem to underpin MUS:
- **Enhanced sense of bodily awareness** Tendency to notice and amplify normal physical sensations such as heartbeat. Over-awareness ↑ anxiety and in turn makes the bodily sensation more likely
- **Misattribution of symptoms** Rather than normalizing symptoms (e.g. 'I have a headache because I've been working too hard'), patients with MUS tend to attribute somatic explanations (e.g. 'I have a headache because I have a brain tumour')

Assessment Consider a diagnosis of MUS in any patient with physical symptoms for >3mo that are affecting functioning but cannot be readily explained. Even if the patient is known to present with MUS, perform your assessment without prejudice. Patients with MUS have the same chance of developing serious new illnesses as any other patient. Ask:
- What are the symptoms? Rule out 'redflags'
- How much and what type of impairment do the symptoms cause?
- What are the patient's concerns about the symptom? Has the patient sought information from other sources, e.g. Internet, friends?
- What made the patient come to the surgery today?
- What would the patient like you to do for him/her?
- Are there any signs of disease on physical examination?
- Does the patient have low mood or any symptoms of anxiety (consider depression and/or anxiety screening questionnaires)?
- Are there any other social/psychological factors that may be triggering symptoms, e.g. family member or close friend who is ill; domestic violence; debt; work problems; past history of child abuse?

Investigation Review patient notes carefully before requesting investigations. Usually investigations are used to clarify diagnosis and reassure the patient and GP. However, in patients with MUS:

- >50% of patients are not reassured following negative investigations
- False positive results lead to ↑ anxiety and further investigation, and
- Colluding with the patient ↑ illness behaviour

❶ Find a balance between appropriate investigation and risk of harm through over-investigation. Prior to doing investigations, explain why they are being done and the meaning of negative results.

Management[G] 4 key areas:

- **Connecting** Go back to the beginning, listen to the patient, acknowledge suffering, use existing knowledge of the individual (or recognize that you have no knowledge of the individual)
- **Summarizing** Allow the patient to summarize problems, recap your understanding of the problem to the patient, give an explanation, and show your interest in the problem
- **Hand over** Develop a shared action plan or personal health plan with realistic goals to improve functioning, and provide reassurance about long-term outcome
- **Safety netting** Share uncertainty, inform patients about red flags indicating serious disease, and offer access should symptoms change

Regular appointments may be helpful, as may a brief physical examination at each visit to check for signs of disease. Offering suggestions for self-management (e.g. doing voluntary work, increasing physical activity levels) can be useful. Avoid referral unless there is a clear medical indication.

General treatment options If self-help is ineffective, try:

- **Antidepressant medication**, e.g. amitriptyline 10mg at 5 p.m. (unlicensed). As response is often not dose-dependent, start with a low dose. Explain that the drug is not being used to treat depression
- **CBT** Allows patients to develop changes in thinking/behaviour that will help them cope more effectively with their problems

Management of specific MUS

- Fibromyalgia 📖 p. 530
- IBS 📖 p. 418
- Chronic fatigue 📖 p. 528
- Atypical facial pain 📖 p. 557
- Chronic pelvic pain 📖 p. 714
- Interstitial cystitis 📖 p. 449
- Tension-type headache 📖 p. 556
- TMJ dysfunction 📖 p. 933
- Globus 📖 p. 384
- Somatization disorder 📖 p. 997

Work Encourage patients to work if possible.

Prognosis 4–10% of patients with MUS go on to have an alternative organic explanation; of those with true MUS, 25% will have ongoing symptoms after 12mo.

Somatization disorder 📖 p. 997

Further information

RCGP/Royal College of Psychiatrists/Trailblazers/National Mental Health Development Unit Guidance for health professionals on MUS (2011) ✎ www.rcgp.org.uk

Normal ageing

The UK is home to 62.3 million people. Median age is 39.9y and rising. By 2012, women aged 65y could expect to live to the age of 85y. Projections suggest that this will ↑ by another 3y by 2021. Over the past 30y, the population aged >65y has grown by 23% from 8.4 to 10.3 million. The largest percentage growth in population is in the >85y age group.

What is ageing? Ageing is a gradual series of changes over time that lead to the loss of function of organs and cells, with the eventual outcome of death. Individuals vary greatly in the rate at which they age. Several factors seem to influence this:

- Genetic make-up
- Psychological health
- Lifestyle—diet, physical exercise, smoking
- Socio-economic factors
- Environment

Normal changes of ageing See Table 9.1

Difficulties assessing the elderly

- Communication problems—hearing, cognition, speech
- Multiplicity of cause—one symptom may be caused by different, concurrent processes, e.g. breathlessness as a result of COPD + heart failure
- Non-specific symptoms/signs—confusion, falls, or 'off legs' may be the only overt sign of underlying disease, e.g. UTI, MI, stroke
- Symptoms may be absent despite disease, and signs harder to elicit
- Polypharmacy (📖 p. 206) may result in side effects and interactions
- Laboratory tests may be unreliable—especially white cell counts and ESR (always check CRP)

Disease The ageing process is compounded by overt disease. This may affect functional capacity, quality of life and independence, cause frailty, ↓ well-being and independence, and result in ↑ care and mobility needs.

Multiple morbidity Older people are more likely to have several ongoing chronic illnesses that can act in combination to cause disability greater than either illness alone and/or result in:

- Direction of care at some problems with relative neglect of others
- Polypharmacy—📖 p. 206
- Involvement of multiple specialist teams which can cause inconvenience to the patient and family, and result in conflicting advice, and opposing opinions on cause/effect of symptoms

Frailty Many elderly people are described as being 'frail'. This term is used to describe individuals who are physically weak and fragile. It can occur on a background of natural ageing or be precipitated by a disease process. It is not a disease or disability in itself, but a vulnerability or inability to withstand physical/psychological stressors. Common features of frailty include:

- Unintentional weight loss (>5kg in a year)
- Feeling of exhaustion
- Weakness—measured by grip strength
- Slow walking speed
- Low levels of physical activity

Table 9.1 Normal changes of ageing

System	Clinical/functional effects
Cardiovascular	Cardiac enlargement/left ventricular hypertrophy
	↓ cardiac output → ↓ exercise capacity
	↓ response of heart rate to exercise
	Systolic hypertension
	Left ventricular failure
Respiratory	↓ FEV$_1$/FVC and ↑ residual volume
	↑ susceptibility to infection
	↑ susceptibility to aspiration
Endocrine	↓ insulin sensitivity → impaired glucose regulation
	↓ thyroid hormone production
Gastrointestinal	↑ in gastric acid production
	Constipation
Genito-urinary	↓ glomerular filtration rate not reflected by ↑ creatinine
	Benign enlargement of the prostate (25–50% of men >65y) → prostatism
	Slowing of sexual function; erectile dysfunction
	Dry vagina and ↑ susceptibility to urinary infections (♀)
Musculoskeletal	Sarcopenia—↓ muscle strength/power, ↓ lean body mass (30–40%), ↑ fat body mass
	↓ mobility
	↑ likelihood of falls
	↑ osteoporosis /susceptibility to fractures
Nervous	Slower thought processes/reaction times
	General decline in performance
	❶ Dementia is *not* a normal change of ageing
Vision	Presbyopia (difficulty focussing on near objects); ↓ visual acuity; cataract; impaired dark adaptation
Hearing	High frequency hearing loss/presbyacusis—deafness affects 80% of 80y olds
	Degenerative changes in the inner ear → impairment of balance causing falls
Immune	Atrophy of the thymus
	Reduced immune function resulting in ↑ infectious disease, reactivation of latent disease (e.g. TB, shingles), ↑ cancer, and ↑ autoimmune disease
Skin/hair	Dry skin, wrinkles, tendency to bruise easily, and slower healing
	Greying of the hair
	↓ sweating, heat generation, and heat conservation → heat stroke; hypothermia
	↓ sensitivity to touch, pain, and temperature discrimination → burns, pressure sores

Elderly care and rehabilitation

'Use strengthens, disuse debilitates'

Hippocrates (460–357 BC)

13–14% of the population has some disability. This is increasing as populations age and people survive longer with disability. Many more are just elderly and frail; 35% of people aged >80y cannot live an independent life.

Role of the GP Most patients are best managed by a multidisciplinary team in their home (if practicable) with a problem-oriented approach. Good interdisciplinary communication and coordination is essential. Psychological and sociocultural aspects are as important as medical aspects of care. Information alone can improve outcome. The GP of any elderly patient or patient receiving rehabilitation in the community is a team member and often the key worker who coordinates care.

Case Management Register (CMR) In England, GP practices must perform risk profiling (see 📖 p. 199) for all registered patients. Those deemed 'high risk' (all patients >75y, those at high risk of admission to hospital or complications of their illnesses, and those requiring end-of-life care) are added to the CMR. Each patient on the CMR must have a personalized care plan, and a named GP responsible for coordinating care and ensuring the care plan is functioning and kept up to date. Same day support must be provided to these patients if needed.

Consider

- Can physical symptoms be improved?
- Can psychological symptoms be improved (including self-esteem)?
- Can functioning within the home be improved (aids and adaptations within the home, extra help)?
- Can functioning in the community be improved? (mobility outside the home, work, social activities)
- Can the patient's or carer's financial state be improved?
- Does the carer need more support?

❶ If progress is slower than expected or stalls, consider other medical problems (e.g. anaemia, hypothyroidism, dementia), a neurological event, depression, or communication problems (e.g. poor vision/hearing).

Principles of rehabilitation and elderly care

- **Use of assessments/measures** Central to the management of frailty/disability. Use validated measures accepted by all team members (e.g. disability scores 📖 p. 584; PHQ-9 📖 p. 1001). Reassess regularly
- **Teamwork** Good outcomes are associated with clinicians working as a team towards a common goal with patients and their families (or carers) included as team members
- **Goal-setting** Goals must be meaningful, challenging but achievable. Use short- and long-term goals. Involve the patient ± carer(s). Regularly renew, review, and adapt
- **Underlying approach to therapy** All approaches focus on modification of impairment with everyday activities and improvement in function

- **Intensity/duration of therapy** How much therapy is needed? Is there a minimum threshold below which there is no benefit at all? Studies on well-organized services show it is rare for patients to receive >2h therapy/d. No one knows what is ideal

Multidisciplinary working A multidisciplinary approach is ideal, for example:
- **DNs** Provide nursing care and equipment, advise on all aspects of nursing care, and teach carers how to do everyday tasks (e.g. emptying catheter bags, lifting). They are sources of information on local services and provide support for carers of patients on their caseload
- **Community physiotherapists** Are invaluable sources of help, advice, and equipment for practical problems relating to mobility
- **Occupational therapists** Can help patients and carers cope with difficulties in everyday living caused by disability by providing for aids and appliances and arranging alterations
- **Speech therapists** Can help with communication problems and swallowing difficulties
- **Dieticians** Can help maintain calorie intake if undernourished, assist with weight ↓ if overweight and advise on special diets

Referral
- **Medical opinion** For clarification of diagnosis (e.g. if diagnosis is in doubt or patient has symptoms/signs incongruous with diagnosis)
- **Specialist rehabilitation services** New or deterioration in existing impairment, disability or handicap, or advances in management that warrant re-referral for specialist care
- **Social services** For assessment of the home for modification, assessment to allow application for mobility aids or services to help the disabled person and/or carer to cope
- **Voluntary organizations and self-help groups** Useful sources of support for patients and carers
- **Citizens Advice Bureau** For independent advice on benefits and services

Common neurological rehabilitation problems 📖 p. 582

Equipment and adaptations 📖 p. 228

Driving 📖 p. 128   **Benefits** 📖 p. 222

Employment 📖 p. 124   **Carers** 📖 p. 220

Patient information and support
Disabled Living Foundation Advice about equipment and appliances ☎ 0845 130 9177 🖰 www.dlf.org.uk
Age UK Wide range of information and factsheets ☎ 0800 169 6565 🖰 www.ageuk.org.uk
Royal Association for Disability and Rehabilitation (RADAR) ☎ 020 7250 3222 🖰 www.radar.org.uk
Citizens Advice Bureau 🖰 www.adviceguide.org.uk
Disablement Information and Advice Line (DIAL) ☎ 01302 310123 🖰 www.scope.org.uk/dial

Prescribing for the elderly

Use of medicines ↑ as people get older; 1 in 3 NHS prescriptions are for patients >65y and 90% of these prescriptions are for repeat medication. Adverse drug events are common reasons for hospital admission in the over-75 age group; many are avoidable. Regular review is essential. Problems commonly encountered:

Polypharmacy Elderly people often have multiple problems. It is easy to keep adding drugs for each new problem → polypharmacy. This ↑ confusion about drug regimes and results in poor concordance and multiple interactions/side effects.

- Before prescribing a new drug, consider whether it is necessary—avoid treating normal changes of ageing; use non-pharmacological therapies wherever possible; avoid 'a pill for every ill' approach and try to treat the underlying condition not the symptoms
- Balance the potential risks of the drug against the benefits. Drug trials of efficacy of medication often exclude older participants—the applicability of evidence to elderly patients cannot be assumed. For prophylactic medication (e.g. warfarin, statins), consider the likelihood of concordance and benefits in the context of the whole person (including other co-morbidities)
- Review medication regularly. Stop ineffective/redundant drugs and consider if the overall drug regime can be simplified

Form of the medicine Swallowing tablets can be difficult for elderly people. Consider using liquid preparations/giving explicit advice to take medication with plenty of water and sitting upright.

Confusion after discharge Up to half of all patients are inadvertently prescribed the wrong medication after hospital discharge. Take care.

Drug hoarding/self-medication Especially if recent changes in medication it is common for elderly people to have a back stock of drugs and continue taking their old drugs alongside new ones. A written list may be helpful. Many elderly people also self-medicate extensively with OTC preparations. If necessary do a home visit to sort out the drugs.

↑ susceptibility to side effects Common due to altered:
- **Pharmacodynamics** ↑ susceptibility to GI side effects (e.g. constipation with opioids; gastric irritation with NSAIDs) and ↑ sensitivity to effects of CNS drugs, e.g. benzodiazepines, opioids—use with care
- **Pharmacokinetics** ↓ renal function is particularly important—always assume any elderly person has moderate impairment if renal function is not known

Social and personal factors Low level of home support; physical factors, e.g. poor vision, poor hearing, or poor manual dexterity; and mental state e.g. confusion/disorientation, depression—can all affect ability of an older person to take medication.

Specific medicines The Beer's list is a list of agents to be avoided/used with extreme caution in elderly patients. It can be accessed via:
℘ www.dcri.duke.edu/ccge/curtis/beers.html

Guidelines for prescribing for the elderly

Think before prescribing
- Is the drug needed?
- Is there another non-pharmacological way of managing the problem?
- Are you treating the underlying condition or the symptoms of it?
- What are the pros and cons of the patient taking this drug?
- What is the evidence base for its use in this age group?
- Will the patient be able to take the drug (formulation; packaging)?
- Will the patient be concordant?
- Will the patient comply with any necessary monitoring?

Limit the range of drugs you use Prescribe from a limited array of drugs that you know well.

Repeats and disposal
- Tell patients how to get more tablets, and monitor frequency of repeat prescriptions
- Review repeat prescriptions regularly (📖 p. 144)
- Tell patients what to do with any leftover if a drug is stopped

↓ the dose
- Start with 50% of the adult dose
- Avoid drugs likely to cause problems (e.g. long-acting antidiabetic agents such as glibenclamide)

Review regularly
- Consider on each occasion whether each drug could be stopped or the regime simplified
- Consider lowering dosage of drugs if renal function is deteriorating
- Involve carers, community pharmacists, and other PHCT members

Simplify regimes
- Use od or bd regimes wherever possible
- Avoid polypharmacy

Explain clearly
- Put precise instructions on the drug bottle—avoid 'use as directed'
- Give written instructions about how the drug should be taken
- Ensure explanations are given to carers as well as patients where appropriate

Consider method of administration
- Bottles with childproof tops are often impossible for arthritic hands to open. Suggest the patient asks the chemist for a standard screw cap
- Drug administration boxes, in which the correct tablets are stored in slots marked with the day and time of administration can be helpful. Available from pharmacists and can be filled by the patient, a carer, friend or relative, or the pharmacist
- Medication reminder charts can also be helpful

Further information
Gallagher P, Ryan C, Byrne S, et al. (2008) STOPP (Screening Tool of Older Persons Prescriptions) and START (Screening Tool to Alert doctors to Right Treatment). Consensus validation. *Int J Clin Pharmacol Ther* 46:72–83.

Falls amongst the elderly

Falls are a major cause of disability and the leading cause of mortality due to injury in people aged >75y. Tendency to fall ↑ with age. Assessment of a patient who has fallen is a common primary care emergency.

Risk factors for falls Recurrence ↑ with number of risk factors:

- ♀:♂ ≈ 2:1 in the over 75s
- ↑ age
- Multiple previous falls
- Disorders of gait or balance
- Visual impairment
- Cognitive impairment
- Low morale/depression
- High level of dependence
- ↓ mobility
- Foot problems
- Lower limb weakness or arthritis
- History of stroke or PD
- Use of psychotropic drugs, sedatives, diuretics, or β-blockers
- Alcohol
- Environmental factors, e.g. loose rugs, poor lighting, ice, high winds
- Infection, e.g. pneumonia, UTI

Assessment Deal with the injuries first—ask about pain, loss of function, headache. Ask carers about behaviour. Check for bruising, ↓ function, confusion, BP, pulse, neurology, and fundi. Consider hypothermia if on the floor for any duration.

Investigate the cause of the fall *Consider:*

- **Physical problems** Neurological problems (e.g. stroke); visual loss; cardiac abnormalities (e.g. arrhythmia, postural hypotension); muscular abnormalities (e.g. steroid-induced myopathy); skeletal problems (e.g. osteoarthritis); infection (pneumonia, UTI)
- **Environmental problems** Climbing ladders to do routine maintenance; loose/holed carpets; slippery floor/bath; chair or bed too low

Management

- Treat any acute injury (20%). Exclude fracture (mainly Colles'/neck of femur). ❶ Subdural haematoma may take days/weeks to reveal itself
- Even if uninjured, older people might not be able to get up off the floor without help. The result may be a prolonged period of lying on the floor until help arrives. Apart from the indignity/helplessness this causes, secondary problems (e.g. pneumonia, pressure sores, hypothermia, UTI, and dehydration) may follow
- Perform/refer to a specialist falls service for a falls assessment
- Undertake measures to ↓ risk of falls or damage from falling

Further actions

- **Refer to A&E** if significant head injury (📖 p. 1112); any suspicion of fracture; any other significant injury, e.g. lacerations
- **Admit to the acute medical or elderly care team** if the cause of the fall was an acute medical problem, e.g. stroke
- **Refer to the intermediate care (rapid response) team** if the patient is unable to cope at home or the patient/carer is worried about the possibility of further falls
- **Refer to the specialist elderly care team or falls clinic** if the cause of recurrent falls remains unclear

Osteoporosis and prevention of fracture 📖 p. 504

Prevention of falls Falls are one of the biggest risk factors for fracture. All elderly people should have risk of falls assessed regularly. ❗ Any fall may seriously undermine an elderly person's confidence and cause worry about the possibility of recurrence. As a result, there may be restriction of activities → ↓ fitness and ↑ dependency on others.

Is a falls assessment needed? Ask if patients fall—they may not volunteer the information spontaneously.

> ***The timed get up and go test*** ❗ May use usual walking aid.
> - Start with the patient sitting in a straight-backed chair of comfortable height with arms
> - Ask the patient to rise from the chair, walk to a line 10 feet (3m) away, turn around, return to the chair, and sit down again
> - Start timing whilst the patient is sitting; end timing when the patient has sat down again
> - A time of ≥13 seconds predicts ↑ falls risk

Falls assessment If available, refer to a specialist falls service. *Record*:
- Frequency and history of circumstances around any previous falls
- Drug therapy: polypharmacy, hypnotics, sedatives, diuretics, antihypertensives may all cause falls
- Assessment of gait and balance, including abnormalities due to foot problems or arthritis, and motor disorders, e.g. stroke, PD
- Examination of basic neurological function, including vision, mental status (impaired cognition and depression), muscle strength, lower extremity peripheral nerves, proprioception, and reflexes
- Assessment of basic cardiovascular status, including BP (exclude postural hypotension), heart rate, and rhythm
- Assessment of environmental risk factors, e.g. poor lighting particularly on the stairs, loose carpets or rugs, badly fitting footwear or clothing, varifocal lenses in glasses (can cause to mis-step), lack of safety equipment such as grab rails, steep stairs, slippery floors, or inaccessible lights or windows

Measures to ↓ risk of falls and damage from falling
- Correct vision, if possible
- Correct postural hypotension—alter medication; consider compression stockings—but many elderly people cannot apply stockings tight enough to be of any use themselves
- Treat other medical conditions, e.g. refer to cardiology if arrhythmia
- Review medication and discontinue/alter inappropriate medication
- Remove environmental hazards—arrange bath at a day centre, refer to OT to identify/correct hazards in the home, e.g. remove loose carpets, wheeled trolley for use indoors, commode/urine bottle at night, etc.
- Liaise with other members of the PHCT and social services to provide additional support if needed; refer to local council or Age UK for 'carephone' or alarm system to call for help if any further falls
- Refer to rehabilitation/physiotherapy to improve confidence after falls and for weight-bearing exercise (focussing on strength and flexibility) and balance training (↓ risk of falls). Use of hip protectors ↓ fracture risk in patients at high risk but compliance is a problem[C]

Assessment of pain

Take a history to ascertain:
- What the patient means when he/she complains of pain
- The cause of the pain
- The severity of the pain

❶ Do not jump to conclusions/make assumptions about a patient's pain.

Assessment questions There are many approaches to assessing pain. The specifics of each scheme are not crucial—but it is important the scheme used has a logical outline which works for the individual clinician. A simple mnemonic approach is detailed in Figure 9.1.

Elderly patients and those with communication difficulty High prevalence of pain in the elderly population is now well recognized. 40–80% of elderly people in institutions are in pain. The reason for this lies in the difficulty in assessing those with communication difficulties. Additionally, the elderly often minimize their pain making it even more difficult to evaluate.

Methods of evaluation Unusual behaviour and its return to normal with adequate analgesia may be the only confirmation of pain in patients with communication difficulties. Examples include:

Verbal expression, e.g.
- Crying when touched
- Shouting
- Becoming very quiet
- Swearing
- Grunting
- Talking without making sense

Facial expression, e.g.
- Grimacing/wincing
- Closing eyes
- Worried expression
- Withdrawn/no expression

Behavioural expression, e.g.
- Jumping on touch
- Hand pointing to body area
- Increasing confusion
- Rocking/shaking
- Not eating
- Staying in bed/chair
- Grumpy mood

Physical expression, e.g.
- Cold
- Pale
- Clammy
- Change in colour
- Change in vital signs if acute pain (e.g. BP, pulse)

Pain assessment tools Sometimes, it is helpful to use pain scales to assess the degree of pain that a patient is in—particularly if communication is difficult. The most commonly used tool is a simple visual analogue pain scale—this consists of a line marked in graduations from 0–10. Ask patients to point to the place on the line which represents how much pain they are in where 10 is the most possible pain and 0 is no pain.

Examine the patient The cause of the problem may be clear to you from history alone but examine the patient to confirm/refute your proposed diagnosis.

S *Site of pain* Where? Any radiation? Numbness where pain felt? Pattern of involvement?

O *Onset* When did it start? How did it start? What started it? Change over time?

C *Character of pain* Type of pain — burning, shooting, stabbing, dull, etc.; pattern of pain, e.g. colicky, constant, etc.

R *Radiation* Does the pain go anywhere else?

A *Associated features* Are there any skin or joint changes, e.g. bruising, redness, or swelling?

T *Timing/pattern* Is it worse at any time of day? Is it associated with any particular activities, e.g. movement, urination, eating, passing stool, coughing?

E *Exacerbating and relieving factors*

S *Severity* Record, especially if the pain is chronic and you want to measure change over time. Consider a patient diary. Ask about:
Pain intensity, e.g. none-mild-moderate-severe; rank on a 1–10 scale.
• Record interference with sleep or usual activities.
• Pain relief e.g. none-slight-moderate-good-complete.

Figure 9.1 Points to consider when taking a history of pain

⚠ Beware of emergency requests for opioids from patients unknown to you or your practice.

Further information
British Pain Society Assessment of pain in older people (2007)
℘ www.britishpainsociety.org

Patient support
Action on Pain ☎ 0845 603 1593 ℘ www.action-on-pain.co.uk
Pain Concern ☎ 0300 123 0789 ℘ www.painconcern.org.uk
Pain Association of Scotland ☎ 0800 783 6059 ℘ www.painassociation.com

Principles of pain control

Acute pain Symptom of injured/diseased tissue. Subsides as the injury heals. Can be worsened by fear. Treat the underlying cause.

Chronic pain Defined as pain persisting for >3–6mo. Affects ~7% of adults in the UK. Cause is often multidimensional—with physical, social, and psychological factors all contributing to the overall feeling of pain.

Goals of chronic pain management

- Set realistic targets—abolition of pain may be impossible—70% have pain despite analgesia
- If analgesia is not helping—stop it
- The aim is often rehabilitation with ↓ in distress/disability

Strategies for pain management A multidisciplinary approach is essential. *Consider:*

- **Prevention**, e.g. wrist splints for carpal tunnel syndrome; analgesia prior to minor surgery
- **Removal of cause** Treat medical causes of pain, e.g. infection, ↓ blood sugar (diabetic neuropathy). Refer surgical causes for surgery if surgery is appropriate, e.g. hip osteoarthritis—joint replacement
- **Pain-relieving drugs** Start with a single drug at low dose and step up dose or add another drug as needed. Especially in situations of acute pain, step down if pain diminishes
- **Physical therapies** Acupuncture, physiotherapy, or TENS
- **Nerve blocks** Consider referral for epidural (low back pain), local nerve block, or sympathectomy (e.g. vascular rest pain)
- **Modification of emotional response** Psychotropic drugs, e.g. anxiolytics, antidepressants
- **Modification of behavioural response,** e.g. back pain—consider referral to a back rehabilitation scheme

The analgesic ladder Use a step-by-step approach (see Figure 9.2).

Step 1: Non-opioid Start treatment with paracetamol. Stress the need for REGULAR dosage. Adult dose is 1g every 4–6h (maximum daily dose 4g). If this is not adequate in 24h, either try an NSAID, e.g. ibuprofen 400mg tds (if appropriate), alone or in combination with paracetamol, or proceed to step 2.

Step 2: Weak opioid + non-opioid Start treatment with a combined preparation of paracetamol + codeine/dihydrocodeine. Combining two analgesics with different mechanisms of action enables better pain control than using either alone. Combinations have ↓ dose-related side effects but the range of side effects is ↑ (additive effects of two drugs). Combinations using 30mg of codeine (e.g. Solpadol®) are more effective than paracetamol alone, but it is cheaper and more flexible if constituents are prescribed separately, e.g. 'paracetamol 500mg/codeine 30mg'. Advise patients to take tablets regularly and not to assess efficacy after only a couple of doses.

❶ There is no proven additional analgesic benefit for preparations containing paracetamol + 8mg of codeine, compared to paracetamol alone.

Step 3: Strong opioid + non-opioid

- Use immediate-release morphine tablets or morphine solution. Two tablets of co-codamol contain 60mg of codeine which is equi-analgesic to ~6mg of oral morphine. If changing to morphine, use a minimum dose of 5mg (6mg is hard to prescribe)
- Chronic pain may be only partially opioid-sensitive. Give for a 2wk trial and only continue if of proven benefit. Worries of tolerance/ addiction are unfounded for patients with true opioid-sensitive pain. If the pain seems responsive to opioids and there are no undue side effects, ↑ the dose upwards by 30–50% every 24 h until pain is controlled—🕮 p. 216

⚠ Take care if the patient is elderly or in renal failure—consider starting with a ↓ dose of morphine.

Addition of co-analgesics and adjuvant drugs In combination with analgesics, can enhance pain control. Examples include:

- **Antidepressants**—In low dose for nerve pain and sleep disturbance associated with pain; in larger doses for secondary depression
- **Anticonvulsants**—Neuropathic pain
- **Corticosteroids**—Pain due to oedema
- **Muscle relaxants**—Muscle cramp pain
- **Antispasmodics**—Bowel colic
- **Antibiotics**—Infection pain
- **Night sedative**—When lack of sleep is lowering pain threshold
- **Anxiolytic**—When anxiety is making pain worse (relaxation exercises may also help in these circumstances)

Referral If unable to remove cause and unable to achieve adequate pain relief consider referral to a specialist pain control clinic or palliative care (depending on the context of the pain).

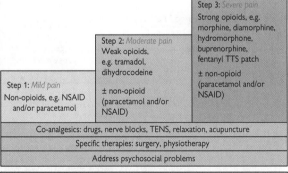

⚠ Be aware of secondary gain from pain if symptoms seem out of proportion (outstanding compensation claims are a significant negative factor in success of pain management).

Figure 9.2 World Health Organization analgesics ladder

Pain-relieving drugs

Paracetamol (*BNF* 4.7.1) As effective a painkiller as ibuprofen. No anti-inflammatory effect but potent antipyretic. Drug of choice in OA where inflammation is absent. Side effects are rare but long-term use may ↑ CVD risk. Dose 1g qds. Overdose (>4g/24 h) can be fatal causing hepatic damage sometimes not apparent for 4–6d. Inadvertent overdose is easy due to presence of paracetamol in most OTC cold preparations—refer to A&E.

Non-steroidal anti-inflammatories (NSAIDs) (*BNF* 10.1.1) See Table 9.2. Anti-inflammatory, analgesic, antipyretic. Start at the lowest recommended dose and do not use >1 NSAID concurrently. 60% respond to any NSAID—for those who do not, another may work.

GI side effects Common (50%) including GI bleeds (25% GI bleeds in UK). ↑ with age. Risks are dose-related and vary between drugs. For the elderly, those on steroids or with past history of GI ulceration or indigestion, protect the stomach with misoprostol or a proton pump inhibitor (PPI). Selective inhibitors of cyclo-oxygenase-2 (COX2) are equally effective but should not be given to any patient with pre-existing or high risk of CVD.

Other side effects Hypersensitivity reactions (5–10% asthmatics have bronchospasm); fluid retention (relative contraindication in patients with ↑ BP/cardiac failure); renal failure (rare—more common in patients with pre-existing renal disease); hepatic impairment (particularly diclofenac).

❶ COX2 inhibitors:
- Have no effect on platelet aggregation, and
- Have no benefit if used in patients on continuous low-dose aspirin

Topical NSAIDs Of proven benefit for acute and chronic conditions and can be as effective as oral preparations. They have lower incidence of GI and other side effects although these still occur.

Table 9.2 Commonly used NSAIDs (*BNF* 10.1.1)

Drug	Dosage	Features
Ibuprofen	1.2–1.8g/d in 3–4 divided doses	Fewer side effects than other NSAIDs. Anti-inflammatory properties are weaker. Do not use if inflammation is prominent, e.g. gout Higher doses (>1.2g/d) are associated with ↑ risk of thrombotic events and MI
Naproxen	0.5–1g/d in 1–2 divided doses	Good efficacy with a low incidence of side, effects. Associated with lower thrombotic risk than other NSAIDs
Celecoxib	200mg od/bd	Selective COX2 inhibitor. As effective as non-selective NSAIDs and shares side effects, but risk of serious upper GI events is lower. Only use it at low risk of CVD. High risk of other GI side effects

❶ Diclofenac carries similar increased risk of CVD as COX2 inhibitors, but has similar risk of GI events to other NSAIDs. It is no longer recommended for anything other than very short-term use.

Codeine (*BNF* 4.7.2) Most commonly used weak opioid in the UK. Dose is 30–60mg every 4h to a maximum of 240mg/24h. Analgesic effect is ↑ by regular ingestion.

Equipotence with morphine 60mg of codeine 4x/d totals 240mg codeine in 24h. 10mg of codeine is equipotent to 1mg of morphine so the equivalent morphine dose would be 24mg/24h.

Side effects The most common side effects of codeine include nausea, vomiting, constipation, and drowsiness (📖 p. 216). Codeine is effective for the relief of mild to moderate pain but is too constipating for long-term use. Always consider prescribing a laxative, e.g. bisacodyl 1–2 tablets nocte, with codeine to prevent constipation.

Reasons for decreased effectiveness
- 5–10% of Caucasians have CYP2D6 genotype. They lack a hepatic enzyme necessary to convert codeine to morphine and will obtain less analgesia when taking codeine-containing analgesics
- Effects of codeine are reduced by concurrent use of:
  - Antipsychotics, e.g. chlorpromazine, haloperidol
  - Metoclopramide
  - Tricyclic antidepressants, e.g. amitriptyline

Dihydrocodeine Has analgesic efficacy and a side effect profile similar to that of codeine. The dose of dihydrocodeine by mouth is 30–60mg every 4h. A 40mg tablet is also available.

Tramadol Is a synthetic analogue of codeine. It is not a controlled drug. Dose is up to 400mg/24h. Produces analgesia by 2 mechanisms:
- An opioid effect, and
- An enhancement of serotonergic and adrenergic pathways

Advantages over codeine and dihydrocodeine
- Rapid absorption of oral doses—analgesia in <1h—peaks at 1–2h
- Metabolized in the liver—safer for the elderly/those with renal failure
- Fewer typical opioid side effects (notably, ↓ respiratory depression, constipation, and addiction potential)
- May have a significant effect on neuropathic pain

Disadvantages
- Psychiatric reactions have been reported
- Nausea and vomiting can be a problem with high doses

Morphine and other strong opioids 📖 p. 216

Further information
British Pain Society 🖰 www.britishpainsociety.org
- Opioids for persistent pain (2010)
- Cancer pain management (2010)

The Oxford Pain Internet Site 🖰 www.medicine.ox.ac.uk/bandolier/booth/painpag/index2.html

Morphine and other strong opioids

Morphine is the strong opioid of first choice for moderate to severe pain in both malignant and non-malignant conditions.

Starting oral morphine Start with 4-hourly immediate release morphine. Give clear instructions. Initial dosage:
- **Adults not pain-controlled with regular weak opioids**
  (e.g. co-codamol 500/30 two tablets qds) 5–10mg every 4h
- **Elderly, cachectic, or not taking regular weak opioids** 2.5–5mg every 4h (2.5mg if very elderly/frail)

Titration of dose ↑ dose as needed by 25–50%/d until pain is controlled/ unacceptable side effects. There is no 'maximum' daily allowance, e.g. 5→10→15→20→30→40→60→80→100→130→160→200mg.

Maintenance Once pain is controlled, consider a long-acting preparation of equivalent dose (e.g MST® bd, MXL® od). Calculate total daily dose of morphine by adding together the 4h doses.

Increasing dose If necessary, use a third to a half dose increments. ↑ dose rather than frequency as tablets are designed for od or bd dosing.

Breakthrough pain Pain of rapid onset and moderate/severe intensity despite background analgesia. *Management:*
- Prescribe immediate release morphine for breakthrough pain—give the equivalent 4-hourly dose as an additional dose
- If pain starts to occur regularly before the next dose of analgesia is due, ↑ the regular background dose

Common side effects of opioid drugs Warn patients:
- **Nausea/vomiting** Affects >1 in 3 patients for the first 2wk of opioid use. Prescribe a regular antiemetic for 2wk, e.g. haloperidol 1.5mg nocte. If nausea/vomiting continues, consider an alternative opioid
- **Constipation** Consider prescribing prophylactic laxatives, e.g. bisacodyl 1–2 tab, nocte. Fentanyl causes less constipation than morphine
- **Drowsiness/cognitive impairment** Usually wears off in <1wk. Advise not to drive, perform other skilled tasks or work with dangerous machinery for ≥1wk after starting morphine (longer if drowsiness persists) or after ↑ in dose. If not improving, consider an alternative opioid or refer for specialist advice

Conversions to other preparations See Table 9.3.

Reasons to choose/switch to an alternative opioid Unacceptable side effects; renal failure (fentanyl is licensed for use; oxycodone is safe in mild/moderate renal failure); patient unable to take oral medication regularly (consider fentanyl or buprenorphine patch, or syringe driver); choice (morphine is unacceptable for some patients).

Alternative strong opioids Diamorphine; oxycodone; fentanyl; buprenorphine; hydromorphone; pethidine (not suitable for severe continuing pain—used for acute pain relief/obstetric pain).

❶ Never attempt dose titration for unstable pain using a fentanyl patch—convert from oral morphine once a stable dose is attained.

Table 9.3 Quick conversions of oral morphine

From	To	Conversion	Example
Oral morphine (total dose) e.g. 10mg morphine 4-hourly = 60mg oral morphine in 24h	sc diamorphine	÷ by 3	60 ÷ 3 = 20mg diamorphine by syringe driver over 24h
	sc morphine	÷ by 2	60 ÷ 2 = 30mg morphine by syringe driver over 24h
	oral oxycodone	÷ by 2	60 ÷ 2 = 30mg oral oxycodone in divided doses over 24h
	oral hydromorphone	÷ by 7.5	60 ÷ 7.5 = (60 x 2)÷15 = 8mg hydromorphone in divided doses over 24h

❶ If total 24h dose is equivalent to 360mg morphine or more—get specialist advice.

Opioid toxicity Intentional or unintentional overdose produces:

- Drowsiness or coma
- Vomiting
- Pinpoint pupils
- Hypotension
- Confusion—including auditory and/or visual hallucinations
- Respiratory depression
  - **If respiratory rate ≥8/min and the patient is easily rousable and not cyanosed**—adopt a policy of 'wait and see'; consider reducing or omitting the next regular dose of opioid. Stop syringe drivers temporarily to allow plasma levels to ↓, then restart at lower dose
  - **If respiratory rate <8/min, and the patient is barely rousable/ unconscious and/or cyanosed**—dilute naloxone 400 microgram to 10mL with sodium chloride 0.9%. Administer 0.5–1mL IV every min until respiratory status is satisfactory. If respiratory function still does not improve, question diagnosis. Further doses may be needed later, as naloxone is shorter acting than morphine
- Muscle rigidity/myoclonus—consider renal failure (can produce myoclonus alone). Treat by rehydration, stopping other medication which may exacerbate myoclonus, switching opioid, or with clonazepam 2–4mg/24h depending on circumstances

Subacute overdosage Slowly progressive somnolence and respiratory depression—common in patients with renal failure. Withhold morphine for 1–2 doses then reintroduce at 25% lower dose.

Opioid toxicity may be ↑ by

- Renal failure
- Dehydration
- Other change in disease status, e.g. hepatic function, weight loss
- Other analgesics, e.g. NSAIDs
- Co-administration of amitriptyline

Syringe drivers 📖 p. 1146.

Further information

British Pain Society 🕉 www.britishpainsociety.org
- Opioids for persistent pain (2010)
- Cancer pain management (2010)

Online converter for fentanyl patches 🕉 www.globalrph.com/fentconv.htm

Neuropathic pain

Neuropathic pain occurs as a result of damage to neural tissue. Examples include post-herpetic neuralgia, following shingles, complex regional pain syndrome (reflex sympathetic dystrophy), peripheral neuropathy (e.g. due to DM), compression neuropathy, and phantom limb pain.

Pain typically occurs in association with altered sensation, e.g. burning, stabbing, or numbness. Pain may also be provoked by non-noxious stimuli (allodynia), e.g. gentle heat or cold.

Management[N] Where possible, treat the underlying cause of the pain. Otherwise, use a stepped treatment regime—see Figure 9.3.

❶ For all drugs listed in Figure 9.3, start at low dose and titrate up the dose according to response. Consider lidocaine patches for people with localized pain who are unable to tolerate oral medication.

* For patients with diabetic neuropathy, step 1 is duloxetine 60–120mg/d—📖 p. 358.

Figure 9.3 Neuropathic pain—steps to pain control[N]

Review

After starting/changing medication Perform an early review after 1–2wk to check dosage titration, tolerability, and adverse effects.

Once established on medication Review regularly every 4–8wk to assess and monitor effectiveness of treatment. Ask about

- Overall perception of improvement
- Adverse effects
- Sleep
- ↓ in pain (pain diaries may help)
- Ability to do everyday activities, e.g. work, driving
- Mood—depression/anxiety screening questionnaires may be helpful

If improvement is sustained over ≥6mo, consider gradual ↓ dose of medication over time.

Refer To a specialist pain clinic or other appropriate specialist service if:

- Severe pain or pain significantly limits activities
- Underlying health condition has deteriorated
- Inadequate response to first- or second-line medication

Tricyclic antidepressants

Amitriptyline First-line treatment for neuropathic pain (unlicensed indication). Start at a dose of 25mg at 5–7 p.m.—10mg if elderly. ↑ dose by 10–25mg at 5–7 p.m. every 5–7d to a maximum of 75mg in a single dose as needed (higher doses under specialist supervision). Some patients do not derive benefit for 4–6 wk.

Alternatives to amitriptyline Nortriptyline and imipramine. Both are given at an initial dose of 10–25mg in the evening; dose can be titrated up to 75mg as needed. May have fewer side effects than amitriptyline.

Anticonvulsants

Pregabalin Licensed for treatment of neuropathic pain. Initially 150mg/d in two divided doses, increased if necessary after 3–7d to 300mg daily in two doses, and increased further if necessary after 7d to a maximum 600mg daily in two divided doses.

Gabapentin Effective for neuropathic pain but has a similar side effect profile, higher NNT for 30% and 50% pain relief, more complicated dosing and titration regime, and is less cost-effective than pregabalin.

Carbamazepine Unlicensed for treatment of neuropathic pain and often poorly tolerated. Traditionally the drug of choice for trigeminal neuralgia. Start with 100–200mg 1–2×/d (less if elderly or frail). Build up dose slowly to minimize adverse effects to the usual dose of 0.8–1.2g daily in divided doses. Oxcarbazepine is an alternative.

❶ Both gabapentin and pregabalin are drugs of abuse; monitor frequency of repeat medication and be careful when issuing prescriptions to temporary residents.

NSAIDs Sometimes effective for neuropathic pain—either because there is mixed nociceptive pain or because they ↓ inflammatory sensitization of nerves. There is considerable variation in individual patient tolerance and response (📖 p. 214).

Opioids Neuropathic pain often responds only partially to opioid analgesics. Of the opioids, oxycodone, tramadol, and methadone are probably the most effective—consider trying tramadol when other measures fail.

Topical lidocaine Plasters impregnated with lidocaine 5% (Versatis™). Licensed for post-herpetic neuralgia. Apply daily for up to 12h, followed by a 12h plaster-free period; discontinue if no response after 4wk. Up to 3 plasters may be used to cover large areas; plasters may be cut.

Trigeminal neuralgia 📖 p. 557   **Shingles** 📖 p. 653

Diabetic neuropathy 📖 p. 358

Further information
NICE Neuropathic pain (2013) ℅ www.nice.org.uk

Information for patients
Neuropathy Trust ℅ www.neurocentre.com

Carers

Who is a carer? A carer is someone of any age who provides unpaid support to family or friends who could not manage without this help. This could be caring for a relative, partner, or friend who is ill, frail, disabled, or has mental health or substance misuse problems. Anyone can become a carer. ~2 million people/y move in/out of caring roles.

Young carers Are children and young people who assume inappropriate responsibilities to look after someone who has an illness, a disability, or is affected by mental ill health or substance misuse. Young carers often take on practical and/or emotional caring responsibilities that would normally be expected of an adult.

> ❶ Some carers do not regard themselves as carers or may dislike the label 'carer', believing that it can detract from their identity as a parent, child, partner, or sibling to the person that they care for. It is also important not to confuse carers with paid care workers.

How many carers are there? 12% of adults in the UK are carers. 1.2 million provide care for >50h/wk; those aged >65y account for 1 in 3 of those providing >50h care each week and many have their own health problems too. There are also around 1 million young carers.

Economic importance Carers save the UK economy ~£119 billion/y in care costs (£18,473/y for every carer in the UK).

Carers as partners in care Carers know the people that they care for better than anyone else. Involving carers is important in order to identify problems that may require intervention; plan patient care and improve concordance with care plans.

What problems do carers have as a result of their roles? Many carers gain great personal satisfaction from their caring role and want to continue caring, but they suffer adverse consequences too:
- **Psychological** ↑ stress and depression/anxiety; abuse from the person being cared for; young carers have ↑ risk of bullying/self-harm
- **Physical health** ↑ mortality; ↑ morbidity from CVD; ↑ risk of back and other musculoskeletal injury
- **Social** Activity restriction, deterioration of relationships with other family members, social isolation
- **Employment/schooling** ↓ ability to work, ↓ promotion prospects, poor performance, and ↑ absenteeism at school
- **Financial** The more care provided the more likely a carer is to be in financial difficulty; 55% are in debt but <50% claim all the benefits they are eligible for

Supporting carers in general practice See Figure 9.4

Benefits For sickness/disability/carers 🕮 p. 222; low income 🕮 p. 104

Social services assessment Every carer has a right to ask for a full assessment of their needs by the social services. *Emergency planning* to provide substitute care in the event of a crisis is part of that assessment.

Further information

RCGP Supporting carers: an action guide for GP and their teams (2011) ℘ www.rcgp.org.uk

Figure 9.4 Practice action plan for supporting carers

Carer support
Carers Direct ☎ 0808 802 0202 🖰 www.nhs.uk/carersdirect/Pages/
CarersDirectHome.aspx
Carers Trust 🖰 www.carers.org
Carers UK 🖰 www.carersuk.org

Pensions and benefits

Retirement pension A state retirement pension is currently payable to people of state pension age, even if still working. Claim forms should be received automatically—if not, request one through the local Benefits office. Pensions are taxable. State pension age is gradually increasing—in women from 60–68y and in men from 65–68y.

Basic pension Flat rate amount—different for single people and married couples. If not enough National Insurance (NI) contributions have been paid, amounts may ↓. >80y, a higher rate is payable which is not dependent on NI contributions.

Increase for dependants Paid if:
- The claimant's spouse is <60y and earns under a set amount/does not receive certain other benefits
- The claimant has children (if claim made before April 2003)

Additional pension State second pension (replaced SERPS). Based on NI contributions and earnings. Workers can opt out of the additional pension scheme, pay into a private or company scheme instead and pay lower NI.

Graduated pension Some people may be entitled to a graduated pension. This is based on earnings between 1961 and 1975.

Extra pension For a person who defers claiming retirement pension for up to 5y. Extra pension is payable when retirement pension is claimed.

❶ If hospitalized, retirement pension is payable for 1y at full rate. After 12mo, basic pension is ↓ but additional pension stays the same.

Pension Credit Apply on form PC1 ☎ 0800 99 1234.

Guarantee credit For anyone older than the women's state pension age with income below the '*appropriate amount*'. Appropriate amount varies according to circumstances. Capital (excluding value of own home) >£6000 is deemed to count as income at the rate of £1/wk/£500 capital. Receipt confers automatic eligibility for additional low income benefits (e.g. housing benefit).

Savings credit ≥ 65y and income > savings credit starting point. Amount received depends on level of income and circumstances. Savings credit will be phased out after 2016 when pension rates are being simplified.

Other benefits just for pensioners
- **Free colour TV licence** All pensioners >75y
- **Winter fuel payment** Annual payment to all pensioners >60y

National insurance credits Protect basic state pension for people who do not work because of childcare responsibilities or because they are carers. If no automatic entitlement, claim on form CF411 (available from HM Revenue and Customs ☎ 0845 302 1479).

Christmas bonus One-off payment made to people receiving a retirement pension a few weeks before Christmas.

Cold weather payment Paid automatically to people with low income or on retirement pension if the temperature is below freezing for seven consecutive days.

Benefits for
- **Low income** 📖 p. 104
- **Disability** See Table 9.5, 📖 p. 225
- **Sickness** See Table 9.4, 📖 p. 224
- **Bereavement** 📖 p. 114
- **Pregnant women** 📖 p. 785
- **Parents and children** 📖 p. 851

Help with mobility See Table 9.6, 📖 p. 227.

Adaptations and equipment See Table 9.7, 📖 p. 228.

War pensions scheme For ex-Service personnel whose injuries, wounds, and illnesses arose prior to 6th April 2005. No time limit for claims. Administered by the Veterans Agency.

War Disablement Pension
- **Basic benefits** Based on percentage disablement: if <20% disabled—lump sum; if >20% disabled—weekly sum (pension)
- **Other benefits** Allowances if severely disabled, e.g. War Pensioners Mobility Supplement—for walking difficulty (holders can apply for the motability scheme and road tax exemption) or Constant Attendance Allowance—for high levels of care

Medical treatment Some services and appliances may be paid for by the Veterans Agency (includes prescription charges, nursing home fees).

War widows and widowers' pensions For spouses/civil partners of Service/ex-Service personnel:
- Where death was a result of Service, or
- Who received War Pensions Constant Attendance Allowance
- Who received a War Disablement Pension at the rate of ≥80% and was getting Unemployability Supplement

War widows' and widowers' allowances Automatic age allowance when widows/widowers reach 65y and further increase at 70y and 80y.

Armed Forces Compensation Scheme (AFCS) Administered by the Veterans Agency. Provides benefits for illness, injury, or death caused by service on or after 6th April 2005. Time limit is 5y from the event, from the time when medical advice was first sought or after retirement—whichever is soonest. There is an exceptions list for late onset conditions. Provides:
- Lump sum for significant illnesses/injuries—15 levels of award
- Tax-free Guaranteed Income Payment (GIP) for life for injuries at the higher tariff levels (1–11) to compensate for loss of earnings capacity
- Guaranteed Income Payment for Survivors (SGIP) where an attributable death occurs

Further information
The Pension Service 🖰 www.thepensionservice.gov.uk
Pensions Advisory Service (TPA) ☎ 0845 601 2923
🖰 www.pensionsad visoryservice.org.uk
Citizens Advice Bureau 🖰 www.adviceguide.org.uk
Veterans Agency ☎ 0800 169 22 77 🖰 www.veterans-uk.info

Table 9.4 Benefits for those unable to work

	Eligibility	How to apply	Amount
Statutory Sick Pay	• Employee age ≥16y and under state pension age • Incapable of work due to sickness or disability • Earning ≥NI lower earnings limit • Unable to work ≥4d and <28wk (including days when would not normally work) • Those ineligible may be eligible for ESA or maternity allowance	Notify employer of illness—self-certification (SC2) for first 7d; Med3 after that time (📖 p. 125)	£86.70/wk. Some employers have more generous arrangements. Paid through normal pay mechanisms
Employment and Support Allowance (ESA)	• Age ≥16y and under state pension age • Not entitled to statutory sick pay • Unable to work due to sickness or disability—SC1 certification for first 7d, then Med3 certification until work capability assessment (done <13wk into period of sickness/disability)—📖 p. 124 • Sufficient NI contributions • Unable to work and claiming ESA for <1y	Claim on form ESA1 from 🖥 www.gov.uk or ☎ 0800 055 6688 (textphone: 0800 023 4888)	*First 3d*—no payment **Assessment phase** (>3d but <14wk) • <25y—£56.80 • ≥25y—£71.70 **Main phase** (≥14wk) • Work-related activity group—up to £100.15 • Support group—up to £106.50
Universal Credit	• Age ≥18y and under state pension age (in exceptional circumstances, students and young people aged 16–17y, may be able to claim) • Not in full-time education • Low income	Claim on form available from 🖥 www.gov.uk or ☎ 0800 055 6688 (textphone: 0800 023 4888)	See 📖 p. 104

Table 9.5 Benefits for disability and illness

	Eligibility	How to apply	Amount
Disability Living Allowance (DLA)▽	• Disability >3mo and expected to last >6mo more* • <16y at time of application **Mobility Component** Help needed to get about outdoors. Two levels. Age restrictions apply **Care Component** Help needed with personal care. Three levels. If terminal illness, highest rate is automatically awarded*	☎ 0800 88 22 00 or ✆ www.gov.uk	**Mobility Component** *Higher rate*—£55.25/wk *Lower rate*—£21/ wk **Care Component** *Higher rate*—£79.15/wk *Middle rate*—£53./wk *Lower rate*—£21/wk
Personal Independence Payment (PIP)▽	• Age 16y to 65y • Disability requiring assistance present >3mo and expected to last >9mo more* • Two payment components assessed against standard criteria: daily living (activities 1–9) and mobility (activities 10–11) **Daily Living Component** Paid at standard rate if ≥8 points from activities 1–9 and at enhanced rate if ≥12 points. Enhanced rate paid automatically if terminal illness* **Mobility Component** Paid at standard rate if ≥8 points from activities 10–11 and at enhanced rate if ≥12 points	☎ 0800 88 22 00 or ✆ www.gov.uk	**Daily Living Component** *Standard rate*—£53/wk *Enhanced rate*—£79.25/wk **Mobility Component** *Standard rate*—£21/wk *Enhanced rate*—£55.25/wk

(continued)

Table 9.5 (Cont.)

	Eligibility	How to apply	Amount
Attendance Allowance (AA)▽	• Disability >3mo and expected to last >6mo more* • ≥65y and not permanently in hospital/local authority accommodation • Needs attention/supervision—higher rate if 24h care required or terminal illness*	☎ 0800 88 22 00 or ℛ www.gov.uk	*Lower rate* £53/wk *Higher rate* £79.25
Local Authority Grants	For people with sickness or disability to: • Re-establish the applicant or a family member in the community • Enable an individual to stay living in the community (e.g. to pay for home modifications) • Ease exceptional pressure on the applicant or a family member • Help with certain travel costs	Apply via local authority—schemes vary	Variable
Carer's Allowance	• Aged ≥16y • Spends ≥35h/wk caring for a person with a disability who is getting AA or Constant Attendance Allowance or middle or higher rate care component of DLA • Earning ≤£100.00/wk after allowable expenses • Not in full-time education • Other benefits (e.g. state pension) may affect eligibility	☎ 0845 608 4321 or ℛ www.gov.uk	£59.75/wk

▽No need to receive help to apply. Not means-tested.

*Terminal illness (not expected to live >6mo)—claim under Special Rules. Claims are processed much faster, and the highest care or daily living rate is automatically awarded. GP or hospital specialist fills in form DS1500 to provide clinical information to support application (fee can be claimed).

🛈 People who need someone's help to get out of the house are entitled to free prescriptions in England 🕮 p. 137.

Table 9.6 Mobility for elderly and disabled people.

	Eligibility	How to Apply	Benefits gained
Blue Badge Scheme	Age >2y and ≥1 of the following: • War Pensioner's Mobility Supplement • Higher rate of the mobility component of DLA/PIP • Motor vehicle supplied by a government health department • Registered blind • Severe disability in both upper limbs, preventing turning of a steering wheel • Permanent and substantial difficulty walking	Apply through local social services department ❶ In most circumstances, the disabled person does not have to be the driver. The badge should not be used if the disabled person is not in the car ⌨ www.dft.gov.uk	Entitles holder to park: • In specified disabled spaces; • Free of charge or time limit at parking meters or other places where waiting is limited • On single yellow lines for up to 3h (no time limit in Scotland)
Motability Scheme	• Higher rate mobility component of DLA/PIP or • War Pension Mobility Supplement ❶ Driver may be someone else	Contact Motability. Application guide available at ⌨ www.motability.co.uk	Registered Charity. Mobility payments can be used to lease or hire-purchase a car, powered scooter, or wheelchair. Grants may also be available for advance payments, adaptations, or driving lessons
Road Tax Exemption	• Higher rate mobility component of DLA/PIP or • War Pension Mobility Supplement or • Person nominated as someone who regularly drives for a disabled person or • Certain types of powered invalid carriages	Usually received automatically. If not and claiming DLA/PIP, ☎ 0845 7123456. If claiming War Pension, ☎ 0800 1692277	Exemption from Road Tax
Seatbelt exemption	Certain medical conditions, e.g. colostomy—but weigh up risks of travelling without a seatbelt	Medical practitioner must complete exemption certificate	Exemption from wearing seatbelt

❶ Local public transport schemes also exist

Table 9.7 Adaptations and equipment for elderly and disabled people

	Eligibility	Applying	Benefits received
Wheelchairs	Anyone requiring a wheelchair(s) for >3mo. Short-term loan of equipment is often available via the Red Cross	Referral by GP or specialist to the wheelchair service centre. Directory of service centres is available at: ℜ www.wheelchairmanagers.nhs.uk	Provision of suitable wheelchair Vouchers enable disabled patients to purchase their chairs privately
Occupational therapy (OT) assessment	All elderly or disabled people	Request a needs assessment by an occupational therapist via the local social services department	Enables provision of equipment and adaptations necessary to maintain an independent lifestyle
Disabled Living Centres / Disability Living Foundation	All elderly or disabled people	49 *Disabled Living Centres* in the UK—list available from ℜ http://assist-uk.org *Disabled Living Foundation* ☎ 0845 130 9177 ℜ www.dlf.org.uk	*Disabled Living Centres:* Look at and try out equipment, with OTs on hand to advise *Disabled Living Foundation:* Information on aids and adaptations
Telephone	People who have physical difficulty using the telephone or communication problems	British Telecom has a helpful website ℜ www.bt.com/includingyou/index.html	Gadgets and services that make it easier for disabled or elderly people to use the telephone
Alarm systems	Any disabled or elderly person who is alone at times, at risk, and mentally capable of using an alarm system	Arrange via local social services or Housing Department. Alternatively, charities for the elderly have schemes (e.g. Age UK Personal Alarm ☎ 0800 011 3846)	Enables a call for help when the phone cannot be reached

ⓘ All purchases related to disability are VAT exempt.

Cardiology and vascular disease

Symptoms and signs of CVD

Chest pain 🕮 p. 1080   Breathlessness or dyspnoea 🕮 p. 294

Blood pressure 🕮 p. 246   Crackles in the chest 🕮 p. 299

Peripheral oedema Swelling of the ankles/legs (or sacrum if bed-bound) occurs when the rate of capillary filtration > rate of drainage.
- Increased capillary filtration occurs due to ↑ venous pressure, hypoalbuminaemia, or local inflammation
- Decreased drainage occurs due to lymphatic obstruction

Consider whether swelling is acute or chronic, symmetrical or asymmetrical, localized, or generalized. Ask about associated symptoms, e.g. breathlessness. Treat according to cause. *Causes:*

Acute
- DVT
- Superficial thrombophlebitis
- Joint effusion/ haemarthrosis
- Cellulitis
- Haematoma
- Baker's cyst
- Arthritis
- Fracture
- Acute arterial ischaemia
- Dermatitis

Chronic
- Gravitational oedema, e.g due to immobility—common in the elderly—advise elevation of feet above waist level when sitting, support stockings (ideally apply stockings before getting out of bed), avoid standing still. Diuretics are not a long-term solution
- Heart failure
- Hypoproteinaemia, e.g. nephrotic syndrome
- Idiopathic oedema
- Reflex sympathetic dystrophy
- Post-thrombotic syndrome
- Chronic venous insufficiency/ venous obstruction
- Lipodermatosclerosis
- Lymphoedema—infection, tumour, trauma
- Congenital vascular abnormalities

Pulmonary oedema Accumulation of fluid in the pulmonary tissues and air spaces. *Causes include:*

Cardiac / vascular
- Left heart failure
- Mitral stenosis
- MI
- Hypertension
- Pulmonary venous obstruction
- IV fluid overload

Other
- High altitude
- Kidney failure
- Nephrotic syndrome
- Cirrhosis
- Lymphatic obstruction, e.g. due to tumour

Lung
- Pneumonia
- PE
- Pneumonitis due to inhalation of toxic substances, e.g. gases, radiation

Cyanosis Dusky blue skin.

Central cyanosis Cyanosis of mucus membranes, e.g. mouth. *Causes:*
- Lung disease resulting in inadequate oxygen transfer (e.g. COPD, PE, pleural effusion, severe chest infection)

- Shunting from pulmonary to systemic circulation (e.g. Fallot's tetralogy, PDA, transposition of the great arteries)
- Inadequate oxygen uptake (e.g. met- or sulf-haemoglobinaemia)

Peripheral cyanosis, e.g. cyanosis of fingers. *Causes:* as for central cyanosis plus
- Physiological (cold, hypovolaemia)
- Local arterial disease (e.g. Raynaud's syndrome)

❶ Feet can be a dusky blue colour due to venous disease. If this occurs without central cyanosis it does not imply abnormal oxygen saturation.

Mitral facies Dusky bluish red flushing of the cheeks (a form of peripheral cyanosis) associated with a low cardiac output.

Clubbing Loss of the angle between nail fold and plate, bulbous finger tip, and the nail fold feels boggy—📖 p. 609.

⚠ Refer any patient with unexplained nail clubbing for urgent CXR[N].

Jugular venous pressure Observe internal jugular vein at 45° with head turned slightly to the left. Vertical height is measured in relation to the sternal angle. Raised if >4cm. Causes of ↑ JVP:
- Fluid overload
- Right heart failure and CCF
- SVC obstruction (non-pulsatile)
- Tricuspid or pulmonary valve disease
- Pulmonary hypertension
- Arrhythmia—AF or atrial flutter, complete heart block
- ↑ intrathoracic pressure e.g. pneumothorax, PE, emphysema

Kussmaul's sign The JVP usually drops on inspiration along with intrathoracic pressure. The reverse pattern is called Kussmaul's sign. Caused by raised intrathoracic pressure or constrictive pericarditis.

Signs of infective endocarditis
- **Infective** Fever, weight ↓, clubbing, splenomegaly, anaemia
- **Cardiac** Murmurs (particularly new murmurs) ± heart failure
- **Embolic** Neurologic deficit due to stroke
- **Vasculitic** Microscopic haematuria, splinter haemorrhages, conjunctival haemorrhages, Roth's spots (retinal vasculitis), Osler's nodes (painful lesions on finger pulps), Janeway lesions (palmar macules)

Signs of hypercholesterolaemia
Corneal arcus Whitish opaque line surrounding the margin of the cornea, separated from it by an area of clear cornea. Rarely congenital—more commonly occurs bilaterally in patients >50y (*arcus senilis*). Sometimes associated with ↑ blood lipids—particularly familial hypercholesterolaemias. Check lipids. If lipids are normal, no treatment is needed.

Xanthomata Localized collections of lipid-laden cells. Appear as yellowish coloured lumps. Often caused by ↑ lipids. Commonly seen on the eyelids (*xanthelasma*), on the skin, or in tendons (appear as mobile nodules in the tendon).

Examining the heart

Apex beat Normal position is in the 5th intercostal space, in the mid-clavicular line. Moved sideways/inferiorly if the heart is enlarged (e.g. CCF) or displaced (e.g. pneumothorax). May not be palpable if the patient is obese, has hyperexpanded lungs (e.g. COPD), or a pericardial effusion. In infants/children apex beat is superior/more lateral.

Parasternal heave Detect by placing the heel of the hand over the left parasternal region. If present, the heel of the hand is lifted off the chest wall with each heart beat. *Causes:* usually right ventricular enlargement—rarely, left atrial enlargement.

Heart sounds See Table 10.2. Low/medium frequency sounds (e.g. 3rd/4th heart sounds) are more easily heard with the bell applied lightly to the skin. High-frequency sounds (e.g. 1st/2nd heart sounds and opening snaps) are more easily heard with a diaphragm.

Heart murmurs Due to abnormalities of flow within the heart and great vessels. Very common. Often incidental findings. Described by:
- **Location** Where heard loudest
- **Quality**, e.g. blowing, harsh
- **Intensity** Graded out of 6 (1—virtually undetectable; 6—heard by an observer with no stethoscope). Grades 4–6 are usually palpable (*thrills*)
- **Timing** Systolic or diastolic, *and*
- **Radiation** Does the murmur spread elsewhere, e.g. to axilla, carotids

⚠ **Red flag symptoms**
- Cyanosis
- Breathlessness
- Lethargy/tiredness
- Collapse
- Weight loss (or failure to thrive)

Always refer for echo. Differential diagnosis—See Table 10.1.

Table 10.1 Differential diagnosis of heart murmurs

Type of murmur	Description	Causes
Ejection systolic murmur	↑ to reach a peak midway between the heart sounds	• Flow murmurs, e.g children, pregnancy, with fever, during/after exercise • Aortic stenosis or sclerosis (🕮 p. 280) • Pulmonary stenosis (🕮 p. 281) • HOCM (🕮 p. 278)
Pan-systolic murmur	Uniform intensity between the two heart sounds. Merges with 2nd heart sound	• Mitral valve regurgitation/prolapse (🕮 p. 280) • Tricuspid regurgitation (🕮 p. 281) • VSD (🕮 p. 282) • ASD (🕮 p. 282)
Early diastolic murmur	Occurs just after the 2nd heart sound. High pitched. Easily missed	• Aortic regurgitation (🕮 p. 281) • Pulmonary regurgitation (🕮 p. 281) • Tricuspid stenosis (mitral stenosis coexists)
Mid-diastolic murmur	Midway between 2nd heart sound of one beat and 1st of the next. Rumbling/low pitch	• Mitral stenosis (🕮 p. 280) • Aortic regurgitation. (Austin Flint murmur—🕮 p. 281)

Table 10.2 Heart sounds, abnormalities, and their causes

Heart sound		Causes
1st heart sound Heard loudest at the apex Caused by closing of the mitral and tricuspid valves	Soft	Mitral regurgitation, low BP, rheumatic carditis, severe heart failure, LBBB
	Loud	AF, tachycardia, atrial premature beat, mitral stenosis
	Variable intensity	Varying duration of diastole, complete AV block
	Split	RBBB, paced beat from the left ventricle, left ventricular ectopics, ASD, Ebstein's anomaly, tricuspid stenosis
2nd heart sound Caused by closure of the aortic (A2) and pulmonary (P2) valves A2 and P2 split on inspiration so that P2 is heard after A2	Soft	• **A2**—calcification of the aortic valve, dilatation of the aortic root • **P2**—pulmonary stenosis
	Loud	• **A2**—↑ BP; thin patients • **P2**—pulmonary hypertension, ASD
	Wide splitting	May be the result of early A2 or delayed P2 • **Early A2**—mitral regurgitation; VSD • **Delayed P2**—RBBB, pulmonary stenosis, ASD, right ventricular failure
	Reversed splitting	A2 is delayed. P2 occurs before A2, so the split between the sounds ↓ on inspiration *Delayed A2*—LBBB, systolic hypertension, HOCM, severe aortic stenosis, PDA, left heart failure
	Single	Calcification of the aortic valve, pulmonary stenosis, Fallot's tetralogy, Ebstein's anomaly, pericardial effusion, large VSD, obesity, emphysema
Clicks and snaps	Early systolic	Caused by opening of the aortic or pulmonary valves • **Aortic**—aortic stenosis, bicuspid valve • **Pulmonary**—pulmonary stenosis, pulmonary hypertension
	Mid/late systolic	Mitral valve prolapse
	Diastolic	Caused by opening of the mitral or tricuspid valves Silent in the healthy heart • **Mitral**—mitral stenosis, rapid mitral flow, e.g. PDA, VSD, severe mitral regurgitation • **Tricuspid** (rare)—rheumatic stenosis, ASD
3rd heart sound Heard in diastole after the 2nd heart sound	Right ventricle	Loudest at lower left sternal edge. Never normal. *Causes:* right heart failure, tricuspid regurgitation, ASD, constrictive pericarditis
	Left ventricle	Loudest at the apex when inclined to the left. Can be normal in children and pregnancy. *Other causes:* LVF, mitral regurgitation, anterior MI
4th heart sound Heard in late diastole		Maximal at the apex or lower left sternal edge. Never normal. *Causes:* ventricular hypertrophy or fibrosis and HOCM

Examination of the arterial system

The main conditions affecting the abdominal and peripheral arteries are:
- Aneurysms (📖 p. 284)
- Atherosclerosis, resulting in ischaemia of the legs and intermittent claudication, atrophic changes and/or rest pain
- Embolization resulting in acute ischaemia of the limbs

General scheme
- Look at the limbs—are there any signs of ischaemia? Are the extremities warm or cold? What colour are they?
- Examine the abdomen looking for a pulsatile mass which might suggest abdominal aortic aneurysm (📖 p. 284). Auscultation may reveal a bruit
- Check the peripheral pulses

⚠ Tenderness on palpation of an abdominal aortic aneurysm suggests need for urgent operative repair.

Blood pressure 📖 p. 246

Carotid pulse Ask the patient to lie supine with head/neck at 45° to the horizontal. When assessing the carotid pulse, consider:

Rate
- **Tachycardia** >100bpm—📖 p. 268
- **Bradycardia** <60bpm—📖 p. 272

Rhythm
- **Irregularly irregular** AF, multiple ectopics
- **Regularly irregular** 2nd degree heart block

Character and volume Always assess with a central pulse, e.g. carotid or femoral.
- **Small volume**—shock, pericardial tamponade, aortic stenosis (slow-rising)
- **Large volume**—hyperdynamic circulation (e.g. pregnancy), aortic incompetence (waterhammer, collapsing pulse), PDA
- **Pulsus paradoxus**—pulse weakens in inspiration by >10mmHg—asthma, cardiac tamponade, pericarditis

Carotid bruits May signify stenosis (>30%) often near the origin of internal carotid. Heard best behind the angle of the jaw. Usual cause is atheroma.

Peripheral pulses
Location See Table 10.3.

Examination Check whether each pulse is present. If present check:
- Rate
- Rhythm
- Amplitude
- Compare pulses in the two legs/two arms

Check for radiofemoral delay—palpate radial and femoral pulses simultaneously—delay suggests coarctation of the aorta.

Table 10.3 Location of the limb pulses

Pulse	Location
Brachial	~2cm medial to the central point of the antecubital fossa over the elbow skin crease
Radial	~½–1cm on the radial (lateral) side of the flexor carpi radialis tendon at the wrist
Femoral	Below inguinal ligament; one-third of the way up from pubic tubercle
Popliteal	With knee flexed at right angles, palpate deep in the midline
Posterior tibial	1cm behind medial malleolus
Dorsalis pedis	Variable—on the dorsum of the foot just lateral to the tendons to the big toe ❶ Many healthy people have only one foot pulse

Check for bruits over the femoral and/or carotid pulses—these indicate disturbed blood flow—usually 2° to narrowing due to atherosclerosis.

⚠ Character and waveform of the pulse should *only* be assessed using the femoral or carotid pulse.

Signs of ischaemia

Acute ischaemia Acutely pale, cold, and pulseless limb—📖 p. 1126. Refer immediately—keep the limb cool in the interim.

Chronic ischaemic changes

• Atrophic skin changes—pallor, cool to the touch, hairless, shiny
• On lowering the leg turns a dusky blue-red colour; on elevation— pallor and venous guttering
• Ulceration—check under the heel and between the toes
• Swelling suggests the patient is sleeping in a chair to avoid rest pain or, rarely, pain from deep infection
• Absent foot pulses—if pulses are present, consider alternative diagnosis
• Ankle–brachial pressure index <0.95

Checking the ankle–brachial pressure index (ABPI)

• Check BP in one arm (📖 p. 246). The systolic measurement is the brachial pressure (B)
• Then inflate a BP cuff around the lower calf just above the ankle
• Using a Doppler ultrasound probe, record the maximum cuff pressure at which the probe can still record a pulse (ankle pressure—A)
• Calculate the ankle–brachial pressure index by dividing the ankle pressure by the brachial pressure, i.e. ABPI = A ÷ B

Interpretation of ABPI results

• ABPI <0.8—ischaemia
• ABPI <0.5—critical ischaemia

❶ Arterial calcification (e.g. due to DM) can result in falsely elevated ankle pressure readings.

Cardiac investigations

Electrocardiogram (ECG)

Graphic recording of electric potentials generated by the heart. Most surgeries now have ECG machines that interpret themselves and print out their findings. Analysis is easier but it is still important to be able to understand the significance of abnormalities and check computer analysis in the clinical context.

Interpreting ECGs Many mistakes in ECG interpretation are errors of omission so a systematic approach is best. *Check:*

- Standardization (calibration) and technical features (including lead placement and artefacts)
- Heart rate—usual speed (25mm/s). Each big square represents 0.2s (small square—0.04s). Rate = 300 ÷ R-R interval (in large squares)
- Rhythm—regular/irregular
- PR interval—normal if <0.2s
- QRS interval—abnormal if >0.12s
- QT interval—varies with rate. At 60bpm normal if 0.35–0.43s
- P waves—present or absent, shape
- QRS voltages—height of complexes—see Table 10.4, 📖 p. 240
- Mean QRS electrical axis—sum of all ventricular forces during ventricular depolarization. Normal axis: −30° to +120°
  - If more −ve = left axis deviation; if more +ve = right axis deviation
  - **Rule of thumb 1** If the majority of the QRS complex is above the baseline (+ve) in leads I and II the axis is normal
  - **Rule of thumb 2** The axis lies at 90° to a QRS complex where the height above the baseline = height below the baseline
- Precordial R-wave progression
- Abnormal Q waves—>25% of the succeeding R-wave and/or >0.04s wide
- ST segments—elevation/depression, shape
- T waves—height, inversion, shape
- U waves—small, rounded deflection (≤1mm), follows T wave and usually has the same polarity

Brief guide to common ECG changes See Table 10.4, 📖 p. 240

24h ambulatory ECG ECG monitoring equipment is worn for 24h. Continuous monitoring may detect intermittent arrhythmia or ischaemia.

Exercise ECG ECG testing whilst the patient undergoes graded exercise on a treadmill/exercise bicycle. Local referral criteria vary. Mortality ~1 in 10,000. Used for:

- Diagnosis of IHD—75% have a +ve test; false +ve rate of ~5%
- Assessment of exercise tolerance
- Response to treatment
- As a prognostic indicator
- Assessment of exercise-related arrhythmias

Contraindications Recent MI (<7d), unstable angina, electrolyte disturbance, aortic stenosis, severe heart failure, known left main coronary artery stenosis, LBBB (may not be possible to interpret the trace).

Cardiac enzymes Biochemical blood assay of molecules released when the heart is damaged. Used in diagnosis of MI.

- **Troponins T and I** Preferred markers as more sensitive/specific than CK, AST, or lactate dehydrogenase. Together with CK, earliest to ↑ after MI
- **Creatine kinase (CK)**↑ in MI, muscle damage (e.g. prolonged running or seizures), after IM injection, and with dermatomyositis (e.g. due to statins). CK-MB assay may help clarify whether a cardiac event has occurred <48h previously
- **AST** 2nd to ↑
- **Lactate dehydrogenase (LDH)** Last to ↑

Echocardiogram (echo) Heart USS. Local referral procedures vary.

- **2-dimensional** Produces a fan-shaped, cross-sectional, moving, real-time image of the heart. May be transthoracic or transoesophageal. Used to assess valvular abnormalities and prosthetic heart valves; aortic aneurysm/dissection; heart failure; pericardial effusion; masses within the heart; myocardial abnormalities (e.g. aneurysms, hypertrophy); IHD; congenital heart disease
- **M-mode** Plotted on a scrolling screen. Stationary structures appear as straight lines across the screen; moving structures appear as undulating lines. Usually displayed with an ECG trace to enable identification of phases of the cardiac cycle. Used to investigate movement of individual structural elements, e.g. valves, chamber walls
- **Doppler** Enables flow across valves and ASD/VSDs to be quantified

Cardiac catheterization Refer via 2° care. Involves passing a catheter, usually via the femoral or brachial artery, to the heart. Used to:

- Measure pressures within the heart and great vessels
- Assess oxygen saturation via blood samples
- Perform coronary angiography—contrast is injected into the coronary arteries to assess their anatomy and/or patency
- Perform intravascular ultrasound
- Perform other procedures, e.g. angioplasty, valvuloplasty, cardiac biopsy

Complications Arrhythmia (0.56%); MI (0.07%); stroke (0.07%); death (0.14%); haemorrhage at the site of insertion (0.56%); thrombo-embolism; trauma to heart and vessels; infection.

Radionucleotide imaging Refer via 2° care. Involves IV administration of a γ-emitting radionucleotide and gamma camera monitoring.

- **Radionucleotide angiography** Uses technetium^{99m}-labelled RBCs to calculate left ventricular ejection fraction/assess ventricular action
- **Myocardial perfusion scintigraphy** Uses thallium^{201} injected IV during exercise testing to demonstrate areas of poorly perfused myocardium

Cardiac MRI/magnetic resonance angiography Used increasingly in 2° care to provide detailed structural information about the heart and rapid angiographic images.

Patient information
British Heart Foundation ☏ 0300 330 3311 ✎ www.bhf.org.uk

Brief guide to common ECG changes

❶ For detailed analysis of ECGs refer to a specialist text, e.g. Hampton JR (2008) *The ECG Made Easy* (7th edn). Churchill Livingstone. ISBN: 0443068178.

Table 10.4 Common ECG abnormalities and their causes

ECG abnormality		Possible causes
Tachycardia	Rate >100bpm	Physiological, AF, atrial flutter, SVT, VT
Bradycardia	Rate <60bpm	Physiological, drugs (e.g. β-blockers, digoxin), heart block (☐ p. 272), sick sinus syndrome
Irregular	Assess whether any pattern or not	AF (no pattern), sick sinus syndrome (no pattern), ventricular ectopics (normally no pattern), heart block (pattern)
P-R interval	Short P-R interval	Nodal rhythm, WPW syndrome (☐ p. 269)
	Prolonged >0.2s	Heart block—☐ p. 272; sick sinus syndrome, drugs (e.g. β-blockers, digoxin)
Left bundle branch block (LBBB)*	QRS >0.12s wide. Last peak is below the isoelectric line in V1	IHD, ↑ BP, cardiomyopathy, aortic valve disease, SVT. Artificial pacemakers may produce a similar QRS complex
Right bundle branch block (RBBB)	QRS >0.12s wide. Last peak is above the iso-electric line in V1	May be normal; congenital heart disease (e.g. ASD), valvular heart disease, IHD, pulmonary hypertension, during SVT
Incomplete bundle branch block	QRS < 0.12s with abnormal-shaped QRS complex	As for RBBB or LBBB
Q-T interval abnormalities	Prolonged Q-T interval	↓K^+, drugs (e.g. TCAs, phenothiazines, amiodarone), SAH or CVA, hypothermia
	Shortened Q-T interval	↑Ca^{2+}, digoxin
Abnormal P-waves	↑ P-wave amplitude (>2.5mm)	Right atrial overload—tricuspid stenosis, pulmonary hypertension, pulmonary stenosis
	Biphasic P-wave in V1 ± broad (>0.12s) often notched P-wave in ≥1 limb lead	Left atrial abnormality—mitral stenosis, aortic stenosis, conduction abnormalities

(Continued)

Table 10.4 (Cont.)

ECG abnormality		Possible causes
Right ventricular hypertrophy (RVH)	Strain pattern—ST depression and T-wave inversion in leads V1–3. Dominant R in V1 with narrow QRS	Pulmonary stenosis, mitral stenosis pulmonary hypertension, ASD (± RBBB). Similar changes seen with inferior MI (T-wave upright); WPW syndrome
Left ventricular hypertrophy (LVH)	Strain pattern—ST↓ and T-wave ↓ in leads V4–6. Large voltages of QRS complex—sum of S in V1 and R in V5 or V6 alone >35mm	↑ BP, aortic stenosis, coarctation of the aorta, HOCM
Right axis deviation	📖 p. 238	RVH/strain (e.g. following PE), cor pulmonale, pulmonary stenosis. Alone with normal QRS = left posterior hemiblock
Left axis deviation	📖 p. 238	LVH /strain (e.g. ↑BP, aortic stenosis, HOCM), VSD, ASD. If occurs alone with normal QRS=left anterior hemiblock
Poor R-wave progression	Small or absent R waves in the R → mid-precordial leads	L or R ventricular enlargement, LBBB, left pneumothorax, dextrocardia, COPD
	Reversed R wave progression—↓in R-wave amplitude from V1 → mid/lateral precordial leads	Right ventricular enlargement
Abnormal Q-waves	>25% of succeeding R-wave and/or >0.04s wide	Normal; left pneumothorax; dextrocardia; MI; myocarditis; hyperkalaemia; cardiomyopathy; amyloid; sarcoid; scleroderma; LVH; RVH; LBBB; WPW syndrome
ST elevation	ST segment raised >1mm above baseline	MI, Prinzmetal angina, pericarditis, ventricular aneurysm
ST depression	ST segment lowered >0.5mm below baseline	Angina, ventricular strain, drugs (digoxin, verapamil), hyperkalaemia, myocarditis, cardiomyopathy, fibrosis, Lyme disease
T-wave inversion	Abnormal if inverted in leads I, II, or V4–6	MI (inverts <24h after MI); ventricular strain (see above); PE (III); digoxin (V5–6)
U-waves	↑ amplitude >1mm	Drugs (e.g. quinidine, procainamide, disopyramide) or ↓ K⁺
Inversion in precordial leads		Subtle sign of ischaemia

* No comment can be made about ST segment or T-wave if LBBB.

❶ Always compare with previous ECGs if available.

Prevention of coronary heart disease

Coronary heart disease (CHD) is the most common cause of death in UK (1 in 4 deaths). Mortality is falling but morbidity rising.

Risk factors for heart disease See Table 10.5.

Primary prevention Aims to stop heart disease developing.

Population strategy Influences factors that ↑ CHD risk in an entire population, e.g. anti-smoking campaigns. GPs can do this by displaying health education posters/literature (e.g. in waiting room, practice leaflet).

Health checks for the over 40s There is a national screening programme for people aged 40–74y in the UK to identify CVD, DM, and cancer earlier through health checks every 5y. The check provides:
- Lifestyle advice
- Information about cancer screening programmes available in the UK
- CVD risk assessment—including demographic information, family history, smoking status, alcohol consumption, BMI, BP, and lipid profile
- DM risk stratification—📖 p. 345

High-risk strategy There are a number of paper-based and computerized risk scores available to estimate CVD risk (📖 p. 244). Most only apply to people aged <75y, who are not diabetic and have no past history of CVD. Most CVD occurs in individuals at medium risk as that is the largest group. However individuals at high risk have the most to gain from risk reduction. This strategy aims to identify individuals with 10y CVD risk ≥20% through opportunistic screening and health checks and ↓ their risk through lifestyle modification ± medication.

❶ Current risk estimation tools give 10y CVD risk; QRisk-Lifetime is a new tool based on the Joint British Societies (JBS3) lifetime risk algorithm. It provides an estimate of lifetime risk but place in management is yet to be determined (℠ www.qrisk2/lifetime).

Selection of patients for intervention Is based on overall risk.
- All patients aged >75y, or with a familial monogenic dyslipidaemia are at high risk
- Most patients with DM are at high risk—📖 p. 354
- Patients with 10y CVD risk ≥20% are at high risk

> ❶ If the risk score is near the threshold for intervention, consider other factors that may predispose to CVD and are not included in the score:
> - Low socio-economic group
> - BMI—risk is ↑ if BMI >40kg/m²
> - Is the person already taking antihypertensive/lipid modification therapy?
> - Has the person recently stopped smoking?
> - Is the person taking antipsychotic medication?
> - Are other conditions present that ↑ risk, e.g. CKD, RA, SLE, HIV?

Secondary prevention Aims to stop progression of symptomatic CHD. 46% people who die from MI are already known to have CHD. There is strong evidence that targeting patients with CHD for risk factor modification is effective in ↓ risk of recurrent CHD.

Table 10.5 Risk factors for heart disease

Non-modifiable	Modifiable (proven benefit)	Modifiable (unproven benefit)
Age—↑ with age	Smoking*—📖 p. 182	Haemostatic factors—↑ plasma fibrinogen
Sex—♂ > ♀ in those < 65y	Hyperlipidaemia—📖 p. 252	
Ethnic origin—in the UK people who originate from the Indian subcontinent have ↑ risk, Afro-Caribbeans have ↓ risk	Hypertension*—📖 p. 248	Apolipoproteins—↑ lipoprotein(a)*
	DM*—📖 p. 354	
	Diet*—📖 p. 174	Homocysteine—↑ blood homocysteine
	Obesity (particularly waist-hip ratio)*—📖 p. 178	Vitamin levels—↓ blood folate, vitamin B_{12} and B_6
Socio-economic position*	Physical inactivity*—📖 p. 180	
Personal history of CVD	Alcohol consumption*—📖 p. 184	Depression
Family history of CVD—< 55y ♂; <65y ♀	Left ventricular dysfunction/heart failure (2° prevention)—📖 p. 262	
Low birthweight (IUGR)	Coronary-prone behaviour—competitiveness, aggression, and feeling under time pressure (2° prevention)—behaviour modification is associated with ↓ risk	

* These 9 factors account for 90% of risk for acute MI.

The GP's role GPs have a role in:
- Identification of patients who would benefit from primary prevention
- Ensuring patients who are at high risk of atherosclerotic disease (established CVD, DM, CVD risk ≥ 20% over 10y, elevated BP with systolic ≥160 and /or diastolic ≥100 and target organ damage, ↑ total cholesterol:HDL ratio ≥6, familial dyslipidaemia) have ongoing follow-up through disease registers, routine recall, and follow-up
- Promoting lifestyle modification in at-risk patients
- Ensuring current best care guidelines are followed and treatment regimes are updated as policies change; this is a major challenge for primary care as guidelines change frequently and often conflict
- Checking the process through audit

Further information

NICE 🖱 www.nice.org.uk
- Cardiovascular risk assessment and the modification of blood lipids for the primary and secondary prevention of cardiovascular disease (2008)
- The management of type 2 diabetes (2009)
- Identifying and supporting people most at risk of dying prematurely (2008)

SIGN Guideline 97: risk estimation and the prevention of cardiovascular disease (2007 and 2012 review) 🖱 www.sign.ac.uk

Patient information
British Heart Foundation 📞 0300 330 3311 🖱 www.bhf.org.uk

Estimating cardiovascular risk

High-risk stategy for primary prevention 📖 p. 242

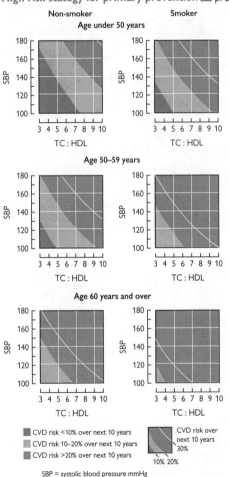

Figure 10.1 CVD risk in non-diabetic men <75y with no previous history of CVD

⚠ If ♂ of south Asian background, ↑ CVD risk ×1.4; if FH of premature heart disease (<55y for ♂; <65y for ♀)—↑ risk ×1.5 if one relative affected; ×2 if >1 relative affected.

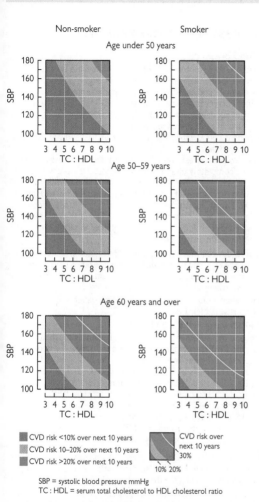

Figure 10.2 CVD risk in non-diabetic women <75y with no previous history of CVD

Computerized risk assessment tools
- Framingham score ✆ http://cvrisk.mvm.ed.ac.uk/calculator/framingham.htm
- QRISK2-2013 ✆ www.qrisk.org
- ASSIGN (Scotland) ✆ www.assign-score.com
- JBS3 Lifetime risk calculator ✆ www.jbs3risk.com

Blood pressure measurement

Taking blood pressure

- Use a validated sphygmomanometer—a list is available on the British Hypertension Society website (&% www.bhsoc.org)
- Regularly maintain and calibrate your sphygmomanometer
- Use a cuff of correct bladder size: most adults—12 x 26cm; large adults (arm circumference >33cm) – 12 x 40cm; thin adults and children with arm circumference ≤26cm—10 x 18cm
- Seat the patient comfortably with arm outstretched and supported at the level of the heart
- Measure BP to the nearest 2mmHg; measure diastolic pressure when heart sounds completely disappear (K_5)—only use the pressure at which they suddenly muffle (K_4) when K_5 cannot be determined
- Measure BP in both arms—if the difference in systolic BP is >10mmHg between the 2 arms, repeat the measurement. A consistent difference of >10mmHg is an independent risk factor for CVD and all-cause mortality; treat identified CVD risk factors. Use the higher of the 2 readings when considering further management of BP

❶ Automated devices may not measure BP accurately if there is pulse irregularity (e.g. AF). Check the radial or brachial pulse before checking BP and measure BP manually using direct auscultation over the brachial artery if pulse is irregular.

'White coat' hypertension Prevalence 10%. Some patients' BP increases in response to having their BP checked.

If BP is ≥140/90mmHg in the consultation

- Take a second measurement—if that measurement is substantially different from the first measurement, take a third measurement; record the lower of these measurements as the BP
- If BP on repeat testing is ≥140/90mmHg and not known to be hypertensive, offer ambulatory BP monitoring (ABPM) or home BP monitoring (HBPM) to confirm the diagnosis; consider ABPM or HBPM monitoring (HBPM) for people on antihypertensive medication who are known to have 'white coat' hypertension
- If hypertension is not confirmed on ABPM/HBPM, measure BP every 5y or more frequently if close to 140/90 mmHg

⚠ If the person has severe hypertension (systolic BP ≥180mmHg or diastolic BP ≥110mmHg, consider starting antihypertensive treatment immediately without waiting for the result of ABPM/HBPM.

Refer for same day specialist assessment if suspected:
- Accelerated hypertension (BP >180/110mmHg ± papilloedema ± retinal haemorrhage) or
- Phaeochromocytoma (labile/postural hypotension, headache, palpitations, pallor, and excessive sweating)

Ambulatory BP monitoring (ABPM) A BP-measuring device is worn on the body for 24h. It takes BP every 20min in the daytime and less frequently (usually hourly) at night. ↑ BP readings on ABPM are more strongly correlated to end-organ damage than one-off measurements. ABPM is used for:

- The diagnosis of hypertension (📖 p. 248)
- Diagnosis or exclusion of 'white coat' hypertension
- Monitoring of response to treatment
- Assessing medication-related postural hypotension

Interpretation ABPM is considered abnormal if:

- Average daytime ABPM is ≥135/85mmHg
- Average night-time ABPM is ≥120/70mmHg

❶ NICE bases the diagnosis of hypertension on average *daytime* ABPM only (minimum 14 readings).

Night-time ABPM BP falls at night in normotensive individuals. Some hypertensive patients are described as 'non-dippers'. This means that their BP does not fall at night and is associated with ↑ risk of target end-organ damage. Conversely, some hypertensive patients have excessive dips in their BP at night (>10%); this is associated with ↑ CVD events.

Home BP monitoring (HBPM) Useful:

- If ABPM facilities are not available within a reasonable time frame for diagnosis of hypertension
- For patients who cannot tolerate ABPM, and
- For monitoring of antihypertensive treatment

Instructions Patients should use a validated and calibrated BP machine.

- Measure BP on at least 4—and preferably 7—consecutive days
- Measure BP 2x/d (morning and evening) when seated; take two readings >1min apart
- Discard the readings taken on day 1 and take an average value of all the remaining measurements

Interpretation HBPM is abnormal if average is ≥135/85mmHg.

Hypertension 📖 p. 248   **Cardiogenic shock** 📖 p. 1074

Postural hypotension BP drops on moving from supine, or sitting, position to standing position. Presents with falls, postural dizziness, and/or light-headedness. Measure BP supine or seated and then ask the patient to stand up. Re-measure BP after 1min standing. Standing usually causes a slight ↓ in the systolic BP (<20mmHg) and a slight ↑ in the diastolic BP (<10mmHg). In postural hypotension there is usually a marked ↓ in both systolic (>20mmHg) and diastolic BP.

- **Review medication** Stop any non-essential medication contributing to symptoms, e.g. night sedation, unnecessary diuretics
- **Optimize treatment** of intercurrent heart disease, Parkinson's disease, or DM
- **Advise** patients to take care when standing—especially if getting up from their beds or out of a hot bath/shower, and after meals

Measure subsequent BP with the patient standing. Consider specialist referral if symptoms persist despite GP management.

Further information

NICE Clinical management of primary hypertension in adults (2011) ℜ www.nice.org.uk

Clark CE, Taylor RS, Shore AC, Campbell JL (2012) The difference in blood pressure readings between arms and survival: primary care cohort study. *BMJ* **344**:e1327.

Hypertension

Hypertension is a major risk factor for CVD. It is normally symptomless until it causes organ damage. Prevalence ↑ with age; 25% of all adults and >50% of people aged >60y have hypertension. Management aims to detect and treat ↑ BP before damage occurs.

Causes

- Unknown ('essential')—95%; alcohol (10%) or obesity may be contributory factors
- Renal disease—📖 p. 438
- Endocrine disease—Cushing's (both syndrome and 2° to steroids); Conn's syndrome; phaeochromocytoma; acromegaly; hyperparathyroidism; DM—📖 p. 355
- Pregnancy—📖 p. 826
- Coarctation of the aorta—📖 p. 282

Presentation

- Usually asymptomatic and found during routine BP screening or incidentally. Occasionally headache or visual disturbance
- May be symptoms of end-organ damage—LVH, TIAs, previous CVA/MI, angina, renal impairment, PVD

Measurement of blood pressure 📖 p. 246

Diagnosis of hypertension BP is a normally distributed continuous variable; each 2mmHg ↑ in systolic BP is associated with a 7% ↑ risk of mortality from IHD and a 10% ↑ risk of mortality from stroke. There is no figure above which hypertension can be diagnosed definitively. Criteria currently in use[N]:

- **Stage 1 hypertension** Clinic BP ≥140/90mmHg and subsequent daytime average ABPM/HBPM ≥135/85mmHg
- **Stage 2 hypertension** Clinic BP ≥160/100mmHg and subsequent daytime average ABPM/HBPM ≥150/95mmHg
- **Severe hypertension** Clinic systolic BP ≥180mmHg or clinic diastolic BP ≥110mmHg

⚠ If the person has severe hypertension (systolic BP ≥180mmHg or diastolic BP ≥110mmHg) consider starting antihypertensive treatment immediately without waiting for the result of ABPM/HBPM.

Refer for same day specialist assessment if suspected:
- Accelerated hypertension (BP >180/110mmHg ± papilloedema ± retinal haemorrhage) or
- Phaeochromocytoma (labile/postural hypotension, headache, palpitations, pallor, and excessive sweating)

Isolated systolic hypertension Systolic BP ≥160mmHg—offer the same treatment as people with ↑ systolic and diastolic blood pressure.

Further assessment Aims to identify target organ damage:
- **Examination** Check heart size, heart sounds, and for heart failure; examine the fundi, looking for silver wiring, AV nipping, flame haemorrhages, and cotton wool spots
- **Blood tests** Creatinine, electrolytes, eGFR, glucose/HbA1c, lipid profile; consider GGT if excess alcohol is a possibility

- **Urine** Dipstick for RBCs and protein; laboratory sample for albumin:creatinine ratio
- **Cardiovascular risk estimation** 📖 p. 244
- **ECG ± echo** (if left ventricular hypertrophy is suspected)

❗ If ↑ BP is not diagnosed but there is evidence of target organ damage (e.g. LVH, proteinuria) look for alternative causes.

Education Patients will not take tablets regularly, be motivated to change lifestyle, or turn up for regular checks if they do not understand why treating their ↑ BP is important. Conversely, some patients who were fit and well prior to their diagnosis will assume a sick role unless it is explained that they are well and treatment is designed to stop illness developing. Back up verbal information with written information that patients can take home; reinforce information at follow-up and offer opportunities for discussion. Do not forget to warn patients about possible side effects of any medications.

Lifestyle advice Offer lifestyle advice to all patients with a diagnosis of hypertension and those with FH of ↑ BP. Reinforce advice with written information:

- Offer smoking cessation advice and help (📖 p. 182)
- ↓ weight to optimum for height (📖 p. 178)
- Encourage regular exercise—dynamic is best, e.g. walking, swimming, cycling (📖 p. 180)
- ↓ alcohol to <21u/wk for ♂ and <14u/wk for ♀ (📖 p. 184)
- ↓ dietary salt intake (aim for <6g salt/d)
- ↑ dietary fruit and vegetable intake—aim for ≥5 portions/d
- ↓ excess coffee consumption and other caffeine-rich products
- Encourage relaxation and stress management
- *Do not* offer Ca^{2+}, Mg^{2+}, or K^+ supplements as a method to ↓ BP

Statin (📖 p. 253). Prescribe:

- If hypertension complicated by CVD irrespective of baseline cholesterol or LDL levels *or*
- For primary prevention in patients >40y with hypertension and 10y CVD risk ≥20%

Initiating antihypertensive drug treatment

Stage 1 hypertension Offer drug treatment if <80y of age and ≥1 of:

- Target organ damage
- Established CVD
- Renal disease
- DM
- 10y CVD risk ≥20%

Stage 2 hypertension Offer drug treatment to all patients.

❗ If aged <40y with stage 1 hypertension and no evidence of target organ damage, CVD, renal disease, or DM, consider specialist referral to exclude 2° causes of hypertension and for detailed estimation of CVD risk.

General rules for antihypertensive drug treatment

- **If a drug is not tolerated** Stop; move to the next line of therapy
- **If a drug is tolerated but the BP target is not met** Add in the next line of therapy
- **Where possible** Recommend treatment with drugs taken only once a day and prescribe non-proprietary drugs which minimize cost

Choice of antihypertensive drug(s) See Figure 10.3, 📖 p. 251.

❶ Side effects of drug treatment for hypertension are common. 40–50% started on an antihypertensive drug discontinue regardless of which class of drug is used. 80% of side effects are seen in first year of treatment.

Treatment targets

Non-diabetic patients without CKD
- Clinic BP <140/90mmHg (<150/90mmHg if aged ≥80y)
- ABPM/HBPM (e.g. for patients with 'white coat' hypertension) average daytime BP <135/85mmHg (<145/85mmHg if aged ≥80y)

Diabetic patients (📖 p. 355)
- <140/80mmHg—uncomplicated type 2 DM
- <135/85mmHg—uncomplicated type 1 DM
- <130/80mmHg—if any renal, foot, eye, or cardiovascular complications of type 1 or type 2 DM

CKD Aim for BP <130/80mmHg (📖 p. 440).

Follow-up Regular review of patients with ↑ BP is essential.

Review interval Depends on stability of BP:
- **After starting treatment** Review after 1mo
- **If BP is controlled** Review after a further 3mo, then every 3–6 mo
- **If BP is not controlled** Bring the patient back to repeat the BP reading and/or ask for ABPM/HBPM. *Do not* alter medication on the strength of a single BP reading. If ↑ BP is sustained, alter medication. Review in the same way monthly until BP is controlled

Format of the annual review
- Check BP and look for signs of end-organ failure—including annual urine test for proteinuria
- Discuss symptoms and medication
- Assess and treat other modifiable risk factors for CHD/CVA
- Reinforce lifestyle advice

Management of hypertension in pregnancy 📖 p. 826

Referral to cardiology/general medicine *E* = Emergency admission; *U* = Urgent; *S* = Soon; *R* = routine.
- Accelerated hypertension—*E*
- Renal impairment—*U/S/R*
- Suspected secondary hypertension—*U/S/R*
- Patients <40y—*R*
- BP difficult to treat (step 4)—*R*
- Pregnancy—to obstetrician—urgency depends on stage of pregnancy and clinical features—📖 p. 826

Reducing or stopping treatment ↓ BP too far (<120/80) may ↑ morbidity (e.g. as a result of postural hypotension and falls)—particularly in the elderly:
- *Do not* stop medication if high CVD risk or end-organ damage
- If diastolic BP <80 and systolic BP <140 consistently, consider ↓ or stopping medication; 1–2y after withdrawal of medication 50% are normotensive and 40% stay off drug therapy permanently
- Continue BP follow-up life-long even if off medication

Figure 10.3 Choice of antihypertensive drug[N]

> **Beta blockers** β-blockers are not recommended as initial therapy for hypertension. *Exceptions:*
> • Younger women of childbearing potential or
> • Patients with hypertension and evidence of ↑ sympathetic drive, or
> • Patients intolerant of or with contraindications to ACE inhibitors/ARBs
> If initial therapy is with a β-blocker and a second drug is required, add a non-rate-limiting calcium channel blocker to ↓ risk of DM.

Further information

NICE ℰ www.nice.org.uk
• Clinical management of primary hypertension in adults (2011)
• Cardiovascular risk assessment and the modification of blood lipids for the primary and secondary prevention of cardiovascular disease (2008)

Patient information

British Heart Foundation ☎ 0300 330 3311 ℰ www.bhf.org.uk

Hyperlipidaemia

Average cholesterol level in a population is a predictor of CVD risk and dependent on diet but, on an individual level, it is a much poorer predictor—only 42% who develop CVD have ↑ cholesterol. However, lowering LDL and raising HDL ↓ progression of coronary atherosclerosis—whatever the age of the patient—and is a valuable tool for both primary and secondary prevention of CVD.

Cholesterol Fatty substance manufactured by the body (mainly liver) which plays a vital role in functioning of cell membranes. Total plasma cholesterol consists of:
- **LDL (low-density lipoprotein) cholesterol** High levels are associated with ↑ risk CVD
- **HDL (high-density lipoprotein) cholesterol** Low levels are associated with ↑ risk CVD
- **Triglycerides (TGs)** Independent risk factor for CVD. If >5 mmol/L, refer for specialist opinion
- **Ratio of total cholesterol:HDL** Used to predict risk. No threshold—the higher the ratio, the greater the risk. High risk if ≥6

Testing for hyperlipidaemia Blood cholesterol concentration is not steady over time. 1 in 4 ↑ cholesterol levels are normal on repeat testing. Check ≥2 samples at different times:
- **Before initiating treatment or if screening for familial dyslipidaemia** Take fasting samples, checking total cholesterol, LDL cholesterol, HDL cholesterol, and triglycerides
- **Screening and routine follow up** Take non-fasting samples, testing total blood cholesterol and total cholesterol:HDL ratio

Primary prevention In the UK, the NHS provides 5-yearly health checks for those aged 40–74y (💷 p. 242). This includes a lipid profile. There are a number of potential problems with this strategy:
- Those most needing a health check are least likely to attend
- There may be less inclination to eat a healthy diet if cholesterol levels are known to be normal
- Those with ↑ cholesterol levels may assume a sick role

Repeat lipid levels with attention to diet if lipid levels are found to be high on screening. Only treat with statin if lipids remain high despite low cholesterol diet and 10y CVD risk is ≥20%. Continue to offer opportunistic screening to those with other risk factors for CVD or signs of ↑ cholesterol (e.g. corneal arcus <50y, xanthelasma, xanthomata).

Screening for familial hyperlipidaemia Screen first-degree blood relatives aged >18y every 5y with fasting lipids if:
- FH of familial hyperlipidaemia
- FH of premature CVD (men <55y, women <65y) or other atherosclerotic disease

Secondary prevention For all those who have proven CVD, check cholesterol levels annually.

Calculating cardiovascular disease (CVD) risk Always consider ↑ cholesterol in the context of other risk factors for CVD—💷 p. 244.

Secondary hyperlipidaemia Conditions associated with secondary hyperlipidaemia include:

- Drugs:
  - Steroids
  - β-blockers
  - Thiazides
  - COC pill
  - Isotretinoin
  - Antipsychotics
  - Tamoxifen
  - Antiretrovirals
- Obesity
- DM*
- Excess alcohol
- Smoking (lowers HDL)
- Pregnancy
- Hypothyroidism**
- Renal failure
- Nephrotic syndrome
- RA/SLE
- HIV
- Cholestasis
- Cushing's syndrome
- Porphyria
- Myeloma
- Lipodystrophies
- Glycogen storage disease

* Treatment of hyperglycaemia in DM ↓ secondary hyperlipidaemia.

** Patients with hypothyroidism should receive adequate thyroid replacement before assessing need for lipid-lowering treatment. Correction of hypothyroidism may resolve the lipid abnormality, and untreated hypothyroidism ↑ risk of myositis with statins.

Non-drug therapy Offer to all patients with ↑ cholesterol and ↑ CVD risk, and those with DM or FH of CHD/CVD. Reinforce advice with written information.

- ↓ intake of fats to <30% of total energy intake (saturated fats <10%) and ↓ cholesterol intake to <300mg/d. Replace saturated fats with monounsaturated/polyunsaturated fats. If cholesterol level >5mmol/L, low-cholesterol diets result in average ↓ in cholesterol of 8.5% at 3mo
- Eat ≥5 portions of fruit or vegetables/d and ≥2 portions of fish/wk including one of oily fish (maximum two portions of oily fish/wk if pregnant)
- ↓ alcohol intake to <3–4u/d (♂) or <2–3u/d (♀)
- Weight ↓—in patients with BMI ≥30kg/m², weight ↓ of 10kg → 7% ↓ in LDL and 13% ↑ in HDL
- ↑ physical activity—enhances cholesterol-lowering effects of diet and weight ↓. Advise 30min moderate exercise ≥5x/wk
- Stop smoking (📖 p. 182)

❶ Foods enriched with plant sterol/stanol esters inhibit cholesterol absorption from the GI tract and can ↓ serum cholesterol in those on an average diet by 10%. Effect on individuals already on a low-fat diet is less and effect on CVD risk is unknown.

Who should be treated with a statin? Consider statin therapy for:

- **Primary prevention** If ≥20% 10y CVD risk (including adjustments for high-risk ethnic groups and family history), aged >75y or DM (aged >40y or with additional risk factors—📖 p. 354)—start treatment after optimizing lifestyle intervention and treatment of other modifiable risk factors/secondary causes of dyslipidaemia
- **Secondary prevention** If history of CVD—start treatment immediately, irrespective of initial cholesterol levels

Before starting treatment Assess:

- Fasting total cholesterol, LDL cholesterol, HDL cholesterol, and triglycerides (if fasting levels not already available)
- Fasting blood glucose
- Renal function
- Liver function (transaminases)
- TSH if dyslipidaemia is present

Factors to consider before starting a statin

- Statins are contraindicated in pregnancy, breastfeeding, and for those with active liver disease. Transaminases that are ↑ but <3x upper limit of normal are not a contraindication
- Important drug interactions—↑ effect warfarin; ↑ risk myositis when taken with other lipid-lowering drugs, macrolide antibiotics (e.g. erythromycin), calcium channel blockers, or ciclosporin
- Statins are most effective taken in the evening

Primary prevention (except DM)

- Start a low-cost statin, e.g. simvastatin 40mg or atorvastatin 20mg nocte
- There is no target level for total or LDL cholesterol for primary prevention
- Check liver function 3mo and 1y after initiating the statin; do not recheck again unless clinically indicated
- Do not recheck lipid levels
- Review drug therapy at least annually; if statins are not tolerated, consider a fibrate, anion exchange resin, or ezitimibe

Secondary prevention and DM

- Start low-cost statin, e.g. simvastatin 40mg od or atorvastatin 20mg od; if acute coronary syndrome, a higher intensity statin may be used
- Aim to ↓ total cholesterol by 25% or to <4mmol/L—whichever is the lower value—*and* to ↓ LDL cholesterol by 30% or to < 2.0 mmol/L—whichever is the lower value
- Measure total cholesterol (non-fasting) 3mo after starting treatment or after any dose change; if stable measure 6–12 monthly
- Consider ↑ dose of statin if target lipid levels are not met
- Check liver function 3mo and 1y after initiating statin therapy. Do not recheck again unless clinically indicated
- If statins are not tolerated, consider fibrate, anion exchange resin, nicotinic acid (not for DM), or ezetimibe

❶ <50% will achieve total cholesterol <4mmol/L or LDL cholesterol <2mmol/L. Use an 'audit' standard of total cholesterol <5mmol/L.

Benefits of statins[M] NNT to prevent 1 adverse event is:

- Primary prevention—34.5
- Secondary prevention—13.8

For each mmol/L ↓ in LDL

- Major coronary events ↓ 23%
- First stroke ↓ 17%
- CHD death ↓19%
- Overall death rate ↓ 12%

Adverse effects of statins

Myositis The most important adverse effect of statins (11/100,000 person years). Ask patients to report unexplained muscle pain/weakness. If this occurs check CK—if >5x upper limit of normal, withdraw therapy.

Peripheral neuropathy Stop statins and seek specialist advice if unexplained peripheral neuropathy develops (12/100,000 person years).

Abnormal liver function Discontinue if serum transaminase ↑ (and stays at) >3x normal.

⚠ **Simvastatin** In 2010 the MHRA issued a warning about ↑ risk of myopathy with 80mg doses of simvastatin. Consider simvastatin 80mg only if severe hypercholesterolaemia and high risk of cardiovascular complications in patients who have not achieved their treatment goals on lower doses, when benefits outweigh risks.

In August 2012, the MHRA issued a further warning about drug interactions with simvastatin that ↑ the likelihood of myopathy:
- Avoid simvastatin completely when treating patients already taking itraconazole, ketoconazole, posaconazole, erythromycin, clarithromycin, telithromycin, HIV protease inhibitors (e.g. nelfinavir), nefazodone, ciclosporin, danazol, or gemfibrozil
- Do not exceed a simvastatin dose of 10mg daily if taking other fibrates (except fenofibrate)
- Do not exceed a simvastatin dose of 20mg daily if taking amiodarone, amlodipine, verapamil, or diltiazem
- Consider temporarily stopping simvastatin if using fusidic acid
- Advise patients taking simvastatin to avoid drinking grapefruit juice completely

Familial hyperlipidaemia There are many types of familial dyslipidaemia. If suspected, refer. Common forms include:
- **Polygenic hypercholesterolaemia** Most common form of familial dyslipidaemia. Presents with FH of premature CHD + ↑ total cholesterol >6.5mmol/L
- **Familial combined hyperlipidaemia** Polygenic hyperlipidaemia affecting 0.5–1% of the population and ~15% of those suffering MI aged <60y. Associated with obesity, insulin resistance/DM, ↑ BP, xanthelasma, corneal arcus, and premature IHD. ↑ total cholesterol (6.5–10 mmol/L); ↑ TGs (2.3–12 mmol/L)
- **Familial hypercholesterolaemia (type IIa)** Autosomal dominant. The heterozygous form is present in 1 in 500 individuals. Associated with tendon xanthomata and FH of premature IHD. ↑ LDL (>4.9mmol/L); ↑ total cholesterol (>7.5mmol/L); normal TGs
- **Familial hypertriglyceridaemia (type IV/V)** Autosomal dominant. Affects ~1% of the general population and ~5% of those having MI < aged 60y. Associated with DM, obesity, gout, eruptive xanthomas, and pancreatitis. Normal (or slightly ↑) total cholesterol; ↑ TGs (2.3–>10mmol/L)

Referral to cardiology/general medicine *R* = routine.
- Familial hypercholesterolaemia (± referral to genetics)—*R*
- High triglycerides—*R*
- Hypercholesterolaemia resistant to treatment or difficult to treat—*R*

Further information

NICE 🖱 www.nice.org.uk
- Cardiovascular risk assessment and the modification of blood lipids for the primary and secondary prevention of cardiovascular disease (2008)
- Familial hypercholesterolaemia (2008)

SIGN Guideline 97: risk estimation and the prevention of cardiovascular disease (2007 and 2012 review) 🖱 www.sign.ac.uk

Patient information British Heart Foundation ☎ 0300 330 3311 🖱 www.bhf.org.uk

Angina

Affects 8% ♂ and 3% ♀ in the UK. Incidence ↑ with age. Coronary artery disease is the most common cause. Rarer causes include HOCM, valve disease, hypoperfusion during arrhythmia, arteritis, anaemia, or thyrotoxicosis. Mortality (usually sudden death or after acute coronary syndrome or LVF) is ~0.5–4%/y—doubled if coexistent left ventricular dysfunction.

Chest pain of recent onset 📖 p. 1080

Presentation of stable angina Diagnosis is usually made on history:
- **Pain** Episodic central-crushing or band-like chest pain that may radiate → jaw/neck and/or one or both arms. Pain in the arms/neck may be the only symptom. Ask about frequency, severity, duration, and timing
- **Precipitating/relieving factors** Precipitated by exertion, cold, emotion, and/or heavy meals. Pain stops with rest or GTN spray
- **Associated symptoms** Pain may be associated with palpitations, sweating, nausea, and/or breathlessness during attacks
- **Presence of risk factors** Smoking history; family history; history of other vascular disease, e.g. CVA/TIA, peripheral vascular disease

Examination There are usually no physical signs although anaemia may exacerbate symptoms. Check BMI and BP. Look for murmurs (especially ejection systolic murmur of aortic stenosis) and evidence of peripheral vascular disease and carotid bruits (especially in patients with DM).

First-line investigations
- **Blood** FBC, fasting lipid profile, fasting blood glucose. Consider checking ESR (to exclude arteritis) and TFTs if clinical suspicion of thyrotoxicosis
- **12-lead resting ECG** Provides information on rhythm, presence of heart block, previous MI, myocardial hypertrophy, and/or ischaemia

❶ A normal ECG does not exclude coronary artery disease, but an abnormal ECG identifies those at higher risk of cardiac events in the next year—consider referral for further investigation.

Differential diagnosis Chest pain—📖 p. 1080.

Referral of patients with suspected stable angina For patients with new onset intermittent chest pains, refer to a rapid access chest pain clinic for prompt specialist assessment to:
- Confirm/refute angina
- Perform an exercise ECG (📖 p. 238) and/or other investigations as appropriate, and
- Provide information on treatment options available, including the merits of revascularization for the individual

❶ Patients with pre-existing cardiac disease (e.g. previous MI, valve disease, cardiomyopathy) are often excluded from rapid access chest pain clinic referral. Refer to cardiology direct.

Management of patients with stable angina

General advice
- **Information about angina and its treatment**
- **Driving** 📖 p. 131

- **Occupation** May not be able to undertake heavy work—give advice/support. Special rules apply to some occupations, e.g. merchant seamen, airline pilots—advise patients to consult occupational health

Non-drug treatment Aimed at secondary prevention of CHD:
- **Smoking cessation**—📖 p. 182
- **Hypertension** Check BP and treat if >140/90—📖 p. 248
- **Diet** Advise healthy diet (oily fish, low cholesterol, ↑ fruit and vegetables, ↓ salt) and, if obese, aim to ↓ weight until BMI <25kg/m²
- **Alcohol** ↓ excess consumption. *Targets:* <3u/d ♂; <2u/d ♀
- **Exercise** ↑ aerobic exercise within the limits set by the disease state
- **Diabetes** Treat any underlying DM—📖 p. 348–53
- **Cardiac rehabilitation** May be helpful for patients with angina and/or after surgery

Drug treatment 📖 p. 258

Referral to cardiology *E* = Admit; *U* = Urgent; *S* = Soon; *R* = Routine.
- Unstable angina/rapidly progressive symptoms—*E*
- Aortic stenosis with angina—*U*
- Angina following MI—*U/S*
- Abnormal ECG at diagnosis—*U/S*
- Angina not controlled by medication with two drugs—*U/S/R*
- If diagnosis is in doubt—*S/R*
- Strong family history—*R*
- Other factors, e.g. occupation affected—*R*

> **Unstable angina** Pain on minimal or no exertion, pain at rest (may occur at night), or angina which is rapidly worsening in intensity, frequency, or duration. *Incidence:* 6/10,000/y; 15% suffer MI in <1mo.
> **Management** Urgent referral to cardiology. Admit if attacks are severe, occur at rest or last >10min even with GTN spray.

Surgical intervention Consider referral for coronary revascularization with bypass surgery (CABG) or percutaneous intervention (PCI) if symptoms are not controlled with anti-anginal drug intervention (two drugs). Both procedures ↓ symptoms, but CABG confers a survival advantage if DM, age >65y, left anterior descending (LAD) artery disease, or complex 3-vessel disease.

Prinzmetal (variant) angina Angina at rest resulting from coronary artery spasm. ECG shows ST elevation. Refer to cardiology to exclude MI and atherosclerotic angina. GTN alleviates immediate episodes. Calcium channel blockers are used to prevent angina. *M. Prinzmetal (1908–87)—US cardiologist.*

Cardiac syndrome X Ongoing angina symptoms despite normal coronary angiography. Treat with β-blockers and/or calcium channel blockers (if effective) but not secondary prevention agents.

Further information

NICE Management of stable angina (2011) ✆ www.nice.org.uk
Cardiac rehabilitation ✆ www.cardiacrehabilitation.org.uk

Patient information

British Heart Foundation ☏ 0300 330 3311 ✆ www.bhf.org.uk

Drug treatment of angina

Symptom control BNF 2.6

As required medication
- Glyceryl trinitrate (GTN) spray is used for 'as required' symptom relief for angina
- Advise 1–2 puffs as needed in response to pain and before engaging in activities that bring on pain
- Warn about side effects—flushing, headaches, and light-headedness (sit down or find something to hold onto if this occurs)

⚠ If used for chest pain, advise patients to repeat the dose of GTN after 5min if the pain has not gone and to call for an emergency ambulance if the pain has not gone 5min after the second dose.

Regular treatment Drugs for regular symptomatic treatment—see Table 10.6. Within any drug class use the cheapest preparation that the patient can tolerate, will comply with, and which controls symptoms. Assess response every 2–4wk after initiating/changing drug therapy.
- **First-line agent** β-blocker or calcium channel blocker—choice depends on co-morbidites, contraindications, and patient preference
- **If treatment is ineffective/not tolerated** Switch to whichever first-line agent has not been tried and/or combine a β-blocker and dihydropyridine calcium channel blocker

Alternative regular treatments Include long-acting nitrates, ivabradine, nicorandil, and ranolazine. Consider:
- Monotherapy if both first-line agents (β-blockers and calcium channel blockers) are contraindicated or not tolerated
- In combination with a first-line agent if symptoms are not controlled with one first-line agent alone and the other first-line agent is contraindicated or not tolerated
- As a third anti-anginal agent if symptoms are not controlled with two anti-anginal drugs and the person is either not suitable for CABG/PCI or is awaiting CABG/PCI

Secondary prevention

Aspirin ↓ mortality by 34%. Unless contraindicated, give 75mg od to *all* patients with angina. Consider clopidogrel 75mg od if aspirin intolerant.

Statin ↓ in total cholesterol and LDL by 25–35% using statin therapy → ↓ CHD mortality by 25–35%. Trial data suggest *all* patients with proven CHD benefit from ↓ in total cholesterol and LDL irrespective of initial cholesterol concentration—📖 p. 253.

ACE inhibitors Significantly ↓ cardiovascular deaths (RR 0.83) and all-cause mortality (RR 0.87) even in the absence of left ventricular dysfunction.

Further information

NICE Management of stable angina (2011) ℘ www.nice.org.uk

Patient information

British Heart Foundation ☏ 0300 330 3311 ℘ www.bhf.org.uk

Table 10.6 Drug treatment of angina

Drug	Treatment notes
β-blockers *BNF 2.4* ❶ May accumulate in patients with renal failure—↓ dose	Effective for symptom control and to prevent vascular events. Check fully β-blocked by monitoring heart rate—resting heart rate ≤65bpm; post-exercise (e.g. walking up two flights of stairs) heart rate ≤90bpm Further ↑ in dose once adequately β-blocked are usually unhelpful Warn patients not to stop suddenly or run out. If the patient needs to stop the drug, tail off over 4wk In patients with asthma/COPD in whom β-blockade is essential, use cardio-selective β-blockers (e.g. atenolol, bisoprolol, metoprolol, nebivolol) with care In patients with left ventricular failure, start at very low dose and titrate dose over weeks/months
Dihydropyridine calcium channel blockers *BNF 2.6.2*	e.g. amlodipine, felodipine All equally effective in symptom control. No evidence of cardioprotective effect *Contraindications:* vary. Do not use if aortic stenosis, <1mo post-MI or uncontrolled heart failure except with specialist advice
Rate-limiting calcium channel blockers *BNF 2.6.2*	e.g. diltiazem, verapamil *Contraindications:* avoid if heart block or heart failure ⚠ Do not combine with β-blockers
Long-acting nitrates *BNF 2.6.1*	e.g. isosorbide mononitrate (ISMO) Oral and patch preparations (dosages ≥10mg/24h) are available. Start with a low dose and ↑ as tolerated. Side effects are common *Side effects:* headache, postural hypotension, and dizziness—wear off with use. Reflex tachycardia may ↓ coronary blood flow and worsen angina *Tolerance:* many patients rapidly develop tolerance with ↓ therapeutic effect. To avoid this allow a nitrate-free period of 4–8h/d overnight by removing patches at night or giving the 2nd dose of ISMO at 4 p.m. *Contraindications:* HOCM, aortic stenosis, constrictive pericarditis, mitral stenosis, severe anaemia, closed-angle glaucoma
Potassium channel activator *BNF 2.6.3*	e.g. nicorandil Headache is common—usually transitory *Contraindications:* left ventricular failure; hypotension
Ivabradine *BNF 2.6.3*	Lowers the heart rate by its action on the sinus node *Contraindications:* avoid if heart rate <60bpm, heart block, or heart failure
Ranolazine *BNF 2.6.3*	Affects sodium-dependent calcium channels *Contraindications:* renal/liver failure; use with caution if CCF or weight <60kg

After myocardial infarction

Acute coronary syndrome 📖 p. 1082

Modification of risk factors after MI Secondary prevention:

- **Cholesterol** All patients with proven CHD benefit from ↓ in total cholesterol and LDL, irrespective of initial cholesterol concentration. ↓ in total cholesterol and LDL by 25–35% using statin therapy reults in 25–35% ↓ in CHD mortality. Serum cholesterol levels ↓ after MI and remain ↓ for several weeks
- **β-blockers** Unless contraindicated, start all patients on an oral β-blocker (e.g.atenolol) soon after MI and continue indefinitely. Estimated to prevent 12 deaths/1,000 treated/y. If β-blockers are contraindicated, a rate-limiting calcium channel blocker (e.g. diltiazem or verapamil) is an alternative

ACE inhibitors ↓ myocardial work and deaths <1mo post-MI by 5/1,000 treated. Survival advantage is sustained >1y even if treatment is not continued long-term. Effects are greater for patients with heart failure at presentation. *Long-term ACE inhibitors:* trials show ↓ mortality for all patients. If ACE inhibitors are not tolerated, use ARB instead.

Antiplatelet medication

Aspirin Starting aspirin 75mg od <24h after MI prevents 80 vascular events over the next 2y/1,000 patients treated. Unless contraindicated, continue life-long.

Clopidogrel 75mg od—prescribe in addition to aspirin for:
- 12mo if non-ST elevation MI (NSTEMI)/unstable angina
- 1mo following ST elevation MI (STEMI) with no coronary stenting
- 3mo following STEMI with bare metal stenting
- 12mo following STEMI with drug-eluting stenting

Alternatives to clopidogrel In certain circumstances, newer antiplatelet agents (e.g. prasugrel or ticagrelor) may be used in combination with aspirin after ACS.

Anticoagulation Occasionally required if AF, left ventricular aneurysm or if clopidogrel/aspirin are not tolerated.

Heart failure/left ventricular dysfunction For patients who have had an acute MI and have symptoms/signs of heart failure and left ventricular systolic dysfunction (ejection fraction <0.4), treatment with an aldosterone antagonist (e.g. spironolactone 25mg od, increasing in <1mo to 50mg od) should be initiated within 3–14d of the MI, preferably after ACE inhibitor therapy.

Treatment of angina 📖 p. 258

Exercise testing Routine exercise testing (usually before discharge from hospital) identifies those likely to have angina post-MI who might benefit from early angiography ± angioplasty/stenting or CABG.

Cardiac rehabilitation ↓ risk of death by 20–25%. Provided by specialist multidisciplinary teams. *Component include:* psychological support, information about CHD, structured exercise programme, and modification of other risk factors.

GP support after discharge

Return to work Guide:
- Sedentary workers: 4–6wk after uncomplicated MI
- Light manual workers: 6–8wk after uncomplicated MI
- Heavy manual workers: 3mo after uncomplicated MI

Physical activity Advise gradual ↑ in activity. Ensure goals given match those given by local cardiac rehabilitation. Guide:
- Up to 2wk—stroll in garden or street
- From 2–6wk—walk 0.5 mile/d aiming to ↑ to 2 miles/d by 6wk
- From 6wk—↑ speed of walking; aim 2 miles in <30min

Sexual activity Resume after 6wk. A leaflet is available from the British Heart Foundation.

Psychological effects ≈ 50% are depressed 1wk after MI and 25% after 1y. Educate about CHD. Check for depression (📖 p. 199), counsel, and treat as needed.

Driving 📖 p. 131

Flying Most airlines will not carry passengers for 2wk after MI and then only if able to climb 1 flight of stairs without difficulty.

Ongoing GP follow-up

Monitoring health Continue regular reviews at least annually life-long. Check for symptoms and signs of cardiac dysfunction (breathlessness, palpitations, angina); depression; carer stress.

Monitoring drug therapy Ongoing prescription of drugs, monitoring of compliance and side effects, changing medication if clinical circumstances or best practice alter.

Secondary prevention
- **Smoking cessation** 📖 p. 182. ↓ risk of death by 50% over 15y
- **Hypertension** Check BP and treat if >140/90—📖 p. 248
- **Diet** Advise healthy diet (low cholesterol, ↑ fruit and vegetables, ↓ salt) and, if obese, aim to ↓ weight until BMI <25. 🔴 The role of fish oil supplements in ↓ risk of further MI is controversial—recent meta-analysis suggests there is no effect
- **Alcohol** ↓ excess consumption. *Targets:* <3u/d ♂; <2u/d ♀
- **Exercise** ↑ aerobic exercise within the limits set by the disease state
- **Diabetes** Treat any underlying DM—📖 pp. 348–53
- Reinforce information given during cardiac rehabilitation

Dressler syndrome (post-MI syndrome) Develops 2–10wk after MI or heart surgery as a result of autoantibodies to heart muscle. Presents with recurrent fever and chest pain ± pleural and/or pericardial effusion. *Management:* refer urgently for cardiology advice. Treatment is with steroids and NSAIDs. *W. Dressler (1890–1969)—US physician.*

Further information

NICE Myocardial infarction: secondary prevention (2007) 🖥 www.nice.org.uk
Cardiac Rehabilitation 🖥 www.cardiacrehabilitation.org.uk

Patient information

British Heart Foundation ☎ 0300 330 3311 🖥 www.bhf.org.uk

Chronic heart failure

Chronic heart failure occurs when output of the heart is inadequate to meet the needs of the body. It is the end stage of all diseases of the heart. 900,000 people in the UK have heart failure; prevalence ↑ with age.

Acute heart failure 📖 p. 1088

Causes of chronic heart failure

High output The heart is working at normal or ↑ rate but the needs of the body are ↑ beyond that which the heart can supply, e.g. hyperthyroidism, anaemia, Paget's disease, AV malformation.

Low output ↓ heart function. Causes:
- ↑ **pre-load**, e.g. mitral regurgitation, fluid overload
- **Pump failure**
  - Cardiac muscle disease—IHD (46%), cardiomyopathy
  - ↓ expansion of heart and restricted filling—restrictive cardiomyopathy, constrictive pericarditis, tamponade
  - Inadequate heart rate—β-blockers, heart block, post-MI
  - Arrhythmia—AF is the most common
  - ↓ power—negatively inotropic drugs, e.g. verapamil, diltiazem
- **Chronic excessive afterload**↑ BP, aortic stenosis

Presentation Clinical diagnosis is difficult. Take a detailed history and do a clinical examination to exclude other disorders.

Algorithm for diagnosing heart failure See Figure 10.4.

Differential diagnosis

- Obesity
- Respiratory disease
- Venous insufficiency in lower limbs
- Drug-induced ankle swelling (e.g. calcium channel blockers) or fluid retention (e.g. NSAIDs)
- Intrinsic renal or hepatic disease
- Pulmonary embolic disease
- Hypoalbuminaemia
- Depression and/or anxiety
- Bilateral renal artery stenosis
- Intrinsic renal or hepatic disease
- Pulmonary embolic disease
- Severe anaemia
- Thyroid disease
- Bilateral renal artery stenosis

Causes of falsely ↑ natriuretic peptide

- Structural or functional cardiac disease of any cause, including MI
- Baseline is ↑ in ♀ and in those >70y
- Lung disease, including COPD and PE
- Renal impairment
- DM
- Liver failure
- Sepsis

Causes of falsely ↓ natriuretic peptide

- Obesity
- Diuretics
- ACE inhibitors/ARBs
- β-blockers
- Aldosterone antagonists

Classification

- **Left ventricular systolic dysfunction**↓ left ventricular ejection fraction (LVEF) on echocardiography
- **Heart failure with preserved ejection fraction** (HFPEF) Also termed diastolic dysfunction—signs/symptoms of heart failure with normal LVEF on echocardiogram

Other tests to consider To exclude aggravating factors/other causes of symptoms—urinalysis, blood (FBC, U&E, creatinine, eGFR, TFTs, FBG/HbA1c), ECG, CXR, and PEFR/spirometry.

Grading of severity The New York Heart Association (NYHA) classification is widely used:

I   No limitation: ordinary physical exercise does not cause undue fatigue, dyspnoea, or palpitations
II Slight limitation of physical activity: comfortable at rest, but ordinary activity results in fatigue, palpitations, or dyspnoea
III Marked limitation of physical activity: comfortable at rest, but less than ordinary activity results in symptoms
IV Unable to carry out any physical activity without discomfort: symptoms of heart failure are present even at rest with ↑ discomfort with any physical activity

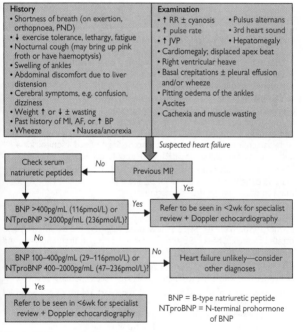

History
• Shortness of breath (on exertion, orthopnoea, PND)
• ↓ exercise tolerance, lethargy, fatigue
• Nocturnal cough (may bring up pink froth or have haemoptysis)
• Swelling of ankles
• Abdominal discomfort due to liver distension
• Cerebral symptoms, e.g. confusion, dizziness
• Weight ↑ or ↓ ± wasting
• Past history of MI, AF, or ↑ BP
• Wheeze   • Nausea/anorexia

Examination
• ↑ RR ± cyanosis   • Pulsus alternans
• ↑ pulse rate   • 3rd heart sound
• ↑ JVP   • Hepatomegaly
• Cardiomegaly; displaced apex beat
• Right ventricular heave
• Basal crepitations ± pleural effusion and/or wheeze
• Pitting oedema of the ankles
• Ascites
• Cachexia and muscle wasting

Suspected heart failure

Previous MI? — No → Check serum natriuretic peptides

Previous MI? — Yes → Refer to be seen in <2wk for specialist review + Doppler echocardiography

BNP >400pg/mL (116pmol/L) or NTproBNP >2000pg/mL (236pmol/L)? — Yes → Refer to be seen in <2wk for specialist review + Doppler echocardiography

No ↓

BNP 100–400pg/mL (29–116pmol/L) or NTproBNP 400–2000pg/mL (47–236pmol/L)? — No → Heart failure unlikely—consider other diagnoses

Yes ↓

Refer to be seen in <6wk for specialist review + Doppler echocardiography

BNP = B-type natriuretic peptide
NTproBNP = N-terminal prohormone of BNP

Figure 10.4 Algorithm for diagnosing heart failure

Further information
NICE Chronic heart failure (2010) ☎ www.nice.org.uk

Patient information
British Heart Foundation ☎ 0300 330 3311 ☎ www.bhf.org.uk

Management of chronic heart failure

❶ Always look for the underlying cause and treat wherever possible. Review the basis for historical diagnosis, and arrange echo to confirm if diagnosis is in doubt.

Regular review Every 6mo or more often, as needed. Check:

- **Clinical state** Functional capacity, fluid status, cardiac rhythm, cognitive and nutritional status
- **Screen for depression** Affects >40%
- **Manage co-morbidities**
- **Medication** Ensure drug record is up to date, review compliance and side effects, change if clinical circumstances/best practice alter
- **Blood** U&E, creatinine, and eGFR

Non-drug measures

- **Educate** About the disease, current/expected symptoms, and need for treatment. Discuss prognosis. Support with written information
- **Discuss ways to make life easier**, e.g. benefits, mobility aids, blue disability parking badge. Consider referral to social services for assessment for services, such as home care
- **Diet** Adequate calories, ↓ salt, ↓ weight if obese, restrict alcohol
- **Lifestyle measures** Smoking cessation (🕮 p. 182); regular exercise
- **Restrict fluid intake** If severe heart failure
- **Vaccination** Pneumococcal and annual influenza vaccination

Diuretics Relieve congestive symptoms/fluid retention in all types of heart failure. Choose a loop diuretic, e.g. furosemide 20–40mg or bumetanide 1–2mg od. Add a thiazide if continued problems with oedema or hypertension. Titrate dose ↑ or ↓ according to need. Monitor for ↓ K⁺ and co-treat with amiloride or K⁺ supplements as needed.

First-line medication for left ventricular systolic dysfunction Start all patients on an ACE inhibitor and a β-blocker. Use clinical judgement to decide which drug to start first.

ACE inhibitors Improve symptoms, ↑ exercise capacity, ↓ progression of disease, ↓ hospital admissions, and ↑ survival in symptomatic and asymptomatic patients. Start at low dose (e.g. ramipril 1.25mg od) and titrate upwards. Check U&E and Cr before starting, at first follow-up, and after each ↑ in dose. Use ARB if not tolerated.

❶ If neither an ACE inhibitor nor ARB is tolerated first-line, combination of hydralazine with a nitrate is an alternative—seek specialist advice.

β-blockers Start a β-blocker licensed for heart failure (e.g. bisoprolol 1.25mg mane) in all those with left ventricular dysfunction regardless of whether symptoms persist. Use in a 'start low, go slow' manner with assessment of pulse, BP, and clinical status after each titration.

Heart failure with preserved ejection fraction (HFPEF) Apart from diuretics, there is no specific treatment for HFPEF. Treat any co-morbidities, e.g. DM, ↑ BP, IHD.

Other drugs to consider

- **Anticoagulation** If heart failure + AF, or history of thromboembolism, left ventricular aneurysm, or intrathoracic thrombus—🕮 p. 672

- **Aspirin** 75–150mg od if heart failure + atherosclerotic arterial disease (including CHD)
- **Statins** Only if other indications—📖 p. 253
- **Amlodipine** Treatment for angina and ↑ BP. ❶ Avoid verapamil, diltiazem, or short-acting dihydropyridine agents

Referral to cardiology (or other suitable specialist) Consider if: (*E* = Emergency admission; *U* = Urgent; *S* = Soon; *R* = Routine)
- Making the initial diagnosis of heart failure—*S/R*
- Heart failure unable to be managed at home—*E*
- Severe heart failure—*U/S*
- Heart failure not controlled by first-line medication—*U/S/R*
- Angina, AF, or other symptomatic arrhythmia—*U/S/R*
- Heart failure due to valve disease or diastolic dysfunction—*R*
- Co-morbidity that may impact on heart failure, e.g. COPD, renal failure, anaemia, thyroid disease, PVD, urinary frequency, gout—*R*
- Woman with heart failure planning pregnancy—*R*

Treatment under specialist supervision

Left ventricular systolic dysfunction Second-line agents that may be started under specialist supervision include:
- Aldosterone antagonists, e.g. spironolactone
- Combination of hydralazine and nitrate
- ARB—used in combination with ACE inhibitor and β-blocker

Digoxin Is anti-arrhythmic and a positive inotrope. It is used for worsening or severe heart failure due to left ventricular systolic dysfunction despite first- and second-line treatment. Only check levels (8–12h after last dose) if suspected toxicity or non-adherence.

Amiodarone May be used to treat arrhythmias associated with heart failure. It requires specialist initiation and close monitoring with TFTs and LFTs at least every 6mo once established on a maintenance dose.

Medical devices
- Implantable cardioverter defibrillator—may be fitted in patients with left ventricular dysfunction and previous episodes of ventricular tachycardia or widened QRS complexes on ECG
- Cardiac resynchronization therapy—considered if severe symptoms on maximal therapy and in sinus rhythm with prolonged QRS complexes

Prognosis Progressive deterioration to death; ~50% die suddenly— probably due to arrhythmias. *Mortality:*
- Mild/moderate heart failure—20–30% 1y mortality
- Severe heart failure—>50% 1y mortality

Palliative care 📖 p. 1028

Further information
NICE Chronic heart failure (2010) ℘ www.nice.org.uk

Patient information
British Heart Foundation ☎ 0300 330 3311 ℘ www.bhf.org.uk

Pulmonary hypertension and cor pulmonale

Normal pulmonary arterial pressure is less than a fifth of that in the systemic circulation. Pulmonary hypertension is defined as pulmonary artery pressure ≥25mmHg. It is classified according to cause:

- **Group 1** Pulmonary arterial hypertension—may be idiopathic or associated with connective tissue disease (mainly scleroderma)
- **Group 2** Left heart disease—severe heart failure (systolic or diastolic), valve disease (e.g. mitral stenosis), congenital heart disease
- **Group 3** Lung disease—COPD, interstitial lung disease
- **Group 4** Chronic thromboembolic pulmonary hypertension—PE, sickle cell disease
- **Group 5** Unclear and multifactorial mechanisms

Cor pulmonale Right heart failure resulting from chronic pulmonary hypertension.

Diagnosis Non-specific symptoms often lead to delayed diagnosis.

Presentation Fatigue and breathlessness on exertion ± angina, palpitations, and pre-syncope. Later, as ventricular failure develops, symptoms include peripheral oedema, ascites, and syncope.

Examination Check for cyanosis, peripheral oedema, ↑ JVP, 4th heart sound, diastolic murmur from pulmonary regurgitation, hepatomegaly ± ascites, crepitations at lung bases ± pleural effusion.

Investigations
- **CXR** Prominent right heart border + enlargement of proximal pulmonary arteries
- **ECG** If abnormal—right axis deviation, tall peaked P-wave in lead II, dominant R-wave in V1, T-wave inversion in anterior leads, *or* RBBB

Management Refer to specialist cardiologist or chest physician.

Specialist investigation
- **Doppler echo** Is used to assess ventricular function and give an estimate of pulmonary arterial pressure
- **Right heart catheterization** and direct measurement of mean pulmonary artery pressure confirms diagnosis, provides information on prognosis, and determines the treatment plan
- **Assessment of functional capacity** The 6min walk test is used to give information about prognosis; <380m at presentation is associated with poor prognosis

Specialist treatment Depending on the underlying cause, treatment is usually through a tertiary specialist centre and includes:
- Oxygen therapy for symptomatic relief
- Diuretic treatment for heart failure
- Vasodilation with calcium channel blockers (in the 10–15% of patients who are responsive)
- Anticoagulation

- Specific drug treatment, and/or
- Surgery

Specific drug treatments for group 1 pulmonary hypertension. Improve symptoms, delay disease progression, and prolong survival. Always initiated in specialist centres:
- Prostanoids, e.g. epoprostenol, iloprost, treprostinil—given IV, sc, or via nebulizer
- Endothelin receptor antagonists, e.g. bosentan, ambrisentan—require monthly monitoring with LFTs
- Phosphodiesterase inhibitors, e.g. sildenafil, tadalafil

Pulmonary endarterectomy Treatment of choice for patients with cardiothromboembolic pulmonary hypertension. The majority can be cured with normalization of pulmonary pressure following surgery (>90% 5y survival).

Bilateral heart/lung transplantation For those who have severe symptoms despite optimal treatment. 5y survival following transplantation is 50–60%.

Further information

British Heart Foundation Factfile Pulmonary hypertension (8/2012) ℘ www.bhf.org.uk

Patient information

Pulmonary Hypertension Association (PHA) UK ☎ 01709 761450 ℘ www.phassociation.uk.com

Tachycardia

Tachycardia is a heart rate >100bpm. It is often felt as palpitations. Tachycardia is common and may be an incidental finding. History and examination can exclude significant problems in most patients.

History Ask about:

- **Palpitations** Duration, frequency and pattern, rhythm (ask the patient to tap it out if not present when seen)
- **Precipitating/relieving factors**
- **Associated symptoms** Chest pain, collapse or funny turns, sweating, breathlessness or hyperventilation
- **Past history**, e.g. previous episodes, heart disease, thyroid disease
- **Lifestyle** Drug history; caffeine/alcohol intake; smoking
- **Occupation** Arrhythmias may affect driving (📖 p. 130) and/or work

⚠ **Red flag symptoms**
- Pre-existing cardiovascular disease
- FH of syncope, arrhythmia, or sudden death
- Arrhythmia associated with falls and/or syncope

Examination

- **General examination** For anaemia, thyrotoxicosis, anxiety, other systemic disease
- **Cardiovascular examination** Heart size, pulse rate and rhythm, JVP, BP, heart sounds and murmurs, evidence of left ventricular failure

Investigations

First-line Resting ECG is all that is needed for many patients.

Further investigations Consider if ECG is abnormal or other concerning features (e.g. syncope, breathlessness, prolonged episodes):

- Blood: TFTs, FBC, ESR/CRP, U&E, FBG/HbA1c, Ca^{2+}, albumin
- Ambulatory ECG or cardiac memo
- Echo if <50y or murmur/heart failure detected
- Exercise tolerance test if exercise-related

Ventricular tachycardia (VT) Broad (>3 small squares) QRS complexes at a rate of >100bpm on ECG. Admit as a 'bluelight' emergency. Meanwhile, give O_2 if available ± 100mg IV lidocaine. If no pulse, treat as VF cardiac arrest (📖 p. 1058).

Recurrent VT May require surgery, insertion of a pacemaker or implantable cardioverter defibrillator.

Ventricular ectopic beats Additional broad QRS complexes, without P-waves, superimposed on regular sinus rhythm. Common and usually of no clinical significance. Rarely may be the presenting feature of viral myocarditis. *Management:*

- **Frequent ectopics (>100/h) on ECG** Urgent cardiology referral
- **R on T phenomenon on ECG** Rarely, ectopics can lead to VF, particularly if they coincide with the T-wave of a preceding beat ('R on T phenomenon'). Admit if this occurs >10x/min on ECG

- **After MI** Ventricular extrasystoles after MI are associated with ↑ mortality—refer to cardiology
- **No sinister features on ECG** Explain benign nature of the condition. Advise avoidance of caffeine, alcohol, smoking, and fatigue. β-blockers can be helpful if unable to tolerate ectopics despite reassurance

Long QT syndrome (LQTS) Heart condition associated with syncope/sudden death due to ventricular arrhythmias, often associated with exercise/excitement. ECG—prolonged QT interval. Genetic form is autosomal dominant or recessive and may be associated with syndactyly or neural deafness. Refer any patient with a family history of sudden cardiac death for specialist assessment. Antenatal screening is possible.

Paroxysmal supraventricular tachycardia (SVT) Narrow QRS complex tachycardia with a regular rate >100bpm on ECG.

Management if seen during an attack
- Get an ECG if possible
- Try carotid sinus massage (unless elderly, IHD, digoxin toxicity, carotid bruit, history of TIAs), the Valsalva manoeuvre, and/or ice on the face (especially effective for children)
- Admit as an emergency if the attack continues

Management if attack terminates or not seen during attack SVT may be diagnosed on 12-lead resting ECG or 24h ECG/cardiac memo. Refer to cardiology for confirmation of diagnosis and initiation of treatment. Urgent referral if chest pain, dizziness, or breathlessness during attacks. Include ECG trace during an attack, if available.

Ongoing care Advise patients to avoid caffeine, alcohol, and smoking. Treatment options are catheter ablation or drug therapy with sotalol, diltiazem, verapamil, or flecainide.

Sinus tachycardia Consider infection, pain, MI, shock, exercise, emotion (including anxiety), heart failure, thyrotoxicosis, drugs.

Atrial fibrillation/flutter 📖 p. 270

No tachycardia and no ECG abnormalities Reassure. Explore the possibility of anxiety disorder (📖 pp. 992–7).

Wolff–Parkinson–White (WPW) syndrome A congenital accessory conduction pathway is present between atrium and ventricle (bundle of Kent). *Clinical features:*
- Predisposes to SVT and AF
- **ECG** Short P-R interval followed by slurred upstroke ('delta wave') into the QRS complex
- **Management** Refer to cardiology. Treatment is with anti-arrhythmics (SVT—verapamil; AF—amiodarone or DC shock) ± ablation of the accessory pathway

L. Wolff (1898–1972) and P.D. White (1886–1973)—US physicians; J. Parkinson (1885–1976)—English physician.

Further information

British Heart Foundation Factfile Palpitations: their significance and investigation (04/2004) 📖 www.bhf.org.uk

Atrial fibrillation

AF is a common disturbance of cardiac rhythm that may be episodic (paroxysmal). Characterized by rapid irregularly irregular narrow QRS complex tachycardia with absence of P-waves. Affects <1% aged <60y but >8% aged >80y. Associated with 5x ↑ risk of stroke (📖 p. 562). *Causes:*

- No cause (isolated AF) ~12%
- ↑ BP (especially if LVH)
- Coronary heart disease
- Cardiomyopathy
- Valvular heart disease (especially mitral valve disease)

Acute AF May be precipitated by acute infection, high alcohol intake, surgery, electrocution, MI, pericarditis, PE, or hyperthyroidism.

Symptoms Often asymptomatic but may cause palpitations, chest pain, stroke/TIA, dyspnoea, fatigue, light-headedness, and/or syncope.

Examination

- **General examination** Check for anaemia, thyrotoxicosis, anxiety, and other systemic disease
- **Cardiovascular examination** Heart size, pulse rate/rhythm (apex rate > radial pulse rate if in AF), JVP, BP, heart sounds/murmurs, LVF

Investigations

- **Routine investigations** Resting ECG, CXR, *Blood:* TFTs, FBC, U&E
- **Further investigations** Ambulatory ECG or cardiac memo if paroxysmal AF; echo if <50y or murmur/heart failure detected; consider exercise tolerance test if exercise-related

Management See Figure 10.5. *Aims to:* relieve symptoms, e.g. palpitations, fatigue, dyspnoea; prevent thromboembolism and ↓ risk of stroke; and maintain cardiac function.

'Pill-in-the-pocket' approach to paroxysmal AF Consider self-medication with a β-blocker prn (e.g. atenolol 50–100mg od) if infrequent symptomatic paroxysms *and* no history of LV dysfunction or valvular/ischaemic heart disease; systolic BP >100mmHg and resting heart rate >70bpm; able to understand when and how to take the medication.

Referral to cardiology E = Emergency admission; U = Urgent; S = Soon; R = Routine.

- Fast rate and compromised by arrhythmia (chest pain, ↓ BP or more than mild heart failure)—*E*
- Candidate for DC or chemical cardioversion—*E/U*
- Uncertainty about diagnosis or treatment—*S/R*
- Symptoms are uncontrolled by standard treatment—*S/R*
- Paroxysmal AF for consideration of sotalol or other anti-arrhythmic drugs when standard β-blockers have failed—*S/R*

Atrial flutter ECG shows regular, sawtooth baseline at rate of 300bpm, with a narrow QRS complex tachycardia superimposed at a rate of 150bpm or 100bpm. Manage in the same way as AF (although specialist drug treatment may differ).

Further information

NICE The management of atrial fibrillation (2006) ℅ www.nice.org.uk

AF

Recent onset (≤7d)?

Yes — No

Treat precipitating causes
e.g. pneumonia, UTI, hyperthyroidism
or
Consider admission for DC or chemical cardioversion if no obvious treatable precipitating cause
or
Admit if fast rate and patient is compromised by the arrhythmia

Address risk factors and treat any underlying illness
↓ excessive alcohol and/or caffeine
Control BP
Treat any thyroid disease
Refer for echo and cardiology assessment if valvular heart disease and/or heart failure

Intermittent?

Yes — No

Paroxysmal AF — Chronic AF

Infrequent, well-tolerated paroxysmal AF, or known precipitants (e.g. caffeine, alcohol) Consider 'no drug treatment' or 'pill-in-the-pocket' strategy. Give patients information and reassure
Frequent symptomatic paroxysms Treat with a β-blocker, e.g. atenolol 50–100mg od. If not controlled, refer for specialist management with flecainide or amiodarone

Anticoagulation
Prevents thromboembolism/CVA
Assess risk and reassess regularly
Warfarin ↓ stroke risk by 60%
Aspirin ↓ stroke risk by 20%
Base decision on which to prescribe on stroke risk and clinical circumstances—Table 16.10 ◻ p. 565

Two treatment approaches
Rhythm control Consider referral/ admission for DC or chemical cardioversion to restore sinus rhythm if:
• Symptomatic or CCF
• Age ≤65y
• First presentation with lone AF
• AF 2° to a treated/corrected precipitant
❶ After treatment, medication (e.g. β-blocker) may be needed to maintain sinus rhythm.

Rate control Consider controlling ventricular rate with a β-blocker (e.g. atenolol 50–100mg od) or rate-limiting calcium channel blocker (e.g. verapamil 40–120mg tds) if:
• Age >65y
• Long duration of AF (>12mo)
• Coronary artery disease
• No CCF
• Structural heart disease which makes AF likely, e.g. mitral stenosis, large left atrium
• History of multiple failed attempts at cardioversion/relapses
• Contraindications to anticoagulation
• Ongoing but reversible cause of AF, e.g. thyrotoxicosis

Aim for a ventricular rate of 60–80bpm at rest and 90–115bpm during moderate exercise. If ineffective during normal activities, combine a β-blocker with digoxin; if ineffective during exercise combine a rate-limiting calcium antagonist with digoxin. If still ineffective/poorly tolerated—refer for consideration of other anti-arrhythmic agents, e.g. sotalol, propafenone, flecainide, or amiodarone.

❶ Consider digoxin as monotherapy for predominantly sedentary patients.

Figure 10.5 Management of AF in primary care[N]

Bradycardia

Heart rate <60 bpm.

Presentation Often an incidental finding but may present with faints or blackouts, drop attacks, dizziness, breathlessness, or lack of energy.

Examination Slow pulse rate; normal/low BP ± evidence of secondary heart failure. There may also be symptoms/signs of associated disease.

Investigations
- **ECG** 12-lead resting ECG; ambulatory ECG may help with diagnosis of intermittent bradycardia (e.g. sick sinus syndrome)
- **Blood** TFTs, FBC, ESR, U&E, LFTs, digoxin levels (if taking digoxin)

Sinus bradycardia Constant bradycardia. P-waves present and P-R interval <0.2s (one large square). *Causes:*

- Physiological, e.g. athletes
- Vasovagal attack
- Drugs, e.g. β-blockers, digoxin
- Inferior MI
- Sick sinus syndrome
- Hypothyroidism
- Hypothermia
- ↑ ICP
- Jaundice

Management Admit acutely if symptomatic. Refer for cardiology opinion if asymptomatic but HR <40bpm despite treatment of reversible causes.

AV node block (heart block) *Causes:*

- IHD
- Drugs (digoxin, verapamil)
- Myocarditis
- Cardiomyopathy
- Fibrosis
- Lyme disease (rare)

Types of heart block
- **1st degree block** Fixed P-R interval >200ms (one large square)
- **2nd degree block**
  - Mobitz type I (Wenckebach)—progressively lengthening P-R interval followed by a dropped beat.
  - Mobitz type II—constant P-R interval with regular dropped beats (e.g. 2:1—every second beat is dropped; consider drug toxicity).
- **3rd degree block** (complete heart block)—P-P intervals are constant and R-R intervals are constant but not related to each other

Management Untreated 2nd and 3rd degree heart block have a mortality of ≈35%. Refer all patients to cardiology, even if asymptomatic. If symptomatic (↓BP <90mmHg systolic, left ventricular failure, heart rate <40bpm), admit as an emergency—give O₂ (if available) whilst awaiting admission.

Stokes Adams attacks Cardiac arrest due to AV block. Results in sudden loss of consciousness ± some limb twitching due to cerebral anoxia. The patient becomes pale and pulseless, but respiration continues. Attacks usually last ~30s although occasionally are fatal. On recovery the patient becomes flushed. Refer to cardiology if suspected. *W. Stokes (1804–1878)—Irish physician and R. Adams (1791–1875)—Irish surgeon.*

Sick sinus syndrome Due to sinus node dysfunction causing brady-cardia ± asystole, sinoatrial block (complete heart block), AF, or SVT alternating with bradycardia (tachy/brady syndrome). Common amongst elderly patients. If symptomatic, heart rate <40bpm, or pauses >3s on ECG refer to cardiology for pacemaker insertion.

Pacemakers Electrically stimulate the heart to beat. *Indications*:
• Symptomatic bradycardia
• 2nd or 3rd degree heart block
• Suppression of resistant tachycardia

Insertion Pacemaker box is attached under the skin of the chest—usually medial to the left axilla under LA. Wires are fed into the great veins of the chest and thus to the heart under X-ray and/or US guidance.

Types Classified according to:
• Chamber paced—atrium, ventricle, or both ('dual')
• Chamber sensed—atrium, ventricle, or both ('dual')
• Mode of response to sensing — inhibited output, triggered, inhibited, and triggered ('dual')

Thus a VVI pacemaker both paces and senses the ventricle in inhibited mode—i.e. if the ventricle beats spontaneously, the pacemaker will not fire.

ECG changes with a pacemaker If the pacemaker is in operation, a pacing 'spike' (vertical line) is seen on ECG.

❶ In devices pacing on demand a spike will not be seen if the natural rate is in excess of the rate set on the pacemaker.

Lifespan Pacemakers last 7–15y. Regular checks are made by pacemaker clinics to ensure the pacemaker remains operational. Reprogramming through the skin is possible. Batteries can be changed via a small surgical procedure under local anaesthetic.

Driving with a pacemaker Inform DVLA and insurance company (📖 p. 130). Stop driving for 1mo after insertion.

⚠ Pacemakers must be removed after death before cremation can occur. A fee is payable.

Further information
NICE Bradycardia: dual chamber pacing (2005) ℘ www.nice.org.uk

Infective endocarditis

⚠ New murmur + fever = endocarditis until proven otherwise.

Infective endocarditis occurs when there is infection of a heart valve (mitral > aortic > tricuspid > pulmonary). The valve may be normal (50%—may be associated with IV drug abuse), rheumatic, degenerative, congenitally abnormal, or prosthetic. Uncommon but consequences may be disastrous and often detected late.

Causes
- **Common organisms** *Strep. viridans* (35–50%); *Staph. aureus* (20%)
- **Non-bacterial causes** SLE, malignancy

Presentation May be acute (acute heart failure) or subacute (course worsening over days/weeks). *Symptoms/signs:*
- **Infective** Fever, weight ↓, night sweats, malaise, lethargy, clubbing, splenomegaly, anaemia, mycotic aneurysms
- **Heart murmurs** ± heart failure
- **Embolic** Stroke, lung abscesses (right heart endocarditis)
- **Vasculitic** Microscopic haematuria, splinter haemorrhages, Osler's nodes (painful lesions on finger pulps), Janeway lesions (palmar macules), Roth's spots (retinal vasculitis), renal failure

High-risk patients Those with:
- Acquired valvular heart disease with stenosis or regurgitation
- Valve replacement
- Structural congenital heart disease, including surgically corrected or palliated structural conditions, but excluding isolated atrial septal defect, fully repaired ventricular septal defect or fully repaired patent ductus arteriosus, and closure devices that are endothelialized
- Hypertrophic cardiomyopathy
- Previous infective endocarditis

When to suspect infective endocarditis[G] Have a high index of suspicion and admit as an emergency for further investigation if:
- Febrile illness and murmur of new valvular regurgitation
- Febrile illness + pre-existing high-risk cardiac lesion and no clinically obvious site of infection
- Febrile illness associated with any of:
  - Predisposition and recent intervention with associated bacteraemia (e.g. dental work or surgical procedure)
  - Evidence of congestive cardiac failure
  - New conduction disturbance
  - Vascular or immunological phenomena, e.g. embolic event, Roth's spots, splinter haemorrhages, Janeway lesions, or Osler's nodes
  - New stroke
  - Peripheral abscesses (renal, splenic, cerebral, vertebral) of unknown cause
- Protracted history of sweats, weight ↓, anorexia or malaise, and at-risk cardiac lesion
- New unexplained embolic event, e.g. CVA, limb ischaemia

Management For patients at ↑ risk, i.e. with valve lesions or prosthetic valves. Admit as an emergency if suspected. Avoid starting antibiotics prior to admission as this might cause delay in diagnosis by rendering the blood cultures sterile.

Investigations in primary care if non-acute presentation
- Blood—non-specific signs of infection, e.g. leukocytosis, ↑ ESR/CRP
- ECG— 10% develop a conduction defect
- CXR

Hospital treatment Once confirmed treatment is with prolonged IV broad-spectrum antibiotics (≥2wk).

Prognosis 80% have major complications during admission, e.g. heart failure. Valve replacement may be required—especially if endocarditis is on a prosthetic valve. 16–27% of those admitted with a diagnosis of infective endocarditis die—those with endocarditis affecting a prosthetic valve have poorer prognosis. Other factors predicting poorer prognosis:
- Infecting organism—*Staph. aureus* 30–40% mortality; streptococci 10% mortality
- ↑ age
- Aortic valve involvement
- Associated heart failure
- CNS complications
- Co-morbidity, e.g. DM

Prevention of infective endocarditis Guidance advises against routine antibiotic prophylaxis because:
- There is no consistent association between having an interventional procedure and development of infective endocarditis
- Regular toothbrushing presents a greater risk of infective endocarditis than a single dental procedure because of repetitive exposure to bacteraemia with oral flora
- Clinical effectiveness of antibiotic prophylaxis is not proven
- Antibiotic prophylaxis against infective endocarditis may lead to a greater number of deaths through fatal anaphylaxis than a strategy of no antibiotic prophylaxis, and is not cost-effective

Advise instead About the:
- Importance of maintaining good oral health
- Symptoms that may indicate infective endocarditis and when to seek expert advice
- The risks of undergoing invasive procedures, including non-medical procedures such as body piercing or tattooing

❶ Do not offer chlorhexidine mouthwash as prophylaxis against infective endocarditis to people at-risk undergoing dental procedures.

Further information

British Society for Antimicrobial Chemotherapy Guidelines for the diagnosis and antibiotic treatment of endocarditis in adults (2012) ℘ www.bsac.org.uk

NICE Prophylaxis against infective endocarditis (2008) ℘ www.nice.org.uk

Rheumatic fever, myocarditis, and pericarditis

Rheumatic fever There has been a dramatic ↓ in incidence of rheumatic fever in industrialized countries since 1950s, but recently numbers of cases have ↑. Rheumatic fever is still an endemic disease in developing countries. *Peak incidence:* age 5–15y.

Cause Rheumatic fever is due to an abnormal immunological response to β-haemolytic streptococcal infection (e.g. 2–4wk after sore throat). Its importance lies in the permanent damage caused to heart valves in some of those affected and subsequent risk of endocarditis.

Diagnosis Can be made if revised Jones criteria are met (see Table 10.7).

Management If suspected refer for specialist care. Specialist management includes: evaluation of heart lesions with echo, bed rest; penicillin; and symptom control (e.g. analgesia, sedatives for chorea). Anti-inflammatory agents such as corticosteroids and aspirin may be used to try to ↓ complications of carditis but their use is controversial.

Prognosis
- 60% develop chronic rheumatic heart disease (70% mitral valve; 40% aortic; 10% tricuspid; 2% pulmonary). Likelihood correlates with severity of initial disease
- Recurrence may occur after further streptococcal infection or be precipitated by pregnancy or combined hormonal contraception

Table 10.7 Revised Jones criteria for diagnosis of rheumatic fever

Requirements for diagnosis of rheumatic fever

Evidence of previous streptococcal infection (scarlet fever, +ve throat swab, and/or ↑ ASO titre >200u/mL)

and

2 major criteria

or

1 major + 2 minor criteria

Major criteria	Minor criteria
Carditis (45–70%)—arrhythmia, new murmur, pericardial rub, heart failure, conduction defects	Prolonged P-R interval on ECG (but not if carditis is one of the major criteria)
Migratory polyarthritis ('flitting' – 75%) red, tender joints	Arthralgia (but not if arthritis is one of the major criteria)
Sydenham's chorea (St Vitus' dance – 10%)	Fever
Subcutaneous nodules (2–20%)	↑ESR or ↑CRP
Erythema marginatum (2–10%)	History of rheumatic heart disease or rheumatic fever

Secondary prevention Penicillin 250mg bd po or sulfadiazine 1g od (500mg od for patients <30kg) for ≥5y to prevent recurrence. Duration of prophylaxis is dependent on whether there was carditis in the initial attack (no carditis—continue for 5y; if cardiac involvement—continue until age 25y or longer).

Acute myocarditis Inflammation of the myocardium. May present in a similar way to MI or with palpitations. *Causes:* viral infection, e.g. Coxsackie virus; diphtheria; rheumatic fever; drugs.

Management Admit for specialist cardiologist care. Treatment is supportive. Some recover spontaneously—others progress to intractable heart failure requiring transplantation.

Pericarditis Sharp, constant sternal pain relieved by sitting forwards. May radiate to left shoulder ± arm or into the abdomen. Worse lying on the left side and on inspiration, swallowing, and coughing. A pericardial rub may be present at the left sternal edge on auscultation. *Causes:*
- Infection, e.g. Coxsackie virus, TB
- Malignancy
- Uraemia
- MI (Dressler's syndrome 🕮 p. 261)
- Trauma
- Radiotherapy
- Connective tissue disease
- Hypothyroidism

Investigations ECG—concave (saddle-shaped) ST elevation in all leads.

Management Refer to cardiology; treat the cause (if possible); symptomatic treatment with NSAID for pain; steroids in resistant cases.

Complications
- **Pericardial effusion** Fluid in the pericardial sac. *Presentation:* heart failure, cardiac tamponade (inability of the heart to dilate in diastole resulting in tachycardia, ↓ BP, ↑ JVP). CXR—large, globular heart. Echo is diagnostic. *Management:* admit for urgent cardiology assessment
- **Constrictive pericarditis** Pericardium becomes fibrosed and non-expansile. Most common cause is TB. *Presentation:* right heart failure, hepatosplenomegaly, ascites, ↓ BP, ↑ JVP. *Management:* refer to cardiologist for confirmation of diagnosis. Treatment involves surgical release of the pericardium

Cardiomyopathy and heart transplant

Cardiomyopathy is primary disease of the heart muscle. Although some cardiomyopathies are 'unclassified' most fall into the following four groups:

Dilated (congestive) cardiomyopathy Prevalence ~35/100,000. ♂ > ♀. Dilation of left ± right ventricle and ↓ contractility. Usually presents with heart failure; may also present with arrhythmia, syncope, peripheral embolism, or abnormalities on ECG/echo. ECG shows non-specific S-T abnormalities; CXR—cardiac enlargement and pulmonary venous hypertension. Echo is diagnostic. *Causes:*

- Idiopathic (50%)
- Familial (20%)
- Cardiovascular—IHD, ↑ BP, congenital heart disease, rheumatic heart disease
- Alcohol
- Infection (Coxsackie virus)
- Endocrine disease—myxoedema, thyrotoxicosis, acromegaly
- Cardiotoxic drugs
- Pregnancy
- Connective tissue disease (SLE, PAN, systemic sclerosis)
- Sarcoidosis
- Amyloidosis
- Haemochromatosis
- Malignancy
- Muscular dystrophy

Management Advise patients to stop drinking alcohol as alcohol may make cardiomyopathy worse. Specialist management is needed in all cases and involves:

- Treatment of heart failure and arrhythmias (may require cardiac resynchronization and/or implantable cardiac defibrillator device)
- Most patients require long-term anticoagulation
- Surgery—cardiomyoplasty or heart transplantation

Mortality 40% in 2y (sudden death, cardiogenic shock).

Hypertrophic cardiomyopathy Familial inheritance (autosomal dominant), though 1 in 2 cases are sporadic—in its most common form causes asymmetrical septal hypertrophy ± aortic outflow obstruction (hypertrophic obstructive cardiomyopathy or HOCM).

Presentation Most cases are diagnosed in childhood (<14y) through echo screening of asymptomatic patients with a FH. *Symptoms/signs:*

- Palpitations—associated with arrhythmias—5% have AF
- Breathlessness on exertion
- Chest pain—may be angina or atypical pain
- Murmur—due to outflow obstruction and/or mitral valve dysfunction
- Faints/collapses

Investigations

- ECG—LVH and ischaemic changes, e.g. T-wave inversion
- CXR—normal until disease is in its late stages
- Echo—diagnostic. Refer if suspicious symptoms or family history

Management and prognosis Ongoing specialist care is essential to provide symptomatic treatment, e.g. β-blockers for chest pain, amiodarone for arrhythmia (digoxin is contraindicated). Implantable cardiac defibrillators improve prognosis for those at high risk of sudden death. Surgical options include alcohol septal ablation and myotomy/myectomy to debulk the septum and relieve obstruction.

Mortality Sudden death is unrelated to severity of symptoms.

Restrictive cardiomyopathy Rare. Stiff ventricle limits filling. Presents with heart failure. Echo is diagnostic. *Causes:* amyloid, sarcoidosis, haemochromatosis. *Management:* specialist management is required. Treatment is symptomatic.

Arrhythmogenic right ventricular cardiomyopathy Rare genetic condition of progressive infiltration of the right ventricular myocardium with fibrofatty tissue. Often asymptomatic until presents with cardiac arrest. Refer any patients with a suspicious family history.

Family history of sudden death Refer first-degree relatives of victims of sudden cardiac death who died aged <40y to cardiology. Antenatal screening for familial cardiomyopathy and LQTS is possible if familial mutation is known. If FH of HOCM and no genetic test:

- Children under <10y—screen with ECG and echo every 3–5y
- Children aged 10–16y—screen every 6–12mo if there is a family history of HOCM; disease is likely to become apparent at this age
- Young people aged 16–20y—screen annually
- >20y—screen every 5y if FH of late-onset hypertrophic cardiomyopathy

❶ Screening intervals are not established for other cardiomyopathies but should be adapted to the pattern of disease within that particular family.

Heart transplantation Considered in patients with estimated 1y survival <50%. *Indications/contraindications*—see Table 10.8.

Assessment Each eligible patient is assessed for psychosocial factors and physical factors (e.g. renal failure, obesity, age, peripheral vascular disease) which affect prognosis before a decision whether to place the patient on the transplant list is made.

Post-operatively Patients require life-long immunosuppression—usually with ciclosporin. Follow-up is undertaken in specialist clinics.

Prognosis 1 in 4 patients die on the transplant list; 60% receive transplant in <2y. Perioperative mortality is <10%; 1y survival 92%; 5y survival 75%; 10y survival 60%. Patients have accelerated graft atherosclerosis. Complications of immunosuppression include ↑ risk of infection and cancer.

Table 10.8 Indications and contraindications for heart transplant

Indications	Contraindications
All patients must have end-stage heart disease. *Causes:*	Systemic disease likely to affect life expectancy (e.g. malignancy)
• IHD (50%)	Active infection (HIV, hepatitis B or C)
• Cardiomyopathy (40%)	Significant pulmonary vascular disease.
• Valvular and congenital heart defects (5%)	Continued excess alcohol consumption
	Significant cerebral/systemic vascular disease

Patient information and support
Cardiomyopathy Association ☎ 0800 018 1024 🖰 www.cardiomyopathy.org
Transplant support network ☎ 0800 027 4490/1
🖰 www.transplantsupportnetwork.org.uk

Valve disease

Heart murmurs 📖 p. 234

⚠ All patients with newly detected valve disease, except those with mitral valve prolapse or aortic sclerosis, require cardiology referral.
- Admit if suspected endocarditis
- Refer urgently/admit if symptomatic valve disease or if valve disease underlies the presenting condition, e.g. heart failure caused by aortic stenosis, AF caused by mitral valve disease

Mitral stenosis Usually due to rheumatic fever.

Presentation
- **Symptoms** Breathlessness, palpitations, fatigue. May result in pulmonary hypertension, which presents with right heart failure, haemoptysis, and/or recurrent bronchitis
- **Signs** Peripheral cyanosis ('malar flush' on cheeks), left parasternal heave, tapping apex beat, AF, rumbling mid-diastolic murmur at the apex

Management Confirm with echo. Refer to cardiology. Treatment is medical (treatment of AF and heart failure, and anticoagulation) ± surgical (valvotomy, balloon valvoplasty, valve replacement).

Mitral regurgitation (incompetence) *Causes:*
- Congenital
- Rheumatic fever
- Mitral valve prolapse
- Ventricular dilatation
- Endocarditis
- Cardiomyopathy
- Ruptured papillary muscle/chordae tendinae following MI
- RA

Presentation
- **Symptoms** Dyspnoea, fatigue
- **Signs** Displaced apex (→ left axilla), pan-systolic murmur at the apex radiating to axilla, AF, left ventricular failure

Management Confirm with echo. Refer to cardiology. Treatment is medical (treatment of AF and heart failure, anticoagulation) ± surgical (valve replacement).

Mitral valve prolapse Prevalence ~1 in 20.

Presentation
- **Symptoms** Usually none. Rarely atypical chest pain, palpitations, syncope, postural hypotension, emboli
- **Signs** Late systolic murmur over apex

Management Confirm with echo. If syncope or palpitations refer to cardiology—a rare complication is ventricular arrhythmia.

Aortic sclerosis Thickening and stiffening of the aortic valve not associated with outflow obstruction that occurs with age. Clinically an ejection systolic murmur is present but no other symptoms or signs. CXR may show a calcified valve. No treatment is required.

Aortic stenosis *Causes:*

- Congenital
- Rheumatic fever
- Bicuspid valve
- Degenerative calcification
- Hypertrophic cardiomyopathy

Presentation
- **Symptoms** Angina, breathlessness, syncope or 'funny turns', dizziness, sudden death
- **Signs** Small volume pulse, low pulse pressure (difference between systolic and diastolic BP), ejection systolic murmur loudest in the aortic area which radiates to carotids and apex

Management Echo is diagnostic and gives an estimate of the gradient across the valve and thus severity of the condition. Refer to cardiology. Surgery (valve replacement or transcutaneous vulvoplasty) is considered for those with syncope or if systolic gradient across the valve is 50mmHg. Avoid treatment with ACE inhibitors.

Aortic regurgitation *Causes:*

- Congenital, e.g. VSD
- Bicuspid aortic valve
- Rheumatic fever
- Aortic dissection
- Endocarditis
- Cardiomyopathy
- Syphilis
- Marfan's or Ehlers–Danlos syndrome

Presentation
- **Symptoms** Dyspnoea, palpitations (extrasystoles)
- **Signs** Prominent pulse ('waterhammer'), wide pulse pressure, visible neck pulsation (Corrigan's sign), head nodding in time with pulse (De Musset's sign), visible capillary pulsations (e.g. in nail bed—Quincke's sign), displaced apex beat, high-pitched early diastolic murmur (easily missed)

Management Confirm with echo. Refer to cardiology for consideration of surgery.

Right heart valve disease Echo is diagnostic. Always requires specialist management.
- **Tricuspid stenosis** Mitral valve disease coexists. *Cause:* rheumatic fever. *Murmur:* early diastolic (left sternal edge in inspiration). Treatment is with diuretics ± surgery (valvotomy or replacement)
- **Tricuspid regurgitation** *Causes:* RV enlargement, endocarditis (IV drug misusers), carcinoid, rheumatic fever, congenital. Presents with oedema, breathlessness, pulsatile hepatomegaly (± jaundice), ascites, pansystolic murmur loudest at left sternal edge. Treatment is with diuretics, vasodilators ± surgery (valve replacement or annuloplasty)
- **Pulmonary stenosis** *Causes:* congenital (Fallot's tetralogy), rheumatic, carcinoid. *Murmur:* ejection systolic murmur (loudest to left of upper sternum, radiating to left shoulder). *ECG:* RVH. *CXR:* dilated pulmonary artery. Treatment (if needed) is with pulmonary valvotomy
- **Pulmonary regurgitation** Due to pulmonary hypertension (📖 p. 266). *Murmur:* decrescendo early diastolic murmur at left sternal edge

⚠ Women planning pregnancy who have known valve disease require review for specialist advice.

Other structural abnormalities of the heart

Coarctation of the aorta Localized narrowing of the descending aorta usually distal to the origin of the left subclavian artery.

Presentation Heart failure, ↑ BP, murmur heard incidentally (ejection systolic murmur over the left side of the chest radiating to the back), lack of femoral pulses or radiofemoral delay. Rarely presentation is with a complication, e.g. subarachnoid haemorrhage or endocarditis. *CXR*—prominent left ventricle. *ECG*—left ventricular hypertrophy.

Management Refer to cardiology—surgery to remove the narrowed portion of the aorta is usually indicated.

Atrial septal defect (ASD) A hole connects the two atria. Holes high in the septum (ostium secundum) are most common (2 in 1,000 live births); holes lower in the septum (ostium primum) are associated with AV valve abnormalities. Blood flows from L → R through the shunt and the right heart takes the burden.

Presentation
- **Ostium secundum defects** Symptoms are rare in infancy and uncommon in childhood. If detected in these groups presents as a murmur (systolic—loudest in the second left interspace) found incidentally, with breathlessness or tiredness on exertion or recurrent chest infections. Presentation is usually in the third or fourth decade with heart failure, pulmonary hypertension, and/or atrial arrhythmias
- **Ostium primum defects** Heart failure commonly develops in infancy/ childhood ± severe pulmonary hypertension. In addition to the ASD murmur, there may be a pansystolic murmur signifying mitral or tricuspid valve regurgitation

Investigation
- **CXR** Cardiomegaly with a prominent right atrium ± pulmonary artery ± pulmonary plethora
- **ECG** Right axis deviation (ostium secundum defect) or left axis deviation (ostium primum defect), RVH ± RBBB
- **Echo** Diagnostic

Management Refer to cardiology. Cardiac surgery to close the defect is usually indicated.

Ventricular septal defect (VSD) A hole connects the 2 ventricles. Blood flows initially from L → R through the hole. May be congenital (2 in 1,000 live births) or acquired (usually septal rupture post-MI).

Acquired VSD Suspect if new pansystolic murmur ± heart failure develop after MI. Investigate as for congenital VSD. Refer to cardiology (speed of referral will depend on state of the patient) for advice on further management.

Congenital VSD

- **Small VSD ('maladie de Roger')** Normally asymptomatic. A thrill may be palpable at lower left sternal border; harsh pansystolic murmur—small holes give loud murmurs. CXR and ECG are normal. Diagnosis is confirmed on echo. Refer to cardiology
- **Moderate VSD** Symptoms usually appear in infancy—breathlessness on feeding/crying, failure to thrive, recurrent chest infections. As the child gets older symptoms improve (relative size of the defect ↓). On examination, there may be cardiomegaly, a thrill palpable at the left sternal edge and a pansystolic murmur. CXR shows cardiomegaly ± prominent pulmonary arteries ± pulmonary plethora. Diagnosis is confirmed on echo. Refer to cardiology
- **Large VSD** Presents with heart failure at ~3mo of age, though there may be symptoms of breathlessness on feeding/crying prior to then. On examination, the baby is obviously unwell—underweight, breathless, pulmonary oedema ± cyanosis, large heart, thrill over left sternal edge ± parasternal heave, murmur (often not pansystolic due to high right ventricular pressures). Admit to paediatrics—medical treatment ± surgery is always needed

Marfan syndrome Autosomal dominant connective tissue disease causing abnormalities of fibrillin (a glycoprotein in elastic fibres). *Features include*:

- Arachnodactyly (long, spidery fingers)
- High-arched palate
- Arm span > height
- Lens dislocation ± unstable iris
- Aortic dilatation (β-blockers appear to slow this)
- Aortic incompetence may occur, e.g. in pregnancy
- Aortic dissection may cause sudden death—echo screening may be helpful for affected individuals

If suspected, refer to cardiology ± genetics. There is currently no antenatal screening test available. *E.J.A. Marfan (1858–1942)—French paediatrician.*

Other congenital heart disease 📖 p. 880

Aneurysms

An arterial aneurysm forms when there is a 50% ↑ in normal diameter of the vessel. Aneurysms may affect any medium/large artery—aorta/iliac arteries > popliteal > femoral > carotid. FH of aneurysm is a risk factor.

Causes Atheroma (most common); injury; infection (e.g. endocarditis, syphilis-mycotic aneurysms).

Abdominal aortic aneurysm (AAA) Prevalence is ~4% in men aged 65–74y (♂:♀≈ 6:1). Acute rupture of AAA in the community has ~90% mortality accounting for 2% of deaths in ♂ aged >65y. Elective surgical repair has ~5–7% mortality.

Risk factors Smoking; ↑ BP; family history (risk ↑ x4–10 if there is an affected first-degree relative).

Factors predisposing to rupture of AAA
- Diameter (risk ↑ with diameter)
- COPD
- Smoking
- ↑ diastolic BP
- FH
- Fast rate of expansion
- Inflammation within the aneurysm wall
- Thrombus-free surface area of aneurysm sac

Presentation Often discovered as an incidental finding on abdominal examination, X-ray (calcification of aneurysm wall in 50% cases) or USS (75% asymptomatic at diagnosis). Otherwise presents with:
- **Local symptoms** Vague abdominal or back pain
- **Distant symptoms** Embolization/acute ischaemia of a limb. Multiple small infarcts (e.g. of toes) with good peripheral pulses suggests an aneurysm proximally
- **Collapse due to rupture** Hypovolaemic shock ± pulsatile abdominal mass ± abdominal or back pain—📖 p. 1074

Investigation USS confirms diagnosis, diameter, site, and extent.

Screening In the UK, all men aged 65y are offered aneurysm screening with a single abdominal USS. Men >65y can self-refer. Screening ↓ death from AAA by 44% over 4y. Possible screening results—see Figure 10.6.

Management of abdominal aortic aneurysm
- **Acute rupture** 📖 p. 1074
- **Elective surgery** Refer if risk of rupture > risk elective repair. The greater the diameter, the more the risk (5.5cm diameter ≈ 10% 1y rupture rate; 10cm diameter >75% 1y rupture rate). AAAs >5.5cm are routinely repaired except if other factors ↑ risk of surgery; there is no survival benefit from treating smaller aneurysms. Refer urgently if symptomatic—may indicate rapid expansion or inflammation, both risk factors for rupture
- **USS surveillance** Patients with AAAs <5.5cm diameter are screened at least annually (see Figure 10.6). Routine repair takes place when and if the aneurysm expands to >5.5cm. 3 in 5 eventually warrant surgery

Inflammatory aneurysms Characterized by inflammatory infiltrate in the aneurysm wall. May be adherent to surrounding structures. *Presentation:* fever, malaise, and abdominal pain. Associated with ↑ mortality at operation.

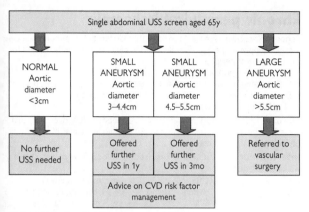

Figure 10.6 Possible AAA screening results

Thoracoabdominal aneurysm Involves thoracic and abdominal aorta—including the origins of the visceral and renal arteries. Surgery is more complex and carries higher mortality.

Dissecting thoracic aortic aneurysm 📖 p. 1074

Popliteal aneurysm 80% peripheral aneurysms. Most are >2cm diameter; 50% are bilateral. Associated with AAA (40%). Presents with acute below-knee ischaemia secondary to aneurysm thrombosis or embolization. Popliteal pulses are pronounced. Diagnosis is confirmed on USS.

Management
• Acute ischaemia—📖 p. 1126
• Elective surgery (popliteal bypass)—when aneurysm >2.5cm diameter

Femoral artery aneurysm *Presentation:* local pressure symptoms, thrombosis, or distal embolization. *Surgical treatment:* bypass surgery.

Carotid artery aneurysm Rare. Presents with pulsatile lateral neck swelling ± carotid territory TIAs. Rarely can rupture. Refer to vascular surgery for surgical treatment.

Carotid body tumour Slow-growing tumour arising in the carotid body at the carotid bifurcation. Presents with a slowly enlarging mass which transmits carotid pulsation. Refer to vascular surgery for angiographic confirmation of diagnosis. Treatment is with surgical excision. If untreated, becomes locally invasive and may eventually metastasize.

Cerebral artery aneurysm 📖 p. 560

Further information

National Screening Aneurysm Screening Programme
🖰 http://aaa.screening.nhs.uk/
British Heart Foundation Factfile Abdominal aortic aneurysms (1/2008)
🖰 www.bhf.org.uk

Patient information and support

Circulation Foundation 🖰 www.circulationfoundation.org.uk

Chronic peripheral ischaemia

Peripheral vascular disease (normally atherosclerotic) commonly affects arteries supplying the legs. *Prevalence:* 20% patients aged >60y. Assess for the presence of peripheral arterial disease if:

- Symptoms suggestive of peripheral arterial disease, *or*
- DM, non-healing wounds on the legs or feet, or unexplained leg pain, *or*
- Being considered for interventions to the leg or foot, or
- Need to use compression hosiery

Natural history Most remain stable. A minority (20% over 10y) progress from intermittent claudication to critical limb ischaemia. Management of CVD risk factors is essential.

Intermittent claudication Restriction of blood flow causes pain on walking. *Risk factors:*

- ♂ > ♀
- ↑ BP
- Physical inactivity
- Smoking
- Hyperlipidaemia
- Hypercoagulable states
- Obesity
- DM
- Post-menopausal

Presentation Presents with muscular, cramp-like pain in the calf, thigh, or buttock on walking that is rapidly relieved on resting. The leg is cool and white, with atrophic skin changes and absent pulses (see Table 10.9):

- **Disease in the superficial femoral artery** Absent popliteal and foot pulses. Causes calf claudication
- **Disease of the aorta or iliac artery** Weak or absent femoral pulse ± femoral bruit. Causes calf, thigh, or buttock claudication

Differential diagnosis Nerve root compression, e.g. sciatica; spinal stenosis—usually bilateral pain which may occur after prolonged standing as well as exercise; not rapidly relieved by rest.

Investigation

- **Blood** FBC, U&E, Cr, eGFR (peripheral vascular disease is associated with renal artery stenosis—📖 p. 443), FBG/HbA1c, lipids
- **Ankle–brachial systolic pressure index (ABPI)** Good history + ABPI <0.95 confirms diagnosis; if good history but normal ABPI (= 1), consider referral for exercise testing*
- **Duplex USS** Used to determine site of disease*

Management

- **Exercise** Offer a supervised programme (ideally 2h/wk for 3mo) to all patients; encourage to exercise to the point of maximal pain
- **↓ risk factors** Patients with claudication have a 3x ↑ risk of death from MI/stroke. Advise to stop smoking, moderate alcohol, and lose weight. Ensure optimum treatment of ↑ BP, lipids, and DM
- **Antiplatelet agents** Treat all patients with aspirin 75mg od (or clopidogrel 75mg od if aspirin-intolerant)
- **Foot care** Regular chiropody

Referral to vascular surgery *E* = Emergency admission; *U* = Urgent; *S* = Soon; *R* = Routine.

- Critical limb ischaemia—*E/U*
- Uncertainty about diagnosis—*R*
- Severe symptoms—*S*
- No better after exercise training—*R*

* May only be available via secondary care referral.

Table 10.9 Location of the pulses of the lower limbs

Pulse	Location
Femoral	Below inguinal ligament; 1/3 of the way up from pubic tubercle
Popliteal	With knee flexed at right angles; palpate deep in the midline
Posterior tibial	1cm behind medial malleolus
Dorsalis pedis	Variable—on the dorsum of the foot just lateral to the tendons to the big toe. ❶ Many healthy people have only 1 foot pulse

Critical limb ischaemia

Presentation Deteriorating claudication and nocturnal rest pain (usually just after fallen asleep—hanging the foot out of bed improves the pain). Ulceration or gangrene results from minor trauma.

Examination Look for:
- Atrophic skin changes—pallor, cool to the touch, hairless, shiny
- On lowering the leg turns a dusky blue-red colour; on elevation— pallor and venous guttering
- Ulceration—check under the heel and between the toes
- Swelling suggests the patient is sleeping in a chair to avoid rest pain or, rarely, pain from deep infection
- Absent foot pulses—if present, consider alternative diagnosis
- ABPI <0.5—❶ arterial calcification can result in falsely high readings

Management Analgesia (often requires opioid); refer for urgent vascular surgical assessment.

The diabetic foot 📖 p. 360

Specialist management of peripheral arterial disease

- **Angiography** To assess extent and position of disease
- **Percutaneous transluminal angioplasty ± stenting** Most suitable for short occlusions/stenoses of the iliac and superficial femoral vessels. 1y patency rate 80–90%
- **Surgery** Most suitable for longer occlusions/multiple stenoses— aortobifemoral bypass grafts have 5y patency rates >90%; femoropopliteal bypass grafting gives 5y patency rates of <70%. Aspirin ↓ risk of re-occlusion. Amputation is a last option

Drug treatment of intermittent claudication
Naftidrofuryl ↑ walking distance but it is unclear whether it influences outcome. Consider only if supervised exercise has not led to improvement and the person does not want or is unsuitable for angioplasty or bypass surgery. Reassess after 3–6mo. Discontinue if no improvement.

Acute limb ischaemia 📖 p. 1126

Further information
NICE Lower limb peripheral arterial disease: diagnosis and management (2012) ✆ www.nice.org.uk

Patient information and support
Circulation Foundation ✆ www.circulationfoundation.org.uk

Varicose veins

Tortuous, twisted, or lengthened veins. *Prevalence:* 17–31%. ♂ > ♀ (≈ 5:4). The vein wall is inherently weak leading to dilatation and separation of the valve cusps so they become incompetent. Blood flows backwards from the deep to superficial venous system, causing back pressure and further dilatation.

Most varicose veins are primary. *Risk factors:* age, parity, occupations requiring a lot of standing, obesity (women only). 2° *causes:* DVT, pelvic tumour, pregnancy, or AV fistula.

Types

- **Trunk** Varicosities of the long or short saphenous vein or their branches. May be symptomatic
- **Reticular** Usually asymptomatic. Dilated tortuous subcutaneous veins not belonging to the main branches of the long or short saphenous vein
- **Telangectasia** Intradermal venules <1 mm—spider veins, thread veins, star bursts, matted veins. Unsightly but otherwise asymptomatic

Presentation *Consider:*

- **Why is the patient consulting now?** Patients are often worried about appearance of varicose veins or prognosis if left untreated but have no other symptoms (1 in 3 consultations)
- **Symptoms** Heaviness, tension, aching (worse on standing and in the evening; improved by elevating the leg and support stockings), itching
- **Complications**
- **PMH** Previous surgery or injection for varicose veins; pregnancy; past history of DVT or thrombophlebitis; CHC or HRT
- **FH** Varicose veins or DVT

Examination

- **Abdominal examination** To exclude secondary causes
- **Veins** With the patient standing, inspect distribution of the veins and any secondary skin changes. Patterns of distribution:
  - *Long saphenous distribution:* thigh and medial aspect of the calf
  - *Short saphenous distribution:* below the knee on the posterior and lateral aspects of the calf

Management Reassurance is often all that is needed.

- **If symptoms are troublesome** Advise support stockings; avoid standing for prolonged periods and if standing do not stand still; walk regularly; ↓ weight (if obese)
- **If any complications or severe symptoms** Refer for vascular surgical assessment. In general, patients with purely cosmetic problems are not treated under the NHS

⚠ Check ABPI to exclude significant arterial disease before recommending compression hosiery (ABPI should be >0.8).

Bleeding varicose veins Bleeding can be stemmed by raising the foot above the level of the heart and applying compression. If the patient is fit for surgery, refer for surgical assessment. Once recovered from the bleed, advise compression hosiery if ABPI >0.8.

Complications

- Haemorrhage
- Varicose eczema
- Skin pigmentation
- Venous ulceration—40% do not have visible varicose veins
- Atrophie blanche—white, lacy scars
- Lipodermatosclerosis—fibrosis of the dermis and subcutis around the ankle, resulting in firm induration

- Thrombophlebitis
- Oedema

CHC and HRT Women with varicose veins taking CHC or HRT are not at ↑ risk of DVT but are at ↑ risk of thrombophlebitis.

Saphena varix Dilatation of the saphenous vein at its confluence with the femoral vein, which transmits a cough impulse. May have bluish tinge and disappears on lying down. A cause of a lump in the groin. Action only needed if symptomatic.

Thrombophlebitis Presents as severe pain, erythema, pigmentation over, and hardening of the vein. Thrombophlebitis in varicose veins results from stasis. Consider underlying malignancy or thrombophilia if thrombophlebitis occurs in normal veins or there is recurrent thrombophlebitis in varicose veins.

Management There is no indication for antibiotics.
- Crepe bandaging to compress vein and minimize propagation of thrombus (if ABPI >0.8)
- Analgesia—preferably NSAID
- Ice packs and elevation
- Low dose aspirin—75–150mg od

⚠ If phlebitis extends up the long saphenous vein towards the saphenofemoral junction, refer for urgent duplex scanning—saphenofemoral ligation may be indicated if thrombus extends into the femoral vein.

Follow-up If the patient is fit for surgery, refer for surgical assessment as thrombophlebitis tends to recur if the underlying venous abnormality is not corrected.

🅿 History of thrombophlebitis is a relative contraindication to CHC (📖 p. 752). Evidence regarding HRT is less clear.

Thrombophlebitis migrans Recurrent tender nodules affecting veins throughout the body. Associated with carcinoma of the pancreas.

Patient information
Circulation Foundation ℡ www.circulationfoundation.org.uk

Deep vein thrombosis

DVT may be proximal—involving veins above the knee—or isolated to the calf veins. It may also occur in the cerebral sinus and veins of the arms, retina, and mesentery. *Incidence:* 1 in 1,000 people/y.

Risk factors

- Age >40y
- Smoking
- Obesity
- Immobility
- Recent long-distance travel
- Pregnancy
- Puerperium
- CHC/HRT use
- Surgery
- Recent trauma
- Malignancy
- Heart failure
- Nephrotic syndrome
- Inflammatory bowel disease
- PMH of venous thromboembolism
- Inherited thrombophilic clotting disorders
- Other chronic illness

❶ Central venous catheters are a common cause of upper limb DVT.

Presentation Unilateral leg pain, swelling, and/or tenderness ± mild fever, pitting oedema, warmth, and distended collateral superficial veins.

Differential diagnosis

- Cellulitis
- Arthritis/muscle tear
- Ruptured Baker's cyst
- Superficial thrombophlebitis
- Chronic venous insufficiency
- Venous obstruction
- Post-thrombotic syndrome
- Acute arterial ischaemia
- Lymphoedema
- Fracture
- Hypoproteinaemia

Immediate action Clinical diagnosis is unreliable. <50% with clinically suspected DVT have diagnosis confirmed on diagnostic imaging. In most areas in the UK, rapid access DVT assessment clinics operate.

⚠ If there will be a delay in investigation to exclude DVT, provide anti-coagulation with low molecular weight heparin (LMWH) in the interim.

Clinical prediction rules (e.g. Wells' score—see Box 10.1) Are used to decide whether patients fall into high or low probability groups for DVT.
- **If low probability** A blood D-dimer test is done. If the D-dimer test is −ve, DVT is excluded. If +ve, the patient is assessed as if medium/high probability
- **If medium/high probability** Compression USS assessment is undertaken ± D-dimer. If USS is negative and low probability or −ve D-dimer, DVT is excluded. If USS is +ve, diagnosis of DVT is confirmed. If USS is −ve and medium/high probability or +ve D-dimer, USS is repeated after 1wk or the patient is assessed with venography, CT, or MRI

D-dimer testing Detects a degradation product of fresh venous thrombus. It may be available as a near-patient test with a result in <15min in some practices—do not delay referral to await result if near-patient testing with rapid result is not available. A normal D-dimer result has a high negative predictive value making DVT unlikely. However raised D-dimer levels are not specific for venous thromboembolism. Other causes of ↑ D-dimer include:
- Malignancy
- Pregnancy
- Wound healing
- Recent trauma
- Inflammation
- Sepsis
- Liver impairment

Management of patients with confirmed DVT

- Initial anticoagulation is with LMWH followed by oral anticoagulation (usually warfarin as an outpatient)
- LMWH should be continued for at least 4d and until INR is in therapeutic range for ≥2d. Target INR 2.5 (range 2–3)
- Oral anticoagulants ↓ risk of further thromboembolism and should be continued for 3–6mo after a single DVT (📖 p. 672)
- Graduated elastic compression stockings—should be worn for >2y as they ↓ risk post-thrombotic leg syndrome by 12–50%

❶ If a patient has a DVT and there is no obvious cause:
- If <45y, consider thrombophilia
- If >45y, consider undiagnosed cancer

Management during pregnancy 📖 p. 824

Complications of DVT

- **Pulmonary embolus** Without treatment 20% with proximal DVT develop PE (📖 p. 1090)
- **Post-thrombotic syndrome** Occurs after DVT. Results in chronic venous hypertension causing limb pain, swelling, hyperpigmentation, dermatitis, ulcers, venous gangrene, and lipodermatosclerosis
- **Recurrent venous thromboembolism** Patients with history of DVT or PE have ↑ risk of recurrence in high-risk situations (trauma, surgery, immobility, pregnancy) and should receive prophylaxis with heparin/oral anticoagulants in such situations

---

Box 10.1 Wells' diagnostic algorithm

Score 1 point if
- Active cancer (ongoing treatment or treatment in the past 6mo, or palliative care)
- Paralysis, paresis, or recent plaster immobilization of the legs
- Recently bedridden for ≥3d or major surgery in the past 12wk (GA or regional anaesthesia)
- Localized tenderness along the distribution of the deep vein system (e.g. back of the calf)
- Entire leg swelling
- Calf diameter of affected leg (measured 10cm below the tibial tuberosity) >3cm greater than that of the unaffected leg
- Pitting oedema of affected, but not unaffected, leg
- Collateral superficial veins (non-varicose)
- Previous DVT

Take away 2 points if an alternative cause is as/more likely than DVT

Interpretation
- If score is <2—DVT is unlikely
- If score is ≥2—DVT is likely

Further information

NICE Venous thromboembolic diseases (2012) ℘ www.nice.org.uk
SIGN Prevention and management of venous thromboembolism (2010) ℘ www.sign.ac.uk

Respiratory medicine

Breathlessness

Dyspnoea Sensation of shortness of breath. Speed of onset helps diagnosis (see Table 11.1). Try to quantify exercise tolerance (e.g. dressing, distance walked, climbing stairs).

Acute breathlessness 📖 p. 1088

Exertional dyspnoea Breathlessness with exercise. Causes are the same as dyspnoea generally. The New York Heart Association classifies four grades of severity:

- **Normal**
- **Moderate** Walking on the level causes breathlessness
- **Severe** Has to stop due to breathlessness when walking on the flat. All but the lightest housework is impossible
- **Gross** Slightest effort → severe breathlessness. The patient is almost bed/chair-bound

Orthopnoea Dyspnoea on lying flat and relieved by sitting up. Associated with left heart dysfunction, e.g. LVF.

Paroxysmal nocturnal dyspnoea Acute form of dyspnoea that causes the patient to awake from sleep. The patient is forced to sit upright or stand out of bed for relief. Associated with pulmonary oedema.

Combined chest pain and dyspnoea Consider:

- MI
- Pericarditis
- Dissecting aneurysm
- PE
- Oesophageal pain
- Musculoskeletal pain
- Chest infection
- Pulmonary malignancy

⚠ Refer any patient with symptoms/signs of superior vena cava obstruction (acute breathlessness, headache worse on stooping, swelling of the face and/or neck with fixed elevation of jugular venous pressure) for immediate medical or oncology assessment[N]. Refer any patient with unexplained dyspnoea of >3wk duration for urgent CXR[N].

Respiratory rate Normal rate for an adult is 14 breaths/min at rest. Higher in children:

- Neonate: 30–60 breaths/min
- Infant: 20–40 breaths/min
- 1–3y: 20–30 breaths/min
- 4–10y: 15–25 breaths/min
- >10y: 15–20 breaths/min

↑ respiratory rate Consider:

- Lung disease, e.g. pneumonia, asthma
- Heart disease, e.g. LVF
- Metabolic disease, e.g. ketoacidosis
- Drugs, e.g. salicylate overdose
- Psychiatric causes, e.g. hyperventilation

↓ respiratory rate Consider:

- CNS disease, e.g. CVA
- Drugs, e.g. opioids

Cheyne–Stokes respiration Breathing becomes progressively deeper and then shallower (± episodic apnoea) in cycles. *Causes:* brainstem lesions/compression (stroke, ↑ ICP); chronic pulmonary oedema; poor cardiac output. It is enhanced by narcotics.

Table 11.1 Causes of dyspnoea

Cause	Acute	Subacute	Chronic
Cardiac disease	Acute LVF Arrhythmia Air hunger due to shock e.g. 2° to MI, dissecting thoracic aneurysm Pericarditis	Arrhythmia Subacute bacterial endocarditis	CCF Mitral stenosis Aortic stenosis Congenital heart disease
Lung disease	Pneumothorax Acute asthma attack PE Acute pneumonitis e.g. inhalation of toxic gas	Asthma Infection Exacerbation of COPD Pleural effusion Pneumonia	COPD Cystic fibrosis Interstitial lung disease Occupational lung disease Mesothelioma Lung cancer
Other	Hyperventilation Foreign body inhalation Guillain–Barré syndrome Altitude sickness Ketoacidosis Polio Musculoskeletal chest pain Oesophageal pain	Aspirin poisoning Myasthenia gravis Thyrotoxicosis	Kyphoscoliosis Anaemia MND MS

Hyperventilation May be fast (>20 breaths/min) or deep (tidal volume ↑). If inappropriate results in palpitations, dizziness, faintness, tinnitus, chest pains, perioral and peripheral tingling (due to plasma Ca^{2+}↓). *Causes include:*

- Anxiety (most common cause)
- Early pulmonary oedema
- PE
- Hyperthyroidism
- Fever
- Lymphangitis
- Weakness of the respiratory muscles

Kussmaul respiration Deep, sighing breathing that is principally seen in metabolic acidosis, e.g. diabetic ketoacidosis and uraemia.

Neurogenic hyperventilation Due to stroke, tumour, or CNS infection.

Hypoventilation Abnormally decreased pulmonary ventilation. Respiration may be too slow or tidal volume ↓. *Causes include:*
- Respiratory depression, e.g. opioid analgesia, anoxia, trauma
- Neurological disease, e.g. Guillain–Barré disease; polio; motor neurone disease; syringobulbia
- Lung disease, e.g. pneumonia, collapse, pneumothorax, pleural effusion
- Respiratory muscle disease, e.g. myasthenia gravis, dermatomyositis
- Limited chest movement, e.g. kyphoscoliosis

Pneumothorax 📖 p. 1090

Further information
NICE Referral guidelines for suspected cancer (2005) ℘ www.nice.org.uk

Cough

A cough is a reaction to irritation anywhere from pharynx to lungs.

Acute cough (<3wk) *Causes:*

- URTI
- Croup
- Tracheitis
- Acute bronchitis
- Pneumonia—productive, loose cough
- Acute exacerbation of normally well-controlled asthma
- Inhaled foreign body—especially in well children

Reserve CXR for patients with marked focal chest signs or where inhalation of foreign body or lung cancer is suspected.

Management Treat the cause where possible; advise OTC cough mixture as needed, e.g. simple linctus; steam inhalation often eases symptoms temporarily; review if not clearing.

Reasons to prescribe antibiotics immediately[N] Investigate further and/or give antibiotics immediately (e.g. amoxicillin 500mg tds/clarithromycin 500mg bd/doxycycline 100mg od) if the patient:

- Is systemically very unwell or has symptoms/signs suggestive of serious illness and/or complications, e.g. pneumonia
- Is at high risk of serious complications because of pre-existing co-morbidity, e.g. significant heart, lung, renal, liver, or neuromuscular disease, immunosuppression, CF, and young children born prematurely
- Is aged >65y with acute cough and ≥2 or more of the following, or aged >80y with acute cough and ≥1 of the following:

- Hospitalization in the previous year
- Type 1 or type 2 DM
- History of congestive heart failure
- Current use of oral glucocorticoids

Chronic cough (>3wk) *Causes:*

- Post-nasal drip
- Post-viral
- COPD/asthma
- Lung cancer
- Pertussis
- TB
- Bronchiectasis
- Pulmonary oedema
- Foreign body
- Vocal cord palsy
- GORD
- LVF
- Drug-induced (e.g. ACE inhibitors)
- Smokers' cough
- Idiopathic
- Ear wax
- Psychogenic

⚠ *Red flags* Weight ↓, night sweats.

Management Refer any patient with a persistent cough for >3wk for urgent CXR[N]. Treat the cause. If no cause is found, refer.

Sputum

- Absolutely clear sputum is probably saliva
- Smoking is the leading cause of excess sputum production—look for black specks of inhaled carbon
- Yellow-green sputum is due to cell debris (bronchial epithelium, neutrophils, eosinophils) and is not always infected
- Bronchiectasis causes copious greenish sputum
- Bloodstained sputum (haemoptysis) always needs full investigation
- Pink froth suggests pulmonary oedema

Haemoptysis Expectoration of blood/bloodstained sputum. *Causes:*

- Infection—bronchitis, pneumonia, lung abscess, TB
- Violent coughing
- Bronchiectasis
- Lung cancer
- PE (blood is not mixed with sputum)
- Inhaled foreign body
- Iatrogenic: anticoagulation, endotracheal tube
- Trauma
- Cardiac: acute LVF, mitral stenosis
- Blood dyscrasia/bleeding diathesis
- Idiopathic pulmonary haemosiderosis
- Bronchial adenoma
- Mycosis, e.g. aspergilloma
- Goodpasture's syndrome
- Collagen vascular disease, e.g. PAN, Wegener's granulomatosis
- Unknown

❶ Differentiate from haematemesis or local bleeding from the nasopharynx or sinuses. Melaena may occur if enough blood is swallowed.

Management Always requires investigation to find the cause.
- Admit as an acute medical emergency if the patient is compromised by the bleeding (i.e. tachycardia, low BP, postural drop) or has symptoms/ signs of a cause requiring acute admission (e.g. PE, acute LVF)
- If not compromised by the bleeding, refer for urgent CXR[N]
- Refer for urgent chest physician assessment if abnormal CXR, persistent haemoptysis with normal CXR, aged >40y and smoker/ ex-smoker, or normal CXR but high suspicion of lung cancer[N]

❶ In patients with lung cancer who have a massive haemoptysis, consider whether it is a terminal event. If so, consider treating with IV morphine/diamorphine and a sedative (e.g. midazolam or rectal diazepam) rather than admitting.

Bronchiectasis Consider in any patient with persistent or recurrent chest infections. Permanently dilated bronchi act as sumps for infected mucus. *Causes:*
- **Congenital** CF, Kartagener syndrome
- **Post-infection** TB, pertussis, measles, pneumonia
- **Other** Bronchial obstruction, aspergillosis (📖 p. 328), hypogammaglobulinaemia (📖 p. 684), gastric aspiration

Presentation
- **Mild cases** Asymptomatic with winter exacerbations consisting of fever, cough, purulent sputum, pleuritic chest pain, dyspnoea
- **More severe cases** Persistent cough and sputum, haemoptysis, clubbing, low-pitched inspiratory and expiratory crackles, and wheeze

Investigations CXR; sputum—M,C&S; spirometry—reversible airways obstruction is common; high-resolution CT detects disease in 97% cases.

Management Refer to a respiratory physician. Treatment includes physiotherapy, antibiotics, bronchodilators, vaccination (influenza and pneumococcal), and (rarely) surgery.

Further information

NICE ☞ www.nice.org.uk
- Referral guidelines for suspected cancer (2005)
- Respiratory tract infections—antibiotic prescribing (2008)

Chest signs

Chest deformity
- **Barrel chest** The antero-posterior diameter of the chest is high compared to the lateral diameter, and expansion is ↓. Ribs move in a pump handle, up-and-down motion. Associated with chronic hyperinflation (e.g. asthma or COPD)
- **Pigeon chest (pectus carinatum)** Prominent sternum and flat chest associated with history of chronic childhood asthma or rickets
- **Funnel chest (pectus excavatum)** The lower end of sternum is depressed. Often inherited or idiopathic and usually harmless
- **Kyphosis** ↑ forward spinal convexity usually affecting thoracic spine
  - *Postural* ('drooping shoulders' or 'roundback'): is common and voluntarily correctable
  - *Structural:* cannot correct voluntarily. *Causes:* osteoporosis, Paget's disease, ankylosing spondylitis, Scheuermann's disease. May cause a restrictive ventilatory defect and eventually respiratory failure
- **Scoliosis** 📖 p. 478
- **Harrison's sulcus** Groove deformity of the lower ribs at the diaphragm attachment site. Suggests chronic childhood asthma or rickets
- **Scars** Are there any scars indicative of previous chest surgery?

Chest expansion Expansion should be symmetrical and equal. If not suspect chest pathology (e.g. consolidation, collapse, pneumothorax, effusion—see Table 11.2) on the side with ↓ movement.

Vocal fremitus or resonance
- **↑ transmission** Implies consolidation. Even whispered sounds are heard clearly with a stethoscope (*whispering pectoriloquy*)
- **↓ transmission** Implies something in the way blocking the transmission of sound. *Consider:* air (e.g. pneumothorax), fluid (e.g. effusion), pleural thickening (e.g. mesothelioma)

Percussion Define any areas of dullness to percussion by percussing from a resonant to dull area. *Interpretation:*
- ↑ resonance—emphysema or pneumothorax (📖 p. 1090)
- ↓ resonance—consolidation, collapse, abscess, tumour, fibrosis
- Stony dullness—pleural effusion

Breath sounds Assess character of breath sounds and added sounds:
- **Bronchial breathing** Breath sounds are harsher than normal and there is an audible gap between inspiration and expiration—often caused by lung consolidation, e.g. due to pneumonia
- **↓ breath sounds** *Consider:* pleural effusion, pneumothorax, emphysema, lung collapse
- **Added sounds** Pleural rub; wheeze; crepitations/crackles

Wheeze Musical sound heard during expiration.
- **Polyphonic wheeze** Indicates narrowing of many small airways—typical of asthma or COPD
- **Monophonic wheeze** Indicates single large airway obstruction, e.g. due to foreign body or tumour

Crackles in the chest Produced by airflow moving secretions.
- **Fine crackles** Consider pulmonary oedema (early inspiratory—usually best heard at the lung bases at the back); early pneumonia; fibrosing alveolitis (late inspiratory)
- **Coarse crackles** Consider TB; resolving pneumonia; bronchiectasis; lung abscess

Pleural rub Creaking sound produced by movement of visceral over parietal pleura when both are inflamed (e.g. pneumonia, infarction).

Pleural effusion Fluid in the pleural cavity. Simple effusions may be transudates (<30g/L protein) or exudates (>30g/L protein). Effusions may also be blood, lymph, or pus (empyema). *Causes of simple effusion:*

- Malignancy, e.g. lung cancer, mesothelioma, Meig's syndrome
- Infection (e.g pneumonia, TB)
- Infarction (PE)
- Heart failure
- Constrictive pericarditis
- Inflammation (SLE, RA, pancreatitis, asbestos exposure)
- Hypoproteinaemia
- Hypothyroidism

Presentation May be incidental finding on CXR. *Symptoms:* dyspnoea, pleuritic pain, symptoms of underlying cause. *Signs:* absent breath sounds, dullness to percussion, ↓ tactile vocal fremitus, ↓ vocal resonance. Above the effusion, there is usually a zone of bronchial breathing. Early on there may be a pleural rub. Large effusions shift the mediastinum away from the affected side and there may be ↓ chest wall movement. Confirm with CXR. If cause is not immediately apparent refer for diagnostic tap.

Management Treat the underlying cause. Refer for drainage if symptomatic. Repeated drainage ± pleurodesis may be necessary.

Surgical emphysema Air in the subcutaneous tissue. Can be caused by spontaneous pneumothorax or trauma to the chest wall. Tissues appear swollen and crackle on palpation

Table 11.2 Chest signs associated with common chest pathology

	Consolidation, e.g. pneumonia	Pleural effusion	Collapsed lung	Pneumothorax
Mediastinum	Not displaced	Normal or displaced away from the effusion	Displaced towards the side of collapse	Displaced away from the side of pneumothorax
Expansion	↓	↓	↓	↓
Percussion	Dull	Stony dull	Dull	Hyperresonant
Breath sounds	Bronchial breathing	↓	↓	↓
Added sounds	Crackles ± rub	Bronchial breathing above effusion	None	None
Other	↑ vocal resonance, whispering pectoriloquy	↓ vocal resonance		↓ vocal resonance

⚠ Refer all patients with unexplained chest signs lasting >3wk for urgent CXR[N].

Other signs of respiratory disease

Weight loss Non-specific symptom or sign. *Consider:*
- **GI causes** Malabsorption, malnutrition, dieting
- **Chronic disease** Hyperthyroidism, DM, COPD, heart failure, renal disease, degenerative neurological/muscle disease, chronic infection (e.g. TB, HIV)
- **Malignancy**
- **Psychiatric causes** Depression, dementia, anorexia

⚠ Refer any patient with unexplained weight loss for urgent CXR[N].

Cachexia Severe generalized muscle wasting. *Causes:* neoplasia, malnutrition, chronic infection (e.g. TB), prolonged inactivity, dementia.

Night sweats *Consider:* TB, lymphoma, leukaemia, solid tumour (e.g. renal carcinoma), menopause, anxiety states.

Erythema nodosum 🕮 p. 600

Peripheral oedema 🕮 p. 232

Horner's syndrome Sympathetic nerve disruption to the iris causes:
- Small (miotic) pupil with lack of pupil dilation in the dark
- Partial lid ptosis
- Anhidrosis of the forehead, *and*
- Enophthalmos

Causes
- Pancoast, cervical cord or mediastinal tumour
- Aortic aneurysm
- Posterior inferior artery or basilar artery occlusion
- Hypothalamic lesion
- Syringomyelia

J. F. Horner (1831–1886), Swiss ophthalmologist.

Pallor Check eyes/mucous membranes for pallor suggesting anaemia.

Cyanosis 🕮 p. 232

Flapping tremor/asterixis Bilateral motor disturbance. Ask the patient to hold his hands straight out in front of him and dorsiflex his hands—this provokes a flapping, asynchronous tremor which is absent at rest. Due to CO_2 retention in severe COPD.

Lymphadenopathy 🕮 p. 938

⚠ Refer any patient with supraclavicular or cervical lymphadenopathy persisting >3wk for urgent CXR[N].

⚠ Refer any unexplained lump in the neck of recent onset, or any previously undiagnosed neck lump that has changed over a period of 3–6wk, for urgent further investigation[N].

Clubbing 📖 p. 605

⚠ Refer any patient with unexplained nail clubbing for urgent CXR[N].

Yellow nails 📖 p. 604

Hoarseness 📖 p. 936

⚠ *Refer urgently for chest X-ray (CXR)*[N] ALL patients with hoarseness for >3wk—particularly smokers aged >50y and heavy drinkers.
• **If there is a POSITIVE finding on CXR** Refer urgently to a team specializing in the management of lung cancer
• **If there is a NEGATIVE finding on CXR** Refer urgently to a team specializing in the management of head and neck cancer

Stridor 📖 p. 937

Jugular venous pressure 📖 p. 233

The trachea
• Palpate the trachea in the supraclavicular notch in the midline
• Deviation to the left or right suggests a shift of the upper mediastinum to that side
• The distance between the suprasternal notch and cricoid cartilage in an adult is 2–3 finger breadths. If it is less than this, the lungs are probably hyperinflated

Further information
NICE Referral guidelines for suspected cancer (2005) 🔗 www.nice.org.uk

Respiratory investigations

Indications for urgent CXR[N]
- Haemoptysis
- Any of the following if unexplained or present for more >3wk:
  - Cough
  - Chest/shoulder pain
  - Dyspnoea
  - Cervical/supraclavicular lymphadenopathy
  - Signs suggesting metastases (brain, bone, liver, skin)
  - Weight loss
  - Chest signs
  - Hoarseness
  - Finger clubbing

Peak flow A simple and cheap test. Peak flow is not a good measure of airflow limitation as it tends to overestimate lung function. It is best used to monitor progress of disease and effects of treatment for patients with asthma. Link with self-management plan (📖 p. 310). Peak flow meters are available on NHS. Peak flow charts are available from NHS supplies (form FP1010) and drug companies.

Measuring peak expiratory flow rate (PEFR)
- Ask the patient to stand up (if possible) and hold the peak flow meter horizontally. Check the indicator is at zero and the track clear
- Ask the patient to take a deep breath in and blow out forcefully into the meter ensuring lips are sealed firmly around the mouthpiece
- Read the PEFR off the meter. The best of three attempts is recorded
- Consider using a low range meter if predicted or best PEFR is <250L/min
- Normal values—see Table 11.4 (📖 p. 304)

Spirometry Measures the volume of air the patient (adult or child >5y) is able to expel from the lungs after a maximal inspiration (see Table 11.3).
- **FEV_1** Volume of air the patient is able to exhale in the first second of forced expiration
- **FVC** Total volume of air the patient can forcibly exhale in one breath
- **FEV_1/FVC** Ratio of FEV_1 to FVC expressed as a %

Measuring FEV_1 and FVC Sit the patient comfortably, then:
- Ask the patient to take a deep breath in
- Ask the patient to blow the whole breath out as hard as possible until there is no breath left to expel and ensuring lips are sealed firmly around the mouthpiece; encourage the patient to keep breathing out
- Repeat the procedure twice (i.e. three attempts in all)
- At least two readings should be within 100mL or 5% of each other
- Normal values—see Table 11.5 (📖 p. 305)

Flow volume measurement Available with some spirometers—see Figure 11.1.

Fractional exhaled nitric oxide concentration Exhaled nitric oxide concentration is ↑ in patients with asthma or other inflammatory respiratory conditions. Measurement of exhaled nitric oxide (usually with hand-held monitor) can be a useful test to support a diagnosis of asthma or assess response to treatment. A normal result does not exclude a diagnosis of asthma.

RCP three questions Useful tool to identify patients with poor asthma control in general practice and monitor effect of changes of treatment. Morbidity categories correlate with lung function.

In the last month
- Have you had any difficulty sleeping because of your asthma symptoms (including cough)?
- Have you had your usual asthma symptoms during the day (cough, wheeze, chest tightness, or breathlessness)?
- Has your asthma interfered with your usual activities, e.g. housework, work/school etc.?

NO to all questions = low morbidity.
1x YES answer = medium morbidity.
2 or 3x YES answers = high morbidity.

❶ Alternatives include the Asthma Control Questionnaire (ACQ) and Asthma Control Test (ACT)/Children's Asthma Control Test. These questionnaires are not designed for use during an acute attack.

Further information
NICE Referral guidelines for suspected cancer (2005) ℘ www.nice.org.uk

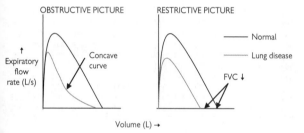

Volume (L) →

Figure 11.1 Flow volume curves for patients with restrictive and obstructive lung disease

Table 11.3 Interpretation of spirometry results

	Restrictive lung disease, e.g. interstitial lung disease	Obstructive lung disease, e.g. COPD
FEV₁ (% of predicted normal)	↓(<80%)	↓(<80%)
FVC (% of predicted normal)	↓(<80%)	Normal or ↓
FEV₁/FVC	Normal (>70%)	↓(<70%)

British Thoracic Society (BTS) Spirometry in practice: a practical guide to using spirometry in primary care (2005). Available from:
℘ www.brit-thoracic.org.uk
ARTP/BTS Certificate in spirometry—further details and list of approved training centres is available from ☎ 0121 354 8200

Table 11.4 Predicted PEFR measurements in L/min (EU scale)

Children Height is the only determinant of PEFR in children. With ↑ age, the pattern of adult values takes over.

Height: ft	3'	3'4"	3'8"	4'	4'4"	4'8"	5'	5'4"	5'8"	6'
m	90 cm	1	1.1	1.2	1.3	1.4	1.5	1.6	1.7	1.8
PEFR L/min	88	105	136	172	220	265	313	371	427	487

Women
Height: →

"	4'10"	4'11"	5'	5'1"	5'2"	5'3"	5'4"	5'5"	5'6"	5'7"	5'8"	5'9"	5'10"
m	1.47	1.5	1.52	1.55	1.57	1.6	1.62	1.65	1.67	1.7	1.72	1.75	1.77
Age													
15y	379	382	385	389	391	394	397	400	402	405	407	411	413
20y	402	406	409	413	416	419	422	425	428	431	434	437	439
25y	415	419	422	426	429	433	435	439	441	445	447	451	453
30y	419	424	427	431	433	437	440	444	446	450	452	456	458
35y	418	423	425	430	432	436	439	443	445	449	451	454	457
40y	413	417	420	424	427	431	433	437	439	443	445	449	451
45y	405	409	412	416	418	422	425	428	431	434	436	440	442
50y	394	399	401	405	407	411	414	417	419	423	425	428	430
55y	383	387	389	393	395	399	401	404	407	410	412	415	417
60y	370	373	376	379	382	385	387	391	393	396	398	401	403
65y	356	360	362	366	368	371	373	376	378	381	383	386	388
70y	343	346	348	351	353	356	358	361	363	366	368	371	372

Men
Height: →

"	5'2"	5'3"	5'4"	5'5"	5'6"	5'7"	5'8"	5'9"	5'10"	5'11"	6'	6'1"	6'2"
m	1.57	1.6	1.62	1.65	1.67	1.7	1.72	1.75	1.77	1.8	1.82	1.85	1.87
Age													
15y	479	485	489	494	498	503	506	511	515	520	523	528	531
20y	534	540	545	551	555	561	565	571	575	580	584	589	593
25y	568	575	580	587	591	598	602	608	612	618	622	628	632
30y	587	594	599	606	611	617	622	628	633	639	643	649	653
35y	594	601	606	613	618	625	629	636	640	646	650	657	661
40y	592	599	604	611	615	622	627	633	637	644	648	654	658
45y	582	590	594	601	606	612	617	623	627	634	638	644	647
50y	568	575	580	586	591	597	601	608	612	618	622	627	631
55y	550	557	561	568	572	578	582	588	592	598	602	607	611
60y	529	536	540	546	550	556	560	566	570	575	579	584	588
65y	507	513	517	523	527	533	536	542	545	551	554	559	562
70y	484	490	493	499	503	508	511	517	520	525	528	533	536

❶ For normal values in age groups/heights not represented on these charts or for conversion from the old Wright scale peak flow meters see ♒ www.peakflow.com

PEFR charts adapted from: Gregg I., Nunn AJ, *BMJ* 1989; 298: 1068–70 and Godfrey S, *et al.* Brit. J. Dis. Chest 1970;64:15

Table 11.5 Predicted FEV$_1$ and FVC measurements (L)

🅞 These values apply for Caucasians. ↓ values by 7% for Asians and 13% for people of Afro-Caribbean origin.

Women

Height ft		4'11"	5'1"	5'3"	5'5"	5'7"	5'9"	5'11"
	m	1.5	1.55	1.6	1.65	1.7	1.75	1.8
Age								
38–41y	FEV$_1$	2.3	2.5	2.7	2.89	3.09	3.29	3.49
	FVC	2.69	2.91	3.13	3.35	3.58	3.80	4.02
42–45y	FEV$_1$	2.2	2.4	2.6	2.79	2.99	3.19	3.39
	FVC	2.59	2.81	3.03	3.25	3.47	3.69	3.91
46–49y	FEV$_1$	2.1	2.3	2.5	2.69	2.89	3.09	3.29
	FVC	2.48	2.7	2.92	3.15	3.37	3.59	3.81
50–53y	FEV$_1$	2	2.2	2.4	2.59	2.79	2.99	3.19
	FVC	2.38	2.6	2.82	3.04	3.26	3.48	3.71
54–57y	FEV$_1$	1.9	2.1	2.3	2.49	2.69	2.89	3.09
	FVC	2.27	2.49	2.72	2.94	3.16	3.38	3.6
58–61y	FEV$_1$	1.8	2	2.2	2.39	2.59	2.79	2.99
	FVC	2.17	2.39	2.61	2.83	3.06	3.28	3.5
62–65y	FEV$_1$	1.7	1.9	2.1	2.29	2.49	2.69	2.89
	FVC	2.07	2.29	2.51	2.73	2.95	3.17	3.39
66–69y	FEV$_1$	1.6	1.8	2	2.19	2.39	2.59	2.79
	FVC	1.96	2.18	2.4	2.63	2.85	3.07	3.29

For women ≥70y, use the formulae:
- FEV$_1$ = (0.0395 × height in m × 100) − (0.025 × age in y) − 2.6
- FVC = (0.0443 × height in m × 100) − (0.026 × age in y) − 2.89

Men

Height ft		5'3"	5'5"	5'7"	5'9"	5'11"	6'1"	6'3"
	m	1.6	1.65	1.7	1.75	1.8	1.85	1.9
Age								
38–41y	FEV$_1$	3.2	3.42	3.63	3.85	4.06	4.28	4.49
	FVC	3.81	4.1	4.39	4.67	4.96	5.25	5.54
42–45y	FEV$_1$	3.09	3.3	3.52	3.73	3.95	4.16	4.38
	FVC	3.71	3.99	4.28	4.57	4.86	5.15	5.43
46–49y	FEV$_1$	2.97	3.18	3.4	3.61	3.83	4.04	4.26
	FVC	3.6	3.89	4.18	4.47	4.75	5.04	5.33
50–53y	FEV$_1$	2.85	3.07	3.28	3.5	3.71	3.93	4.14
	FVC	3.5	3.79	4.07	4.36	4.65	4.94	5.23
54–57y	FEV$_1$	2.74	2.95	3.17	3.38	3.6	3.81	4.03
	FVC	3.39	3.68	3.97	4.26	4.55	4.83	5.12
58–61y	FEV$_1$	2.62	2.84	3.05	3.27	3.48	3.7	3.91
	FVC	3.29	3.58	3.87	4.15	4.44	4.73	5.02
62–65y	FEV$_1$	2.51	2.72	2.94	3.15	3.37	3.58	3.8
	FVC	3.19	3.47	3.76	4.05	4.34	4.63	4.91
66–69y	FEV$_1$	2.39	2.6	2.82	3.03	3.25	3.46	3.68
	FVC	3.08	3.37	3.66	3.95	4.23	4.52	4.81

For men ≥70y, use the formulae:
- FEV$_1$ = (0.043 × height in m × 100) − (0.029 × age in y) − 2.49
- FVC = (0.0576 × height in m × 100) − (0.026 × age in y) − 4.34

Spirometry normal values reproduced with permission from the British Thoracic Society

Bronchodilators and steroids

Bronchodilators Cause relaxation of bronchial smooth muscle.

Short-acting β_2 agonists (e.g. salbutamol, terbutaline). Safest, most effective β_2 agonists for use as quick relievers in asthma and COPD.
• Duration of action: ~3–5h. Oral preparations are less effective than inhaled preparations. Prescribe as 1–2 puffs prn
• Warn patients to seek medical advice if usual dose does not relieve symptoms or relieves symptoms for <3h
• Regular treatment with bronchodilators alone may be linked with worsening of asthma and asthma deaths. If the patient has asthma and is using a β_2 agonist inhaler >2x/wk, consider prophylaxis—📖 p. 312

Longer-acting β_2 agonists (e.g. salmeterol, formoterol)
• **Asthma** (e.g. salmeterol 50–100 micrograms bd), as an adjunct to existing corticosteroid treatment—📖 p. 312. Particularly useful for night time asthma. Duration of action is ~12h. Not for relief of acute attacks
• **COPD**—📖 p. 316

Steroids Short- and long-term treatment of inflammatory conditions.
• **Oral steroids** Prescribe as a single dose in the morning. Often started at high dose (e.g. 40–50mg od) to suppress disease process and then stopped after improvement. If used as maintenance therapy, use the minimum dose that controls disease. Supply with a 'steroid card'
• **Inhaled steroids** Use regularly to obtain maximum benefit. Alleviation of symptoms occurs 3–7d after initiation. If causes coughing, try a short-acting β_2 agonist before use. Common unwanted effects are oral candidiasis (5%) and hoarseness—↓ by use of a large volume spacer or mouthwashing after use

❶ Beclometasone inhalers should be prescribed by brand name.

Side effects
• ↑ BP
• Osteoporosis ± fracture
• Proximal muscle wasting
• Euphoria
• Paranoid states/depression—especially if PMH
• Peptic ulceration—soluble or enteric-coated versions may ↓ risk
• Suppression of clinical signs—may allow diseases, e.g. septicaemia, to reach advanced stage before being recognized
• Spread of infection, e.g. chickenpox
• DM/worsening of diabetic control
• Cushing's syndrome—moon face, striae, and acne
• Adrenal atrophy—can persist years after stopping long-term steroids—illness/surgical emergencies may need to be covered with steroid supplements
• Growth suppression in children
• Na^+ and water retention; K^+ loss

Steroid cards Should be carried by patients on oral/high doses of inhaled steroids. The card informs other practitioners that the patient is on steroids and gives the patient advice on use of steroids and risk of infection. Steroid cards can be obtained from: ☎ 0161 6832189 E-mail: nhsforms@spsl.uk.com

Withdrawal of steroids Stop abruptly if disease is unlikely to relapse, the patient has received treatment for ≤3wk and is not included in the patient groups described in the following list. Withdraw gradually if disease is unlikely to relapse and the patient has:

• Recently had repeated steroid courses (particularly if taken for >3wk)
• Taken a short course <1y after stopping long-term therapy
• Other possible causes of adrenal suppression
• Received >40mg od of prednisolone (or equivalent)
• Been given repeat doses in the evening
• Received treatment with steroids for >3wk

During corticosteroid withdrawal, ↓ dose rapidly to physiological levels (~7.5mg od prednisolone)—thereafter ↓ more slowly. Assess the disease during withdrawal to ensure relapse does not occur.

Use of spacers with metered-dose inhalers (MDIs)

Advantages of using a spacer Allows more time for evaporation of propellant so a larger proportion of active drug is deposited in the lungs; there is no need to coordinate actuation with inhalation; results in less oropharyngeal side effects (e.g. thrush, hoarseness with inhaled steroids).

Use of spacers Both large Volumatic® spacers and medium-volume devices (e.g. AeroChamber®) are widely available, acceptable, and portable. Inhale the drug from the spacer immediately after actuation as effect of the drugs is short-lived. Spacers should be washed and air-dried weekly to prevent build-up of electrostatic charge affecting drug delivery, and replaced every 6–12mo.

Home nebulizer therapy In England and Wales nebulizers are not available via the NHS (but are free of VAT). Some nebulizers are available in Scotland on form GP10A. Nebulizers convert a solution of drug into an aerosol for inhalation. They are used to deliver a higher dosage of drug than is usual with inhalers over a short period of time (5–10min). List of available devices—*BNF* 3.1.5. *Indications:*

• Acute exacerbations ± regular treatment of asthma/COPD
• Antibiotic treatment—for patients with chronic, purulent infection, e.g. CF, bronchiectasis; prophylaxis and treatment of pneumocystis pneumonia with pentamidine in patients with AIDS
• Palliative care—palliation of breathlessness and cough, e.g. bronchodilators, lidocaine, or bupivacaine for dry, persistent cough

Use in asthma/COPD Before suggesting long-term use:

• Review diagnosis, technique using handheld device ± spacer, and compliance
• Try ↑ dose of bronchodilator via a handheld device for at least 2wk
• Perform a 2wk trial of nebulizer therapy and monitor therapeutic effect (e.g. with PEFR in asthma or dyspnoea score with COPD)
• Provide clear instructions on the use of the nebulizer, monitoring and when to seek help. Follow up regularly

Further information

European Respiratory Society Guidelines on the use of nebulizers (2001) *European Respiratory Journal* **18**:228–42.

Asthma in adults

Symptoms/signs of a severe asthma attack
- PEFR 33–50% predicted or best
- Oxygen saturation ≥92%
- Unable to talk in sentences
- Intercostal recession
- Tachypnoea (respiratory rate ≥25 breaths/min)
- Tachycardia (heart rate ≥110bpm)

Life-threatening signs
- PEFR <33% predicted or best
- Oxygen saturation <92%
- Arrhythmia
- Hypotension
- Cyanosis
- Exhaustion
- Poor respiratory effort
- Silent chest (inaudible wheeze)
- Altered consciousness

Management of an acute asthma attack 📖 pp. 1092–7

Asthma is a condition of paroxysmal, reversible airways obstruction with 3 characteristic features:
- Airflow limitation—usually reversible spontaneously or with treatment
- Airway hyper-responsiveness to a wide range of stimuli
- Inflammation of the bronchi

Prevalence European Respiratory Health Survey figures:
- 25% adults aged 20–44y suffer from wheeze ± breathlessness
- 7% have doctor-diagnosed asthma (1–2% occupational asthma)

Asthma in special groups
- **Children** 📖 pp. 882–7
- **Occupational asthma** 📖 p. 336
- **Pregnancy** 📖 p. 822

Diagnosis of asthma Is based on recognition of a characteristic pattern of symptoms/signs in the absence of an alternative explanation.

Clinical features that ↑ probability of asthma >1 of:
- Wheeze
- Breathlessness
- Chest tightness
- Cough

Particularly if:
- Symptoms are worse:
  - At night/early morning
  - With exercise, allergen and/or cold air exposure
  - After aspirin/β-blockers
- PMH of atopy
- FH asthma and/or atopy
- Widespread wheeze
- Unexplained low FEV_1 or PEFR
- Unexplained eosinophilia

Clinical features that ↓ probability of asthma
- Prominent dizziness, light-headedness, peripheral tingling
- Chronic productive cough without wheeze/breathlessness
- Normal examination of chest when symptomatic
- Voice disturbance
- Symptoms with colds only
- Smoking history (>20 pack y)
- Cardiac disease
- Normal PEFR/spirometry when symptomatic

❶ Normal spirometry when asymptomatic does not exclude asthma.

Tests Spirometry is the preferred initial test. Interpret PEFR records with caution. They are more useful for monitoring established asthma.

Differential diagnosis Airflow obstruction = FEV_1/FVC <0.7.

Airflow obstruction	*No airflow obstruction*
• COPD	• Chronic cough syndromes
• Bronchiectasis*	• Hyperventilation syndrome
• Inhaled foreign body*	• Vocal cord dysfunction
• Obliterative bronchiolitis	• Rhinitis
• Large airway stenosis	• Gastro-oesophageal reflux
• Lung cancer*	• Heart failure
• Sarcoidosis*	• Pulmonary fibrosis

* May also be associated with non-obstructive spirometry.

Action

High probability of asthma Give trial of treatment with inhaled beclometasone 200 micrograms bd (or equivalent) for 6–8wk. If response is poor despite adequate inhaler technique/concordance, investigate further.

❶ If significant airflow obstruction, there may be inhaled steroid resistance. Treat with oral prednisolone 30mg od for 2wk instead.

Intermediate probability of asthma
- If FEV_1/FVC <0.7 (i.e. significant airways obstruction)—offer reversibility testing and/or trial of treatment. If significant reversibility and/or trial of treatment is beneficial, treat as asthma. If insignificant reversibility and treatment trial is not beneficial, consider tests for alternative diagnoses
- If FEV_1/FVC >0.7 (i.e. no evidence of airways obstruction), arrange further investigations before commencing treatment ± refer

Low probability of asthma Consider alternative diagnoses and investigate/manage accordingly. Reconsider asthma if no response.

Reversibility testing For patients with diagnostic uncertainty:
- If airflow obstruction is present at the time of assessment—assess FEV_1 (or PEFR) and/or symptoms before and after 400 micrograms of inhaled salbutamol via MDI and spacer
- If no airflow obstruction is present or response to inhaled salbutamol is uncertain—assess FEV_1 (or PEFR) and/or symptoms after trial of treatment with inhaled (beclometasone 200 micrograms bd or equivalent) or oral steroids (prednisolone 30mg od for 14d)

>400mL ↑ in FEV_1 suggests asthma. If smaller improvement—decide whether to continue treatment based on assessment of symptoms. Trial of treatment withdrawal may be helpful if there is doubt.

Other investigations to consider in primary care CXR—consider if atypical/additional symptoms; exhaled nitrous oxide testing, eosinophil count.

Reasons for referral *E* = Emergency; *U* = Urgent; *S* = Soon; *R* = Routine
- Severe asthma exacerbation—*E*
- Monophonic wheeze/stridor—*E/U*
- CXR shadowing—*U*
- Prominent systemic features (myalgia, fever, weight loss)—*U/S*
- Diagnosis unclear—*S/R*
- Unexpected clinical findings (e.g. crackles, clubbing, cyanosis)—*S/R*
- Constant breathlessness—*S/R*
- Poor response to treatment—*S/R*
- Unexplained restrictive spirometry—*R*
- Suspected occupational asthma—*R*
- Chronic sputum production—*R*
- Eosinophilia (>1 x 10^9/L)—*R*

Asthma management in practice

Aims of treatment To:

- ↓ symptoms and impact on lifestyle (e.g. absence from work/school)
- Minimize the need for reliever medication
- Prevent severe attacks/exacerbations

GP services Routine asthma care should be carried out in a specialized clinic. Doctors/nurses involved need appropriate training and regular updates. Practices should keep an asthma register to ensure adequate follow-up and allow audit. ❶ Not all patients want to attend a pre-arranged appointment. Telephone reviews may be as effective as face-to-face consultations.

Reviews and monitoring Frequency depends on needs. Aim to review all patients with asthma at least annually (see Figure 11.2).

- Check symptoms since last seen. Use objective measures, e.g. RCP three questions (📖 p. 303)
- Record smoking status and advise smokers to stop
- Record any exacerbations/acute attacks since last seen
- Check medication—use, concordance (prescription count—📖 p. 142), inhaler technique, problems, side effects
- Check influenza/pneumococcal vaccination received
- Review objective measures of lung function e.g. home PEFR chart, PEFR/spirometry at review
- Address any problems or queries and educate about asthma
- Agree management goals and date for further review

Self-management All patients should receive:

- **Self-management education** Brief, simple education linked to patient goals is most likely to be successful. Include information about: nature of disease, nature of the treatment and how to use it, self-monitoring/self-assessment, recognition of acute exacerbations, allergen/trigger avoidance, patients' own goals of treatment
- **Written action plan** Focus on individual needs. Include information about symptom triggers and peak flow levels that indicate when asthma is worsening, and guidance about what to do under those circumstances. Action plans ↓ morbidity and health costs from asthma[S]
- **PEFR monitoring** Record PEFR at asthma review and if acute exacerbation. Home monitoring + action plan can be useful, especially for patients with severe asthma, brittle asthma (i.e. rapid development of acute asthma attacks) and/or if poor perceivers of symptoms

⚠ Be aware that those from ethnic minorities, socially disadvantaged groups, those with communication problems, adolescents, and the elderly have complex needs.

Management of acute asthma 📖 pp. 1092–7

Non-pharmacological measures

- **Smoking** Smoking may ↑ symptoms of asthma—advise to stop
- **Weight** There is some evidence that weight ↓ in obese patients with asthma results in ↑ asthma control[R]

- **Allergen avoidance**
  - *House dust mite* There is little evidence that ↓ house dust mite results in clinical improvement[C]. In committed families advise: complete barrier bed coverings; removal of carpets; removal of soft toys from bed; high-temperature washing of bed linen; acaricides to soft furnishings; dehumidification. There is no evidence that air ionizers have any beneficial effect
  - *Pets* There is no evidence that removing pets from a home results in improved symptoms but many experts still advise removal of the pet for patients with asthma who also have an allergy to the pet

Drug therapy 📖 p. 312

Patient information and support
Asthma UK ☎ 08457 01 02 03 🖱 www.asthma.org.uk

Figure 11.2 Summary of the annual asthma review

Drug treatment of asthma

Management of acute asthma 📖 pp. 1092–7

Use a stepwise approach[G] (see Figure 11.3). Start at the step most appropriate to the initial severity of symptoms. The aim is to achieve early control of the condition and then to ↓ treatment by stepping down.

> Exacerbations Treat early. In adult patients on 200 microgram doses of inhaled steroids, a 5x ↑ in dose reduces severity of exacerbations. Alternatively, and in all other cases, use prednisolone 30–40mg od for 1–2wk.

Selection of inhaler device If possible use an MDI. Inadequate technique may result in drug failure. Patients must inhale slowly and hold their breath for 10s after inhalation. Demonstrate inhaler technique before prescribing and check at follow-ups. Spacers/breath-activated devices are useful if patients find activation difficult. Dry powder inhalers are an alternative.

Short-acting β_2 agonists 📖 p. 306 (e.g. salbutamol). Work more quickly and with fewer side effects than alternatives. Use prn unless shown to benefit from regular dosing. Using ≥2 canisters/mo or >10–12 puffs/d is a marker of poorly controlled asthma.

❶ A budesonide/formoterol combination inhaler is an alternative rescue medication.

Inhaled corticosteroids (📖 p. 306) Effective preventer. May be beneficial even for patients with mild asthma. Consider if: exacerbation of asthma in the last 2y requiring steroids; using inhaled β_2 agonists ≥3x/wk; or symptomatic ≥ 3x/wk or ≥1 night/wk.

Oral steroids 📖 p. 306

Add-on therapy Aims to improve lung function/symptoms. Before initiating a new drug, check compliance, inhaler technique, and eliminate trigger factors. Only continue if of demonstrable benefit.

- **Inhaled long-acting β_2 agonists (LABA)** 📖 p. 306 (e.g. salmeterol). Do not use without inhaled steroids. Combination inhalers (steroid + LABA) improve compliance
- **Leukotriene receptor agonists** (e.g. montelukast) ↓ exacerbations
- **Theophylline** Side effects are common

Stepping down Review and consider stepping down at intervals ≥3mo. Maintain on the lowest dose of inhaled steroid controlling symptoms. When reducing steroids, cut dose by 25–50% each time.

Omalizumab Monoclonal antibody that binds to circulating IgE. Useful for adults and children >6y if allergy is a factor in asthma, on high-dose inhaled steroid + LABA, and frequent exacerbations. Given sc every 2–4wk. Always specialist-initiated.

Complementary therapies Buteyko breathing technique ↓ symptoms/bronchodilator use. Immunotherapy in specialist clinics is effective for patients with specific allergies. Other complementary therapies—no convincing evidence of effectiveness.

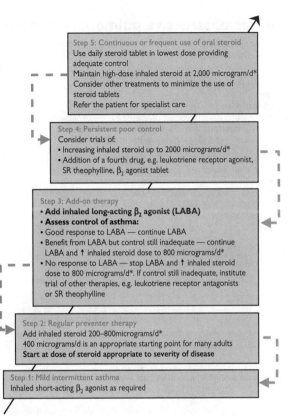

Step 5: Continuous or frequent use of oral steroid
Use daily steroid tablet in lowest dose providing adequate control
Maintain high-dose inhaled steroid at 2,000 microgram/d*
Consider other treatments to minimize the use of steroid tablets
Refer the patient for specialist care

Step 4: Persistent poor control
Consider trials of:
• Increasing inhaled steroid up to 2000 micrograms/d*
• Addition of a fourth drug, e.g. leukotriene receptor agonist, SR theophylline, β₂ agonist tablet

Step 3: Add-on therapy
• **Add inhaled long-acting β₂ agonist (LABA)**
• **Assess control of asthma:**
• Good response to LABA — continue LABA
• Benefit from LABA but control still inadequate — continue LABA and ↑ inhaled steroid dose to 800 micrograms/d*
• No response to LABA — stop LABA and ↑ inhaled steroid dose to 800 micrograms/d*. If control still inadequate, institute trial of other therapies, e.g. leukotriene receptor antagonists or SR theophylline

Step 2: Regular preventer therapy
Add inhaled steroid 200–800micrograms/d*
400 micrograms/d is an appropriate starting point for many adults
Start at dose of steroid appropriate to severity of disease

Step 1: Mild intermittent asthma
Inhaled short-acting β₂ agonist as required

* All doses given refer to hydrofluoroalkane-beclometasone dipropionate (BDP-HFA) equivalent inhalers. For other drugs/formulations adjust dose accordingly (see *BNF* Section 3).

Figure 11.3 Summary of stepwise management in adults
Reproduced from British Guideline on the management of asthma (May 2008, rev. Jan 2012), p48 with permission from the Scottish Intercollegiate Guidelines Network.

Difficult asthma Persistent symptoms and/or frequent exacerbations despite treatment at step 4/5. Check diagnosis and exacerbating factors. Assess adherence to medication. Find out about family, psychological, or social problems that may be interfering with effective management.

Further information

British Thoracic Society/SIGN British guideline on the management of asthma (2011) ✆ www.sign.ac.uk
BNF Section 3 ✆ www.bnf.org

Chronic obstructive pulmonary disease

Chronic obstructive pulmonary disease (COPD) is a slowly progressive disorder characterized by airflow obstruction. Affects ~16% of the population in the 40–68y age group (~3 million people in the UK—two-thirds undiagnosed). ♂ > ♀. Responsible for ~5% of deaths.

Causes
- Cigarette smoking
- Genetic—bronchial hyperresponsiveness; α1-antitrypsin deficiency
- Race—Chinese and Afro-Caribbeans have ↓ susceptibility
- Diet—poor diet and low birthweight

Diagnosis Is suggested by history, signs, and baseline spirometry. Consider in any patient >35y with a risk factor for COPD (generally smoking) and ≥1 of:
- Shortness of breath on exertion—use an objective measure, e.g. MRC dyspnoea scale (see Table 11.6) to grade breathlessness
- Chronic cough
- Wheeze
- Regular sputum production
- Frequent winter 'bronchitis'

Table 11.6 MRC dyspnoea scale

Grade	Degree of breathlessness related to physical activity
1	Not troubled by breathlessness, except on strenuous exercise
2	Short of breath when hurrying or walking up a slight hill
3	Walks slower than contemporaries on level ground because of breathlessness or has to stop for breath when walking at own pace
4	Stops for breath after walking 100m or after a few minutes on level ground
5	Too breathless to leave the house or breathless on dressing/undressing

If diagnosis is suspected also ask about weight ↓, effort intolerance, waking at night, ankle swelling, fatigue, and occupational hazards.

⚠ Chest pain or haemoptysis are uncommon in COPD—if present consider an alternative diagnosis.

Signs May be none. *Possible signs:*
- Hyperinflated chest ± poor chest expansion on inspiration
- ↓ cricosternal distance
- Hyperresonant chest with ↓ cardiac dullness on percussion
- Wheeze or quiet breath sounds
- Paradoxical movement of lower ribs
- Use of accessory muscles
- Tachypnoea
- Pursing of lips on expiration (purse lip breathing)
- Peripheral oedema
- Cyanosis
- ↑ JVP
- Cachexia

Spirometry (📖 p. 302) Predicts severity (see Table 11.7) and prognosis but not disability/quality of life. Diagnose airflow obstruction if:
- FEV_1/FVC <0.7 (<70%), and
- FEV_1 <70% predicted (QOF criterion), and
- <15% response to a reversibility test

Table 11.7 Severity of COPD and expected clinical picture

Severity	Spirometry (FEV$_1$/FVC <0.7)	Clinical picture
Stage 1 Mild	FEV$_1$ ≥80%	Cough. Little/no breathlessness. No abnormal signs. No ↑ use of services
Stage 2 Moderate	FEV$_1$ 50–80% predicted	Breathlessness, wheeze on exertion, cough ± sputum. Some abnormal signs. Known to GP—intermittent exacerbations
Stage 3 Severe	FEV$_1$ 30–49% predicted	SOBOE. Marked wheeze/cough. Usually other signs. Known to GP and specialist with frequent exacerbations/admissions
Stage 4 Very severe	FEV$_1$ <30% predicted or <50% + respiratory failure	As for stage 3 but more breathless and severely restricted in activities of daily living

Differential diagnosis Asthma (see Table 11.8), bronchiectasis, heart failure, lung cancer.

Table 11.8 Comparison of COPD and asthma

	COPD	Asthma
Symptoms <35y	Rare	Common
Smoking history	Nearly all	Maybe
Breathlessness	Persistent and progressive Poor response to inhaled therapy—if good reconsider diagnosis	Variable throughout the day and from day to day. Good response to inhaled therapy is typical
Chronic productive cough	Common	Uncommon
Waking at night with cough/wheeze	Uncommon	Common

Reversibility testing Can be misleading. Not routinely recommended:
- >400mL ↑ in FEV$_1$ following trial of bronchodilator or prednisolone (30mg od for 2wk) suggests asthma
- Clinically significant COPD is *not* present if FEV$_1$ and FEV$_1$/FVC return to normal after drug therapy

PEFR (📖 p. 302) Patients with COPD have little variability in PEFR. Serial home PEFR measurements can help distinguish between asthma and COPD. PEFR may underestimate severity of airflow limitation and a normal PEFR does not exclude airflow obstruction.

Other investigations organized in primary care
- **CXR** Indicated to exclude other diagnoses, e.g. lung cancer
- **FBC** To identify polycythaemia or anaemia
- **BMI**
- **α1-antitrypsin** If early onset COPD or family history
- **ECG/echo** If cor pulmonale is suspected
- **Sputum culture** If purulent sputum is persistent

Management of COPD

Record values of spirometric tests performed at diagnosis and review. At each review record current symptoms, problems since last seen, exercise tolerance, and smoking status. Calculate BODE score if possible. Educate the patient/family about COPD, medication, and self-help strategies.

Non-drug therapy

- **Smoking cessation** Most important. Improves outcome (see Table 11.9).
- **Vaccination** Offer pneumococcal and annual influenza vaccination
- **Exercise** Lack of exercise ↓ FEV_1. Pulmonary rehabilitation is of proven benefit—refer directly or via respiratory physicians
- **Nutrition** Weight ↓ in obese patients improves exercise tolerance

Screening for depression 📖 p. 199

Drug therapy Treat according to severity (Table 11.7); document effects of each drug treatment on symptoms, quality of life, and lung function as tried—see Figure 11.4.

Management of acute exacerbations 📖 p. 318

Referral for specialist care

- Uncertain diagnosis
- Age <40y
- Severe COPD
- Rapid decline in FEV_1
- Cor pulmonale
- Frequent infections
- Haemoptysis
- α1-antitrypsin deficiency
- Assessment for:
  - LTOT
  - Long-term oral steroids
  - Withdrawal of long-term steroids
  - Long-term nebulizer therapy
  - Pulmonary rehabilitation
  - Surgery, e.g. lung transplant

Long-term oxygen therapy (LTOT) *Only* prescribe after evaluation by a respiratory physician. Refer patients with:

- Severe airflow obstruction (FEV_1 <30%—consider if 30–49%)
- Hypoxaemia (oxygen saturation ≤92% breathing air)
- Cyanosis
- Polycythaemia
- Peripheral oedema
- ↑ JVP

Treatment for >15h/d ↑ survival and quality of life. Ambulatory oxygen therapy can ↑ exercise tolerance in some patients. 🛈 Always warn patients about the fire risks of having pure oxygen in their homes.

O_2 cylinders and associated equipment Arrangements for supply of oxygen are different in England and Wales, Scotland, and Northern Ireland—see *BNF* section 3.6. Specify amount of O_2 required (h/d) and flow rate. O_2 concentrators are more economical for LTOT. Supply back-up cylinders in case of breakdown or power cut.

Prognosis The BODE index (see Table 11.10—BMI, airflow obstruction, dyspnoea, and exercise capacity) can be used to assess prognosis:

Score	0–2	3–4	4–6	7–10
• *1y mortality*	2%	2%	2%	5%
• *2y mortality*	6%	8%	14%	31%
• *52mo mortality*	19%	32%	40%	80%

Figure 11.4 Drug treatment of COPD
Adapted from NICE COPD (2010), with permission.

Table 11.9 Smoking and COPD

	FEV₁ as % of value aged 25y	
	Age 60y	**Age 75y**
Non-smoker	85%	80%
Ex-smoker: quit aged 40y	60%	45% (symptoms)
Ex-smoker: quit aged 60y	33% (severe symptoms)	15% (severe disability)
Ongoing smoker	33% (severe symptoms)	Dead

Table 11.10 The BODE index

	Points on BODE index			
	0	**1**	**2**	**3**
FEV₁ (% predicted)	≥65	50–64	36–49	≤35
6 minute walk test (m)	≥350	250–349	150–249	≤149
MRC dyspnoea scale	0–1	2	3	4
BMI (kg/m²)	>21	≤21		

Further information
NICE Chronic obstructive pulmonary disease (2010) ✆ www.nice.org.uk
Patient support
British Lung Foundation ☎ 03000 030 555 ✆ www.lunguk.org

Acute exacerbations of COPD

Presentation Worsening of previous stable condition. *Features:* ≥1 of:

- ↑ dyspnoea—marked dyspnoea, tachypnoea (>25 breaths/min), use of accessory muscles at rest and purse lip breathing are signs of severe exacerbation
- ↓ exercise tolerance—marked ↓ in activities of daily living is a sign of severe exacerbation
- ↑ fatigue
- ↑ fluid retention—new-onset oedema is a sign of severe exacerbation
- ↑ wheeze
- Chest tightness
- ↑ cough
- ↑ sputum purulence
- ↑ sputum volume
- Upper airways symptoms, e.g. colds, sore throats,
- New-onset cyanosis—severe exacerbation
- Acute confusion—severe exacerbation

❶ Fever and chest pain are uncommon presenting features—consider alternative diagnosis.

Causes of exacerbations 30% have no identifiable cause
- **Infections** Viral upper and lower respiratory tract infections, e.g. common cold, influenza; bacterial lower respiratory tract infections
- **Pollutants**, e.g. nitrous oxide, sulphur dioxide, ozone

Differential diagnosis

- Pneumonia
- LVF/pulmonary oedema
- Lung cancer
- Pleural effusion
- Recurrent aspiration
- Pneumothorax
- PE
- Upper airway obstruction

Investigations

- **Pulse oximetry** Can be used to assess severity (saturation ≤92% breathing air suggests hypoxaemia—consider admission) and to monitor progress
- **CXR** Consider if diagnostic doubt and/or to exclude other causes of symptoms
- **Sputum culture** Not recommended routinely in the community[G]

Management Decide whether to treat at home or admit to hospital—see Table 11.11.

Home treatment of acute exacerbations

- **Add or ↑ bronchodilators** Consider if inhaler device and technique are appropriate
- **Start antibiotics** Use broad-spectrum antibiotic, e.g. clarithromycin 500mg bd or doxycycline 100mg od/bd if sputum becomes more purulent *or* clinical signs of pneumonia *or* consolidation on CXR
- **Oral corticosteroids** Start early in the course of the exacerbation if ↑ breathlessness which interferes with daily activities. Dosage: 30–40mg/d of prednisolone for 1–2wk. Consider osteoporosis prophylaxis with a bisphosphonate if frequent courses are required (📖 p. 509)

Follow-up

- Reassess as necessary. If the patient deteriorates, reconsider the need for hospital admission. If not fully improved within 2wk consider CXR and/or hospital referral
- Reassess patients who have been admitted 4–6wk after discharge Assess their ability to cope at home. ~1 in 3 are readmitted in <3mo
- Reassess inhaler technique and understanding of treatment regime
- In severe cases, reassess the need for LTOT and/or home nebulizer
- Check FEV_1
- Emphasize the potential benefit of lifestyle modification—smoking cessation, exercise, weight loss if obese
- Arrange ongoing regular follow-up

Table 11.11 Deciding to treat exacerbations at home or in hospital
The more features in the 'treat in hospital' column, the more likely the need for admission.

	Treat at home	Treat in hospital*
Ability to cope at home	Yes	No
Breathlessness	Mild	Severe
General condition	Good	Poor—deteriorating
Level of activity	Good	Poor/confined to bed
Cyanosis	No	Yes
Worsening peripheral oedema	No	Yes
Level of consciousness	Normal	Impaired
Already receiving LTOT	No	Yes
Social circumstances	Good	Living alone/not coping
Acute confusion	No	Yes
Rapid rate of onset	No	Yes
Significant co-morbidity (e.g. cardiac disease, DM)	No	Yes
Changes on CXR (if available)	No	Present

* Hospital-at-home schemes and assisted discharge schemes are a suitable alternative.
Reproduced with permission of BMJ journals.

Further information

NICE Chronic obstructive pulmonary disease (2010) ℘ www.nice.org.uk

Lung cancer

Referral for suspected lung cancer

Immediate referral/acute admission
- Stridor
- Superior vena cava obstruction (swelling of face/neck with fixed ↑ JVP)

Urgent referral
To a team specializing in management of lung cancer:
- Persistent haemoptysis (in smokers/ex-smokers aged ≥40y)
- CXR suggestive of lung cancer (including pleural effusion and slowly resolving consolidation)
- Normal CXR where there is high suspicion of lung cancer
- History of asbestos exposure and recent onset of chest pain, shortness of breath, or unexplained systemic symptoms where a CXR indicates pleural effusion, pleural mass, or any suspicious lung pathology

Urgent referral for CXR
- Haemoptysis
- Any of the following if unexplained or present for >3wk*:
  - Cough
  - Chest/shoulder pain
  - Dyspnoea
  - Weight loss
  - Chest signs
  - Hoarseness (refer urgently to ENT if CXR is normal)
  - Finger clubbing
  - Cervical or supraclavicular lymphadenopathy
  - Features suggestive of metastases from a lung cancer, e.g. secondaries in the brain, bone, liver, or skin

* Do not delay for 3wk if high risk of lung cancer, i.e. smoker/ex-smoker, COPD, history of asbestos exposure, previous history of cancer (especially head/neck cancer).

Lung cancer is the most common cancer and third most common cause of death in the UK. Incidence ↑ with age—85% are aged >65y and 1% <40y at presentation. ♂:♀ ≈ 2:1 but incidence is increasing in women.

Types
- **Small cell lung cancer** Accounts for ~25% all cases. Often disseminated at diagnosis. Spreads to liver, bones, brain, and adrenals
- **Non-small cell lung cancer** Mainly adenocarcinoma or squamous cell carcinoma. Not always smoking-related

Screening A 2003 Cochrane review concluded that current evidence does not support screening for lung cancer with chest radiography or sputum cytology. Frequent chest X-ray screening might be harmful. Results of trials of screening with CT scanning are awaited from the US but preliminary results do not suggest this will be an effective screening strategy.

Prevention
- **Smoking cessation** 90% of lung cancer patients are smokers or ex-smokers. The younger a person is when he/she starts smoking the greater the risk of developing lung cancer. Risk also ↑ with amount smoked (duration of smoking and number of cigarettes smoked/d)

- **Diet** ↑ consumption of fruit, carrots, and green vegetables may
  ↓ incidence, but there is no evidence that vitamin supplements are
  beneficial and they might be harmful[C]

Presentation >90% have symptoms at the time of diagnosis. Common
presenting features:

- Cough (56%)
- Chest/shoulder pain (37%)
- Haemoptysis (7%)
- Dyspnoea
- Hoarseness
- Weight ↓
- Finger clubbing
- General malaise
- Distant metastases
- Incidental finding on CXR

Pancoast syndrome Apical lung cancer + ipsilateral Horner's syndrome. *Cause:* invasion of the cervical sympathetic plexus. *Other features:*
shoulder and arm pain (brachial plexus invasion C8–T2) ± hoarse voice/
bovine cough (unilateral recurrent laryngeal nerve palsy and vocal cord
paralysis). *H.K. Pancoast (1875–1939)—US radiologist.*

Paraneoplastic syndromes (e.g. ectopic ACTH production, SIADH,
hypercalcaemia, hypercoagulability) Affect 10–20% of patients with lung
cancer—particularly small cell. Have a high index of suspicion and refer
for specialist management if suspected.

Management Once the diagnosis has been confirmed, liaise with the
chest physician, specialist lung cancer team, primary healthcare team, and
specialist palliative care services (e.g. Macmillan nurses). Active treatment
options depend on type and extent of tumour and include surgery, radiotherapy, and/or chemotherapy. Follow-up regularly. 80% die in <1y.

Palliative radiotherapy Radiotherapy is a key component of symptomatic
treatment for:

- Haemoptysis
- Chest pain
- Breathlessness due to bronchial occlusion
- Pain from bone metastasis
- Symptoms from brain metastasis

Radiotherapy may be combined with palliative chemotherapy, particularly
for patients with non-small cell lung cancer.

Mesothelioma 📖 p. 337

Palliative care 📖 pp. 1028–47

Further information

NICE 🖰 www.nice.org.uk
- Referral guidelines for suspected cancer (2005)
- The diagnosis and treatment of lung cancer (2011)
SIGN Management of lung cancer (2005) 🖰 www.sign.ac.uk

Information and support for patients

The Roy Castle Lung Cancer Foundation ☎ 0800 358 7200
🖰 www.roycastle.org
Macmillan Cancer Support ☎ 0808 808 0000 🖰 www.macmillan.org.uk
Cancer Research UK ☎ 0808 800 4040 🖰 www.cancerhelp.org.uk
British Lung Foundation ☎ 03000 030 555 🖰 www.lunguk.org

Colds and influenza

The common cold Acute, usually afebrile, respiratory tract infection.
- **Causes** Rhino (30–50%), picorna, echo, and Coxsackie viruses. At any one time only a few viruses are prevalent
- **Spread** Contaminated secretions on fingers and droplet infection. Most people are infected 2–3x/y
- **Management** Advise patients to take plenty of fluids and paracetamol for symptom relief. Usually symptoms resolve in <1.5wk
- **Complications** Exacerbation of asthma/COPD; secondary infection (bronchitis, pneumonia, conjunctivitis, OM, sinusitis, tonsillitis). Similar symptoms are caused by the adeno and parainfluenza viruses

Acute bronchitis Inflammation of major bronchi. Often follows viral URTI especially in winter months. Symptoms include cough ± sputum, breathlessness, and wheeze. If signs are present they include wheeze and scattered coarse crepitations.

Management Self-limiting illness (settles in <3wk) in normally healthy people. *Consider:* bronchodilators if wheeze is heard; antibiotics—may shorten symptoms but weigh benefits against possible side effects (↑ in community antibiotic resistance and 'medicalizing' a self-limiting condition). If recurrent bronchitis, consider a diagnosis of COPD.

Reasons to prescribe antibiotics immediately[N] Investigate further and/or give antibiotics (e.g. amoxicillin 500mg tds) if:
- Systemically very unwell
- Symptoms/signs of serious illness or complications, e.g. pneumonia
- At high risk of serious complications because of pre-existing co-morbidity, e.g. significant heart, lung, renal, liver, or neuromuscular disease, immunosuppression, CF, or young children born prematurely
- Aged >65y with acute cough and ≥2 or more of the following, or aged >80y with acute cough and ≥1 of the following:
- Hospitalization in the previous year • History of CCF
- Type 1 or type 2 DM • Current use of oral steroids

Influenza Sporadic respiratory illness during autumn and winter, causing ~600 deaths/y with epidemics every 2–3y leading to a 10x ↑ in deaths, and worldwide pandemics every 30–40y killing many more. *Causes:* influenza viruses A, B, or C. *Spread:* droplet infection, person-to-person contact, or contact with contaminated items. *Incubation:* 1–7d.

Presentation In mild cases symptoms are like those of a common cold. In more severe cases fever begins suddenly accompanied by prostration and generalized aches/pains. Other symptoms may follow: headache, sore throat, respiratory tract symptoms (usually cough ± coryza). Acute symptoms resolve in <5d but weakness, sweating, and fatigue may persist longer. Secondary chest infection with *Staphylococcus aureus* or *Streptococcus pneumoniae* is common. Rarely patients with influenza A (Asian flu) develop severe viral pneumonia.

Management Rest, fluids, and paracetamol for fever/symptom control. Treat complications, e.g. antibiotics for chest infection; treatment of exacerbations of COPD or asthma.

Antivirals: Zanamivir (10mg bd for 5d by inhalation) and oseltamivir (75mg bd for 5d) are not a 'cure' for influenza but shorten symptoms and ↓ incidence of complications if started <72h after onset. Zanamivir is for adults only; oseltamivir can be used for adults and children. Only use:
• For treatment of high-risk groups (see Box 11.1—except pregnancy) and
• When influenza is prevalent in the community— determined by community-based virological surveillance schemes

⚠ Zanamivir may cause bronchospasm—avoid in severe asthma, and ensure a short-acting bronchodilator is available.

Prevention
• Influenza vaccine is prepared each year from viruses of the three strains thought most likely to cause 'flu' that winter. It is ~70% effective (range 30–90%). Protection lasts 1y. Give to high-risk groups—see Box 11.1
• Oseltamivir is recommended for prophylaxis in high-risk patients >13y who are not effectively vaccinated or who live in residential care where a staff member has influenza-like symptoms (only when influenza is prevalent in the community). Use at a dose of 75mg od for 7–10d from diagnosis of the latest case in the establishment[N]

Box 11.1 Risk factors for severe disease with influenza

• Aged ≥65y, *or*
• With ≥1 of the following conditions:
  • Chronic respiratory disease, including COPD and asthma, or weak respiratory muscles, e.g. MS, MND, CVA
  • Significant cardiovascular disease, excluding hypertension
  • Immunosuppression, (including hyposplenism)
  • Chronic renal disease   • DM

Indications for influenza vaccination
• ≥65y
• Pregnant women
• DM
• Chronic renal disease
• Chronic lung disease, e.g. asthma, COPD
• Chronic liver disease
• Cardiovascular disease (except ↑ BP alone)
• Immunocompromised or asplenic patients
• Carers of patients with disabilities
• Patients living in long-stay residential care establishments
• Health professionals expected to be in contact with influenza

❶ In 2013, annual intranasal influenza vaccine was introduced for *all* children aged 2–3y in the UK; plans to extend this programme to all children aged 2–16y are under way.

Further information
HM Government Pandemic flu: a national framework for responding to an influenza pandemic (2011) ℘ www.dh.gov.uk
NICE ℘ www.nice.org.uk
• Guidance on the use of zanamivir, oseltamivir, and amantadine for the treatment of influenza (2009)
• Respiratory tract infections—antibiotic prescribing (2008)

Pneumonia in adults

Common condition with annual incidence of ~8 cases/1,000 adult population. Incidence ↑ with age and peaks in the winter. Mortality for those managed in the community is <1% but 1 in 4 patients with pneumonia are admitted to hospital and mortality for those admitted is ~9%.

Presentation Acute illness is characterized by:
- Symptoms of an acute lower respiratory tract illness (cough + ≥1 other lower respiratory tract symptom, e.g. purulent sputum, pleurisy)
- New focal chest signs on examination (consolidation or ↓ air entry, coarse crackles, and/or pleural rub)
- ≥1 systemic feature:
  - Sweating, fevers, shivers, aches and pains, *and/or*
  - Temperature ≥38°C
- No other explanation for the illness

❶The elderly may present atypically, e.g. 'off legs' or acute confusion.

Common causative organisms
- Pneumococcus (*S. pneumoniae*–36%)—◻ p. 654
- *H. influenzae* (10%)—more common amongst the elderly (◻ p. 656)
- *Influenza A and B* (8%)—annual epidemics during the winter months—~3% develop pneumonia (◻ p. 332)
- *Mycoplasma pneumoniae* (1.3%)—less common in the elderly; epidemics occur every 4y in the UK (◻ p. 328)
- Gram –ve enteric bacteria (1.3%)
- *C. psittaci* (1.3%)—~20% have history of bird contact (◻ p. 328)
- *S. aureus* (0.8%)—more common in the winter months; may be associated with viral infection, e.g. flu (◻ p. 655)
- *Legionella* spp. (0.4%)—most common in September/October; >50% related to travel

TB ◻ p. 326   **Immunocompromised patients** ◻ p. 650

Prevention
- Influenza vaccination: ◻ p. 323
- Pneumococcal vaccination: ◻ p. 654

Differential diagnosis Pneumonitis, e.g. secondary to radiotherapy, chemical inhalation; pulmonary oedema (may coexist in the elderly); PE.

Investigations Often unnecessary in general practice. *Consider:*
- **Pulse oximetry** Use to assess severity. If oxygen saturation is ≤92% in air, the patient is hypoxic and requires admission
- **CXR** If diagnostic uncertainty or symptoms not resolving. CXR changes may lag behind clinical signs but should return to normal <6wk after recovery. Persistent changes on CXR >6wk after recovery require further investigation
- **Sputum culture** If not responding to treatment. If weight ↓, malaise, night sweats or risk factors for TB (ethnic origin, history of TB exposure, social deprivation, or elderly), request mycobacterium culture
- **Blood** *FBC*—↑ WCC; ↑ ESR; acute and convalescent titres to confirm 'atypical' pneumonia (*Legionella, C. psittaci, M. pneumoniae*)

Any of:
• Confusion*
• Respiratory rate ≥30 breaths/min
• Blood pressure (systolic <90mmHg; diastolic ≤60mmHg)
• Age ≥65y
Score 1 point for each feature present

CRB-65 score

| 0 | 1 or 2 | 3 or 4 |

Likely suitable for home treatment | Consider hospital referral | Urgent hospital admission

* Defined as a mental test score of ≤8/or new disorientation in person, place, or time.

Figure 11.5 Assessment of severity and management of pneumonia.
Reproduced from Guidelines for the management of community acquired pneumonia in adults: update 2009. *Thorax* 2009; 64 (Supppl III): 1–55, with permission from the British Thoracic Society.

Management
• **Consider the need for admission** See Figure 11.5. Have a low threshold for admission if ill but apyrexial, concomitant illness (e.g. heart failure, chronic lung, renal or liver disease, DM, cancer), or poor social situation. If life-threatening infection or considerable delay (>2h) consider administering antibiotics before admission
• **If a decision is made to treat at home**
  • Advise not to smoke, to rest, and drink plenty of fluids
  • Start antibiotics, e.g. amoxicillin 500mg–1g tds, doxycycline 100–200mg od, or clarithromycin 500mg bd
  • Treat pleuritic pain with simple analgesia, e.g. paracetamol 1g qds
  • Review within 48h. Reassess clinical state. If deteriorating or not improving consider CXR or admission

Complications Require specialist management—refer.
• Pleural effusion (may be reactive or empyema—pus in the lung cavity)
• Lung abscess (presents with swinging fever and worsening pneumonia)
• Septicaemia   • Respiratory failure
• Metastatic infections   • Jaundice

Further information

British Thoracic Society Guidelines for the management of community-acquired pneumonia in adults (2009) ℘ www.brit-thoracic.org.uk
Robinson S, Stradling G, West J, Chapman S. (2014) *Oxford Handbook of Respiratory Medicine.* Oxford: Oxford University Press. ISBN: 9780198703860.

Tuberculosis[ND]

Caused by *Mycobacterium tuberculosis*. Worldwide 1.5 billion people have tuberculosis (TB). In the UK 9,000 cases of TB are reported each year and ~350 patients die. Incidence is increasing.

Risk factors In the UK:
- 40% cases of TB occur in London; TB is an urban disease
- 70% cases occur in ethnic minority populations—60% in those born abroad (half are diagnosed <5y after entering the country)
- Contacts—if living in the same house, risk is 1 in 3; if school/work contact, risk is 1 in 50; casual social contact risk is 1 in 100,000
- Immunosuppression—especially patients with HIV
- Homelessness

Primary TB Initial infection. Transmitted by droplet infection. A lesion forms (usually pulmonary) which drains to local LNs. Immunity develops and the infection becomes quiescent. There may be no symptoms. Possible symptoms include:

- Fever
- Night sweats
- Persistent cough ± sputum
- Haemoptysis
- Pneumonia
- Pleural effusion
- Anorexia
- Weight ↓
- Erythema nodosum

Investigations and management
- CXR
- Sputum samples for culture (state on the form that you are looking for acid-fast bacilli)
- Tuberculin test +ve (may be –ve if immunocompromised)
- If diagnosis is confirmed, refer for treatment and contact tracing.

Post-primary TB Reactivation of a primary infection. Initial lesions (usually in the upper lobes of the lung) progress and fibrose. Other sites may develop disease. Multiple small lesions throughout the body result in miliary TB which is common in immunocompromised patients. Symptoms and signs relate to the organs infected. In all cases refer for specialist treatment. *Extrapulmonary disease sites:*

- CNS
- Lymph nodes
- Spine (rarely other bones/joints)
- Peripheral cold abscess
- Pericardium
- Miliary

Screening TB is a notifiable disease. After notification, contact tracing is initiated—usually through chest clinics. All contacts are screened for TB with a tuberculin test (see Table 11.12).

Tuberculin skin test Useful in diagnosis of TB and must be carried out before BCG immunization, except for infants <3mo old who have not had any recent contact with TB. Interpretation—see Table 11.13. The tuberculin test can be suppressed by:

- Hodgkin's disease
- Glandular fever
- Viral infections
- Corticosteroid therapy
- Sarcoidosis
- Live viral vaccines—do not do a tuberculin test <3wk after vaccination
- Immunosuppressant treatment or diseases, including HIV.

⚠ If a patient has a +ve tuberculin test—DO NOT give BCG vaccination.

Table 11.12 Tuberculin testing and interpretation of results

Heaf test	Mantoux test	Grade
No induration at puncture sites	0mm induration	0—negative
Discrete induration at ≥4 sites	1–4mm induration	1—negative
Ring of induration with clear centre	5–14mm induration	2—positive*
Disc of induration 5–10mm wide	≥15mm induration	3—refer to chest clinic
Solid induration >10mm wide ± vesiculation or ulceration		4—refer to chest clinic

* In school children, a grade 2 response requires no further action. In other circumstances, refer to a chest clinic.

Treatment[N] ❶ Always refer to the chest clinic; 10% of infections are antibiotic-resistant.

Asymptomatic patients If +ve tuberculin skin test (Mantoux >10mm) but normal CXR, treatment is with isoniazid for 6mo or isoniazid + rifampicin for 3mo to prevent development of the clinical disease.

Treatment of symptomatic patients Combination of 3–4 antibiotics for the first 2mo, then two antibiotics for a further 4mo. Antibiotics used are rifampicin, isoniazid, pyrazinamide, and ethambutol. All have potentially serious side effects and require blood monitoring. Compliance is imperative to prevent antibiotic resistance. Those found to be non-compliant are treated with directly observed therapy (DOT)—drugs are dispensed by and taken in the presence of a health professional.

Prevention Bacille Calmette–Guérin (BCG) is a live attenuated strain of bacteria derived from *M. bovis*. BCG vaccination provides immunity lasting ≥15y to 70–80% of recipients. It is given by intradermal injection into the left upper arm. Target groups:

- All infants living in areas where incidence of TB is ≥40/100,000 and infants whose parents or grandparents were born in a country with TB incidence of ≥40/100,000
- Previously unvaccinated new immigrants from countries where there is a high prevalence of TB
- Those at risk due to their occupation, e.g. healthcare workers, veterinary staff, prison staff
- Contacts of known cases or those living or working in high prevalence countries for extended periods (generally ≥1mo)

⚠ Do not give other immunizations into the same arm for 3mo.

Further information

Health Protection Agency (HPA) Topics A–Z: tuberculosis. ℰ www.hpa.org.uk
NICE Clinical diagnosis and management of tuberculosis (2011) ℰ www.nice.org.uk

Information for patients

NHS Choices UK vaccination schedule ℰ www.nhs.uk/Conditions/vaccinations
British Lung foundation ☎ 03000 030 555 ℰ www.lunguk.org

Other respiratory infections

Mycoplasma *Mycoplasma pneumoniae* causes epidemics of lower respiratory tract infection every 3–4y. Spread by droplet infection.
- **Incubation** 12–14d
- **Presentation** Dry, persistent cough ± arthralgia. CXR shows bilateral, patchy consolidation. Infection is confirmed with serology
- **Management** Clarithromycin 500mg bd for 2wk or doxycycline 100–200mg daily for 2wk. Relapse is common. Severe infections may require hospital admission

Respiratory chlamydial infection
- **C. pneumoniae** Responsible for 6–19% of community-acquired pneumonia—especially in children and young adults. May be clinically indistinguishable from pneumonia caused by *Mycoplasma*. Treat with doxycycline 100–200mg/d or clarithromycin 500mg bd for 2wk (azithromycin 500mg od for 3d is an alternative)
- **C. psittaci** Infects many animals, but human infection is closely related to contact with birds. Treat as for *C. pneumoniae*

Pertussis (whooping cough)[ND] Caused by *Bordetella pertussis*
- **Incubation** 7d
- **Symptoms**
  - Catarrhal stage—symptoms and signs of URTI; lasts 1–2wk
  - Coughing stage—increasingly severe and paroxysmal cough with spasms of coughing followed by a 'whoop'; associated with vomiting, cyanosis during coughing spasms, and exhaustion; lasts 4–6wk, then cough improves over 2–3wk
- **Examination** Chest is clear between coughing bouts
- **Investigation** Microscopy and culture of pernasal swabs (special swab and culture medium available from the lab); FBC—lymphocytosis
- **Management** Erythromycin in the catarrhal stage. Once coughing stage has started, treatment is symptomatic
- **Complications** Pneumonia, bronchiectasis, convulsions, subconjunctival haemorrhages, and facial petechiae

Prevention
- **Proven contacts** Treat with erythromycin
- **Vaccination** Routinely given in childhood (📖 p. 645). Children with a personal or family history of febrile convulsion, FH of epilepsy, and children with well-controlled epilepsy can be vaccinated—give advice on fever prevention. Defer vaccination for children with any undiagnosed or evolving neurological condition or poorly controlled epilepsy until the condition is stable—if in doubt refer to paediatrics. A temporary pertussis vaccination programme was launched in 2012 in the UK for pregnant women (28–38wk) to protect newborn babies.

❶ Pertussis immunity wanes 4–20y after vaccination—do not rule out the possibility of pertussis because a person has been vaccinated

Aspergillosis A spectrum of diseases. *Cause:* Aspergillus fungus present in the soil and decaying vegetation. Its spores can be inhaled any time of the year but reach peak levels in autumn and winter. Inhaled fungal spores colonize bronchial mucosa and nasal sinuses.

Presentations
- **Extrinsic asthma** 📖 p. 308
- **Allergic bronchopulmonary aspergillosis** Grows in the walls of the bronchi. Presents with episodes of eosinophilic pneumonia (characterized by wheeze, cough, fever, and malaise) throughout the year but worse in late autumn. CXR shows fleeting lung shadows (cleared by expectorating firm, brown plugs of mucus). Untreated → upper lobe fibrosis and 'proximal' bronchiectasis
- **Invasive aspergillosis** Only occurs in the immunocompromised. Aspergillus disseminates from the lung → brain, kidneys, and other organs. Carries very poor prognosis
- **Aspergillus sinusitis** Nasal congestion, headache, and facial pain
- **Aspergilloma** Growth within existing lung cavities (e.g. from previous TB or sarcoidosis). A ball of fungus forms. CXR shows a round lesion with air halo above it. Occasionally results in haemoptysis

Management If suspected, refer for specialist management.

Pneumocystis jiroveci (formerly known as PCP) May be classified as a protozoan or fungus. Causes pneumonia in immunocompromised patients.
- **Presentation** Fever, breathlessness, tachypnoea, dry cough, respiratory failure (± cyanosis)
- **Investigation** CXR normal or 'ground glass' appearance; sputum culture may be diagnostic
- **Management** If suspected refer for specialist care. Treatment is with co-trimoxazole or dapsone
- **Prevention** Prophylactic antibiotics (usually co-trimoxazole) are given to AIDS patients with CD4 counts <200 cells/mm^3

SARS (sudden acute respiratory syndrome) SARS was first reported in China in 2002. Since then there have been several further clusters in far east Asia and one in Canada. SARS is caused by a corona virus (SARS-CoV) and spread by direct contact with an infected individual or rarely aerosol transmission. Incubation is 2–10d.

Two stages
- **Prodrome**—fever (>38°C), malaise, headache, myalgia
- **Respiratory phase**—develops after 3–7d—dry cough and breathlessness. A high proportion progress to respiratory failure. 70% also develop diffuse watery diarrhoea

❶ Cases in the UK are most likely to occur within 10d of return from an affected area—especially one where transmission is thought to be continuing. Admit to a specialist infectious diseases unit. Symptomatic suspected cases should wear a surgical mask during transit.

Further information
Health Protection Agency (HPA) Topics A–Z: Aspergillus; Pertussis, Pneumocystis, SARS ℘ www.hpa.org.uk
The Aspergillus Website ℘ www.aspergillus.man.ac.uk

Cystic fibrosis and Kartagener syndrome

Cystic fibrosis (CF) is the most common inherited disorder in the UK (prevalence: 1 in 2500). Median survival has ↑ dramatically and is now >40y but, of the 7500 CF patients in the UK, 6000 are <25y old.

Genetics Results from mutation of a single gene on chromosome 7 (cystic fibrosis transmembrane conductance regulator) essential for salt and water movement across cell membranes → thickened secretions. >1200 different mutations have been described. Autosomal recessive inheritance—1 in 4 chance of having a child with CF if both parents are carriers. ~1 in 25 adults in the UK carries the CF gene. Most common in Caucasians—rare in people of Afro-Caribbean origin.

Screening Several possibilities:
- **Preconceptual screening** Buccal smears to karyotype prospective parents
- **Antenatal screening** Chorionic villous sampling at ~10wk—for parents with an affected child already or where both parents are +ve on karyotyping
- **Neonatal screening**— 📖 p. 850

Common problems associated with CF Figure 11.6.

Diagnosis
- Screening
- If clinical suspicion of CF, refer to paediatrics. A +ve sweat test (Na$^+$ > 70mmol/L; Cl$^-$ >60mmol/L on 2 occasions) is diagnostic as is ↑ potential difference across the nasal respiratory epithelium

Management CF is a multisystem disease requiring a holistic approach to care which aims to maintain patients' independence, improve quality of life *and* extend life expectancy. A multidisciplinary team in a specialist CF centre is best placed to achieve this. Patients usually have direct access. Management involves:
- Treatment of lung disease e.g. with exercise, physiotherapy, antibiotics, and mucolytics
- Maintaining good nutritional state e.g pre-meal oral pancreatic enzymes, high calorie diet and fat soluble vitamin supplements (A, D, & E)
- Treatment of complications e.g. DM, osteoporosis

Further information for patients and professionals
CF Trust 🏠 www.cysticfibrosis.org.uk

Kartagener syndrome (immotile cilia syndrome) Combination of bronchiectasis, chronic sinusitis and male infertility plus situs inversus (transposed heart and abdominal organs). Caused by a defect in cilia function. Otitis media and salpingitis are frequent. *M. Kartagener (1897–1975)—Swiss physician.*

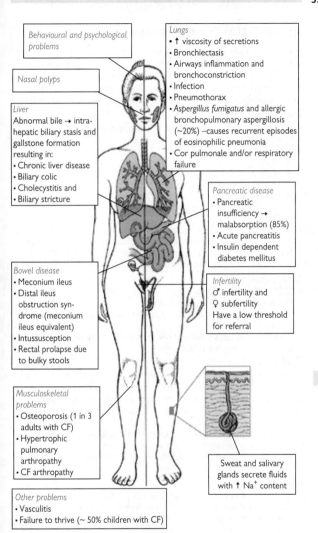

Behavioural and psychological problems

Nasal polyps

Liver
Abnormal bile → intra-hepatic biliary stasis and gallstone formation resulting in:
• Chronic liver disease
• Biliary colic
• Cholecystitis and
• Biliary stricture

Lungs
• ↑ viscosity of secretions
• Bronchiectasis
• Airways inflammation and bronchoconstriction
• Infection
• Pneumothorax
• *Aspergillus fumigatus* and allergic bronchopulmonary aspergillosis (~20%) –causes recurrent episodes of eosinophilic pneumonia
• Cor pulmonale and/or respiratory failure

Pancreatic disease
• Pancreatic insufficiency → malabsorption (85%)
• Acute pancreatitis
• Insulin dependent diabetes mellitus

Bowel disease
• Meconium ileus
• Distal ileus obstruction syndrome (meconium ileus equivalent)
• Intussusception
• Rectal prolapse due to bulky stools

Infertility
♂ infertility and ♀ subfertility
Have a low threshold for referral

Musculoskeletal problems
• Osteoporosis (1 in 3 adults with CF)
• Hypertrophic pulmonary arthropathy
• CF arthropathy

Sweat and salivary glands secrete fluids with ↑ Na^+ content

Other problems
• Vasculitis
• Failure to thrive (~ 50% children with CF)

Figure 11.6 Features of cystic fibrosis
Image without annotations is reproduced from Beers MH (2004) *The Merck Manual of Medical Information* (2nd home edn), with permission from Wiley-Blackwell.

Interstitial lung disease

Also known as diffuse parenchymal lung disease. Comprises >200 different diseases (many rare) in which inflammation affects the alveolar wall, leading to fluid in the alveolar air spaces.

Presentation Increasing dyspnoea ± cough. More rarely wheeze, pleurisy, and/or haemoptysis. May present incidentally with changes on CXR.

Further assessment

- History of the condition—acute, episodic, chronic?
- Severity—exercise tolerance
- Possible causes:
  - Smoking
  - Hobbies and occupation
  - Usual environment (e.g. lives on a farm) and travel
  - Past medical history (particularly rheumatological symptoms and immunosuppression, e.g HIV) and family history
  - Drugs
- Examine looking for fine inspiratory crackles in the chest and evidence of systemic disease, e.g fever, rashes or other skin changes, eye signs (particularly red eye), hepatomegaly and/or splenomegaly, arthritis
- Pulse oximetry—decreased saturations

Investigations
- **CXR** Diffuse shadowing
- **Urine dipstick** For protein and blood
- **Blood** FBC, ESR, liver and kidney function tests, thyroid function tests, autoimmune profile
- **Lung function tests** Usually show restrictive picture—rarely no abnormalities or obstructive picture

Classification See Table 11.13.

Hypersensitivity pneumonitis Also known as extrinsic allergic alveolitis, farmer's lung, and bird fancier's lung. Inhaled particles (e.g. fungal spores, avian proteins) cause an allergic reaction in lungs of hypersensitive individuals. May present as an acute or chronic reaction, or both may occur together.

- **Acute reaction** 2–4h post-exposure. Fever, malaise, dry cough, shortness of breath
- **Chronic reaction** Malaise, weight ↓, exertional dyspnoea, fine crepitations in both lung fields

Investigations
- **Blood** *FBC:* ↑ neutrophils (acute reaction); ↑ *ESR* (acute reaction)
- **CXR** May be normal or show typical changes (shadowing, widespread small nodules, or ground glass appearance)
- Diagnosis is based on history and high-resolution CT scan findings. Serum precipitins to the provoking factor are found in ≥90%

Management If possible prevent further exposure to the allergen. In all cases, refer for specialist advice. Treatment is usually with corticosteroids. If occupational exposure, may qualify as industrial disease and be eligible for compensation—📖 p. 116.

Table 11.13 Classification of interstitial lung disease

Classification	Causes
Acute	Infective: • Bacterial (TB) • Viral (chickenpox, measles) • Fungal Allergy—drugs, fungi, helminths Toxins—drugs, gases Haemodynamic—LVF, fluid overload, renal failure Vasculitis Adult repiratory distress syndrome
Episodic	Eosinophilic pneumonia, e.g. allergic bronchopulmonary aspergillosis Vasculitis, e.g. Churg–Strauss syndrome Hypersensitivity pneumonitis Cryptogenic organizing pneumonia
Chronic due to occupational or environmental exposure	Dust-induced (📖 p. 336)—asbestosis, silicosis, coal worker's pneumoconiosis, siderosis (iron) Farmer's lung Bird fancier's lung Radiation Drugs, e.g. nitrofurantoin, sulfasalazine, gold, penicillamine, aspirin, amiodarone, bleomycin, methotrexate, hydralazine, heroin, methadone, oxygen
Chronic with evidence of systemic disease	Connective tissue disease, e.g. RA, Sjögren's syndrome, SLE Neoplastic, e.g. lymphoma Vasculitis, e.g. Wegener's granulomatosis, Goodpasture's syndrome Sarcoidosis Inherited disorders, e.g. tuberous sclerosis, neurofibromatosis Miscellaneous, e.g. HIV, inflammatory bowel disease, post-bone marrow transplant, amyloidosis
Chronic without evidence of systemic disease	Idiopathic pulmonary fibrosis Chronic aspiration

⚠ Advise all patients with interstitial lung disease to stop smoking. This results in better prognosis for their interstitial lung disease. Furthermore, patients with chronic interstitial lung disease are at substantially increased risk of lung cancer.

Idiopathic pulmonary fibrosis (IPF) Incidence ↑ with age. Most patients are >50y. Progressive condition of unknown cause with insidious onset. Can only be diagnosed if other causes of interstitial lung disease have been excluded and symptoms present >3mo.

Presentation
- Progressive exertional dyspnoea
- Dry cough
- Clubbing (>50%)
- Fine 'Velcro-like' crepitations
- Malaise
- Weight ↓
- Central cyanosis and right heart failure (advanced cases)

Investigations
- **CXR** Diffuse shadowing (although may be normal)
- **Lung function tests** Restrictive picture

Differential diagnosis
- LVF
- COPD
- Drugs
- Other causes of lung fibrosis—dust exposure (coal, asbestos, silica, farmer's lung, bird fancier's lung)
- Inhalant exposure (O_2, NO_2)
- Radiation

Management Refer to a respiratory physician for diagnosis and advice on management. Treatment, where appropriate, is with oral steroids + azathioprine. Pulmonary rehabilitation may be helpful. Lung transplant is a last option. Most patients have poor prognosis, with median survival 3y (5y survival 10–15%), but the subgroup with fibrotic, non-specific interstitial pneumonia (NSIP) has substantially better prognosis with >50% surviving 5y.

❶ Patients with IPF have a 10x ↑ risk of lung cancer. This risk is multiplicative with that from smoking. Patients with IPF who smoke 20 cigarettes a day may have a 200x ↑ risk of lung cancer compared with non-smokers without IPF.

Sarcoidosis Multisystem inflammatory disease of unknown cause characterized by non-caseating granuloma. Incidence in the UK is 3/100,000/y. Typically presents with lung granuloma in a young adult. ♀ > ♂.

Non-respiratory manifestations of sarcoidosis
- Fever and malaise
- Erythema nodosum
- Lupus pernio (blue red nodules on the nose, face, and/or hands)
- Scar infiltration
- Enlarged lacrimal glands
- Hypopyon
- Uveitis
- Arthralgia
- Arrhythmias
- Heart failure
- Pericardial effusion
- Cranial and/or peripheral nerve palsies
- Seizures
- Hypercalcaemia
- Renal stones
- Lymphadenopathy
- Hepatosplenomegaly

Acute sarcoidosis (Löfgren syndrome)
- Polyarthralgia
- Swinging fever
- Erythema nodosum
- Bilateral hilar lymphadenopathy on CXR

Insidious onset CXR shows hilar lymphadenopathy—incidental finding in 30–50%. If symptomatic, usually presents with tiredness, malaise, weight ↓ and/or arthralgia. 15% have lung symptoms with gradual onset of progressive exertional dyspnoea and dry cough.

Management Refer any patient with bilateral hilar lymphadenopathy for further investigation. For patients with confirmed sarcoidosis, specialist management is needed. Steroids are the first-line treatment but should only be used if:
• Progressive disease (on imaging or lung function testing)
• Significant symptoms, or
• Extrapulmonary disease requiring treatment

Rarely, if steroids are not controlling disease progression or symptoms, methotrexate will be added. Inhaled steroids may be helpful to control cough but do not influence disease progression. For patients with severe symptoms, pulmonary rehabilitation may be helpful. Lung transplant may be considered for patients with end-stage pulmonary sarcoidosis.

Prognosis Remits without treatment in 2:3 cases. Acute sarcoidosis has good prognosis with most resolving in <2y. ~30% have chronic progressive disease. Mortality is <3%—usually death is due to CCF and/or cor pulmonale.

Occupational lung disease 📖 p. 336

Further information

British Thoracic Society Interstitial lung disease (2008) *Thorax* **63**: v1–v58 ℘ www.brit-thoracic.org.uk
NICE Idiopathic pulmonary fibrosis (2013) ℘ www.nice.org.uk

Patient support
British Lung Foundation ☏ 03000 030 555 ℘ www.lunguk.org

Occupational lung disease

Exposure to gases, vapours, and dusts at work can lead to lung disease.

Coal worker's pneumoconiosis 90% of all compensated industrial lung disease in the UK. 'Pneumoconiosis' means accumulation of dust in the lungs and tissue reaction to its presence. Incidence is related to total dust exposure. Divides into:

- **Simple pneumoconiosis** Deposition of coal dust in the lung. Graded on CXR appearance. Grading determines whether disability benefit is payable in the UK. Effect on lung function is debated. Predisposes to progressive massive fibrosis
- **Progressive massive fibrosis** Round fibrotic masses several cm in diameter form in the upper lobes. Presents with exertional dyspnoea, cough, black sputum, and, eventually, respiratory failure. Symptoms progress (or even start) after exposure to coal dust has ceased. Lung function tests show a mixed restrictive and obstructive picture with loss of lung volume, irreversible airflow limitation, and ↓ gas transfer

Asbestosis Before legislation banning its use, exposure was widespread and occurred particularly in naval shipyards and power stations. Effects of asbestos exposure—see Table 11.14. Also consider diagnosis in relatives who came into contact with asbestos, for example whilst washing clothes—they can claim compensation if affected.

Silicosis Uncommon. Affects stonemasons, pottery workers, workers exposed to sandblasting, and fettlers (remove sand from metal casts). Caused by inhalation of silica. CXR appearance is distinctive. Presents with exertional dyspnoea ± cough. *Lung function tests:* as for progressive massive fibrosis. Associated with ↑ risk of lung cancer and TB.

Byssinosis Affects cotton mill workers. Symptoms (tightness in the chest, cough, and breathlessness) start on the first day back at work after a break (Monday sickness) with improvement as the week progresses. CXR is normal.

Berylliosis Rare. Long latent period. Affects workers in the aerospace, nuclear power, and electrical industries, and their close relatives. Presents similarly to sarcoidosis (📖 p. 334).

Iron (siderosis), barium (baritosis), and tin (stannosis) dust inhalation Result in dramatic dense nodular shadowing on the CXR but effects on lung function and symptoms are often minimal.

Occupational asthma >200 industrial materials cause occupational asthma. Important causes are recognized occupational diseases in the UK—patients may be eligible for statutory compensation if they apply <10y after leaving the occupation in which asthma developed. Suspect if a patient has symptoms which improve on days away from work/holiday.

Hypersensitivity pneumonitis ('farmer's lung') 📖 p. 332

Management In all cases, refer to a respiratory physician for confirmation of diagnosis (essential if seeking compensation) and advice on management.

Table 11.14 Conditions caused by asbestos exposure

Condition	Asbestos exposure	Features/management
Benign pleural effusion	Usually occurs <20y after exposure	Increasing dyspnoea ± pleuritic pain Refer for drainage of effusion May be recurrent and require pleurodesis
Bilateral diffuse pleural thickening*	Follows light or moderate exposure to asbestos May progress, even in the absence of further exposure	Defined as pleural thickening >5mm thick covering >¼ of the chest wall **Symptoms:** exertional dyspnoea **Lung function tests:** restrictive picture Treatment is symptomatic
Asbestosis*	Follows heavy exposure after a 5–10y interval	Presents with progressive dyspnoea, finger clubbing, and basal end-expiratory crackles **CXR:** 'honeycomb lung'—diffuse streaky shadowing **Lung function tests:** severe restrictive defect and ↓ gas transfer Treatment is symptomatic
Mesothelioma*	Can follow even light exposure to asbestos 20–40y time lag between exposure and appearance of disease	Presents with increasing shortness of breath ± pleuritic pain Examination and CXR reveal unilateral (rarely bilateral) effusion There is no effective active treatment Palliative care— 📖 pp. 1027–47 Median survival is 2y from diagnosis
Asbestosis-related lung cancer*	Patients exposed to asbestos, who have evidence of that exposure (pleural plaques, bilateral pleural thickening, or asbestosis), have an ↑ risk of bronchial carcinoma—usually adenocarcinoma. Smokers exposed to asbestos have a 5× ↑ risk compared to non-smokers exposed to asbestos. Manage as for lung cancer— 📖 p. 320	

* Eligible for industrial injuries benefit in the UK.

Benefits 📖 p. 117

Notification and compensation 📖 p. 116. Some individuals with employment-related lung disease may be able to seek compensation directly from their employers. Expert legal advice is needed.

Patient support
British Lung Foundation ☎ 03000 030 555 🖱 www.lunguk.org

Snoring and obstructive sleep apnoea

Snoring During sleep, the pharyngeal airway narrows due to ↓ dilator muscle tone. Snoring is vibratory noise generated from the pharynx and soft palate as the air passes through this narrowed space. Further narrowing produces louder snoring, laboured inspiration and eventually apnoeic episodes. Social consequences are the usual reason for the patient to seek help. They can be distressing: banishment from the bedroom, marital disharmony, no holidays, fear of travelling, or falling asleep in a public place, etc.

❶ Snoring may be used by the spouse as an excuse to leave the marital bed and may actually be trivial/absent. If suspected, ask the patient to bring a cassette recording of the offending noise.

Obstructive sleep apnoea Occurs when the pharyngeal airway completely closes during sleep resulting in apnoeic episodes. ↑ inspiratory effort is sensed by the brain and a transient arousal provoked. A few of these arousals don't matter—but many (sometimes hundreds) per night → fragmented sleep and consequent daytime sleepiness.

Clinical features
- **Dominant features** Excessive daytime sleepiness (not tiredness—Epworth Sleepiness Scale is a useful assessment tool), impaired concentration, snoring (see Figure 11.7)
- **Other features** Unrefreshing sleep, choking episodes during sleep, witnessed apnoeic episodes, restless sleep, irritability/personality change, nocturia, ↓ libido

Causes of snoring and sleep apnoea Overweight (neck circumference >16"), nasal congestion, evening alcohol/sedatives, large tonsils, receding lower jaw, smoking, hypothyroidism, menopause.

Management
Snoring without sleep apnoea
- **Initial approaches** Suggest changing sleeping position (discourage from sleeping on back); elevate head of the bed (e.g. prop up on bricks—can ↓ nasal congestion); limit number of pillows to one thick/two thin pillows to maximize pharyngeal size; ↓ weight if obese; ↓ or stop evening alcohol/sleeping tablets; suggest partner tries ear plugs (purchase from chemist—takes several nights to get used to wearing them)
- **If clinically indicated**
  - Nasal congestion—start beclometasone nasal spray (applied head downwards) 2 puffs bd ± ipratropium bromide nasal spray 2 puffs nocte
  - Check TFTs to exclude hypothyroidism
  - Discuss the use of HRT in menopausal women
- **If simple measures fail** Refer to:
  - Dentist or ENT for a mandibular advancement device
  - ENT for surgery—septal straightening, polypectomy, turbinate reduction, tonsillectomy, or uvulopalatopharyngoplasty

Sleep apnoea
- Advise patients to: ↓ weight if obese; ↓ or stop evening alcohol/ sleeping tablets, *and*
- Refer to a sleep unit or physician with a special interest in sleep problems. If diagnosis is proven and causing significant daytime sleepiness, usual treatment is with CPAP therapy at night. Mandibular advancement devices are alternatives for patients who cannot tolerate CPAP or have very mild symptoms with no daytime sleepiness. Occasionally, if large tonsils, referral to ENT for surgery is warranted

⚠ **Driving** Warn patients NOT to drive if sleepy. Once diagnosis of sleep apnoea is confirmed, they must inform the DVLA and their insurance company (📖 p. 130).

 Sleep apnoea in children Common in children aged 2–7y in association with tonsil enlargement during URTI. Sleep disruption can cause daytime sleepiness, hyperactivity, poor attention span, and bad behaviour. If tonsils are big enough to produce sleep apnoea in the absence of current infection, refer to ENT for consideration of tonsillectomy.

How likely are you to doze off or fall asleep in the following situations, in contrast to feeling just tired?

This refers to your usual way of life in recent times. Even if you have not done some of these things recently try to work out how they would have affected you.

Situation	Chance of dozing
Sitting and reading	☐
Watching TV	☐
Sitting inactive in a public place (e.g. a theatre or a meeting)	☐
As a passenger in a car for an hour without a break	☐
Lying down to rest in the afternoon when circumstances permit	☐
Sitting and talking to someone	☐
Sitting quietly after a lunch without alcohol	☐
In a car, while stopped for a few minutes in traffic	☐

0—no chance of dozing　　　　　　　　　*2—moderate chance of dozing*
1—slight chance of dozing　　　　　　　*3—high chance of dozing*

If score > 10 – consider sleep apnoea

Figure 11.7 The Epworth Sleepiness Scale

Reproduced from: Johns MW (1991) A new method for measuring daytime sleepiness: the Epworth Sleepiness Scale. *Sleep* **14**:540–5, with permission from Associated Professional Sleep Societies, LLC.

Further information

SIGN/British Thoracic Society Management of obstructive sleep apnoea/ hypopnoea syndrome in adults (2003) ℘ www.sign.ac.uk

Patient support

The Sleep Apnoea Trust (SATA) ℘ www.sleep-apnoea-trust.org

Endocrinology

Symptoms of endocrine disease

Hormones secreted by the endocrine system perform a wide range of functions. Therefore, clinical presentation of different endocrine disorders varies widely from non-specific symptoms such as tiredness, to very specific signs such as delayed puberty. Specific features depend on the gland and hormones involved.

Polydipsia Over-frequent drinking of fluid—often associated, for logical reasons, with polyuria. Ask if associated with thirst. Take a history of fluid intake. If no history of excess fluid intake and BM/fasting blood glucose/ HbA1c is normal, investigate further with U&E, Cr, and Ca^{2+}.

Common causes
- Change in lifestyle: diet/activity/exercise level—may be associated with polyuria but no other symptoms. No history of thirst
- DM—usually accompanied by a history of thirst

Other causes Diarrhoea, diabetes insipidus, ↑ Ca^{2+}, compulsive water drinking (may be a feature of psychotic illness), phosphorus poisoning.

Polyuria Passage of excessive urine. Check the patient does not mean frequency of urination. It can be difficult to distinguish the two. Causes are similar to those of polydipsia and the 2 symptoms are related. Take a history of fluid intake. If no history of excess fluid intake and BM/fasting blood glucose/ HbA1c is normal, investigate further with MSU (for M,C&S), U&E, Cr, and Ca^{2+}.

Consider
- DM—always check a BM and/or fasting blood glucose if a patient complains of polyuria
- Diabetes insipidus
- Hypercalcaemia
- Excessive intake—due to change in lifestyle or psychiatric conditions, e.g. schizophrenia
- Chronic renal failure
- Drugs—diuretics, caffeine, alcohol

Glycosuria Often detected incidentally on urine dipstick. *Causes:*
- DM
- Pregnancy
- Sepsis
- Renal tubular damage
- Low renal threshold

In all cases, check HbA1c/fasting blood glucose (+ glucose tolerance test if pregnant). Check immediate BM if other symptoms suggestive of DM.

Hirsutism Affects 10% ♀. Excess hair in androgenic distribution. *Causes:*
- Most cases are idiopathic; there may be a family history
- Drugs—phenytoin; corticosteroids; ciclosporin; androgenic oral contraception; anabolic steroids; minoxidil; diazoxide
- Polycystic ovarian syndrome (PCOS)
- Late-onset congenital adrenal hyperplasia (rare)
- Cushing's syndrome
- Ovarian tumours (rare)

Assessment
- **History** Long-standing or recent onset, family history, ethnic origin (more common in Mediterranean countries), menstrual history
- **Examination** Distribution of excess hair

Investigation Women with longstanding hirsutism (since puberty) and regular periods need no further investigation unless abnormal signs.

Otherwise: blood—testosterone (↑ in PCOS, androgen-secreting tumour, late-onset congenital adrenal hyperplasia); LH/FSH ratio (>3:1 suggests PCOS).

Refer to gynaecologist or endocrinologist if recent onset, abnormal blood tests, virilism, galactorrhoea, menstrual disturbance, infertility, and/or pelvic mass.

Treatment of idiopathic hirsutism
- Cosmetic—bleaching, shaving, waxing, depilatory creams, electrolysis
- Weight ↓ in obese individuals
- Psychological support
- Topical eflornithine ↓ growth of unwanted facial hair. Continuous use for >8wk is required before benefit is seen. Must be used indefinitely to prevent regrowth. Discontinue if no improvement in 4mo
- Oral medication—all must be taken for ≥6mo to take effect and none abolishes the problem. In all cases, continue treatment until acceptable level of hair growth then stop. Relapse usually follows withdrawal and repeat courses are then required. *Drugs used:* COC pill containing desogestrel or co-cyprindiol; spironolactone

Menopause 📖 p. 710

Delayed or precocious puberty 📖 p. 893

Obesity 📖 p. 178

Metabolic syndrome (syndrome X; insulin resistance syndrome) Impaired glucose tolerance or DM, insulin resistance (in patients on insulin, suggested by insulin doses >1u/kg/d) + other risk factors for CVD including:
- Truncal obesity—waist circumference >0.9m (♀); >1.0m (♂), use 0.1m lower figures for people of south Asian extraction
- ↑ BP—>135/80
- Dyslipidaemia—serum HDL <1.2mmol/L (♀) or <1.0 (♂); fasting serum triglycerides >1.8mmol/L

Associated with high risk of CVD. Treat risk factors aggressively.

Tiredness and lethargy 📖 p. 528

Diabetes mellitus

Diabetes mellitus (DM) is a common syndrome caused by lack, or ↓ effectiveness, of endogenous insulin. It affects 3% of the UK population and is characterized by ↑ blood sugars + abnormalities of carbohydrate/lipid metabolism.

Classification of primary diabetes

Type 1 Occurs at any age but more common in those aged <30y. Autoimmune disease—islet cell antibodies may initially be present. Associated with other autoimmune disease and certain genotypes (HLA DR3/4—although identical twin concordance ≈30%.). Patients are prone to profound weight ↓ and ketoacidosis. Insulin is needed from diagnosis.

Type 2 80–90% patients with DM. ♂:♀≈ 3:2. Prevalence is rising. Lifetime risk of developing type 2 DM is >10% and ~50% remain undiagnosed. *Risk factors:*

- Age >65
- Obesity
- FH of DM (identical twin concordance ≈ 100%)
- Impaired glucose tolerance
- Ethnic group—South Asians/Afro-Caribbeans have 5–10x ↑ risk
- PMH of gestational diabetes or a baby >4kg at birth

Progressive disease resulting from impaired insulin secretion *and* insulin resistance. Life expectancy is ↓ by 30–40% in the age range 40–70y—a ↓ of 8–10y of life. Onset is often insidious; 50% have complications at diagnosis.

Latent autoimmune diabetes in adulthood (LADA) 6–10% of patients with type 2 DM. Characterized by anti-glutamic acid decarboxylase (GAD) antibodies. Associated with higher risk of ketoacidosis and ↑ risk of progression to insulin dependence. Suspect if type 2 DM and:

- Absence of metabolic syndrome features
- Uncontrolled hyperglycaemia despite oral agents, and/or
- Other autoimmune diseases (e.g. thyroid disease, pernicious anaemia)

Maturity onset diabetes of the young (MODY) 1–2% of patients with DM. Present <25y and there is a family history. Genetic syndrome with autosomal dominant inheritance. Gene mutations involved: HNF1-α (70%); HNF1-β; HNF4-α; glucokinase. Gene testing is important to identify the type of MODY, as treatment differs according to type.

Diabetes and pregnancy 📖 p. 828

Other (secondary) causes of DM

- **Drugs** Steroids, thiazides
- **Pancreatic disease** Pancreatitis, surgery, pancreatic cancer, haemochromatosis, cystic fibrosis
- **Endocrine disease** Cushing's disease, acromegaly, thyrotoxicosis, phaeochromocytoma
- **Others** Glycogen storage diseases, insulin receptor antibodies

⚠ Blood glucose may be temporarily ↑ during acute illness, after trauma or surgery or during short courses of blood glucose-raising drugs (see 2° causes). If HbA1c >48mmol/mol DM is likely.

Presentation

- **Acute** Ketoacidosis or hyperosmolar non-ketotic coma (📖 p. 1100)
- **Subacute** Weight ↓, polydipsia, polyuria, lethargy, irritability, infections (candidiasis, skin infection, recurrent infections slow to clear), genital itching, blurred vision, tingling in hands/feet
- **With complications** Skin changes, neuropathy, nephropathy, arterial or eye disease (📖 pp. 354–61)
- **Asymptomatic** Incidental finding or through risk stratification

Risk stratification[N] Use a risk stratification tool (e.g. Diabetes Risk Score or QDiabetes) to assess all patients:

- >40y, or
- >25y of South Asian, Chinese, Afro-Caribbean, or black African origin, from hard-to-reach populations (e.g. homeless) or with other medical conditions that predispose to DM (e.g. pancreatitis)

If low/intermediate risk, give lifestyle advice and reassess in 5y. If high risk or of South Asian/Chinese ethnic origin and BMI >23kg/m², check FBG or HbA1c:

- FBG <5.5mmol/L or HbA1c <42mmol/mol—provide lifestyle advice and reassess every 3y
- FBG 5.5–6.9mmol/L or HbA1c 42–47mmol/mol—provide interventions to ↓ risk (e.g. weight management, dietary advice, help with smoking cessation, BP and lipid management) and reassess annually
- FBG ≥7.0mmol/L or HbA1c ≥48mmol/mol—consider type 2 DM

Diagnosis of diabetes

If symptomatic ↑ plasma glucose (random ≥11.1mmol/L; fasting ≥7.0mmol/L) or ↑ HbA1c ≥48mmol/mol. For all children and adults with suspected ketoacidosis or who are unwell, do not delay to get a laboratory sample, but admit or refer for same-day specialist assessment on BM alone. Otherwise only diagnose with laboratory samples.

If asymptomatic

- ↑ plasma glucose (random ≥11.1mmol/L; fasting ≥7.0mmol/L) *or* ↑ HbA1c ≥48mmol/mol on two separate measurements on different days
- ↑ plasma glucose (random ≥11.1mmol/L; fasting ≥7.0mmol/L) and ↑ HbA1c ≥48 mmol/mol at the same testing

Pre-diabetes (non-diabetic hyperglycaemia) FBG ≥6.1 and <7mmol/L or HbA1c of 42–47mmol/mol. Risk factor for DM and CVD. Follow-up with annual FBG or HbA1c. 4%/y develop DM. Treat CVD risk factors aggressively.

Further information

WHO Use of glycated haemoglobin (HbA1c) in the diagnosis of diabetes mellitus (2011) ⅏ www.who.int/diabetes
NICE ⅏ www.nice.org.uk

- Type 1 diabetes: diagnosis and management (2004)
- Type 2 diabetes (2009)
- Preventing type 2 diabetes: risk identification and interventions for individuals at high risk (2012)

Patient advice and support

Diabetes UK ☎ 0845 120 2960 ⅏ www.diabetes.org.uk

Organization and monitoring of care

Aims of diabetic care
- Alleviation of symptoms
- Minimization of complications
- ↓ in early mortality
- Quality of life enhancement
- Education of the patient and family/carers

Features of well-organized care
- Use of a register and structured records (available as part of in-house computer software)
- 6-monthly review, with recall system and follow-up of defaulters
- Protocol for patient-centred care, including provision of personal care plans tailored to each individual and including self-management plans
- Provision of protected time for the clinic
- Availability of good quality written information for patients
- Open access for patients to receive advice
- Multidisciplinary team covering all aspects of diabetes care—GPs, diabetes nurse specialists/assistants, educators, dieticians, and podiatrists
- Quality monitoring through audit and patient feedback
- Continuing education for professional staff

Routine diabetic review Each diabetic patient requires 6-monthly review (or more frequent, as necessary). This should include a thorough annual review of all aspects of disease and care. Reviews should cover:
- **Problems** Recent life events; new symptoms; difficulties with management since last visit
- **Review of:**
  - Indices of control, e.g. HbA1c
  - Self-monitored results and discussion of their meaning
  - Lifestyle—dietary behaviours; physical activity; smoking
  - Diabetes education—including referral to a structured education programme for those newly diagnosed and information on lifestyle, self-care, support, and when to step up treatment/seek further medical help
  - Skills, e.g. injection technique
  - Foot care
  - Blood glucose, lipid and BP therapy, and results
  - Other medical conditions and therapy affecting DM
  - Immunizations—influenza ± pneumococcal vaccination
  - Depression screening (📖 p. 199)
- **Review of complications** Annual review—more frequent if established complications. Cardiovascular disease; nephropathy; neuropathy; eye disease; foot problems; erectile dysfunction
- **Review of services** Annual review—more frequent if problems
- **Analysis and planning** Agreement on the main points covered, targets for coming months, changes in therapy, interval to next review
- **Recording** Completion of structured record ± patient-held record

❶ 7–10% of patients in long-term residential care have DM. Patients in residential care with DM tend to be neglected. Agree a diabetes care plan for each affected resident, and ensure at least annual diabetic review.

Monitoring blood glucose All patients can achieve good levels of control (see Table 12.1). Poorer control is acceptable in the elderly or others with limited life expectancy as long as they are symptom-free.
- **Fingerprick capillary glucose monitoring** Essential for all patients using insulin. Useful for patients taking sulfonylureas/glinides
  - Explain the range of suitable monitoring devices available (*BNF* 6.1.6), and train in the use of the selected method
  - Frequency of self-monitoring varies according to need
  - Set targets for preprandial glucose levels
  - Assess skills (and meters) yearly or if problems self-monitoring
  - Evaluate reliability of results by comparison with HbA1c results and results obtained at review
- **Glycosylated haemoglobin (HbA1c)** Measure at least 2x/y. Represents average blood glucose control over the previous 6–8wk

❶ Patients with type 2 DM who have a Group 2 driving licence and are taking sulfonylureas or glinides must check blood glucose twice daily so will need blood glucose meters and a supply of testing sticks.

Table 12.1 Indices of control

Measure	Target
Blood glucose (mmol/L)	4–7 fasting (post-prandial <9)—adults 4–8 fasting (post-prandial <10)—children
Urine	−ve (postprandial sugars <0.5%)
HbA1c (normal 20–42 mmol/mol)—measure every 2–6mo depending on control	48–58mmol/mol* If HbA1c remains high but pre-meal self-monitoring levels remain well controlled (<7.0mmol/L), consider self-monitoring to detect postprandial hyperglycaemia (>8.5mmol/L).
Serum cholesterol (mmol/L)	↓ total cholesterol by 25% or to <4—whichever is the lower value *or* ↓ LDL cholesterol by 30% or to <2—whichever is the lower value
BMI (kg/m²)	25–30
BP (mmHg)	<140/80—uncomplicated type 2 DM <135/85—uncomplicated type 2 DM <130/80—if any renal, foot, eye or cardiovascular complications of type 1 or type 2 DM

* Adjust target to the individual.

Further information
NICE Diabetes in adults quality standards (2011) ॐ www.nice.org.uk

Management of diabetes: education

Education is an essential aspect of diabetic care. Diabetes is a chronic condition, and however well it is managed in the clinic, the patient has to manage his or her own disease the rest of the time. Everyone with DM should receive education through a structured, quality-controlled education programme, e.g. diabetes education and self-management for ongoing and newly diagnosed (DESMOND). Education enables patients and their carers to become equal partners in the management of their disease. *Topics to cover during routine reviews:*

General knowledge Information about:
- DM, its progressive nature, and complications
- Aims of management
- Structure of diabetic services and ways to access them
- Equipment required and usage instructions—syringes, needles, blood testing equipment, etc.
- Free prescriptions for patients requiring drugs or insulin to control their diabetes
- Problems of pregnancy (women of childbearing age only)
- Alert bracelets/tags—Medic-Alert (☎ 0800 581 420) or Medi-Tag (☎ 0121 200 1616) provide engraved jewellery, watches, and tags

Diet Patients do *not* need a separate diet from the rest of the family or expensive 'diabetes' food products. A diabetic diet is a healthy diet.
- Aim for ≥50% of calorie intake from fibre-rich carbohydrate, with minimum fat (especially saturated), refined carbohydrate, and alcohol
- Adjust total calorie intake according to desired BMI
- Recommend ≥5 portions of fresh fruit or vegetables/d
- Spread food intake evenly across the day for patients controlled with tablets or diet
- Diet sheets are available from Diabetes UK and should be provided
- Ready-made meals, processed foods, and alcohol are often sources of hidden sugar

Immunizations Offer influenza and pneumococcal vaccine to all patients with diabetes.

Psychological problems Discuss concerns about the diagnosis of DM or development of complications. Arrange counselling/refer to self-help resources as needed. Teenagers with diabetes can be a particularly difficult group to manage. Often control is poor due to a combination of rapid bodily changes and rebellion against the diagnosis of DM. Support information and advice given in specialist clinics.

Exercise Encourage regular exercise.
- Review activity at work and in getting to and from the workplace, hobbies, and physical activity in the home
- Advise physical activity can ↑ insulin sensitivity, ↓ BP, and improve blood lipid control
- If appropriate, suggest regular physical activity tailored to individual ability (e.g. brisk walking for 30min/d; exercise prescription)

Smoking Advice on and assistance with smoking cessation (🕮 p. 182).

Driving Advise all drivers that they must notify their car insurance company and the DVLA, unless their diabetes is controlled by diet alone. Be aware of insurers who cater for diabetic drivers.
• Type 1 DM—must be aware of hypoglycaemic episodes
• All type 1 DM and those with type 2 DM taking sulfonylurea or glinide: group 1 licence—<2 hypoglycaemic episodes/y requiring assistance of another person; group 2 licence—no hypoglycaemic episodes requiring assistance of another person and must monitor blood glucose 2x/d

Foot care 📖 p. 360

Employment Advise those on insulin that certain jobs are no longer possible:
• Working on scaffolding or with dangerous machinery
• Joining the police or the armed services
• Driving a heavy goods or public service vehicle

Jobs without these hazards should pose no problems though the patient might wish to tell his/her employer. Special advice may be needed for shift work.

Travel Give advice on:
• Management of change in time zones (📖 p. 133)
• Transport of insulin
• Keeping monitoring and injection equipment in hand-luggage
• Differences in insulin types and concentrations between countries
• Travel related illness (especially gastroenteritis)
• Need for immunization and travel insurance

Be aware of insurers who cater for diabetic travellers.

Further information
DH Structured patient education in diabetes: report from the Patient Education Working Group (2005) ℘ www.dh.gov.uk
NICE ℘ www.nice.org.uk
• Type 2 diabetes (2009)
• Diabetes in adults quality standards (2011)

Patient advice and support
Diabetes UK ☎ 0845 120 2960 ℘ www.diabetes.org.uk

Treatment of type 2 diabetes

△ *Always* combine treatment of hyperglycaemia with modification of other risk factors for vascular complications—📖 p. 354.

Healthy eating and exercise Diet is the cornerstone of treatment. Diet sheets are available from Diabetes UK. ↑ physical activity is beneficial (↓ weight, ↓ lipids, and ↑ insulin sensitivity) but not always possible.

First-line oral hypoglycaemic agents[N] See Figure 12.1 and *BNF* 6.1.2.

Biguanides Metformin 500mg–1g bd. ↓ gluconeogenesis and ↑ peripheral utilization of glucose. Only effective if some endogenous insulin production. Initiate metformin for all patients if HbA1c remains ≥48mmol/mol after a trial of diet/lifestyle interventions. Avoid in very elderly patients and those with serious heart disease, liver/renal failure, or high alcohol intake, as ↑ risk of lactic acidosis. Hypoglycaemia is not a problem. Start with the minimum dose and ↑ monthly until control is achieved/maximum dose reached.

Sulfonylureas (e.g. gliclazide 80–160mg bd) Consider first-line if not overweight, hyperglycaemic symptoms requiring rapid response, and/or metformin is contraindicated/not tolerated. Augment insulin secretion, so only effective if residual endogenous insulin production. All are equally effective. If one sulfonylurea does not work—another is not likely to either. Advise patients to take before meals—warn about hypoglycaemia if meals are omitted (and need for blood monitoring if group 2 driving licence). Start at the minimum dose, and ↑ until blood sugar is controlled/maximum dose is reached. Wait ≥1mo between adjustments. Main side effect is weight ↑.

Second-/third-line oral hypoglycaemic agents[N] (*BNF* 6.1.2)

Pioglitazone 15mg od. ↑ insulin secretion/sensitivity, slightly ↓ BP, and ↓ total cholesterol. Does not cause hypoglycaemia. May cause weight ↑. Use in combination with metformin and/or sulfonylurea for patients with poor glycaemic control. ❶ Associated with ↑ risk of bladder cancer, fluid retention, and heart failure.

DPP-4 inhibitors (e.g. sitagliptin 100mg od, saxagliptin 5mg od, vildagliptin 5mg od/bd, linagliptin 5mg od) ↑ incretin levels. Do not cause weight ↑ or hypoglycaemia. Use with metformin and/or sulfonylurea if poor glycaemic control. Linagliptin is useful for patients with renal failure as excreted via the gall bladder.

Other treatments[N]

- **Exenetide** (bd/weekly injection), **lixisenatide** (od injection) and **liraglutide** (od injection)—may be an alternative to insulin in obese patients. Stimulate insulin production and ↓ rate of glucose absorption from the gut. Licensed for use in addition to metformin and/or a sulfonylurea. Continue after 6mo only if HbA1c has ↓ >1mmol/mol and weight ↓ is >3% of initial body weight
- **Rapid-acting insulin secretagogues** (nateglinide, repaglinide)—stimulate insulin release. Rapid onset and short duration of activity. May be useful as second-line treatment with metformin for those with erratic lifestyle

Starting insulin (📖 p. 352) If on dual therapy (metformin + sulfonylurea) and markedly hyperglycaemic, start insulin in preference to adding other drugs unless very good reasons not to. Continue metformin and sulfonylurea except if planning pregnancy. Review the use of sulfonylurea if hypoglycaemia occurs.

Drug treatment of obesity 📖 p. 179.

Figure 12.1 Using oral hypoglycaemic agents in type 2 DM (HbA1c units are in mmol/mol)[N]

Further information
NICE Type 2 diabetes (2009) 🖱 www.nice.org.uk

Treatment with insulin

First-line treatment for type 1 DM and used when diet + oral therapy have failed for type 2 DM. Local guidelines govern who does what.

⚠ All drivers must notify the DVLA and their insurance company.

Types of insulin

- **Rapid-acting analogues** (e.g. insulin lispro—fastest acting; peak 0–3h after injection; last 2–5h; give just prior to meals)
- **Soluble (clear) human, porcine, or bovine** (e.g. Actrapid®—short-acting; peak 2–6h after injection; last 8h; give 15–30min before meals)
- **Intermediate- or longer-acting (cloudy) human, porcine, or bovine** (e.g. Humulin I®)—peak 4–12h after injection; last up to 30h. Taken alone, od/bd to provide background insulin, or with short/rapid-acting insulin
- **Long-acting insulin analogues** (e.g. insulin glargine)—last 24h; provide background insulin; as no peak, associated with ↓ risk of hypoglycaemia
- **Pre-mixed**—combination of short- + long-acting insulin, e.g. 30%:70%

Examples of injection regimes[*]

- Intermediate ± short-acting insulin od/bd (mane ± pre-evening meal)
- Short- + intermediate-acting insulin mane, short-rapid-acting[*] insulin before evening meal, and intermediate-acting insulin before bed
- Short-rapid-acting[*] insulin tds pre-meals + intermediate-acting pre-bed
- Combinations of oral therapy + od/bd long-intermediate-acting insulin
- Rarely, continuous sc infusion of short-acting insulin is needed to achieve control—needs specialist supervision

[*] Use rapid-acting insulin as an alternative to mealtime soluble insulin where nocturnal or late interprandial hypoglycaemia is a problem or to eliminate the need for snacks between meals.

Administration

- Deep sc injection into upper arm, thigh, buttock, or abdomen
- Fat hypertrophy/scarring are minimized by rotation of injection sites
- 'Pen' devices and syringe/needle are equally effective. In all cases prime the needle using an 'air shot' (an empty needle ↓ insulin dose by ~2u)
- Rock 'pens' containing premixed insulins to mix contents before use
- ↑ absorption can occur if a limb is exercised following injection

Monitoring

- Check blood glucose pre-prandially ≥1x/d at different times—more often if multiple injection regimes, after dose changes or during intercurrent illness; ask patients to keep a timed/dated diary of readings
- Record episodes of hypoglycaemia
- *Target:* blood glucose 4–7mmol/L pre-meals, with hypoglycaemic episodes kept to a minimum (4–8mmol/L pre-meals if <18y old)

Starting insulin for patients with type 2 DM Use a structured programme. Appropriate training is needed for all practice staff involved.

- Before starting—teach home blood glucose monitoring; reinforce diet
- Continue metformin ± sulfonylurea
- Teach insulin injection technique—start 10u of long-acting insulin od
- Teach patients/carers about safe disposal of sharps and hypoglycaemia

- Give instructions to ↑ dose every 3–7d until target levels are reached e.g. average fasting glucose >10mmol/L—↑ by 6–8u/d; 8–10mmol/L—↑ by 4–6u/d; 6–8mmol/L—↑ by 2–4u/d
- Provide a contact telephone number for advice; follow up after 2–3d and then as needed; check HbA1c every 3mo until stable

Exercise ↓ insulin dose acting at the time of exercise *or* take 1–2 glucose tablets before exercise, then check blood glucose afterwards. Adjust alterations/glucose dose with experience of effects of exercise.

Intercurrent illness Continue insulin in usual dose and keep a regular check (≥qds) of blood sugar. Maintain glucose intake even if not eating (e.g. with Lucozade or milk).

- If glucose >13mmol/L, ↑ insulin by 2u/d until control is achieved or use top-up injections of short-acting insulin qds prn
- Admit to hospital if: condition warrants admission; unable to take glucose; persistent vomiting and/or dehydration; ketotic (check urine if blood sugar >13mmol/L)

Poor control
- Exclude intercurrent illness
- Consider psychosocial factors
- Consider diet and/or gastroparesis
- Check insulin is being used correctly
- Check injection sites are not scarred or hypertrophic
- Consider changing insulin dose—ask the patient to record a glucose profile (blood sugar pre-meals and before bed); if using >1 insulin, adjust one at a time ↑ or ↓ as needed; alter by ≤10% each time; allow ≥48h between dose adjustments; alter dose of insulin acting at the time blood sugar is most out of control

Hypoglycaemia

Emergency management 📖 p. 1100

Advice for patients
- Check blood sugar before driving and every 2h during a long journey
- Carry glucose everywhere and sandwiches on long journeys
- If hypoglycaemia occurs, stop hazardous activities and take action
- Wait until fully recovered before resuming activities

In case of severe hypoglycaemia Supply a responsible member of the family with glucose gel (e.g. GlucoGel®) and glucagon injection—teach him/her to use it. Response is short-lived—give oral glucose (e.g. Lucozade, glucose tablets, milk) as soon as the patient is conscious.

Recurrent hypoglycaemia
- If hypoglycaemia occurs in a regular pattern check pattern of meals and activity and alter insulin to match needs
- If erratic consider erratic lifestyle, alcohol, problems with absorption, errors in administration, gastroparesis
- If no obvious cause, consider change in underlying insulin sensitivity (e.g. age, renal impairment)

Hypoglycaemia unawareness To restore warning signs adjust insulin/food intake to stop glucose levels dropping to <4mmol/L. Consider undetected night-time hypoglycaemia if HbA1c < expected from blood sugar diary. Driving is not permitted if hypoglycaemic awareness has been lost or >1 hypoglycaemic episode requiring assistance from another individual in the past year (no episodes permitted for group 2 licence).

Diabetic complications: cardiovascular

Diabetic patients are at ↑ risk of MI (2–5x), stroke (2–3x), and peripheral vascular disease. Protective effect of female sex is lost. Atherosclerotic disease accounts for most of the excess mortality due to DM. Check arterial risk factors annually:

- Age
- Family history of arterial disease
- Abdominal adiposity
- BP
- Lipid profile (LDL, HDL cholesterol, and triglycerides)
- Albumin excretion rate
- Blood glucose control
- Smoking—give smoking cessation advice at every opportunity. Help patients who want to give up with advice, medication, and support

⚠ **High-risk groups**

Type 1 Consider patients at increased risk if:
- >35y
- Originate in the Indian subcontinent
- Family history of premature heart disease
- Pre-existing CVD
- ≥2 features of the metabolic syndrome (🔲 p. 343)
- Abnormal lipids
- ↑ BP
- Microalbuminuria/proteinuria

Type 2 Consider to be at high CVD risk *unless all* the following apply:
- Not overweight for ethnic group
- Normotensive (BP <140/80mmHg without antihypertensive therapy)
- No microalbuminuria
- Non-smoker
- No high-risk lipid profile
- No history of cardiovascular disease
- No family history of cardiovascular disease

Aspirin Control systolic BP to <145/90mmHg before starting treatment. Give 75mg od to all those with a prior history of CVD. Do not use for primary prevention.

Statin Give a statin (e.g. simvastatin or atorvastatin) to:
- All type 1 diabetics with ↑ risk of arterial disease
- All type 2 diabetics aged >75y
- Type 2 diabetics of any age with any high-risk factors
- Type 2 diabetics >40y with no high risk factors, but who have 10y CVD risk >20%, calculated using special diabetic risk tables, e.g. UKPDS risk engine (🖰 www.dtu.ox.ac.uk/riskengine)

Choice of statin depends on cost and other medication the patient is taking. Start with a mid-range dose (e.g. simvastatin 40mg or atorvastatin 20mg nocte). Recheck lipid profile 1–3mo after starting treatment. Aim to ↓ total cholesterol to <4mmol/L *or* ↓ LDL cholesterol to <2.0mmol/L. If treatment does not bring lipids within target levels, ↑ the statin dose or change to an alternative statin ($\triangle$ simvastatin at a dose of 80mg is no longer recommended; avoid 40mg dose in combination with amlodipine, diltiazem, verapamil, or amiodarone).

Triglycerides

- If triglycerides are >4.5mmol/L despite optimal glycaemic control, start a fibrate (e.g. fenofibrate) to ↓ risk of pancreatitis. If this is ineffective, consider a trial of high-concentration omega-3 fish oils
- If high CVD risk and triglycerides are 2.3–4.5mmol/L despite statin treatment, consider adding a fibrate

Blood glucose Target HbA1c is <48mmol/mol if type 1 DM or type 2 DM treated with lifestyle measures or one/two oral agents. Otherwise target HbA1c is <58mmol/mol.

BP Any ↓ in average BP ↓ risk of cardiovascular complications. Measure BP annually if not hypertensive and no renal disease. If BP is higher than target, consider 24h ambulatory blood pressure monitoring ($\square$ p. 246).

- **Type 1 DM**[N] Treat if systolic BP >135 or diastolic BP >85mmHg, *unless* microalbuminuria/proteinuria or ≥2 features of the metabolic syndrome ($\square$ p. 343) when treat if systolic BP >130 or diastolic BP >80mmHg
- **Type 2 DM**[N] Treat if systolic BP ≥140 or diastolic BP ≥80mmHg, regardless of absolute risk of CVD. Aim to ↓ BP to <140/80mmHg (or <130/80mmHg if kidney, eye, or cardiovascular disease)

Choice of antihypertensive[N]

- In all cases, discuss lifestyle modifications ($\square$ p. 249)
- If already on antihypertensives at the time of diagnosis of DM, review BP and medication use. Change only if BP is poorly controlled or current medication is inappropriate
- For those with new hypertension, start with an ACE inhibitor (unless possibility of becoming pregnant when start with Ca^{2+} channel blocker). Titrate dose to the maximum tolerated. If side effects with ACE inhibitor, ARB is an alternative. For people of Afro-Caribbean descent offer ACE inhibitor + Ca^{2+} channel blocker. Monitor BP every 1–2mo until stable within target
- If BP remains above target add a calcium channel blocker (e.g. amlodipine 5mg od)
- If BP still remains above target, add a diuretic (e.g. indapamide M/R 1.5mg od)
- Fourth-line agents include alpha-blockers, beta-blockers, or further diuretic therapy, e.g. spironolactone 25mg od. Consider referral

Monitoring Monitor BP every 4–6mo once stable on treatment. Check for possible adverse side effects of medication (including postural drop).

Further information

NICE $\wp$ www.nice.org.uk
- Type 1 diabetes: diagnosis and management (2004)
- Type 2 diabetes (2009)
- Hypertension in adults (2011)

Diabetic complications: renal and eye

Renal disease

Urinary tract infections More common in patients with poorly controlled DM. May exacerbate renal failure and lead to renal scarring. Consider papillary necrosis if recurrent (more common in DM).

Nephropathy

- Most common cause of end-stage renal failure in adults starting dialysis in the UK. 25% diabetics have renal damage—more common if of Asian or African ethnic origin
- Nephropathy is characterized by proteinuria, ↑ BP, and progressive ↓ in renal function
- Before overt nephropathy occurs, there is a phase (microalbuminuria or incipient nephropathy) in which the urine contains traces of protein not detected by standard protein dipstick. Presence of ↑ urine albumin levels and/or ↑ serum creatinine is associated with ↑ risk of premature cardiovascular events and renal failure
- Check renal function annually (first-pass urine specimen for albumin:creatinine ratio; dipstick for protein and haematuria; serum creatinine and eGFR)

Interpretation of albumin:creatinine ratio

- Microalbuminuria is defined as albumin:creatinine ratio ≥2.5mg/mmol (♂) or ≥3.5mg/mmol (♀) or albumin concentration ≥20mg/L in the absence of overt proteinuria or urinary tract infection
- If albumin:creatinine ratio is abnormal, repeat the test 2x over the next 3–4mo. Microalbuminuria is confirmed if ≥1 of the repeat results is also abnormal

Suspect other renal disease if

- Albumin:creatinine ratio is ↑ *without* retinopathy
- BP is particularly high or resistant to treatment
- Heavy proteinuria (albumin:creatinine ratio >100mg/mmol) but previously documented as normal
- Significant haematuria
- GFR has worsened rapidly
- The person is systemically unwell

Management of nephropathy

- Optimize blood glucose control
- Monitor and treat ↑ BP (target BP <130/80mmHg) and treat other arterial risk factors aggressively
- Modify diet (↓ salt intake, ↓ protein intake with target of 0.8g/kg)
- Treat all patients with DM and microalbuminuria or CKD with an ACE inhibitor (or ARB), titrating the dose to the maximum tolerated. This protects renal function and ↓ proteinuria, even if the patient is not hypertensive
- Refer to a nephrologist if proteinuria (albumin:creatinine ratio >70mg/mmol, or total protein:creatinine ratio >100mg/mmol, and UTI excluded); eGFR <30 or eGFR drops by >15% between tests (see CKD 📖 p. 440)

Eye disease ~1:3 diabetics have eye problems at the time of diagnosis.

Blurred vision May occur if blood glucose control is poor—caused by osmotic changes in the lens, and corrects with normalization of blood sugar. Wait before changing glasses.

Cataract Juvenile 'snowflake' cataracts are more common and can develop rapidly (over days). Senile cataracts occur ~10y earlier in DM.

Glaucoma DM is a risk factor for developing glaucoma.

Retinopathy Most common cause of blindness in people of working age in industrialized countries (risk is ↑ x20 compared to non-diabetics). 20–40% type 2 diabetics have retinopathy at diagnosis. 20y after diagnosis, 95% type 1 diabetics and 60% type 2 diabetics have retinopathy—sight-threatening in 5–10%.

Pathogenesis of retinopathy Small retinal blood vessels become blocked, swollen (aneurysms) or leaky causing exudate formation, oedema or new vessels. Laser treatment (photo-coagulation) halts progression but does not restore vision.

- Good diabetic control slows development of retinopathy. Aim for HbA1c of <58 mmol/mol
- Monitor and treat risk factors—BP, lipids (hard exudates), smoking
- Fenofibrate ↓ risk of retinopathy and retinopathy progression[R]. Place in routine management is yet to be determined

> ❶ Digital retinal photography is available throughout the UK. Screen at least annually to detect retinopathy before visual loss occurs.

Refer to ophthalmologist if
- Sudden loss of vision—*E*
- Rubeosis iridis—*E*
- Pre-retinal or vitreous haemorrhage—*E*
- Retinal detachment—*E*
- New vessel formation—*U*
- Maculopathy—*R*
- Pre-proliferative retinopathy—*R*
- Cataract affecting visual acuity—*R*
- Unexplained drop in visual acuity—*R*

E = Emergency; *U* = urgent; *R* = routine

Further information

NICE ℘ www.nice.org.uk
- Type 1 diabetes: diagnosis and management (2004)
- Type 2 diabetes (2009)

ACCORD Study Group and ACCORD Eye Study Group (2010) Effects of medical therapies on retinopathy progression in type 2 diabetes. *New England Journal of Medicine* **363**:233–44

Diabetic complications: nerve and skin

Neuropathy Enquire annually about painful and other symptomatic neuropathy, impotence in men and manifestations of autonomic neuropathy especially if renal complications or erratic blood glucose control. Optimize blood sugar control.

Symmetrical sensory progressive polyneuropathy Affects 40–50% of patients with DM. Starts distally feet>hands. Glove-and-stocking distribution. May be asymptomatic or cause numbness, tingling, or neuropathic pain. Pain can be depressing and disabling. Be supportive. If simple analgesia with paracetamol or NSAID is ineffective try neuropathic painkillers (Figure 12.2). When pain is controlled, review regularly and consider reducing dose/stopping.

Mononeuropathies/mononeuritis multiplex Especially cranial nerves III and VI—🕮 p. 536.

Amyotrophy Painful wasting of quadriceps muscles—reversible with improved blood sugar control.

Autonomic neuropathy
- **Postural ↓ BP** Common especially in the elderly. Increasing dietary salt intake may help. Other treatments are all unlicensed. They include fludrocortisone 100–400 micrograms od (uncomfortable oedema is a common side effect) ± flurbiprofen or ephedrine hydrochloride (30–60mg tds to relieve oedema), and midodrine (alpha agonist)
- **Urinary retention** 🕮 p. 454
- **Diabetic diarrhoea** Exclude other causes of change in bowel habit—🕮 p. 406. Diabetic diarrhoea can be treated with 2 or 3 doses of tetracycline (250mg—unlicensed). Otherwise treat with codeine phosphate 30mg tds/qds prn
- **Erectile dysfunction** 🕮 p. 776
- **Gastric paresis** Treat with an antiemetic which promotes gastric transit e.g. domperidone 30mg tds. When this fails, erythromycin may be used but evidence of effectiveness is lacking
- **Gustatory sweating** Can be treated with an antimuscarinic such as propantheline bromide but side effects are common. Hyperhidrosis—🕮 p. 603

Depression Some physical illnesses, including DM, predispose patients to depression. Screen for depression as part of the annual diabetic check (🕮 p. 199)

Skin changes associated with DM Numerous skin problems are associated with DM. These include:
- Predisposition to infection e.g. candidiasis, staphylococcal infection (folliculitis, boils)
- Pruritus
- Xanthomas
- Vitiligo (type 1 DM)
- Neuropathic and/or ischaemic ulcers—see the diabetic foot—🕮 p. 360

- Fat atrophy/hypertrophy at insulin injection sites
- Necrobiosis lipoidica—50% associated with DM. Small, dusky red nodules with well-circumscribed borders; can be single or multiple. Usually on the outside of the shin. Enlarge slowly becoming brownish yellow, irregular, and flattened/depressed. Long-standing lesions may ulcerate. No effective treatment
- Diabetic dermopathy—pigmented scars over shins
- Granuloma annulare —asymptomatic dermal nodules; association with DM is controversial
- Diabetic cheiroarthropathy—waxy skin thickening over the dorsum of the hand with restricted mobility

Refer to pain clinic or endocrinology

If pain is not controlled, try adding/replacing with tramadol (50–100mg qds)

If amitriptyline is ineffective, consider changing to/adding pregabalin (75–300mg bd)

If duloxetine is ineffective or not tolerated, switch to amitriptyline (10–75mg) taken at 5–7 p.m.

Start with duloxetine (60–120mg/d)

Figure 12.2 Diabetic neuropathy—steps to pain control[N]

❶ For all drugs listed in Figure 12.2, start at low dose and titrate up the dose according to response. Consider lidocaine patches for people with localized pain who are unable to tolerate oral medication.

Further information
NICE www.nice.org.uk
- Type 1 diabetes: diagnosis and management (2004)
- Type 2 diabetes (2009)
- Neuropathic pain (2010)
- Depression in adults with a chronic physical health problem (2009)

The diabetic foot

Foot problems are common amongst people with diabetes—5% develop a foot ulcer in any year (see Table 12.2). Foot problems are due to:
- Peripheral neuropathy (affects 20–40% diabetic patients) → ↓ foot sensation, *and*
- Peripheral vascular disease (affects 20–40% diabetic patients) → pain and predisposition to ulceration

Table 12.2 Clinical features of neuropathic and vascular foot ulcers

Neuropathic	Vascular
Warm foot	Cool foot
Bounding pulses, normal ABPI	Absent pulses, ↓ ABPI
Located at pressure points	Located at extremities (e.g. between toes)
Painless	Painful
Clearly defined or 'punched out'	Less clearly delineated
Surrounded by callus	

Information about foot care

- Self-care and self-monitoring:
  - Daily examination of the feet for problems—colour change; swelling; breaks in the skin
  - Footwear—importance of well-fitting shoes and hosiery
  - Hygiene (daily washing and careful drying) and nail care
  - Dangers associated with procedures, e.g. corn/verruca removal
  - Methods to help self-monitoring, e.g. mirrors if ↓ mobility
- When to seek advice from a health professional—if any colour change, swelling, breaks in the skin, or numbness, or if self-monitoring is not possible (e.g. due to mobility problems)
- For patients at increased or high risk or with ulcers, additionally, advise no barefoot walking and that, due to ↓ sensation, extra care and attention is needed
- If skin lesions, advise patients to seek help if any change in the lesion, or if ↑ swelling, pain, odour, colour change, or systemic symptoms

Risk factors

- Neuropathy
- Peripheral vascular disease
- Previous ulceration or amputation
- Age >70y
- Plantar callus
- Foot deformities
- Poor footwear
- Long duration of DM
- Social deprivation and isolation
- Poor vision
- Smoking

The foot check Check the feet as part of the annual review.

History

- Foot problems since last review
- Visual or mobility problems affecting self-care of feet
- Self-care behaviours and knowledge of foot care
- History of numbness, tingling, or burning—may be worse at night

Examination
- Foot shape, deformity, joint rigidity, and shoes
- Foot skin condition—fragility, cracking, oedema, callus, ulceration, sweating, presence of hair
- Foot and ankle pulses
- Sensitivity to 10g monofilament or vibration

Management

General points
- Optimize diabetic control and risk factors for vascular disease (including smoking cessation)
- Review drug therapy—stop β-blockers if peripheral vascular disease
- Educate about foot care

Specific management Classification—Table 12.3
- **Low risk** Foot care education
- **Increased risk** Foot care education. Refer to the foot protection team. Check feet every 3–6mo. Consider referral for vascular assessment. Consider regular podiatry if poor vision, immobility, or poor social conditions/foot hygiene. If previous foot ulcer, deformity, or skin changes manage as high risk
- **High risk** Stress importance of foot care. Refer to the foot protection team for specialist podiatry. Inspect feet every 3–6mo. Review need for vascular assessment. Treat fungal infection
- **Foot ulcer** Refer to the multidisciplinary specialist foot care team urgently. Assess ischaemia using Dopplers. Consider referral for angiography. Treat infection. If new ulceration, cellulitis or discoloration refer to a specialized podiatry/foot care team within 24h

Table 12.3 Classification of foot risk

Foot risk	Features
Low current risk	Normal sensation, palpable pulses
Increased risk	Neuropathy, absent pulses, or other risk factors
High risk	Neuropathy or absent pulses + deformity or skin changes or previous ulcer
Ulcerated foot	Foot ulcer on examination

❶ Patients with diabetes may have coexisting peripheral neuropathy and peripheral vascular disease. ABPI may be artificially ↑ due to calcification of vessels.

Charcot osteoarthropathy (Charcot's joint) Neuropathic foot damaged because of trauma 2° to loss of pain sensation. If suspected refer immediately to the multidisciplinary foot care team for immobilization and long-term management.

Further information

NICE ◌ www.nice.org.uk
- Type 1 diabetes: diagnosis and management (2004)
- Type 2 diabetes (2008)

Lumps in the thyroid gland and goitres

Faced with a lump in the pre-tracheal region of the neck, ask:
- Is it in the thyroid (moves up and down on swallowing)?
- Is it a solitary lump or more generalized (a goitre)?
- Is the patient thyrotoxic, euthyroid, or hypothyroid?
- Is the trachea being compressed (patient is breathless)?

Management of thyroid lumps[N]

Refer immediately to a thyroid surgeon If symptoms of tracheal compression, including stridor due to thyroid swelling.

Refer urgently to a thyroid surgeon If thyroid swelling + *any* of:
- Patient aged ≥65y
- Solitary nodule increasing in size
- History of neck irradiation
- FH of an endocrine tumour
- Unexplained hoarseness/voice changes
- Cervical lymphadenopathy
- Very young (pre-pubertal) patient

Investigation of patients who do not require urgent referral Request TFTs if thyroid swelling *without* stridor or any of the features listed above. ❶ Do not request USS or isotope scanning
- **Refer non-urgently to endocrinology** Patients with hyper- or hypothyroidism and an associated goitre
- **Refer non-urgently to a thyroid surgeon** Patients with goitre and normal thyroid function tests without any of the features listed above

Solitary thyroid nodules Investigate *all* solitary nodules. Check TFTs and refer as above. Differential diagnosis:
- **Benign** (90%): cyst, adenoma, discrete nodule in a nodular goitre
- **Malignant** (10%): *primary*—thyroid adenocarcinoma, lymphoma, medullary carcinoma; *secondary*—direct spread from local tumour, metastatic spread from breast, colon/rectum, kidney, lung, lymphoma

Carcinoma of the thyroid

Primary tumours
- **Papillary adenocarcinoma** (60%) Typical age: 10–40y. ♀ > ♂ Low-grade malignancy. Rarely fatal. Spreads to local LNs and/or lung. Sensitive to TSH. Treated with thyroidectomy then life-long thyroxine
- **Follicular carcinoma** (25%) Typical age range: 40–60y. ♀ > ♂. May arise in a pre-existing multinodular goitre. Spreads via bloodstream. Bony secondaries are common. Treatment is with surgery and thyroxine suppression therapy and/or radioactive iodine
- **Lymphoma** (5%) Occurs at any age. May be 1° or 2°. Associated with Hashimoto's thyroiditis. Staged/treated as for lymphomas elsewhere (📖 p. 680). Prognosis is good
- **Anaplastic carcinoma** (rare) Typical age: 50–60y. ♀ > ♂. Aggressive tumour. Grows rapidly and infiltrates tissues of the neck. Tracheal compression is common. Metastasizes locally to LNs and via lymphatics. Poor response to treatment
- **Medullary carcinoma** (rare) Occurs at any age. ♀ = ♂. Familial incidence; associated with adenomas elsewhere. Often secretes calcitonin (used as tumour marker). Spreads to local LNs. Treated by excision then chemotherapy ± radiotherapy

Goitre There are 4 main types of goitre—see Table 12.4.

Thyroid cyst Usually degenerative part of a nodular goitre, though true cysts do occur. Rapid enlargement/pain may be caused by haemorrhage into a cyst. Refer for confirmation of diagnosis.

Thyroid adenoma 4 types classified according to histological appearance—papillary, follicular, embryonal, hurtle cell. A few produce thyroxine → thyrotoxicosis. Haemorrhage is rare and results in rapid ↑ in size. Refer for confirmation of diagnosis ± surgery.

Table 12.4 Types of goitre—presentation and management

Type	Features	Management
Congenital	Enlarged thyroid gland present at birth ± hypo- or hyperthyroidism	Hypothyroid babies are treated with thyroxine; if there is tracheal compression or hyperthyroidism, treatment is surgical
Physiological	Occurs at puberty, during pregnancy, and in conditions of iodine deficiency	Usually requires no treatment. If iodine deficient, treat with iodine supplements
Nodular	Benign enlargement of the thyroid gland with areas of hyperplasia and involution	No treatment is necessary unless: • Thyrotoxic • Compression of the neck structures → dyspnoea or dysphagia • Worried by cosmetic appearance • Focal ↑ in size or recurrent laryngeal nerve palsy (hoarseness)—suggests malignant change If treatment is needed, refer to surgery or endocrinology, depending on symptoms
Toxic	*Graves' disease*—smooth thyroid enlargement + thyrotoxicosis	See management of hyperthyroidism—📖 p. 364
Inflammatory	*Hashimoto's thyroiditis:* ♀>♂. Antibodies to thyroid tissue are produced. Initially goitre and thyrotoxicosis. Later myxoedema	
	De Quervain's thyroiditis: Inflammation due to viral infection—usually Coxsackie virus. Acutely swollen, tender thyroid gland and transient thyrotoxicosis often preceded by sore throat/malaise. Settles spontaneously	In all cases, refer to endocrinology for confirmation of diagnosis and management guidance
	Riedel's thyroiditis: Rare. Infiltrated by scar tissue → hypothyroidism ± recurrent laryngeal nerve palsy ± stridor	

Further information

NICE Referral guidelines for suspected cancer (2005) ⏎ www.nice.org.uk

Thyroid disease

Interpretation of thyroid function tests See Table 12.5

Hyperthyroidism Affects 2% ♀ and 0.2% ♂. *Peak age: 20–49y.* Causes:

- Graves' disease
- Toxic nodular goitre—older women with past history of goitre
- Thyroiditis
- Amiodarone
- Kelp ingestion

Presentation

- Weight loss
- Tremor
- Palpitations
- Hyperactivity
- AF
- Hyperhidrosis
- Eye changes
- Infertility
- Alopecia

❶ In elderly patients, symptoms may be less obvious and include confusion, dementia, apathy, and depression.

Management Refer to endocrinology at presentation. *Treatment:*

- **β-blockers** (e.g. propranolol, atenolol) Useful for symptom control until antithyroid drug therapy takes effect
- **Carbimazole** Inhibits synthesis of thyroid hormones. Ineffective for treatment of thyroiditis. May be given short-term to render a patient euthyroid prior to surgery or treatment with radioactive iodine, or long-term (12–18mo) in an attempt to induce remission (but >50% relapse). 3/1,000 patients have serious adverse effects—agranulocytosis, hepatitis, aplastic anaemia, or lupus-like syndromes
- **Radioactive iodine** (^{131}I) Effects take 3–4mo to become apparent. Withdraw carbimazole >4d prior to treatment, and do not restart until >3d after. Advise women of childbearing age to avoid pregnancy for 4mo. Most become hypothyroid at some point (sometimes years) after treatment. Continue monitoring TFTs long-term. Associated with small ↑ risk of thyroid malignancy
- **Surgery** Partial or total thyroidectomy—reserved for patients with large goitres or who decline radioactive iodine. Carries risk of damage to recurrent laryngeal nerve or parathyroids

⚠ Warn *all* patients starting carbimazole to stop the drug and seek urgent medical attention if they develop sore throat or other infection.

Thyrotoxic crisis/storm 📖 p. 1101

Graves' disease Most common cause of hyperthyroidism. ♀:♂ ≈ 5:1. *Peak age: 30–50y.* Associated with smoking and stressful life events. Autoimmune disease in which antibodies to the TSH receptor are produced. *R.J. Graves (1797–1853)—Irish physician.*

Clinical features

- Hyperthyroidism
- Diffuse goitre ± thyroid bruit due to ↑ vascularity
- Extrathyroid features: thyroid eye disease—25–50% (bilateral in >90%); pretibial myxoedema—5%; thyroid acropathy (clubbing, finger swelling)—rare; onycholysis—rare

Management As for hyperthyroidism.

Table 12.5 Interpretation of thyroid function test results

Results of TFTs	Interpretation	Notes
TSH ↓, T$_4$↑	Thyrotoxic	Occasionally T$_4$ is normal but T$_3$↑
TSH ↑, T$_4$↓	Hypothyroid	TSH ↓ if hypothyroidism is secondary to pituitary failure (rare)
TSH ↑, T$_4$↔	Subclinical hypothyroidism	If any symptoms (including depression and non-specific symptoms or hyper-cholesterolaemia) consider a trial of treatment
		If no symptoms monitor annually

Thyroid eye disease Presents with:
- Double vision
- Eye discomfort ± protrusion (exophthalmos and proptosis)
- Lid lag
- Ophthalmoplegia (especially of upward gaze)
- TFTs can be ↑ or normal

Management Refer to ophthalmologist. If ↓ acuity or loss of colour vision—refer urgently as there may be optic nerve compression.

Hypothyroidism (myxoedema) Common—10% ♀ >60y, ♀:♂≈ 8:1.

Causes Chronic autoimmune thyroiditis, post-^{131}I, thyroidectomy.

Presentation Onset tends to be insidious and may go undiagnosed for years. *Always* consider hypothyroidism when a patient has non-specific symptoms, depression, fatigue, lethargy, or general malaise. Other symptoms—weight ↑, constipation, hoarse voice, or dry skin/hair. Signs are often absent—there may be a goitre, slow-relaxing reflexes, or non-pitting oedema of the hands, feet, or eyelids.

Screening Check TFTs in patients:
- With persistent symptoms of tiredness/lethargy without clear cause
- On amiodarone or with a history of ^{131}I administration
- With hypercholesterolaemia, infertility, Turner's or Down's syndrome, depression, dementia, obesity, DM, or other autoimmune disease

Management Patients taking thyroxine replacement are entitled to apply for free prescriptions in England (🔲 p. 137).
- **<65y and healthy** 100 micrograms od levothyroxine. Recheck TFTs after 4–6wk. Adjust dose to keep TSH in the normal range. Once dose is stable and TSH is within normal range monitor annually and if symptomatic or worries about compliance. ❶ Over-replacement is associated with AF and osteoporosis
- **If elderly or pre-existing heart disease** Start 25 micrograms od levothyroxine and ↑ dose every 4–6wk according to TFTs. Consider adding propranolol if history of CHD as levothyroxine can provoke angina

Withdrawal of levothyroxine Usually needed life long. If diagnosis is in doubt stop and remeasure TFTs after 4–6wk.

Hypothyroid coma 🔲 p. 1101

Information for patients
British Thyroid Foundation ☎ 01423 709707 🖰 www.btf-thyroid.org

Hyper- and hypocalcaemia

Checking Ca²⁺ Take an *uncuffed* sample (to avoid falsely high readings) and correct for serum albumin—for every mmol/L less than 40, a correction of 0.02mmol/L should be added. For example:

Calcium   2.40   Corrected calcium   = $(40 - 24) \times 0.02 + 2.4$
Albumin   24   = $0.32 + 2.4 = \mathbf{2.72}$

Hypocalcaemia ↓ serum calcium (<2.15mmol/L). *Causes:*

• **If phosphate ↑** CRF, hypoparathyroidism (may be congenital or 2° to thyroid or parathyroid surgery, or malignant infiltration), pseudohypoparathyroidism (insensitivity to parathyroid hormone)
• **If phosphate normal or ↓** Vitamin D deficiency (osteomalacia, rickets), malabsorption, overhydration, pancreatitis

Presentation May be subtle. Includes:

• Tetany
• Irritability, depression, or psychosis
• Perioral paraesthesia
• Carpo-pedal spasm (wrist flexion and fingers drawn together)
• Neuromuscular excitability (tapping over parotid causes facial muscles to contract—Chvostek's sign)

❶ Apparent hypocalcaemia may be an artefact of hypoalbuminaemia.

Management Check vitamin D levels. Supplement with calcium. Referral may be needed to investigate/treat the underlying cause.

Hypercalcaemia ↑ level of serum calcium (>2.55mmol/L). *Prevalence* ≈1:500; ♂:♀ ≈1:3. Rare < age 50y.

Common causes (90%)
• Primary hyperparathyroidism
• Malignancy (10% tumours— usually myeloma, breast, lung, kidney, thyroid, prostate, ovary, or colon)

Uncommon causes
• Chronic renal failure
• Familial benign hypercalcaemia
• Sarcoidosis
• Thyrotoxicosis
• Milk alkali syndrome
• Vitamin D treatment

Presentation Often very non-specific. May be an incidental finding. Other symptoms: *'bones, stones, groans, and abdominal moans'*.

• Tiredness
• Lethargy
• Weakness
• Mild aches and pains
• Anorexia
• Weight loss
• Low mood
• Stone formation
• Nausea/vomiting (often intractable)
• Polyuria and polydipsia
• Abdominal pain
• Constipation
• Confusion
• Corneal calcification

Management
• Treat according to cause (see Figure 12.3)—malignancy (📖 p. 1030); hyperparathyroidism (📖 p. 367)
• If diagnosis is unclear, refer to endocrinology. Urgency depends on serum Ca²⁺ and severity of symptoms

⚠ Hypercalcaemia can be fatal. If Ca²⁺ >3.5mmol/L or severe symptoms, admit for lowering of Ca²⁺ with forced diuresis and IV bisphosphonate.

Hyperparathyroidism ↑ secretion of parathyroid hormone (PTH).

- **1° hyperparathyroidism** Incidence 0.5/1,000. Peak age 40–60y. ♀:♂≈ 2:1. Circulating level of PTH is inappropriately high. Most patients are hypercalcaemic (but may be normocalcaemic if coexistent vitamin D deficiency). Due to ↑ secretion of PTH from one or both parathyroid glands. Refer. Treatment is usually surgical
- **2° hyperparathyroidism** ↑ PTH in response to chronic hypocalcaemia or hyperphosphataemia. Treat cause
- **Tertiary hyperparathyroidism** Inappropriately ↑ PTH →↑ Ca^{2+}. Follows prolonged 2° hyperparathyroidism. Most common in patients with chronic renal failure (especially if on dialysis) or chronic malabsorption. Treatment is usually surgical

Familial benign hypercalcaemia Asymptomatic. Inherited condition in which serum calcium concentrations are mildly ↑ throughout life. Confirm (if possible) by demonstrating ↑ Ca^{2+} in other family members. No adverse consequences and no treatment needed.

Milk alkali syndrome Usually due to ingestion of OTC indigestion remedies (e.g. Rennies®). Ca^{2+} levels revert to normal on stopping. Investigate the reason why the patient is taking these remedies (? peptic ulcer). Sometimes also caused by calcium supplements taken with bisphosphonates for prophylaxis of osteoporosis—stop the calcium supplement.

Figure 12.3 Guide to the diagnosis of cause of hypercalcaemia (must be taken in clinical context)

Adrenal disorders

Disorders of the adrenal cortex The adrenal cortex produces three classes of steroids:
- Glucocorticoids, e.g. cortisol
- Mineralocorticoids, e.g. aldosterone, and
- Sex hormones, e.g. androstenedione, testosterone, and oestrogen

Symptoms result from disturbance in production of these steroids.

Cushing's syndrome In the majority of cases, Cushing's syndrome is iatrogenic—caused by exogenous administration of prednisolone or other corticosteroids. Non-iatrogenic Cushing's syndrome is much rarer with annual incidence of 1–2/million ($\female$:$\male$ ≈3:1):
- 80% have a pituitary adenoma which secretes adrenocorticotrophic hormone (ACTH) causing hypersecretion of glucocorticoids and sex hormones (Cushing's disease)
- 20% are due to ectopic ACTH secretion by other tumours (e.g. small cell lung cancer) or hypersecreting tumours of the adrenal cortex

H.W. Cushing (1869–1939)—US neurosurgeon.

Presentation Cushing's syndrome has high morbidity and mortality. Clinical features include:
- Moon face (90%)
- Truncal obesity (85%)
- Hypertension (80%)
- Menstrual disturbance (80%)
- Striae and bruising (60%)
- Osteoporosis (60%)
- Lethargy/depression (60%)
- Hirsuitism
- Acne
- Pigmentation
- Feminization in men
- Polyuria and polydipsia
- Psychosis

Management
- Stop/minimize exogenous steroids
- If no exogenous steroids and Cushing's syndrome is suspected, request a dexamethasone suppression test—dexamethasone 1mg po at midnight, then serum cortisol measured at 9 a.m. If <50mmol/L exclude diagnosis unless cortisol secretion is episodic. If ≥50mmol/L check ACTH level and 24h urinary free cortisol and seek expert advice

Adrenal insufficiency (Addison's disease) May be:
- Primary—resulting from adrenal disease/failure, or
- Secondary—resulting from inadequate pituitary or hypothalamic stimulation of the adrenal glands

In the UK, most cases result from autoimmune disease, surgery, cessation of therapeutic corticosteroids, or failure to ↑ steroid dose to cover stress. Worldwide TB and AIDS are major causes. *T. Addison (1795–1860)—English physician.*

Clinical features
- Tiredness (95%)
- Weakness (95%)
- Anorexia (95%)
- Weight loss (90%)
- Pigmentation (buccal, palmar creases, new scars—90%)
- Abdominal pain (30%)
- Myalgia/arthralgia (20%)
- Postural hypotension/fainting (15%)
- Nausea

Presentation
- Can be dramatic with coma and severe hypoglycaemia (📖 p. 1101—admit as an emergency) or insidious
- 50% patients with autoimmune Addison's disease have or will develop another autoimmune disease (e.g. Graves' disease, pernicious anaemia) and 5% of women develop premature ovarian failure

Short Synacthen® test Take 9 a.m. blood for serum cortisol levels; inject 250 micrograms Synacthen® IV or IM; take a further blood sample for serum cortisol levels half an hour later. If 30min cortisol level is:
- >600nmol/L—adrenal insufficiency is excluded
- 400–590nmol/L—the result is equivocal; repeat
- <400nmol/L—adrenal insufficiency is confirmed; check ACTH (if ↓, investigate pituitary function; if ↑ investigate cause of adrenal disease)

Other investigations
- Biochemical abnormalities—↑ K^+, ↓ Na^+, ↓ glucose (may not be symptomatic), uraemia, ↑ Ca^{2+}, abnormal LFTs
- FBC—normocytic anaemia, eosinophilia, lymphocytosis

Management Refer to endocrinology. Treatment usually involves replacing deficient steroids with hydrocortisone and fludrocortisone.

❗ Warn patients not to stop steroids abruptly, to tell any doctor treating them about their condition and wear Medic-Alert/Medi-Tag bracelet in case of emergency. Double dose of hydrocortisone prior to dental treatment or if intercurrent illness (e.g. URTI). If vomiting, replace hydrocortisone po with IM hydrocortisone.

Hyperaldosteronism Suggested by presence of ↑ BP resistant to treatment together with ↓ K^+—but normokalaemic cases are also described. May be primary (two out of three have an aldosterone-secreting adenoma) when termed Conn's syndrome, or secondary to excess renin secretion (e.g. due to renal artery stenosis). If suspected, refer for endocrine assessment. Treatment depends on the cause.

Congenital adrenal hyperplasia 📖 p. 894

Disorders of the adrenal medulla

Phaechromocytoma Rare but serious disorder affecting 0.1% hypertensive patients. Usually caused by catecholamine-secreting tumours—10% are bilateral; 10% are extra-adrenal; 10% occur in children; 10% are malignant. May present with a huge array of symptoms and signs. ↑ BP may be sporadic or sustained. Suspect in patients who:
- Are young with ↑ BP
- Have very labile BP or sudden onset hypertension
- Have ↑ BP and associated headaches, sweating, and/or palpitations
- Have other associated conditions (e.g. neurofibromatosis)

Check 24h urine catecholamine/metabolite levels (follow local laboratory protocol). If confirmed or strong suspicion despite –ve test, refer for specialist opinion. Treatment is usually surgical if tumour is found.

Patient advice and support
The Pituitary Foundation ☎ 0845 450 0375 🖰 www.pituitary.org.uk
Addison's Disease Self Help Group 🖰 www.addisons.org.uk

Pituitary problems

Hypopituitarism ↓ production of all pituitary hormones (ACTH, growth hormone, FSH, LH, TSH, and prolactin). *Causes:*

- Surgery
- Irradiation
- Tumour (may be non-secreting or secrete one pituitary hormone with ↓ secretion of the others)
- Infection—TB
- Sheehan's syndrome—pituitary necrosis after post-partum haemorrhage *(H.L. Sheehan—English pathologist)*

Presentation

- Hypothyroidism
- Hypogonadism
- Anorexia
- Headache
- Depression
- Hair loss
- Hypotension
- Visual field defect

Management If suspected refer to neurology or endocrinology for further investigation and advice on treatment.

Pituitary tumours 10% intracranial tumours. Almost all are benign. Classified by histological type (chromophobic, acidophilic, or basophilic) or by the hormone secreted:

- No hormone (30%)
- Prolactin (35%)
- Growth hormone (20%)
- ACTH (7%)
- Prolactin and growth hormone (7%)
- LH, FSH, and TSH (1%)

Presentation Present with symptoms caused by:

- Local pressure—bilateral hemianopia, cranial nerve palsies, headache
- Hormone secretion, and/or
- Hypopituitarism

Management If suspected refer for further investigation and treatment.

Pituitary apoplexy Rapid expansion of a pituitary tumour due to infarction or haemorrhage. Suspect if sudden onset of headache in a patient with a known pituitary tumour. Admit as a medical/neurosurgical emergency.

Craniopharyngioma Tumour originating from Rathke's pouch. 50% present with local pressure effects in children. Refer as for pituitary tumours.

Hyperprolactinaemia The most common pituitary disorder resulting from pituitary adenoma.

Presentation Tends to present earlier in women than men. Symptoms are due to pressure effects or ↑ prolactin. Symptoms of ↑ prolactin:

- ♀: loss of libido, weight gain, apathy, vaginal dryness, menstrual disturbance, infertility, galactorrhoea
- ♂: impotence, ↓ facial hair

Investigation Check basal plasma prolactin (ask the laboratory for conditions under which they would like the sample taken).

Management If suspected refer for specialist opinion.

Other causes of ↑ prolactin
- Pregnancy
- Breastfeeding
- Stress
- Sleep
- Hypothyroidism
- Drugs—phenothiazines, metoclopramide, domperidone, SSRIs, methyldopa, oestrogens
- Chronic renal failure
- Sarcoidosis

Acromegaly Rare condition due to a growth-hormone-secreting pituitary tumour. *Typical age at presentation:* 30–50y.

Presentation
- Local pressure symptoms
- Changes in appearance—coarse oily skin; change in facial appearance with coarsening of features; ↑ foot size; ↑ teeth spacing
- Other effects—deepening of voice, sweating, paraesthesia, proximal muscle weakness, progressive heart failure, goitre
- *Complications*—DM, ↑ BP, cardiomyopathy, large bowel tumours

Investigation and management Refer to endocrinology.

Diabetes insipidus (DI) Caused by impaired water resorption by the kidney. Two mechanisms:
- **Cranial DI** ↓ ADH secretion from the posterior pituitary. 50% idiopathic. *Other causes:* head injury, tumour, infection, sarcoidosis, vascular, inherited
- **Nephrogenic DI** Impaired response of the kidney to ADH. *Causes:* drugs (e.g. lithium), hypercalcaemia, pyelonephritis, hydronephrosis, pregnancy (rare)

Presentation Polydipsia, polyuria, dilute urine, dehydration.

Investigations U&E (Na$^+$↑), plasma and urine osmolality (plasma ↑, urine ↓—ratio >1). Specialist investigations (e.g. water deprivation test) confirm diagnosis.

Management Treat the cause.
- Cranial DI may be treated with intranasal desmopressin or surgery
- Nephrogenic DI may be treated with dietary restriction of protein and salt and/or bendroflumethiazide

Syndrome of inappropriate ADH (SIADH) Important cause of hyponatraemia. Diagnosis is made by finding a concentrated urine (sodium >20mmol/L) in the presence of hyponatraemia (<125mmol/L) or low plasma osmolality (<260mmol/kg) in the absence of hypovolaemia, oedema, or diuretics. Always requires specialist management. *Causes:*
- **Malignancy,** e.g. small cell lung cancer; pancreas; lymphoma
- **CNS disorders,** e.g. stroke; subdural haemorrhage; vasculitis (SLE)

Patient advice and support
The Pituitary Foundation ☎ 0845 450 0375 ✆ www.pituitary.org.uk

Gastrointestinal medicine

Assessment of abdominal pain

ⓘ Signs may be unclear in elderly patients, children, or those on steroids.

History Consider:
- Site of pain—see Figure 13.1
- Onset: how long? How did it start? Change over time?
- Character of pain: colicky pain comes and goes in waves—results from GI obstruction, renal/biliary colic, gastroenteritis, or IBS
- Radiation
- Associated symptoms, e.g. nausea, vomiting, diarrhoea
- Timing/pattern, e.g. constant, colicky, relationship to food
- Exacerbating/relieving factors—including previous treatments tried
- Severity

Examination
- Temperature, pulse, BP, respiratory rate
- Anaemia or jaundice?
- Abdomen—site of pain (see Figure 13.1); guarding/rebound tenderness?
- Rectal/vaginal examination as needed
- Consider urine dipstick/finger prick blood glucose testing as needed

Management Treat the cause (see Table 13.1).

⚠ If acute or subacute onset of severe pain, admit as a surgical emergency to hospital.

Table 13.1 Differential diagnosis of abdominal pain

Renal/urological	Gastrointestinal	Other intra-abdominal
Renal colic	*Surgical*	Sickle cell crisis
UTI	Perforated bowel	Ruptured spleen
Pyelonephritis	Bowel obstruction	Leaking/ruptured AAA
Urinary retention/ hydronephrosis	Intussusception	Mesenteric ischaemia
Henoch–Schönlein purpura	Strangulated hernia	Mesenteric adenitis
Torsion of the testis	Volvulus	Subphrenic abscess
	Appendicitis	
Gynaecological	Meckel's diverticulum	**Metabolic**
Ectopic pregnancy	Gall bladder disease	DM—ketoacidosis
Dysmenorrhoea	Pancreatitis	Porphyria
Endometriosis	GI malignancy	Addison's disease
Pelvic inflammatory disease		Lead poisoning
Ovarian torsion	*Medical*	
Ovarian cyst—bleed/ rupture	Gastritis	**Other extra-abdominal**
Gynaecological malignancy	Peptic ulcer	Shingles/post-herpetic neuralgia
	Gastroenteritis	Spinal arthritis
	Crohn's/UC	Muscular pain
	IBS	MI
	Constipation	CCF
	Diverticular disease	Pneumonia
	Liver disease	

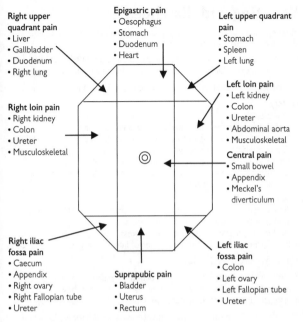

Right upper quadrant pain
• Liver
• Gallbladder
• Duodenum
• Right lung

Epigastric pain
• Oesophagus
• Stomach
• Duodenum
• Heart

Left upper quadrant pain
• Stomach
• Spleen
• Left lung

Right loin pain
• Right kidney
• Colon
• Ureter
• Musculoskeletal

Left loin pain
• Left kidney
• Colon
• Ureter
• Abdominal aorta
• Musculoskeletal

Central pain
• Small bowel
• Appendix
• Meckel's diverticulum

Right iliac fossa pain
• Caecum
• Appendix
• Right ovary
• Right Fallopian tube
• Ureter

Suprapubic pain
• Bladder
• Uterus
• Rectum

Left iliac fossa pain
• Colon
• Left ovary
• Left Fallopian tube
• Ureter

Figure 13.1 Location of pain and organs likely to be involved

Pelvic pain 📖 p. 714

Anal/perianal pain Treat the cause. *Consider*:

• Anal fissure
• Haemorrhoids/perianal haematoma (thrombosed pile)
• Perianal abscess
• Anal/perianal fistula
• Pilonidal sinus
• Skin infection (e.g. hidradenitis suppurativa)
• Functional pain (proctalgia fugax)
• Rectal/anal carcinoma

Tenesmus Sensation of incomplete rectal emptying following defecation— as if something has been left behind which cannot be passed. Common in irritable bowel syndrome. Can be also be caused by proctitis/inflammatory bowel disease and tumour.

> **Abdominal migraine or periodic syndrome** Seen in children. Presents as stereotyped attacks in which nausea, vomiting, and headache accompany abdominal pain. Treat as for migraine. Some of these children develop classical migraine later.

Vomiting and diarrhoea

Most episodes of acute vomiting and diarrhoea are due to viral infection, short-lived (2–5d), and self-limiting.

Nausea Unpleasant symptom. The patient feels as if he/she might vomit. Most conditions which cause vomiting can also cause nausea.

Vomiting Common symptom. Causes—see Table 13.2.

History
- Duration
- Ability to retain food and fluids/relationship to eating
- Nature of vomitus, e.g. presence of blood or 'coffee grounds'; bilious
- Other associated symptoms, e.g. fever, abdominal pain, diarrhoea
- Other illnesses, e.g. DM, Ménière's disease, migraine, cancer
- Medication, e.g. opioids, chemotherapy

Examination
- Assess hydration status—BP, pulse rate; dry mouth, ↓ skin turgor, sunken eyes, or sunken fontanelle (babies) are all late signs
- Abdomen—masses, distension, tenderness, bowel sounds
- For children—look for other sources of infection, e.g. ENT, chest, UTI

Haematemesis 📖 p. 1076

Slimy stool Caused by overproduction of mucus in the large bowel. Almost always associated with colonic disease/irritable bowel syndrome. Investigate, unless all other features are typical of IBS and age is <40y.

Diarrhoea Establish what the patient means by diarrhoea. Diarrhoea is the abnormal passage of loose or liquid stools. Causes—see Table 13.2.

History
- Duration—termed 'chronic' if persists >4wk
- Nature of the diarrhoea—colour, consistency, blood/mucus
- Contact with anyone else with similar symptoms?
- Occupation and travel history
- Associated symptoms, e.g. fever, abdominal pain, vomiting, weight ↓
- Association with other factors (e.g. food intolerance, stress)
- Past medical history—surgery (especially ileal resection or cholecystectomy); pancreatic disease; systemic disease (e.g. DM, thyrotoxicosis)
- Family history—inflammatory bowel or coeliac disease; bowel cancer
- Alcohol consumption—high intake is associated with diarrhoea
- Medication, e.g. antibiotics, regular medications (4% chronic diarrhoea)

Examination
- Assess hydration status—BP, pulse rate; dry mouth, ↓ skin turgor, sunken eyes, or sunken fontanelle (babies) are all late signs
- Abdomen—masses, distension, tenderness, bowel sounds, stool

Investigation Send a stool sample for M,C&S if any of the following:

• Fever	• Recent return from	• Resident in an
• Blood in stool	a tropical climate	institution
• Food worker	• Immunocompromise	• Persists >7d

Table 13.2 Causes of vomiting and diarrhoea

Vomiting	Diarrhoea
Physiological e.g. possetting in babies	**Acute diarrhoea**
Travel/motion sickness	– Dietary indiscretion
GI infection, e.g. viral gastroenteritis, food poisoning	– Infection, e.g. food poisoning, travellers' diarrhoea
Other infection (particularly children)— tonsillitis, otitis media	– Constipation with overflow
Other GI causes: GI obstruction, pyloric stenosis, 'acute abdomen'	– Pseudomembranous colitis— recent history of oral antibiotics
CNS causes: raised intracranial pressure, head injury, migraine, vertigo	– Onset of inflammatory bowel disease or other chronic diarrhoea
Metabolic causes: pregnancy, uraemia, ketoacidosis	**Chronic diarrhoea**
Psychiatric causes: anorexia, bulimia	See Table 13.11, 📖 p. 407
Malignancy	
Drugs and toxins, e.g. alcohol, opioids, cytotoxic agents	

Management of acute diarrhoea and/or vomiting

- Treat any identified cause
- Rehydration—encourage clear fluid intake (small amounts frequently) ± rehydration salts (use a commercial preparation, e.g. Dioralyte®)
- Food—stick to a bland diet, avoiding dairy products until symptoms have settled. Babies who are breastfed or have not been weaned should continue their normal milk
- If dehydrated and unable to replace fluids, e.g. diarrhoea with concomitant vomiting or child/elderly person refusing to drink—admit

⚠ Never give children antidiarrhoeal agents.

❶ *If no cause is found and diarrhoea lasts >4wk or any atypical features, consider referral for urgent investigation—📖 p. 406.*

Gastroenteritis 📖 p. 410

Chronic diarrhoea and malabsorption 📖 p. 406

Faecal incontinence 📖 p. 408

Melaena or rectal bleeding 📖 p. 1076

Factitious diarrhoea 📖 p. 407

- Some children may become cow's milk intolerant after a bout of gastroenteritis—📖 p. 889
- Think of haemolytic uraemic syndrome in any child with diarrhoea who passes blood in the stool

Further information

NICE Diarrhoea and vomiting in children under 5 (2009) ℘ www.nice.org.uk

Constipation

3 million GP consultations/y in the UK result from constipation. Differentiate normal stools a few days apart (normal, needs no treatment) and infrequent hard stools (suggests constipation).

Definition Two or more of the following for ≥3 mo:
- Straining at defecation ≥25% of the time
- A sensation of incomplete evacuation ≥25% of the time
- ≤2 bowel movements /wk
- Lumpy and/or hard stools ≥25% of the time

❶ Most patients consulting in general practice do not meet these criteria.

Children with constipation 📖 p. 888

Young patients <40y with lone constipation ♀:♂≈ 9:1. Establish symptoms—constipation is usually long-standing in this group. Include drug and diet history. Ask about health beliefs—80% believe their bowels should open daily. Explore concerns about underlying disease. If long-standing ask why the patient is consulting now. Examine the abdomen. Investigate if symptoms/signs suggestive of organic disease (see Table 13.3).

Management Treat organic causes. Otherwise:
- Give lifestyle advice—↑ fluid intake to ≥2L/d (8–10 cups); avoid alcohol; ↑ exercise if possible; add fibre to diet (↑ fruit/vegetables, eat wholegrain foods, add coarse bran to food); open bowel when needed
- If lifestyle advice alone fails and symptoms are causing distress, start an osmotic laxative, e.g. magnesium hydroxide 15mL bd
- If an osmotic laxative fails, try a short course of stimulant laxative e.g. senna 1–2 tablets at 5 p.m. either alone or in combination with an osmotic laxative. Long-term use of some stimulant laxatives is reported to cause cathartic atonic colon. Although there is no evidence that senna causes this, in young, fit patients only use short courses or use intermittently, e.g twice weekly
- If still constipated specialist referral is warranted

Irritable bowel syndrome with constipation 20% develop symptoms of irritable bowel syndrome (IBS) in their lifetime (📖 p. 418). Constipation is the predominant symptom in 30%, but other symptoms are usually present. Establish symptoms. Examine the abdomen. Investigation includes FBC, CRP, and coeliac serology to exclude organic causes.

Management If <40 y, examination and investigations are normal and fulfill IBS criteria (📖 p. 418), manage as for young patients with lone constipation but avoid osmotic laxatives as they make bloating worse.

Constipation in the over 40s Any sustained change in bowel habit for >6wk should be taken seriously and investigated if appropriate. Establish symptoms and onset. Specifically ask about tenesmus, blood in stool, abdominal pain, and diarrhoea. Check current medication. Examine the abdomen for masses and hepatomegaly. Rectal examination is essential to exclude low rectal or anal carcinoma and detect faecal impaction.

Table 13.3 Organic causes of constipation

Colonic disease	Carcinoma	Stricture
	Diverticular disease	Intussusception
	Crohn's disease	Volvulus
Anorectal disease	Anterior mucosal prolapse	Anal fissure
	Distal proctitis	Perianal abscess
Pelvic disease	Ovarian tumour	Endometriosis
	Uterine tumour	
Endocrine/metabolic disorders	Hypercalcaemia	DM with autonomic
	Hypothyroidism	neuropathy
Drugs	Opioids	Antiparkinsonian drugs
	Antacids containing calcium	Anticholinergics
	or aluminium	Anticonvulsants
	Antidepressants	Antihistamines
	Iron	Calcium antagonists
Other	Pregnancy	Poor fluid intake
	Immobility	

Management

- Check FBC, ESR, renal function tests, LFTs, TFTs, and serum glucose
- Image the lower bowel by colonoscopy or CT colography if new symptoms that persist >6wk
- Treat any reversible, underlying organic cause—see Table 13.3
- Give lifestyle advice (see management of young people with lone constipation)
- Treat symptomatically if no cause is found/cause is untreatable
- Laxatives—consider an osmotic (e.g. lactulose, magnesium hydroxide) or bulk-forming laxative (e.g. ispaghula, sterculia) ± a stimulant laxative (e.g. senna). Titrate dose to response
- Long-term use of stimulant laxatives including co-danthrusate is acceptable in the very elderly. Otherwise, use prn or intermittently
- If oral laxatives are ineffective consider adding rectal measures. If soft stool, try bisacodyl suppositories (❶ must come into direct contact with rectum); if hard stools try glycerin suppositories (act in 1–6h)
- If still not cleared/faecal impaction—refer to the district nurse for lubricant ± high phosphate (stimulant) enema (acts in ~20min)
- Once constipation has been cleared, leave the patient with clear instructions about what to do if symptoms recur

⚠ **High-risk patients,** e.g. patients on opioids; those who are immobile or have medical conditions which predispose them to constipation. Pre-empt constipation by putting high-risk patients on regular aperients.

Occult presentations of constipation are common in the elderly and include:
- Confusion
- Urinary retention
- Abdominal pain
- Overflow diarrhoea
- Loss of appetite and nausea

Other abdominal symptoms and signs

Dyspepsia 📖 p. 382

Abdominal distension Consider abdominal/pelvic masses and:

- Fluid—ascites or full bladder
- Fat
- Faeces
- Flatus—intestinal obstruction; air swallowing
- Fetus
- Food, e.g. malabsorption

Abdominal masses Distinguished from pelvic masses by the ability to get beneath them. *Causes:* Malignancy—any intra-abdominal organ or kidney; stool; abdominal aortic aneurysm; hepato- and/or splenomegaly; appendix mass/abscess; Crohn's mass; lymph nodes or TB mass. ❶ A hernia may present as a mass in abdominal wall/groin lump—📖 p. 392.

Pelvic masses *Causes:* fetus; full bladder; fibroids; gynaecological malignancy; bladder cancer.

Splenomegaly *Causes:*

- **Haematological** Lymphoma, leukaemia, myeloproliferative disorders, sickle cell disease (children usually), thalassaemia
- **Inflammatory** RA or Sjögren's syndrome, sarcoid, amyloid
- **Infection** Glandular fever, malaria, SBE, TB, leishmaniasis

Hepatomegaly *Causes:*

- **Apparent** Reidel's lobe, low-lying diaphragm
- **Tumours** Secondary (most common), primary
- **Venous congestion** Heart failure, hepatic vein occlusion
- **Haematological** Leukaemia, lymphoma, myeloproliferative disorders, sickle cell disease
- **Biliary obstruction** Particularly extrahepatic
- **Inflammation** Hepatitis, abscess, schistosomiasis
- **Metabolic** Fatty liver, amyloid, glycogen storage disease
- **Cysts** Polycystic liver, hydatid

Ascites Free fluid in the peritoneal cavity. *Signs:* abdominal distension, shifting dullness to percussion, fluid thrill. *Causes:* Malignancy—any intra-abdominal organ, ovary, or kidney; hypoproteinaemia, e.g. nephrotic syndrome; right heart failure; portal hypertension.

Fistula Abnormal communication between one organ and another—usually due to cancer or complication of surgery. Presentation—Table 13.4. Refer urgently if suspected.

Table 13.4 Presentation of fistula

Connection	Presentation
Bowel → skin	Faecal discharge through surgical wound
Bladder/ureters → skin	Clear, watery discharge which smells of urine
Bowel → vagina	Faeculent material in vagina
Bladder → vagina	Leakage of urine per vaginum
Bowel → bladder	Air or faeculent material in urine; recurrent UTI

Urgent referral for upper GI symptoms[N] Consider checking FBC when referring, depending on local protocols.

Urgent referral to a team specializing in upper GI malignancy Patients presenting with:
- Dysphagia
- Unexplained upper abdominal pain and weight ↓ ± back pain
- Upper abdominal mass without dyspepsia
- Obstructive jaundice (depending on clinical state)—consider urgent USS if available

Consider urgent referral to a specialist in upper GI malignancy Patients presenting with:
- Persistent vomiting and weight ↓ in the absence of dyspepsia
- Unexplained weight ↓ or iron deficiency in the absence of dyspepsia
- Unexplained worsening of dyspepsia and Barrett's oesophagus; known dysplasia, atrophic gastritis, or intestinal metaplasia; or peptic ulcer surgery >20y ago

Consider urgent specialist referral or referral for urgent endoscopy Patients of any age with dyspepsia and:
- Chronic GI bleeding
- Dysphagia
- Progressive unintentional weight ↓
- Persistent vomiting
- Iron deficiency anaemia
- Epigastric mass
- Suspicious barium meal result

Urgent referral for endoscopy Any patient ≥55y and with unexplained (i.e. no obvious cause, e.g NSAIDs) and persistent, recent-onset dyspepsia alone. GPs should not allow symptoms to persist >4–6wk before referral.

❶ *Helicobacter pylori* status should not affect the decision to refer for suspected cancer. Consider checking FBC to exclude iron deficiency anaemia in all patients presenting with new-onset dyspepsia.

Urgent referral for lower GI symptoms[N] Refer urgently to a team specializing in lower GI malignancy if:

Any age with:
- Right lower abdominal mass consistent with involvement of large bowel
- A palpable rectal mass (intraluminal, not pelvic; a pelvic mass outside the bowel would warrant an urgent referral to a urologist)
- Unexplained iron deficiency anaemia (Hb ≤110g/dL for ♂ ≤100g/dL for a non-menstruating ♀)

Aged ≥40y Reporting rectal bleeding with a change of bowel habit towards looser stools and/or increased stool frequency persisting ≥6wk.

Aged ≥60y with:
- Rectal bleeding persisting for ≥6wk without a change in bowel habit and without anal symptoms
- Change in bowel habit to looser stools and/or more frequent stools persisting for ≥6wk without rectal bleeding

❶ In a patient with equivocal symptoms who is not unduly anxious, it is reasonable to 'treat, watch, and wait'.

Dyspepsia and *H. pylori*

In any year, up to 40% of the adult population suffer from dyspepsia—1:10 seek their GP's advice; ~10% of these are referred for endoscopy.

Causes
- Gastro-oesophageal reflux disease (GORD)—15–25% (📖 p. 386)
- Peptic ulcer (PU)—15–25% (📖 p. 388)
- Stomach cancer—2% (📖 p. 390)
- The remaining 60% are classified as *non-ulcer dyspepsia* (NUD, 'functional' dyspepsia)—manage as for uninvestigated dyspepsia
- *Rarer causes:* oesophagitis from swallowed corrosives, oesophageal infection (especially in the immunocompromised)

Differential diagnosis Cardiac pain (difficult to distinguish), gallstone pain, pancreatitis, bile reflux.

Presentation Common symptoms include retrosternal or epigastric pain, fullness, bloating, wind, heartburn, nausea, and vomiting. Examination is usually normal though there may be epigastric tenderness. Check for clinical anaemia, epigastric mass/hepatomegaly, and LNs in the neck.

Management See Figure 13.2.

Helicobacter pylori Infection is associated with:
- **GI disease**—peptic ulcer disease; gastric cancer; non-ulcer dyspepsia; oesophagitis
- **Non-GI disease**—ranging from cardiovascular disease and haematological malignancy to cot death

Testing for H. pylori[N] 'Test and treat' all patients with dyspepsia who do not meet referral criteria (see Figure 13.2). In practice choice of test is limited by availability, ease of access, and cost. Options in the community are: serology, urea breath test, and faecal antigen test. A 2wk washout period following proton pump inhibitor (PPI) use is necessary before testing for *H. pylori* with a breath test or a stool antigen test.

Eradication[N] Clears 80–85% *H. pylori* infections. Options:
- **PAC$_{500}$ regimen** Full-dose PPI (e.g. omeprazole 20mg bd) + amoxicillin 1g bd + clarithromycin 500mg bd for 1wk, *or*
- **PMC$_{250}$ regimen** Full-dose PPI (e.g. omeprazole 20mg bd) + metronidazole 400mg bd + clarithromycin 250mg bd for 1wk

❶ Do not re-test even if dyspepsia remains unless there is a strong clinical need. Re-test if needed using a urea breath test.

Lifestyle advice Give advice on healthy eating, weight ↓, and smoking cessation. Advise patients to avoid precipitating factors, e.g. alcohol, coffee, chocolate, fatty foods. Raising the head of the bed and having a main meal well before going to bed may help some people. Promote continued use of antacids/alginates.

Further information
NICE Management of dyspepsia in adults in primary care (2004) ℰ www.nice.org.uk

Figure 13.2 Algorithm for management of uninvestigated dyspepsia in general practice

Oesophageal conditions

Oesophagitis Common condition. Reflux of acid from the stomach to the oesophagus causes mucosal damage resulting in inflammation and ulceration. *Other causes:* drugs (e.g. NSAIDs); infection (e.g. CMV, HSV, candida—especially in the immunocompromised); ingestion of caustic substances.

Management Treat reflux-induced oesophagitis as for GORD—🕮 p. 386. Otherwise treat the cause.

Barrett's oesophagus 🕮 p. 387.

Chronic benign stricture Recurrent oesophagitis (e.g. 2° to GORD, NSAIDs, K⁺ preparations) scars the oesophagus resulting in stricture formation. Most common in elderly women.

Presentation Long history of reflux with more recent dysphagia. If obstruction is severe undigested food may be regurgitated immediately after swallowing. May be associated with night-time coughing paroxysms due to aspiration of gastric contents into the chest. Examination is usually normal.

Management Refer for urgent endoscopy to confirm diagnosis and exclude carcinoma. Treatment is by endoscopic dilatation of the stricture.

Carcinoma of the oesophagus 🕮 p. 390

Presbyoesophagus Common among the elderly. Intermittent sensation that food is getting stuck—usually at the back of the throat. Examination is normal as is endoscopy. Barium swallow or oesophageal motility studies may reveal oesophageal spasm. Reassure.

Globus pharyngis (or hystericus) Sensation of a lump in the throat without difficulty swallowing is common. It may indicate anxiety. Reassure if no organic signs and treat any dyspepsia. If not responding refer to ENT for exclusion of an organic cause.

Oesophageal achalasia Failure of relaxation of the circular muscles at the distal oesophagus. *Peak incidence:* 30–40y; ♀ slightly >♂.

Presentation Gradual onset of dysphagia over years accompanied by regurgitation of stagnant food and foul belching. Night-time coughing fits are due to aspiration which can result in recurrent chest infections. Examination is usually normal although there may be signs of aspiration pneumonia.

Management CXR to exclude aspiration pneumonia; endoscopy confirms diagnosis. Refer for surgery.

Plummer–Vinson syndrome Iron deficiency anaemia + dysphagia due to a post-cricoid web in the oesophagus. ♀ > ♂. *Peak incidence:* 40–50y. Presents with high dysphagia with food sticking in the back of the throat ± retching/choking sensation. This is a pre-malignant condition so refer for biopsy and dilatation of pharyngeal web; replace iron.

H.S. Plummer (1874–1936); P.P. Vinson (1890–1959)—US physicians.

Pharyngeal pouch Pulsion diverticulum of the pharyngeal mucosa through Killian's dehiscence (area of weakness between the 2 parts of the inferior pharyngeal constrictor). ♂ > ♀; ↑ with age. Usually develops posteriorly then protrudes to one side—L > R. As the pouch gets larger the oesophagus is displaced laterally.

Presentation Dysphagia—the first mouthful is swallowed easily, then fills the pouch which makes further swallowing difficult. Accompanied by regurgitation of food from the pouch ± symptoms of aspiration (night-time coughing, recurrent chest infection). A swelling is palpable in the neck in two-thirds of cases.

Management Refer for further investigation. Diagnosis is confirmed with endoscopy/barium swallow. Treatment is surgical.

Oesophageal varices Result from portal hypertenion (📖 p. 425) and can bleed massively—admit as a 'blue light' emergency if bleeding.

Impacted oesophageal foreign body Usually the patient notices something has stuck resulting in pain, difficulty swallowing ± retching. If suspected refer immediately to A&E for further investigation ± removal of the foreign body.

Oesophageal perforation Rare—usually a complication of endoscopy. Less commonly due to violent vomiting. The patient becomes very distressed with pain relating to the site of perforation which is worse on swallowing. Examination reveals tachycardia, shock ± pyrexia ± breathlessness ± surgical emphysema in neck. Admit as a surgical emergency.

Oesophageal atresia and/or tracheo-oesophageal fistula 1:2,500 live births. 5% have oesophageal atresia alone; 5% tracheo-oesophageal fistula (TOF) alone; the remainder have both. Risk factor for sudden infant death syndrome.

Presentation
- **Antenatal**: at routine USS or following investigation of polyhydramnios
- **Post-natal**: cough or breathing difficulties in a newborn infant, choking on the first feed, inability to swallow saliva → bubbling of fluid from the mouth, developing soon after birth
- **Later in childhood**: 'H type' fistulas where there is no atresia, but just a fistula may present late with recurrent chest infections

Management Diagnosis is confirmed with X-ray. Treatment is surgical. Post-operatively children may have a barking cough (*'TOF cough'*) and/or dysphagia—both settle before 2y.

Gastro-oesophageal reflux and gastritis

Gastro-oesophageal reflux disease (GORD) Caused by retrograde flow of gastric contents through an incompetent gastro-oesophageal junction. It affects ~5% of the adult population.

Risk factors

- Smoking
- Alcohol
- Coffee
- Fatty food
- Big meals

- Obesity
- Hiatus hernia
- Tight clothes
- Pregnancy
- Systemic sclerosis

- Drugs (NSAIDs, TCAs, SSRIs, iron supplements, anticholinergics, nitrates, alendronic acid)
- Surgery for achalasia

Conditions caused by GORD

- Oesophagitis (defined by mucosal breaks) ± oesophageal ulcer
- Benign oesophageal stricture—📖 p. 384
- Intestinal metaplasia: Barrett's oesophagus
- Oesophageal haemorrhage
- Anaemia

Presentation

- **Heartburn:** most common symptom. Burning retrosternal or epigastric pain which worsens on bending, stooping or lying, and with hot drinks. Relieved by antacids
- **Other symptoms:**
  - Waterbrash—mouth fills with saliva
  - Reflux of acid into the mouth—especially on lying flat
  - Nausea and vomiting
  - Nocturnal cough/wheeze due to aspiration of refluxed stomach contents
- **Examination:** usually normal. Check for clinical anaemia, epigastric mass/hepatomegaly, and LNs in the neck

Investigation Endoscopy if indicated—see Figure 13.2, 📖 p. 383.

❶ Symptoms are poorly correlated with endoscopic findings. Reflux may remain silent in patients with Barrett's oesophagus but heartburn can severely affect quality of life of patients with −ve endoscopy results.

Initial management[N]

- In all cases, give lifestyle advice (📖 p. 382)
- If diagnosis is clinical (i.e. patient presents with 'reflux-like' symptoms), treat as for uninvestigated dyspepsia (see Figure 13.2, 📖 p. 383)
- For patients with reflux confirmed on endoscopy, offer treatment with a PPI (e.g. omeprazole 20mg od) for 1–2mo. If oesophagitis at endoscopy and the patient remains symptomatic on PPI, double the dose of PPI for a further 1mo
- If inadequate response to PPI, try an H_2 receptor antagonist (e.g. ranitidine 150mg bd) and/or add a prokinetic (e.g. domperidone 10mg tds) for 1mo

Long-term management of endoscopically/barium-confirmed GORD[N].

- Patients who have had dilatation of an oesophageal stricture should remain on long-term full-dose PPI therapy
- For all other patients, if symptoms recur following initial treatment, offer a PPI at the lowest dose possible to control symptoms, with a limited number of repeat prescriptions. Discuss using the treatment on an as-required basis to manage symptoms
- Refer for consideration of surgery if quality of life remains significantly impaired despite optimal treatment. Surgery of any type is >90% successful although results may deteriorate with time

Hiatus hernia Common (30% of over 50s); 50% have GORD. Obesity is a risk factor. The proximal stomach herniates through the diaphragmatic hiatus into the thorax

- 80% have a 'sliding' hiatus hernia where the gastro-oesophageal junction slides into the chest
- 20% have a 'rolling' hernia where a bulge of stomach herniates into the chest alongside the oesophagus. The gastro-oesophageal junction remains in the abdomen

Management Treat as for GORD.

Barrett's oesophagus Usually found incidentally at endoscopy for symptoms of GORD and caused by chronic GORD. The squamous mucosa of the oesophagus undergoes metaplastic change, and the squamocolumnar junction appears to migrate away from the stomach. The length affected varies. It carries a ×40 ↑ risk of adenocarcinoma of the oesophagus, so regular endoscopy is essential. Treatment is with long-term PPIs (e.g omeprazole 20–40mg od) ± laser therapy ± resection. *N.R. Barrett (1903–1979)—British surgeon.*

Acute gastritis Mucosal inflammation of the stomach with no ulcer.
- **Type A:** affects the entire stomach; associated with pernicious anaemia; pre-malignant
- **Type B:** affects antrum ± duodenum; associated with *H. pylori*
- **Type C:** due to irritants, e.g. NSAIDs, alcohol, bile reflux

Presentation and investigation Dyspepsia—📖 p. 382

Management
- Treat the cause where possible (e.g. vitamin B_{12} injections; *H. pylori* eradication; avoidance of alcohol)
- Acid suppression—H_2 receptor antagonist (e.g. ranitidine, nizatidine) or PPI for 4–8wk
- Re-endoscope to confirm healing

Complications Haemorrhage, gastric atrophy ± gastric cancer (type A only).

Peptic ulceration

Peptic ulceration (PU) is a term which includes both gastric and duodenal ulceration. Most patients present with dyspepsia (📖 p. 382). Specific features of gastric and duodenal ulcers are listed in Table 13.5.

Management

For patients not taking NSAIDs

- **Eradicate H. pylori if present** (📖 p. 382). Speeds ulcer healing and ↓ relapse; confirm eradication with a urea breath test (duodenal ulcer) or repeat endoscopy (gastric ulcer), and retreat if still present
- **If H. pylori negative** Treat with full-dose PPI (e.g omeprazole 20mg od) for 1–2mo. If gastric ulcer, re-endoscope to check ulcer is healed

For patients taking NSAIDs

- Stop NSAIDs where possible. If not possible consider changing to a safer alternative (e.g. paracetamol, ↓ dose of NSAID, COX2-selective NSAID) and adding gastric protection with a PPI or misoprostol
- Offer full-dose PPI or H_2 receptor antagonist (H_2RA) therapy for 2mo and, if H. pylori is present, subsequently offer eradication therapy
- Check eradication with repeat endoscopy (gastric ulcer) or urea breath test (duodenal ulcer)

For all patients

- **Lifestyle measures** Avoid foods (or alcohol) which exacerbate symptoms; eat little and often; avoid eating <3h before bed. Stop smoking
- **If symptoms recur following initial treatment** Offer a PPI at lowest dose to control symptoms, with a limited number of repeat prescriptions. Discuss using the treatment on a prn basis
- **Offer H_2RA therapy** If there is an inadequate response to a PPI
- **In patients with unhealed ulcer or continuing symptoms** Despite adequate treatment, exclude non-adherence, malignancy, failure to detect H. pylori, inadvertent NSAID use, other ulcer-inducing medication, and rare causes, e.g. Zollinger–Ellison syndrome, Crohn's disease
- **Once symptoms are controlled** Review at least annually to discuss symptom control, lifestyle advice, and medication
- **Refer** If gastric ulcer fails to heal or if symptoms do not respond to medical treatment. Possible surgical procedures include: gastrectomy, vagotomy, and drainage procedure; highly selective vagotomy

Zollinger–Ellison syndrome Association of peptic ulcer with a gastrin-secreting pancreatic (rarely duodenal) adenoma—50–60% are malignant, 10% are multiple, and 30% are associated with multiple endocrine neoplasia (MEN I). *Incidence:* 0.1% of patients with duodenal ulcer disease. Suspect in those with multiple peptic ulcers resistant to drugs, particularly if associated with diarrhoea ± steatorrhoea or a family history of peptic ulcers (or islet cell, pituitary, or parathyroid adenomas). Refer for further investigation. Treatment is with PPIs (e.g omeprazole 10–60mg bd) ± surgery.

R.M. Zollinger (1903–1992); E.H. Ellison (1918–1970)—US surgeons.

Table 13.5 Features of gastric and duodenal ulcers

	Gastric ulcer (GU)	Duodenal ulcer (DU)
Population	Typically affects middle-aged/elderly ♂	Typically affects young–middle-aged ♂, although can affect any adult. ♂ > ♀
Risk factors	H. pylori (70–90%) NSAID use (↑ risk x3–4) Delayed gastric emptying Reflux from the duodenum (↑ by smoking)	H. pylori (>90%) NSAID use Gastric hyperacidity Rapid gastric emptying Smoking Stress (◆)
Presentation	May be asymptomatic Epigastric pain worsened by food and helped by antacids or lying flat ± weight loss With complications	May be asymptomatic or spontaneously relapse and remit Epigastric pain typically relieved by food and worse at night ± weight ↑ ± waterbrash (saliva fills the mouth) With complications
Examination	In uncomplicated gastric ulceration, examination is usually normal, though there may be epigastric/left upper quadrant tenderness	In uncomplicated duodenal ulceration, examination is usually normal, though there may be epigastric tenderness
Investigation	As for dyspepsia (🔲 p. 382)	
Complications	*Bleeding:* Acute GI bleeding—🔲 p. 1076; iron deficiency anaemia—🔲 p. 664 *Perforated peptic ulcer:* DU > GU; GUs may perforate posteriorly into the lesser sac; DUs usually perforate anteriorly into the peritoneal cavity. There may not be a past history of indigestion. Presents with sudden onset severe epigastric pain which rapidly becomes generalized. When a GU perforates into the lesser sac symptoms may remain localized or be confined to the right side of the abdomen. *Examination:* generalized peritonism with 'board-like rigidity'. *Management:* acute surgical admission *Pyloric stenosis in adults:* duodenal stenosis 2° to scarring from a chronic DU. Characterized by copious vomiting of food 1–2 days old. There may not be a past history of indigestion. *Examination:* if prolonged vomiting may be evidence of dehydration ± weight ↓. Succussion splash may be audible. *Management:* surgical referral for confirmation of diagnosis and surgical relief	

Further information
NICE Management of dyspepsia in adults in primary care (2004)
🕸 www.nice.org.uk

Gastro-oesophageal malignancy

Carcinoma of the oesophagus Common cancer accounting for 7,500 deaths/y in the UK. Most common in patients >60y. Overall, ♂:♀ ≈5:1. Usually presents late when prognosis is poor. Two types:
- **Squamous cell carcinoma** (50%)—predominant form in upper two-thirds of the oesophagus
- **Adenocarcinoma** (50%)—predominant in lower third of the oesophagus. Incidence is increasing. ♂:♀ ≈5:1

Common risk factors

Squamous cell carcinoma
- Smoking*
- Alcohol
- Low fruit/vegetable intake

* Risk ↓ to that of a non-smoker 10y after giving up

Adenocarcinoma
- Smoking*
- Obesity
- Low fruit/vegetable intake
- GORD—particularly Barrett's oesophagus (risk ↑ >30x—the longer the affected segment, the higher the risk)

Other risk factors
- Previous mediastinal radiotherapy (↑ x2 for patients treated for breast cancer; ↑ x20 for patients treated for Hodgkin's lymphoma)
- Plummer–Vinson (or Patterson–Kelly) syndrome—oesophageal web and iron deficiency anaemia
- Tylosis—rare, inherited disorder with hyperkeratosis of the palms; 40% develop oesophageal cancer

Presentation Short history of rapidly progressive dysphagia affecting solids initially then solids and liquids ± weight loss ± regurgitation of food and fluids (may be bloodstained). Retrosternal pain is a late feature. Other symptoms include hoarseness and/or cough (due to aspiration or fistula formation). Examination may be normal. Look for evidence of recent weight loss, hepatomegaly, and cervical lymphadenopathy.

Management Refer for urgent endoscopy if suspected. Rapid access dysphagia clinics are run in most areas. Specialist management involves resection (treatment of choice but only 1:3 patients are suitable), chemotherapy, radiotherapy, and/or palliation with a stenting tube. Tubes commonly become blocked. Good palliative care is essential—refer early (📖 p. 1028). Overall 8% 5y survival.

Stomach cancer Stomach cancer causes ~5,000 deaths/y in the UK; 95% are adenocarcinomas. Disease affecting older people, with 92% diagnosed >55y; ♂ > ♀ (5:3). Incidence has more than halved over the past 30y in the UK probably due to improved diet.

Other risk factors Include:
- Geography—common in Japan
- Blood group A
- *H. pylori* infection (not clear if eradication ↓ risk)
- Atrophic gastritis
- Pernicious anaemia
- Smoking
- Adenomatous polyps
- Social class
- Previous partial gastrectomy

Presentation Often non-specific. Presents with dyspepsia, weight ↓, anorexia or early satiety, vomiting, dysphagia, anaemia, and/or GI bleeding. Suspect in any patient >55y with recent onset dyspepsia (within 1y) and/or other risk factors. Examination is usually normal until incurable. Look for epigastric mass, hepatomegaly, jaundice, ascites, enlarged supraclavicular LN (Virchow's node), acanthosis nigricans.

Management If suspected, refer for urgent endoscopy. In early stages total/partial gastrectomy may be curative. Most present at later stage. Overall 5y survival is 15%.

Post-gastrectomy syndromes

Abdominal fullness A feeling of early satiety ± weight loss. Advise to take small, frequent meals.

Bilious vomiting Affects ~10% patients post-gastrectomy. Intermittent, sudden attacks of bilious vomiting 15–30min after eating ± epigastric cramping pain relieved by vomiting. Usually settles spontaneously. Metoclopramide or domperidone may be helpful in the interim. If symptoms are severe or fail to settle, request surgical review. Surgical bile diversion or stomach reconstruction may alleviate symptoms.

Dumping Abdominal distension, colic, and vasomotor disturbance (e.g. sweating, fainting) after meals. Affects 1–2% of gastrectomy patients (more common early after surgery—most settle within 6mo). 2 types:

- **Early dumping** Due to rapid gastric emptying. Starts immediately after a meal. *Consists of:* sweating, flushing, tachycardia, palpitations, epigastric fullness, nausea. Occasionally there may be vomiting, diarrhoea ± colicky abdominal pain. *Advise:* small, dry meals with restricted carbohydrate. Take drinks between meals. If severe, re-refer
- **Late dumping** Due to rapid gastric emptying → hyperglycaemia. The resultant hyperinsulinaemia causes a rebound hypoglycaemia. Starts 1–2h after meals. *Consists of:* faintness, sweating, tremor, and nausea. Advise patients to ↓ the sugar content of meals, rest for 1h after each meal, and take glucose if symptoms occur. If severe, re-refer

Diarrhoea post-gastrectomy 50% of patients who have had a truncal vagotomy or gastrectomy suffer some frequency of defecation; 5% require treatment. The diarrhoea is typically episodic and unpredictable. The exact mechanism is not clear. Treatment is with codeine phosphate or loperamide prn. Antibiotic treatment is occasionally successful—seek expert advice. Surgical measures are rarely necessary.

Anaemia Gastrectomy can result in both vitamin B_{12} deficiency and iron deficiency anaemia. Prophylactic B_{12} injections may be advised by the operating surgeon. Many advise iron supplements for life. An annual FBC to monitor for anaemia is advisable. Treat with iron/B_{12} supplements.

Stomach cancer Risk of stomach cancer is ↑ after partial gastrectomy (2x after 20y, and 7x after 45y).

Advice and support for patients

Cancer Research UK ☎ 0808 800 4040 🖰 www.cancerhelp.org.uk
Macmillan Cancer Support ☎ 0808 808 0000 🖰 www.macmillan.org.uk

Hernias

Irreducible hernia
- Most types of hernia may become irreducible
- It may be the first presentation of a hernia or a complication of a longstanding hernia
- If obstructed (incarcerated) or strangulated (blood supply to bowel contained within the hernia sac is compromised) the hernia is tender and there are symptoms/signs of small bowel obstruction

⚠ If you are unable to reduce a hernia, admit for surgical assessment.

Inguinal hernia Protruberance of peritoneal contents through the abdominal wall where it is weakened by the presence of the inguinal canal. Common condition (♂ > ♀) which can occur at any age.

Presentation Lump in the groin ± discomfort on straining/standing for any length of time. There may be a distinct precipitating event (e.g. heavy lifting). *Risk factors*: chronic cough (e.g. COPD), constipation, urinary obstruction, heavy lifting, ascites, previous abdominal surgery. *2 types*:
- **Indirect (80%)** Follow the course of the spermatic cord or round ligament down the inguinal canal through the internal inguinal ring (located at the mid-point of the inguinal ligament, 1.5cm above the femoral pulse), and sometimes out through the external inguinal ring into the scrotum/vulva
- **Direct (20%)** Passes through a defect in the abdominal wall into the inguinal canal. Rare in children and more common in the elderly

Differential diagnosis of groin lumps See Table 13.6.

Examination Examine the patient standing up. Look for a bulge in the groin above the line of the inguinal ligament. Unless incarcerated the lump should have a cough impulse. Check that you are able to reduce the hernia—sometimes, it is easier if the patient lies down. Ask the patient to reduce the hernia if you cannot.

Management Small hernias often require no treatment. For larger hernias and smaller hernias that are symptomatic, consider referral for surgical repair. Various methods are used—all have a high level of success (<2% recurrence). Trusses can be useful for symptomatic hernias in elderly patients, those unfit for surgery, or whilst awaiting surgery (prescribe on NHS prescription).

Inguinal hernias in children 📖 p. 890

Femoral hernia Less common than inguinal hernia. ♂ > ♀. The patient is usually elderly, although can occur at any age. Peritoneal contents protrude down the femoral canal. Risk of strangulation is high. Presents as a painful lump in the groin and/or small bowel obstruction.

Examination Rounded swelling medially in the groin and lateral to the pubic tubercle; if reducible a soft palpable lump remains after reduction.

Management Always refer for urgent surgical repair. Admit as surgical emergency if obstructed or irreducible.

Incisional hernia Breakdown of the muscle closure in an abdominal wound sometime after surgery. There may be a history of wound sepsis, haematoma, or breakdown. Presents with a bulge at the site of the operation scar ± discomfort.

Examination The hernia is usually visible when the patient stands—it can be made more obvious by asking the patient to cough or straight leg raise whilst lying flat. The margins of the muscular defect are palpable under the skin. Note whether fully reducible or not.

Management Often reassurance suffices. If obstructed/strangulated or causing discomfort, then refer for surgical assessment.

Umbilical hernia Most common in infants (🕮 p. 890). In adults para-umbilical hernias, presenting as a bulge adjacent to the umbilicus, may occur due to weakness in the linea alba. ♀ > ♂. Refer adults for surgical assessment—usually repaired as risk of strangulation is high. Admit as a surgical emergency if obstructed/irreducible.

Epigastric hernia Midline hernia through a defect in the linea alba above the umbilicus. Never contains bowel. Usually symptomless, though occasionally causes epigastric pain ± vomiting. *Examination:* epigastric mass with cough impulse. Refer for surgical repair.

Spigelian hernia A hernial sac protrudes lateral to the rectus sheath midway between the umbilicus and pubic bone. Presents with discomfort ± vomiting. Refer for surgical repair.

Obturator hernia Hernia protrudes out from the pelvis through the obturator canal. Usually presents with strangulation ± pain referred to the knee. Admit for surgery.

Richter hernia A knuckle of the side wall of the gut gets caught in a hernia sac and becomes strangulated but the bowel is not obstructed. Presents with abdominal pain which rapidly becomes worse ± shock. Admit as for acute abdomen; diagnosis is usually made at surgery.

Table 13.6 Differential diagnosis of groin lumps

Position relative to the skin	Groin lump	Position relative to the inguinal ligament	
		Above	Below
In the skin	Lipoma, fibroma, haemangioma, and other skin lumps	✓	✓
Deep to the skin	Femoral or inguinal lymph nodes	✓	✓
	Saphena varix of the femoral vein	✗	✓
	Femoral artery aneurysm	✗	✓
	Femoral hernia	✗	✓
	Inguinal hernia	✓	✗

❶ The inguinal ligament runs from the pubic tubercle medially to the anterior superior iliac spine laterally.

Appendicitis and small bowel disease

Acute appendicitis Most common surgical emergency in the UK. *Peak age:* 10–30y. Presents with central abdominal colic that progresses to localize in the right iliac fossa. Pain is worse on movement (especially coughing, laughing) and associated with anorexia, nausea ± vomiting, dysuria, constipation or rarely diarrhoea.

Assessment Watch for discomfort on walking (walk stooped). May be flushed and unwell—pyrexial (~37.5°C); furred tongue and/or foetor oris; tenderness, rebound tenderness and guarding in the right iliac fossa (especially over McBurney's point—two-thirds of the distance between the umbilicus and anterior superior iliac spine); pain in the right iliac fossa on palpation of the left iliac fossa (Rovsing's sign). Urinalysis is normal or +ve for protein and/or leucocyte esterase but –ve for nitrites.

Differential diagnosis
- Mesenteric adenitis
- Gastroenteritis
- Meckel's diverticulum
- Intussusception
- Crohn's disease
- Urological cause, e.g. UTI, testicular torsion
- Gynaecological cause (e.g. pelvic inflammatory disease; ectopic pregnancy)
- Non-abdominal cause, e.g. otitis media, diabetic ketoacidosis, pneumonia

Management Admit as a surgical emergency—expect to be wrong ~50% the time. *Complications:* generalized peritonitis 2° to perforation; appendix abscess; appendix mass; subphrenic abscess; female infertility.

Subphrenic abscess Rarely follows 7–21d after generalized peritonitis—particularly after acute appendicitis. Presents with general malaise, swinging fever, nausea, and weight ↓ ± pain in the upper abdomen radiating to the shoulder tip. Breathlessness can be associated due to reactive pleural effusion or lower lobe collapse. *Examination:* subcostal tenderness ± liver enlargement. FBC—↑ WCC. If suspected admit for surgical assessment.

⚠ **Appendicitis in pregnancy** Appendicitis affects 1:1,000 pregnancies. Mortality is ↑ and perforation more common (15–20%). Fetal mortality is 5–10% for simple appendicitis; 30% when there is perforation. Due to the pregnancy, the appendix is displaced—pain is often felt in the paraumbilical region or subcostally. Admit immediately if suspected.

 Children with appendicitis Symptoms/signs of appendicitis may be atypical—especially in very young children—as children localize pain poorly and signs of peritonitis can be difficult to elicit.
- If unsure of diagnosis and the child is unwell, admit
- If unsure of diagnosis and the child is well, either arrange to review a few hours later, or ask the carer to contact you if there is any deterioration, or change in symptoms

Mesenteric adentitis Inflammation of the mesenteric LNs, causing abdominal pain in children. May follow URTI. Can mimic appendicitis. Check MSU to exclude UTI. If guarding/rebound tenderness, refer for acute surgical assessment. Settles spontaneously with simple analgesia and fluids. If not settling in 1–2wk refer for paediatric assessment.

Meckel's diverticulum Remnant of the attachment of the small bowel to the embryological yolk sac. It is 2 inches (~5cm) long, ~2ft (60cm) proximal to the appendix and present in 2% of the population. A Meckel's diverticulum may not cause any problems or cause an appendicitis-like picture; acute intestinal obstruction, or GI bleeding. Symptoms can occur at any age but are most common in children.

J.F. Meckel (1781–1833)—German anatomist.

Adhesions Arise as a result of intra-abdominal inflammation. Bowel loops become adherent to each other, omentum, mesentery, and the abdominal wall. Fibrous bands may form connecting adjacent structures. Presents with abdominal pain ± obstruction. *Causes:* surgery; intra-abdominal sepsis (e.g. appendicitis, cholecystitis; salpingitis); inflammatory bowel disease; endometriosis. Refer to a surgeon. Treatment is difficult, as any surgery may result in new adhesions; conservative management with analgesia and stool softeners is preferred. Laparoscopic, or rarely open division of adhesions is occasionally necessary.

Intestinal non-Hodgkin's lymphoma The majority of intestinal NHLs are B-cell type lymphomas, but coeliac disease is associated with T-cell intestinal lymphoma. *Abdominal symptoms:* non-specific abdominal pain (70–80%); perforation (up to 25%); bowel obstruction; abdominal mass; intussusception; malabsorption (usually lymphoma associated with coeliac disease), or alteration in bowel habit (small intestine NHL may present like Crohn's disease). *Systemic symptoms:* weight ↓ (30%), fatigue, sweats, unexplained fevers. ❶ Lymphadenopathy and hepatosplenomegaly are usually absent.

Management (📖 p. 680) Gastric lymphoma may remit with treatment of *H. pylori* infection.

Carcinoid tumours Slow-growing tumours of low malignancy, which arise from neuroendocrine cells or their precursors. *Incidence:* 3–4/100,000. *Peak age:* 61y. ♀ > ♂. 60% are in the midgut (especially appendix and terminal ileum). Examination may reveal an abdominal mass and/or enlarged liver. Rarely presents with bowel obstruction. Ileal carcinoids are multiple in 30%. *Non-intestinal sites:* lung, testes, and ovary.

Carcinoid syndrome Affects <10% of patients with a carcinoid tumour. Develops when serotonin (5HT) is released by the tumour and not degraded by the liver due to hepatic metastases. *Features:*

• Paroxysmal flushing, e.g. following alcohol or certain foods
• Watery, explosive diarrhoea   • Bronchoconstriction (like asthma)
• Abdominal pain   • Right heart failure
• Rash—symmetrical, pruritic erythematous rash which blisters/crusts

Management Refer for urgent assessment if suspected. Therapeutic options include surgery, somatostatin analogues such as octreotide, or radiofrequency ablation of liver metastases. Prognosis—if no metastases, median survival is 5–8y; with metastases median survival is 38mo.

Colorectal cancer screening

Screening for colorectal cancer is available throughout the UK. Patients presenting with tumour confined to the bowel wall have >90% long-term survival. Without screening, most tumours are detected at advanced stages and overall 5y survival is ≈50%. Screening aims to detect colorectal cancer at an early stage to ↑ survival chances.

Screening test Faecal occult blood (FOB) test kits are sent every 2y to all patients aged 60–74y with instructions for completion/return. The test kit has 3 flaps, each with 2 windows underneath. 2 samples are taken from a bowel motion and spread onto the 2 windows under the first flap using the cardboard sticks provided. The flap is then sealed and the process repeated using the remaining 2 flaps for the subsequent 2 bowel motions. Once all 6 windows have been used, the kit is returned. Kits must be returned <14d after the first sample is taken. Results are sent to the patients in <2wk.

Screening outcomes (See Tables 13.7 and 13.8) If 60% of those aged 60–69y do the FOB test, 1,200 deaths will be prevented each year in the UK.

Family history If a patient has one first-degree relative (mother, father, sister, brother, daughter, or son) with colorectal cancer, risk of developing colorectal cancer is ↑ 2–3x.

Refer for colonoscopy At presentation or aged 35–40y (whichever is later), and repeat colonoscopy aged 55y if:
- 2x first-degree relatives with a history of colorectal cancer, *or*
- 1x first-degree relative with a history of colorectal cancer aged <45y

Refer for specialist follow-up and genetic counselling if:
- >2x first-degree relatives with a history of colorectal cancer, *or*
- Family history of:
  - **Familial adenomatous polyposis (FAP)**—usually develop cancer aged <40y. Lifetime risk of colorectal cancer is 1:2.5
  - **Juvenile polyposis**—lifetime risk of colorectal cancer is 1:3
  - **Peutz–Jegher syndrome**—autosomal dominant disorder. Benign intestinal (usually small intestine) polyps in association with dark freckles on lips, oral mucosa, face, palm and soles. May cause GI obstruction or GI bleeding. Malignant change occurs in ~3%
  - **Hereditary non-polyposis colorectal cancer**—≥3 family members with colorectal cancer where ≥2 generations have been affected and ≥1 affected family member developed the disease <50y of age; 40% lifetime risk of colorectal cancer
  - **MMR (mismatch repair) oncogene**

Ulcerative colitis ↑ risk of colorectal cancer. Offer all patients a follow-up plan agreed with their specialist. In some cases, prophylactic colectomy is appropriate.

Previous colorectal cancer ↑ risk of developing a second colorectal primary. After successful treatment, younger patients are routinely followed up with colonoscopy every 5y until 70y. Remain vigilant for recurrences, and re-refer urgently if suspected.

Table 13.7 FOB test outcomes

FOB result	Explanation	Action
Normal	0 +ve spots	Screening offered again in 2y if <70y
Unclear ~4% tested	1–4 +ve spots	Test repeated If the second test is abnormal, colonoscopy is offered If the second test is normal, a third test is requested If the third test is normal, repeat screening in 2y is offered if <70y If the third test is abnormal, colonoscopy is offered
Abnormal	5–6 +ve spots	Colonoscopy is offered
Technical failure or spoilt kit	Laboratory or patient error	Repeat testing is offered

Table 13.8 Colonoscopy outcomes

- ~2% of those FOB tested are referred on for colonoscopy—uptake of colonoscopy is ~80%
- Sensitivity of colonoscopy to detect significant abnormalities is ~90%
- Polyps found during colonoscopy are usually removed
- Complications of colonoscopy include heavy bleeding (1:150); bowel perforation (1:1,500); death (1:10,000)

Colonoscopy result		Explanation	Action
Normal (~50%)		No abnormalities detected	FOB screening offered again in 2y if <70y
Polyp (~40%)	Low risk	1–2 small (<1cm) adenomas	FOB screening offered again in 2y if <70y
	Intermediate risk	3–4 small (<1cm) adenomas *or* ≥1 adenoma ≥1cm	3-yearly colonoscopy until 2x negative examinations
	High risk	≥5 adenomas *or* ≥3 adenomas of which at least 1 is ≥1cm	Colonoscopy at 12mo, *then* 3-yearly colonoscopy until 2x negative examinations
Cancer (~10%)		Colorectal cancer detected at colonoscopy	Refer urgently for further treatment
Other pathology		Other pathology (e.g. UC) detected at colonoscopy	Refer/treat/advise as necessary
Technical difficulty		Unable to perform the procedure adequately	Repeat colonoscopy or alternative imaging

Further information

NICE Referral guidelines for suspected cancer (2005) ℘ www.nice.org.uk
NHS Bowel Cancer Screening Programme ℘ www.cancerscreening. nhs.uk/bowel/index.html

Information for patients

Bowel cancer screening—the Facts ℘ www.cancerscreening.nhs.uk

Colorectal cancer

Lifetime risk of developing colorectal cancer is 1:15 for ♀ and 1:19 for ♂. Colorectal cancer accounts for 14% of all cancers and 16,000 deaths/y in the UK. Two-thirds arise in the colon and a third in the rectum; 72% of tumours occur in patients >65y and >95% are adenocarcinomas.

Adenomatous polyps Bowel cancers arise from polyps over many years. Polyps may be removed because of risk of malignant change. Follow-up surveillance with repeated colonoscopy may be necessary depending on the number of polyps and their size (📖 p. 397).

Protective and risk factors

Lifestyle factors
- Obesity—↑ risk by 15% if overweight and 30% if obese
- Dietary factors—diets with less red and processed meat, and more vegetables, fibre, fish, and milk are associated with ↓ risk (diet is thought to explain geographic variations)
- Alcohol—↑ risk for heavy drinkers, especially if also low folate
- Physical activity—↑ physical activity can ↓ risk by 30%

Medication history
- HRT—risk ↓ by 20% if ever taken; ↓ by 30% if taking HRT currently
- COC pill—risk ↓ by 18% if ever taken
- Statins—risk is ↓ after 5y use
- Aspirin—75mg od taken for >5y ↓ risk by 40%

Other medical history
- History of gall bladder disease and/or cholecystectomy—50% ↑ in risk
- Type 2 (non-insulin-dependent) diabetes—30% ↑ risk
- UC or Crohn's disease—↑ risk (📖 p. 414)

Family history 📖 p. 396

Bowel cancer screening 📖 p. 396

Presentation May be found at bowel cancer screening. Clinical presentations depends on site involved:
- **Change in bowel habit:** diarrhoea ± mucus, constipation or alternating diarrhoea and constipation, tenesmus
- **Intestinal obstruction:** pain, distension, absolute constipation ± vomiting. May be an acute, sudden event (20% of patients not detected by screening present with an acute obstruction) or gradually evolve
- **Rectal bleeding:** bright red rectal bleeding or +ve faecal occult blood test—60% rectal tumours. Rarely melaena if high tumour
- **Perforation:** causing generalized peritonitis or into an adjacent viscus (e.g. bladder), resulting in a fistula
- **Spread:** abdominal distension 2° to ascites, jaundice, rectal/pelvic pain
- **General effects:** weight ↓, anorexia, anaemia, malaise

Examination and investigation
- General examination—cachexia, jaundice, anaemia (check FBC)
- Abdominal mass   • Hepatomegaly   • Ascites
- Rectal examination—detects >75% of rectal tumours

Suspicious lower GI symptoms and signs Refer urgently (to be seen in <2wk) to a team specializing in lower GI malignancy.

Any age with:
- Right lower abdominal mass consistent with involvement of large bowel
- A palpable rectal mass (intraluminal, not pelvic; a pelvic mass outside the bowel would warrant an urgent referral to a urologist)
- Unexplained iron deficiency anaemia (Hb ≤11g/dL for ♂; ≤10g/dL for a non-menstruating ♀)

Aged ≥40y Reporting rectal bleeding with a change of bowel habit towards looser stools and/or ↑ stool frequency persisting ≥6wk.

Aged ≥60y with:
- Rectal bleeding persisting for ≥6wk without a change in bowel habit and without anal symptoms
- Change in bowel habit to looser stools and/or more frequent stools persisting for ≥6wk without rectal bleeding

❶ In a patient with equivocal symptoms who is not unduly anxious, it is reasonable to 'treat, watch, and wait'.

Specialist management Confirmation of diagnosis with sigmoidoscopy/colonoscopy and/or CT colonography. If diagnosis is confirmed further investigations include LFTs, tumour markers (carcino-embryonic antigen or CEA is produced in >80% advanced tumours), CXR, CT/MRI, and USS to evaluate spread.

Treatment Laparoscopic or open surgical resection when possible. Staging based on findings at surgery dictates further management with chemotherapy. For patients with more advanced disease, resection or radioablation of hepatic metastases may be an option.

Adverse pathological features
- Presence/number of involved LNs
- Lymphovascular, perineural, or venous invasion
- Depth of bowel wall penetration
- Positive resection margin
- Mucinous histology

Adverse clinical features
- Emergency presentation with bowel obstruction or perforation
- Incomplete resection
- Metastatic disease
- Presentation aged <50y

Further information

NICE Ꮑ www.nice.org.uk
- Referral guidelines for suspected cancer (2005)
- Colorectal cancer (2011)

SIGN Diagnosis and management of colorectal cancer (2011)
Ꮑ www.sign.ac.uk

Patient advice and support

Cancer Research UK ☎ 0808 800 4040 Ꮑ www.cancerhelp.org.uk
Macmillan Cancer Support ☎ 0808 808 0000 Ꮑ www.macmillan.org.uk
British Colostomy Association ☎ 0800 328 4257
Ꮑ www.colostomyassociation.org.uk

Other large bowel conditions

Intestinal obstruction Blockage of the bowel due to either mechanical obstruction or failure of peristalsis (ileus). *Causes:*

- **Obstruction from outside the bowel** Adhesions/bands; volvulus; obstructed hernia (📖 p. 392); neighbouring malignancy (e.g. bladder)
- **Obstruction from within the bowel wall** Tumour; infarction; congenital atresia; Hirschsprung's disease; inflammatory bowel disease (📖 p. 414); diverticulitis
- **Obstruction in the lumen** Impacted faeces/constipation (📖 p. 378); bolus obstruction (e.g. swallowed foreign body); gallstone ileus; intussusception; large polyps
- **Ileus/functional obstruction** Post-op; electrolyte disturbance; uraemia; DM; back pain; anticholinergic drugs

Presentation Anorexia; nausea; vomiting (may be faeculent) gives relief; colicky central abdominal pain and distension; absolute constipation for stool and gas (though if high obstruction constipation may not be absolute). *Examination:* uncomfortable and restless; abdominal distension ± tenderness (though no guarding/rebound); active tinkling bowel sounds or quiet/absent bowel sounds (later).

Management Admit as surgical emergency.

Diverticulosis Common condition of the colon associated with muscle hypertrophy and ↑ intraluminal pressure. Mucosa-lined pouches are pushed out through the colonic wall usually at the entry points of vessels. These pouches are the diverticula; 95% are in the sigmoid colon although they may occur anywhere in the bowel. They are present in >1:3 people >60y in the UK. Risk factors include low-roughage diet and age. Diverticular disease implies the diverticula are symptomatic—see Table 13.9.

Ischaemic bowel Interruption of the blood supply of the bowel.

- *1° ischaemia:* usually due to either mesenteric embolus from the right side of the heart, or venous thrombosis and typically occurs in elderly patients who might have pre-existing heart or vascular disease
- *2° ischaemia:* usually due to intestinal obstruction (e.g. strangulated hernia, volvulus, intussusception)

Presentation Sudden onset of abdominal pain which rapidly becomes severe. There may be a prior history of pain worse after meals (mesenteric angina). Rarely presents with PR bleeding. *Examination:* very unwell; shocked; may be in AF; generalized tenderness but normally no guarding/rebound. Often signs are out of proportion to symptoms.

Management Give opioid analgesia. Admit as surgical emergency.

Sigmoid volvulus Occurs in people who have redundant colon on a long mesentery with a narrow base. The sigmoid loop twists, causing intestinal obstruction. The loop may become ischaemic. *Risk factors:* constipation, laxatives, tranquillizers. Presents with acute onset of abdominal distension and colicky abdominal pain with complete constipation and absence of flatus. There may be a history of repeated attacks.

Management Admit acutely to hospital. Treatment is release by passing a flatus tube and/or surgery. Once treated, ↓ recurrences by preventing constipation and stopping tranquillizers if possible.

Hirschprung's disease Caused by absence of the ganglion cells of the myenteric plexus in the distal bowel. Presents with delay in passing meconium, abdominal distension, vomiting, and poor feeding in a neonate. If only a short segment is affected, presentation may be much later with chronic constipation. Diagnosis is confirmed with rectal biopsy. Refer to surgery. Treatment is surgical removal of the affected area of bowel.
H. Hirschprung (1830–1916)—Danish paediatrician.

Table 13.9 Presentation and management of diverticular disease

	Presentation	Management
Chronic diverticulitis (painful diverticular disease)	Presents with altered bowel habit, abdominal pain (often colicky and left-sided), nausea, and flatulence. Symptoms are often improved by defecation.	Investigate for change in bowel habit (📖 p. 399) Once diverticular disease is confirmed, treat with high-fibre diet ± antispasmodics (e.g. mebeverine 135mg tds) Refer if severe symptoms
Acute diverticulitis	Presents with: • Altered bowel habit • Colicky left-sided abdominal pain—may become continuous and cause guarding/peritonism in the left iliac fossa • Fever • Malaise ± nausea • Flatulence ❗ There may be few abdominal signs in the elderly	Treat with oral antibiotics (e.g. co-amoxiclav 250mg tds or cefaclor 250–500mg tds and metronidazole 400mg bd or ciprofloxacin 500–750mg bd) There may also be some benefit from a low-residue diet If severe symptoms, uncertain diagnosis, or not settling, admit as an acute surgical emergency
Diverticular abscess	Presents with swinging fever, general malaise ± other localizing symptoms, e.g. pelvic pain	Refer for urgent surgical assessment/admit as a surgical emergency
Perforated diverticulum	Presents with ileus, peritonitis and shock	Admit as an acute surgical emergency
Fistula formation	A fistula may form if a diverticulum perforates into bladder, 'vagina' or small bowel—📖 p. 380	Refer for surgical assessment Treatment is usually surgical
Haemorrhage from a diverticulum	Common cause of rectal bleeding—usually sudden and painless.	Gain IV access Admit as an acute surgical emergency (📖 p. 1076)
Post-infective stricture	Fibrous tissue formation following infection can cause narrowing of the colon → obstruction	Keep stool soft If recurrent problems, refer for surgery

Carcinoma of the colon 📖 p. 398   **Anal conditions** 📖 p. 402
Inflammatory bowel disease 📖 p. 414

Anal and perianal problems

Haemorrhoids ('piles') Common in all age groups from mid-teens onwards. Represent distension of the submuscosal plexus of veins in the anus. Three main groups situated at 3, 7, and 11 o'clock positions (relative to the patient viewed in lithotomy position). *Risk factors:* constipation; FH; varicose veins; pregnancy; ↑ anal tone (cause not understood); pelvic tumour; portal hypertension. *Classification:*

- **1st degree** Piles remain within the anal canal
- **2nd degree** Prolapse out of anal verge but spontaneously reduce
- **3rd degree** Prolapse out of anus and require digital reduction
- **4th degree** Permanently prolapsed

Presentation Discomfort or discharge ± fresh red rectal bleeding (blood on toilet paper, coating stool, or dripping into pan after defecation); feeling of incomplete emptying of the rectum; mucus discharge; pruritus ani. *Rectal examination:* prolapsing piles are obvious, 1st degree piles are not visible or palpable.

Management If piles are not obvious on examination, arrange proctoscopy ± sigmoidoscopy for all patients >40y. *Treatment:* soften stool (bran, ispaghula husk) and recommend topical analgesia (e.g. lidocaine 5% ointment or OTC preparation). If not responding to treatment, uncertainty over diagnosis, or severe symptoms (e.g. soiling of underwear), refer for surgical assessment. *Complications:*

- **Strangulation** Circulation to the pile is obstructed by the anal sphincter. Results in intense pain + anal sphincter spasm. Treat with analgesia. If severe pain or symptoms are not settling, admit
- **Thrombosis** Pain/anal sphincter spasm—analgesia, ice packs, and bed rest; consider referral for surgery to prevent recurrence

Perianal haematoma (thrombosed external pile) Due to a ruptured superficial perianal vein causing a subcutaneous haematoma. Presents with sudden onset of severe perianal pain. A tender, 2–4mm 'dark blueberry' under the skin adjacent to the anus is visible. Give analgesia. Settles spontaneously over ~1wk. If <1d old can be evacuated via a small incision under LA.

Rectal prolapse Occurs in 2 age groups—the very young and those >60y. Presents with mass coming down through the anus ± anal discharge. In adults there are 2 types:

- **Mucosal** Adults with 3rd degree piles—bowel musculature remains in position but redundant mucosa prolapses from the anal canal
- **Complete** Descent of the upper rectum into the lower anal canal. Usually due to weak pelvic floor from childbirth. Bowel wall is inverted and passed out through the anus. May be associated uterine prolapse

Refer for surgery. A supporting ring may be used if unfit for surgery.

Anal fissure The anal mucosa is torn—usually on the posterior aspect of the anal canal. May occur at any age. Presents with pain on defecation ± constipation ± fresh rectal bleeding ('blood on toilet paper'). The fissure is often visible as is a 'sentinel pile' (bunched up mucosa at the base of the tear). Rectal examination is very tender due to muscle spasm.

Management Soften stool (e.g. ispaghula husk); try analgesic suppositories (e.g. 5% lidocaine ointment; OTC haemorrhoid preparations). If unsuccessful add glyceryl trinitrate 0.4% ointment bd which relieves pain and spasm but may cause headache; 2% topical diltiazem cream bd is a third-line option (unlicensed). If interventions fail refer to surgeon.

Perianal abscess Usually caused by infection arising in a perianal gland. Tends to lie between the internal and external sphincters and points towards the skin at the anal margin. May affect patients of any age and presents with gradual onset of perianal pain which becomes throbbing and severe; defecation and sitting are painful—characteristically patients sit with one buttock raised off the chair. *Examination:* abscess in the skin next to the anus. Refer as an acute surgical emergency for drainage.

Perianal fistula Abnormal connection between the lumen of the anus (or rectum) and skin. Usually develops from a perianal abscess. Fistulae are either 'high' (open into the bowel above the deep external anal sphincter) or 'low' (open into the bowel below this point). High fistulae are rare and usually due to UC, Crohn's disease, or tumour—they are more complex to repair. Presents with persistent perianal discharge and/or recurrent abscess. The external opening is usually visible lateral to the anus; the internal opening may be palpable on rectal examination. Refer for surgical repair.

Pilonidal sinus Obstruction of a hair follicle in the natal cleft. The ingrowing hair triggers a foreign body reaction → pain, swelling, abscess, and/or fistula formation ± foul-smelling discharge. Refer for surgery.

Pruritus ani Itching around the anus. Occurs if the anus is moist or soiled, e.g. poor personal hygiene; anal leakage or faecal incontinence; fissures; nylon/tight underwear. *Other causes:* dermatological conditions (e.g. contact dermatitis, lichen sclerosus); threadworm infection; anxiety; other causes of generalized pruritus (📖 p. 594). Treat cause if possible; avoid spicy food; moist wipe post-defecation.

Anal ulcers Rare. Consider Crohn's disease, syphilis, tumour.

 Threadworm Common in the UK—especially in children. *Enterobius vermicularis* causes anal itch, as it leaves the bowel to lay eggs on the perineum. Often seen as silvery thread-like worms at the anus of children. *Treatment:* mebendazole (available OTC). Treat household contacts as well as the index case.

Anal cancer Usually squamous cell cancer (>50%). *Risk factors:* anal sex; syphilis; anal warts (HPV). Presents with bleeding, pain, anal mass or ulcer, pruritus, stricture, change in bowel habit. A mass may be palpable on rectal examination. Check for inguinal LNs.

Management Refer for urgent surgical review and confirmation of diagnosis. Treatment is usually with a combination of radiotherapy ± chemotherapy. Abdominoperineal resection is reserved for salvage therapy after chemo- or radiotherapy failure.

Patients with ostomies

❶ Specialist stoma nurses are an extremely useful source of advice and help. If in doubt about the correct stoma appliances and accessories to supply or a patient has a problem with a stoma, wherever possible liaise with your local specialist stoma nurse.

The first iatrogenic stoma was constructed in France in 1776 for an obstructing rectal cancer. Stomas (from the Greek meaning 'mouth') may be temporary or permanent (see Table 13.10).

Stoma retraction can → leakage and severe skin problems. Most common reason for re-operation. Refer for specialist advice.

Prolapse Seen most frequently with loop colostomy. If persists and disrupts pouching, refer for consideration of revision.

Peristomal hernia Common complication. Symptomatic cases require referral for repair.

Stenosis Narrowing of the stoma may result in difficulty or pain passing stool and/or obstruction. If problematic refer for revision.

Skin complications Skin irritation can be due to:
- Leakage onto the skin
- Allergic reactions to the adhesive material in a skin barrier
- Fungal infection, or
- Inadequate hygiene

Prevention of skin complications
- Advise patients to clean, rinse, and pat the skin dry between pouch changes
- Avoid using an oily soap, which can leave a film that interferes with proper adhesion of the skin barrier
- Ensure the pouch system fits
- Treat any infection with oral antibiotics and/or oral or topical antifungals
- Apply skin barrier cream
- If the skin is uneven (e.g. due to scarring), fill irregularities with stoma paste to give a better fit
- Consider the use of convex discs or stoma belts (refer to specialist stoma nurse for advice)

Drugs Enteric-coated and modified-release preparations are unsuitable for people with bowel stomas—particularly for patients with ileostomy.

Diet
- Avoid foods that cause intestinal upset or diarrhoea
- For descending/sigmoid colostomy, avoid foods that cause constipation. If constipation does occur, ↑ fluid intake and/or dietary fibre
- Certain foods, e.g. beans, cucumbers, and carbonated drinks, can cause gas, along with certain habits such as talking or swallowing air while eating, using a straw, breathing through the mouth, and chewing gum

- A daily portion of apple sauce, cranberry juice, yogurt, or buttermilk can help control odour. If odour is strong and persistent, consider use of charcoal filters or pouch deodorizers (seek advice from a specialist stoma nurse)

Psychosocial problems Self-help groups provide information and tips on lifestyle and stoma care; specialist stoma nurses can provide support and counselling.

Activities Advise patients to avoid rough contact sports and heavy lifting as these might → herniation around the stoma. Patients with stomas may swim. Water will not enter a stoma due to peristalsis so stomas do not need to be covered when bathing. A body belt (available on FP10) to hold the stoma bag in place against the body may stop rustling/leakage for those doing aerobic exercise—seek advice from a specialist stoma nurse.

Travel Advise patients to pack sufficient supplies of their stoma products and carry supplies with them in case baggage is misplaced. Avoid storing supplies in a very hot environment as heat may damage pouches.

Patient advice and support
British Colostomy Association ☎ 0800 328 4257
⌖ www.colostomyas sociation.org.uk

Table 13.10 The three main types of stoma

Colostomy	Ileostomy	Urostomy
Age Most >50y	*Peak age range* 10–50y	*Age* Most >50y
Output Depends on site: • Transverse colostomy—soft stool • Descending/sigmoid colostomy—formed stool	*Output* Soft/fluid stool	*Output* Urine—continent procedures using bowel to fashion a bladder which is then drained with a catheter through the stoma are becoming common
Reasons for colostomy Carcinoma Diverticular disease Trauma Radiation enteritis Bowel ischaemia Hirschprung's disease Congenital abnormalities Obstruction Crohn's disease Faecal incontinence	*Reasons for ileostomy* Ulcerative colitis Crohn's disease Familial polyposis coli Obstruction Radiation enteritis Trauma Bowel ischaemia Meconium ileus Carcinoma	*Reasons for urostomy* Carcinoma Urinary incontinence Fistulas Spinal column disorders

Chronic diarrhoea and malabsorption

Chronic diarrhoea Diarrhoea persisting >4wk. Patients' perceptions of diarrhoea vary widely. Clarify what is meant. Chronic diarrhoea affects ~4–5% of adults in the UK. There are many causes (see Table 13.11), and all patients require investigation. Careful history is vital.

Symptoms suggestive of organic disease
- History of <3mo duration
- Mainly nocturnal or continuous (as opposed to intermittent) diarrhoea
- Significant weight ↓
- Liquid stools with blood and/or mucus

Symptoms suggestive of malabsorption
- Pale and/or offensive stools
- Steatorrhoea—excess fat in faeces. The stool is pale-coloured and foul-smelling and floats ('difficult to flush')

Examination and investigation Full examination. Look for signs of systemic disease and examine abdomen thoroughly. Check:
- **Blood:** FBC, ESR, Ca^{2+}, LFTs, haematinics, TFTs, coeliac serology
- **Stool:** M,C&S

Management
- If obvious identifiable cause, e.g. GI infection, constipation, drug side effect, then treat and review. Refer to gastroenterology if treatment does not relieve symptoms
- If symptoms suggestive of functional bowel disease and <45y with normal investigations, irritable bowel syndrome is likely. Reassure, offer advice, and review as necessary. Refer to gastroenterology if atypical symptoms appear or the patient is unhappy with the diagnosis
- Otherwise refer to gastroenterology for assessment. Speed of referral depends on age and severity of symptoms

⚠ **Refer urgently** to a team specializing in lower GI malignancy if:

Any age with:
- Right lower abdominal mass consistent with involvement of large bowel
- A palpable rectal mass (intraluminal, not pelvic; a pelvic mass outside the bowel would warrant an urgent referral to a urologist)
- Unexplained iron deficiency anaemia (Hb ≤11g/dL for ♂; ≤10g/dL for a non-menstruating ♀)

Aged ≥40y Reporting rectal bleeding with a change of bowel habit towards looser stools and/or increased stool frequency persisting ≥6wk.

Aged ≥60y with:
- Rectal bleeding persisting for ≥6wk without a change in bowel habit and without anal symptoms
- Change in bowel habit to looser stools and/or more frequent stools persisting for ≥6 wk without rectal bleeding

❶ In a patient with equivocal symptoms who is not unduly anxious, it is reasonable to 'treat, watch and wait'.

Table 13.11 Causes of chronic diarrhoea

Colon	Small bowel	Pancreas
Colonic cancer	Crohn's disease	Pancreatic cancer
Ulcerative colitis	Coeliac disease	Chronic pancreatitis
Crohn's disease	Other enteropathies, e.g. Whipple's disease	CF
Constipation with overflow diarrhoea	Bile acid malabsorption	**Other**
	Ischaemia	Bowel resection
Endocrine	Enzyme deficiencies, e.g. lactase deficiency	Bile salt malabsorption
DM (autonomic neuropathy)	Radiation damage	Intestinal fistula
Hyperthyroidism	Bacterial overgrowth	Drugs
Hypoparathyroidism	Lymphoma	Alcohol
Addison's disease	Infection (e.g. giardiasis, *Cryptosporidium*)	Autonomic neuropathy
Hormone-secreting tumours, e.g. carcinoid	Irritable bowel syndrome	'Factitious' diarrhoea

Malabsorption Presents with chronic diarrhoea, weight ↓, steatorrhoea, vitamin/iron deficiencies, and/or oedema due to protein deficiency. Refer to gastroenterology for investigation/treatment of the cause.

Usual causes
- Coeliac disease—📖 p. 412
- Chronic pancreatitis—📖 p. 430
- Crohn's disease—📖 p. 414

Rarer causes
- CF
- Pancreatic cancer—📖 p. 432
- Whipple's disease
- Biliary insufficiency
- Bacterial overgrowth
- Chronic infection (e.g. giardiasis, tropical sprue)
- Following gastric surgery

Whipple's disease A cause of malabsorption which usually occurs in ♂ >50 y. *Other features:* arthralgia, pigmentation, weight ↓, lymphadenopathy, ± cerebellar or cardiac signs. *Cause:* Tropheryma whippelii. Refer for gastroenterology assessment. Jejunal biopsy is characteristic. *Treatment:* long-term broad-spectrum antibiotics.

Malabsorption in children 📖 p. 888

Factitious diarrhoea Responsible for 4% referrals to gastroenterology departments and 20% of tertiary referrals. Due to laxative abuse or adding of water or urine to stool samples. Difficult to spot—have a high index of suspicion especially in patients with history of eating disorder or somatization.

Further information

British Society of Gastroenterology Guidelines for the investigation of chronic diarrhoea (2003) ☞ www.bsg.org.uk
NICE ☞ www.nice.org.uk
- Referral guidelines for suspected cancer (2005)
- Diarrhoea and vomiting in children under 5 (2009)

Faecal incontinence

Affects ~2% of all ages, causing great personal disability. It is a common reason for carers to request placement in a nursing home.

Causes

- Age and frailty
- Constipation (overflow incontinence)
- Childbirth
- Colonic resection/anal surgery
- Rectal prolapse/haemorrhoids
- Loose stools or diarrhoea from any cause, e.g. inflammatory bowel disease
- After radiotherapy
- Systemic sclerosis
- Neurological disorders
- Cognitive deficit
- Congenital disorders (e.g. anal atresia, Hirschsprung's disease)
- Emotional problems, e.g. encoparesis in children

History Aimed at establishing the underlying causes of the incontinence (may be >1) and other factors that might be contributing to it. *Ask about:*

- Onset and nature of symptoms ❶ Always consider faecal incontinence when patients present with anal soreness and/or itching
- Bowel habit including timing and frequency of incontinence
- Difficulties with toileting and help available
- Other medical conditions
- Medication
- Diet
- Social circumstances

⚠ Persistent change in bowel habit to looser stools may be a sign of GI malignancy—📖 p. 399.

Examination General and rectal examination (to detect abnormalities of anal tone, local anal pathology, e.g. rectal prolapse, and constipation causing overflow incontinence). Further examination depends on age group and history, e.g. cognitive assessment if suspected cognitive deficit; neurological examination if ↓ anal tone.

Primary care management

Treatment of cause

- Clear any constipation/faecal loading (📖 p. 378)—use rectal preparations initially to clear faecal load. If unsuccessful/rectal preparations are inappropriate, then switch to oral laxatives. Take steps to prevent recurrence, e.g. add fibre to diet, ↑ fluid intake, consider regular laxatives
- Treat other reversible causes, e.g. infective diarrhoea, UC
- Consider alternatives to any contributing medications, e.g. tranquillizers

General measures where cause cannot be treated

- Advise fluid intake of at least 1.5L/d
- Encourage bowel emptying after a meal—advise patients to assume a seated/squatting position and not to strain
- Ensure that toilet facilities are private, accessible, and safe—refer for OT assessment if needed

- Manipulate diet to promote optimal stool consistency and predictable bowel emptying. A food/fluid diary may be helpful. Only change one food at a time. Consider referral to a dietician
- If stool must be in the rectum at a set time (e.g. when a carer is there), manipulate bowel action with pr/po laxatives and/or loperamide
- If loose stools, consider treatment with loperamide, co-phenotrope, or codeine phosphate, prn or continuously. When using loperamide, introduce at a very low dose (consider syrup for doses <2mg) and ↑ dose until desired stool consistency is reached. Dose and/or frequency can be adjusted ↑ or ↓ in response to stool consistency and lifestyle
  ❶ Do not use if hard stools, undiagnosed diarrhoea, or flare-up of UC
- Review regularly. If no improvement with simple strategies, consider referral for specialist care

Patients with faecal incontinence from enteral feeding Discuss with the patient's dietician. Modifying type/timing of feeds may help.

Patients with spinal injury or disease Bowel function is a reflex action which we learn to override as children. If the lesion is above the level of this reflex pathway (T_{12} for bowel function) then automatic emptying will still occur when the bladder or bowel is full, although there is no control. If the lesion is below this level there is no emptying reflex. Bowel care programmes reflect this. Useful leaflets are available from the spinal injuries association (☏ 0800 980 0501 🖰 www.spinal.co.uk).

Referral Consider if symptoms are not controlled:

- To continence adviser—for advice on skin care/hygiene and supplies of incontinence pads. Pelvic floor muscle training, bowel retraining, biofeedback, electrical stimulation, and/or rectal irrigation may be useful. Devices e.g. anal plugs or faecal collectors can help in some situations
- To surgeon—for sphincter repair if significant sphincter defect; for consideration of implanted sacral nerve stimulation device; for appendicostomy/continent colonic conduit for anterograde irrigation in patients with colonic motility disorders; for stoma formation (last resort)
- To old age psychiatry—if cognitive deficit and incontinence
- To paediatrics—if encoparesis due to chronic constipation, or child psychiatry if encoparesis due to emotional distress

Encopresis in children 📖 p. 915

Further information

NICE Faecal incontinence (2007) 🖰 www.nice.org.uk

Patient information

Bladder and Bowel Foundation Provides information and support as well as 'Just can't wait' or JCW cards. This card allows patients with bowel problems access to staff toilet facilities in many high street stores on production of their access card. ☏ 0845 345 0165
🖰 www.bladderandbowelfoundation.org

RADAR Keys The National Key Scheme (NKS) offers independent access to disabled people to around 7,000 locked public toilets around the country. Keys are available to purchase from 🖰 www.radar-shop.org.uk. If the patient has an ongoing disability, purchase can be made VAT-free.

Gastroenteritis and food poisoning

Ingestion of viruses, bacteria, or their toxins commonly causes diarrhoea and/or vomiting (see Table 13.12). ❶ Suspected food poisoning is a notifiable disease.

Prevention Handwashing after using the toilet; longer cooking and rewarming times; prompt consumption of food.

Presentation

- *History* Severity and duration of symptoms, food eaten and water drunk, time relationship between ingestion and symptoms, other affected contacts, recent foreign travel
- *Examination* Usually normal. Dehydration may prompt admission

Investigation and management See Vomiting and diarrhoea—🕮 p. 376. Advise fluid replacement. Only give antibiotics if recommended following stool culture (exception is *Giardia* diarrhoea—🕮 p. 649).

Campylobacter Most common bacterial cause of infectious diarrhoea in the UK. Two species (*C. jejuni* and *C. coli*) are responsible for most cases. Symptoms occur 2–5d after ingestion of infected food (usually milk or poultry). Malaise followed by abdominal pain and diarrhoea—often bloody. Rarely associated with arthritis. Usually clears spontaneously. If needed, treatment is with erythromycin or ciprofloxacin.

Salmonella Common cause of infectious diarrhoea. Usually ingested in infected meat, poultry, or eggs. *Symptoms*: vomiting, diarrhoea, abdominal pain, and fever—develop from 12h–2d after ingestion. Rarely associated with arthritis 2–3 wk after acute infection. In <1%, a carrier state develops. Only use antibiotics on microbiologist advice.

Escherichia coli Many different strains of *E. coli* cause diarrhoea via a variety of mechanisms. In most cases, treatment is supportive with fluid replacement. Rarely, for enterohaemorrhagic strains, antibiotics may be recommended, but use is controversial, as antibiotic treatment has been linked with haemolytic uraemic syndrome.

Cryptosporidium Protozoan causing diarrhoeal disease. Infections are usually spread in water. Responsible for ~5% of all gastroenteritis in both industrialized and developing countries. Presents with profuse watery diarrhoea, abdominal cramp ± nausea, anorexia, fever, and malaise. Treatment is supportive. Usually symptoms last 1–2wk (rarely >1mo). Immunocompromised patients develop profuse intractable diarrhoea which is difficult to clear and may continue intermittently for life.

Norovirus ('winter vomiting virus') Most common cause of infectious gastroenteritis in the UK—particularly in communal settings, e.g. schools, hospitals. Illness is generally mild and lasts 2–3d. There are no long-term effects. Infections can occur at any age because immunity is not long-lasting. Scrupulous hygiene is needed to contain outbreaks.

Further information

Health Protection Agency (HPA) Infections: topics A–Z: gastrointestinal disease ॐ www.hpa.org.uk

Table 13.12 Common causes of gastroenteritis in the UK

Organism/source	Incubation	Symptoms				Food
		D	V	P	F	O	

Organism/source	Incubation	D	V	P	F	O	Food
B. cereus	1–5h	✓	✓				Rice
Campylobacter	48h–5d	✓		✓	✓	Blood in stool	Milk, poultry
C. botulinum	12–36h		✓			Paralysis	Canned food
C. perfringens	6–24h	✓		✓			Meat
E. coli	12–72h	✓		✓	✓	Blood in stool	Food, water
Salmonella species	12–48h	✓	✓	✓	✓		Meat, eggs, poultry
Shigella[ND]	48–72h	✓		✓	✓	Blood in stool	Any food
Staph. aureus	1–6h	✓	✓	✓		↓ BP	Meat
V. para-haemolyticus	12–24h	✓	✓	✓			Fish
Y. enterocolitica	24–36h	✓		✓	✓		Milk, water
Giardia lamblia	1–4wk	✓					Water
Entamoeba histolytica	1–4wk	✓		✓	✓	Blood in stool	Food, water
Cryptosporidium	4–12d	✓		✓	✓		Water
Listeria						Flu-like illness, pneumonia, miscarriage	Milk products, pâtés, raw vegetables
Norovirus	24–48h	✓	✓		✓	Malaise	Food, water
Rotavirus	1–7d	✓	✓		✓	Malaise	Food, water
Mushrooms	15min–24h	✓	✓	✓		Fits, coma, renal/liver failure	
Scrombrotoxin	10–60min	✓				Flushes, erythema	Fish
Heavy metals, e.g. zinc	5min–2h		✓	✓			

D = diarrhoea; V = vomiting; P = abdominal pain; F = fever; O = other.

Rotavirus Most common cause of gastroenteritis in children. Most are immune by 5y. Presents with malaise, abdominal pain, diarrhea, and vomiting. Common cause of hospital admission. Treatment is supportive. Babies in the UK are offered rotavirus vaccination within the childhood immunization programme (📖 p. 645)

❶ Some children may become cow's milk-intolerant after a bout of gastroenteritis—📖 p. 889.

Coeliac disease

Gluten sensitivity results in inflammation of the bowel and malabsorption. Coeliac disease is a common disorder (UK prevalence 0.5–1%, ♀:♂ ≈3:1) although only a minority have recognized disease. Peak incidence in adults is in the fifth decade; in children at ~4y. Associated with HLA-DQ2 or DQ8; first-degree relatives have a 1:10 chance of being affected.

Investigation

- **Serological testing** With IgA anti-tissue transglutaminase antibodies (TTG) or anti-endomysial antibodies (EMA) if any symptoms/signs listed in Table 13.13. Consider testing if associated condition or genetic predisposition. ❶ Test only if the patient has eaten >1 meal/d containing gluten for ≥6wk
- **Other tests** Also consider FBC, ESR/CRP, B_{12}, folate, ferritin, LFTs, Ca^{2+}, TFTs, and stool sample for M,C&S (if diarrhoea)

⚠ Selective IgA deficiency is more common amongst people with coeliac disease (2.6%) than the general population (0.4%). People who are IgA-deficient have false –ve results with IgA TTG/EMA testing. When there is strong clinical suspicion and coeliac serology is negative, check serum IgA levels; if deficient, request IgG TTG/EMA antibody testing.

Initial management Refer for specialist review if:
- +ve serology—duodenal biopsy showing villous atrophy is diagnostic
- Strong clinical suspicion of coeliac disease but –ve serology
- Unwilling to reintroduce gluten to diet to enable serological testing

Gluten-free diet Is the cornerstone of the management of coeliac disease and should be followed life-long. Patients should avoid proteins derived from wheat, rye, or barley. ♦ Avoidance of oats is controversial. Refer to a dietician for specialist advice. Coeliac UK provides a directory of approved products as well as recipes for those on gluten-free diets.

Prescriptions for gluten-free foods Prescribe adequate gluten-free foods (see Table 13.14), marking prescriptions 'ACBS'. Add deficient nutrients, e.g. iron, folic acid, calcium until established on a gluten-free diet.

Failure to respond to diet The most common reason is continued ingestion of gluten (intentional or inadvertent). Re-refer to dieticians. If symptoms recur after a period of remission, re-refer for specialist review.

Pneumococcal vaccination Pneumococcal infection is more common 2° to hyposplensim—advise vaccination.

Follow-up Every 6–12mo in a specialist clinic or by a GP under shared care arrangements. Routine checks include: symptoms, weight, and blood tests (Hb, B_{12}, folate, iron, albumin, Ca^{2+}, TTG or EMA antibodies).

Long-term complications Are almost eliminated by strict diet:
- Osteoporosis—consider DEXA scan at diagnosis, after 3y on a gluten-free diet (if abnormal baseline DEXA), at menopause for ♀, aged 55y for ♂, or if fragility fracture[G]
- Malignancy—lymphoma or carcinoma of the small intestine. Rare—if suspected, refer urgently for specialist review

Table 13.13 Presentation of coeliac disease

Symptoms and signs	Associated conditions	
Chronic/intermittent diarrhoea (50%)	*GI*	*Endocrine*
	Dental enamel defects	Type 1 DM
Failure to thrive/faltering growth in children	Mouth ulcers	Autoimmune thyroid disease
	Irritable bowel syndrome	
Recurrent abdominal pain/cramping/bloating	Microscopic colitis	Addison's disease
	Persistent/unexplained constipation	Amenorrhoea
Other persistent unexplained GI symptoms, e.g. nausea/vomiting	Unexplained, persistent ↑ in liver enzymes (usually normalize in <6mo on gluten-free diet)	*Other*
Sudden or unexpected weight ↓		Unexplained alopecia
		Dermatitis herpetiformis
Unexplained anaemia (iron deficiency or other)	Autoimmune liver disease	Depression or bipolar disorder
	Musculoskeletal	Polyneuropathy
Genetic predisposition	↓ bone mineral density	Epilepsy
First-degree relative (parent, sibling, child)	Low trauma fracture	Autoimmune myocarditis
	Metabolic bone disease (e.g. rickets, osteomalacia)	Chronic TTP
Down's/Turner syndrome	Sjögren's syndrome	Lymphoma
	Sarcoidosis	Recurrent miscarriage
		Unexplained subfertility

Table 13.14 Guide to the amount of gluten-free products to prescribe monthly for patients with coeliac disease

Child age	Units/mo	♂ age	Units/mo	♀ age	Units/mo
1–3y	10	19–59y	18	19–74y	14
4–6y	11	60–74y	16	75+y	12
7–10y	13	75+y	14	Breastfeeding	Add 4 units
11–14y	15			3rd trimester pregnancy	Add 1 unit
15–18y	18	High activity level (♂ or ♀)—add 4 units			

400g of bread or rolls or baguette = 1 unit   250g of pasta = 1 unit
500g of bread or flour = 2 units   2 pizza bases = 1 unit
200g of sweet or savoury biscuits, crackers, or crispbread = 1 unit

Further information
NICE Recognition and assessment of coeliac disease (2009)
⌖ www.nice.org.uk
British Society of Gastroenterology The management of adults with coeliac disease (2010) ⌖ www.bsg.org.uk

Patient advice and support
Coeliac UK ☎ 0845 305 2060 ⌖ www.coeliac.co.uk

Inflammatory bowel disease

Ulcerative colitis (UC) and Crohn's disease (*B.B. Crohn (1884–1983)—US gastroenterologist*) are collectively termed inflammatory bowel disease. Both are chronic, relapsing-remitting diseases characterized by acute, non-infectious inflammation of the gut. In UC, inflammation is limited to the colorectal mucosa. Extent varies from disease limited to the rectum (proctitis) to disease affecting the whole colon (pancolitis). In Crohn's, any part of the gut from mouth to anus can be affected with normal bowel between affected areas (*skip lesions*).

Cause Unknown. Both diseases are thought to result from an environmental trigger on genetically susceptible individuals. Factors implicated (none proven) include:

- Smoking—protective against UC (95% are non-smokers or ex-smokers) but a causative factor in Crohn's disease (two-thirds are smokers, and smoking cessation halves the relapse rate)
- Gut flora or other infections, e.g. *Mycobacterium paratuberculosis*
- Food constituents

Features See Table 13.16.

Differential diagnosis

- Irritable bowel syndrome
- Coeliac disease
- Anal fissure
- Gut infection, e.g. giardiasis
- Diverticulitis
- Colonic tumour
- Food sensitive colitis (infants)
- Pseudomembranous colitis
- Ischaemic colitis
- Microscopic colitis

Suspected diagnosis ~50% of severe attacks of UC are first attacks in patients who do not have a prior diagnosis. If bloody diarrhoea + fever >37.5°C or tachycardia >90bpm, admit as an acute emergency. If persistent, unexplained diarrhoea lasting >4wk and/or persistent abdominal pain, refer for urgent further investigation to exclude GI malignancy and establish diagnosis.

Table 13.15 Assessing the severity of ulcerative colitis

Severity	Symptoms
Mild	<4 liquid stools/d
	Little/no rectal bleeding
	No signs of systemic disturbance
Moderate	4–6 liquid stools/d
	Moderate rectal bleeding
	Some signs of systemic disturbance
	Mild disease that does not respond to treatment
Severe	>6 liquid stools/d
	Severe rectal bleeding
	Any systemic disturbance (↑ pulse rate >90bpm, pyrexia >37.5°C, ↑ ESR, ↑ WCC, ↓ Hb <10g/dL)
	Signs of malnutrition (e.g. hypoalbuminaemia <35g/dL)
	Weight loss >10%

Table 13.16 Features of inflammatory bowel disease

	UC	Crohn's disease
Incidence	10–20/100,000/y	5–10/100,000/y and increasing
Prevalence	100–200/100,000	50–100/100,000
Peak age	40–60y (85% <60y)	
Gender	♂ = ♀	
Risk factors	Smoking is protective	Smoking is a risk factor
GI symptoms	Diarrhoea + blood/mucus (stool may be solid if rectal disease only) Faecal urgency/incontinence Tenesmus Lower abdominal pain	Diarrhoea ± blood/mucus Malabsorption Abdominal pain (crampy) Mouth ulcers Bowel obstruction due to strictures Fistulae (often perianal) Abscesses (perianal and intra-abdominal)
Systemic symptoms	Tiredness and/or malaise Weight ↓ or failure to thrive/grow (children) Fever	
Associated conditions	_Joint disease_—arthritis, sacroiliitis, ankylosing spondylitis _Eye disease_—iritis or uveitis _Skin changes_—erythema nodosum, pyoderma gangrenosum (UC > Crohn's) _Liver disease_—autoimmune hepatitis (UC), gallstones (Crohn's), sclerosing cholangitis (UC > Crohn's) _Miscellaneous_—thromboembolism, osteoporosis (Crohn's); amyloidosis (Crohn's)	
Examination	_Abdominal + rectal examination_—abdominal tenderness. Anal and perianal lesions (pendulous skin tags, abscesses, fistulae) and/or mass in the right iliac fossa are characteristic of Crohn's disease _General examination_—clubbing, aphthous ulcers in the mouth (Crohn's), signs of weight loss, anaemia, or hypoproteinaemia	
Investigation	_Blood:_ FBC (anaemia, ↑ WCC), ESR (↑ when disease is active), eGFR, LFTs (including serum albumin). In severe UC, CRP >45g/dL after 3d steroid treatment indicates high (~85%) risk for colectomy. _Stool:_ M,C&S (including _C. difficile_) to exclude infection _AXR:_ consider to clarify extent of disease, exclude toxic megacolon (transverse colon diameter >5cm) or bowel obstruction, and/or identify proximal constipation _Proctoscopy:_ inflammation and shallow ulceration extending proximally from the anal margin suggests UC	

 UC and Crohn's disease are rare in childhood. Presentation is variable and can be with non-specific features (e.g. failure to thrive), GI symptoms (e.g. malabsorption, bloody diarrhoea, acute abdomen) or complications (e.g. arthropathy or iritis). If suspected refer for confirmation of diagnosis and specialist management.

Management of ulcerative colitis See *BNF* 1.5.

Assessing severity See Table 13.15, 🕮 p. 414.

Active disease
- Mesalazine 2–4g daily. Topical 5-ASA derivatives are a useful adjunct if troublesome rectal symptoms
- Add steroids (prednisolone 40mg od po + rectal preparation) if prompt response is needed or mesalazine is unsuccessful. Review frequently and ↓ dose over 8wk. Rapid withdrawal ↑ risk of relapse
- Azathioprine is added if the patient is having recurring attacks despite mesalazine maintenance frequent steroids (≥2 courses/y), disease relapses as dose of steroid is ↓, or relapse <6wk after stopping steroids. Requires regular supervision
- Ciclosporin or infliximab (anti-TNF antibody)—consultant supervised; may be effective as acute therapy for severe, steroid-refractory disease

⚠ ***Admit acutely if***
- Severe abdominal pain (especially if associated with tenderness)
- Severe diarrhoea (>8x/d) ± bleeding
- Dramatic weight loss
- Fever >37.5°C, tachycardia >90bpm, or other signs of systemic disease

Maintenance treatment Follow-up in 2° care is routine. Most patients require life-long therapy. Mainstays of treatment are 5-ASA derivatives (e.g. mesalazine 1–2g/d or balsalazide 3g/d). Use a rectal formulation (e.g mesalazine 1g/d PR) if disease is confined to the rectum or descending colon. Long-term treatment ↓ risk of colonic cancer by 75%. 10% are intolerant to 5-ASA derivatives—alternative is azathioprine (consultant supervision required). Treat proximal constipation with stool-bulking agents or laxatives. NSAIDs can precipitate relapse so avoid.

Surgery Last resort—but should not be delayed if severe colitis and failing to respond to medical therapy. 20–30% of patients with pancolitis require colectomy—1:3 develop pouchitis (non-specific inflammation of the ileal reservoir) within 5y of surgery.

Prognosis At any time 50% are asymptomatic, 30% have mild symptoms, and 20% moderate/severe symptoms. <5% are free from relapse after 10y. Relapses usually affect the same part of the colon.

Complications See Table 13.17.

Management of Crohn's disease

Active ileal and/or colonic disease
- Treat with mesalazine 4g daily. Less effective than for UC
- Add steroids (prednisolone 40mg od po or budesonide 9mg daily) if unresponsive to mesalazine. Review frequently, and ↓ dose over 8wk. Rapid withdrawal ↑ risk of relapse. ❶ Steroids are associated with ↑ risk of severe sepsis and mortality in Crohn's disease, so alternatives to steroid therapy are increasingly sought and steroid maintenance for >3mo should always be avoided
- Elemental or polymeric diets for 4–6wk can be a useful adjunct or alternative to steroid treatment—take consultant advice

- Other treatments (consultant supervision) include metronidazole, azathioprine, anti-tumour necrosis factor (infliximab or adalimumab)
- Surgery is an option if medical treatment has failed. 50% need surgery <10y after onset. Surgery is not curative and 50% will require a further operation at a later stage. After ileal resection check B_{12} levels annually

⚠ *Admit acutely if*
- Severe abdominal pain (especially if associated with tenderness)
- Severe diarrhoea (>8x/d) ± bleeding
- Dramatic weight loss
- Bowel obstruction
- Fever/other signs of systemic disease

🅵 For disease elsewhere, take specialist advice.

Maintenance treatment Follow-up in 2° care is routine. Treatment is aimed at ↓ impact of the disease. The most effective measure is to stop smoking. Mesalazine has limited benefit. It is ineffective at doses <2g/d. Other agents used include azathioprine, methotrexate, and 2-monthly infliximab. All require consultant supervision. Treat diarrhoea symptomatically with codeine phosphate or loperamide unless it is due to active colonic disease. C-olestyramine (4g 1–3x/d) ↓ diarrhoea due to terminal ileal disease/resection. NSAIDs can precipitate relapse so avoid.

Prognosis 75% are back to work after the first year but 15% remain unable to work long term. Complications—see Table 13.17.

Table 13.17 Complications of inflammatory bowel disease

UC	Crohn's
Toxic megacolon Colon distends and may perforate	*Intra-abdominal* abscess
Colonic cancer Risk ↑ if disease >8y, onset in childhood/adolescence, age >45y, FH of colon cancer, extensive colitis, sclerosing cholangitis. *Prevention:* screening with colonoscopy	*Intestinal stricture* Common—may require surgery
	Toxic megacolon Rare (see UC)
Frequency depends on severity of the disease and duration of symptoms	*Bowel obstruction*
Sclerosing cholangitis Fibrosis and stricture of intra- and extrahepatic bile ducts. Presents with obstructive jaundice	*Fistula formation*
	Perianal disease
	Malignancy Large and small bowel cancer—5% 10y after diagnosis
	Osteoporosis
Psychological effects Chronic, life-long conditions which have major impact on work and domestic life. Self-help groups can be useful	

Further information
NICE Crohn's disease (2012) 🖱 www.nice.org.uk
British Society of Gastroenterology Guidelines for the management of inflammatory bowel disease in adults (2004) 🖱 www.bsg.org.uk

Advice and support for patients
Crohn's and Colitis UK ☎ 0845 130 2233 (info); 0845 130 3344 (support) 🖱 www.crohnsandcolitis.org.uk

Irritable bowel syndrome

Irritable bowel syndrome (IBS) is a chronic (>6mo) relapsing and remitting condition of unknown cause, with symptoms including: Abdominal pain or discomfort; Bloating; and Change in bowel habit.

It is a diagnosed on symptoms with no confirmatory test and no cure. Extremely common. Lifetime prevalence ≥20%, although ~50% never consult a GP. ♀ > ♂ (2.5:1). Symptoms can appear at any age.

Diagnosis of IBS Abdominal pain or discomfort that is:
- Relieved by defecation, or
- Associated with altered bowel frequency or stool form

and ≥2 of the following:
- Altered stool passage (straining, urgency, incomplete evacuation)
- Abdominal bloating (♀ > ♂), distension, tension, or hardness
- Symptoms made worse by eating
- Passage of mucus

Other commonly associated symptoms include Lethargy, nausea, backache, and bladder symptoms.

Differential diagnosis
- Colonic carcinoma
- Coeliac disease
- Inflammatory bowel disease (Crohn's disease or UC)
- Pelvic inflammatory disease
- Endometriosis
- GI infection
- Thyrotoxicosis

Investigation A diagnosis of exclusion. How far to investigate is a clinical judgement weighing risks of investigation against possibility of serious disease. Judgement is based on age of the patient, family history, length of history, and symptom cluster.
- *Patients <40y* Check FBC, ESR, and antibody testing to exclude coeliac disease (TTG/EMA)
- *Patients >40y* Colonic cancer must be excluded for any patient with a persistent, unexplained change in bowel habit—particularly towards looser stools (📖 p. 399)
- *Other investigations to consider*
  - Thyroid function tests if other symptoms/signs of thyroid disease
  - Stool samples to exclude GI infection if diarrhoea
  - Endocervical swabs for chlamydia
  - Colonoscopy to exclude inflammatory bowel disease
  - Laparoscopy to exclude endometriosis

Referral To gastroenterology/colorectal surgery if:
- Passing blood (except if from an anal fissure or haemorrhoids)—*U*
- Abdominal, rectal, or pelvic mass—*U*
- Unintentional/unexplained weight loss—*U/S*
- Positive inflammatory markers and/or anaemia—*U/S*
- >40y with new symptoms—*U (if age >60y)/S/R*
- Change in symptoms, especially if >40y—*U (if age >60y)/S/R*
- Atypical features (i.e. not those listed above)—*U/S/R*
- Family history of bowel or ovarian cancer—*R*
- Patient is unhappy to accept a diagnosis of IBS despite explanation—*R*

U = urgent; *S* = soon; *R* = routine.

Treatment Reassure. Information leaflets are helpful. Encourage lifestyle measures, stress ↓, leisure time, and regular physical exercise.

Diet Encourage patients to have regular meals and take time to eat. Avoid missing meals or leaving long gaps between eating.

- Drink ≥8 cups of fluid/d, especially water. Restrict tea/coffee to 3 cups/d. ↓ intake of alcohol and fizzy drinks
- ↓ intake of high-fibre foods (e.g. wholemeal/high-fibre flour and breads, cereals high in bran, and whole grains such as brown rice)
- ↓ intake of 'resistant starch' found in processed or re-cooked foods
- Limit fresh fruit to 3x 80g portions/d
- For diarrhoea, avoid sorbitol, an artificial sweetener
- For wind and bloating consider increasing intake of oats (e.g. oat-based breakfast cereal or porridge) and linseeds (≤1 tablespoon/d)
- Up to 50% may be helped by exclusion of certain foods (especially patients with diarrhoea—predominant disease). Diaries may help identify foods that provoke symptoms. Common candidates are dairy products, citrus fruits, caffeine, alcohol, tomatoes, gluten, and eggs. Refer to dietician for exclusion diet

Specific measures
- **Probiotics** Some evidence of effectiveness. Try a 4wk trial
- **Fibre/bulking agents** Constipation-predominant IBS. Bran can make some patients worse. Ispaghula husk is better tolerated. Laxatives are an alternative but avoid use of lactulose
- **Antispasmodics** (e.g. mebeverine, peppermint oil) All equally effective. If no response in a few days, switch to another—different agents suit different individuals. Once symptoms are controlled use prn
- **Antidiarrhoeal preparations** (e.g. loperamide) Avoid codeine phosphate as may cause dependence. Use prn for patients with diarrhoea-predominant disease. Use pre-emptive doses to cover difficult situations (e.g. air travel)
- **Antidepressants** There is evidence that low-dose amitriptyline, e.g. 10mg nocte, is effective. SSRIs are less effective unless the patient is overtly depressed. Withdraw if no response after 4–6wk
- **Psychotherapy and hypnosis** Some effect in trials. Reserve for cases that have failed to respond to more conventional treatment

Failure to respond to treatment Consider another diagnosis—review history and examination ± refer for further investigation.

Prognosis >50% still have symptoms after 5y.

Further information

NICE Irritable bowel syndrome in adults: diagnosis and management of irritable bowel syndrome in primary care (2008) ℘ www.nice.org.uk

Advice and support for patients

The IBS Network ☏ 0872 300 4537 ℘ http://theibsnetwork.org

Jaundice and abnormal liver function

Jaundice Yellow pigmentation of the tissues due to excessive bile pigment. Clinical jaundice appears when serum bilirubin >35micromol/L.

Causes
- ↑ **production of bilirubin (pre-hepatic)** Haemolytic anaemia, drug-induced haemolysis, malaria, Gilbert's/Crigler–Najjar syndrome
- **Defective processing (hepatic)** Hepatitis, cirrhosis
- **Blocked excretion (obstructive)** Gallstones, pancreatic cancer, primary biliary cirrhosis, primary sclerosing cholangitis, cholangiocarcinoma, sepsis, enlarged porta hepatis (e.g. 2° to lymphoma)

History Patients presenting with jaundice may have no other symptoms. General symptoms include tiredness, nausea, and pruritus. Ask about colour of the stools and urine (dark urine suggests conjugated hyperbilirubinaemia and hepatobiliary disease). Check alcohol consumption.

Examination Mild jaundice is best seen by examining the sclerae in natural light. Look for signs of chronic liver disease and examine the abdomen for masses and hepatomegaly.

Investigations Initially check FBC and liver function tests—see Table 13.18. Further investigations depend on the results.

Management Treat the cause of the jaundice. Most patients (except those with Gilbert's syndrome or self-limiting viral hepatitis) will require specialist referral. Refer patients with pre-hepatic and hepatic jaundice to a hepatologist or gastroenterologist; refer patients with post-hepatic (obstructive or cholestatic) jaundice to a general or hepatobiliary surgeon.

Neonatal jaundice 📖 p. 868

Abnormal liver function

Raised AST/ALT/GGT in isolation Liver enzymes can ↑ transiently as a result of viral infection, drugs, or alcohol. ALT tends to be more raised in viral and autoimmune hepatitis; AST tends to be more raised in patients with fatty liver; raised GGT is particularly associated with alcohol excess.
- Check medication including herbal medicines
- Stop alcohol
- Repeat LFTs:
  - In 1mo if AST/ALT are <3x upper limit of normal
  - In 1wk if AST/ALT is ≥3x upper limit of normal
- If still raised request hepatitis screen and USS, or refer to hepatology or gastroenterology depending on clinical state
- If ALT is <2x upper limit of normal and hepatitis screen is negative:
  - If USS is normal, repeat LFTs every 3–6mo to see if abnormalities settle—may be due to drugs, alcohol, or early fatty liver disease
  - If USS shows fatty liver and consuming excess alcohol—advise abstinence from alcohol and recheck LFTs every 3–6mo
  - If USS shows fatty liver and alcohol consumption is within normal limits, advise weight loss and low-fat diet; treat metabolic syndrome, and recheck LFTs every 3–6mo
- In all other cases, refer for specialist opinion

Table 13.18 Distinguishing different types of jaundice

	Type of jaundice		
	Pre-hepatic	Hepatic	Cholestatic
Tests			
Bilirubin	↑↑	↑↑	↑↑
AST/ALT	Normal	↑↑	↑
Alkaline phosphatase	Normal	↑	↑↑↑
Hb	↓	Normal	Normal
Jaundice	Mild, lemon yellow	May be marked jaundice	May be marked jaundice
Other symptoms	Urine is *not* darkened	Tender, enlarged liver	Enlarged liver, itching skin, pale stools

❶ A mixed picture is common and can be confusing.

Raised bilirubin Possible causes include:
- Hepatitis/biliary obstruction—if ALT/AST are ↑, refer for liver USS and do a hepatitis screen or refer as for jaundice
- Haemolysis—check FBC/reticulocyte count—refer to haematology if abnormal
- Gilbert's disease—likely if serum bilirubin is <40mmol/L and ALT/AST and RBC/reticulocytes are normal. Bilirubin levels ↑ after a fast
- If isolated ↑ bilirubin >40mmol/L—probably still Gilbert's syndrome, but refer

Raised alkaline phosphatase Usually originates from liver or bone. Bone is more likely if serum Ca^{2+} and phosphate are raised and GGT is normal. ↑ may be associated with any liver disease but is particularly marked in patients with biliary obstruction and primary biliary cirrhosis.

Medications that cause raised AST/ALT

- Most penicillins (especially co-amoxiclav) and minocycline
- Antifungals
- Statins
- Anti-epileptics
- NSAIDs
- Some herbal medicines
- Some recreational drugs

Statins and abnormal liver function Statins cause a biochemical abnormality only but do not cause liver failure and are not contra-indicated in compensated liver disease. May improve fatty liver disease. Measure liver function tests pre-treatment and after 1–3mo. Thereafter measure each 6m for 1y. Discontinue if AST/ALT ↑ and stays at >3x normal.

Hepatitis screen Check as appropriate:

- Hepatitis A, B, and C serology
- EBV serology
- Liver autoantibodies
- Iron studies and transferrin saturation to exclude haemochromatosis
- α1-antitrypsin level
- Serum copper and caerulo-plasmin levels (if <40y)
- αFP
- Fasting blood glucose and lipids
- HbA1c

Hepatitis

Acute hepatitis May be asymptomatic or present with fatigue, flu-like symptoms, fever, light stools, dark urine, and/or jaundice. Causes:

- Viral hepatitis, e.g. HBV, HAV, EBV
- Alcohol
- Drugs (e.g. diclofenac, co-amoxiclav)
- Toxins
- Obstructive jaundice
- Other infections—malaria, Q fever, leptospirosis, yellow fever

Management Check LFTs, FBC, U&E, eGFR, hepatitis serology. Treat the cause. Admit if condition is poor or rapidly deteriorating; refer for investigation if sustained abnormalities in liver function with unclear cause (☐ p. 420). *Complications:* chronic hepatitis, acute liver failure.

Hepatitis A (HAV) Common. *Spread:* faecal–oral route. Patients are infectious 2wk before feeling ill. Incubation is 2–7wk (average 4wk). *High-risk groups:* travellers to high-risk areas, institutional inhabitants and workers, IV drug abusers, patients with high-risk sexual practices. May be asymptomatic (especially young children) or present with fever, malaise, fatigue, anorexia, nausea/vomiting, abdominal pain, diarrhoea, tender hepatomegaly, pale stools, dark urine, and/or jaundice (70–80% adults).

Management Check LFTs (hepatic jaundice—☐ p. 420) and hepatitis serology—IgM antibodies signify recent infection, IgG remains detectable life-long. Management is supportive. Avoid alcohol until LFTs are normal. Most recover in <2mo. There is no carrier state and hepatitis A does not cause chronic liver disease. After infection immunity is life-long.

Prevention Vaccination is indicated for travellers to high-risk areas, people with chronic liver disease, or those working in high-risk situations. Preparations available include monovalent vaccine (e.g. Havrix®), hepatitis A and B combined vaccine (Twinrix®) and hepatitis A and typhoid combined vaccine (e.g. Hepatyrix®). Passive immunization with human immunoglobulin gives protection for ≤3mo and is used for short-term travel or protecting household contacts of sufferers.

Hepatitis E (HEV) Similar to HAV infection. Usually acquired in developing countries. Incubation is 2–9 wk (average 40d). Diagnosis is made with serology. Treatment is supportive. There is no chronic state. Mortality in pregnancy can be as high as 20%. No vaccine exists.

Hepatitis B (HBV) ☐ p. 742   **Hepatitis C (HCV)** ☐ p. 742

Chronic hepatitis Hepatitis lasting >6mo. May be asymptomatic or present with fatigue; RUQ pain; jaundice; arthralgia; signs of chronic liver disease—gynaecomastia, testicular atrophy, clubbing, palmar erythema, leuconychia, peripheral oedema, spider naevi, portal hypertension, recurrent infection; and/or complications—acute liver failure, cirrhosis, hepatocellular carcinoma. *Causes:*

- Viral hepatitis
- Alcohol
- Drugs (e.g. nitrofurantoin, methyldopa, isoniazid)
- Chronic autoimmune hepatitis
- Primary biliary cirrhosis
- Wilson's disease
- Haemochromatosis
- α1-antitrypsin deficiency
- Sarcoidosis

Management Check LFTs; FBC; U&E; eGFR; and hepatitis screen (📖 p. 421). Refer for specialist care.

Chronic autoimmune hepatitis Typically young women. Associated with personal/family history of autoimmune disease (e.g. RA, vitiligo). Diagnosis is confirmed with liver biopsy and autoimmune markers. Specialist management is with steroids ± immunosuppressants.

Primary biliary cirrhosis Slow progressive cholangiohepatitis eventually resulting in cirrhosis. ♀:♂ ≈9:1. *Peak age at presentation:* 45y. *Cause:* probably autoimmune. *Associations:*

- Thyroid disease
- Sjögren's syndrome
- CREST syndrome
- Coeliac disease
- Hepatic and extrahepatic malignancy
- Pancreatic hyposecretion

Presentation 50% are asymptomatic at presentation. *Symptoms/signs:*

- Fatigue
- Pruritus
- Arthralgia
- Osteoporosis/ osteomalacia
- Hirsutism
- Obstructive jaundice (late)
- Symptoms/signs of cirrhosis or liver failure

Investigation and management Blood: LFTs (↑ alk phos, ↑ ALT, ↑ GGT). Liver biopsy is diagnostic. Refer for specialist care. If asymptomatic, 1:3 remain symptom-free—the rest develop symptoms in 2–4y. Median survival is 7–10y. Liver transplant is an option. Prognosis following transplant is good but recurrence may occur in the transplanted liver.

Primary haemochromatosis Autosomal recessive condition of excess gut absorption of iron → iron deposition and damage to heart, liver, pancreas, joints, and pituitary. ~1:400 people are homozygous for the condition but expression is highly variable. ♂ > ♀ (women present ~10y later). Often an incidental finding, or found by screening relatives of affected individuals (genetic testing or serum ferritin). *Symptoms/signs:*

- Tiredness
- Arthralgia/arthritis
- Skin pigmentation
- Hepatomegaly ± signs of cirrhosis
- DM
- Impotence/ testicular atrophy
- Cardiomyopathy

Investigation and management Blood: ↑ ferritin; ↑ iron; transferrin saturation >70%; total iron binding capacity ↓. Refer. Liver biopsy is diagnostic. Venesection returns life expectancy to normal.

Secondary haemochromatosis Iron overload from frequent transfusions, e.g. for haemolysis. Specialist management with chelation therapy to ↑ iron excretion is required.

α1- antitrypsin deficiency 📖 p. 425

Wilson's disease (hepatolenticular degeneration) Rare, autosomal recessive disorder. Defective biliary copper excretion → accumulation of copper in the liver, brain, kidney, and cornea. Treatment is with penicillamine. Liver transplantation is the only treatment if presentation is with acute liver failure. *S.A.K. Wilson (1878–1937)—British neurologist.*

Information and support for patients

British Liver Trust ☎ 0800 652 7330 ✍ www.britishlivertrust.org.uk
Primary Biliary Cirrhosis Organization ✍ www.pbcers.org
Wilson's Disease Association ✍ www.wilsonsdisease.org

Liver failure and portal hypertension

'Jaundice is the disease that your friends diagnose'

Aphorisms, Sir William Osler (1849–1920)

Cirrhosis The liver is replaced by fibrotic tissue and regenerating nodules of hepatocytes.

Causes

- Unknown (30%)
- Alcohol (25%)
- Viral hepatitis
- Primary biliary cirrhosis
- Haemochromatosis
- Wilson's disease
- Budd–Chiari syndrome
- Chronic active hepatitis
- α1-antitrypsin deficiency

Presentation Variable. May be an incidental finding. *Symptoms/signs:*

- Hepatomegaly (although liver becomes small and hard in late stages)
- Spider naevi
- Dupuytren's contracture
- Palmar erythema
- Gynaecomastia
- Testicular atrophy
- Clubbing
- Xanthelasma/xanthomata
- Portal hypertension
- Splenomegaly

Acute liver failure Presents with sudden onset of severe illness.

- Jaundice
- Hypoglycaemia
- Hepatic encephalopathy—ranges from mild confusion and irritability, through drowsiness and increasing confusion, to coma
- Haemorrhage—due to deranged clotting factors
- Ascites—hepatosplenomegaly and ascites are not usually prominent
- Infection
- Nausea ± vomiting
- ↑ BP
- Foetor hepaticus (sweet smell on the breath)

Causes

In previously healthy patients:

- Viral hepatitis
- Weil's disease
- Paracetamol overdose
- Halothane
- Idiosyncratic drug reactions
- Fungal/plant toxins
- Malignant infiltration
- Chemical exposure (e.g. carbon tetrachloride)
- Heatstroke

- Budd–Chiari syndrome
- Pregnancy
- Wilson's disease
- Reye's syndrome

In patients with chronic liver disease:

- Infection
- GI bleeding
- Sedation
- Diuretics and/or electrolyte imbalance
- Alcohol binges
- Constipation

Management Admit as emergency to a hepatologist/gastroenterologist unless an expected terminal event. Prognosis is poor (<60% survive).

Late signs Occur when the liver can no longer compensate for the damage to it—jaundice, hepatic encephalopathy, leuconychia, and oedema (due to hypoalbuminaemia).

Investigation

- **Blood**—FBC, LFTs (may be normal until late stages), GGT, U&E, Cr, eGFR, hepatitis screen (📖 p. 421)
- **Liver** *USS*

Management

- Refer to gastroenterology/hepatology for expert advice
- Treat the cause where possible
- Avoid alcohol and refer to dietician for advice on nutrition
- Pruritus 2° to jaundice may respond to cholestyramine
- Give flu and pneumococcal vaccination

Complications

- Portal hypertension (± bleeding oesophageal varices)
- Encephalopathy
- Hepatocellular carcinoma
- Ascites (bacterial peritonitis complicates 1:4 cases—consider prophylaxis with ciprofloxacin)
- Renal failure

Prognosis Very variable—half survive 5y.

α1-antitrypsin deficiency Autosomal recessive disorder. Defective α1-antitrypsin production → lung, and more rarely, liver damage. 📌 Treatment with IV α1-antitrypsin ↓ progression of COPD. Paracetamol may protect the liver. Encourage use for minor illness. Liver transplantation may eventually be needed.

Portal hypertension Portal venous pressure is raised due to obstruction of the portal system before, within, or after the liver. In western countries the most common cause is cirrhosis.

- Elevated portal venous pressure → collaterals between the portal and systemic circulation (including oesophageal varices). Usually presents with haematemesis and/or melaena from bleeding varices
- Ascites develops if there is coexistent liver failure with hypoproteinaemia and hyperaldosteronism
- Splenomegaly is common → thrombocytopaenia and leucopenia
- *Signs:* splenomegaly (80–90%), ascites, dilated veins around the umbilicus (rare); purpura; signs of chronic liver disease—jaundice, clubbing, spider naevi, palmar erythema, gynaecomastia, testicular atrophy; encephalopathy
- Refer to gastroenterology/hepatology. Specialist management is essential. If GI bleeding, refer as a 'blue light' emergency

Information and support for patients
British Liver Trust ☎ 0800 652 7330 🖰 www.britishlivertrust.org.uk
Alpha-1 Support for people with α1-antitrypsin deficiency
🖰 www.alpha1.org.uk

Other liver disease

Fatty liver Reversible condition affecting up to 1:4 adults in the UK. Large vacuoles of triglyceride accumulate in liver cells.

Presentation
- Usually asymptomatic. >50% present as a result of investigation for abnormal LFTs (📖 p. 420). Characteristic 'bright' appearance on liver USS
- Less frequently presents with a smoothly enlarged liver or symptoms— nausea, vomiting, abdominal pain, fat embolus (may be fatal)

Broadly divides into 2 forms:

Alcohol associated fatty liver disease
- Defined as fatty liver disease with daily ethanol consumption >20g (♀) or 30g (♂)
- Typically serum AST and ALT are ↑, but serum AST > serum ALT
- GGT may be ↑, and alk. phos may also be ↑ but usually <2x upper limit of normal
- Predisposes to alcoholic hepatitis and cirrhosis (irreversible)
- Abstinence from alcohol results in resolution

Non-alcoholic fatty liver disease (NAFLD)
- Associated with obesity (present in 35% of obese patients), insulin resistance, and metabolic syndrome (📖 p. 343)
- Typically, serum AST and ALT are ↑, but serum ALT > serum AST
- GGT may be ↑ and ALP may also be ↑ but usually <2x upper limit of normal
- More severe disease results in *non-alcoholic steatohepatitis (NASH)* and is thought to be one of the major causes of cryptogenic cirrhosis— liver failure is uncommon
- A high proportion of patients develop DM long-term
- Treatment is with weight ↓, metformin, and/or thiazolidinediones
- Treatment with statins is ineffective

Other rarer causes of fatty liver disease
- Drugs, e.g. amiodarone, tamoxifen, valproate
- Pregnancy
- Malnutrition
- Inflammatory bowel disease

Gilbert's syndrome Inherited metabolic disorder causing unconjugated hyperbilirubinaemia. *Prevalence:* ~1–2%. Onset is shortly after birth—but the condition may go unnoticed for years. Jaundice occurs during intercurrent illness. ↑ bilirubin on fasting can confirm the diagnosis. Liver biopsy is normal. No treatment is required and prognosis is excellent.

N.A. Gilbert (1858–1927)—French physician

Benign tumours Hepatomegaly ± RUQ pain or an incidental finding.

Common types Hepatic adenoma, fibroma, leiomyoma, lipoma, haemangioma, focal nodular hyperplasia (e.g. with cirrhosis).

Management Refer to gastroenterology to exclude malignancy and confirm diagnosis. Urgency depends on clinical picture and findings on USS.

Hepatocellular cancer (HCC) Rare in the UK (100 new cases and 100 deaths/y). Much more common in areas of the world where hepatitis B is endemic (e.g. China, India). Usually arises from regenerating nodules in a cirrhotic liver. *Peak age:* 60–70y. Intra- and extrahepatic spread is common and occurs early.

Presentation In a patient with known cirrhosis:
- Fatigue
- Fever
- Anorexia and/or weight ↓
- Ascites
- Rapid deterioration in liver function
- Haemorrhage into the peritoneal cavity (often fatal)
- Budd–Chiari syndrome (occlusion of the hepatic vein resulting in jaundice, epigastric pain, and shock)
- *Examination*—may reveal an abdominal mass, hepatomegaly ± an arterial bruit over the tumour

Management If suspected check αFP and refer for urgent assessment. αFP >500ng/mL in a patient with known cirrhosis is almost certainly diagnostic. The most important prognostic factors are the number and size of the liver lesions and the presence of vascular involvement. 95% of patients with cirrhosis have disease too extensive for curative surgery, or their severely compromised liver function makes radical surgery inappropriate. 50% of patients without cirrhosis have resectable tumours. Surgery may be combined with liver transplantation. Inoperable tumours may be treated with hepatic artery ligation or embolization. Tumours respond poorly to chemo- or radiotherapy.

Overall prognosis Patients with cirrhosis—median survival 3mo; patients without cirrhosis—median survival 1y.

Cholangiocarcinoma Rare adenocarcinoma of the biliary tract. May be associated with UC. Typically presents in patients >60y with jaundice, RUQ pain and weight loss. The only effective treatment is surgery, which is only possible in ~10–20% of patients. Selected fit patients with unresectable disease may be offered palliative chemotherapy or enrolment in a clinical trial. Median survival 4–6mo.

Secondary tumours The most common type of liver tumours—usually signalling late disease. *Presentation:* hard, enlarged, knobbly liver ± RUQ pain ± jaundice (late). If found and no history of malignancy refer to oncology/general surgery for urgent referral to find the primary.

1° tumours commonly metastasizing to the liver Lung, breast, large bowel, stomach, uterus, pancreas, carcinoid, lymphoma, leukaemia.

Advice and support for patients

Cancer Research UK ☎ 0808 800 4040 ✆ www.cancerhelp.org.uk
Macmillan Cancer Support ☎ 0808 808 0000 ✆ www.macmillan.org.uk
British Liver Trust ☎ 0800 652 7330 ✆ www.britishlivertrust.org.uk

Gallbladder disease

Gallstones Gallstones are increasingly common. 9% of 60y olds have them and prevalence ↑ with age.

Other risk factors
- Gender (♀ > ♂)
- Body weight—prevalence ↑ with weight; also associated with rapid weight ↓
- Race—in the USA, Native American > Hispanic > white > black
- Affluency
- Pregnancy (and possibly HRT but not COC pill)
- Alcohol is protective
- Diet—vegetarian diet is protective

Associated conditions
- Haemolysis
- DM
- Hypertriglyceridaemia
- Cirrhosis
- Crohn's disease
- Partial gastrectomy

Drugs which cause gallstones Clofibrate (and other fibric acid derivatives); octreotide (somatostatin analogue).

Presentation Gallstones are blamed for many digestive symptoms—they are probably innocent in most cases. 70% of stones in the gall bladder do not cause symptoms. Common presentations—see Table 13.19.

Management of gallstones
- Advise the patient to stick to a low-fat diet
- Refer for surgical review ± further evaluation (e.g. ERCP—endoscopic retrograde cholangiopancreatography)
- Gallstones can be removed by cholecystectomy (laparoscopic or open) or ERCP or may be dissolved with ursodeoxycholic acid (stones <5mm diameter—40% recur in <5y) or shattered with lithotripsy (1:3 develop biliary colic afterwards)
- Persistent digestive symptoms after surgery are common (50% after cholecystectomy) and difficult to treat

Gallbladder cancer Rare. ♀ > ♂. Gallstones are a predisposing factor. Typically presents in patients >40y with right upper quadrant pain, anorexia, weight ↓, and jaundice. Surgical resection offers the only hope of cure but disease is usually advanced at presentation. Selected fit patients with unresectable disease may be offered palliative chemotherapy or enrolment in a clinical trial. Prognosis is poor.

Information and support for patients
British Liver Trust ☎ 0800 652 7330 🖰 www.britishlivertrust.org.uk

Table 13.19 Presentation and management of gallstone disease

	Presentation	Management
Biliary colic	Clear-cut attacks of severe upper abdominal pain which may radiate → back/shoulder tip, lasting ≥30min and causing restlessness ± jaundice ± nausea or vomiting *Examination:* tenderness ± guarding in the right upper quadrant (↑ on deep inspiration—Murphy's sign)	**Treat** acute attacks with pethidine (50mg IM/po) or naproxen (500mg po) + prochlorperazine 12.5mg IM or domperidone 10mg po/PR for nausea **Admit if:** uncertain of diagnosis, inadequate social support, persistent symptoms despite analgesia, suspicion of complications, and/or concomitant medical problems (e.g. dehydration, pregnant, DM, Addison's) **Investigate:** for gallstones with abdominal USS to prove diagnosis when the episode has settled **Differential diagnosis:** any cause of acute abdomen **Treat:** gallstones to prevent recurrence
Acute cholecystitis/ cholangitis	Pain and tenderness in the right upper quadrant/epigastrium ± vomiting *Examination:* tenderness ± guarding in the right upper quadrant ± fever ± jaundice	*Treatment:* broad-spectrum antibiotic (e.g. ciprofloxacin) and analgesia as for biliary colic **Admit if:** generalized peritonism, diagnosis uncertain, very toxic, concomitant medical problems (e.g. dehydration, DM, Addison's, pregnancy), inadequate social support, or not responding to medication **Empyema** occurs when the obstructed gall bladder fills with pus. Presents with persistent swinging fever and pain. Usually requires cholecystectomy ± surgical drainage **Investigate** and follow up to prevent recurrence as for biliary colic
Pancreatitis	📖 p. 430	📖 p. 430
Gallstone ileus	Occurs usually after an attack of cholecystitis. A stone perforates from the gall bladder into the duodenum and impacts in the terminal ileum causing bowel obstruction	📖 p. 400
Chronic cholecystitis	Vague intermittent abdominal discomfort, nausea, flatulence, and intolerance of fats	Investigate for gallstones with abdominal USS to prove the diagnosis **Differential diagnosis:** reflux, IBS, upper GI tumour, PU Refer for treatment of gallstones
Jaundice	Obstructive jaundice—📖 p. 420 ± right upper quadrant pain	Refer for same day or urgent specialist surgical assessment (depending on clinical state)

Pancreatitis

Acute pancreatitis Premature activation of pancreatic enzymes results in autodigestion and tissue damage. Most episodes are mild and self-limiting but 1:5 patients have a severe attack. Overall mortality ~5–10%. May be recurrent.

Causes In 10% patients no cause is identified.
- **Common causes (80%):** gallstones, alcohol
- **Rarer causes:**
  - Drugs (e.g. azathioprine)
  - Trauma
  - Pancreatic tumours
  - Post-ERCP
  - Viral infection (mumps, HIV, Coxsackie B)
  - Mycoplasma infection
  - Hypercalcaemia
  - Hyperlipidaemia
  - Pancreas divisum (normal variant in 7–8% of the white population)
  - Familial pancreatitis
  - Vasculitis
  - Ischaemia or embolism
  - Pregnancy
  - End-stage renal failure

Presentation
- Poorly localized, continuous, boring epigastric pain which ↑ over ~1h—often worse lying down ± radiation to the back (50%)
- Nausea ± vomiting

Examination
- **General** Tachycardia, fever, shock, jaundice
- **Abdominal** Localized epigastric tenderness or generalized abdominal tenderness; abdominal distension ±↓ bowel sounds; evidence of retroperitoneal haemorrhage (periumbilical and flank bruising—rare)

Management Admit as an acute surgical emergency. Prior to transfer, give analgesia with pethidine (morphine may induce spasm of the sphincter of Oddi).

Complications Delayed complications may present in general practice—suspect if persistent pain or failure to regain weight or appetite. Complications include:
- Pancreatic necrosis
- Pseudocyst—localized collection of pancreatic secretions
- Fistula/abscess formation
- Bleeding or thrombosis

Prevention of further attacks
- Avoid factors that may have caused pancreatitis, e.g. alcohol, drugs
- Advise patients to follow a low-fat diet
- Treat reversible causes, e.g. hyperlipidaemia, gallstones

Chronic pancreatitis Chronic inflammation of the pancreas results in gradual destruction and fibrosis of the gland ± loss of pancreatic function → malabsorption and DM.

Cause Alcohol is responsible for most cases. *More rarely:* familial; CF; haemochromatosis; pancreatic duct obstruction (gallstones/pancreatic cancer); hyperparathyroidism.

Presentation
- Constant or episodic epigastric pain, radiating to the back and relieved by sitting forwards
- Vomiting
- Weakness
- Jaundice
- Steatorrhoea
- Weight ↓
- DM
- Chronic poor health

Management Refer to gastroenterology. *Treatment*:
- **Diet** Low-fat, high-protein, high-calorie diet with fat-soluble vitamin supplements. Refer to dietician
- **Pancreatic enzyme supplementation** (e.g. Creon® capsules pre-meals) May improve diarrhoea
- **Alcohol abstinence**
- **Pain control** Provide analgesia—beware of opioid abuse. Consider referral for coeliac plexus block
- **Surgery** Pancreatectomy or pancreaticojejunostomy for pancreatic duct stricture, obstructive jaundice, unremitting pain, or weight loss
- **Diabetes management**

Pancreatic insufficiency Global ↓ function of the pancreas. *Causes*:
- **Child** Cystic fibrosis
- **Adult** Chronic pancreatitis, pancreatic tumour, pancreatectomy, total gastrectomy

Presentation Malabsorption (frequent loose, odorous stools ± abdominal pain), weight loss or failure to thrive, DM.

Management Take specialist advice. Treat the underlying cause. Treat associated DM. Suppplement digestive enzymes (e.g. with Creon®).

Pancreatic tumours

Pancreatic cancer accounts for 3% of all malignancies, causing 7,800 deaths/y in the UK. 80% of cases occur in patients >60y. ♂ > ♀ (3:2).

Risk factors

- Smoking—causes 25–30% of pancreatic cancers in the UK. Risk returns to non-smoker levels 10–20y after cessation
- Chronic pancreatitis—usually related to excess alcohol
- Type II (non-insulin-dependent) DM—relative risk ≈ 1.8
- Obesity—↑ risk by 19%
- Genetic—5% pancreatic cancers are hereditary; characterized by presentation aged <30y. and +ve FH
- Occupation—cancer is ↑ among nickel workers and workers exposed to insecticides, radiation, lead, iron, or chromium

Tumour characteristics

- The majority of pancreatic tumours develop in the exocrine part of the gland. 95% of tumours are adenocarcinomas. Rarely tumours develop from the endocrine part—these have better prognosis
- 75% arise in the head of the pancreas, 15% from the body, and 10% from the tail. Tumours arising in the head of the pancreas tend to present earlier and are easier to remove
- Spread to local LNs occurs early and metastatic spread to the peritoneum, liver, and lungs is frequently found at presentation

Presentation Non-specific with:
- Gradual deterioration in health or fatigue
- Anorexia or weight ↓
- Pain—epigastric ± radiation → back—may be relieved by sitting forward
- Diarrhoea/steatorrhoea due to malabsorption
- Early satiety, dyspepsia, or nausea/vomiting (gastric outlet obstruction)
- Obstructive jaundice
- Pancreatitis
- New DM
- Spontaneous venous thrombosis

Examination Check for weight ↓, epigastric or left upper quadrant mass, hepatomegaly, jaundice. If jaundice is present the gall bladder may be palpable as a small, rounded mass beneath the liver.

Management Refer for urgent surgical assessment. Diagnosis is confirmed using a combination of USS, CT, MRI, and/or ERCP. The only potentially curative treatment for pancreatic cancer is surgery but <15% of patients are suitable for surgery at presentation. The operation of choice is a Whipple's procedure (pancreaticoduodenectomy). Surgery is associated with significant morbidity; mortality 5–15%.

Prognosis Those undergoing surgical resection have 5y survival of 7–25% (median survival 11–20mo) but those that survive 5y are likely to survive long-term. Median survival for those with irresectable locally advanced disease is 6–11mo, and 2–6mo if metastatic disease.

Palliative treatment Patients with locally advanced/metastatic disease may benefit from surgical bypass of common bile duct and/or duodenal obstruction. An alternative is a biliary stent. Chemotherapy may give some survival benefit. Refer for palliative care support early.

Endocrine tumours In all cases specialist management is required.

Glucagonoma Islet cell tumour of the pancreas. Most are malignant and 90% have liver or LN metastases at presentation. 5–20% of tumours occur as part of multiple endocrine neoplasia (MEN I) syndrome. *Presents with:*
- Attacks of hyperglycaemia (DM in >50%)
- Skin changes—sore mouth, necrolytic migratory erythema (70%—rash which starts as an erythematous rash then blisters before crusting)
- Weight ↓/cachexia (60%)
- Tendency to venous thrombosis (11%)
- Anaemia
- Diarrhoea
- Depression/psychosis

Insulinoma Tumour of the APUD cells of the Islets of Langerhans. >90% are benign. 7–8% are associated with MEN I syndrome. Presents with episodes of hypoglycaemia, especially when exercising or fasting. ↑ appetite and frequent food intake to avoid hypoglycaemia often results in substantial weight gain.

Somatostatinoma Uncommon islet cell tumour. Most are large tumours (>5cm) in the head/body of the pancreas. Presents with gallstones, steatorrhoea, and DM.

❶ Extrapancreatic somatostatinomas can present in association with neurofibromatosis type I and phaeochromocytoma.

Verner–Morrison syndrome An intestinal vasointestinal peptide (VIP)-producing tumour results in profuse watery diarrhoea → dehydration, metabolic acidosis, and ↓ K⁺. Also associated with insulin resistance and impaired glucose tolerance. VIPomas account for <10% islet cell tumours. 60% are malignant. *J.V. Verner, (b.1927)—US physician; A.B. Morrison, (b.1922)—US pathologist.*

Advice and support for patients
Cancer Research UK ☎ 0808 800 4040 🖰 www.cancerhelp.org.uk
Macmillan Cancer Support ☎ 0808 808 0000 🖰 www.macmillan.org.uk

Renal medicine and urology

Creatinine, urea, and electrolytes

Serum creatinine Commonly ordered test to detect renal dysfunction. Rough guide to glomerular filtration rate (GFR) when corrected for age, gender, and weight—↓ in GFR is associated with ↑ in serum creatinine. Causes of an abnormal serum creatinine—see Table 14.1.

Estimated glomerular filtration rate (eGFR) More sensitive measure than serum creatinine to assess renal function. *Calculated from:*

- Serum creatinine
- Age
- Gender, *and*
- Ethnicity—people of Afro-Caribbean origin tend to have ↑ muscle mass so their eGFR must be multiplied by 1.21

Changes in eGFR can be used to monitor changes in kidney function.
- Normal eGFR is >90mL/min/1.73m^2
- eGFR 60–90mL/min/1.73m^2 does not indicate CKD unless additional markers of damage are present—persistent microalbuminuria, persistent proteinuria, persistent microscopic haematuria, or structural abnormality, e.g. polycystic kidneys
- eGFR <60mL/min/1.73m^2 indicates CKD (☐ p. 440)

> Renal function ↓ with age (approximately 1mL/min/y >40y). Many elderly patients have a GFR <60mL/min which, because of ↓ muscle mass, may not be indicated by a ↑ serum creatinine. Measuring eGFR gives a better indication of renal function.

Urea Commonly ordered test to detect renal dysfunction. While ↓ in GFR is associated with ↑ in serum urea, serum urea may also vary independently of the GFR. Causes of abnormal serum urea—see Table 14.1.

Hyperkalaemia High serum potassium (>5mmol/L). *Causes:* See Table 14.2. Treat the cause.

> ⚠ Plasma potassium >6.5mmol/L needs urgent treatment.
> - Check it is not an artifact, e.g. due to haemolysis inside the bottle
> - Admit for investigation of cause and treatment

ECG changes associated with hyperkalaemia Tall tented T-waves; small P-wave; wide QRS complex becoming sinusoidal VF.

Hypokalaemia Low serum potassium (<3.5mmol/L). Presents with muscle weakness, hypotonia, cardiac arrhythmias, cramps, and tetany. *Causes:* see Table 14.2. If K$^+$ >2.5mmol/L and no symptoms, give oral potassium supplement. ❶ If the patient is taking a thiazide diuretic, hypokalaemia >3.0mmol/L rarely needs treating.

> ⚠ Plasma potassium <2.5mmol/L needs urgent treatment—admit.

ECG changes associated with hypokalaemia Small/inverted T-waves; prominent U-wave; prolonged P-R interval; depressed ST segment.

Hyponatraemia Low serum sodium (<135mmol/L). Rarely symptomatic in general practice. May present with signs of water excess— confusion, fits,

↑ BP, cardiac failure, oedema, anorexia, nausea, muscle weakness. *Causes:* see Table 14.2. *Management:* treat the cause. If unwell admit for investigation.

Hypernatraemia Excess serum sodium (>145mmol/L). Rare in general practice. *Presentation:* thirst, confusion, coma, fits, signs of dehydration—dry skin, ↓ skin turgor, postural hypotension, and oliguria if water deficient. *Causes:* see Table 14.2. *Management:* admit for investigation.

Table 14.1 Causes of an altered serum creatinine and urea

↑ creatinine (>150micromol/L)	↓ creatinine (<70micromol/L)	↑ urea (>6.7mmol/L)	↓ urea (<2.5mmol/L)
Renal disease/renal failure	Muscular dystrophy (late stage)	Renal failure	Liver disease (↓ urea production)
Drugs (e.g. trimethoprim, probenecid, cimetidine, potassium-sparing diuretics)	Myasthenia gravis	GI bleeding	Anabolic state
Large muscle bulk		High-protein diet	High ADH levels (high GFR)
Muscle breakdown (e.g. muscular dystrophy)		Drugs—high-dose steroids, tetracycline	Starvation or low-protein diet
		Dehydration	Pregnancy

Table 14.2 Causes of altered serum electrolytes

↑ potassium (>5mmol/L)	↓ potassium (<3.5mmol/L)	↑ sodium (>145mmol/L)	↓ sodium (<135mmol/L)
Renal failure	Diuretics	Fluid loss without water replacement (e.g. diarrhoea, vomiting, burns)	Diuretic excess—especially thiazides
Drugs (e.g. ACE inhibitors, excess K+ therapy, K+ sparing diuretics)	Cushing's syndrome/ steroids	Diabetes insipidus—suspect if large urine volume	Renal failure or nephrotic syndrome
Addison's disease	Vomiting and/or diarrhoea	Osmotic diuresis	Diarrhoea/vomiting
Metabolic acidosis (DM)	Conn's syndrome	Primary aldosteronism—suspect if ↑ BP, ↓ K+, alkalosis	Fistula
Artefact (haemolysed sample)	Villous adenoma of the rectum		Rectal villous adenoma
	Purgative or liquorice abuse		Small bowel obstruction
	Intestinal fistula		CF (□ p. 330)
	Renal tubular failure		Heat exposure
	Hypokalaemic periodic paralysis—intermittent weakness lasting <72h		SIADH (□ p. 371)
			Water overload (e.g. polydipsia)
			Severe hypothyroidism
			Addison's disease
			Glucocorticoid deficiency
			Cardiac failure
			Cirrhosis

Presentation of renal disease

See Table 14.3. Renal disease may present with:

- Haematuria (📖 p. 446) or proteinuria
- UTI/pyelonephritis (📖 p. 448)
- Outflow tract obstruction (📖 p. 454)
- Nephrotic syndrome
- Nephritic syndrome (📖 p. 439)
- Renal failure (📖 p. 440)
- Hypertension (📖 p. 248)

Proteinuria Normally detected with urine dipstick. If +ve, then repeat with another sample to exclude spurious results, and send sample for M,C&S to exclude UTI. Treat the cause where necessary. *Causes:*

- UTI
- Vaginal mucus
- DM
- ↑ BP
- Glomerulonephritis
- Pyrexia
- Pregnancy (and PET)
- Postural proteinuria—2–5% adolescents; rare >30y
- Haemolytic uraemic syndrome
- CCF
- SLE
- Myeloma
- Drugs, e.g. gold, penicillamine
- Amyloid

Microalbuminuria Albuminuria in the range 30–200 mg/L. Not detectable with standard urine dipsticks. Special sticks are available for routine screening of high-risk groups, e.g. diabetics. *Causes:*

- **DM** Microalbuminuria precedes frank proteinuria—📖 p. 356
- **Arteriopathy** Microalbuminuria may be present in patients with CCF or ↑ BP. Presence of microalbuminuria predicts ↑ risk of MI, CVA, CCF, and cardiovascular and all-cause mortality
- **Other chronic illness** Malignancy, COPD
- **Acute illness** Inflammatory bowel disease, MI, acute pancreatitis, trauma, burns, meningitis

Haematuria 📖 p. 446   **Glycosuria** 📖 p. 342

Nephrotic syndrome Proteinuria, hypoalbuminaemia, and oedema. Often associated with ↑ cholesterol. *Causes:*

- Minimal change GN (90% children, 30% adults)
- Membranous GN
- Focal segmental glomerulosclerosis
- Membrano-proliferative GN
- DM
- Amyloid
- Neoplasia
- Endocarditis
- PAN
- SLE
- Sickle cell disease
- Malaria
- Drugs (penicillamine, gold)

Presentation Swelling of eyelids and face; ascites, peripheral oedema; urine froth due to protein. *Nephrotic crisis:* unwell with oedema, anorexia, vomiting, pleural effusions, and muscle wasting.

Investigation Urine—total protein:creatinine ratio (TPCR) >200mg/mmol; microscopy for red cells, casts; *Blood*—U&E, creatinine, eGFR, albumin (<25g/L), cholesterol, FBC, ESR.

Management Refer all suspected cases of nephrotic syndrome to a renal physician. *Complications include:*

- Thromboembolism
- Infection—especially pneumococcal; if persistent nephrotic syndrome, offer vaccination
- Hypovolaemia and renal failure
- Hypercholesterolaemia

- Loss of specific proteins, e.g. transferrin (causes hypochromic anaemia, which is iron-resistant)

Nephritic syndrome Central feature is blood and protein in the urine from glomerular inflammation.

- **Causes** Glomerulonephritis (may occur after throat, ear, or skin infection with group A β-haemolytic streptococci), vasculitis.
- **Features** Oliguria, haematuria and proteinuria, fluid retention, ↑ BP, uraemia, and ↑ creatinine
- **Management** Refer suspected cases immediately to renal medicine
- **Risks** Hypertensive encephalopathy, pulmonary oedema, acute kidney injury
- **Prognosis** Excellent in children; in adults some proteinuria/urine sediment may persist. CKD is rare

Nephrocalcinosis Deposition of Ca^{2+} in the kidneys. *X-ray—*calcification. May cause symptoms of UTI or renal stones. *Causes:*

- **Medullary** (95%). Hyperparathyroidism, distal renal tubular acidosis, medullary sponge kidney, idiopathic calciuria, papillary necrosis, oxalosis
- **Cortical** Serious renal disease or chronic GN

Pyelonephritis/UTI 📖 p. 448   **Hypertension** 📖 p. 248

Strangury Distressing desire to pass something per urethra that will not pass, e.g. stone.

Table 14.3 Presentation of renal disease

	GN	Interstitial disease			Vascular disease			Outflow tract obstruction
		AIN	ATN	CIN	Small	Large	RVT	
Nephrotic syndrome	++	0	0	0	(+)	0	+*	0
Nephritic syndrome	++	(+)	0	0	(+)	0	+	0
Acute kidney injury	+	+	++**	0	+	+	(+)	++
Chronic kidney disease	++	(+)	0	++	(+)	+	0	++
Pyelonephritis/ UTI	0	0	0	0	0	0	+	+
Hypertension	(+)	(+)	(+)	0	(+)	(+)	0	+

GN: glomerulonephritis—📖 p. 442   *RVT*: renal vein thrombosis—📖 p. 443
CIN: chronic interstitial nephritis—   *AIN*: acute interstitial nephritis—📖 p. 442
📖 p. 442
ATN: acute tubular necrosis

* Renal vein thrombosis is a complication not a cause of nephrotic syndrome.

** Acute tubular necrosis is the most common cause of acute renal failure.

Patient support and information
UK National Kidney Federation ☎ 0845 601 02 09 🖰 www.kidney.org.uk
Kidney Patient Guide 🖰 www.kidneypatientguide.org.uk

Renal failure

Oliguria Urine output <400mL/24h. *Causes:* dehydration, cardiac failure, ureteric obstruction, renal failure.

Acute kidney injury (AKI) Also known as acute renal failure (ARF). ↓ renal function over hours/days ± oliguria/anuria. Refer immediately if acute ↑ in urea/creatinine *or* ↓ in eGFR (to <60mL/min/1.73m² if normal in last 3mo, or ↓ of >15% over 5d). *Causes:* acute tubular necrosis (80%—due to acute circulatory compromise); renal tract obstruction (5%); GN.

Chronic kidney disease (CKD)[N] Also known as chronic renal failure (CRF). Slow ↓ renal function over months/years. *Causes:*

- DM
- SLE
- Polycystic kidneys
- Amyloid
- ↑ BP
- ↑ Ca²⁺
- Glomerulonephritis
- Myeloma
- Urinary tract obstruction
- Renovascular disease
- PAN
- Chronic pyelonephritis
- Interstitial nephritis

Presentation
- **History** FH (polycystic kidneys); UTI; drugs (especially analgesics)
- **Symptoms** Often no symptoms. Nausea, anorexia, lethargy, itch, nocturia, impotence. *Later:* oedema, dyspnoea, chest pain (from pericarditis), vomiting, confusion, fits, hiccups, neuropathy, coma
- **Signs** Pallor, 'lemon tinge' to skin, pulmonary/peripheral oedema, pericarditis, pleural effusions, metabolic flap, ↑ BP, retinopathy

Investigation
- **Urine** M, C&S, microalbuminuria, albumin:creatinine ratio (ACR) or TPCR, RBCs, glucose
- **Blood** U&E, creatinine, eGFR, glucose, Ca²⁺, PO₄⁻ urate, protein, FBC, ESR, serum electrophoresis.
- **Renal tract USS** If progressive or advanced (stage 4/5) disease, refractory ↑ BP, haematuria, or palpable bladder/lower urinary tract signs

Management classification—see Table 14.4
- Treat reversible causes. Stop/avoid nephrotoxic drugs (e.g. NSAIDs). Consider ↓ dose of other drugs as excretion/metabolism may be impaired. ❶ Metformin should be stopped if eGFR <30 mL/min/1.73m²
- Monitor Cr/eGFR and dipstick urine (see Table 14.4). If proteinuria, send urine for M,C&S. If no infection but proteinuria persists, test TPCR or ACR in early morning urine. If TPCR >100mg/mmol or ACR >70mg/mmol, refer
- Manage CVD risk. Monitor/treat ↑ cholesterol and ↑ BP (target 130/80—ACE/ARB is first-line). Treat DM. Smoking cessation
- Monitor and treat anaemia and renal bone disease

❶ If sudden ↓ in renal function (↓ eGFR of >15% between tests *or* >5mL/min/1.73m² in <1y *or* >10mL/min/1.73m² in <5y) suspect infection, dehydration, uncontrolled ↑ BP, metabolic disturbance (e.g. ↑ Ca²⁺), obstruction, nephrotoxins (e.g. drugs). If unable to find cause or treatment does not ↑ renal function, refer.

Refer To a renal physician if:
- Stage 4/5 CKD
- Significant proteinuria (TPCR >100mg/mmol or ACR >70mg/mmol)

- Sudden ↓ in eGFR (>15%) and UTI excluded
- Persistent microscopic haematuria and <50y (to urologist if >50y)
- Functional consequences of CKD, i.e. anaemia (<11g/dL), bone disease, or refractory hypertension (>140/90 on 4 agents)

End-stage renal disease (ESRD) 80 new patients/million population/y. Irreversible. Dialysis starts when GFR is 10–15% normal. Dialysis is needed lifelong unless a kidney transplant becomes available. Refer back to the renal unit managing the patient if you have any problems.

Haemodialysis Blood flows opposite dialysis fluid and substances are cleared along a concentration gradient across a semi-permeable membrane. *Problems:* pulmonary oedema; infection (HIV, hepatitis, bacteria); U&E imbalance; BP ↓ or ↑; problems with vascular access; dialysis arthropathy (especially shoulders and wrists); aluminium toxicity; time.

Continuous ambulatory peritoneal dialysis (CAPD) A permanent catheter is inserted into the peritoneum via a subcutaneous tunnel. ~2L dialysis fluid is introduced and kept in the peritoneum. This is changed for fresh fluid up to 5x/d at home. Does not tie the patient to a dialysis machine. *Problems:* peritonitis; catheter blockage (refer as an emergency); weight ↑; poor DM control; pleural effusion; leakage.

Anaemia and erythropoietin 2° anaemia due to ↓ kidney erythropoietin production is universal amongst people with ESRD. Exclude other causes. Recombinant erythropoietin is given if Hb <10.5g/dL (75%).

Renal transplantation Transplanted kidneys are usually sited in an iliac fossa. 5y graft survival is ~88% for adults. Closer genetic matches have better survival rates. *Problems:*

- Rejection
- Persistent ↑ BP and ↑ cholesterol
- Atherosclerosis (5x ↑ risk MI death)
- Renal artery stenosis at 3–9mo post-op
- Obstruction at ureteric anastmosis
- Ciclosporin-induced nephropathy
- Infection 2° to immunosuppression
- Malignancy from immunosuppressants

Table 14.4 Classification of chronic kidney disease

Stage	GFR mL/min	Description	Prevalence %	Complications	Testing frequency
1	>90	Kidney damage with normal or ↑ GFR	3.3	↑ BP	Yearly
2	60–89	Kidney damage with mild ↓ GFR	3	↑ BP	Yearly
3A	45–59	Moderate ↓ GFR	4.3	↑ BP, Ca^{2+} and PO_4^- changes, renal anaemia, LVF	6mo
3B	30–44				
4	15–29	Severe ↓ GFR	0.2	As above + ↑ K^+	3–6mo
5	<15	Established renal failure	0.2	As above + salt/water retention	6wk

Further information
NICE CKD (2008) ℘ www.nice.org.uk

Kidney diseases

Interstitial nephritis Important cause of renal failure. Associated with inflammatory cell infiltration of the renal interstitium/tubules. *Causes:*

- **Acute interstitial nephritis** Idiosyncratic reaction to drugs (penicillin, NSAIDs, furosemide) or infection (*Staphylo-* or *Streptococcus*)
- **Chronic interstitial nephritis** Idiopathic (most), drugs, sickle-cell disease, analgesic nephropathy.

Presentation and prognosis Presents with AKI/CKD, raised temperature, arthralgia, eosinophilia. Patients with AKI have good prognosis. Those with CKD have gradual deterioration over time.

Diabetic nephropathy 📖 p. 356

Analgesic nephropathy Caused by prolonged heavy use of analgesics (including NSAIDs). Presents with an interstitial nephritis-like picture. Associated with ↑ incidence of UTI. Carcinoma of the renal pelvis is a rare complication. Investigate promptly if the patient develops haematuria.

Glomerulonephritis Types and presentation—see Table 14.5. Refer all suspected cases urgently to a renal physician. *Terminology:*

- **Focal** Some glomeruli affected
- **Diffuse** All glomeruli affected
- **Segmental** Part of each glomerulus affected
- **Global** All of each glomerulus affected

Chronic pyelonephritis Presents as CKD or one of its complications. Probably arises from UTIs, vesico-ureteric reflux and consequent renal scarring in childhood (📖 p. 878). Refer to a renal physician.

Table 14.5 Types of glomerulonephritis

Type	Features
Minimal change	Most common in children. Presents with nephrotic syndrome
Membranous	30% adult nephrotic syndrome. Underlying malignancy in 10% of adults. 1 in 3 enter remission, 1 in 3 are proteinuric, 1 in 3 progress to ESRD
Focal segmental glomerulosclerosis	Proteinuria or nephrotic syndrome. May be associated with heroin abuse. >50% progress to CKD
Membrano-proliferative	50% present as nephrotic syndrome. Associations—endocarditis, C3 nephritic factor (autoantibody), hepatitis C, measles
Proliferative	Presents with nephritic syndrome. Classically seen 2wk after *Strep.* infection. Prognosis is excellent
IgA disease (Berger's disease)	Causes recurrent haematuria in young men. A similar histological picture is seen in Henoch–Schönlein purpura (📖 p. 526). 30% progress to ESRD
Rapidly progressive/ crescentic	Presents with haematuria, oliguria, ↑ BP, acute renal failure. Vigorous treatment may preserve renal function. *Causes:* anti-glomerular basement membrane disease (Goodpasture's disease), Wegener's granulomatosis, Henoch–Schönlein purpura

Haemolytic uraemic syndrome Most common cause of AKI in children. Usually follows gastroenteritis. Due to *E. coli* toxin. Have a high index of suspicion in any child with bloody diarrhoea. Occasionally occurs without diarrhoea. *Other features:*

- Dehydration
- Oliguria (though may be polyuria)
- Proteinuria/haematuria
- Haematological features—anaemia, thrombocytopenia ± purpura
- CNS symptoms—irritability, drowsiness, ataxia, coma
- ↑ BP (associated with non-diarrhoeal disease)

Management Admit for specialist care—often including dialysis. If associated with diarrhoeal illness, >80% make full recovery. Mortality is 1.8%. Poor prognostic indicators are age >5y at onset and dialysis for >2wk. Disease in the absence of diarrhoea has poorer prognosis.

Adult polycystic kidney disease Autosomal dominant disease (1:1,000). Cysts develop in the kidney causing gradual ↓ in renal function. Common cause of CKD. Presents with haematuria, UTI, abdominal mass (30% have cysts in the liver/pancreas too), lumbar/abdominal pain, and/or ↑ BP. May be associated with mitral valve prolapse and SAH/berry aneurysms. USS shows large kidneys with multiple cysts. Refer to a renal physician if CKD 3–5. Treat infections and ↑ BP. Check family members (though cysts may not be seen <30y). 45% progress to ESRD by 60y.

Medullary sponge kidney Developmental abnormality of the medullary pyramids of the kidney, characterized by dilatation of the renal collecting tubules. ♂ > ♀. There may be a family history. Most are asymptomatic and the condition is an incidental finding. If symptomatic, presents with UTIs, renal stones, haematuria. Refer if symptomatic. Usually prognosis is very good and most require no treatment.

Renal vein thrombosis (RVT) *Causes:* nephrotic syndrome (15–20% develop RVT); membranous GN (30%); acute dehydration. Presentation varies from no symptoms to severe pain and loin tenderness. Suspect in at-risk individuals if unexplained loss of renal function and RBCs in urine. Refer to a renal physician for further investigation.

Renal artery stenosis *Causes:* atheroma, fibromuscular hyperplasia (in the young). Presents with ↑ BP (may be severe or drug-resistant); vascular disease elsewhere; abdominal bruit; ↑ Cr, ↓ eGFR, and proteinuria. If bilateral or extensive, renal failure may be precipitated by dehydration, ↓ BP, or drugs (ACE/ARB initiation; NSAIDs). Refer to a renal physician (if diagnosis is unsure) or vascular surgeon (if diagnosis is known).

Alport's syndrome X-linked or autosomal inherited disease. Congenital sensorineural deafness, haematuria, proteinuria, and renal failure. Associated with lens abnormalities, platelet dysfunction, and ↑ BP. Causes ESRD by third decade in ♂; ♀ rarely develop ESRD. Renal failure does not recur after transplantation. *A.C. Alport (1880–1959)—South African physician.*

Patient support and information
UK National Kidney federation ☎ 0845 601 02 09 🖰 www.kidney.org.uk

Renal stones

12% of ♂ and 3% of ♀ will develop a renal stone at some point; peak age 20–50y. Symptoms are not dependent on size of the stone.

Risk factors

- Family history—↑ risk x3. *Specific conditions:* X-linked nephrolithiasis, cystinuria, hyperoxaluria
- Anatomically abnormal kidneys, e.g. horseshoe kidney, medullary sponge kidney
- Metabolic disease, e.g. gout, hypercalcaemia/hypercalciuria, cystinuria, renal tubular acidosis or other acidosis (ileostomy, adenomatous polyp), oxaluria, aminoaciduria
- Dehydration   • Immobilization   • Chronic UTI

Drugs predisposing patients to stone formation Acetazolamide, allopurinol, aspirin, steroids, indinavir, nelfinavir, loop diuretics, probenecid, quinolones, sulfonamides, theophylline, thiazides, triamterene, antacids, calcium/vitamin D supplements, high-dose vitamin C.

Presentation Usually presents with pain ± nausea/vomiting. Location and type of pain gives clues about the site of the stone:

- **Loin pain**—kidney stone   • **Strangury**—bladder stone
- **Renal colic**—ureteric stone   • **Interruption of flow**—urethral stone

Renal colic

- **Symptoms** Severe pain with waves of ↑ severity. Usually starts abruptly as flank pain which then radiates around the abdomen to the groin as stone progresses down the ureter. May be referred to testis/tip of penis in men or labia majora in women
- **Signs** Patient is obviously in pain—usually unable to sit still and keeps shifting position to try to get comfortable (in contrast to peritonitis where patients tend to sit still). May be pale and sweaty. May be mild tenderness on deep abdominal palpation or loin tenderness, though often minimal signs. If fever suspect infection

Other presentations UTI, haematuria, retention, renal failure (rare).

Differential diagnosis Pyelonephritis; ruptured AAA; cholecystitis; pancreatitis; appendicitis; diverticulitis; obstruction; strangulated hernia; testicular torsion; pethidine addiction.

Immediate investigations Dipstick urine if possible. Absence of RBCs does not exclude renal colic but consider alternative diagnosis.

Immediate management Stones usually pass spontaneously. Give pain relief (diclofenac 75mg IM/100mg PR) ± antiemetic. Consider admission to hospital if:

- Fever   • Pregnant   • Analgesia ineffective /
- Oliguria   • Lives alone   short-lived
- Poor intake of fluid • Uncertain diagnosis • Symptoms >24h

If not admitted Encourage ↑ fluid intake; sieve urine for stones. Monitor/review pain relief and for complications.

Further investigations Can wait until the next working day and include:
- **Blood** U&E, creatinine, eGFR, Ca^{2+}, PO_4^{3-}, alkaline phosphatase, uric acid, albumin
- **Urine** M,C&S; RBCs. Consider checking 'spot' test for urine cystine, and TPCR, Ca^{2+}, PO_4^{3-}, uric acid, and sodium excretion
- **Radiology** X-ray of kidneys, ureters, and bladder—90% of renal stones are radio-opaque—only urate and xanthine stones are radio-transluscent; renal tract USS

Follow-up 50% recur in 5–7y. Give general advice on prevention of stones (see Table 14.6). If investigations show any loss of renal function, renal obstruction, or remaining stones—refer to urology. Dependent on composition of stones, give dietary advice/refer to dietician (see Table 14.6).

Hyperoxaluria May be 1° (autosomal recessive condition) or 2° to gut resection/malabsorption or dietary excess of spinach or vitamin C. Take specialist advice on management. There are two types of 1° hyperoxaluria:
- **Type 1 hyperoxaluria** Calcium oxalate stones are widely distributed throughout the body. Presents as renal stones and nephrocalcinosis in children. 80% have chronic renal failure in <20y.
- **Type 2 hyperoxaluria** More benign but less common—nephrocalcinosis but no chronic renal failure.

Cystinuria Most common aminoaciduria. Usually presents with stones at age 10–30y. *Urine:* cystine ↑, ornithine ↑, arginine ↑, lysine ↑. Take specialist advice on management.

Hypercalcaemia 📖 p. 366

❶ Hypercalciuria may occur without hypercalcaemia and is found in ~ 80% of patients with calcium oxalate stones.

Table 14.6 Prevention of renal stones

Type of stone	Preventative measures
All types	↑ fluid intake (>2–2.5L/24h), especially in hot weather; ↓ weight if obese; ↓ animal protein and ↑ fruit/vegetables in diet; ↓ salt intake
Calcium oxalate	Urinary alkalinization with potassium citrate; avoid chocolate, tea, rhubarb and spinach, nuts, beans, beetroot; ↓ citrus fruits; bendroflumethiazide 2.5mg od may help if hypercalciuria; hyperoxaluria is treated with pyridoxine
Calcium phosphate	Low Ca^{2+} diet; avoid vitamin D supplements. Bendroflumethiazide 2.5mg od may help if hypercalciuria
Staghorn/triple phosphate (calcium, magnesium, and ammonium)	Associated with UTI due to *Proteus* species and urinary stasis, e.g. due to anatomical abnormality. Treat UTI with antibiotics
Urate	Avoid beer as has uricosuric effect; allopurinol; urinary alkalinization with potassium citrate (pH >6.5)
Cystine	Urinary alkalinization with potassium citrate

Haematuria, bladder and renal cancer

Haematuria Blood in the urine. *Causes*—see Table 14.7.
- May be frank (visible) or microscopic (up to 20% population).
- Investigate *all* cases of haematuria further
- Check MSU for M,C&S, and blood for U&E, creatinine, and eGFR. Free Hb and myoglobin make urine test sticks +ve in absence of red cells
- Urine discoloration can result from beetroot ingestion, porphyria, or rifampicin
- If cause is identified (e.g. sample taken when menstruating, UTI)—repeat the check for blood in urine once treated/resolved
- Refer if no cause is found. Rapid access one-stop clinics are now operated in most areas

Table 14.7 Causes of haematuria

Kidney	Stones	Infection
	Tumour	Glomerulonephritis
Ureter	Stones	Tumour (rare)
Bladder	UTI	Tumour
	Stones	Chronic inflammation
Prostate	Prostatitis	Tumour
Urethral inflammation		

Sterile pyuria Presence of white cells in the urine in the absence of UTI. *Causes:*

- Inadequately treated UTI
- Appendicitis
- Calculi
- Prostatitis
- Bladder tumour
- Renal TB
- Papillary necrosis
- UTI with failure to culture organism
- Interstitial nephritis or cystitis
- Polycystic kidney
- Chemical cystitis, e.g. due to radiotherapy

Management Initially repeat with clean-catch MSU. If finding persists refer to urology.

Management of haematuria[N]

Urgent referral Patients:
- Of any age with painless macroscopic haematuria
- Aged ≥40y with recurrent/persistent UTI associated with haematuria
- Aged ≥50y with unexplained microscopic haematuria
- With an abdominal mass identified clinically or on imaging that is thought to arise from the urinary tract

Non-urgent referral Patients <50y with microscopic haematuria. If proteinuria, ↑ serum creatinine, or ↓ eGFR, refer to a renal physician. Otherwise refer to urology.

❶ In male patients with symptoms suggestive of UTI and macroscopic haematuria, diagnose and treat the infection before considering referral. If infection is not confirmed, refer urgently.

Wilms' nephroblastoma 📖 p. 906

Bladder cancer *Incidence:* 10,540 cases/y in the UK; ♂:♀ ≈5:2. Transitional cell carcinoma (TCC) is most common in the UK—squamous cell carcinoma (SCC) is most common worldwide. *Risk factors:*
- Smoking (50% male cases are attributable to smoking)
- Aromatic amine exposure (textile or rubber industries)
- Schistosomiasis (SCC)   • Chronic UTI
- Stasis of urine

Presentation Haematuria—painless or painful. *Less commonly:*
- Recurrent UTI   • Loin pain   • Bladder outflow
- Frequency   • Pelvic pain   obstruction

Investigation MSU—excludes UTI and detects sterile pyuria and/or microscopic haematuria.

Management Refer urgently to urology to be seen in <2wk. Treatment depends on stage at diagnosis—see Table 14.8.

Table 14.8 Stage of bladder cancer, treatment, and prognosis

Stage	Description and treatment	Prognosis
T1 (80%)	Disease confined to mucosa/submucosa. Treated with transurethral resection of the tumour (TURBT) ± single intravesical chemotherapy treatment. Follow-up is with regular cystoscopy	Very good—most die from other causes
T2	Invasion into connective tissue surrounding the bladder. Treatment is with TURBT ± radiotherapy. Follow-up as for T1	60% survive 5y
T3	Invasion through the muscle into the fat layer. Radical cystectomy and/or radiotherapy	40–50% 5y survival
T4	Spread beyond the bladder. TURBT for local symptoms. Palliative radiotherapy ± chemotherapy. Palliative care	20–30% 5y survival—less if para-aortic nodes are involved

Hypernephroma Clear cell adenocarcinoma of renal tubular epithelium. Incidence: 9,300 cases/y in the UK. *Typical age:* 50y. ♂:♀ ≈1.5:1. Spread can be local or haematogenous (bone, liver, lung—causes cannon ball metastases seen on CXR).

Presentation
- Haematuria   • Abdominal mass   • Left varicocele
- Loin pain   • Anaemia   • Occasionally night sweats

Investigations Urine: RBCs. Blood:↑ PCV (2%), anaemia, hypercalcaemia. Radiology: USS, CXR.

Management Refer to urology urgently to be seen in <2wk. Treatment includes surgery where possible ± chemotherapy, radiotherapy, and/or biological therapy. Overall 50% 5y survival.

Further information

NICE Referral guidelines for suspected cancer (2005) ॐ www.nice.org.uk

Information and support for patients

Cancer Research UK ☎ 0808 800 4040 ॐ www.cancerhelp.org.uk
Macmillan Cancer Support ☎ 0808 808 0000 ॐ www.macmillan.org.uk

Urinary tract infection

Urinary tract infection (UTI) is one of the most common conditions seen in general practice, accounting for up to 6% of consultations (one case/average surgery). ♀ > ♂. 20% of women at any time have asymptomatic bacteriuria and 20–40% of women will have a UTI in their lifetime.

Infecting organisms E. coli (>70%), *Proteus* spp., *Pseudomonas* spp., streptococci, staphylococci.

Risk factors

- Prior infection
- DM
- Stones
- Pregnancy
- Dehydration
- GU instrumentation
- Catheterization
- ↓ oestrogen (menopause)
- Sexual intercourse
- Diaphragm use
- GU malformation
- Urinary stasis (e.g. obstruction)
- Delayed micturition (e.g. on long journeys)

Presentations of UTI

- **Cystitis** Frequency, dysuria, urgency, strangury, low abdominal pain, incontinence of urine, acute retention of urine, cloudy or offensive urine, and/or haematuria
- **Pyelonephritis** Loin pain, fever, rigors, malaise, vomiting, and/or haematuria

Dysuria and urgency Painful micturition resulting from urethral or bladder inflammation. *Causes:* UTI, urethral syndrome, inflammation (e.g. interstitial cystitis, radiation-induced cystitis), intravesical lesion (tumour, stone), atrophy (menopause).

Frequency Passage of urine more often than usual. *Causes:*

- UTI
- Urethral syndrome
- Detrusor instability
- Inflammation (e.g. interstitial cystitis)
- Fibrosis (e.g. post-radiotherapy)
- Atrophy (menopause)
- Neurogenic bladder (e.g. MS)
- External pressure (e.g. pregnancy, fibroids)
- Bladder tumour or stone
- Enlarged prostate
- Drugs (e.g. diuretics)
- DM
- Excessive fluid intake
- Habit

Initial investigation If uncomplicated UTI in an otherwise healthy woman, test urine with a leucocyte and nitrite dipstick. If +ve, treat for UTI. *Reasons to send MSU for M,C&S:*

- Unresolved infection after antibiotics
- Recurrent UTI
- Uncatheterized man with UTI
- Catheterized man or woman with symptomatic UTI
- Child—📖 p. 878
- Pregnant woman—📖 p. 812
- Suspected pyelonephritis
- Haematuria—microscopic or macroscopic; always investigate further (📖 p. 446)

❶ For women with severe or 3 or more symptoms of cystitis, start treatment without urine dipstick. Take MSUs prior to starting antibiotics—send to the laboratory fresh. Consider chlamydia infection in young men or women with symptoms of UTI.

Further investigation Consider further investigation with blood tests (U&E, Cr, eGFR, and/or PSA if >40y and ♂) and/or radiology (e.g. renal tract USS, KUB) if:

- UTI in a man
- UTI in a child (📖 p. 879)
- Recurrent UTI in a woman
- Pyelonephritis
- Unclear diagnosis (e.g. persisting symptoms but negative MSU)
- Unusual infecting organism
- Sterile pyuria (📖 p. 446)

Management

Catheterized patients—📖 p. 453   *Pregnant women*—📖 p. 812

Children—📖 p. 878

All other patients

- ↑ fluid intake (>3L/24h). Alkalinize urine (e.g. potassium citrate solution) to ease symptoms
- Prescribe oral antibiotics, e.g. trimethoprim 200mg bd (80% organisms are sensitive). Use a 3d course for women with uncomplicated UTI, a 7d course for men, patients with GU malformations or immunosuppression, relapse (same organism) or recurrent UTI (different organism). Use a 7d course of a quinolone (e.g. ciprofloxacin 500mg bd) for patents with pyelonephritis
- Refer to urology if any abnormalities are detected on further investigation or unable to resolve symptoms. Admission is rarely needed

Prevention of recurrent cystitis Reinfection after successful treatment of infection (90%) or relapse after inadequate treatment.

- **General advice** Advise patients to urinate frequently; ↑ fluid intake; double void (i.e. go again after 5–10min) and void after intercourse. ♦ Efficacy of cranberry juice is controversial
- **Prophylactic antibiotics** Consider prescribing either post-coitally (e.g. nitrofurantoin 50mg stat) or continuously (trimethoprim 100mg nocte or nitrofurantoin 50mg nocte)
- **Men with BPH** Finasteride or dutasteride and/or doxazosin ↓ incidence of UTI
- **HRT** Topical oestrogen ↓ recurrent UTI in women of all ages[R]
- **Vaccines** Results of large-scale trials are awaited

Prostatitis 📖 p. 456   **Chronic pyelonephritis** 📖 p. 442

Urethral syndrome Symptoms of cystitis with −ve MSU. Unknown cause. Associated with cold, stress, nylon underwear, CHC, and intercourse. Advise fluids ++ and to wear cotton underwear. Consider changing/stopping CHC or trying topical oestrogen if post-menopausal. Tetracyclines (e.g doxycycline 100mg bd for 14d) or azithromycin (500mg od for 6d)[R] are helpful in some. If not settling, refer to urology. Urethral dilatation/massage may be helpful.

Interstitial cystitis Predominantly middle-aged women. Can cause fibrosis of the bladder wall. Main symptoms—frequency, urgency, and pelvic/suprapubic pain especially when the bladder is full. Often misdiagnosed as recurrent UTI. MSU—no bacteriuria. Refer to urologist for confirmation. There is no satisfactory treatment, though antispasmodics, amitriptyline, and bladder stretching under GA may help some patients.

Incontinence of urine

Involuntary loss of urine which is objectively demonstrable and a social or hygienic problem. 1 in 3 with incontinence consult at outset, 1 in 3 consult later, 1 in 3 suffer in silence. Opportunistic questioning can identify sufferers.

History

- Frequency of complaint
- Volume passed
- Degree of incapacity
- Whether occurs with standing/coughing/sneezing
- Urgency/dysuria/frequency of micturition
- Past obstetric and medical history
- Medication
- Mobility and accessibility of toilets

Examination

- **Abdominal including DRE**—enlarged bladder, masses, loaded colon, faecal impaction, anal tone
- **Pelvic**—prolapse, atrophy, neurological deficit, retention of urine, and pelvic masses

Investigation *Intake/output diary* (at least 3d, including working and leisure days)—evaluates problem and benchmark for progress—record drinks and passage of urine; *urine*—RBCs, MC&S; consider blood for U&E, eGFR, FBC, FBG/HbA1c if renal impairment/DM is suspected.

Drugs that exacerbate/cause incontinence Diuretics, antihistamines, anxiolytics, α-blockers, sedatives and hypnotics, anticholinergic drugs, TCAs.

GP management ❶ 30% have a mixed pattern. Treat according to dominant symptom. Try general measures before referring to urology/gynaecology or for further investigations (see Table 14.9).

General measures

- Manipulate fluid intake: amount, type (avoid tea, coffee, alcohol), timing
- Promote weight ↓
- Alter medication, e.g. timing of diuretics
- Treat UTI and chronic respiratory conditions
- Avoid constipation
- Consider HRT (topical or systemic) for oestrogen deficiency
- Consider scheduled voiding if cognitive deficit

Aids and appliances 📖 p. 452

Nocturnal enuresis in children 📖 p. 914

Stress incontinence

- **Symptoms** Small losses of urine without warning throughout the day related to coughing/exercise
- **Causes** Prostatectomy; childbirth; deterioration of pelvic floor muscles/nerves
- **Treatment** Pelvic floor exercises (📖 p. 841) continued >3mo help 60% (taught by physiotherapists/continence advisors; leaflets available)—may be assisted by vaginal cones and/or electrical stimulation. Mechanical devices (e.g. Contrelle Activguard®, FemSoft®) may help.

Urge incontinence (overactive bladder syndrome) Detrusor instability or hyperreflexia cause the bladder to contract unintentionally
- **Symptoms** Frequency, overwhelming desire to void (often precipitated by stressful event), large loss, nocturia
- **Causes** Idiopathic, neurological problems (stroke, MS, DM, spinal cord injury, dementia, PD), local irritation (bladder stones, bladder cancer, infection), obstruction (BPH), surgery (TURP)
- **Treatment** Bladder training—resist the urge to pass urine for ↑ periods. Start with an achievable interval based on diary evidence and ↑ slowly—continue for >6wk. If bladder training is ineffective, try oxybutinin first-line[N] (alternatives: darifenacin, solifenacin, tolteridone, trospium). Spontaneously remits/relapses, so reassess every 3–4mo

Overflow Constant dribbling loss day and night. *Causes:* BPH, prostate cancer, urethral stricture, faecal impaction, neurological (LMN lesions), side effect of medication. Treatment is aimed at relieving the obstruction (📖 p. 454).

Urinary fistula Communication between bladder and the outside—normally through the vagina. Results in constant dribbling loss day and night. Refer to gynaecology/urology. *Causes:* congenital, malignancy, complication of surgery.

Functional incontinence No urological problem. Caused by other factors, e.g. inaccessible toilets/immobility, behavioural problems, cognitive deficit. Treat the cause.

Table 14.9 Referral for incontinence problems

Specialist continence advisor/DN	• Advice on aids or appliances • Advice on primary care management • Patient support
Urodynamic studies	• If type of incontinence is uncertain • Atypical features of incontinence • After unsuccessful surgery • If a neurological problem is suspected
Gynaecology or urology opinion	• GP management has failed • Severe symptoms and/or pain • Recurrent UTI • Concomitant gynaecological problems (e.g. prolapse) • Concomitant urological problems (e.g. chronic retention, prostate abnormality on rectal examination) • Failed incontinence surgery • Pelvic radiotherapy • Vesico-vaginal fistula • Haematuria 📖 p. 446

Further information
European Association of Urology Guidelines on urinary incontinence (2012) ℘ www.uroweb.org
NICE Urinary incontinence (2006) ℘ www.nice.org.uk
Patient information and support
Bladder and Bowel Foundation ☎ 0845 345 0165
℘ www.bladderandbowelfoundation.org

Aids and appliances for incontinence

Pads Many different types. DNs or continence advisors are best aware of those available via the NHS locally. They are not available on FP10 and supplied by local NHS Trusts on a 'daily allowance' basis. This varies across the country.

Bed covers Absorb 1–4L of urine. Good laundry facilities are needed. If left wet can cause skin breakdown. Available via NHS Trusts.

Sheaths or external catheters Can be prescribed on NHS prescription. Approved appliances are listed in part IXB of the UK Drug Tariff. Used for men who have intractable incontinence and who are highly physically dependent, do not have urine retention and do not require an internal catheter. Assessment and fitting by a DN or continence adviser is essential.

Used in association with a drainage bag. Sheaths may be non-adhesive, self-adhesive or attached with adhesive strips. Adhesive sheaths can last several days but daily changing is recommended. Replace non-adhesive sheaths 2–3x/d (some are reusable).

Problems Include ↑ susceptibility to UTI, sores on penis, and skin irritation due to the adhesive.

Catheters Can be prescribed on NHS prescription. Approved appliances are listed in part IXA of the UK Drug Tariff.

Indwelling catheters Only use catheters in patients who have:
• Urinary retention or neurogenic bladder dysfunction
• Severe pressure sores
• Inoperable obstructions that prevent the bladder emptying
• Terminal illness
• Housebound without adequate carer support

Types Only long-term Foley catheters are suitable for use in primary care. They last 3–12wk.

Catheter size Unless specified a 12 or 14Ch catheter is supplied. Use the smallest diameter of catheter that drains urine effectively. Catheters >16Ch are more likely to cause bypassing of urine around the catheter and urethral strictures.

Catheter length Men require longer catheters than women. Specify 'male' or 'female' on the prescription.

Catheter balloon 10mL balloons are supplied unless specified otherwise. Pre-filled catheters contain sterile water which inflates the retaining balloon with water. They are more expensive but quicker to insert and there are no costs for syringes or sterile water.

Insertion 📖 p. 455

Drainage Usually attached to a leg bag, although catheter valves are also available allowing the patient to use his/her bladder as a urine reservoir. The valve must be released every 3–4h to drain out the urine.

Common problems
- **Leakage** Check no constipation, check catheter not blocked, try smaller gauge catheter
- **Infection** 90% develop bacteriuria <4wk after insertion. Always confirm suspected UTI with MSU—only treat if symptomatic or *Proteus* species grown. May prove difficult to eliminate. No good evidence bladder instillations help
- **Encrustation** (50%) Deposition of minerals and other materials from the urine onto the catheter. Worse if there is infection with *Proteus* species. May cause catheter blockage or pain changing the catheter. Check pH of urine regularly in patients with problems. Citric acid patency solutions may help if pH >7.4, or a daily dose of vitamin C
- **Inflammation** Results from physical presence of a catheter in the urethra. Exacerbated by encrustation and infection. There is no easy solution—try a different brand catheter (e.g. hydrogel catheter rather than silicone)
- **Blockage** Change catheter. The interval of routine changes should be altered if there is regular blockage towards the end of the life of a catheter

Intermittent self-catheterization Patient inserts a catheter into his/her bladder 4–5x/d to drain urine. ↓ problems of infection and blockage. Useful for neurological bladder dysfunction. *Types:*
- Reusable silver or stainless steel
- Reusable PVC—washed and reused for 1wk. Usually supply 5/mo
- Single use—need 125–150/mo. Expensive. Only use on consultant advice

Collecting bags Can be prescribed on NHS prescription. Approved appliances are listed in part IXB of the UK Drug Tariff.
- **Leg bags** Drainable bags last 5–7d. Usually 500/750mL. Larger capacity bags are too heavy for mobile patients. A variety of attachment systems are available on prescription. Long tubes are needed to wear a bag on the calf
- **Night drainage bags** Connect to night bag attachment of day bags Single use, disposable non-draining bags are recommended. Bag hangers are not available on NHS prescription

Enuresis alarms 📖 p. 915

Further information
NHSBSA Electronic drug tariff ℘ www.nhsbsa.nhs.uk/prescriptions

Patient advice and support
Bladder and Bowel Foundation ☎ 0845 345 0165
℘ www.bladderandbowelfoundation.org

Urinary tract obstruction

Causes of obstruction (See Figure 14.1) Obstruction may be unilateral (kidney, pelvi-ureteric junction, or ureter) or bilateral (bladder, urethra, prostate). Unilateral obstruction may present late if the other kidney remains functioning. Suspect if loin ache worsened by drinking. Confirm with USS and refer to urology. Obstructing lesions may be in the lumen (e.g. stones) in the wall (e.g. tumours) or impinging from outside (e.g. retroperitoneal fibrosis).

Acute retention of urine Sudden inability to pass urine → lower abdominal discomfort with inability to keep still. Differentiate from AKI. ♂ > ♀. *Risk factors:* age >70y; symptoms of prostatism/poor urinary stream.

Causes Prostatic obstruction (82%); constipation; alcohol; drugs (anticholinergics, diuretics); UTI; operation (e.g. hernia repair). *Rarer causes:* urethral stricture; clot retention; spinal cord compression; bladder stone.

Examination Abdomen—palpable bladder; DRE—enlarged ± irregular prostate; perineal sensation to exclude neurological cause.

Investigation MSU to exclude infection. Blood for U&E, Cr, and eGFR. *Only* investigate if catheterizing in the community.

Management Catheterize (record initial volume drained) or refer to urology for catheterization—local policies vary. Treat infection. Refer to DN for instruction on management of the catheter. Refer to urology for further assessment and treatment.

Chronic retention of urine Insidious onset. *Causes:* benign prostatic hypertrophy; pelvic malignancy; CNS disease. May present as:
• Nocturnal enuresis   • Acute on chronic retention   • UTI
• Overflow incontinence   • Lower abdominal mass   • Renal failure

Examination and investigation As for acute retention. Bladder is enlarged (may contain >1.5L) but usually non-tender.

Management Refer to urology for further assessment and treatment. Refer urgently or acutely if pain, UTI or renal failure (eGFR <60mL/ min/1.73m^2). *Do not* catheterize in the community.

Retroperitoneal fibrosis Ureters become embedded in dense fibrous plaques in the retroperitoneal space. Associations:
• Drugs, e.g. methysergide   • Connective tissue disease
• Carcinoma   • Raynaud's syndrome
• Crohn's disease   • Fibrotic diseases (e.g. alveolitis)

Presentation and management Typically middle-aged men presenting with fever, malaise, sweating, leg oedema, ↑ BP, palpable mass, and/or acute/chronic renal failure. Refer for specialist care. Options include steroids and nephrostomies.

Horseshoe kidney Congenital abnormality. Kidneys are fused in the midline to form a horseshoe-shaped mass. The kidney may function normally or may present with obstructive nephropathy or UTIs.

Unilateral:

Pelvi-ureteric junction
- *Tumour*
- *Calculus*

Ureter
- *Calculus*
- *Tumour*
- *Impacted sloughed papilla*
- *Retroperitoneal fibrosis*
- *Compression by LNs*

Bladder
- *Tumour*
- *Clot*
- *Pelvic malignancy*
- *Calculus*

Bilateral:

Both ureters
- *Retroperitoneal fibrosis*

Bladder
- *Tumour*
- *Clot*
- *Pelvic malignancy*
- *Calculus*

Prostate
- *Benign prostatic hypertrophy*
- *Prostate cancer*

Urethra
- *Urethral stricture*
- *Urethral valves*

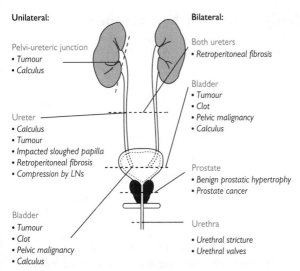

Figure 14.1 Causes of urinary tract obstruction

Passing a urethral catheter ❶ Technique learned through supervised experience. Only attempt alone if you are competent to do so.

Prepare the equipment needed
- Sterile rubber gloves, plastic sheet to prevent spills, paper sheet to provide sterile field, cleansing materials—cotton swabs, cleansing fluid
- Local anaesthetic/lubricating gel e.g. 1% lidocaine + 0.25% chlorhexidine
- Catheter—usually 12Ch or 14Ch; ensure the catheter is a long catheter if catheterizing a man (📖 p. 452); and if the catheter is not pre-filled—sterile syringe + 10mL of sterile water
- Kidney dish/other receptacle to catch the urine before connecting the drainage bag; drainage tube and bag

Inserting the catheter
- Ensure the patient is comfortable; protect against spills with a plastic sheet; cover area with a sterile paper sheet
- Ensure strict aseptic technique. Cleanse the penis/vulva and squeeze lubricant/local anaesthetic gel into the urethra—allow to work
- Gently but firmly, push the catheter into the urethra. Ensure the end of the catheter is over the receptacle. When the catheter enters the bladder, urine flows into the receptacle. Inflate the balloon with sterile water (if needed) once the catheter is inside the bladder. Connect the catheter to the collecting tube and bag
- If male, pull the foreskin over the glans again to prevent paraphimosis

❶ If you are unable to pass a catheter, refer to urology.

Benign prostatic hypertrophy

10–30% of men in their early 70s have symptomatic benign prostatic hypertrophy (BPH). There is no relation between size of the prostate and symptoms. *Assessment*—see Table 14.10.

Symptoms of prostatism

- **Obstructive** ↓ and intermittent urinary stream, double micturition, hesitancy, terminal dribbling, feeling of incomplete emptying, and straining to void. *Differential diagnosis:* prostatic enlargement, strictures, tumours, urethral valves, bladder neck contracture
- **Irritative** (due to detrusor muscle hypertrophy)—Urinary frequency, urgency, dysuria, and nocturia. *Differential diagnosis:* enlarged prostate, UTI, polydipsia, detrusor instability, hypercalcaemia, uraemia

Complications 10% at presentation:

- Recurrent UTI
- Bladder stones
- Haematuria
- Acute retention of urine (± prior obstructive symptoms)—📖 p. 454
- Chronic retention—📖 p. 454
- Overflow incontinence—📖 p. 451
- Obstructive nephropathy

GP management Symptoms can improve spontaneously but overall progress slowly. 1–2%/y develop urinary retention. *Options:*

Watchful waiting Patients with mild to moderate symptoms at presentation, with no complications of BPH and who are not severely troubled by their symptoms. Self-help includes: ↓ evening fluid intake, ↓ caffeine intake, bladder retraining, and prevention of constipation.

Drug therapy Those with mild/moderate symptoms who are troubled by their symptoms. *Consider:*

- **α-adrenoceptor antagonists,** e.g. prazosin, doxazosin—watch for postural hypotension. ↓ symptomatic worsening
- **5α-reductase inhibitors,** e.g. finasteride—best for patients with bulky prostates; takes up to 6mo to work. ↓ risk of urinary retention
- **Combination therapy**—α-adrenoceptor agonist and 5α-reductase inhibitor ↓ progression by 66% more than either agent alone

❶ Serenoa repens (saw palmetto) has no benefit over placebo[c].

Referral to a urologist *E* = Emergency admission; *U* = Urgent; *S* = Soon; *R* = Routine.

- Complicated BPH (e.g. acute retention)—*E/U*
- Nodular/firm prostate on DRE—*U*
- Failure to respond to drug therapy after 3–12mo (α-blocker) or 6–12mo (5α-reductase inhibitor)—*R*
- ↑ PSA (📖 p. 459)—*U*
- Severe symptoms—*S*

Acute bacterial prostatitis Consider in men presenting with suspected UTI. *Other features:* fever; arthralgia/myalgia; low back, perineal, penile ± rectal pain. DRE reveals swollen, tender prostate. If suspected, check MSU and treat with 4wk course of oral antibiotic which penetrates prostatic tissue, e.g. ciprofloxacin 500mg bd, ofloxacin 200mg bd. Refer for specialist advice if not settling. *Complications include:* acute retention of urine, chronic bacterial prostatitis, and prostate abscess.

Table 14.10 Assessment of BPH

Assessment	Comments
History	• General well-being • Obstructive symptoms • Irritative symptoms • Haematuria • Pain • Polyuria and polydipsia • Neurological symptoms • Past history of urological instrumentation or STIs
Frequency-volume chart	Assess pattern and type of fluid consumption (e.g. alcohol/caffeine at night ↑ nocturia)
Symptom score (IPSS— 🕮 p. 458)	Objectively grade symptoms, giving measure of severity. IPSS scores: • 0–7 mild • 8–19 moderate • 20–35 severe A general quality of life measurement can be used to assess impact of symptoms
Abdominal examination	Look for distended bladder, palpable kidneys. Examine external genitalia
Digital rectal examination	Anal tone, size, shape, and consistency of prostate (normal prostate—size of a chestnut with smooth, rubbery consistency)
Serum urea, creatinine, and eGFR	Renal function assessment
MSU	Dipstick for blood and glucose. M,C&S
Ultrasound measurement of post-micturition residual*	
Maximum voiding flow rate*	<15mL/s for voided volume >100mL is abnormal
Serum PSA	High values can indicate prostate cancer (🕮 p. 459)

*May be available through open-access prostate assessment clinics

Chronic prostatitis (chronic pelvic pain syndrome) 2–14% lifetime prevalence. Cause is unknown. Presents with >3mo history of:
• Urological pain—lower abdomen, pelvis/perineum, penis (especially tip ± on ejaculation), testicles, rectum, low back ±
• Irritative/obstructive symptoms and/or ejaculatory disturbance

Diagnosis is based on history with exclusion of other causes. Suitable investigations include DRE, MSU, urine cytology, STI screen (🕮 p. 739), PSA ± urodynamic studies. Treatment is difficult—provide information and support; try α-blockers (e.g. doxazosin 4mg od for 6mo). Spontaneous improvement/remission often occurs.

Patient support

Prostatitis Foundation ℗ www.prostatitis.org

Further information

BASHH Management of prostatitis (2008) ℗ www.bashh.org.uk
Cochrane Tacklind J, MacDonald R, Rutks I, et al. (2012) Serenoa repens for benign prostatic hyperplasia. *Cochrane Database of Systematic Reviews*, Issue 12. Art. No.: CD001423. DOI: 10.1002/14651858.CD001423.pub3.

Table 14.11 The International Prostate Symptom Score

	Not at all	Less than 1 time in 5	Less than half the time	About half the time	More than half the time	Almost always	Your score
Over the past month, how often have you had a sensation of not emptying your bladder completely after you finish urinating?	0	1	2	3	4	5	☐
Over the past month, how often have you had to urinate again <2h after you finished urinating?	0	1	2	3	4	5	☐
Over the past month, how often have you stopped and started several times when you urinated?	0	1	2	3	4	5	☐
Over the past month, how often have you found it difficult to postpone urinating?	0	1	2	3	4	5	☐
Over the past month, how often have you had a weak urinary stream?	0	1	2	3	4	5	☐
Over the past month, how often have you had to push or strain to begin urinating?	0	1	2	3	4	5	☐
Over the past month, typically from the time you went to bed to the time you got up in the morning, how many times did you get up to urinate?	0	1	2	3	4	5+	☐
Total IPSS score							☐

	Delighted	Pleased	Mostly satisfied	Equally satisfied/dissatisfied	Mostly dissatisfied	Unhappy	Terrible
If you were to live the rest of your life with your urinary condition the way it is now, how would you feel about it?	0	1	2	3	4	5	6

0–7 = mildly symptomatic

8–19 = moderately symptomatic

20–35 = severely symptomatic

The International Prostate Symptom Score is reproduced with permission from the American Urological Association.

Prostate-specific antigen (PSA) testing There is no prostate screening programme in the UK but men can request a PSA test. The government has introduced a PSA Informed Choice Programme. Warn patients about the poor specificity of the test, before performing the test and provide information about the pros and cons of testing.

In addition, PSA is routinely measured in men with urological symptoms. Abnormal PSA is a common reason for referral to a urologist. Its sensitivity and specificity are poor.

Pros and cons of PSA testing

Benefits of PSA testing	Downside of PSA testing
• It may provide reassurance if the test result is normal	• It can miss cancer and provide false reassurance
• It may find cancer before symptoms develop and at an early stage when treatments could be beneficial	• It may lead to unnecessary anxiety and medical tests when no cancer is present
• If treatment is successful, the consequences of more advanced cancer are avoided	• It might detect slow-growing cancer that may never cause any symptoms or shortened lifespan
	• The main treatments of prostate cancer have significant side effects, and there is no certainty that treatment will be successful

Reasons for increased PSA

- Prostate cancer
- Benign prostatic hypertrophy
- Acute or chronic prostatitis
- Physical exercise
- Acute urinary retention
- Prostate instrumentation (includes prostate biopsy and urinary catheterization)
- Old age

! PSA may be *normal* when early prostate cancer is present.

Performing a PSA test Digital rectal examination may cause a transient ↑ in PSA levels (◆), so do the PSA test before doing a digital rectal examination. If that is not possible, delay the test for 1wk after the examination. Exclude urinary infection before PSA testing. Do NOT do a PSA test if the man has:

- A proven UTI—treat the UTI and postpone the PSA test for ≥1mo
- Ejaculated within 48h
- Exercised vigorously in the previous 48h
- Had a prostate biopsy <6wk ago

PSA cut-offs that should prompt referral

Age (y)	Refer to urology if PSA (ng/mL)
50–59	≥3.0
60–69	≥4.0
≥70	>5.0

! Finasteride and dutasteride ↓ PSA by ~50%.

Prostate cancer

Prostate cancer is the sixth most common cancer worldwide. It is the second most common cancer affecting men and 10,720 men/y die from the disease in the UK. 1 in 6 men have clinical prostate cancer in their lifetime and the incidence is rising.

Classification

Non-metastatic prostate cancer

Can be divided into:

- Clinically localized disease—cancer thought, after clinical examination, to be confined to the prostate gland
- Locally advanced disease—cancer that has spread outside the capsule of the prostate gland but has not yet spread to other organs

Metastatic prostate cancer Cancer that has spread outside the prostate gland to local, regional, or systemic LNs, seminal vesicles, or other body organs (e.g. bone, liver, brain).

Risk factors

- **Age** Uncommon <50y; 85% are diagnosed aged >65y
- **Genetic** ↑ incidence if first-degree relative affected
- **Racial** Incidence varies according to location in the world and ethnic group. Highest rates are in men of black ethnic group in the USA—lowest in Chinese men
- **Dietary** Links are proposed between prostate cancer, low intake of fruit (particularly tomatoes) and high intake of fat, meat, and Ca^{2+}

Screening A large-scale trial of screening for prostate cancer is underway in the UK. *Problems with screening:*

- Incidental post-mortem evidence of prostate cancer is high (~75% men >75y); very few become clinically evident, so many more men would be found with prostate cancer by screening than would die or have symptoms from it
- Natural history of prostate cancer is not understood—there is no means to detect which 'early' cancers become more widespread
- Inadequate screening tests
- It is not clear if early treatment enhances life expectancy
- Peak incidence of morbidity and mortality is in old age (75–79y), so potential years of life saved by screening are small

Screening tests

- **Prostate-specific antigen (PSA)** 🕮 p. 459
- **Digital rectal examination (DRE)** Operator-dependent, fails to detect early prostate cancers, and lacks specificity. Annual screening in the USA and Germany has not ↓ mortality
- **Transrectal ultrasound (TRUS)** Too expensive

The most effective screening regime involves rectal examination and PSA testing followed by TRUS for suspicious lesions[5]. Optimal screening interval is unknown but serial screening does ↑ detection.

Symptoms and signs

Early cancer Symptomless. Usually detected following an incidental finding of ↑ PSA. Hard nodule sometimes felt in prostate on DRE.

Local disease

- Prostatism
- Urinary retention
- Haematuria
- Lower extremity oedema
- On rectal examination, the prostate is hard and non-tender and sulci lose definition

Metastatic disease

- Malaise
- Weight loss
- Bone pain
- Pathological fractures
- Spinal cord compression
- Ureteric obstruction may cause renal failure
- Signs depend on site of metastases

Investigation[N] A digital rectal examination and PSA test (after counselling) are recommended for patients with any of the following unexplained symptoms:

- Erectile dysfunction
- Haematuria
- Lower back pain
- Bone pain
- Inflammatory or obstructive lower urinary tract symptoms
- Weight loss, especially in the elderly

! Exclude UTI before PSA testing and postpone digital rectal examination until after the PSA test is done.

Urgent referral[N]

- Rectal examination—hard, irregular prostate typical of prostate cancer. PSA result should accompany the referral
- Rectal examination—normal prostate, but rising/raised age-specific PSA ± lower urinary tract symptoms*
- Symptoms and high PSA levels
- Asymptomatic men with borderline, age-specific PSA results repeat PSA after 1–3mo. If the PSA level is rising, refer the patient urgently

* Consider discussion with specialist and patient ± carer before referral for very elderly patients/those compromised by other co-morbidities.

! Referral is not needed if the prostate is simply enlarged and the PSA is in the age-specific reference range.

Further information for GPs

NICE ℠ www.nice.org.uk
- Referral guidelines for suspected cancer (2005)
- Prostate cancer: diagnosis and treatment (2008)
Cancer research UK ℠ www.cancerresearchuk.org
National screening ℠ www.cancerscreening.nhs.uk

Information for patients on PSA testing and prostate cancer

National screening ℠ www.cancerscreening.nhs.uk
Cancer Research UK ☎ 0808 800 4040 ℠ www.cancerhelp.org.uk
Macmillan Cancer Support ☎ 0808 808 0000 ℠ www.macmillan.org.uk
Prostate Cancer Charity ☎ 0800 074 8383 ℠ www.prostatecancer.org.uk
Prostate Cancer Support Association ☎ 0845 601 0766
℠ www.prostatecancersupport.co.uk

Treatment of prostate cancer

Symptomless local disease Treatment is controversial. There are two arguments:

Benefits of treatment are outweighed by risks	*or*	Aggressive treatment before spread is the only way to ensure cure

>50% of men >50y who die from other causes are found post-mortem to have prostate cancer—prostate cancer kills only a small minority of men who have it. The personal and economic cost of treating men whose cancer would never have caused them any problems must be considered.

Options

- **Watchful waiting or active surveillance** Monitor with PSA and regular rectal examination. ↑ in PSA or size of nodule triggers active treatment. At 10y follow-up <10% with moderately well-differentiated cancer will have died from their cancer. Progression rates are higher in patients with poorly differentiated cancer. Some men find the uncertainty of waiting difficult to cope with
- **Radical prostatectomy** Has potential for cure, but in the age group most affected by prostate cancer mortality is 1.4%. Other common complications: impotence (50%), incontinence (25%)
- **Radiotherapy** May not be effective—persistent cancer is found in 30% on biopsy. Brachytherapy (radioactive treatment in implanted seeds or wires) has proven efficacy in early prostate cancer
- **Hormone treatment** No convincing evidence that this gives survival benefit in early disease
- **Others** Minimally invasive treatments, e.g. cryotherapy and microwave therapy, are as yet unproven

Symptomatic disease 30% 5y survival. Hormone manipulation is the mainstay of treatment and gives 80% ↓ in bone pain, PSA, or both, and a lower incidence of serious complications (e.g. spinal cord compression) if treatment starts at the time of diagnosis. *Options:*

Luteinizing hormone releasing hormone (LHRH) analogues (e.g. goserelin) sc injection every 4–12wk (depending on the preparation used). Testosterone levels ↓ to levels of castrated men in <2mo. *Side effects:* impotence, hot flushes, gynaecomastia, local bruising, and infection around injection site. When starting LHRH analogues, LH level initially ↑ which can cause increased tumour activity or 'flare'. Counteracted by prescription of anti-androgens (e.g. flutamide) for a few days before administration of the first dose of LHRH and concurrently for 3wk. Response in most patients lasts for 12–18mo.

Anti-androgens (e.g. cyproterone acetate, flutamide, bicalutamide). Do not suppress androgen production completely. Used to prevent side effects due to testosterone flare during initiation of LHRH analogues, as monotherapy (e.g. bicalutamide 150mg od) and in combination with LHRH analogues to produce maximum androgen blockade.

Surgical castration ↓ testosterone secretion permanently without the need for medication. However, rarely used.

Bony metastases In addition to hormone therapy, local radiotherapy and corticosteroids are used for bone pain. Radioactive strontium ↓ the number of new sites of bone pain developed. Mean survival <5y.

Hormone-resistant disease No agreed treatment. Involve the multidisciplinary team-including urology, oncology, and palliative care. Dexamethasone 0.5mg daily or docetaxel may be helpful.

Prognosis See Table 14.12.

Table 14.12 Factors affecting prognosis of prostate cancer

Stage	Tumour		Lymph nodes involved?		Metastases?
T1	Inpalpable	N0	No	M0	No spread outside the pelvis
T2	Tumour completely within the prostate gland	N1	1 +ve LN <2cm diameter	M1	Spread outside the pelvis
T3	Tumour has breached the capsule of the prostate	N2	>1 +ve LN or 1 LN of 2–5cm diameter		
T4	Spread within the pelvis, e.g. to bladder or bowel	N3	Any +ve LN >5cm diameter		

Gleason score Histological grade. Cells are graded 1–5 the less differentiated they are. The two areas of the biopsy with the highest grade cells are added together. Low-grade tumours likely to grow slowly have low scores (2–4); high-grade tumours have high scores (7–10).

Age Older patients with low-grade tumours are likely to die from something other than their prostate cancer.

PSA
• PSA >40: high chance of nodal or metastatic spread
• PSA >100: metastatic spread is very likely

Prognosis 5y survival rates for tumour stage:
• 1 or 2—tumour confined within the prostate (65–98%)
• 3—tumour has breached the capsule of the prostate (60%)
• 4—spread to LNs, within the pelvis or elsewhere (20–30%)

Further information
NICE Prostate cancer: diagnosis and treatment (2008) ℘ www.nice.org.uk
Cancer Research UK ℘ www.cancerresearchuk.org
National screening ℘ www.cancerscreening.nhs.uk

Conditions of the penis

Posterior urethral valves Folds of mucosa inhibit or block passage of urine causing urethral, bladder, ureter, and renal pelvis dilatation.

Presentation Usually detected on antenatal USS. Can present in neonates with urinary retention or dribbling urine + distended bladder, UTI or uraemia, or later in childhood with recurrent UTI or incontinence.

Investigation and management MCUG confirms diagnosis. In all cases refer to urology for surgical disruption of the valves.

Hypospadias 1 in 400 male births. The urethral meatus opens on the ventral side of the penis. There is often hooding of the foreskin and ventral flexion of the penis. Refer to urology. Treated with corrective surgery, ideally preschool.

Non-retractile foreskin Usually noted by parents. May be history of recurrent balanitis. *Examination*: foreskin adherent.

Management Age <4y—do nothing unless recurrent balanitis. If >4y and/or recurrent balanitis, consider treatment with topical steroids (e.g. betamethasone 0.1% od) for 3–4mo. If ineffective, refer to paediatric surgery for circumcision.

Phimosis Foreskin obstructs urine flow. Common in small children. Time usually obviates the need for circumcision. Treat as for non-retractile foreskin if recurrent balanitis.

Peyronie's disease Hard lumps in the shaft of the penis. Unknown cause. 4% ♂ >40y. 1 in 3 have pain/bending of the penis when erect. Associated with erectile dysfunction (📖 p. 776). 5% have Dupuytren's contracture. *F.G. de la Peyronie (1678–1747)—French surgeon.*

Management Reassurance usually suffices. No proven medical treatments. Refer to urology for surgery if pain or severe bending on erection so that intercourse is not possible.

Paraphimosis Foreskin is retracted then (because of oedema) unable to be replaced. Commonly occurs in catheterized patients when the catheter is changed.

Management Try to replace foreskin using ice packs (↓ swelling) and lubrication (e.g. KY jelly). If unable to replace the foreskin, admit for surgery.

Balanitis Acute inflammation of glans and foreskin. Common organisms—staphylococci, streptococci, coliforms, candida. Can occur at any age. Most common in young boys when associated with non-retractile foreskin/phimosis. In elderly patients consider DM.

Management Oral antibiotics (e.g. flucloxacillin) or topical antifungals (e.g. clotrimazole). If recurrent or secondary to phimosis consider referral for circumcision.

Balanitis xerotica et obliterans Chronic fibrosing condition of the foreskin which may become adherent to the glans. Treatment is with topical steroid creams, e.g betamethasone 0.1%. Consider referral for circumcision.

Trauma to the foreskin Torn frenulum—seen after poorly lubricated intercourse or if caught in a zip. No treatment required. If recurrent, consider referral for circumcision.

Erectile dysfunction 📖 p. 776

Priapism Persistent painful erection not related to sexual desire.

Cause Medication for erectile dysfunction, idiopathic, leukaemia, sickle cell disease, or pelvic tumour.

Management Ask the patient to climb stairs (arterial 'steal' phenomenon), apply ice packs. If unsuccessful refer to A&E for aspiration of corpora. Rarely surgery is needed.

Erythroplasia of Queryat Pre-malignant condition of glans. Moist velvety-looking patches. Refer to urology. Treatment is surgical.

Carcinoma of the penis Squamous cell carcinoma (95%) or malignant melanoma. Usually elderly men. Rare in the UK.

Management[N] Refer urgently patients with symptoms or signs of penile cancer. These include:
• Progressive ulceration in the glans, prepuce, or skin of the penile shaft
• Mass in the glans, prepuce, or skin of the penile shaft

❶ Lumps within the corpora cavernosa can indicate Peyronie's disease, which does not require urgent referral.

Penile discharge Associated with urethritis, e.g. due to chlamydia or gonorrhoea. Refer to GUM clinic.

Further information
BASHH Management of balanitis (2008) ℘ www.bashh.org.uk
NICE Referral guidelines for suspected cancer (2005) ℘ www.nice.org.uk

Testicular disease

Testicular pain Treat the cause:
- Epididymo-orchitis
- Torsion of the testis
- Trauma and haematoma formation
- Varicocele
- Testicular tumour (rarely painful)

> **Torsion of the testis** Peak age 15–30y. Presents with sudden onset of severe scrotal pain. May be associated with right iliac fossa pain, nausea, and vomiting. *Examination:* tender, hard testis riding higher than contralateral testis. Admit urgently to surgical/urology team.

Torsion of the hydatid of Morgagni Small embryological remnant at the upper pole of the testis. Presents similarly to torsion of the testis. Refer as an emergency to exclude torsion of the testis.

Epididymo-orchitis Inflammation of the testis and epididymis due to infection. May occur at any age. The most common viral cause is mumps. The most common bacterial causes are chlamydia or gonococci (<35y) and coliforms (>35y). Chronic infection with TB or syphilis is rare.

Presentation Acute onset pain in testis; swelling and tenderness of testis/epididymis; fever ± rigors; may be urethritis, dysuria, and/or ↑ frequency.

Management May be difficult to distinguish from torsion of the testis. If in doubt, admit for urology/surgical opinion. Otherwise investigate and treat for the underlying cause.

Testicular lumps and swellings See Figure 14.2.

Hydrocele Collection of fluid in the tunica vaginalis. Occurs at any age.
- 1° **hydrocele**—no predisposing cause in scrotum
- 2° **hydrocele**—reaction to pathology in testis or covering (infection, tumour, torsion). In adults presenting with hydrocele always consider impalpable tumour beneath

Presentation Swelling in the scrotum. The examiner should be able to get above the swelling. Smooth surface, transilluminates; testis is within the swelling and not palpable separately.

Management Investigation is not required in children; refer adults for USS if testis is not palpable. Options for adults:
- Conservative management—reassurance; small hydroceles
- Tapping—may be suitable for large hydroceles where surgery is inappropriate; 2° infection and recurrence are common
- Surgery—refer to urologist

> Hydroceles in children are usually congenital. May be unilateral or bilateral. Most resolve spontaneously in the first year of life. Refer to urology if persists >1y.

Hydrocele of the cord Arises in part of the processus vaginalis in the spermatic cord above the testis. Rounded lump which slips up and down the inguinal canal. No action needed.

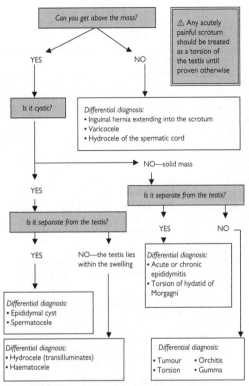

Figure 14.2 Diagnosis of testicular lumps

Referral guidelines[N]

- Refer urgently patients with a swelling or mass in the body of the testis
- Consider an urgent ultrasound in men with a scrotal mass that does not transilluminate and/or when the body of the testis cannot be distinguished

Further information

NICE Referral guidelines for suspected cancer (2005) ℗ www.nice.org.uk
BASHH Management of epididymo-orchitis (2010) ℗ www.bashh.org.uk

Haematocele Damage to the testis (e.g. due to a direct blow, vasectomy) can result in the testis rupturing and the tunica vaginalis filling with blood. Refer as an emergency for urological assessment.

Varicocele Collection of varicose veins in the pampiniform plexus of the cord and scrotum. Can be 2° to obstruction of the testicular veins in the abdomen. L > R. Associated with infertility (thought due to ↑ temperature of testis). Presents with a dull ache in the testis especially at the end of the day or after exercise. Usually visible when the patient is standing. No treatment is needed—reassure. Occasionally surgery or radiological embolization may help if symptoms are severe.

Epididymal cyst Common and often multiple. Found in middle-aged/elderly men. Usually presents when the patient finds a painless lump.
- **Examination** Smooth-walled cyst in epididymis (palpable above and behind testis), often bilateral
- **Investigation** If unsure of diagnosis refer for USS
- **Management** Reassurance. Refer to urology if painful

Spermatocele Cyst containing sperm. Typically situated in the head of the epididymis—more rarely in the spermatic cord. Clinically presents in the same way as epididymal cyst. Management is the same.

Testicular gumma 📖 p. 749

Benign testicular tumours Rare (<2% tumours). Sertoli cell adenomas; Leydig cell adenomas. Produce sex hormones and cause feminization/masculinization respectively. Refer.

Testicular cancer Most common malignancy in men age 20–34y. Devastating disease as sufferers tend to be young and fit and do not expect to be ill. Screening is not effective. Education to ensure men check their testes for lumps regularly and present early is preferable.

Risk factors Undescended testes—bilateral undescended testis → 10x ↑ risk; past history of testicular cancer—4% risk second cancer.

Presentation Painless lump in testis; occasionally testicular pain or hydrocele; may present with metastases—back pain/dyspnoea.

Management Testicular lumps are tumours until proven otherwise. Refer for urgent urological opinion. USS can help diagnosis but *do not* delay referral. Definitive diagnosis is only made at biopsy. Specialist treatment depends on tumour type and extent (see Table 14.13). Sperm banking is routinely offered in case of ↓ fertility due to treatment.

❶ Children conceived of men treated for testicular cancer are not at ↑ risk of congenital abnormality.

Empty scrotum If the scrotum has never contained a testis, it is hypoplastic. If the scrotum has contained a testis in the past, it is normally developed but empty.

Causes of an empty scrotum Undescended or retractile testis; surgical removal, e.g. for torsion, trauma, or tumour; testicular atrophy (e.g. due to mumps or trauma); ambiguous genitalia; testicular agenesis—diagnosis of exclusion.

Table 14.13 Types and features of testicular cancer

	Seminoma (60%)	Teratoma
Typical age	30–40y	<30y
Tumour markers	None	β-HCG αFP LDH—correlates with volume of metastatic disease
Nature of tumour	Solid	Solid/cystic components 40% occur within seminomas Mixed tumours are treated like teratomas
Growth speed	Slow-growing	Fast-growing—can ↑ x2 in size in days
Stage of presentation	90% stage 1 (tumour confined to testis)	60% stage 1 (tumour confined to testis)
Treatment	Treated with inguinal orchidectomy + radiotherapy Relapses are treated with chemotherapy More advanced disease is treated with radio- or chemotherapy	Treatment of stage 1 disease is with inguinal orchidectomy and surveillance of tumour markers. 25% relapse in <18mo Treatment of relapses and metastatic disease is with chemotherapy
Survival	98% 5y survival for stage 1 disease. Overall >85% 5y survival	Prognosis depends on stage and degree of differentiation

Carcinoma of the scrotal skin SCC or melanoma. Uncommon <50y. Painless lump/ulcer of the scrotal skin ± enlarged inguinal LNs. If suspected, refer urgently to urology or dermatology.

Fournier's gangrene Necrotizing fasciitis of the scrotal skin and/or penis. Patients are usually elderly and often have a hydrocele. Starts as a black spot and spreads rapidly. Early diagnosis is critical to survival so, if suspected admit as an acute urological emergency. Treatment is with surgical debridement and IV antibiotics.

 Undescended testis Affects 2–3% of ♂ neonates—but most descend during the first year. Refer those that do not for surgical descent/fixation to avoid ↑ risk of malignancy and later infertility.

Retractile testis Usually young boys with active cremasteric reflex. No treatment needed.

Examination Scrotum is usually well developed. Try to find the testis, and milk it down into scrotum. May be found anywhere from the scrotum to the internal inguinal ring. If not found or you are unable to bring the testis down into the scrotum assume it is undescended.

Information and support for patients with testicular cancer
Cancer Research UK ☎ 0808 800 4040 ⌨ www.cancerhelp.org.uk
Macmillan Cancer Support ☎ 0808 808 0000 ⌨ www.macmillan.org.uk

Musculoskeletal problems

Symptoms of musculoskeletal disease

Bone pain *Consider:*
- **Fracture** Due to injury, stress fracture, or pathological fracture
- **Arthritis** Referred pain from affected joints
- **Malignancy** Primary bone malignancy, haematological malignancy, e.g. multiple myeloma, or secondaries (usually from breast, prostate, lung, thyroid, kidney—more rarely bowel, melanoma)
- **Benign bone tumour**
- **Osteomyelitis**
- **Metabolic causes,** (e.g. hypercalcaemia)

Pain in one joint Common. Ask:

Is the problem articular or periarticular?
- Articular disease (e.g. osteoarthritis) is suggested by joint line tenderness and pain at the end of the range of movement in any direction
- Periarticular problems (e.g. ligamentous injury)—point tenderness over the involved structure and pain exacerbated by movements

If articular Is the problem inflammatory or mechanical? Look for:
- Signs of inflammation—warmth, redness, effusions; may indicate joint infection or inflammatory arthritis
- Features of a mechanical problem—locking or catching, e.g. cartilage tear

If periarticular Which structure is causing pain? *Options:* bursa; tendon; tendon sheath; ligament; soft tissue.

> ⚠ **Red flags** Features which should prompt early/urgent referral:
> - Inflamed joint with associated fever or constitutional disturbance—beware of infection
> - Any joint which is 'locked' or so painful that movement is impossible
> - Severe pain at rest or at night
> - Pain that gets relentlessly worse over a period of days or weeks

Pain in multiple joints
- Differentiate between articular or periarticular disease, and whether the condition is inflammatory or not as for pain in one joint. Screening with blood tests (ESR or CRP, FBC ± autoimmune profile) may help
- Look for the pattern of disease—joint sites involved and other symptoms/signs

Common arthropathies 📖 pp. 512–23
- Osteoarthritis
- Rheumatoid arthritis
- Ankylosing spondylitis
- SLE
- Reactive arthritis
- Psoriatic arthritis
- Enteropathic arthropathy
- Gout or pseudogout
- Sicca syndrome
- Malignancy

⚠ *Red flags* Features which should prompt early/urgent referral:
- Severe systemic symptoms—high fevers, significant weight loss, or a very ill patient (suggests rheumatoid arthritis, sepsis, or malignancy)
- Focal systemic signs, e.g. rashes, nodules, or GI disturbances
- Severe pain and/or inability to function

Myalgia Isolated myalgia can be a result of overuse or soft tissue injury. Generalized myalgia is associated with many diseases including:
- Infection
- Statin use (check CK)
- Fibromyalgia
- Chronic fatigue syndrome
- PMR (shoulder and hip girdle)
- Vasculitis e.g. Wegener's granulomatosis, PAN

Dystonia 📖 p. 546

Short stature 📖 p. 892

Tall stature 📖 p. 893

Chest deformity 📖 p. 298

 Children with musculoskeletal pain of unknown cause Take a history and examine carefully. Investigate further with FBC, blood film, and ESR ± X-ray if bone pain, rest pain, or persistent or unexplained back pain[N]. If no cause is found, treatment is with analgesia and reassurance. Advise to return for reassessment ± orthopaedic referral if pain worsens, continues >6wk, changes in nature, or other symptoms develop.

Nocturnal musculoskeletal pains (growing pains) Episodic, muscular pains, usually in the legs, lasting ~30min and waking the child from sleep. Rubbing the limb brings rapid relief. There is no pain or disability in the morning. Diagnosis can be made on history if there are no associated symptoms and examination is normal. If in doubt, check FBC and ESR—which should be normal. In most cases reassurance ± analgesia are all that is needed. In resistant cases, physiotherapy may help.

The limping child 📖 p. 491

Further information
NICE Referral guidelines for suspected cancer (2005) ℘ www.nice.org.uk

Neck pain

⚠ **Neck trauma** Any significant cervical trauma requires neck immobilization with a hard collar and referral to A&E for cervical spine X-rays to exclude vertebral fracture or instability that could threaten the spinal cord.

Neck pain is common (lifetime incidence 50%) and contributes to 2% of GP consultations. Prevalence is highest in middle age. Most neck pain is acute and self-limiting (within days/weeks) but 1 in 3 have symptoms lasting >6mo or recurring pain.

History

- Pain—onset, site, radiation, aggravating and relieving factors, timing
- Stiffness—timing (continuous? worse in the mornings?)
- Deformity (e.g. torticollis)—onset, changes
- Neurological symptoms—numbness, paraesthesiae, weakness
- Other symptoms—weight loss, bowel/bladder dysfunction, sweats

❶ Pain is often poorly localized and neck problems commonly present with shoulder pain and/or headache (cervicogenic headache).

Examination

- **Look** Posture; deformity, e.g. torticollis, asymmetry of scapulae; arms and hands—wasting, fasciculation? Leg weakness?
- **Feel** Tenderness? Midline tenderness may be due to supraspinous or spinous process damage following a whiplash injury. Paraspinal tenderness ± spasm radiating into the trapezius ± crepitation is common with cervical spondylosis
- **Move/measure** Normal ranges: flexion/extension—130° total range; lateral flexion—45° in each direction from a neutral position; rotation—80° in each direction from a neutral position
- **Neurology** Weakness in the upper limbs in a segmental distribution, with loss of dermatomal sensation and altered reflexes indicates a root lesion (see Table 15.1). If cervical cord compression is suspected, examine the lower limbs looking for upgoing plantars and hyperreflexia

Cervical spondylosis Degenerative disease of the cervical spine can cause pain, but minor changes are normal (especially >40y) and usually asymptomatic. Pain is generally intermittent and related to activity. Examination reveals ↓ neck mobility. Severe degeneration can cause nerve root signs. Treat with analgesia ± cervical collar. X-ray only if conservative measures fail, troublesome pain, nerve root signs, or the patient has psoriasis (? psoriatic arthropathy).

Nerve root irritation or entrapment Secondary to degeneration, vertebral displacement/collapse, disc prolapse, local tumour, or abscess. Causes neck stiffness, pain in arms or fingers, ↓ reflexes, sensory loss, and ↓ power. The level of entrapment can usually be determined clinically (see Table 15.1). Treat with analgesia ± cervical collar. X-ray cervical spine—lateral or oblique views. Refer for physiotherapy. Refer for further investigations (e.g. MRI) if conservative management fails and there is objective evidence of a root lesion.

Table 15.1 Neurology associated with cervical nerve root entrapment

Root	Sensory changes	Motor weakness	Reflex changes
C5	Lateral arm	Shoulder abduction/flexion Elbow flexion	Biceps
C6	Lateral forearm Thumb Index finger	Elbow flexion Wrist extension	Biceps Supinator
C7	Middle finger	Elbow extension Wrist flexion Finger extension	Triceps
C8	Medial side of lower forearm Ring and little fingers	Finger flexion	None
T1	Medial side of upper forearm	Finger abduction/ adduction	None

⚠ Refer urgently if there are signs of spinal cord compression:
- Root pain and lower motor neurone signs at the level of the lesion, *and*
- Spastic weakness, brisk reflexes, upgoing plantars, loss of coordination and sensation below the lesion

Spasmodic torticollis (wry neck) Common. Sudden onset of painful stiff neck due to spasm of trapezius and sternocleidomastoid muscles. Self-limiting. Heat, gentle mobilization, muscle relaxants, and analgesia can speed recovery. A cervical collar may help in the short term but can prolong symptoms. Often caused by poor posture, e.g. computer-seating position; carrying heavy, uneven loads.

Cervical rib Congenital condition of C7 vertebra costal process enlargement. Usually asymptomatic but can cause thoracic outlet compression → hand or forearm pain, weakness or numbness, and thenar or hypothenar wasting. Radial pulse may be weak. X-ray of thoracic outlet may show cervical rib—but symptoms are sometimes due to fibrous bands that are not seen on X-ray. Refer to upper limb orthopaedic surgeon for further assessment.

Whiplash injuries Neck pain resulting from stretching or tearing of cervical muscles and ligaments due to sudden extension of the neck—often due to a RTA. Pain and ↓ neck mobility typically starts several hours or days after injury. Pain may radiate to shoulders, arms, and head.

Management Examine carefully to exclude bony tenderness requiring X-ray. Treat with analgesia and early mobilization—collar may help initially but avoid long-term use. Recovery is often slow and 40% patients suffer long-lasting symptoms. As a general rule of thumb, the quicker the symptoms develop, the longer they will take to disappear. Early physiotherapy, if available, can improve recovery rate. Psychological problems and medicolegal issues can affect progress.

Low back pain

Definitions

- **Acute low back pain** New episode of low back pain of <6wk duration. Common—lifetime prevalence 58%
- **Chronic low back pain** Back pain lasting >3mo

Causes of back pain See Table 15.2.

History Ask:

- Circumstances of pain—history of injury; duration
- Nature/severity of pain—pain/stiffness mainly at rest/at night, easing with movement suggests inflammation, e.g. discitis, spondylarthropathy
- Associated symptoms—numbness, weakness, bowel/bladder symptoms
- PMH—past illnesses (e.g. cancer), previous back problems
- Exclude pain not coming from the back (e.g. GI or GU pain)

Examination

- Deformity, e.g. kyphosis (typical of ankylosing spondylitis), loss of lumbar lordosis (common in acute mechanical back pain), scoliosis
- Palpate for tenderness, step deformity, and muscle spasm
- Assess flexion, extension, lateral flexion, and rotation whilst standing
- Ask to lie down—this gives a good indication of severity of symptoms
- In lower limbs look for muscle wasting and check power, sensory loss, and reflexes (knee jerk and ankle jerk). See Table 15.3. Assess straight leg raise (SLR)—sciatica is present if SLR on one side elicits back/buttock pain (usually ipsilateral but can be either side) compared to SLR on the other side

> ⚠ **'Red flags'**
> - <20 or >55y
> - Non-mechanical pain
> - Pain that worsens when supine
> - Night-time pain
> - Thoracic pain
> - Past history of cancer
> - HIV
> - Immune suppression
> - IV drug use
> - Taking steroids
> - Unwell
> - Weight ↓
> - Widespread neurology (see Table 15.3)
> - Structural deformity

Management of acute pain in the community Triage according to history and examination—see Figure 15.1, 📖 p. 479.

For patients who do not require immediate referral Prescribe analgesia, e.g. paracetamol ± NSAIDs ± amitriptyline (10–25mg nocte) and use the Keele STarT back screening tool (see Box 15.1):

- If total score ≤3, explain likely natural history of the pain and advise to avoid bed rest and maintain normal activities as far as possible (↓ chance of chronic pain). Suggest self-help exercises
- If total score is ≥4, check question 5–9 sub-score:
  - If ≤3—if not resolved in 4wk, refer for physical therapy. Options include: back exercise classes, physiotherapy, chiropractic, osteopathy, or acupuncture, if available.
  - If ≥4—if not resolved in 4wk, refer directly for specialist intervention, sooner if worsening or severe pain
- In all cases, challenge any 'yellow flag' factors (see Figure 15.1, 📖 p. 479) that may inhibit recovery and delay return to normal functioning

Table 15.2 Causes of back pain: age suggests the most likely cause

Age (y)	Causes		
15–30	• Postural • Mechanical • Prolapsed disc	• Trauma • Fracture • Ankylosing spondylosis	• Spondylolisthesis • Pregnancy
30–50	• Postural • Prolapsed disc	• Spondylarthropathies • Discitis	• Degenerative joint disease
>50	• Postural • Degenerative • Paget's disease	• Malignancy (lung, breast, prostate, thyroid, kidney)	• Osteoporotic collapse • Myeloma
Other causes	• Referred pain • Spinal stenosis	• Cauda equina tumours	• Spinal infection

Table 15.3 Neurology with lumbosacral nerve root entrapment

Root	Sensory changes	Motor weakness	Reflex changes
L2	Front of thigh	Hip flexion/adduction	None
L3	Inner thigh	Knee extension	Knee
L4	Inner shin	Knee extension Foot dorsiflexion	Knee
L5	Outer shin Dorsum of foot	Knee flexion Foot inversion Big toe dorsiflexion	None
S1	Lateral side of foot/sole	Knee flexion Foot plantarflexion	Ankle

Box 15.1 Keele STarT Back Pain Scoring Tool

Ask patients to consider the following statements and state whether they agree or disagree with them. *Thinking about the past 2wk:*

1. My back pain has spread down my leg(s) at some time in the last 2wk
2. I have had pain in the shoulder or neck at some time in the last 2wk
3. I have only walked short distances because of my back pain
4. In the last 2wk, I have dressed more slowly than usual because of back pain
5. It's not really safe for a person with a condition like mine to be physically active
6. Worrying thoughts have been going through my mind a lot of the time
7. I feel that my back pain is terrible and it's never going to get any better
8. In general I have not enjoyed all the things I used to enjoy

If the patient agrees with a statement, score 1; if disagrees, score 0.

9. Overall, how bothersome has your back pain been in the last 2wk?
   • *Not at all, slightly, or moderately*—score 0
   • *Very much or extremely*—score 1

❶ *Do not X-ray for back pain routinely* X-rays require a high radiation dose, and clinically meaningful findings are rare. *Exceptions:*
- Young (<25y)—X-ray SI joints to exclude ankylosing spondylitis
- Elderly—if vertebral collapse/malignancy suspected
- History of trauma

Cauda equina syndrome Compression of the cauda equina below L2, e.g. by disc protrusion at L4/5. Presents with:
- Numbness of the buttocks and backs of thighs
- Urinary/faecal incontinence
- Lower motor neurone weakness:
  - L4—loss of dorsiflexion of the foot (and toes—L4/5)
  - S1—loss of ankle reflex, plantarflexion, and eversion of the foot

Management Refer/admit as a neurological emergency. Rapid surgical intervention ↑ the chance of full motor and sphincter recovery.

Spinal cord compression Affects 5% of cancer patients—70% in the thoracic region. Maintain a *high* level of suspicion if history of cancer and new back pain—especially if known bony metastases or tumour likely to metastasize to bone. Presents with:
- Back pain, worse on movement—often appears before neurology
- Neurological symptoms/signs—can be non-specific, e.g. constipation, weak legs, urinary hesitancy. Lesions above L1 (lower end of spinal cord) produce upper motor neurone signs (e.g. ↑ tone/reflexes) and a sensory level; lesions below L1 produce lower motor neurone signs (↓ tone/reflexes) and perianal numbness (cauda equina syndrome)

Management Prompt treatment (<24–48h from first neurological symptoms) is needed; once paralysed, <5% walk again. Treat with oral dexamethasone 16mg/d and refer for same-day assessment and surgery/radiotherapy unless in final stages of disease.

Osteoporotic vertebral collapse 📖 p. 508

Scoliosis Lateral curvature of the spine associated with rotation of vertebrae ± ribs or wedging of vertebrae. Early treatment prevents progression and complications, e.g. cardiopulmonary disturbance. *Causes:*
- Idiopathic
- Congenital (butterfly vertebra)
- Infection—TB of spine
- Metabolic, e.g. bone dysplasias
- Neuromuscular problems, e.g. cerebral palsy, neurofibromatosis, Friedreich's ataxia, muscular dystrophy, polio
- Trauma → damage in vertebral growth plate and uneven growth
- Neoplasm 1°, 2°, or as a result of radiotherapy

Clinical features Difference in shoulder height; spinal curvature; difference in the space between the trunk and upper limbs. ❶ Scoliosis which disappears on bending is postural and of no clinical significance.

Management In all cases where structural scoliosis is suspected, refer for an orthopaedic opinion. If associated with pain, especially at night, consider spinal tumour and refer urgently.

Further information
NICE Low back pain (2009) ॐ www.nice.org.uk

Figure 15.1 Triage of acute back pain

Patient information and support
Arthritis Research UK ☎ 0300 790 0400 🖰 www.arthritisresearchuk.org

Shoulder problems

History

- **Pain and stiffness** Joint pain is felt anteriorly and may radiate down the arm; pain on top of the shoulder suggests acromioclavicular joint problems or cervical spine disorders. ❶ Pain in the shoulder may be referred from the neck, heart, mediastinum, or diaphragm
- **Deformity** Swelling of the shoulder; prominence of the acromioclavicular (AC) joint; winging of the scapula
- **Loss of function** Difficulty reaching behind back (e.g. doing up bra strap), brushing hair, or dressing

Examination

- **Look** Posture; asymmetry; muscle wasting; swelling (large effusions can be seen anteriorly); scars
- **Feel** Tenderness; warmth; swelling; crepitus
- **Move/measure** Compare sides. Check range of movement; complex movements (e.g. scratching opposite scapula in 3 ways, hands behind head, arm across front of chest to top of opposite shoulder); power

General rules Intra-articular disease—painful limitation of movement in all directions; tendonitis—painful limitation of movement in one plane only; tendon rupture or neurological lesions—painless weakness.

> ⚠ **Red flags**
> - Past history of carcinoma
> - Constitutional symptoms, e.g. fever, chills, or unexplained weight ↓
> - Recent bacterial infection
> - IV drug use
> - Immune suppression
> - Constant/worsening rest pain
> - Structural deformity

Causes of a stiff, painful shoulder joint

- Adhesive capsulitis—1° or 2° to DM or intrathoracic pathology
- Inflammation—inflammatory arthritis (e.g. RA, psoriatic), infection
- Osteoarthritis
- Prolonged immobilization, e.g. hemiplegia, strapping after dislocation
- Polymyalgia rheumatica

Shoulder OA Often occurs after a history of trauma. Less common than knee or hip OA. Often associated with crystal-induced inflammation and 2° causes of OA (e.g. gout, haemochromatosis). Imaging for synovitis (USS/MRI) is important to rule out disease that may benefit from steroid injection. Shoulder replacement may be considered in severe cases.

Frozen shoulder (adhesive capsulitis) Overdiagnosed in primary care. Affects patients aged 40–60y. Painful, stiff shoulder with global limitation of movement—notably external rotation. Pain is often worse at night. Cause unknown, but ↑ in diabetics and those with intrathoracic pathology (MI, lung disease) or neck disease.

Management If not known to be diabetic, check fasting blood glucose. NSAIDs, physiotherapy, and local steroid injection can all be helpful. May take >1y to recover and long-term outcome is uncertain. If restricted movements are slow to return consider orthopaedic referral.

Rotator cuff injury The shoulder is the most mobile joint in the body and relies on the musculo-tendinous rotator cuff to maintain stability. Disorders of the rotator cuff account for most shoulder pain.

- **Acute tendinitis** Often caused by excessive use/trauma in patients <40y. Presents with severe pain in the upper arm. Patients hold the arm immobile and are unable to lie on the affected side. Usually starts to resolve spontaneously after a few days. In middle age can be caused by inflammation around calcific deposits—requires steroid injection
- **Rotator cuff tears** May accompany subacromial impingement pain and is difficult to diagnose clinically unless the tear is large—suspect if impingement pain is recurrent. Refer
- **Subacromial impingement** Pain occurs in a limited arc of abduction (60–120°—*painful arc syndrome*) or on internal rotation due to acromial or ligament pressure on a damaged rotator cuff tendon. In patients <40y, associated with glenohumeral instability from generalized connective tissue laxity or labral injury. In older patients, often due to chronic rotator cuff tendinitis or functional cuff weakness/tear

Investigations X-ray may show calcification of the supraspinatus tendon in acute tendinitis and irregularities/cysts at the humeral greater tuberosity if chronic cuff tendinitis.

Treatment Rest followed by mobilization and physiotherapy, NSAIDs, and/or subacromial steroid injection (📖 p. 166). If conservative measures fail refer for imaging, arthroscopy, and consideration for surgery.

Shoulder dislocation Usually due to fall on arm or shoulder—anterior dislocation is most common. Shoulder contour is lost (flattening of deltoid) and the head of the humerus is seen as an anterior bulge. Axillary nerve may be damaged → absent sensation on a patch below the shoulder. Refer to A&E for X-ray and reduction. In young patients, ~30% have recurrent dislocations afterwards due to labral tear. Dislocation is associated with rotator cuff tear in ~25% of elderly patients.

Recurrent dislocation Usually anterior and follows trauma—but 5% recurrent dislocations are in teenagers with no trauma but general joint laxity. Refer for specialist physiotherapy and consideration of surgery.

Acromioclavicular joint problems Pain on the top of the shoulder or in the suprascapular area suggests a problem with the acromioclavicular (AC) joint or neck. AC joint pain is usually due to trauma or OA—joint tenderness and pain are present on palpation and passive horizontal adduction. *Management:* NSAIDs ± local steroid injection.

Fractured clavicle 📖 p. 1111

Cleido-cranial dysostosis Inherited autosomal dominant condition. Part/all of the clavicle is missing and ossification of the skull is delayed—sutures remain open. Associated with short stature. No treatment.

Rupture of the long head of biceps Discomfort in the arm on lifting and a feeling of 'something going'. A lump appears in the body of biceps muscle on elbow flexion. May be associated with other shoulder pathology. *Management:* exclude distal rupture of the tendon at the elbow. Reassure. No treatment necessary.

Elbow problems

History

- **Pain and stiffness** Joint pain is diffuse; pain well localized over the medial or lateral epicondyles may be due to tendinitis
- **Deformity** Swelling? Nodules? Structural deformity?
- **Loss of function** May be limitation of flexion, extension, pronation, and/or supination. This can affect function, e.g. causing difficulty eating (can't get hand to mouth) or with personal care
- **Neurology** Numbness and paraesthesiae distal to the elbow—particularly in the ulnar nerve distribution

Examination

- **Look** Carrying angle (~11° for ♂ 13° for ♀). Effusion may be visible either side of the olecranon. A discrete swelling over the olecranon could be RA nodule, gouty tophus, olecranon bursa, or other nodule. Check for muscle wasting
- **Feel** Tenderness? Swellings? Warmth? If indicated test neurology and check pulses distal to the elbow
- **Move** Active and passive movements. Compare both sides. Normal range is from 0° in full extension to 145° in full flexion. Check pronation/supination. Normal range is 75° and 80° respectively

Tennis elbow and golfer's elbow (epicondylitis) Common extensor tendon inflammation at the epicondyle. *Cause:* repeated strain.

- **Tennis elbow**—tenderness over the lateral epicondyle and lateral elbow pain on resisted wrist extension
- **Golfer's elbow**—tenderness over the medial epicondyle and medial elbow pain on resisted wrist pronation

Management Stop trigger movements if possible. Often settles with time ± NSAIDs. Recovery is speeded by local steroid injection (📖 p. 166), although relapse is more common after injection. Physiotherapy may help, as may an epicondylar clasp. Rarely referral for autologous blood injection or surgical release is indicated.

Dislocated elbow Usually due to fall on outstretched hand with flexed elbow. Ulna is displaced backwards, elbow is swollen and held in fixed flexion. May have associated fracture. Refer to A&E for reduction.

Olecranon bursitis Traumatic bursitis due to repeated pressure on the elbow. Pain and swelling over olecranon. Aspirate fluid from bursa—send for microscopy to exclude sepsis and gout (request polarized light microscopy). Fluid may reaccumulate—if sepsis has been excluded, inject hydrocortisone to help settle. Refer septic bursitis for surgical drainage.

Ulnar neuritis Narrowing of the ulnar grove (from OA, RA, or post-fracture) causes pressure on the ulnar nerve → ulnar neuropathy. Clumsiness with the hand is often the first symptom, then weakness ± wasting of hand muscles innervated by the ulnar nerve and ↓ sensation in the little finger and medial half of the ring finger. Rule out metabolic and autoimmune causes of a mononeuritis and refer for consideration of surgical decompression ± nerve conduction studies if entrapment is likely.

Pulled elbow Common in children <5y. Traction injury to elbow causes subluxation of radial head. Often occurs when the child is pulled up suddenly by the hand. Child will not use the arm. No clinical signs. ♂ > ♀. Left arm > right. X-rays are unhelpful.

Management Apply anterior pressure with the thumb on the radial head whilst supinating and extending the forearm. Immediate recovery is seen after reduction.

Further information for patients
Arthritis Research UK ☎ 0300 790 0400 🖰 www.arthritisresearchuk.org

Wrist and hand problems

History

Wrist

- **Pain/stiffness** Pain is often well localized in the wrist. Five conditions are associated with point tenderness: De Quervain's disease; old scaphoid fracture; carpometacarpal OA; Kienböck's disease (avascular necrosis of the lunate); tenosynovitis of the extensors. Wrist pain may also be associated with RA, OA, and ganglia. Carpal tunnel syndrome is associated with pain in the hand
- **Deformity** May be swelling of tendon sheaths or wrist. Bony deformity is a late feature of arthritis or secondary to trauma
- **Function** Ask about weakness and numbness in the hand

Hand

- **Pain/stiffness** Pain from the hand is felt in the fingers and/or palm. A diffuse ache may be referred from the neck, shoulder, or mediastinum
- **Deformity** May occur acutely, e.g. due to tendon rupture or slowly due to bone or joint pathology. The pattern and symmetry of joint involvement can be diagnostic
- **Function** Good hand function is essential for everyday tasks, e.g. turning keys, doing buttons up, writing. Ask about limitations

Examination

Wrist

- **Look** Symmetry; swelling; deformity (ulnar deviation, volar subluxation; rheumatoid nodules; ganglia); muscle wasting in forearm/hand
- **Feel** Temperature; nature of any swellings; tenderness of the radiocarpal, midcarpal, or distal radio-ulnar joint
- **Move/measure** Range of movement (normal range—extension >75°, flexion >75°, pronation >75° from the vertical, supination >80° from the vertical); crepitation?
- **Neurology** Check for ulnar and median nerve function

Hand

- **Look** Posture of the hand; swellings (rheumatoid nodules; Heberden's and Bouchard's nodes; ganglions; tophi); nail signs, e.g. pitting of psoriasis; scars; deformity (mallet finger; swan neck deformity; Boutonnière deformity; Dupuytren's contracture); ulnar deviation. If there is joint disease note distribution and whether it is symmetrical
- **Feel** Temperature; condition of the skin, e.g. dryness, sweating; nature of swellings; muscle bulk, e.g. small muscles of the hand; tenderness
- **Move/measure** Ask the patient to make a fist, spread his fingers out, and then test each individual joint. Then test opposition, pinch grip, key grip, palmar grasp of ball, and practical tasks, e.g. picking up a coin

Fractures 📖 p. 1111.

Ganglion Smooth, firm, painless swelling—usually around the wrist. No treatment is needed unless causing local problems. May resolve spontaneously; can be drained (large-bore needle)/excised but often recurs.

For all hand injuries Check for:

Nerve injury Can occur due to trauma or lacerations of the hand or wrist. Examine sensory and motor function. Always ensure no other structures are damaged before suturing skin wounds. Refer all nerve injuries for specialist assessment and management—surgery can improve the outcome considerably in some cases. Intensive hand physiotherapy is important to regain function. *Types of nerve injury:*

- **Neurapraxia** Temporary loss of nerve conduction—often caused by pressure causing ischaemia
- **Axonotmesis** Damage to the nerve fibre, but nerve tube is intact— the chance of successful nerve regrowth and a good recovery is high
- **Neurotmesis**—Divided nerve—lack of guidance to the regrowing fibrils gives ↓ chance of a good recovery, and a neuroma may develop

Median nerve damage The median nerve controls grasp. Damage causes inability to lift the thumb out of the plane of the palm (abductor pollicis brevis failure) and loss of sensation over the lateral side of the hand.

Ulnar nerve damage Injury distal to the wrist causes a claw hand deformity, loss of abduction/adduction of the fingers, and sensory loss over the little finger and a variable area of the ring finger.

Radial nerve damage The radial nerve opens the fist—injury produces wrist drop and variable sensory loss including the dorsal aspect of the root of the thumb.

Tendon injury Can occur due to attrition or lacerations of the hand or wrist. Examine hand function. Always ensure no other structures are damaged before suturing skin wounds. Extensor or flexor tendons can be affected. Refer—primary surgical repair is usually the treatment of choice.

Vascular injury Can occur due to trauma/lacerations of the hand or wrist. Check perfusion and temperature of fingers and examine pulses. Ensure no other structures are damaged before suturing skin wounds. Refer all vascular injuries for specialist assessment and management.

Work-related upper limb pain Work-related pain in the arm ± wrist, e.g. due to keyboard use. Overuse syndrome. Often termed repetitive strain injury (RSI). Diagnosis of exclusion—no physical signs. Exclude other conditions, e.g. carpal tunnel syndrome (CTS), tennis elbow.

Management Reassure—condition is curable, continue work, but avoid the aggravating activity, liaise with work to ensure evaluation of workstation ergonomics. Gradually reintroduce activity. Physiotherapy may help. Explore psychological and work-related issues. A multidisciplinary approach is needed. ❶ Work-related upper limb pain is a notifiable industrial disease.

☞ Existence of RSI has been challenged—rigorous assessment often reveals undiagnosed causes of pain.

Complex regional pain disorder (also known as reflex sympathetic dystrophy or algodystrophy). Pain ± vasomotor changes in a limb → loss of function. Most common in the hand and wrist. Usually follows trauma—but the trauma may be trivial and signs may appear weeks/months later. *Signs:* pain at rest exacerbated by movement and light touch, swelling, discoloration, temperature changes, abnormal sensitivity, sweating, and loss of function. X-ray may show osteopenia.

Management Physiotherapy improves prognosis if started early; analgesia (NSAIDs, opioids, and/or nerve painkillers). Refer to pain clinic or rheumatology for specialist treatments, e.g. nerve block, spinal cord stimulation, CBT, and/or graded motor imagery.

Tenosynovitis Inflammation of the tendon sheath—often due to unaccustomed activity (e.g. gardening). May affect extensor or flexor tendons. Pain is often worse in the morning. Presents with swelling and tenderness over the tendon sheath and pain on using the tendon. Treat with rest and NSAIDs. If not settling, an injection of steroid into the tendon sheath may help. ❶ Notifiable industrial disease if work-related.

De Quervain's tenosynovitis Tenosynovitis of thumb extensor and abductor tendon sheaths. Pain over radial styloid and on forced adduction/flexion of the thumb. Treat with thumb splint ± local steroid injection. Refer if not settling. *F. de Quervain (1868–1940)—Swiss surgeon.*

Carpal tunnel syndrome Pain in the radial 3½ digits of the hand ± numbness, pins and needles, and thenar wasting. Due to compression of the median nerve as it passes under the flexor retinaculum. Worse at night. Symptoms are improved by shaking the wrist. *Associations:* pregnancy, hypothyroidism, DM, obesity, and carpal arthritis.

Investigations Phalen's test—hyperflexion of wrist for 1min triggers symptoms; Tinel's test—tapping over the carpal tunnel causes paraesthesiae; request nerve conduction studies if diagnosis is in doubt.

Management GP treatment—night splints may help ± carpal tunnel steroid injection (📖 p. 166). Less likely to help if age >50y or symptoms >10mo. If GP treatment fails, constant paraesthesiae and/or triggering of fingers, refer to orthopaedics for division of the flexor retinaculum.

Kienböck's disease The lunate bone develops patchy necrosis after acute or chronic injury. The patient is usually a young adult complaining of aching and stiffness of one wrist. *Examination:* tenderness in the centre of the back of the wrist ± limitation of wrist extension. X-ray is normal at first but later shows ↑ density of the lunate ± deformity. Refer for orthopaedic opinion. *R. Kienböck (1871–1953)—Austrian radiologist.*

Osteoarthritis in the hand
- Heberden's nodes—swellings of DIP joints. No treatment needed
- Bouchard's nodes—swellings of PIP joints. No treatment needed

First carpometacarpal OA Pain and swelling at the base of the thumb. Thumb becomes stiff. A splint or steroid injection can be helpful. If pain persists surgery (trapeziectomy) may help.

Dupuytren's contracture Palmar fascia contracts so that the fingers (typically the right fifth finger) cannot extend. *Prevalence:* 10% ♂ > 65y (more if family history). Less common in women. *Associations:* smoking; alcohol; heavy manual labour; trauma; DM; phenytoin; Peyronie's disease; AIDS. Often simple reassurance suffices. Consider referral for surgery (fasciotomy or fasciectomy) if MCP joint contracture >30° or PIP/DIP joint contracture >10°. *G. Dupuytren (1777–1835)—French surgeon.*

Trigger finger Nodules on the tendon can occur spontaneously and in RA and DM. Most common in ring and middle fingers. The nodule can be palpated moving with the tendon. Pain and triggering (the finger is in fixed flexion and needs to be flicked straight by the other hand) occur because the nodule jams in the tendon sheath. *Management:* local steroid injection or refer for surgical release.

Mallet finger The fingertip droops due to avulsion of the extensor tendon attachment to the terminal phalanx (see Figure 15.2). Refer for X-ray. *Management:* a plastic splint which holds the terminal phalanx in extension is worn for 6wk to help union (must not be removed). Arthrodesis may be needed if healing does not occur.

Gamekeeper's thumb Forced thumb abduction causes rupture of the ulnar collateral ligament. Can occur on wringing a pheasant's neck—hence the name, or, more commonly, by catching the thumb in the matting on a dry ski slope. The thumb is very painful and pincer grip weak. Refer—open surgical repair is the most effective treatment.

Nail injuries

Avulsed nail Protect the nail bed of an avulsed nail with soft paraffin and gauze, check tetanus status, and give antibiotic prophylaxis (e.g. flucloxacillin 500mg qds for 7d). Partially avulsed nails need removing under ring block to exclude an underlying nail bed injury—the nail is replaced to act as a splint to the nail matrix.

Subungual haematoma A blow to the finger can cause bleeding under the nail—very painful due to pressure build-up. Relieve by trephining a hole through the nail using a 19 gauge needle (no force required; just twist the needle as it rests vertically on the nail) or a heated point (e.g. of a paper clip or cautery instrument). Of benefit up to 2d after injury.

 Polydactyly Extra digits can vary from small fleshy tags to complete duplications. They may be an isolated defect or associated with syndromes. Small fleshy tags are removed in the first few months. For extra digits that are firmly fixed or involving tendons or joints, surgery is delayed until the child is >1y. Refer to orthopaedics or plastic surgery.

Syndactyly Digits may be joined by a web of skin or more firmly fused. Webbing is usually mild and treatment is for cosmetic reasons if at all. Where digits are fused separation and skin grafting is carried out at ~4y. Refer to plastic surgery.

Hip and pelvis problems

History Pain on walking? Pain at rest? Hip joint pain is usually felt in the groin (see Table 15.4). Referred pain is often felt in the knee. Hip disease results in ↓ walking distance, difficulty climbing stairs and getting out of low chairs.

Examination

- **Look** Watch the patient walk—hip disease → limp or waddling gait
- **Feel** Joint tenderness is just distal to the midpoint of the inguinal ligament
- **Move** Passive movement with the patient lying supine. Check range of movement—pain reproduced on movement? Crepitus?
- **Measure** Hip disease is often associated with shortening of the affected leg—true leg length: anterior superior iliac spine → medial malleolus; apparent leg length: umbilicus → medial malleolus
- **Trendelenburg test** Ask the patient to stand on one leg and lift the foot on the contralateral side off the ground. Place your fingers on the anterior superior iliac spines. If the pelvis sags on the unsupported side (+ve Trendelenburg sign) the hip on which the patient is standing is painful or has a weak/mechanically disadvantaged gluteus medius ❶ False +ve in 10%.

Malignancy Hip and pelvis are common sites for 2° malignancy. Pain is severe and unremitting, day and night. Often accompanied by weight loss. X-ray may show no abnormalities or reveal lytic or sclerotic deposits. Bone scan is diagnostic but may miss myeloma. Depending on clinical circumstances either refer for specialist advice (oncologist, radiotherapist) or to palliative care. Treat with analgesia meanwhile. High risk of pathological fracture.

Osteoarthritis of the hip Major cause of hip pain and disability. Incidence ↑ with age; ♂ ≈ ♀. *Predisposing factors:* past hip disease (e.g. Perthes') or trauma; unequal leg length.

Presentation Pain may be diffuse and felt in hip region, thigh, or knee. Relieved by rest in early stages of disease. *Signs:* ↓ internal rotation and abduction of hip, with pain at extremes of movement; antalgic gait; eventually fixed flexion of the hip. *Investigation:* X-ray may confirm diagnosis but is often not needed. There is poor correlation between X-ray changes and pain felt. Perform Oxford Hip Score (see Table 15.5).

Table 15.4 Causes of pain around the hip

Pain	Causes
Buttock pain	PMR, sacroiliitis, vascular insufficiency, referred from back
Groin pain	Hip joint disease (OA, RA, Paget's, osteomalacia), fracture, osteitis pubis, hernia, psoas abscess
Lateral thigh pain	Trochanteric bursitis, referred pain from back, enthesitis (spondylarthropathies), gluteus medius tear, meralgia paraesthetica, fascia lata syndrome

Table 15.5 Oxford Hip Score

1. **During the past 4 weeks**... How would you describe the pain you <u>usually</u> have from your hip?

   None (4)   Very mild (3)   Mild (2)   Moderate (1)   Severe (0)

2. **During the past 4 weeks**... Have you had any trouble with washing and drying yourself (all over) <u>because of your hip</u>?

No trouble at all (4)	Very little trouble (3)	Moderate trouble (2)	Extreme difficulty (1)	Impossible to do (0)

3. **During the past 4 weeks**... Have you had any trouble getting in and out of a car or using public transportation <u>because of your hip</u>? (whichever you tend to use)

No trouble at all (4)	Very little trouble (3)	Moderate trouble (2)	Extreme difficulty (1)	Impossible to do (0)

4. **During the past 4 weeks**... Have you been able to put on a pair of socks, stockings or tights?

Yes, easily (4)	With little difficulty (3)	With moderate difficulty (2)	With extreme difficulty (1)	No, impossible (0)

5. **During the past 4 weeks**... **Could** you do the household shopping <u>on your own</u>?

Yes, easily (4)	With little difficulty (3)	With moderate difficulty (2)	With extreme difficulty (1)	No, impossible (0)

6. **During the past 4 weeks**... For how long have you been able to walk before <u>pain from your hip</u> becomes **severe** (with or without a stick)?

No pain/ for ≥30 min (4)	16–30 min (3)	5–15 min (2)	Around the house only (1)	Not at all (0)

7. **During the past 4 weeks**... Have you been able to climb a flight of stairs?

Yes, easily (4)	With little difficulty (3)	With moderate difficulty (2)	With extreme difficulty (1)	No, impossible (0)

8. **During the past 4 weeks**... After a meal (sat at a table), how painful has it been for you to stand up from a chair <u>because of your hip</u>?

Not at all painful (4)	Slightly painful (3)	Moderately painful (2)	Very painful (1)	Unbearable (0)

9. **During the past 4 weeks**... Have you been limping when walking <u>because of your hip</u>?

Rarely/never (4)	Sometimes or just at first (3)	Often, not just at first (2)	Most of the time (1)	All of the time (0)

10. **During the past 4 weeks**... Have you had any sudden, severe pain - 'shooting', 'stabbing' or 'spasms' - <u>from the affected hip</u>?

    No days (4)   1 or 2 days (3)   Some days (2)   Most days (1)   Every day (0)

11. **During the past 4 weeks**... How much has <u>pain from your hip</u> interfered with your usual work (including housework)?

    Not at all (4)   A little bit (3)   Moderately (2)   Greatly (1)   Totally (0)

12. **During the past 4 weeks**... Have you been troubled by <u>pain from your hip</u> in bed at night?

    No nights (4)   1 or 2 nights (3)   Some nights (2)   Most nights (1)   Every night (0)

Reproduced with permission from Isis Innovation Limited, 1998.

Management of hip osteoarthritis Analgesia (e.g. regular paracetamol, NSAIDs), education, weight ↓, exercise, correction of unequal leg length. Walking stick ± shock-absorbing shoe insoles can help. Consider referral for physiotherapy (muscle strengthening exercises may ↓ pain) or, if significant impairment in functioning (e.g. Oxford Hip Score ≤20) to orthopaedics for hip resurfacing or replacement .

Total hip replacement >90% achieve good result. Most last >15y. *Post-op care:* risk of dislocation in the first 6wk—advise to avoid crossing legs; take care with transfers; use a walking stick; no driving for 6wk. Physiotherapy is usually arranged via secondary care.

Hip dislocation Occurs in front seat passengers in car accidents as the knee strikes the dashboard. Reduction under anaesthetic is required.

Greater trochanter pain (trochanteric bursitis) Can mimic ± coexist with hip OA. May be associated with muscle weakness around the hip. *Diagnosis:* point tenderness over the greater trochanter.

Management Consider local steroid injection if trochanteric bursitis is likely. Refer to physiotherapy for exercises to strengthen hip musculature to prevent recurrence.

Meralgia paraesthetica Burning/numbness in the upper lateral aspect of the thigh due to compression of the lateral cutaneous nerve of the thigh. *Risk factors:* pregnancy, obesity, DM. *Examination:* extension of the hip or deep palpation just below the anterior superior iliac spine provokes symptoms. *Treatment:* analgesia (including neuropathic painkillers), TENS ± local steroid injection. Rarely surgical decompression is needed.

Fascia lata syndrome Inflammation of the fascia lata causing pain in the lateral thigh. Often due to overuse or weak musculature around the hip. Treatment is with rest ± referral to physiotherapy.

Hip infection Presents with hip pain, ↓ weight, night sweats, and rigors. Be aware of infection in patients with RA, hip prosthesis, or immunocompromise. Refer for investigation. X-rays are often unhelpful—bone scan is non-specific. Admit for USS-guided drainage, bed rest, and IV antibiotics.

Avascular necrosis May present with hip pain. Have a high level of suspicion in patients with risk factors—SLE, sickle cell disease, high alcohol consumption, pregnancy, or corticosteroids. X-ray or bone scan may confirm diagnosis but MRI is most sensitive. Specialist management is needed. Usually progresses to cause OA.

Pubic symphysis dehiscence Painful condition occuring in late pregnancy that may persist after delivery. The pubic symphysis separates resulting in low abdominal pain which may be accompanied by low back pain and radiate down both thighs. Pain is constant and worse on movement. It resolves on rest. Examination reveals a soft abdomen and obstetric examination is normal. Advise simple analgesia (paracetamol 1g qds). Rest in a semi-recumbent position when in pain. Refer for physiotherapy, especially if still a problem in the puerperium. Most resolve spontaneously within several months of delivery. Some persist and need specialist referral.

The limping child

- If a child is limping, take it seriously. Look for a problem
- Children find it difficult to localize pain. Pain can be referred from the hip to the knee. Examine the whole limb carefully
- Other causes of referred pain include: spinal pathology, psoas spasm from GI pathology (e.g. appendicitis)
- Limping without pain is uncommon and may be due to undiagnosed developmental dysplasia of the hip—📖 p. 854

Transient synovitis of the hip (irritable hip) The most common reason for limping in childhood. *Peak age:* 2–10y. ♂ > ♀. The child is usually well but complains of pain in the hip or knee and may refuse to weight-bear. Often occurs after a viral infection. Cause is unknown. Exclude septic arthritis—refer to orthopaedics. Usually resolves in 7–10d without treatment.

Perthes' disease Pain in the hip or knee, limp, and limited hip movement developing over ~1mo. Due to avascular necrosis of the femoral head. Bilateral in 10%. *Peak age:* 4–7y (range 3–11y). ♂ : ♀≈ 4:1.

Management If suspected refer for X-ray and to orthopaedics. Treatment is with rest, X-ray surveillance, bracing, and/or surgery depending on severity. Usually heals over 2–3y. Joint damage may cause early arthritis. Risk factors for poor outcome include:

- ♀
- Onset >8y
- Involvement of the whole femoral head
- Pronounced metaphyseal rarefaction
- Lateral displacement of the femoral head

G.C. Perthes (1869–1927)—German surgeon.

Slipped upper femoral epiphysis The upper femoral epiphysis slips with respect to the femur, usually in a postero-inferior direction. Bilateral in 20%. *Incidence:* 1:100,000. *Peak age:* 10–15y. ♂:♀≈ 3:1. Typically affects obese, underdeveloped children or tall, thin boys.

Presentation Pain at rest in the groin, hip, thigh, or referred to the knee; limp and/or pain on movement; ↓ hip movements—particularly abduction and medial rotation. The affected leg may be externally rotated and shortened.

Management Confirm diagnosis on X-ray (include lateral views)—shows backwards and downwards slippage of the epiphysis. Refer to orthopaedics—surgical pinning or reconstructive surgery is needed. Monitoring of the other hip is essential. Complications include: avascular necrosis; coxa vara; early OA; slipped epiphysis on the contralateral side.

Developmental dysplasia of the hip 📖 p. 854

Further information for patients

Arthritis Research UK ☎ 0300 790 0400 🖰 www.arthritisresearchuk.org
Steps Support for patients with lower limb conditions and their families
☎ 01925 750271 🖰 www.steps-charity.org.uk

Knee problems

History

- **Trauma** History of injury—ask about degree and direction of force
- **Pain/stiffness** Attempt to distinguish well-localized mechanical pain and diffuse inflammatory/degenerative pain
- **Deformity** Swelling? If injury, time of onset of swelling in relation to history (immediate effusion suggests haemarthrosis; post-traumatic effusions appear later). Knock-knees or bow-legs?
- **Function** Do the Oxford Knee Score (see Table 15.6)

Examination Always compare the two knees.

- **Look** Watch the patient walk. Look at the knees whilst standing—varus/valgus deformity? Ask the patient to lie down. Note quadriceps wasting, scars, skin changes, swelling, and deformity. A space under the knee viewed laterally suggests a fixed flexion deformity. With legs extended, lift both feet off the bed to demonstrate hyperextension
- **Feel** Feel the quadriceps for wasting and palpate the knee for warmth. Check the joint line, collateral ligaments, tibial tubercle, and femoral epicondyles for tenderness. Palpate the popliteal fossa for a Baker's cyst. Check for an effusion. Test for patellofemoral lesions by sliding the patella sideways across the underlying femoral condyles
- **Move** With the patient lying on his back check active and passive range of movement—pain reproduced on movement? Crepitus? Test the medial and lateral collateral ligaments and cruciate ligaments
- **Measure** Quadriceps diameter 18cm up from the joint line in adults

❶ Knee pain can be referred from the hip so examine the hip as well.

Osteoarthritis of the knee Very common; X-ray evidence of OA is even more common. *Treatment:* education; glucosamine; analgesia (paracetamol ± NSAIDs); exercise (refer to physiotherapy). Suggest using a walking stick. Steroid injection can be helpful in some patients. If pain and disability are severe (e.g. Oxford Knee Score ≤16), refer to orthopaedics for consideration of total or partial knee replacement. Knee replacement is a very successful procedure resulting in ↓ pain and ↑ mobility. 95% prostheses last >10y.

Infection of the knee joint Most commonly infected joint. *Signs:* hot, red, swollen, painful knee. *Differential diagnosis:* Reiter's disease, gout, pseudogout, traumatic effusion, RA. If infection is suspected refer as an emergency to rheumatology or orthopaedics for investigation. ❶ Do not give antibiotics until the joint has been aspirated.

Non-traumatic knee effusion *Common causes:* gout, RA, calcium pyrophosphate dehydrate disease (pseudogout), spondylarthropathies (including reactive arthritis). Consider FBC, ESR, rheumatoid factor, anti-nuclear antibody, LFTs, bone biochemistry, and thyroid function tests. Drain effusion (or refer to rheumatology to drain) and send fluid for polarized light miscroscopy (for crystals) and microbiology (?infection).

Management If no infection, inject with long-acting steroid (📖 p. 164). If recurrent and no cause found, refer to rheumatology.

Table 15.6 Oxford Knee Score

1. **During the past 4 weeks**...How would you describe the pain you <u>usually</u> have from your knee?

None (4)   Very mild (3)   Mild (2)   Moderate (1)   Severe (0)

2. **During the past 4 weeks**...Have you had any trouble with washing and drying yourself (all over) <u>because of your knee?</u>

| No trouble at all (4) | Very little trouble (3) | Moderate trouble (2) | Extreme difficulty (1) | Impossible to do (0) |

3. **During the past 4 weeks**...Have you had any trouble getting in and out of a car or using public transport <u>because of your knee?</u> (whichever you tend to use)

| No trouble at all (4) | Very little trouble (3) | Moderate trouble (2) | Extreme difficulty (1) | Impossible to do (0) |

4. **During the past 4 weeks**...For how long have you been able to walk before <u>pain in your knee</u> becomes **severe** (with or without a stick)?

| No pain/ for ≥60 min (4) | 16–30 min (3) | 5–15 min (2) | Around the house only (1) | Not at all (0) |

5. **During the past 4 weeks**...After a meal (sat at a table), how painful has it been for you to stand up from a chair <u>because of your knee?</u>

| Not at all painful (4) | Slightly painful (3) | Moderately painful (2) | Very painful (1) | Unbearable (0) |

6. **During the past 4 weeks**...Have you been limping when walking, <u>because of your knee?</u>

| Rarely/never (4) | Sometimes or just at first (3) | Often, not just at first (2) | Most of the time (1) | All of the time (0) |

7. **During the past 4 weeks**...Could you kneel down and get up again afterwards?

| Yes, easily (4) | With little difficulty (3) | With moderate difficulty (2) | With extreme difficulty (1) | No, impossible (0) |

8. **During the past 4 weeks**...Have you been troubled by <u>pain from your knee</u> in bed at night?

No nights (4) 1 or 2 nights (3) Some nights (2) Most nights (1) Every night (0)

9. **During the past 4 weeks**...How much has <u>pain from your knee</u> interfered with your usual work (including housework)?

Not at all (4)   A little bit (3)   Moderately (2)   Greatly (1)   Totally (0)

10. **During the past 4 weeks**...Have you felt that your knee might suddenly 'give way' or let you down?

| Rarely/never (4) | Sometimes or just at first (3) | Often, not just at first (2) | Most of the time (1) | All of the time (0) |

11. **During the past 4 weeks**...Could you do the household shopping <u>on your own?</u>

| Yes, easily (4) | With little difficulty (3) | With moderate difficulty (2) | With extreme difficulty (1) | No, impossible (0) |

12. **During the past 4 weeks**...Could you walk down one flight of stairs?

| Yes, easily (4) | With little difficulty (3) | With moderate difficulty (2) | With extreme difficulty (1) | No, impossible (0) |

Reproduced with permission from Isis Innovation Limited, 1998.

Bipartite patella Detected on X-ray. Usually asymptomatic incidental finding but can cause pain due to excessive mobility of a patella fragment. If troublesome refer for fragment excision.

Patellar dislocation Lateral dislocation of the patella and tearing of the medial capsule/quadriceps can occur due to trauma. More common in young people and if joint hypermobility syndrome. Patient is in pain and unable to flex knee. Refer via A&E or orthopaedics for reduction.

Recurrent subluxation of the patella Medial knee pain + knee 'gives way' due to lateral subluxation of the patella. Most common in girls with valgus knees. *Associations:* familial, hypermobility, high-riding patella. *Signs:*↑ lateral patella movement and +ve apprehension test (pain and reflex contraction of quadriceps on lateral patella pressure). Refer to physiotherapy for vastus medialis exercises. If that is unhelpful, refer to rheumatology to exclude a hereditary connective tissue disorder and/or to orthopaedics for consideration of lateral retinacular release.

Patella tendinitis Small tear in the patella tendon causes pain. Most commonly seen in athletes. Differential includes inferior patellar pole enthesitis (spondylarthropathies), fat-pad syndrome, anterior cartilage lesion, and bursitis. Diagnosis is with USS. Treatment is with rest, NSAIDs ± steroid injection around (not into) the tendon.

Bursitis Prepatellar bursitis (housemaid's knee) is associated with excess kneeling. Vicar's knee (infrapatellar bursitis) is associated with upright kneeling. Avoid aggravating activity, aspirate ± steroid injection (↓ recurrence). If infected treat with antibiotics ± refer for drainage.

Baker's cyst Popliteal cyst (herniation of joint synovium) can cause swelling and discomfort behind the knee. Usually caused by a degenerative knee. Rupture may result in pain and swelling in the calf mimicking DVT. Treat underlying knee synovitis. Surgical cyst removal may be necessary if persistent problems. *W.M. Baker (1839–96)—English surgeon.*

Collateral ligament injury Common in contact sports. Causes knee effusion if severe ± tenderness over the injured ligament. Collateral ligaments provide lateral stability to the knee. Normally there is <5° of movement—if >5° the ligament may be ruptured. Treat with rest, knee support, analgesia. Refer to orthopaedics if rupture is suspected.

Cruciate ligament injury Cruciate ligaments provide anterior/posterior knee stability. Assessment can be difficult.
- **Anterior cruciate tears** Result from a blow to the back of tibia ± rotation when the foot is fixed on the ground. *Signs:* effusion and +ve drawer test (supine with foot fixed and knee at 90°, pull the tibia forward—test is +ve if the tibia moves forward on the femur)
- **Posterior cruciate tears** Caused, e.g. when the knee hits the dashboard in car accidents. Reverse drawer test is +ve (supine with knee at 90°; apply pressure to push the tibia backwards—test is +ve if the tibia moves backward on the femur)

Management Refer to orthopaedics if suspected. Splinting and then physiotherapy helps most (60%) but some require reconstructive surgery—consider urgent referral if keen sportsman.

Loose bodies in the knee May result in locking of the joint and/or effusion. *Causes:* OA, chip fractures, osteochondritis dissecans, synovial chondromatosis. If problematic refer for removal.

Osteochondritis dissecans Necrosis of articular cartilage and underlying bone. Can cause loose body formation. Cause unknown. Seen in young adults → pain after exercise and intermittent knee swelling ± locking. Predisposes to arthritis. Refer for expert management.

Meniscal lesions Twisting with the knee flexed can cause medial (bucket handle) meniscal tears and adduction with internal rotation can cause lateral cartilage tears. *Symptoms/signs:*

- Locking of the knee—extension is limited due to cartilage fragment lodging between the condyles
- Giving way of the knee
- Tender joint line
- +ve McMurray's test—rotation of the tibia on the femur with flexed knee followed by knee extension causes pain and a click, as the trapped cartilage fragment is released. 🔖 Reliability of this test is debated

Management Refer for MRI ± arthroscopy. Treated by removal of the torn meniscal fragment.

Meniscal cyst Pain + swelling over the joint line due to a meniscal tear. Lateral cysts are more common than medial. The knee may click and give way. Refer for arthroscopy—removal of damaged meniscus relieves pain.

 Chondromalacia patellae Common in teenage girls. Pain on walking up or down stairs or on prolonged sitting. *Signs:* pain on stressing the undersurface of the patella. Arthroscopy (indicated only in severe cases) reveals degenerative cartilage on the posterior surface of the patella. Treat with analgesia + physiotherapy (vastus medialis strengthening ↓ pain in 80%). If persistent, exclude spondylarthropathy (📖 p. 518) and refer to orthopaedics for arthroscopy.

Osgood–Schlatter disease Seen in athletic teenagers. Pain and tenderness ± swelling over the tibial tubercle. X-rays not required. Avoid aggravating activities. Usually settles over a few months. If not settling refer to orthopaedics or rheumatology for further assessment. *R.B. Osgood (1873–1956)—US orthopaedic surgeon; C.B. Schlatter (1864–1934)—Swiss physician.*

Bow-legs and knock-knees in children

- **Genu varum (bow-legs)** Outward curving of the tibia usually associated with internal tibial torsion. Except in severe cases always resolves spontaneously. Severe cases raise the possibility of rickets or other rare developmental disorders—refer for orthopaedic opinion.
- **Genu valgum (knock-knees)** Common amongst 2–4y olds. Innocent if symmetrical and independent of any other abnormality. Severe, progressive cases suggest rickets—refer for X-ray.

Further information for patients
Arthritis Research UK ☎ 0300 790 0400 🖥 www.arthritisresearchuk.org
Steps Support for patients with lower limb conditions and their families ☎ 01925 750271 🖥 www.steps-charity.org.uk

Ankle and foot problems

History Trauma; ↑ activity, e.g. walking or running a long way for the patient; feeling of instability; pain/stiffness (relation to weight-bearing; localized/diffuse); deformity (problems getting shoes, shoes wear in odd places, or shoes are always uncomfortable); interference with activities.

Examination Compare one foot with the other:
- **Look** Watch the patient walk normally and on tiptoe. Look at the foot with the patient seated. Check for deformities, the colour of the foot, and any skin/nail changes. Check the shoes for any abnormal patterns of wear (wear is normally under the ball of the foot medially and posterolaterally at the heel)
- **Feel** Is there any tenderness? Palpate any swellings. Check pulses and skin temperature
- **Move** Assess active and passive movements of the ankle, subtalar, mid-tarsal, and toe joints systematically. Check range of movement of joints and pain
- **Neurology** Check sensation if patient reports any loss of sensation

Ankle, foot, and toe fracture p. 1110

Achilles tendonitis Inflammation of the Achilles tendon may be related to overuse or a spondylarthropathy. Presents as a painful local swelling of the tendon. Advise rest. NSAIDs, heel padding, physiotherapy ± steroid injection may help (never inject into the tendon). If persistent refer to rheumatology.

Ruptured Achilles tendon Presents with a sudden pain in the back of the ankle during activity (felt as a 'kick'). The patient walks with a limp. There is some plantar flexion, but the patient cannot raise the affected heel from the floor when standing on tiptoe. A 'gap' can usually be felt in the tendon. Calf squeeze test is −ve (squeezing the calf muscles results in movement of the foot if the Achilles tendon is intact). Refer immediately for consideration of repair. The alternative is immobilization in a splint with the foot plantar flexed.

Pes cavus High foot arches may be idiopathic, due to polio, spina bifida, or other neurological conditions. Toes may claw. Padding under the metatarsal heads relieves pressure. Operative treatment—soft tissue release or arthrodesis—straightens toes. Can lead to tarsal bone OA causing pain—refer for fusion.

Foot drop Patients trip frequently or walk with a high stepping gait. On examination, patients are unable to walk on their heels and cannot dorsiflex their foot. Check ankle jerk. *Causes:*
- Common peroneal palsy, e.g. due to trauma—normal ankle jerk
- Sciatica—ankle jerk absent
- L4, L5 root lesion—ankle jerk may be absent
- Peripheral motor neuropathy, e.g. alcoholic—ankle jerk weak or absent
- Distal myopathy—ankle jerk weak or absent
- Motor neurone disease—↑ ankle jerk

Club foot (talipes) Consists of inversion of the foot, adduction of forefoot relative to hindfoot, and equinus (plantar flexion).

Positional talipes Moulding deformity seen in neonates. The foot can be passively everted and dorsiflexed to the normal position. Treatment is with physiotherapy. Follow-up to check the deformity is resolving.

True talipes The foot *cannot* be passively everted and dorsiflexed to the normal position. Refer to orthopaedics. Treatment is with physiotherapy, splints ± surgery.

Flat feet (pes planus) Low medial arch. All babies and toddlers have flat feet. The arch develops after 2–3y of walking. Persistent flat feet may be familial or due to joint laxity. If pain-free, foot is mobile, and the patient develops an arch on standing on tiptoe ('flexible' foot), no action is required. If painful may be helped by analgesia, exercises, or insoles. For severe pain, hind foot fusion is an option. Refer if the arch does not restore on tiptoeing ('rigid').

In-toe and out-toe gait
- **In-toe** Originates in the femur (persistent anteversion of the femoral neck), tibia (tibial torsion), or foot (metatarsus varus). Does not cause pain or affect mobility. Usually resolves by age 5–6y
- **Out-toe** Common <2y. May be unilateral. Corrects spontaneously

Sever's disease Apophysitis of the heel. *Peak age:* 8–13y. Treated with analgesia, raising the heel of the shoe a little, calf-stretching, and avoiding strenuous activities for a few weeks.

Osteochondritis See Table 15.7.

Syndactyly and polydactyly 📖 p. 487

Table 15.7 Osteochondritis of the foot in children and young adults

	Bone(s) involved	Features	Treatment
Kohler's disease	Navicular bone	*Peak age:* 3–5y Presents with pain and tenderness over the dorsum of the mid-foot X-ray—small navicular bone of ↑ density	Pain usually resolves with simple analgesia and rest
Freiberg's disease	Second and third metatarsal heads	Most common in teenagers and young adults ♀ > ♂ Presents with pain in the foot on walking. The head of the metatarsal is palpable and tender X-ray shows a wide, flat metatarsal	Treatment is usually conservative with cushioning of shoes and simple analgesia. If severe refer to orthopaedics. Excision of the metatarsal head may relieve pain

Tender heel pad Dull throbbing pain under the heel. Develops a few months after heel trauma. May be due to plantar fasciitis, bursitis, or tendinitis. Treat with rest and heel padding. Refer to physiotherapy—ultrasound treatment can help. Blind steroid injections into the fat pad are not recommended. In persistent cases refer to rheumatology.

Plantar fasciitis/bursitis Common cause of inferior heel pain, especially amongst runners. Pain is worst when taking the first few steps after getting out of bed. Usually unilateral and generally settles in <6wk. Advise shoes with arch support, soft heels, and heel padding (e.g. trainers). Achilles tendon-stretching exercises can help; NSAIDs and steroid injection are also helpful. In persistent cases refer to podiatry (for fitting of an insole) ± orthopaedics.

Metatarsalgia (forefoot pain) May be due to synovitis, stress fractures, sesamoid fracture, injury or ↑ pressure on the metatarsal heads due to mechanical dysfunction (e.g. in RA). Treat with insoles and padding under the metatarsal heads. Surgery may be helpful in RA—discuss with rheumatologist.

Morton's metatarsalgia (interdigital neuroma) Pain due to entrapment of the interdigital nerve between the third/fourth metatarsal heads (usually). Gradual onset of sudden attacks of pain or paraesthesia during walking. Refer to orthopaedics. Treatment is with steroid injection and advice on footwear. Some need surgical excision of the neuroma. *T.G. Morton (1835–1903)—US surgeon.*

Hammer and claw toes See Figure 15.2.
- **Hammer toes** Extended MTP joint, hyperflexed PIP joint, and extended DIP joint. Most common in second toes
- **Claw toes** Extended MTP joint, flexion at PIP and DIP joints. Due to imbalance of extensors and flexors (e.g. after polio)

If causing pain or difficulty with walking/footwear, refer for surgery.

Hallux valgus (bunion) Lateral deviation of the big toe at the MTP joint exacerbated by wearing pointed shoes ± high heels. A bunion develops where the MTP joint rubs on footwear. Arthritis at the MTP joint is common. Bunion pads can help but severe deformity requires surgery.

Hallus rigidus Arthritis at first MTP joint causes a stiff, painful big toe. Refer severe cases to podiatrist or orthotist for offloading or custom-made rocker-bottom foot orthoses. Resistant pain requires surgery.

Ingrowing toe nail Most common in the big toe. Ill-fitting shoes and poor nail cutting predispose to the nail growing into the toe skin → pain. The inflamed tissue is prone to infection. Advise about cutting nails (cut straight with edges beyond the flesh). Refer to podiatry. Treat infection with antibiotics (e.g. flucloxacillin 250–500mg qds). If recurrent infection, consider referral for surgery (e.g. wedge resection of the nail).

Information for patients
British Orthopaedic Foot and Ankle Society ℘ www.bofas.org.uk

Hammer toe

Claw toes

Figure 15.2 Hammer and claw toes

Achilles-tendon-stretching exercises

Towel stretch Sit on the floor with your legs stretched out in front of you. Loop a towel around the top of the injured foot. Slowly pull the towel towards you keeping your body straight. Hold for 15–30s then relax—repeat ×10.

Calf/Achilles stretch Stand facing a wall. Place your hands on the wall, chest high. Move the injured heel back and with the foot flat on the floor. Move the other leg forward and slowly lean toward the wall until you feel a gentle stretch through the calf; hold for 15–20s and repeat.

Stair stretch Stand on a step on the balls for your feet, hold the rail or wall for balance. Slowly lower the heel of the injured foot to gently stretch the arch of your foot for 15–20s.

Toe stretch Sit on the floor with knee bent. Pull the toes back on the injured foot until stretch across the arch is felt. Hold for 15–20s and repeat.

Frozen can roll Roll your bare injured foot back and forth from the tip of the toes to the heel over a frozen juice can (not fizzy) or small plastic water bottle. This is a good exercise after activity because it both stretches the plantar fascia and provides cold therapy to the injured area.

Sports medicine

Fitness to perform sporting activities GPs are commonly asked to certify fitness to perform sports. Normally the patient will come with a medical form. If there is a form, request to see it before the medical. If there is no form and you are unsure what to check, telephone the sport's governing body or the event organizer. A fee is payable by the patient.

Many gyms/sports clubs also ask older patients/patients with pre-existing conditions or disabilities to check with their GP before they will sign them on. Assuming that a suitable regime is undertaken most people can participate. Consider the patient's baseline fitness, check BP and medications and recommend gradual introduction to new forms of exercise.

❶ Remember—signing a form may result in legal action against you should the patient NOT be fit to undertake an activity. Where possible, include a caveat, e.g. 'based on information available in the medical notes the patient appears to be fit to... although it is impossible to guarantee this.' If unsure, consult your local LMC/medical defence organization.

⚠ **Hypertrophic obstructive cardiomyopathy** Can cause sudden death during sport. It is difficult to exclude on clinical examination—if there is a FH or systolic murmur, refer to cardiology before recommending new intense activity.

Benefits of exercise 📖 p. 180

> **Children and sport**
> - Exercise is good for children—it stimulates development of the musculoskeletal and cardiovascular systems
> - It should be fun and not physically or emotionally over-demanding
> - Children are more prone to sports injuries due to continuing growth (bone growth plates are prone to damage) but are more flexible so have ↓ injury rate
> - Children's temperature control is not as good as adults
> - Equipment must be checked regularly to ensure it fits
> - Encourage warm up and stretching exercises before sport
> - Refer children with suspected overuse or sports injuries, that do not recover rapidly with simple analgesia, for specialist assessment

Nutrition Recommend a normal varied diet (📖 p. 174).
- **Special circumstances** Particular sports have special requirements (e.g. ↑ protein for strength athletes); increasing muscle glycogen stores before exercise can ↓ fatigue during prolonged heavy exercise, e.g. 'carbohydrate loading'—3–4d of ↑ carbohydrate (8–10g/kg body weight) and a carbohydrate meal 3–4h before competing
- **Fluids** Sufficient fluid during exercise is vital to good performance and health especially in hot conditions. Rehydration fluids containing carbohydrate and electrolytes are absorbed faster than plain water
- **Supplements** (e.g. vitamins, minerals, amino acids, carnitine, creatine) A good diet generally supplies sufficient nutrients

Drugs and sport Most regulating bodies have strict codes regarding drug use. Regulations may differ between different sports. Status of a particular medicine may be checked in the Global Drug Reference Online (℘ www.globaldro.com).

Prohibited classes of drugs
- **Stimulants**—e.g. amphetamine, caffeine (above 12micrograms/mL), ephedrine, certain β_2-agonists (inhaled medication for asthma is allowed)
- **Narcotics**—e.g. morphine, diamorphine, pethidine, methadone (codeine is allowed)
- **Anabolic agents**—e.g. nandrolone, DHEA, testosterone
- **Diuretics**—e.g. furosemide, bendroflumethiazide
- **Hormones, hormone antagonists, and related substances**—e.g. growth hormone, erythropoietin
- **Cannabinoids**

Classes of drugs subjected to restrictions
- **Alcohol and marijuana** Restricted in certain sports
- **Local anaesthetics** Local or intra-articular injections only are allowed (provide written notification of administration)
- **Corticosteroids** Topical, inhaled, or local/intra-articular injections only are allowed (provide written notification of administration)
- **β-blockers**—Restricted in certain sports

Drugs for pain relief Generally paracetamol, all NSAIDs, and codeine are allowed for pain relief. Stronger opioids and drugs containing caffeine are banned. If in doubt, check on the Global Drug Reference before prescribing.

Anabolic steroid misuse Significant problem in the UK (5% in gyms and fitness clubs). Drugs are often used in complicated regimes at high doses to ↑ lean muscle mass and ↓ body fat. *Side effects include:*
- ↑ cholesterol
- ↑ BP
- Gynaecomastia
- ↑ LFTs
- Testicular atrophy
- Baldness
- Acne
- Mood changes

❶ Other drugs may be taken in conjunction with anabolic steroids to ↓ these side effects.

⚠ Doctors who prescribe or collude in the provision of drugs or treatment with the intention of improperly enhancing an individual's performance in sport, risk losing their GMC registration. This does not preclude the provision of any care or treatment where the doctor's intention is to protect or improve the patient's health.

Further information
UKAD Antidoping in Sport ℘ www.ukad.org.uk
Global Drug Reference Online ℘ www.globaldro.com
British Association of Sport and Exercise Medicine ℘ www.basem.co.uk
MacAuley D (2012) *Oxford Handbook of Sports and Exercise Medicine* (2nd edn). Oxford: Oxford University Press. ISBN: 0199660158

Management of sporting injuries

Principles of managing sporting injuries
- **First aid** (**A**irway, **B**reathing, **C**irculation). Refer severe injuries to A&E.
- **R I C E**
  - **Rest** Relative rest of affected part whilst continuing other activities to maintain overall fitness
  - **Ice and analgesia** Use immediately after injury (wrap ice in a towel and use for maximum 10min at a time to prevent acute cold injury)
  - **Compression** Taping or strapping can be used to treat (↓ swelling) and also to prevent acute sprains and strains
  - **Elevation** ↓ local swelling and dependent oedema, enabling quicker recovery
- **Confirm the diagnosis** Clinical examination, X-ray
- **Early treatment** According to cause. Do not delay
- **Liaise** With sports physician, sports physio, and coach if elite athlete
- **Rehabilitation** Regaining fitness, strength, and flexibility, examine and correct the cause of the injury (e.g. poor technique, equipment)
- **Graded return to activity** Discuss with coach
- **Prevention** Suitable preparation and training (e.g. suitable footwear, warm-up and warm-down exercises, safety equipment) can ↓ likelihood of injuries

Muscle injuries
- **Haematoma** Within or between muscles can → dramatic whole limb bruising (due to tracking of blood) and stiffness. Treat with RICE regime, encourage movement in pain-free range
- **Strain** (e.g. hamstring injury) Refer to physiotherapy. A secondary injury is likely if the patient returns to sport too soon

Ligament injuries (sprains)
- **Grade 1** Local tenderness, normal joint movement. Give NSAIDs, support strain, encourage mobilization
- **Grade 2** Slightly abnormal joint movement. More joint protection, NSAIDs, elevate limb, encourage middle of the range movement
- **Grade 3** Abnormal joint movement. Refer to orthopaedics

Groin pain in athletes Consider:
- Conjoint tendon pathology (Gilmour's groin)
- Symphysitis (footballers notably), and
- Adductor tendonitis

Liaise with a sports medicine physician or physiotherapist early.

Overuse injuries Incidence is increasing due to increasingly intensive training regimes, especially in young adults—even amongst amateurs.
- **Causes** Load too great for conditions, poor technique or posture, faulty or poor-quality equipment
- **Types of injury** Stress fractures, joint tenderness or effusion, ligament and tendon strains, muscle stiffness

- **Management** Rest, NSAIDs, physiotherapy, improved training regime
- **Prevention** Recognize and correct poor posture or technique, check equipment is appropriate and fits, warm-up and stretching before exercise, gradually ↑ intensity and duration of training

Shin splints Exercise-related shin pain may be due to a stress fracture of the tibia, compartment syndrome, or periostitis. Fractures are not always seen on X-ray—bone scan is more sensitive and shows periostitis. Treat with rest and analgesia. Consider referral to sports physiotherapist.

Iliotibial tract syndrome Pain due to inflammation of the synovium under the iliotibial tract from rubbing of the tract on the lateral femoral condyle. Seen in runners. Treat with rest, NSAIDs, specialist physiotherapy ± steroid injection.

Over-training syndrome Poor performance, fatigue, heavy muscles, and depression due to excessive sports training or competing without sufficient rest. Usually diagnosed from history. Exclude other causes of fatigue (📖 p. 528). Manage with rest, reassurance, and alteration of training programme.

'Scrumpox' (herpes gladiatorum) Herpes simplex virus is very contagious and outbreaks among sporting teams are common, e.g. spread by close contact and facial stubble grazes whilst scrumming. *Treatment:* aciclovir (cream or tablets) and exclusion of infected players. Impetigo, erysipelas, and tinea barbae can be transmitted in the same way.

Environmental factors
- **Heat cramps** Painful spasm of heavily exercised muscles (calves and feet)—due to salt depletion. *Treatment:* rest, massage of affected muscle, and fluid and salt replacement (e.g. Dioralyte®)
- **Heat stroke/exhaustion** Exercising in excessive heat → salt and water depletion, dehydration, and metabolite accumulation. *Signs:* headache, nausea, confusion, incoordination, cramps, weakness, dizziness, and malaise. Eventually thermoregulatory mechanisms fail → seizures and coma. *Signs:* flushing, sweating, and dehydration. Temperature may be normal (mild cases) or ↑. *Treatment:* rest, fluid and salt replacement (e.g. Dioralyte®). Admission for IV fluids and supportive measures in severe cases
- **Hypothermia** Ensure appropriate clothing and limit time in the cold *Signs:* behaviour change, incoordination, clouding of consciousness *Treatment:* remove from cold environment, wrap in blankets (including the head), and transfer to hospital. Do not use direct heat
- **Frost bite** Freezing of the peripheries (usually feet, hands, ears, or nose). Tissues become hard, insensitive, and white. *Treatment:* gentle re-warming. Refer if significant dead tissue. Debridement is usually delayed to allow natural recovery
- **Diving** Decompression illness is due to rapid ascent causing nitrogen dissolved in blood to form gas bubbles. Usually <1–36h after surfacing. *Presentation:* deep muscle aches, joint pains, skin pain, paraesthesia, itching and burning, retrosternal pain, cough and breathlessness, neurological symptoms. Refer suspected cases urgently to A&E

Bone disorders

Osteogenesis imperfecta Inherited condition with autosomal dominant inheritance (rarely recessive). Several types but all have an underlying problem with collagen metabolism resulting in fragile bones that break easily. Other features include lax joints, thin skin, blue sclerae, hypoplastic teeth, and deafness. Presentation varies according to severity. May be obvious at birth or present early with fractures. Less severe cases present later and may be mistaken for NAI. Mild cases may not present until adolescence with thin bones on X-ray. Treatment is supportive.

Osteopetrosis (marble bone disease) Inherited condition with autosomal dominant or recessive inheritance. Dominant form presents in childhood with fractures, osteomyelitis ± facial paralysis. Recessive form is more severe causing bone marrow failure and death. Bone marrow transplantation has been tried but is of limited success.

Paget's disease of bone Abnormal osteoclast activity causes accelerated disorganized bone remodelling. Affects 1–2% of UK adults; 15% have a FH. ♂:♀≈ 3:1. Most common in the elderly—only a minority are symptomatic. Affects just one bone in 1 in 3 cases.

Presentation Pain—dull ache aggravated by weight-bearing often remains at rest; deformity—bowing of weight-bearing bones, especially tibia (sabre), femur, and forearm usually asymmetrical; frontal bossing of the forehead; distinctive changes on X-ray; ↑ bone-specific alk phos; normal Ca^{2+}, PO_4^{3-}, and PTH.

Management Refer to rheumatology. Give analgesia. Oral/IV bisphosphonates ↓ pain and long-term complications. *Complications:* pathological fracture; OA of adjacent joints; high-output CCF; hydrocephalus and/or cranial nerve compression → neurological symptoms, e.g. deafness; spinal stenosis; bone sarcoma (rare—0.1–1.15%).

Osteomyelitis Infection of bone. May spread from abscesses or follow surgery. Often no primary site is found. More common in those with DM, sickle cell disease, impaired immunity, and/or poor living standards. *Organisms involved:* S. aureus, streptococci, E. coli, Salmonella, Proteus, and Pseudomonas species, TB. Presents with pain, unwillingness to move affected part, warmth, effusions in neighbouring joints, fever, and malaise. Blood cultures are +ve in 60%; ↑ ESR/CRP; ↑ WCC.

Management Refer suspected cases for same-day orthopaedic opinion. Diagnosis is confirmed with imaging, e.g. MRI or bone scan (X-ray changes can take days to appear). *Treatment:* is with IV then po antibiotics (≥6wk) and surgery to drain abscesses. *Complications:* septic arthritis, pathological fracture, deformity of growing bone, chronic infection.

Chronic osteomyelitis Occurs after delayed/inadequate treatment of acute osteomyelitis. *Signs:* pain, fever, and discharge of pus from sinuses. Follows a relapsing/remitting course over years. Needs specialist management.

Referral guidelines for suspected sarcoma[N]

Refer for immediate X-ray Any patient with suspected spontaneous fracture. If the X-ray:
- Indicates possible bone cancer, refer urgently
- Is normal but symptoms persist, follow up and/or request repeat X-ray, bone function tests, or referral

Refer urgently If a patient presents with a palpable lump that is:
- >5cm in diameter
- Increasing in size
- Deep to fascia, fixed, or immobile
- Painful
- A recurrence after previous excision

❶ If a patient has HIV, consider Kaposi's sarcoma and make an urgent referral if suspected.

Urgently investigate increasing, unexplained, or persistent bone pain or tenderness, particularly pain at rest (and especially if not in the joint), or an unexplained limp. In older people metastases, myeloma or lymphoma, as well as sarcoma, should be considered.

Sarcoma Is cancer of the bone or connective tissue. 2,300 patients/y are diagnosed with sarcoma in the UK, and it causes 1,000 deaths. There are 2 peaks of incidence—1 in teenagers and another in old age. 5 types of sarcoma account for >80% of tumours:

Osteosarcoma and the Ewing's family of tumours Present with aching bone pain, swelling ± pathological fracture. If X-ray is normal, but symptoms persist, consider checking bone function tests, re-X-raying, discussing the patient with a specialist or referral. Treatment involves surgery and chemotherapy. Overall 5y survival is 50–80%.

Adult soft tissue sarcoma of limb or trunk Usually presents with a palpable lump. The most common tumours are leiomyosarcoma, liposarcoma, and synovial sarcoma. Treated with surgery ± radiotherapy (high-grade tumours). Chemotherapy is reserved for palliation.

Kaposi's sarcoma 📖 p. 746

Intra-abdominal sarcoma Usually presents late. Often arises in the retroperitoneum. If possible, surgery is the main treatment. Local relapse is common and often not responsive to cytotoxic therapy.

 Rhabdomyosarcoma Originates from striated muscle. Presents usually in children <2y with a lump. Responds to intensive multi-modal therapy; outlook is generally good (>60% long-term survival).

Further information
NICE Referral guidelines for suspected cancer (2005) 🖳 www.nice.org.uk

Patient information and support
Brittle Bone Society ☎ 01382 204446 🖳 www.brittlebone.org
Paget's Association ☎ 0161 799 4646 🖳 www.paget.org.uk
Sarcoma UK ☎ 020 7250 8271 🖳 www.sarcoma.org.uk

Rickets and osteomalacia

Vitamin D deficiency causes rickets in children and osteomalacia in adults. The body needs ~10 micrograms of vitamin D per day to maintain healthy bones. The body makes its own vitamin D when sunlight falls on the skin in the summer months but a diet with adequate vitamin D is needed to maintain the supply in the winter—especially for people who do not get out or for cultural or religious reasons are completely shielded from the sun by their clothing. For dietary sources of vitamin D and calcium see Tables 15.8 and 15.9.

Clinical features of rickets

- Bone pain/tenderness: arms, legs, spine, pelvis
- Skeletal deformity: bow-legs, pigeon chest (forward projection of the sternum), rachitic rosary (enlarged ends of ribs), asymmetrical/odd-shaped skull due to soft skull bones, spinal deformity (kyphosis, scoliosis), pelvic deformities
- Pathological fracture
- Dental deformities—delayed formation of teeth, holes in enamel, ↑ cavities
- Muscular problems—progressive weakness, ↓ muscle tone, muscle cramps
- Impaired growth → short stature (can be permanent)

Clinical features of osteomalacia

- Bone pain—diffuse, particularly in hips
- Muscle weakness
- Pathological fractures
- Low calcium → perioral numbness, numbness of extremities, hand and feet spasms, and/or arrhythmias

Causes and management

Dietary deficiency (<30nmol/L) Particularly in children with pigmented skin in northern climes. Give vitamin D and Ca^{2+} supplements.

Age-related deficiency (<30nmol/L) Vitamin D metabolism deteriorates with age and many >80y are deficient. Consider giving vitamin D (800iu/d) to all elderly >80y.

Secondary rickets/osteomalacia Due to other disease, e.g. malabsorption, liver disease, renal tubular disorders, or chronic renal failure. Treat underlying cause/supplement Ca^{2+} and vitamin D.

Vitamin D-dependent rickets Rare autosomal recessive inherited disorder resulting in an enzyme deficit in the metabolism of vitamin D. Refer for specialist care. Treated with vitamin D and Ca^{2+} supplements.

Hypophosphataemic rickets (vitamin D-resistant rickets) X-linked dominant trait resulting in ↓ proximal renal tubular resorption of phosphate. Parathyroid hormone and vitamin D levels are normal. Specialist management is needed. Treatment is with phosphate replacement ± calcitriol.

Table 15.8 Approximate vitamin D content of common foods*

Food	Serving	Vitamin D (micrograms)
Margarine	10g (¹/₂oz)	0.8
Eggs	1 size 3	1.1
Cheese	60g (2oz)	0.2
Milk	0.15L (¹/₄ pint)	0.05
Butter	10g (¹/₂oz)	0.1
Fortified cereals	30g (1oz)	0.5
Herring	100g (3¹/₂oz)	16.5
Mackerel	100g (3¹/₂oz)	8
Sardines	100g (3¹/₂oz)	7.5
Tinned tuna	100g (3¹/₂oz)	4
Tinned salmon	100g (3¹/₂oz)	12.5
Kipper	100g (3¹/₂oz)	13.5

*Recommended daily intakes: birth to 50y—5 micrograms; 50 to 70y—10 micrograms; >70y—15 micrograms

Table 15.9 Approximate calcium content of common foods**

Food	Serving	Calcium (mg)
Whole milk	0.2L (¹/₃ pint)	220
Semi-skimmed milk	0.2L (¹/₃ pint)	230
Hard cheese	30g (1oz)	190
Cottage cheese	115g (4oz)	80
Low-fat yoghurt	150g (5oz)	225
Sardines (including bones)	60g (2oz)	310
Brown or white bread	3 large slices	100
Wholemeal bread	3 large slices	55
Baked beans	115g (4oz)	60
Boiled cabbage	115g (4oz)	40

**Recommended daily intakes: birth to 6mo—210mg; 7mo to 1y—270mg; 1 to 3y—500mg; 4 to 8y—800mg; 9 to 18y—1300mg; 19 to 50y—1,000mg; >50y—1,200mg.

Patient information and support

Arthritis Research UK ☎ 0300 790 0400 🖰 www.arthritisresearchuk.org

Osteoporosis

Lifetime risk of osteoporotic fracture is 1:3 in ♀ and 1:5 in ♂ (>200,000 fractures/y in the UK). The main morbidity and financial costs of osteoporosis relate to hip fracture where incidence ↑ steeply >70y. Treatment aims to prevent fracture.

Definitions

- **T-scores** compare bone mineral density (BMD) of the subject with the young adult mean (age 30y)
- **Osteoporosis** is defined as BMD >2.5 standard deviations (SD) below the young adult mean (T-score of −2.5). There is ↑ relative risk of fracture x2–3 for each SD ↓ in BMD
- **Osteopenia** is diagnosed if T-score is between −1 and −2.5
- **Z-scores** compare BMDs of subjects and age-matched normal controls, i.e. they measure whether BMD is normal for the patient's age. They cannot be used to diagnose osteoporosis or osteopenia, but may be useful in young patients to predict osteoporosis risk for the future

Causes Osteoporosis may be 1° or 2° to other medical conditions:

- **Endocrine** Hypogonadism (e.g. premature menopause, anorexia, androgen blockade, taking aromatase inhibitors), hyperthyroidism, hyperparathyroidism, hyperprolactinaemia, Cushing's disease, type 1 DM
- **GI** Coeliac disease or other causes of malabsorption, inflammatory bowel disease, chronic liver disease, chronic pancreatitis
- **Rheumatological** RA, other inflammatory arthropathies
- **Other** Immobility, multiple myeloma, haemoglobinopathy, systemic mastocytosis, CF, COPD, CKD, homocystinuria

Fragility fracture Fracture sustained falling from ≤ standing height—includes vertebral collapse (may not be as a result of a fall). Previous fracture is a risk for future fracture. *Common fractures:*

- **Hip** Associated with ↑ mortality   • **Wrist** Colles' fracture
- **Osteoporotic vertebral collapse** causes pain, ↓ height, and kyphosis. Pain can take 3–6mo to settle and requires strong analgesia. Calcitonin is useful for pain relief for 3mo after vertebral fracture if other analgesics are ineffective

Predicting fracture risk[N] 2 validated fracture risk prediction tools are available: FRAX (available from ℘ www.shef.ac.uk/FRAX) and Qfracture (available from ℘ www.qfracture.org). Qfracture does not require BMD measurement; FRAX can be performed without BMD measurement. Both provide information on 10y probability of hip or other osteoporotic fracture. Case-finding and further actions—see Figure 15.3.

Bone mineral density (BMD) measurement X-rays cannot be used to measure BMD but are useful if vertebral fracture or metastases are suspected. Hip and lumbar spine BMD is measured using dual-energy X-ray absorptiometry (DEXA). Do not request without prior use of a risk prediction tool, e.g. FRAX (without BMD measurement) or Qfracture.

Glucocorticoid use Steroid use is a risk factor for osteoporosis. Minimize steroid dose. For patients taking oral/high-dose inhaled steroids for >3mo or frequent courses of steroids, in addition:

- Add bone protection agent (e.g. bisphosphonate) for patients >65y or with history of fragility fracture, *or*
- Refer patients <65y without history of fragility fracture for DEXA scan and add a bone protection agent if T-score is ≤−1.5

Figure 15.3 Use of fracture risk predction tools

Further information

NICE Fragility fracture risk (2012) ℘ www.nice.org.uk
National Osteoporosis Guideline Group Diagnosis and management of osteoporosis in postmenopausal women and men from the age of 50y (2010) ℘ www.shef.ac.uk/NOGG

Treatment options for osteoporosis

Lifestyle advice Provide to all at-risk patients.

Adequate nutrition
- Maintain body weight so BMI >19kg/m²
- Advise adequate intake of calcium and vitamin D (food rich in calcium and vitamin D—see Tables 15.8 and 15.9, ☐ p. 507)
- Give Ca²⁺ and/or vitamin D supplements to post-menopausal women with dietary deficiency; also consider if on long-term steroids, >80y, housebound, or institutionalized

Regular exercise Weight-bearing activity >30min/d ↓ fracture rate

Stop smoking Women that stop smoking pre-menopause have a 25% ↓ fracture rate post-menopause

↓ alcohol consumption To <21u/wk (♂) or <14u/wk (♀)

Bisphosphonates (e.g. alendronic acid 70mg once weekly) ↓ bone loss and fracture rateᶜ. Mainstay of treatment for osteoporosis. Avoid if severe CKD or woman of child bearing age (possible teratogenic effects).

Instructions for use Take on an empty stomach first thing in the morning, ≥30min before food/other medication; take in an upright position washed down with plenty of water; sit upright for 30min after taking.

Osteonecrosis of the jaw Rare complication of bisphosphonate therapy (IV > po preparations). Causes non-healing gum lesions. The only treatment is surgical excision of the affected bone. Risk of osteonecrosis ↑ after dental work—advise patients to have a dental check-up and any necessary dental work done before starting bisphosphonate treatment, and to report any oral symptoms when on treatment to their dentist.

Atypical femoral fracture Prolonged bisphosphonate treatment >5y → oversuppression of bone turnover and ↑ bone fragility. Acute sub-trochanteric or mid-shaft femoral fractures are most common. ☛ To prevent this, a 'drug holiday' of 1–5y has been proposed for low-risk patients after 5y use—follow local guidance.

Strontium ranelate No longer recommended for 1° or 2° prevention of osteoporosis due to concerns regarding skin/hypersensitivity reactions and ↑ risk of venous thromboembolism and CVD. May still be of benefit for those at high risk of fracture, who have no history of CVD and are intolerant of other medication. Patients taking strontium ranelate should have regular screening/monitoring to exclude CVD.

Raloxifene 60mg od. Selective oestrogen receptor modulator (SERM).
- For patients with previous fragility fracture if bisphosphonates are contraindicated/not tolerated or there is an unsatisfactory response with bisphosphonates (further fracture and/or ↓ in BMD after ≥1y treatment). SERMs are not recommended for primary prevention of osteoporotic fractureᴺ
- Avoid if past history of DVT/PE, cholestasis, endometrial cancer, or undiagnosed vaginal bleeding

Denosumab 60mg sc every 6mo. Monoclonal antibody that ↓ osteoclast activation and ↓ bone resorption.
- For post-menopausal osteoporosis when bisphosphonates are contraindicated/not tolerated and severe osteoporosis[N]
- Can be used for women with severe CKD; correct hypocalcaemia before starting treatment. May cause osteonecrosis of the jaw

HRT (📖 p. 712) Postpones post-menopausal bone loss and ↓ fractures[C]. Optimum duration of use is uncertain (>5–7y) but benefit disappears <5y after stopping. ↑ in breast cancer and cardiovascular risk limits use[R].

> ⚠ *CSM guidance (2003)*
> - **Premature menopause** HRT is recommended for the prevention of osteoporosis until women reach 51y
> - **>51y** HRT should *not* be considered first-line therapy for long-term prevention of osteoporosis. HRT remains an option where other therapies are contraindicated, cannot be tolerated, or if there is a lack of response; risks and benefits should be carefully assessed

Teriparatide Third-line for postmenopausal women and second-line for men with past history of fragility fracture if other treatments are not tolerated/ineffective and specific T-score and clinical criteria are met. Given by daily injection. Maximum duration of use is 18mo. Consider referral for consultant initiation if other treatment options are exhausted.

Osteoporosis in men Currently only bisphosphonates and teriparatide are recommended for treatment of osteoporosis in men.

Monitoring There is no consensus about duration of treatment for osteoporosis or monitoring of BMD during treatment. Circumstances in which repeat DEXA scanning might be necessary include:
- Fragility fracture on treatment
- If considering a change in treatment
- When considering restarting therapy after a drug holiday

Referral Consider referral to an appropriate specialist if:
- Another cause for fragility fracture is suspected (e.g. metastasis)—*U*
- Fragility fracture on treatment—*R*
- Unusual presentation of osteoporosis, e.g. pre-menopausal woman—*R*
- For consideration of treatment with IV bisphosphonate, denosumab, or teriparatide—*R*

U = urgent referral; *R* = routine referral.

Osteopenia If T-score of between −1 and −2.5, provide lifestyle advice. Repeat DEXA scan in ~2y.

Further information

NICE 🖰 www.nice.org.uk
- Osteoporotic fractures—denosumab (2010)
- Alendronic acid, etidronate, risedronate, raloxifene, strontium ranelate and teriparatide for the primary and secondary prevention of osteoporotic fragility fractures in postmenopausal women (2011)

CSM Guidance Further advice on safety of HRT (12/2003)
🖰 www.mca.gov.uk

Osteoarthritis

Osteoarthritis (OA) is the most important cause of locomotor disability. It used to be considered 'wear and tear' of the bone/cartilage of synovial joints but is now recognized as a metabolically active process involving the whole joint—i.e. cartilage, bone, synovium, capsule, and muscle.

The main reason for patients seeking medical help is pain. Level of pain and disability are greatly influenced by the patient's personality, anxiety, depression, and activity, and often do not correlate well with clinical signs.

Risk factors ↑ age (uncommon <45y); ♀ > ♂;↑ in black and Asian populations; genetic predisposition; obesity; abnormal mechanical loading of joint, e.g. instability; poor muscle function; post-meniscectomy; certain occupations, e.g. farming.

Symptoms and signs Joint pain ± stiffness, synovial thickening, deformity, effusion, crepitus, muscle weakness and wasting, and ↓ function. Most commonly affects hip, knee, and base of thumb. Typically exacerbations occur that may last weeks to months. Nodal OA, with swelling of the distal interphalangeal joints (Heberden's nodes), has a familial tendency.

Investigations X-rays may show ↓ joint space, cysts, and sclerosis in subchondral bone, and osteophytes. OA is common and may be a coincidental finding. Exclude other causes of pain, e.g. check FBC and ESR if inflammatory arthritis is suspected (normal or mildly ↑ in OA—ESR >30mm/h suggests RA or psoriatic arthritis).

Management of osteoarthritis in primary care Employ a holistic approach. Assess effect of OA on the patient's functioning, quality of life, occupation, mood, relationships, and leisure activities. Formulate a management plan with the patient that includes self-management strategies, effects of co-morbidities, and regular review.

Information and advice Give information and advice on all relevant aspects of osteoarthritis and its management. Arthritis Research UK produces a range of leaflets for patients. Use the whole multidisciplinary team, e.g. refer to:
• Physiotherapist for advice on exercises, strapping, and splints
• OT for aids
• Chiropodist for foot care and insoles
• Social worker for advice on disability benefits and housing
• Orthopaedics for surgery if significant disability/night pain

↓ **load on the joint** Weight reduction can ↓ symptoms and may ↓ progression in knee OA. Using a walking stick in the opposite hand to the affected hip and cushioned insoles/shoes (e.g. trainers) can also help.

Exercise and improving muscle strength ↓ pain and disability, e.g. walking (for OA knee), swimming (for OA back and hip but may make neck worse), cycling (for OA hip or knee but may worsen patellofemoral OA). Refer to physiotherapy for advice on exercises especially isometric exercises for the less mobile.

Pain control
- Use non-pharmacological methods first (activity, exercise, weight ↓, footwear modification, walking stick, TENS, local heat/cold treatments)
- Regular paracetamol (1g qds) is first-line drug treatment for all OA and/or topical NSAIDs for knee/hand OA only. Topical NSAIDs have less side effects than oral NSAIDs and are more acceptable to patients
- Use opioids, oral NSAIDs, or COX2 inhibitors as second-line agents in addition to, or instead of paracetamol. Use the lowest effective dose for the shortest possible time. Co-prescribe a proton pump inhibitor (e.g. omeprazole 20mg od) with NSAIDs
- Low-dose antidepressants, e.g. amitriptyline 10–75mg nocte (unlicensed), are a useful adjunct especially for pain causing sleep disturbance
- Capsaicin cream can also be helpful for knee/hand OA[N]

Aspiration of joint effusions and joint injections Can help in exacerbations. Some patients respond well to long-acting steroid injections—it may be worth considering a trial of a single treatment. Hyaluronic acid knee injections are not recommended by NICE.

Complementary therapies ~60% of sufferers from OA are thought to use CAM, e.g. copper bracelets, acupuncture, food supplements, dietary manipulation. There is good evidence chiropractic/osteopathy can be helpful for back pain, but otherwise evidence of effectiveness is scanty. Advise patients to find a reputable practitioner with accredited training who is a member of a recognized professional body and carries professional indemnity insurance.

☞ Other drugs/supplements
- **Glucosamine** It is controversial whether glucosamine modifies OA progression. It is available OTC but not recommended by NICE
- **Strontium ranelate** ↓ progression of OA, ↓ pain, and ↑ mobility[R]. Place in OA management is yet to be determined

Psychological factors have a major impact on the disability from OA. Education about the disease, and emphasis that it is not progressive in most people, is important. Seek and treat depression and anxiety with screening tools—📖 p. 199

Refer
- **To rheumatology** To confirm diagnosis if coexistent psoriasis (psoriatic arthritis mimics OA and can be missed by radiologists); rule out 2° causes of OA (e.g. pseudogout, haemochromatosis) if young OA or odd distribution; if joint injection is thought worthwhile but you lack expertise or confidence to do it
- **To orthopaedics** If symptoms are severe for joint replacement. Refer as an emergency if you suspect joint sepsis

Further information
NICE Osteoarthritis: the care and management of osteoarthritis in adults (2008) ॐ www.nice.org.uk

Information and support for patients
Arthritis Research UK ☎ 0300 790 0400 ॐ www.arthritisresearchuk.org
Arthritis Care ☎ 0808 800 4050 ॐ www.arthritiscare.org.uk

Rheumatoid arthritis

Rheumatoid arthritis (RA) is the most common disorder of connective tissue affecting ~1% of the UK population. It is an immunological disease, triggered by environmental factors, in patients with genetic predisposition. Disease course is variable with exacerbations and remissions.

⚠ Refer all suspected cases of rheumatoid arthritis to rheumatology—early treatment with disease-modifying drugs can significantly alter disease progression. Refer urgently[N] if:
- Small joints of the hands/feet are affected
- >1 joint is affected
- There has been a delay of ≥3mo between onset of symptoms and seeking medical advice

Presentation
- Can present at any age—most common in middle age. ♀:♂ ≈3:1
- Variable onset—often gradual but may be acute
- Usually starts with symmetrical small joint involvement—i.e. pain, stiffness, swelling, and functional loss (especially in the hands); joint damage and deformity occur later
- Irreversible damage occurs early if untreated and can → deformity and joint instability
- Other presentations—monoarthritis, migratory (palindromic) arthritis; PMR-like illness; systemic illness of malaise, pain, and stiffness

Symptoms and signs Predominantly peripheral joints are affected—symmetrical joint pain, effusions, soft tissue swelling, early morning stiffness. Progression to joint destruction and deformity. Tendons may rupture. Specific features—see Table 15.10.

Differential diagnosis Diagnosis may not be easy—consider:
- Psoriatic arthritis
- Nodal OA
- SLE (especially in ♀ <50y)
- Bilateral carpal tunnel syndrome
- Other connective tissue disorders
- Polymyalgia rheumatica if >50y

Investigations
- Check FBC (normochromic, normocytic or hypochromic, microcytic anaemia), ESR and/or CRP (↑). May have ↑ platelets, ↓ WCC
- Rheumatoid factor and anti-CCP antibodies are +ve in the majority. A minority have a +ve ANA titre
- X-rays—normal, periarticular osteoporosis or soft tissue swelling in the early stages; later—loss of joint space, erosions, and joint destruction

Management A multidisciplinary team approach is ideal, e.g. GP, medical and surgical teams, physiotherapist, podiatrist, OT, nurse specialist and social worker.

Screening for depression 📖 p. 199.

General support Provision of information about the disease, treatments, and support available (including equipment and help with everyday activities, self-help and carers groups, disabled parking badges, financial support—📖 p. 222).

Physical therapy Exercises, splints, appliances, and strapping help to keep joints mobile, ↓ pain, and preserve function.

Table 15.10 Specific features of rheumatoid arthritis

Hands	• Ulnar deviation of the fingers • 'z' deformity of the thumb • Swan neck (hyperextended PIP and flexed DIP joints) and boutonnière (flexed PIP and extended MCP joints, hyperextended DIP joint) deformities of the fingers (see Figure 15.4) • ↓ grip strength and ↓ hand function causes disability
Legs and feet	• Subluxation of the metatarsal heads in feet and claw toes → pain on walking • Baker's cysts (🔲 p. 494) at the knee may rupture mimicking DVT
Spine	Especially cervical spine—causing neck pain, cervical subluxation, and atlanto-axial instability leading to a risk of cord compression. X-rays are required prior to general anaesthesia
Non-articular features	• Common. Weight ↓, fever, malaise • **Rheumatoid nodules** (especially extensor surfaces of forearms) • **Vasculitis**—digital infarction, skin ulcers, mononeuritis • **Eye**—Sjögren's syndrome, episcleritis, scleritits • **Lungs**—pleural effusions, fibrosing alveolitis, nodules • **Heart**—pericarditis, mitral valve disease, conduction defects • **Skin**—palmar erythema, vasculitis, rashes • **Neurological**—nerve entrapment, e.g. carpal tunnel syndrome, mononeuritis, and peripheral neuropathy • **Felty's syndrome** Combination of RA, splenomegaly, and leucopenia. Occurs in patients with long-standing RA. Recurrent infections are common. Hypersplenism → anaemia and thrombocytopenia. Associated with lymphadenopathy, pigmentation, and persistent skin ulcers. Splenectomy may improve the neutropenia

C-reactive protein (CRP) Acute phase protein that ↑ ≤6h after an acute event. Follows clinical state more rapidly than ESR (🔲 p. 665). Not ↑ by SLE, leukaemia, UC, pregnancy, OA, anaemia, polycythaemia, or heart failure. Highest levels are seen in bacterial infections (>10mg/L).

Figure 15.4 Boutonnière and swan neck deformities of the fingers

Information and support for patients
Arthritis Research UK 📞 0300 790 0400 🔗 www.arthritisresearchuk.org
Arthritis Care 📞 0808 800 4050 🔗 www.arthritiscare.org.uk

Medication

NSAIDs and simple analgesics (e.g. regular paracetamol). Provide symptomatic relief but do not alter the course of disease. Patients' response to NSAIDs is individual—start with the least gastric-toxic, e.g. ibuprofen 200–400mg tds and alter as necessary, e.g. to naproxen 500mg bd. If the patient has a history of indigestion/gastric problems consider adding gastric protection, e.g. PPI, or, if there is no history of CVD, using a COX2 inhibitor, e.g. celecoxib 100mg bd.

Corticosteroids Intra-articular injections of steroids (e.g. triamcinolone) can settle localized flares (e.g. knee or shoulder) and can be used up to 3x/y in any particular joint. Depot IM injections or IV infusions (pulses) can also help to settle an acute flare but offer short-term benefits with the risk of systemic side effects. Daily low-dose oral steroids help symptoms and there is some evidence that they can modify disease progression, but concerns about adverse side effects have limited use.

Disease-modifying drugs (DMARDs)

- Methotrexate
- Sulfasalazine
- Penicillamine
- Gold
- Azathioprine
- Leflunomide
- Hydroxychloroquine
- Ciclosporin
- Cyclophosphamide
- Biologic therapies, e.g. rituximab, infliximab, etanercept, adalimumab

Use only under consultant supervision. ↓ disease progression by modifying the immune response and inflammation. Used individually or in combination, they are now started very early in the disease (i.e. first 3–6 mo)—hence the need for early referral. DMARDs can take several months to show any effect. Before starting check baseline U&E, Cr, eGFR, LFTs, FBC, and urinalysis. Side effects and monitoring—see Table 15.11.

⚠ *Results requiring action*

- Total WBC <3.5 x 10⁹/L
- Neutrophils <2 x 10⁹/L
- Persistent proteinuria (>1+ x2) or haematuria
- Platelets <150 x 10⁹/L
- LFTs (ALT/AST) >2x baseline

Discuss with rheumatologist ± stop medication

Surgery Aims to relieve pain and improve function. Consideration of the risks, benefits, and the most appropriate timing of surgery is vital. Common procedures include: joint fusion, replacement, and excision; tendon transfer and repair; and nerve decompression.

Complications of RA Physical disability, depression, osteoporosis, ↑ infections, lymphoma, cardiovascular disease, amyloidosis (10%), side effects of treatment.

Further information

NICE Rheumatoid arthritis (2009) ℘ www.nice.org.uk
British Society for Rheumatology ℘ www.rheumatology.org.uk
- Guidelines for DMARD therapy (2008)
- Management of RA (after first 2 years) (2009)
BNF ℘ www.bnf.org
Primary Care Rheumatology Society ℘ www.pcrsociety.org.uk

Table 15.11 Specific disease-modifying drugs—side effects and monitoring

⚠ Before starting, check baseline U&E, Cr, eGFR, LFTs, FBC, and urinalysis.

Drug	Routine monitoring	Side effects to monitor
Methotrexate 7.5–25mg weekly It is common practice to give folic acid 5mg the day after methotrexate (i.e. weekly) as well	FBC, U&E, eGFR, and LFT weekly until dose and monitoring are stable. Then monthly for at least 1y Frequency of monitoring may be ↓ by specialist if disease/ dose stable after 1y CXR within 1y of start of treatment. Check baseline lung function if lung disease	Ask to report symptoms/signs of infection—especially sore throat If severe respiratory symptoms <6mo after starting, refer to A&E If MCV >105fL, check B₁₂/folate

⚠ Advise patients NOT to self-medicate with aspirin or ibuprofen. Avoid alcohol.

Sulfasalazine 1g bd/tds maintenance	FBC and LFT monthly for first 3mo. Then every 3mo Urgent FBC if intercurrent illness during initiation If stable after a year, frequency of monitoring may be ↓ by specialist	Rash (1%) Nausea/diarrhoea—often transient Bone marrow suppression in 1–2% in the first months If MCV >105fL, check B₁₂/folate
Intramuscular gold (Myocrisin®) 50mg monthly	FBC and urinalysis at the time of each injection CXR within 1y of start of treatment	*Ask patients to report:* Symptoms/signs of infection— especially sore throat, bleeding/bruising, breathlessness/cough, mouth ulcers/metallic taste, or rashes
Penicillamine 500–750mg/d maintenance	FBC, urinalysis 2-weekly for 3mo and 1wk after any ↑ dose Then monthly	Altered taste (can be ignored), rash
Azathioprine 1.5–2.5mg/kg/d maintenance	FBC and LFT weekly for 6wk, then every 2wk until dose/ monitoring stable for 6wk Then monthly	GI side effects, rash, bone marrow suppression Avoid live vaccines

⚠ If allopurinol is co-prescribed, ↓ dose to 25% of the original

Ciclosporin 1.25mg/kg bd maintenance	FBC and LFT monthly until dose/monitoring stable for 3mo, then every 3mo U&E, Cr/eGFR every 2wk until dose stable for 3mo, then monthly Lipids 6-monthly	Rash, gum soreness, hirsutism, renal failure/↑ Cr (if ↑ by >30% from baseline, withhold and discuss with rheumatologist), ↑ BP Monitor BP
Hydroxychloroquine 200–400mg/d maintenance	Baseline eye check and annual check of visual symptoms and visual acuity	Rash, GI effects, ocular side effects (rare)
Leflunomide 10–20mg/d maintenance	FBC and LFT monthly for 6mo then, if stable every 2mo	Rash, GI, ↑ BP, ↑ ALT Check weight and BP at each review

The spondylarthropathies

A group of inflammatory rheumatic diseases characterized by predominant involvement of axial and peripheral joints and entheses (areas where tendons, ligaments, or joint capsules attach to bone). Includes:

- Ankylosing spondylitis
- Psoriatic arthritis
- Reactive arthritis and Reiter's syndrome
- Behçet's disease
- Arthritis that accompanies inflammatory bowel disease
- Whipple's disease (📖 p. 407)

Sacroiliitis and spondylitis occur with all of them, and they are all associated with the HLA B27 genotype.

Ankylosing spondylitis (AS) Prevalence 1:2,000. ♂:♀ ≈2½:1. 95% HLA B27 +ve—prevalence in a population mirrors the frequency of the HLA B27 genotype. Risk of developing AS if HLA B27 +ve ≈1:3.

Presentation Typically presents with morning back pain/stiffness in a young man. Progressive spinal fusion (ankylosis) leads to ↓ spinal movement, spinal kyphosis, sacroiliac (SI) joint fusion, neck hyperextension, and neck rotation. *Other features:*

- ↓ chest expansion
- Chest pain
- Hip and knee arthritis
- Plantar fasciitis and other enthesopathies
- Iritis

- Crohn's or UC
- Heart disease—carditis, aortic regurgitation, conduction defects
- Osteoporosis
- Psoriaform rashes

Tests
- **Blood** FBC—normochromic or microcytic hypochromic anaemia, ↑ ESR (may be normal), rheumatoid factor is usually –ve
- **X-ray** Initial signs are widening of the SI joints and marginal sclerosis— later, SI joint fusion and a 'bamboo spine' (vertebral squaring/fusion)

Management Aims to ↓ inflammation, pain, and stiffness; alleviate systemic symptoms, e.g. fatigue; and slow or stop long-term progression of the disease. Exercise helps back pain. NSAIDs (e.g. naproxen 500mg bd) also help pain. Refer to a rheumatologist early for confirmation of diagnosis, education, disease-modifying drugs (📖 p. 517), and advice on appropriate exercise regimes to maintain mobility.

Psoriatic arthritis Inflammatory arthritis associated with psoriasis (~40% psoriasis patients. ♂ = ♀). 75% patients have a pre-existing history of psoriasis before the arthropathy; in 15% the rash appears simultaneously with the joint symptoms; in 10% the arthritis precedes the skin changes. Presentation is variable. Patterns include:
- **Distal arthritis** DIP joint swelling of hands/feet, nail dystrophy ± flexion deformity. Sausage-shaped fingers are characteristic of psoriatic arthritis affecting the hand
- **Rheumatoid-like polyarthropathy** Similar to rheumatoid arthritis but less symmetrical and rheumatoid factor is –ve

- **Mutilans** Associated with severe psoriasis. Erosions in small bones of hands/feet → progressive deformity
- **Ankylosing spondylitis/sacroiliitis** Usually HLA B27 +ve

Investigations WBC—usually ↑; ESR/CRP—usually ↑; rheumatoid factor –ve; X-ray appearances can be diagnostic.

Management Education; physiotherapy; NSAIDs. Refer to rheumatology for confirmation of diagnosis, advice on management, and disease-modifying drugs (📖 p. 517). Medication, e.g. methotrexate, may improve both skin and musculoskeletal symptoms.

Reactive arthritis Often asymmetrical aseptic arthritis in ≥1 joint. Occurs 2–6wk after bacterial infection elsewhere—e.g. gastroenteritis (*Salmonella*, *Campylobacter*), GU infection (chlamydia, gonorrhoea). ↑ incidence in HLA B27 +ve individuals.

Management NSAIDs, physiotherapy, and steroid joint injections. Recovery usually occurs within months. A minority develop chronic arthritis requiring disease-modifying drugs. Refer to rheumatology.

Reiter's syndrome Polyarthropathy, urethritis, iritis, and a psoriaform rash. Affects men with HLA B27 genotype. Commonly follows genito-urinary or bowel infection. Joint and eye changes are often severe. Refer for specialist management. *H.C. Reiter (1881–1969)—German public health physician.*

Behçet's disease Multi-organ disease of unknown cause (although thought to be infective). ♂:♀ ≈ 2:1. *Clinical picture* (only some features): arthritis; ocular symptoms and signs—pain, ↓ vision, floaters, iritis; scarring, painful ulceration of mouth and/or scrotum; colitis; meningoencephalitis. Refer to GUM clinic, ophthalmologist or general physician depending on symptom cluster. Treatment is usually with steroids ± azathioprine or ciclosporin. Topical steroids may be useful for ulcers. *H. Behçet (1889–1948)—Turkish dermatologist.*

Enteropathic spondylarthropathy Oligoarticular or polyarticular arthritis linked to inflammatory bowel disease. Presentation is variable and includes: sacroiliitis, plantar fasciitis, inflammatory spinal pains, and other enthesitides (insertional ligament/tendon inflammation). Arthritis may evolve and relapse/remit independently of bowel disease.

Management NSAIDs may help joint pain but aggravate bowel disease. Refer to rheumatology for confirmation of diagnosis, advice on management, and disease-modifying drugs.

Information and support for patients
National Ankylosing Spondylitis Society (NASS) ☎ 020 8948 9117 🖳 www.nass.co.uk
Psorasis and Psoriatic Arthritis Alliance (PAPAA) ☎ 01923 672837 🖳 www.papaa.org
Arthritis Research UK ☎ 0300 790 0400 🖳 www.arthritisresearchuk.org

Crystal-induced arthritis

Hyperuricaemia Increased serum uric acid. *Causes:*

- **Drugs** Cytotoxics; thiazides; ethambutol
- ↑ **cell turnover** Lymphoma; leukaemia; psoriasis; haemolysis; muscle necrosis
- ↓ **excretion** Primary gout; chronic renal failure; lead nephropathy; hyperparathyroidism

In addition Associated with ↑ BP and hyperlipidaemia. Urate may also be ↑ in disorders of purine synthesis, e.g. Lesch–Nyhan syndrome.

Acute gout Intermittent attacks of acute joint pain due to deposition of uric acid crystals. *Prevalence:* 3–8/1,000. ↑ with age; ♂:♀ ≈5:1. *Predisposing factors:*

- FH
- Obesity
- Excess alcohol intake
- High-purine diet
- Diuretics
- Acute infection
- Ketosis
- Surgery
- Plaque psoriasis
- Polycythaemia
- Leukaemia
- Cytotoxic treatment
- Renal failure

Presentation Painful swollen joint (big toe, feet, and ankles most commonly); red skin which may peel ± fever. Can be polyarticular—especially in elderly ♀. May mimic septic arthritis.

Investigation

- **Blood** ↑ WCC; ↑ ESR; ↑ blood urate (but may be normal)
- **Microscopy of synovial fluid** Not usually required—reveals sodium monourate crystals on polarized light microscopy
- **X-rays** Not usually required—show soft tissue swelling only, unless severe disease when an erosive pattern is seen

Management Resolves in <2wk—often after 2–7d if treated.

- Exclude infection
- Rest and elevate joint—apply ice packs
- NSAIDs are helpful—e.g. naproxen 500mg bd—caution if GI problems
- Alternatively, if NSAIDs are contraindicated, try colchicine 500 micrograms bd, increased slowly to qds until pain is relieved or side effects, e.g. nausea, vomiting, or diarrhoea (max 6mg—do not repeat in <3d)
- Steroid joint injection or IM steroid (e.g. Depo-Medrone® 80–120mg) are also effective

Prevention of further attacks

- ↓ weight; avoid alcohol and purine-rich foods (e.g. offal, red meat, yeast extracts, pulses, and mussels)
- Avoid thiazide diuretics and aspirin
- Consider prophylactic medication if recurrent attacks. First-line treatment is allopurinol 100–300mg daily—wait until 1mo after acute attack and co-prescribe colchicine (500 micrograms bd) or NSAID for first 1–3mo to try to avoid precipitation of another acute attack. Check serum urate level after 2mo—aim for low normal range
- If allopurinol is not effective/not tolerated, febuxostat is an alternative
- Alternatively or in addition try a uricosuric, e.g. sulfinpyrazone

> **❶**
> - Gout may be linked to ↑ risk of hypertension and coronary heart disease—screen patients
> - Refer any patient with gout and kidney stones or recurrent UTI to urology

Chronic gout Recurrent attacks, tophi (urate deposits) in pinna, tendons and joints, and joint damage. Refer to rheumatology.

Calcium pyrophosphate deposition disease (CPPD) Also known as *pseudogout*. Inflammatory arthritis due to deposition of pyrophosphate crystals. Associated with OA, hyperparathyroidism, and haemochromatosis.

Presentation Attacks are less severe than gout and may be difficult to differentiate from other types of arthritis. Knee, wrist, and shoulder are most commonly affected. Acute attacks can be triggered by intercurrent illness and metabolic disturbance.

Investigation Chondrocalcinosis may be seen on X-ray (calcification of articular cartilage). Presence of joint crystals confirms diagnosis.

Management
- Treat acute attacks like acute gout
- A chronic form also occurs—frequently erosive. Refer to rheumatology for confirmation of diagnosis, advice on management and disease-modifying drugs

⚠ **Septic arthritis** This is the most important differential diagnosis for acute gout. It is most common in children <5y old and most commonly affects the hip or knee, but septic arthritis can occur at any age and affect any joint. The patient is usually systemically unwell and holds the affected joint completely still. The joint may be swollen, hot, and tender. This is an orthopaedic emergency—if suspected admit. Treatment is with IV antibiotics ± surgical washout of the joint.

Connective tissue diseases

Group of overlapping diseases that affect many organs and are associated with fever, malaise, chronic (often relapsing/remitting) course, and response to steroids. Often difficult to diagnose.

Systemic lupus erythematosus (SLE) Autoimmune disease with prevalence 1:3,000; ♀:♂ ≈ 9:1. ↑ in Afro-caribbeans and Asians. Onset 15–40y. Presentation—see Table 15.12. There *must* be multisystem involvement.

Investigations Check an autoimmune profile—95% are ANA (anti-nuclear antibody) +ve. *Other immunological abnormalities*—↑ double-stranded DNA, RhF +ve (40%), ↓ complement (C3, C4). *FBC:* ↓ Hb, ↓ WCC, ↑ ESR.

Management Refer to rheumatology. Use NSAIDs for symptom control. Sunscreens protect skin (ACBS). Steroids are the mainstay of treatment of acute flares (always discuss with a rheumatologist). Hydroxychloroquine can improve skin and joint symptoms. Cyclophosphamide, methotrexate, and ciclosporin are also used.

⚠ Sulfonamides and hormonal contraceptives/HRT may worsen SLE.

Drug-induced lupus Occurs with:

- Minocycline
- Isoniazid
- Hydralazine
- Procainamide
- Chlorpromazine
- Sulfasalazine
- Losartan
- Anticonvulsants

Remits slowly when the drug is stopped, but steroids may be needed.

Discoid lupus erythematosus (LE) ♀:♂ ≈2:1. ≥1 well-defined, red, round/oval plaques on the face, scalp, or hands. Scarring may → scalp alopecia and skin hypopigmentation. Internal involvement is not a feature. Confirm with lesion biopsy. Investigate with an autoimmune profile as for SLE. Treat with potent topical steroids and sunscreen. Remission occurs in 40%. 5% develop SLE.

Antiphospholipid syndrome ↑ clotting tendency occurring with SLE or alone. Associated with thrombosis, stroke, migraine, miscarriage, myelitis, MI, and multi-infarct dementia. If suspected start aspirin 150mg od and refer to rheumatology. May need anticoagulation.

Sjögren's syndrome

- **Primary Sjögren's syndrome** Under-recognized cause of fatigue and dryness of skin/mucous membranes (may present with dyspareunia). Often presents with nodal OA. Long-term, associated with lymphoma. Autoimmune profile is characteristic
- **Secondary Sjögren's syndrome** Association of any connective tissue disease (50% have RA) with keratoconjunctivitis sicca (↓ lacrimation → dry eyes) or xerostomia (↓ salivation → dry mouth)

Management Refer to rheumatology. Provide information/support. Use artificial tears for dry eyes. Xerostomia may respond to frequent cool drinks, artificial saliva sprays, e.g. Glandosane®, or sugar-free gum. Inform dentist of the diagnosis. Rashes may respond to antimalarials.

H.S.C. Sjögren (1899–1986)—Swedish ophthalmologist.

Raynaud's syndrome Intermittent digital ischaemia precipitated by cold or emotion. Fingers ache and change colour: pale → blue → red on rewarming. Usually presents <25y of age and is idiopathic. *Prevalence:* 3–20%; ♀ > ♂; often abates at the menopause; 5% develop autoimmune rheumatic disease—mainly scleroderma and SLE.

Differential diagnosis
- Other rheumatology conditions—scleroderma; SLE; RA
- Haematology conditions—leukaemia; polycythaemia; thrombocytosis; cold agglutinins; monoclonal gammopathy; mixed cryoglobulinaemia
- Drugs, e.g. β-blockers
- Thoracic outlet obstruction
- Smoking/arteriosclerosis
- Trauma, e.g. use of vibrating tools

Management Keep warm—woolly socks/gloves/hats in cold weather, hand warmers, stay inside if cold. Avoid drugs that worsen symptoms, e.g. β-blockers. Stop smoking. Nifedipine 10–20mg tds, amlodipine 5mg od, or fluoxetine 20mg od (unlicensed) may help. If associated/severe symptoms. refer to rheumatology (urgently if critical ischaemia—e.g. ulceration/ infarcts on fingers). *A.G.M. Raynaud (1834–1881)—French physician.*

Systemic sclerosis Spectrum of disorders causing fibrosis and skin tightening (scleroderma). Raynaud's is usually present ± ↑ BP, lung fibrosis, GI symptoms, telangiectasia, polyarthritis, and/or myopathy. Provide education/support. Treat symptoms. Early specialist referral is vital. *CREST* (Calcinosis of subcutaneous tissues; Raynaud's; oEsophageal motility problems; Sclerodacyly; and Telangiectasia) has better prognosis.

Table 15.12 Presentation of SLE

System	% of patients	Presenting complaints	
Joints	95	• Arthritis	• Myalgia
		• Arthralgia	• Tenosynovitis
Skin	80	• Photosensitivity	• Hair loss
		• Facial 'butterfly' rash	• Urticaria
		• Vasculitic rash	• Discoid lesions
Lungs	50	• Pleurisy	• Pleural effusion
		• Pneumonitis	• Fibrosing alveolitis
Kidney	50	• Proteinuria	• Glomerulonephritis
		• ↑ BP	• Renal failure
Heart	40	• Pericarditis	• Endocarditis
CNS	15	• Depression	• Fits
		• Psychosis	• Cranial nerve lesions
		• Infarction	
Blood	95	• Anaemia (very common)	• Splenomegaly
		• Thrombocytopenia	
Fatigue	95		

Information and support for patients
Lupus UK ☎ 01708 731251 🖰 www.lupusuk.org.uk
Raynaud's and Scleroderma Association ☎ 01270 872776
🖰 www.raynauds.org.uk
British Sjögren's Association ☎ 0121 478 1133 🖰 www.bssa.uk.net

Polymyalgia and giant cell arteritis

Polymyalgia rheumatica (PMR) and giant cell (or temporal) arteritis (GCA) are two clinical syndromes that are part of the same spectrum. *Key features:*
- Both PMR and GCA affect the elderly (rare <50y); ♀:♂ ≈3:1
- 50% of patients with GCA also have PMR; 15% with PMR have GCA
- Both conditions usually respond rapidly and dramatically to corticosteroids

Presentation Diagnosis is clinical. Both PMR and GCA may present with malaise, anorexia, fever, night sweats, weight ↓, and depression. Check ESR/CRP on presentation.

Diagnosis of PMR A person may be regarded as having PMR if the following criteria are present^G:
- Age >50y; duration >2wk
- Bilateral shoulder or pelvic girdle aching, or both
- Morning stiffness duration of >45min
- Evidence of acute phase response, i.e. ↑ ESR (usually >30mm/h) or ↑ CRP) ❶ Diagnosis can be made without ↑ inflammatory markers if classical clinical picture and rapid response to steroid treatment

Diagnosis of GCA A person may be regarded as having GCA if ≥3 of the following criteria are met^G:
- Age ≥50y
- New headache—unilateral throbbing headache, facial pain, scalp tenderness, e.g. on brushing hair and/or jaw claudication (↑ likelihood of visual symptoms)
- Temporal artery abnormality (tenderness, thickening, ↓ pulsation)
- ↑ ESR >50mm/h (or ↑ CRP)
- Abnormal temporal artery biopsy compatible with GCA

❶ Visual symptoms (amaurosis fugax, diplopia, or sudden loss of vision) are early complications of GCA and may be the presenting feature.

Differential diagnosis

PMR
- Inflammatory arthritis, e.g. RA
- Connective tissue disease/ vasculitis, e.g. SLE
- OA
- Septic arthritis
- Shoulder disease
- Neoplasia, e.g. myeloma
- Occult sepsis, e.g. endocarditis
- Inflammatory myopathy
- Fibromyalgia
- Endocrinopathy/metabolic bone disease

GCA
- Herpes zoster
- Migraine
- Intracranial pathology
- Other causes of acute vision loss, e.g. amaurosis fugax
- Cluster headache
- Cervical spondylosis or other cervical spine disease
- Sinus/ear disease
- TMJ pain
- Connective tissue disease/ vasculitis

Further investigation Intended to exclude other diagnoses:
- Full blood count—normocytic anaemia may be seen in PMR/GCA
- Urea and electrolytes/eGFR
- Liver function tests
- Bone profile
- TFTs
- Creatine kinase
- Dipstick urinalysis
- Protein electrophoresis (also consider urinary Bence Jones protein)
- Rheumatoid factor (consider ANA and anti-CCP antibodies too)
- Consider CXR and/or hip/pelvis/shoulder/cervical spine X-ray

Further management of PMR If typical symptoms/signs management in primary care is appropriate.
- Start prednisolone 15mg od—there should be a rapid response (≥70% ↓ of symptoms in <1wk); if not question the diagnosis. ESR/CRP should return to normal in <4wk
- Continue prednisolone 15mg od for 3wk then ↓ dose to 12.5mg od for 3wk, then 10mg od for 4–6wk, then by 1mg every 4–8wk. Tailor steroid regime to the individual—a longer time at each dose may be needed
- If there is relapse of symptoms, go back to the previous higher dosage
- At the start of treatment give osteoporosis prophylaxis (📖 p. 509) and supply with a steroid card (📖 p. 306)
- Usually 1–2y of treatment is needed. The need for ongoing treatment >2y should prompt referral for specialist assessment

Referral for rheumatology assessment
- Red flag features: prominent systemic features, weight ↓, night pain, neurological signs (urgent referral)
- Symptoms of GCA
- Younger patient <60y
- Chronic onset (over >2mo)
- Lack of shoulder involvement
- Lack of inflammatory stiffness
- Normal or very high ESR/CRP
- Peripheral arthritis or other features of connective tissue/muscle disease
- Treatment dilemmas e.g. incomplete/non-response to steroids; treatment required >2y

Further management of GCA
- Corticosteroids prevent vascular complications, particularly blindness, and rapidly relieve symptoms (70% improvement in <1wk); prescribe prednisolone 40–60mg daily to start immediately if a diagnosis of GCA is suspected
- At the start of treatment give osteoporosis prophylaxis (📖 p. 509) and supply with a steroid card (📖 p. 306)
- Consider starting aspirin 75mg od
- Refer urgently to ophthalmology or rheumatology depending on local referral pathways for temporal artery biopsy and ongoing management (same day if visual symptoms)

❶ Temporal artery biopsy may be –ve even in cases of GCA due to skip lesions. Do not withhold treatment whilst waiting for biopsy—but if the patient has had steroids ≥2wk +ve biopsy is less likely.

Further information

British Society for Rheumatology 🖱 www.rheumatology.org.uk
- Management of polymyalgia rheumatica (2009)
- Management of giant cell arteritis (2010)

Vasculitis

Characterized by inflammation within or around blood vessels ± necrosis. Severity depends on size and site of vessels affected. Systemic vasculitis can be life-threatening. *Causes:*

• Idiopathic (50%)
• Connective tissue disease (e.g. RA, SLE)
• Infection (e.g. rheumatic fever, infective endocarditis, Lyme's disease)
• Drugs (e.g. NSAIDs, antibiotics)
• Neoplasia (e.g. lymphoma, leukaemia)

Presentation Variable—may be confined to the skin or systemic involving joints, kidneys, lungs, gut, and nervous system.

• **Skin signs** Palpable purpura (often painful)—usually on lower legs/buttocks
• **Systemic effects** Fever, night sweats, malaise, weight ↓, myalgia, and arthralgia may occur in all types of vasculitis

Conditions See Table 15.13—many are rare.

Patient information and support

Arthritis Research UK ☎ 0300 790 0400 ♒ www.arthritisresearchuk.org
Vasculitis UK (Stuart Strange Trust) ♒ www.vasculitis-uk.org
European Vasculitis Study Group ♒ www.vasculitis.org
Kawasaki Support Group ☎ 024 7661 2178 ♒ www.kssg.org.uk

Table 15.13 Vasculitic conditions

Condition	Features	Management
Erythema nodosum	📖 p. 596	📖 p. 596
Henoch–Schönlein purpura (HSP)	More common in children than adults; ♂ > ♀ Presents with a purpuric rash over buttocks and extensor surfaces. Platelet count is normal Often follows a respiratory infection *Other features:* urticaria, nephritis, joint pains, abdominal pain (may mimic acute abdomen)	Refer to paediatrics for confirmation of diagnosis Most recover fully without treatment over a few months
Polyarteritis nodosa (PAN)	Uncommon in the UK. ♂:♀ ≈ 4:1 Peak incidence in middle age Multisystem necrotizing vasculitis → aneurysms of medium-sized arteries *Presents with:* tender subcutaneous nodules along the line of arteries, coronary arteritis, ↑ BP, mononeuritis multiplex, renal failure, and gastrointestinal symptoms Sometimes associated with hepatitis B	Refer to rheumatology for angiography to confirm diagnosis and for advice on management Treatment is with control of ↑ BP, high-dose steroids, and cyclophosphamide

(Continued)

Table 15.13 (Cont.)

Condition	Features	Management
Churg–Strauss syndrome	Associated with asthma Affects coronary, pulmonary, cerebral, and splanchnic circulations Skin manifestations and mononeuritis can also occur Diagnosis is based on clinical features and biopsy	Refer for specialist treatment with high-dose prednisolone ± cyclophosphamide Avoid leukotriene receptor agonist drugs for control of asthma as may worsen symptoms
Wegener's granulomatosis	Granulomatous vasculitis Any organ may be involved and symptoms/signs relate to those affected, e.g. mouth ulcers; nasal ulceration with epistaxis/rhinitis; otitis media; cranial nerve lesions; lung symptoms and shadows on CXR; ↑ BP; eye signs (50%) Often long prodrome of 'limited Wegener's granulomatosis'—nasal stuffiness, headaches, hearing difficulties, and nose bleeds	Refer to rheumatology/general medicine for investigation ANCA helps diagnostically and in disease monitoring Treatment is with high-dose steroids, methotrexate, mofetil, and cyclophosphamide
Kawasaki's disease	Predominantly affects children <5y Cause unknown *Diagnosis:* diseases with similar presentations have been excluded *and* ≥5 of: • Fever for ≥5d • Bilateral conjunctivitis • Polymorphous rash • Changes in lips/mouth—red, dry, or cracked lips; strawberry tongue; diffuse redness of mucosa • Changes in extremities: reddening of palms/soles; oedema of hands/feet; peeling of skin of hands, feet, and/or groin • Cervical lymphadenopathy >15mm diameter (usually single and painful) ↑ suspicion if poor response to anti-pyretics	If suspected, refer for urgent paediatric assessment Early treatment (<10d after onset) with IV immunoglobulin and aspirin ↓ incidence and severity of aneurysm formation as well as giving symptom relief *Complications:* Coronary arteritis with formation of aneurysms; accelerated atherosclerosis

Tiredness and chronic fatigue syndrome

Tired all the time Fatigue is common. 1:400 sustained episodes of fatigue generate a GP consultation. GPs see 30 patients/y whose main complaint is fatigue and it may be a 2° symptom in many others. 2% of consultations result in 2° care referral. Almost any disease processes can cause tiredness—whether physical or psychological. Physical causes account for ~9% of cases; 75% have symptoms of emotional distress.

Assessment
- **Onset/duration**—short history/abrupt onset suggest post-viral or DM
- **Pattern of fatigue**—on exertion relieved by rest suggests organic cause; worst in the morning and never goes suggests depression
- **Associated symptoms**—e.g. breathlessness, weight ↓, or anorexia suggest underlying organic disease. Chronic pain may cause fatigue
- **Sleep patterns**—early morning wakening/unrefreshing sleep suggest depression; snoring, pauses of breathing in sleep, and daytime sleepiness suggest sleep apnoea
- **Psychiatric history**—symptoms of depression, anxiety, and stress
- **Alcohol and medication**—including OTC and illicit drugs
- **Patient's worries**—what does the patient think is wrong?
- **Examination**—usually normal

Common organic causes of fatigue in general practice
- Anaemia
- Infections (EBV, CMV, hepatitis)
- DM
- Hypo- or hyperthyroidism
- Perimenopausal
- Asthma
- Carcinomatosis
- Sleep apnoea

Investigation If sustained fatigue with no obvious cause, check:
- **Urine** Dipstick for protein, blood, and glucose
- **Blood** FBC (all children should have FBC/blood film checked on presentation with fatigue[N]); ESR/CRP; U&E, Cr, and eGFR; LFTs and Ca^{2+}; TFTs; random blood glucose; anti-endomysial antibody test (to exclude coeliac disease); CK

 In addition, check serum ferritin if the patient is a child/young person. Do not check ferritin in adults unless FBC suggests iron deficiency.

Use clinical judgement to decide on additional tests to exclude other diagnoses (e.g. serological testing if history suggestive of infection).

Management Treat organic causes. In most no physical cause is found—reassure. Explaining the relationship of psychological and emotional factors to fatigue can help patients deal with symptoms. If lasts >6–12wk and symptoms/signs of depression, consider a trial of antidepressants, e.g. sertraline 50mg od.

Chronic fatigue syndrome (CFS, ME) A debilitating and distressing condition. *Prevalence:* 0.2–2.6%; ♀:♂ ≈3:2. Cause is unknown though viral infections (≈10% after EBV), immunization, chemical toxins (e.g. organophosphates, chemotherapy drugs) have all been implicated.

❶ Fatigue must have been present for ≥4mo for adults and ≥3mo for children and young people for a diagnosis of CFS to be made.

Clinical features Unexplained persistent and/or recurrent fatigue of new/ definite onset, not explained by other conditions and resulting in ↓ activity (often starting 1–2d after mental/physical exertion and lasting >24h) and ≥1 of:

- General malaise
- Dizziness/nausea
- Palpitations without cardiac dysfunction
- Cognitive dysfunction, e.g. impaired concentration/memory
- Tender cervical/axillary LNs without enlargement
- Physical/mental exertion makes symptoms worse
- Headaches of new type, pattern, or severity
- Multi-site muscle/joint pain without inflammation
- Sore throat
- Difficulty with sleeping

Additional symptoms Must not have pre-dated fatigue. Symptoms may fluctuate or change in nature over time. Include:

- Postural dizziness
- Vertigo
- Altered temperature sensation
- Paraesthesiae
- Sensitivity to light/ sound
- Palpitations
- IBS
- Food intolerance
- Fibromyalgia
- Feelings of dyspnoea
- Mood swings
- Panic attacks
- Depression

❶ Infection/immunization, drugs, caffeine, alcohol, and stress cause setbacks.

⚠ Red flag symptoms that suggest another diagnosis

- Significant weight ↓
- Localizing/focal neurological signs
- Signs/symptoms of inflammatory arthritis or connective tissue disease
- Signs/symptoms of cardiorespiratory disease
- Sleep apnoea
- Clinically significant lymphadenopathy

Children presenting with sustained fatigue of any duration with no obvious cause should *always* be referred for paediatric review.

Reconsider diagnosis if none of the following are present Cognitive difficulties; chronic pain; post-exertional fatigue/malaise; sleep disturbance.

Management Provide support and reassurance—explanation, information ± self-help groups. Avoid exacerbating factors, e.g. caffeine, alcohol. Advise graded exercise and regular, limited rest periods (e.g. 30min 4–5x/d). Treat symptoms, e.g. amitriptyline 10–50mg nocte to help sleep ± relieve headache/neuropathic pain; SSRI for depression. Refer adults if severe symptoms or symptoms persist >6mo. Specialist treatments include CBT and rehabilitation programmes.

Prognosis Variable. 55% of adults have symptoms >6mo. Risk ↑ x3 if history of anxiety/depression. Prognosis in children is better.

Further information

NICE Diagnosis and management of CFS/ME in adults and children (2007) ℘ www.nice.org.uk

Information and support for patients

ME Association ☎ 0844 576 5326 ℘ www.meassociation.org.uk
Action for ME ☎ 0845 123 2314 ℘ www.actionforme.org.uk

Miscellaneous conditions

Neuropathic arthritis Charcot's disease is a rapidly progressive degeneration in a joint which lacks position sense and protective pain sensation. Upper limb disease is usually associated with syringomyelia. Lower limb disease is usually associated with diabetic neuropathy or cauda equina lesions. The joint may be very deformed but is usually painless. Treat the underlying condition (e.g. DM). The joint cannot recover, but refer to orthopaedics for advice on stabilization.

Fibromyalgia Painful, non-articular condition of unknown cause, predominantly involving muscles. Fibromyalgia is common and often results in significant disability. Peak age 40–50y—90% female.

Diagnostic criteria

- History of widespread pain (defined as pain on both left and right sides, above and below the waist, together with axial skeletal pain, e.g. neck or back pain), *in combination with:*
- Pain in ≥11 out of 18 tender sites (see Figure 15.5) on digital palpation

Other clinical features

- Clinical findings are unremarkable
- Pain is worsened by stress, cold, and activity and associated with generalized morning stiffness; analgesics, NSAIDs, and local physical treatments are ineffective and may worsen symptoms
- Sleep patterns are poor—patients tend to wake exhausted and complain of poor concentration; anxiety and depression scores are high
- Associated symptoms include unexplained headache, paraesthesiae of hands/feet, urinary frequency, and abdominal symptoms

Investigation Exclude other causes of pain and fatigue (e.g. hypothyroidism, SLE, Sjögren's, psoriatic arthritis, inflammatory myopathy, hyperparathyroidism, osteomalacia)—check FBC, ESR, TFTs, U&E, eGFR, Ca^{2+}, CK, PO_4^{3-}, ANA, RhF, and immunoglobulins.

Management Multidisciplinary approach is helpful.

- Be supportive—reassurance that there is no serious pathology, explanation and information are vital
- Low-dose amitriptyline 25–75mg nocte may help with sleep/pain. SSRI, e.g. sertraline 25–50mg od, may help anxiety, depression, and sleep—stop if no improvement after a month's trial
- Graded exercise regimes improve pain, lethargy, mood, and malaise
- Counselling/learning coping strategies/CBT can be beneficial
- ◆ Some patients benefit from injection of hyperalgesic trigger points with steroid or acupuncture to trigger points

Hypermobility Children/young adults with lax joints; <50% are symptomatic. Those that have symptoms present with recurrent joint pains—mainly affecting the knees. Other symptoms include joint effusion, dislocation, ligamentous injuries, low back pain, and premature OA. The condition is benign, and joints become stiffer with age. Treatment, when needed, is with physiotherapy. Rarely associated with congenital disorders, e.g. Ehlers–Danlos syndrome.

1. Insertion of nuchal muscles into the occiput
2. Upper border of trapezius mid-portion
3. Muscle attachments to upper medial border of scapula
4. Anterior aspects of the C_5, C_7 intertransverse spaces
5. Second rib space ~3cm lateral to the sternal border
6. Muscle attachments to the lateral epicondyle at the elbow
7. Upper outer quadrant of gluteal muscles
8. Muscle attachments just posterior to the greater trochanter
9. Medial fat pad of the knee just proximal to the joint line

Figure 15.5 Tender point sites for diagnosis of fibromyalgia

Reproduced from Davies R, Everitt H, Simon C (2006) *Musculoskeletal Problems*, with permission from Oxford University Press.

Tietze's syndrome Idiopathic costochondritis. Pain is enhanced by motion, coughing, or sneezing. The second rib is most commonly affected. *Examination:* marked localized tenderness. *Differential diagnosis:* muscular sprain; rarely inflammatory chest wall enthesitis/osteitis 2° to spondylarthropathy. When affects lower ribs (L>R), sometimes termed *slipped rib syndrome*.

Management Explanation and reassurance that nothing serious is happening; simple OTC analgesia, e.g. ibuprofen 400mg tds. If pain persists, local steroid or marcaine injections can be helpful. If not settling consider referral to rheumatology.

A.Tietze (1864–1927)—German surgeon.

Further information

European League Against Rheumatism (EULAR) Evidence-based recommendations for the management of fibromyalgia syndrome (2007).

Patient information and support

Arthritis Research UK ☎ 0300 790 0400 🖱 www.arthritisresearchuk.org
Fibromyalgia Association UK ☎ 0844 887 2444
🖱 www.fibromyalgia-associationuk.org
Hypermobility Syndrome Association (HMSA) 🖱 www.hypermobility.org

Neurology

Reflexes and muscle power

Automatic responses. The reflex arc goes from the stimulus via a sensory nerve to the spinal cord and then back along a motor nerve to cause muscle contraction, without brain involvement.

Key reflexes See Table 16.2. Record whether absent, present with reinforcement, normal, or brisk ± clonus.

Absent or ↓ reflex Implies a breach in the reflex arc at:
- Sensory nerve or root, e.g. neuropathy, spondylosis
- Anterior horn cell, e.g. MND, polio
- Motor nerve or root, e.g. neuropathy, spondylosis
- Nerve endings, e.g myasthenia gravis, or
- Muscle, e.g. myopathy

↑ reflex Implies lack of higher control—an upper motor neurone lesion, e.g. post-stroke.

Clonus Rhythmic involuntary muscle contraction due to abrupt tendon stretching, e.g. by dorsiflexing the ankle—associated with an UMN lesion.

Reinforcement Method of accentuating reflexes. Use if a reflex seems absent. Ask patients to clench their teeth (to reinforce upper limb reflexes) or clench their hands and pull in opposite directions (to accentuate lower limb reflexes). This effect only lasts ~1s, so ask patients to perform the manoeuvre simultaneously with the tap from the tendon hammer.

Testing for muscle power See Table 16.1

Table 16.1 Quick screening test for muscle power

Joint	Movement	Nerve roots	Joint	Movement	Nerve roots
Shoulder	Abduction	C5,6	Hip	Flexion	L1–3
	Adduction	C6–8		Extension	L4,5 & S1
Elbow	Flexion	C5,6	Knee	Flexion	L5 & S1
	Extension	C7,8		Extension	L3,4
Wrist	Flexion	C7,8	Ankle	Dorsiflexion	L4,5
	Extension	C6,7		Plantarflexion	S1,2
Fingers	Flexion	C8	Toes	Extensors	L5,S1
	Extension	C7		Flexors	S2
	Abduction	T1			

❗ Test proximal muscle power by asking the patient to sit from lying, pull you towards him/herself, or rise from squatting.

Table 16.2 Key reflexes and nerve roots involved

Reflex	Test	Expected result	Nerve roots
Jaw	Ask the patient to let his mouth open slightly. Place a finger on the chin and tap the finger with a tendon hammer	Contraction of masseters and closure of mouth	Vth cranial nerve
Gag	Touch the back of the patient's pharynx on each side with a spatula, If absent, ask the patient whether he can feel the spatula—if he can, then Xth nerve palsy	Contraction of the soft palate	IXth/Xth cranial nerve
Biceps	Tap a finger placed on the biceps tendon by letting the tendon hammer fall on it	Contraction of the biceps + elbow flexion	C5, C6
Supinator	Tap the lower end of the radius just above the wrist with the tendon hammer	Contraction of brachioradialis + elbow flexion	C5, C6
Triceps	Support elbow in flexion with one hand. Tap the triceps tendon with a tendon hammer held in the other hand	Contraction of triceps + elbow extension	C7, C8
Knee	Support the knees so that relaxed and slightly bent. Let the tendon hammer fall onto the infrapatellar tendon	Contraction of quadriceps + extension of knee	L3, L4
Ankle	Externally rotate the thigh and flex the knee. Let the tendon hammer fall onto the Achilles tendon	Contraction of gastrocnemius + plantar flexion of the ankle	S1
Abdominal	Lightly stroke the abdominal wall diagonally towards the umbilicus in each of the four abdominal quadrants	Abdominal wall contractions. When absent can be normal or indicate UMN or LMN lesion	T7–T12
Cremaster	♂ patients only. Pre-warn the patient. Stroke the superior and medial aspect of the thigh in a downwards direction	Contraction of cremasteric muscle → raising of scrotum and testis on the side stroked. Absent in UMN and LMN lesions	L1
Anal	Scratch the perianal skin	Reflex contraction of the external sphincter. Absent in UMN and LMN lesions	S4, S5
Plantar	Pre-warn the patient. Run a blunt object up the lateral side of the sole of the foot, curving medially before the MTP joints	Flexion of big toe (if >1y old). Extension implies UMN lesion	S1

Cranial nerve lesions

Table 16.3 summarizes cranial nerve lesions and their causes. Figure 16.1 shows the cutaneous innervation of the head and neck. Cranial nerves may be affected at any point from the nerve nucleus within the brainstem to the point of innervation. Think systematically about the level of the lesion.
Potential sites:
- Muscle
- Neuromuscular junction
- Along the course of the nerve outside the brainstem
- Within the brainstem

❶ Any cranial nerve may be affected by DM, MS, tumours, sarcoid, vasculitis or syphilis and >1 nerve may be affected by a lesion. Refer according to cause to ENT, ophthalmology, or neurology.

Table 16.3 Cranial nerve lesions and their causes

Nerve	Clinical test	Causes
I Olfactory	**Smell**—test each nostril for the ability to differentiate different smells	Trauma, frontal lobe tumour, meningitis
II Optic	**Acuity**—Snellen chart **Visual fields**—compare with your own visual fields by standing directly in front of the patient with your head at the same level as theirs **Pupils**—size, shape, reaction to light, and accommodation **Ophthalmoscopy**—darken room, dilate pupil with 1 drop tropicamide 0.5% if needed, view optic disc (? pale, swollen), follow each vessel outwards to view each quadrant, track outwards to check lens and cornea	**Monocular blindness**—lesion in one eye or optic nerve (e.g. MS, giant cell arteritis) **Bitemporal hemianopia**—optic chiasm compression, e.g. pituitary adenoma, craniopharyngioma, internal carotid artery aneurysm **Homonymous hemianopia**—affects half the visual field on the side opposite the lesion. Caused by lesion beyond the optic chiasm, e.g. stroke, abscess, tumour
III	Ptosis, large pupil, eye looks down- and outwards ❶ Diplopia from a 3rd nerve lesion may cause nystagmus	DM, giant cell arteritis, syphilis, posterior communicating artery aneurysm, idiopathic If pupil normal size, results fom DM or other vascular cause
IV	Diplopia on looking down and in; may compensate by tilting head	Rare in isolation. May occur as a result of trauma to the orbit
V Trigeminal	**Motor**—open mouth. Jaw deviates to the side of the lesion **Sensory**—corneal reflex lost first. Check all three divisions	**Motor**—bulbar palsy (📖 p. 549), acoustic neuroma **Sensory**—trigeminal neuralgia (📖 p. 549); herpes zoster; nasopharyngeal carcinoma
VI	Horizontal diplopia on looking outwards	MS, pontine CVA, ↑ ICP

(continued)

Table 16.3 (Cont.)

Nerve	Clinical test	Causes
VII Facial	Causes facial weakness and droop Ask to raise eyebrows, show teeth, puff out cheeks. • **LMN lesion:** all one side of face affected • **UMN lesion:** lower two-thirds of the face affected only	**LMN**—Bell's palsy, polio, otitis media, skull fracture, cerebello pontine angle tumour, parotid tumour, herpes zoster (Ramsay Hunt syndrome 📖 p. 538) **UMN**—stroke, tumour
VIII Vestibulo-auditory	**Auditory**—ask to repeat a number whispered in 1 ear whilst you block the other **Vestibular**—ask about balance, check for nystagmus (📖 p. 950)—ask patient to fix on finger ¾ m away—check gaze upwards, downwards, lateral (both directions), keeping finger <30° from midline	Noise, Paget's disease, Ménière's disease (📖 p. 951), herpes zoster, acoustic neuroma, brainstem CVA, drugs (e.g. furosemide)
IX, X	Gag reflex, palate moves → normal side on saying 'Aah'	Trauma, brainstem lesions, neck tumours
XI	**Trapezii**—shrug shoulders against resistance **Sternomastoid**—turn head to right/left against resistance	Rare. Polio, syringomyelia, tumours near jugular foramen, stroke, bulbar palsy (📖 p. 549), polio, trauma, TB
XII	Tongue deviates to the side of the lesion	Trauma, brainstem lesions, neck tumours

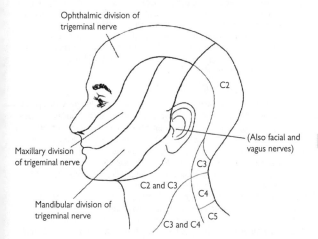

Figure 16.1 Cutaneous innervation of the head and neck

Reproduced from Simon C (2006) *Neurology*, with permission from Oxford University Press.

Neuropathy

Dermatomes and peripheral nerve distribution See Figure 16.2 (📖 p. 540) and Figure 16.3 (📖 p. 541).

Mononeuropathy Lesions of individual peripheral (including cranial) nerves. *Causes:* trauma, compression, DM, leprosy. If >1 peripheral nerve is involved, the term *mononeuritis multiplex* is used. *Causes:* DM, sarcoid, cancer, PAN, amyloid, leprosy.

Common mononeuropathies See Table 16.4.

Bell's palsy Facial palsy without other signs. Unknown cause—possibly viral. *Peak age:* 10–40y. ♂ = ♀. *Lifetime incidence:* ~1:65. Affects left and right side of the face equally often. Usually sudden onset—may be preceded by pain around the ear. *Other possible symptoms:* facial numbness; ↓ noise tolerance; disturbed taste on the anterior part of the tongue.

Management ~70% recover completely; 13% have insignificant sequelae; the remainder have permanent deficit. 85% improve in <3wk—reassure. Give prednisolone (25mg bd for 10d) if <72h after onset of symptoms[R]. Protect eye—tape lid shut and pad at night; glasses in the day ± artificial tears if drying. *Refer:*

- If recovery is not starting after 3wk
- For tarsorraphy if complete or long-standing palsy
- If unacceptable cosmetic result—may benefit from plastic surgery

C. Bell (1774–1842)—*Scottish anatomist and surgeon*

Ramsay Hunt syndrome (herpes zoster oticus) Severe pain in the ear precedes facial nerve palsy. Zoster vesicles appear around the ear, in the external ear canal, on the soft palate, and in the tonsillar fossa. Often accompanied by deafness ± vertigo which are slow to resolve and may result in permanent deficit. Pain usually abates after 48h but post-herpetic neuralgia can be a problem. If detected <24h after the rash appears, treatment with antivirals (e.g. aciclovir 800mg 5x/d for 1 wk) may be effective. J. Ramsay Hunt (1872–1937)—*US neurologist.*

Morton's metatarsalgia 📖 p. 498

Autonomic neuropathy Postural hypotension (dizziness or syncope on standing, after exercise or a large meal), impotence, inability to sweat, vomiting and dysphagia, diarrhoea or constipation, urinary retention or incontinence, Horner's syndrome (📖 p. 300). Check BP lying and standing—a postural drop of ≥30/15mmHg is abnormal. *Causes:*

- **Primary autonomic failure** No known cause. Occurs alone or as part of multisystem atrophy. Typically middle-aged/elderly men. Onset is insidious. Survival—rarely >10y after diagnosis
- **Ageing** 25% >74y have postural hypotension. Review medication, discourage prolonged bed rest. Often associated with disordered thermoregulation, making elderly people prone to hypothermia. Exclude other disorders (e.g. DM, multisystem atrophy, drugs) before putting down to ageing alone

Table 16.4 Common mononeuropathies

Nerve involved	Nerve roots	Presentation	Common causes
Median	C5–T1	Loss of sensation over lateral 3½ fingers and palm. Wasting of the thenar eminence Inability to flex the terminal phalanx of the thumb implies involvement of the anterior interosseous branch	Trauma (especially wrist lacerations), carpal tunnel syndrome (📖 p. 486)
Ulnar	C7–T1	Weakness and wasting of interossei muscles (weakness of abduction of fingers) and claw hand deformity. Wasting of hypothenar eminence, sensory loss over medial 1½ fingers and ulnar side of the hand. Flexion of 4th and 5th fingers is weak if proximal lesion	Trauma or compression at the elbow (📖 p. 482), trauma at the wrist
Radial	C5–T1	Sensory loss is variable but always includes the dorsal aspect of the root of the thumb. Wrist drop and weak extension of thumb and fingers	Compression against the humerus, trauma
Sciatic	L4–S2	Weakness of hamstrings and all muscles below the knee (foot drop). Loss of sensation below the knee laterally	Back injury, pelvic tumour
Common peroneal	L4–S2	Inability to dorsiflex the foot (foot drop), evert the foot, or extend the toes. Sensory loss over dorsum of the foot	Trauma
Tibial	S1–S3	Inability to stand on tiptoe, invert the foot or flex toes Sensory loss over sole	Trauma or entrapment

- **Drugs** Common culprits—antihypertensives (e.g. thiazides), diuretics (over-diuresis), L-dopa, TCAs, phenothiazines, benzodiazepines
- **Polyneuropathies** May be part of more general polyneuropathy, e.g. DM, Guillain–Barré syndrome, or alcoholic/nutritional neuropathy
- **Other causes** Craniopharyngioma, vascular lesions, spinal cord lesions, tabes dorsalis, Chagas' disease, HIV, familial dysautonomia

Management Treat any underlying cause. Advise patients to stand slowly, raise the head of the bed at night, eat little and often, and ↓ carbohydrate and alcohol intake. Fludrocortisone (0.1mg/d, increasing prn–unlicensed) may help those most severely affected. An alternative (also unlicensed) is midodrine. Refer if diagnosis is unclear or simple measures are ineffective.

Polyneuropathy 📖 p. 542

Figure 16.2 Dermatomes and peripheral nerve distribution

Figure 16.3 Dermatomes and peripheral nerve distribution

Polyneuropathy

Generalized disorder of peripheral nerves, including cranial and autonomic nerves. Distribution is bilateral, symmetrical, and widespread.

Sensory neuropathy Presents as numbness, tingling, or burning sensation often affecting the extremities first (*glove and stocking distribution*) or causing clumsiness handling fine objects (e.g. needle).

Motor neuropathy Presents as progressive weakness or clumsiness of hands, stumbling/falls on walking, respiratory difficulty (can progress rapidly). *Examination:* wasting and weakness most marked distally; reflexes are ↓ or absent.

Causes See Table 16.5.

Initial investigations Exclude common causes—check blood glucose, FBC, ESR, U&E, Cr and eGFR, LFTs, TFTs, plasma B$_{12}$, autoimmune profile, syphilis serology.

Management Treat cause if possible. Involve physiotherapists and OT. If sensory neuropathy care of the feet is important to minimize trauma and consequent disability. Refer if a cause is not found.

⚠ If rapid deterioration admit as acute medical emergency as ventilation may be needed.

Specific polyneuropathies

Charcot–Marie–Tooth syndrome (peroneal muscular atrophy) Presents at puberty or in early adult life and begins with foot drop and weak legs. The peroneal muscles are the first to atrophy. The disease spreads to the hands then arms. Sensation and reflexes are also ↓. Unknown cause. Once diagnosis is confirmed treatment is supportive.
J.M. Charcot (1825–93) and P. Marie (1853–1940)—French neurologists; H.H. Tooth (1856–1925)—English neurologist.

Guillain–Barré polyneuritis Develops within a few weeks of surgery, flu vaccination or infection (URTI, flu, VZ, HSV, CMV, EBV, *Campylobacter*, *Mycoplasma*). In 40% no precipitating event is found.

Presents with ascending motor neuropathy which may advance fast. Proximal muscles are more affected than distal muscles. Trunk, respiratory muscles, and cranial nerves are commonly affected.

If suspected admit immediately to hospital as an emergency. Ventilation on ITU is frequently required; 85% make a complete or near-complete recovery; 10% are unable to walk alone at 1y; mortality is 10%.
C. Guillain (1876–1961) and J.A. Barré (1880–1967)—French neurologists.

Polio 📖 p. 579

Refsum's syndrome Rare autosomal recessive disorder which presents in the second decade or later with sensorimotor polyneuropathy, ataxia, visual, and/or hearing problems. Treatment involves dietary restriction (avoidance of chlorophyll-containing foods) and plasmapheresis.
S. Refsum (1907–1991)—Norwegian physician.

Table 16.5 Causes of polyneuropathy

Inflammatory	Guillain–Barré syndrome (mostly motor) Chronic inflammatory demyelinating polyneuropathy (CDP) Sarcoidosis
Metabolic	DM (mainly sensory) Renal failure (mainly sensory) Hypothyroidism Hypoglycaemia Mitochondrial disorders
Vasculitis	Polyarteritis nodosa Rheumatoid arthritis Wegener's granulomatosis
Malignancy	Paraneoplastic syndromes (especially small cell lung cancer) Polycythaemia rubra vera
Infection	HIV Syphilis Lyme disease Leprosy (mainly sensory)
Vitamin deficiency	Lack of B_1, B_6, B_{12} (e.g. alcoholic)
Inherited	Refsum's syndrome Charcot–Marie–Tooth syndrome (mostly motor) Porphyria
Toxins	Lead (mostly motor) Arsenic
Drugs	Alcohol Cisplatin Isoniazid Vincristine Nitrofurantoin *Less frequently:* metronidazole, phenytoin
Others	Paraproteinaemias, e.g. multiple myeloma, amyloidosis

Walking problems

 Walking difficulty ('off legs') Common symptom in the elderly. *Causes:*
- **Musculoskeletal** Osteoarthritis or RA, osteoporotic fractures, fractured neck of femur, osteomalacia, Paget's disease, polymyalgia rheumatica
- **Psychological** Depression, bereavement, fear of falling
- **Neurological** Stroke, Parkinson's disease, peripheral neuropathy
- **Spinal cord compression**
- **Systemic** Pneumonia, UTI, anaemia, hypothyroidism, renal failure, infection, hypothermia

Management Treat according to cause. Refer (e.g. to rapid response team, social services, or elderly care) if inadequate support at home, cause warrants referral, or no cause is found.

Abnormal gait Gait means manner of walking. Abnormal gait can give clues to the underlying problem.

Abnormal movements Normal gait is interrupted by abnormal movements, e.g. choreiform movements, athetoid movements or hemiballismus. May indicate underlying neurological problem, e.g. cerebral palsy, Huntington's chorea.

Antalgic gait Gait adjusts to try to minimize pain in a joint—usually OA hip. The patient leans towards the affected side and takes a rapid step on that side followed by a slower step on the contralateral side—check Trendelenburg's sign (🕮 p. 488).

Drunken gait Apart from alcohol, the other major cause of drunken gait is a cerebellar lesion. *Features:*
- Wide-based gait or reeling gait on a narrow base
- Feet are often raised too high and placed over carefully, with the patient looking ahead
- If a cerebellar lesion, the patient falls to the side of the lesion

Foot drop Patients trip frequently or walk with a high stepping gait. On examination, patients are unable to walk on their heels and cannot dorsiflex their foot. Check ankle jerk. *Causes:*
- **Common peroneal palsy**, e.g. due to trauma—normal ankle jerk
- **Sciatica**—ankle jerk absent
- **L4, L5 root lesion**—ankle jerk may be absent
- **Peripheral motor neuropathy**, e.g. alcoholic—ankle jerk weak or absent
- **Distal myopathy**—ankle jerk weak or absent
- **Motor neurone disease**—↑ ankle jerk

Hemiplegic gait Style of walking seen in patients with UMN lesions. *Features:*
- Arm adducted and internally rotated, elbow flexed and pronated ± finger flexion
- Foot is plantar flexed and the leg swings in a lateral arc

Frontal lesions Marked unsteadiness—the feet appear stuck to the floor causing a wide-based, shuffling gait.

Parkinsonian gait Seen in patients with Parkinson's disease and other causes of parkinsonism. *Features:*

- **Shuffling gait** Short steps, with the feet barely leaving the ground, producing an audible shuffling noise. May trip over small obstacles
- **Turning 'en bloc'** Keeping the neck and trunk rigid, and requiring multiple small steps to accomplish a turn
- **Gait freezing** Inability to move feet. May worsen in tight, cluttered spaces or when attempting to initiate gait
- **Festinant gait** Flexed posture as if hurrying to keep up with feet
- **Lack of normal arm swing**

Scissor gait As the name implies, the patient walks as if his/her legs were like a pair of scissors. Associated with spastic paraplegia

- Both legs are held rigid with plantar flexion of the ankle, extension of the knee, and adduction/internal rotation of the hips
- The patient walks on tiptoe and the knees rub together/cross during the walking cycle
- Often accompanied by complex movements of the upper limbs to assist the walking movements

Sensory ataxic gait Loss of proprioception due to peripheral neuropathy or spinal cord disease (e.g. cervical spondylosis, MS, syphilis, combined degeneration of the cord) results in an ataxic gait similar to that seen with cerebellar disease. Check Romberg's test. *Features:*

- Broad-based gait with a tendency to stamp feet down clumsily
- Patient tends to look at feet throughout the walking cycle
- Romberg's sign +ve

Waddling gait Typically seen in patients with proximal myopathy, e.g. due to muscular dystrophy. *Other causes:* pregnancy, congenital dislocation of the hip. *Features:*

- Broad-based gait. The pelvis drops to the side of the leg being raised
- The patient moves his/her body and hips to accommodate this, resulting in a duck-like waddle in the swing phase
- Commonly accompanied by ↑ forward curvature of the lower spine

---

Examining gait Note abnormalities and any aids/assistance required.

- Make sure that you can see the legs well
- Ask the patient to stand up from a chair without support. If able to do that, repeat with feet together and/or with eyes closed
- Ask the patient to stand still with feet together. If able to do that ask the patient to close his eyes and see what happens (*Romberg's sign*)
- Ask the patient to walk normally for ~5m, turn round, and walk back
- Ask the patient to walk heel-to-toe (testing for cerebellar disease)
- Ask the patient to stand with the feet together
  - With eyes open—testing cerebellar and posterior column function
  - With eyes closed—testing posterior column function
  - On toes alone—impossible with S1 lesions
  - On heels alone—impossible if L4/L5 lesion

Other movement problems

Abbnormal gait 📖 p. 544

Cramp Painful muscle spasm. Common—especially at night and after exercise. Rarely associated with disease—salt depletion, muscle ischaemia, myopathy. Forearm cramps suggest motor neurone disease. Night cramps in the elderly may respond to quinine bisulphate 300mg nocte twice weekly.

Dystonia Prolonged muscle contraction producing abnormal postures or repetitive movements.

- **Spasmodic torticollis** Head is pulled to one side and held there by a contracting sternomastoid muscle. Treat with physiotherapy
- **Blepharospasm** Involuntary contraction of the orbicularis oculi. If troublesome, consider treatment with diazepam (but be careful to avoid dependence) or refer for treatment with botulinum toxin
- **Writer's cramp** Spasm of the hand and forearm muscles on writing
- **Generalized dystonia** Primary generalized dystonia is usually genetic. Specialist treatment from a neurologist is essential. First-line drug treatment is with levodopa. If that is ineffective, an anticholinergic drug (e.g. trihexyphenidyl) can be helpful in controlling muscle spasms and tremor. Second-line treatments may include clonazepam, tetrabenazine, baclofen, botulinum toxin injections. Deep brain stimulation may also be helpful
- **Secondary dystonia** Symptoms of dystonia that result from drugs or other medical conditions. Includes: drug-induced dystonia (acute dystonia or tardive dyskinesia); dystonia associated with cerebral palsy; dystonia assosicated with Parkinson's disease; dystonia associated with other brain injury or disease; and dystonia associated with metabolic conditions (e.g. Wilson's disease)

Tardive dyskinesia Involuntary chewing and grimacing movements, resulting from long-term neuroleptic treatment (metoclopramide and prochlorperazine are also possible causes). Withdraw neuroleptic—if no improvement after 3–6mo consider tetrabenazine 25–50mg tds po.

Patient information and support
The Dystonia Society ☎ 020 7793 3650 ⬥ www.dystonia.org.uk

Myoclonus Sudden, involuntary focal or general jerks. May be normal, especially if occurs when falling asleep. *Other causes:*
- Neurodegenerative disease (e.g. CJD)
- Myoclonic epilepsy
- Benign essential myoclonus (generalized myoclonus beginning in childhood as muscle twitches, may be inherited as autosomal dominant)
- Asterixis (metabolic flap—e.g liver failure, uraemia)

Treatment If needed treat with sodium valproate or clonazepam.

Dyspraxia Impairment of performance of complex movements despite preservation of ability to perform their individual components. Test by asking the patient to perform everyday tasks (e.g. ask to dress/undress), copy complex hand movements and do familiar sequences of movements (e.g. 'head, shoulders, knees, and toes').

Childhood p. 916

Adults Most common causes are stroke or space-occupying lesion. Involve rehabilitation services and OT.

- **Dressing dyspraxia** Patient is unsure of the orientation of clothes on his/her body.
- **Constructional dyspraxia** Difficulty in assembling objects or drawing (ask to draw 5-pointed star)
- **Gait dyspraxia** Gait disorder although the lower limbs function normally—more common amongst the elderly

Tremor

- **Resting tremor** Present at rest but abolished on voluntary movement. Most common cause—PD when tremor is rhythmic
- **Intention tremor** Irregular large amplitude tremor worse on movement, e.g. reaching for something. Typical of cerebellar disease
- **Tremors on movement** Thyrotoxicosis, anxiety, benign essential tremor (inherited), and drugs (e.g. β-agonists) cause a fine tremor abolished at rest. Alcohol and β-blockers may help

Asterixis Intermittent lapses of an assumed posture. May involve arms, neck, tongue, jaw, and eyelids. Usually bilateral, absent at rest, and asynchronous on each side. *Causes:* liver failure (flapping tremor), heart failure, respiratory failure, renal failure, hypoglycaemia, barbiturate intoxication.

Athetosis Slow, confluent, often rhythmic, purposeless movements of hands, tongue, fingers, or face. *Causes:* cerebral palsy, kernicterus.

Chorea Non-rhythmic, jerky, purposeless movements (especially hands), with voluntary movements possible in between. *Most common causes:* cerebral palsy, Huntington's chorea, Sydenham's chorea.

Ballismus/hemiballismus Large-amplitude, involuntary flinging movements of limbs. May occur after stroke, in Huntington's disease or with high doses of levodopa for PD.

Tics Brief, repeated, and stereotyped movements which are able to be suppressed voluntarily for a while. Common in children and usually resolve spontaneously. Consider clonazepam or clonidine if tics are severe.

Gilles de la Tourette syndrome p. 911

Speech problems

Hoarseness 📖 p. 936

Stammer Disorder of rhythm and fluency of speech in which syllables, words, or phrases are repeated. ♂:♀ ≈4:1. *Cause:* unknown. Can result in stress and embarrassment.
• **Younger children** Often short-lived; usually resolves spontaneously
• **Older children/adults** Refer to speech therapy

Dysarthria Difficulty with articulation due to incoordination or weakness of the musculature of speech. Language is normal. Ask to repeat 'baby hippopotamus' or 'British constitution'. Treat the cause if possible otherwise support with speech therapy and aids to communication. *Causes:* see Table 16.6.

Dysphasia Impairment of language due to brain damage to the dominant hemisphere. The left hemisphere is dominant for 99% of right-handed people and 60% of left-handers. In most cases, due to stroke or brain tumour. Rarely due to head injury or dementia. *Assessment and classification:* see Table 16.7. Mixed pictures are common. *Treatment:*
• Speech therapy may, or may not, be helpful
• Support, e.g. dysphasia groups
• Aids to communication, e.g. computers, picture boards

Myasthenia gravis Autoimmune disease. Antibodies to the acetylcholine receptor cause a deficit of receptors at the neuromuscular junction → muscle weakness. Antibodies are detectable in 90%. ♀:♂ ≈2:1. Associated with thymic tumours and other autoimmune disease, e.g. RA, SLE, hyperthyroidism. Generally follows a relapsing or slowly progressive course. If thymoma present, 5y survival ≈ 30%.

Presentation Young adults with easy fatigability of muscles. Commonly affected muscles are the:
• Orbital muscles causing ptosis and diplopia, *and*
• Bulbar muscles causing slurring of speech—ask to count to 50

Weakness is exacerbated by pregnancy, infection, drugs (e.g. β-blockers, opiates, tetracycline, quinine), climate change, emotion, and exercise.

Management If suspected refer for confirmation by a neurologist and specialist treatment. *Treated with:*
• Anticholinesterase, e.g. pyridostigmine
• Immunosuppression with prednisolone, methotrexate, or azathioprine
• Thymectomy → remission in 30% and benefit in another 40%
• Plasmapheresis

Lambert–Eaton syndrome (or myasthenic syndrome) Occurs in association with small cell carcinoma of the lung or rarely autoimmune disease. Differs from myasthenia gravis by the tendency to hyporeflexia. Autonomic involvement is common. Proximal limb muscles/trunk are most commonly involved. Specialist treatment is essential.

Patient support
Myaesthenia Gravis Association UK 🕸 www.mgauk.org

Table 16.6 Causes of dysarthria

Cause	Characteristics
Cerebellar disease	Slurring of speech as if drunk Speech is irregular in volume and scanning in quality
Extrapyramidal disease, e.g. Parkinson's disease	Soft, indistinct, and monotonous speech
Pseudo-bulbar palsy, e.g. stroke (bilateral), MS, MND	Alteration of speech—typically nasal speech sounding like Donald Duck Difficulty swallowing or chewing Tongue is spastic and jaw jerk ↑
Bulbar palsy, e.g. MND, Guillain–Barré, alcoholic brainstem myelinolysis, 1° or 2° brainstem tumours, syringobulbia, polio, hyponatraemia	Speech—quiet, hoarse or nasal Loss of function of the tongue, muscles of chewing/swallowing ± facial muscles Flaccid, fasciculating tongue Jaw jerk normal or absent
Palate paralysis	Nasal speech Asymmetric or absent gag reflex
Myasthenia gravis	Slurring of speech when fatigued

Table 16.7 Assessment and classification of dysphasia

Assessment:
Is speech fluent, grammatical, meaningful, and apt? If yes, dysphasia is unlikely.
Comprehension: can the patient follow one, two, or multiple step commands?
Repetition: can the patient repeat a phrase after you?
Naming: can the patient name common and uncommon items?
Reading and writing? Usually affected too. If not, question the diagnosis of dysphasia.

Characteristics of dysphasia	Broca's (expressive)	Wernicke's (receptive)	Conduction	Transcortical
Fluent?	✗	✓	✓	✓ or ✗
Repetition normal?	✗	✗	✗	✓
Understanding impaired?	✗	✓	✗	✓ or ✗

Fits, faints, and funny turns

Blackouts, faints, and funny turns are all common presentations to general practice. The major questions which should be asked seeing an individual who has had a funny turn are:

- Is it epilepsy?
- If it is epilepsy, then what kind?
- If it is not epilepsy, then is there another serious underlying cause, e.g. heart disease?

History A good history from the patient and ideally from a witness is essential in the correct diagnosis. *Ask:*

- What happened?
- When and where? Particularly, did it start during sleep?
- Were there any precipitating events?
- Were there any warning signs (e.g. aura, feeling going to faint, etc.)?
- Does the patient remember the whole episode? If not, which bits are missing and how long are the gaps?
- Did the patient lose consciousness? Quite frequently, patients describe episodes of dizziness or unsteadiness/falling as 'funny turns'
- Did the patient jerk his/her limbs? If so, was the jerking generalized or restricted to one area of the body?
- What did the patient look like during the attack? An eye witness account is helpful
- Did anything else happen during the attack (e.g. tongue biting, incontinence)?
- What happened after the attack? Was the patient conscious straight away? Was there disorientation, drowsiness, or headache?

Also check

- General medical history, including cardiac history and history of other neurological symptoms
- Psychiatric history—anxiety, depression, panic attacks?
- Past medical history—birth trauma, febrile convulsions in childhood, significant head injury, and/or meningitis/encephalitis
- Family history—epilepsy
- Substance abuse? Drugs or alcohol?

Examination Complete general and neurological examination. Particularly check for:

- **Skin changes** Café-au-lait spots (neurofibromatosis); adenoma sebaceum (tuberous sclerosis); trigeminal capillary haemangioma (Sturge–Weber syndrome)
- **Cardiovascular abnormalities** Heart rate and rhythm, murmurs, carotid bruits, BP
- **Focal neurological deficits** Suggest presence of a structural neurological lesion

Funny turns in small children 📖 p. 896

Epilepsy 📖 p. 574

Syncope Abrupt and transient loss of consciousness due to a sudden ↓ in cerebral perfusion. Common—prevalence ~6% adults. It has many causes, ranging from benign (vasovagal syncope) to fatal (sustained ventricular tachycardia); the prognosis depends on the cause.

Diagnosis A typical attack takes the following pattern:
- **Prodromal symptoms** Nausea, clammy sweating, blurring, greying and possible loss of vision, light-headedness, dizziness and tinnitus, yawning. The collection is characteristic
- **Anoxic phase** Loss of consciousness, pallor, sweating, pupil dilatation, tachypnoea, bradycardia. Muscle tone is ↓, causing eyes to roll up and the patient to fall. May be accompanied by a few myoclonic jerks as the patient falls
- **Recovery** In the horizontal position, skin colour, pulse, and consciousness usually return within seconds. ❶ If the patient is unable to fall and is kept upright a 2° anoxic seizure may occur
- **After-effects** Confusion, amnesia, and drowsiness are not prolonged. Injury and incontinence are rare but may occur. Tongue biting is very rare

Presyncope Is the term applied to a less severe attack with partial loss of consciousness and a near fall.

Simple faint/vasovagal attack Common. Peripheral vasodilatation, bradycardia, and venous pooling → postural hypotension. Often cause is unclear, though ♀ > ♂. *Known precipitants:* fright (e.g. during venesection) or emotion. Exclude other reasons for loss of consciousness. No treatment needed—reassure.

Dizziness and giddiness Distinguish between true vertigo (the illusion of rotatory movement—the room spinning) and a feeling of unsteadiness or light-headedness:
- **Vertigo** 📖 p. 950
- **Imbalance** Implies difficulty in walking straight, e.g. from disease of peripheral nerves, posterior columns, or cerebellum
- **Faintness** The feeling of being about to pass out. Associated with some seizure disorders and a variety of non-neurological conditions (e.g. postural hypotension, vasovagal fainting; hyperventilation; hypoglycaemia; arrhythmias; cough syncope). Sometimes >1 element coexists

Hyperventilation and panic attacks 📖 p. 1120
❶ Usually history is diagnostic but occasionally, seizures of temporal lobe origin may have similar symptomatology.

Hypoglycaemia Affects patients with DM—particularly those taking insulin or oral hypoglycaemic agents. Produces autonomic changes, e.g. pallor, sweating and tachycardia, and behavioural changes (confusion, altered personality). If action is not taken to ↑ blood sugar, coma ± fitting ensues—📖 p. 1100.

Abnormal perceptions (e.g hallucinations—📖 p. 988).

Assessment of headache

Common presenting complaint. The skill lies in deciding which headaches are benign, needing no intervention, and which require action.

History

- **Is there >1 type of headache?** Take a separate history for each.
- **Time** When did the headaches start? New or recently changed headache calls for especially careful assessment. How often do they happen? Do they have any pattern? (e.g. constant, episodic, daily) How long do they last? Why is the patient coming to the doctor now? A headache diary over >8wk may help if long-standing headaches
- **Character** Nature/quality, site, and spread of the pain. Associated symptoms, e.g. nausea/vomiting, visual disturbance, photophobia, neurological symptoms
- **Cause** Predisposing and/or trigger factors; aggravating and/or relieving factors; relationship to menstrual cycle; family history
- **Response** Details of medication used (type, dose, frequency, timing). What does the patient do, e.g. can the patient continue work?
- **Health between attacks** Do headaches go completely or is the patient unwell between attacks? Other past/current medical problems
- **Anxieties and concerns** Of the patient/family

Examination *In acute, severe headache,* examine for fever and purpuric skin rash. *In all cases* check BP, brief neurological examination including fundi, visual acuity, and gait, palpation of the temporal region/sinuses for tenderness, and examination of the neck. *In young children,* measure head circumference and plot on a centile chart.

⚠ **Red flags**

- Fever and worsening headache ± purpuric rash/meningism
- Thunderclap headache (reaching peak intensity in <5min)
- Progressive headache, worsening over weeks
- Headache associated with postural change, sneezing, coughing, or exercise
- Recent head injury (<3mo)
- Papilloedema
- Change in personality/new cognitive or neurological deficit
- New onset in a patient with a history of HIV or cancer.
- Headache with atypical aura (>1h ± motor weakness)
- Aura for first time and using CHC

Investigation Often not needed. ESR if temporal arteritis is suspected.

Differential diagnosis and management See Table 16.8. ↑ BP may cause acute or chronic headache. Direct treatment at the cause.

Meningism Headache, stiff neck, and photophobia. Associated with meningitis. May also be seen with encephalitis and SAH.

Further information

NICE Headaches in young people and adults (2012) ℘ www.nice.org.uk

Table 16.8 Differential diagnosis of headache

	Cause	Features	Management
Acute new headache	Meningitis	Fever, photophobia, stiff neck, rash	IV/IM penicillin V and immediate admission (📖 p. 1078)
	Encephalitis	Fever, confusion, ↓ conscious level	Immediate admission (📖 p. 1078)
	Subarachnoid haemorrhage	'Thunder-clap' or very sudden onset headache ± stiff neck	Immediate admission (📖 p. 560)
	Head injury	Bruising/injury; ↓ conscious level, periods lucidity, amnesia	Consider admission (📖 p. 1112)
	Self-limiting viral illness	Vary. Often associated with other symptoms, e.g. coryza, sore throat, low-grade fever	Paracetamol/ NSAID—review if worsens or if not settling in 2–3d
	Sinusitis	Tender over sinuses ± history of URTI	📖 p. 942
	Dental caries	Facial pain ± tenderness	📖 p. 932
	Tropical illness	History of travel, fever	📖 p. 648
Acute recurrent headache	Migraine	Aura, visual disturbance, nausea/vomiting, triggers	📖 p. 554
	Cluster headache	Nightly pain in 1 eye for 2–3mo, then pain-free for >1y	📖 p. 556
	Exertional or coital headache	Suggested by history of association	NSAID or propranolol before attacks
	Trigeminal neuralgia	Intense stabbing pain lasting seconds in trigeminal nerve distribution	📖 p. 557
	Glaucoma	Red eye, haloes, ↓ visual acuity, pupil abnormality	📖 p. 976
Subacute headache	Giant cell arteritis	>50y, scalp tenderness, ↑ ESR, rarely ↓ visual acuity	📖 p. 524
Chronic headache	Tension type headache	Band around the head, stress, low mood	📖 p. 556
	Cervicogenic headache	Unilateral or bilateral; band from neck to forehead; scalp tenderness	📖 p. 474
	Medication overuse	Rebound headache on stopping analgesics	📖 p. 557
	↑ intracranial pressure	Worse on waking/ sneezing, ↓ pulse, ↑ BP, neurological signs	📖 p. 558
	Paget's disease	>40y, bowed tibia, ↑ alk phos	📖 p. 504

Migraine

Migraine affects 15% of the UK population. ♂:♀ ≈1:3. One in three experiences significant disability. Caused by disturbance of cerebral blood flow under the influence of 5HT.

Aura Occurs with or without headache. Symptoms arise over ≥5min and last 5–60min before resolving completely. Diagnose if:
- Visual symptoms, e.g. flickering lights, spots, lines; partial loss of vision
- Sensory symptoms, e.g. numbness; paraesthesia and/or
- Speech disturbance

Atypical aura Consider referral for further investigation if: motor weakness; double vision; visual symptoms affecting only one eye; poor balance or ↓ level of consciousness.

Migraine headache Moderate to severe unilateral or bilateral throbbing/pulsating headache that lasts 4–72h (1–72h in children) and prevents usual activities. May occur with or without aura and be associated with nausea/vomiting ± ↑ sensitivity to light/noise.
- **Episodic** Occurs on <15d/mo
- **Chronic** Occurs on ≥15d/mo over >3mo

History, examination, and differential diagnosis 📖 p. 552

Management of an acute attack[N] Combination therapy with:
- **Triptan** (e.g. sumatriptan 50–100mg po)—choice depends on cost. Not effective if taken before the headache develops. Stops 70–85% attacks. Start with lowest dose and ↑ as needed. If consistently ineffective try an alternative triptan. Consider nasal triptan as first-line if aged 12–17y
- **NSAID** (e.g. naproxen 500mg bd) *or* **paracetamol** (1g qds) ± antiemetic (e.g. prochlorperazine 5mg, metoclopramide 10mg, or domperidone 10–20mg)—even if no nausea/vomiting

If oral preparations are ineffective/not tolerated, offer metoclopramide 10mg pr or buccal prochlorperazine 3–6mg and consider adding a non-oral NSAID (e.g. diclofenac 100mg pr) or triptan (e.g. sumatriptan 20mg nasal spray or 6mg sc).

⚠ Do not offer ergots or opioids for the acute treatment of migraine.

Treatment of recurrence within the same attack Repeat symptomatic treatments within their dose limitations—pre-emptively if recurrence is usual/expected. If using triptans, a second dose may be effective, but repeated dosing can cause rebound headache. Naratriptan and eletriptan are associated with relatively low recurrence rates.

Management of chronic migraine[G] Aims to control symptoms and minimize impact on the patient's life. Cure is not a realistic aim.

Trigger factors Half have a trigger for their migraine. *Consider:*
- **Psychological factors** Stress/relief of stress; anxiety/depression; extreme emotions, e.g. anger or grief
- **Environmental factors** Loud noise, bright/flickering lights, strong perfume, stuffy atmosphere, VDUs, strong winds, extreme heat/cold

- **Food factors** Lack of food/infrequent meals; foods containing monosodium glutamate, caffeine, and tyramine; specific foods, e.g. chocolate, citrus fruits, cheese; alcohol, especially red wine.
- **Sleep** Overtiredness (physical/mental); changes in sleep patterns (e.g. late nights, weekend lie-in, shift work, holidays); long-distance travel
- **Health factors** Hormonal changes (e.g. monthly periods, CHC, HRT, the menopause); ↑ BP; toothache or pain in the eyes, sinuses, or neck; unaccustomed physical activity

Assessing severity Assessment scales, e.g Migraine Disability Assessment Score (MIDAS—see Box 16.1 📖 p. 585), can be useful in assessing impact of symptoms on daily life and monitoring response to treatment.

General measures Reassure. Instruct about management of acute attacks. A diary can be used to identify trigger factors, assess headache frequency, severity, medication usage/overusage, and response to treatment. Avoid trigger factors where possible. Give advice on relaxation techniques and stress management. Do not offer CHC to women with migraine, especially if aura (📖 p. 753).

Prophylaxis[N] Consider if ≥4 attacks/mo or severe attacks. ↓ attacks by ~50%. Try a drug for 2mo before deeming it ineffective. If effective, continue for 6mo then review to consider ↓ dose slowly before stopping.
- **1st-line** Propranolol S/R 80–160mg od/bd or topiramate 25–50mg od/bd—start at low dose and ↑ dose every 2–4wk; ❶ Topiramate is teratogenic and may interact with hormonal contraception
- **2nd-line** Gabapentin (up to 1200mg/d in divided doses) or acupuncture (up to 10 sessions over 5–8wk)
- **3rd-line** Botulinum type A toxin may be helpful for patients who have chronic migraine, do not have medication-overuse headache and have not responded to ≥3 different prophylactic medications[N]

Alternative therapies Riboflavin 400mg od may ↓ frequency/intensity of headaches[N]; feverfew 200mg daily may↓ symptoms after 6wk use[C].

Menstrual migraine[N] Suspect if migraine occurs from 2d before to 3d after start of period on at least 2 out of 3 consecutive months (use headache diary). If predictable menstrual-related migraine that does not respond to standard acute treatment, consider frovatriptan (2.5mg bd) or zolmitriptan (2.5 mg bd/tds) on the days that migraine is expected.

❶ >1 type of headache may coexist—50% migraine sufferers develop tension type headache resulting in background pain between attacks. Consider each separately.

Further information
NICE ● www.nice.org.uk
- Headaches in young people and adults (2012)
- Migraine (chronic)—botulinum toxin type A (2012)

Patient information and support
Migraine Action Association ● 0116 275 8317 ✆ www.migraine.org.uk
Migraine Trust ● 020 7631 6970 ✆ www.migrainetrust.org

Other headaches and facial pain

Assessment and differential diagnosis of headache 📖 p. 552

Migraine 📖 p. 554

Chronic daily headache Prevalence 4%. Defined as any headache that occurs >15d/mo. *Common causes:* tension-type headache, cervicogenic headache (📖 p. 474), medication-overuse headache, migraine, errors of refraction (usually headache is mild, frontal, in the eyes themselves, and absent on waking). Treat the cause (may be >1).

Tension type headache[N] Associated with stress and anxiety and/or functional or structural abnormalities of the head or neck. Prevalence ≈2%. ♀:♂ ≈2:1. Symptoms begin aged <10y in 15% patients. Prevalence ↓ with age. Family history of similar headaches is common (40%), but twin studies do not suggest a genetic basis. Distinguish between episodic and chronic tension-type headache:

* **Episodic** Defined as headache lasting 30min–7d and occurring <180d/y (<15d/mo)
* **Chronic** Headaches on ≥15d/mo (≥180d/y) for ≥3mo

In both cases pain:
* Is bilateral, pressing, and/or tightening in quality
* Of mild/moderate intensity
* Does not prohibit activities
* Is not associated with vomiting
* Is not aggravated by physical activity

Non-drug management Reassure no serious underlying pathology. Try measures to alleviate stress—relaxation; massage; yoga; exercise. Treat musculoskeletal symptoms with physiotherapy.

Drug therapy Analgesics are of limited value and might make matters worse (see Medication-overuse headache).
* **Acute management** Simple analgesia, e.g. paracetamol, ibuprofen. Avoid codeine-containing preparations and other opioids
* **Prophylaxis** Acupuncture—up to 10 sessions over 5–8wk

Cluster headaches Extremely painful headaches focussed around 1 eye with associated autonomic symptoms on that side (drooping eyelid, constricted pupil, red watery eye, runny or blocked nose, forehead sweating). Rare <20y of age. ♂:♀ ≈6:1. More common in smokers. Pain lasts 15–180min and occurs from 1x every 2d to 8x/day. Recurrences affect the same side. Onset is often predictable (1–2h after falling asleep; after alcohol). 2 patterns:
* **Episodic** Remissions of >1mo
* **Chronic** Remissions of <1mo in a 12mo period

Management Refer for specialist advice/neuroimaging for first bout of cluster headache. *Drug treatments:*
* **Acute attack** 100% oxygen (>12L/min) for 10–20min; $5HT_1$ agonists, e.g. sumatriptan (6mg sc or 20mg nasal)—stops 75% in <15min
* **Prophylaxis** Consider verapamil 80mg tds/qds if attacks are frequent (needs ECG monitoring—seek specialist advice if unfamiliar with use). More effective if initiated early at the start of a new cluster. Refer for specialist advice if no response to verapamil.

Medication overuse (analgesic) headache[N] Persistent headache in patients with other causes of pain who are overusing analgesics. Affects 1 in 50 adults; ♀:♂ ≈5:1. Consider if headache develops/worsens when taking analgesic medication for ≥3mo. Implicated drugs include:
- Triptans, opioids, ergots, or combination analgesics on ≥10d/mo
- Paracetamol, aspirin, or NSAID on ≥15d/mo

Management Explain the condition to the patient. Advise stopping overused medication abruptly for at least 1mo. Provide follow-up and support over 4–8wk; warn that symptoms may worsen initially (day 3–7) before improving. Review treatment of any underlying problem (e.g. migraine or chronic musculoskeletal pain). Consider specialist referral if taking strong opioids or recurrent, failed attempts to stop medication overuse.

Facial pain Treat the cause. *Common causes include:* trigeminal neuralgia; temporomandibular joint disorders; dental disorders; sinusitis; migrainous neuralgia; shingles and post-herpetic neuralgia. No cause is found in many patients—it is then termed *atypical facial pain*. Atypical facial pain may respond to simple analgesia with paracetamol or NSAID. If this fails, try nerve painkillers, e.g. amitriptyline 10–75mg nocte. If troublesome symptoms, refer to ENT, maxillofacial surgery, or neurology.

Trigeminal neuralgia Paroxysms of intense stabbing, burning, or 'electric shock' type pain, lasting seconds to minutes in the trigeminal (V) nerve distribution; 96% unilateral. Mandibular/maxillary > ophthalmic division. Between attacks there are no symptoms. Frequency of attacks ranges from hundreds/d to remissions lasting years. Pain may be provoked by movement of the face (talking, eating, laughing) or touching the skin (shaving, washing). Can occur at any age but more common >50y. ♀ > ♂. Unknown cause but associated with MS.

Management Spontaneous remission may occur.
- **Carbamazepine** Start at low dose, e.g. 100mg od/bd, and ↑ dose over weeks until symptoms are controlled. Usual dose ≈200–400mg tds. Oxcarbazine is an alternative
- **Pregabalin** Start with 75mg bd. Increase as needed to a maximum of 300mg bd. If ineffective, consider combining with amitriptyline
- **Amitriptyline** Start at a dose of 25mg at 5–7 p.m.—10mg if elderly. ↑ dose by 10–25mg every 5–7d to a maximum of 75mg in a single dose as needed. Consider combining with pregabalin if ineffective alone

Refer to neurology if <50y; neurological deficit between attacks; treatment with first-line agents fails—specialist options include lamotrigine, duloxetine, baclofen, phenytoin, or surgical intervention.

Further information
NICE ℘ www.nice.org.uk
- Neuropathic pain (2013)
- Headaches in young people and adults (2012)

Patient information and support
Organization for the Understanding of Cluster Headaches (OUCH UK)
☎ 01646 651 979 ℘ www.ouchuk.org
Trigeminal Neuralgia Association UK ☎ 01883 370214 ℘ www.tna.org.uk

Raised intracranial pressure

Raised intracranial pressure (↑ ICP) usually presents with increasing headache associated with drowsiness, listlessness, vomiting, focal neurology, and/or seizures. *Causes include:* 1° or 2° tumours, head injury, intracranial haemorrhage, hydrocephalus, meningitis, encephalitis, brain abscess, and cerebral oedema (2° to tumour, trauma, infection, ischaemia).

Clinical features of ↑ ICP ⚠ If suspected, admit as an emergency.
- Drowsiness
- ↓ conscious level
- Irritability
- VI nerve palsy
- Papilloedema
- Dropping pulse
- Rising BP
- Focal neurological signs—due to underlying pathology
- Pupil changes—constriction, then dilatation

Benign intracranial hypertension Symptoms/signs of a space-occupying lesion, but none is found. Usually occurs in young, obese women. Cause unknown. Treated with repeat lumbar puncture, ventriculo-peritoneal shunt, diuretics, or dexamethasone. Usually resolves—but 10% recur later.

Brain abscess May be single or multiple. Organisms reach the brain via the blood stream, direct implantation, or local extension from adjacent sites (e.g. sinusitis). Presents with ↑ ICP, focal neurological signs, systemic effects of infection, and/or local effects due to the cause. Usually, features develop over 2–3 wk—occasionally, more slowly; in the immunosuppressed, onset is rapid. If suspected, admit as an emergency. Treatment is with IV antibiotics ± surgical drainage. Mortality is 20–30%. 50% of survivors have long-term neurological deficit; 30% epilepsy.

Intracranial tumours

- **1° tumours** 70%. Classified by whether they are benign/malignant and cell type. Glioma is an umbrella term meaning tumour of nervous system origin. *Common subtypes:* astrocytoma, oligodendroglioma, glioblastoma multiforme, and ependymoma. Tumours of the meninges (*meningiomas*) and cerebral blood vessels (*cerebellar haemangioblastomas*) can also occur.
- **2° brain tumours** 30%—usually from carcinoma of breast, lung, or melanoma—in 50%, tumours are multiple

Presentation ❶ <1% of patients with headache have a brain tumour.

- **↑ ICP** 23–50% have papilloedema at presentation; headache 25–35%
- **Seizures** 25–30%. Suspect in all adults who have a first seizure—especially if focal or with localizing aura. Refer for urgent assessment[N]
- **Evolving focal neurology** Depends on the site. >50% have focal neurology at presentation. Frontal lobe lesions tend to present late
- **False localizing signs** Caused by ↑ ICP. VI nerve palsy (causing double vision) is most common due to its long intracranial course
- **Subtle personality change** 16–20% at presentation—irritability, lack of application, lack of initiative, socially inappropriate behaviour
- **Local effects** Skull base masses, proptosis, epistaxis

Differential diagnosis Stroke, MS, head injury, vasculitis, encephalitis, Todd's palsy (🕮 p. 574), metabolic/electrolyte disturbance, other causes of space-occupying lesion—aneurysm, abscess, chronic subdural haematoma, granuloma, cyst.

Prognosis Gliomas all have <50% 5y survival. Depending on site, meningiomas and haemangioblastomas have better prognosis.

⚠ Referral guidelines for suspected brain tumour[N]

Refer urgently (to be seen in <2wk) Patients in whom a brain tumour is suspected with:

- Symptoms related to the CNS, including:
  - Progressive neurological deficit
  - New-onset seizures
  - Unilateral sensorineural deafness
  - Headaches
  - Mental changes
  - Cranial nerve palsy
- Headaches of recent onset accompanied by features suggestive of raised intracranial pressure, e.g.:
  - Vomiting
  - Drowsiness
  - Posture-related headache
  - Pulse-synchronous tinnitus

  or accompanied by other focal or non-focal neurological symptoms, e.g. blackout, change in personality, or memory
- A new, qualitatively different, unexplained headache that becomes progressively severe
- Suspected recent-onset seizures

Consider urgent referral In patients with rapid progression of:
- Subacute focal neurological deficit
- Unexplained cognitive impairment, behavioural disturbance or slowness, or a combination of these
- Personality changes confirmed by a witness and for which there is no reasonable explanation even in the absence of the other symptoms and signs of a brain tumour

Consider non-urgent referral Or discussion with specialist for unexplained headaches of recent onset:
- Present for ≥1 mo
- Not accompanied by features suggestive of ↑ intracranial pressure

Hydrocephalus Dilatation of the cerebral ventricles and accumulation of CSF. May be:
- **Communicating** Due to ↓ reabsorption of CSF. *Causes:* post-meningitis; SAH (80% develop some degree of hydrocephalus); trauma; neoplastic infiltration in the subarachnoid space
- **Non-communicating** CSF flow is blocked due to an obstruction within the ventricles. Due to congenital malformations, tumour, brain abscesss, SAH, meningeal scarring due to meningitis, or cranial trauma

Presentation and management In infants presents with macrocephaly (📖 p. 893); convulsions; developmental delay; and/or spasticity. In adults presents with ↑ ICP. Refer for urgent neurological assessment. ❗ All patients with a CSF shunt should have pneumococcal vaccination.

Further information
NICE Referral guidelines for suspected cancer (2005) ℘ www.nice.org.uk

Information and support for patients
Brain & Spine Foundation ☎ 0808 808 1000 ℘ www.brainandspine.org.uk

Intracranial bleeds

Haemorrhagic stroke 📖 p. 562

Subarachnoid haemorrhage (SAH) Spontaneous bleeding into the subarachnoid space. Incidence 15/100,000. ♀ > ♂. Peak age 35–65y. Frequently fatal. *Causes:*

- No cause (15%)
- Rupture of congenital berry aneurysm (70%)
- Arteriovenous malformation (15%)
- Bleeding disorder
- Mycotic aneurysm 2° to endocarditis (rare)

Risk factors Smoking, alcohol, ↑ BP, less common pre-menopause. Berry aneurysms may run in families and are associated with polycystic kidneys, coarctation of the aorta, and Ehlers–Danlos syndrome.

Presentation

- Typically presents as a sudden devastating headache—'thunderclap headache'—often occipital
- Rarely (6%) preceded by a 'sentinel headache' representing a small leak ahead of a larger bleed
- Vomiting and collapse with loss of consciousness ± fitting ± focal neurology follow

Examination May be nothing to find initially. Neck stiffness takes 6h to develop. In later stages:

- Papilloedema
- Retinal and other intraocular haemorrhages
- Focal neurology
- ↓ level of consciousness

Action If suspected admit immediately as a medical emergency. Only 1 in 4 admitted with suspected SAH turn out to have one. In most no cause for the headache is found.

Subdural haemorrhage Bleeding is from bridging veins between cortex and venous sinuses, resulting in accumulation of blood between dura and arachnoid. *Causes:* trauma (may be trivial); idiopathic.

Risk factors Age, alcohol, falls, epilepsy, anticoagulant therapy.

Presentation Often insidious and history may go back several weeks:

- Fluctuation of conscious level (35%)
- Physical and intellectual slowing
- Sleepiness
- Headache
- Personality change
- Unsteadiness on feet
- Slowly evolving stroke (e.g. hemiparesis)
- Symptoms/signs of ↑ ICP

Differential diagnosis Stroke, cerebral tumour, dementia.

Action If suspected, admit as a medical emergency for further investigation. Evacuation of clot is possible even in very elderly patients and often results in full recovery.

Extradural haemorrhage Blood accumulated between the dura and bone of the skull. Usually occurs after head injury.

Presentation Deterioration of level of consciousness after head injury that initially produced no loss of consciousness or after initial post-injury drowsiness has resolved. This 'lucid' interval may last anything from a few hours to a few days. May be accompanied by worsening headache, vomiting, confusion ± focal neurological signs.

Action If suspected, admit as an emergency for further investigation. Early evacuation of clot carries excellent prognosis. Outlook is less good if coma pre-op.

Acute stroke

Clinical syndrome typified by rapidly developing signs of focal or global disturbance of cerebral functions, lasting >24h or leading to death, with no apparent causes other than of vascular origin. Common and devastating condition—most common cause of adult disability in the UK. Half of all strokes occur in people >70y.

Causes

- **Cerebral infarction** (~70%). Atherothrombotic occlusion or embolism. *Sources of embolism:* left atrium (AF) or left ventricle (MI or heart failure). Ischaemia causes direct injury from lack of blood supply
- **Intracerebral or subarachnoid haemorrhage** (~19%). Haemorrhage causes direct neuronal injury and pressure exerted by the blood results in adjacent ischaemia
- **Rare causes** Sudden ↓ BP, vasculitis, venous-sinus thrombosis, carotid artery dissection

Risk factors

- Age
- ↑ BP
- DM
- AF
- Previous stroke or TIA
- MI
- Artificial heart valves
- Hyperviscosity syndromes
- Smoking
- Alcohol
- Obesity
- Low physical activity

Presentation

- **History** Sudden onset of CNS symptoms or stepwise progression of symptoms over hours or days
- **Examination** Conscious level—may be ↓ or normal; neurological signs (including dysphagia and incontinence); BP; heart rate and rhythm; heart murmurs; carotid bruits; systemic signs of infection or neoplasm

Differential diagnosis Decompensation after recovery from previous stroke (e.g. due to infection, metabolic disorder); SOL—1° or 2° cerebral neoplasm; cerebral abscess; trauma—subdural haematoma, traumatic brain injury; epileptic seizure; migraine; MS.

Acute management Admit all patients who have suffered an acute stroke to hospital. Treatment of stroke in a stroke unit ↓ mortality and morbidity[C]. Thrombolysis early after stroke results in better outcome, so do not delay referral until the patient is seen. If stroke is suspected admit directly to hospital by emergency ambulance.

⚠ Do not give aspirin prior to admission.

Transient ischaemic attack (TIA) History is as for stroke but recovery takes place within 24h of initial symptoms. Patients with a history of TIA have a 20% risk of stroke in the following month with highest risk in the first 72h. Risk can be predicted using the ABCD2 scoring system (see Table 16.9).

Management of TIA

- Admit if >1 TIA in <1wk. Consider admission/specialist assessment in <24h if the patient falls into a high/medium-risk group

- If not admitting, once all symptoms have stopped, start aspirin 75mg od. Check blood for FBC, ESR, U&E, Cr, eGFR, lipids, and glucose. Consider clotting screen ± thrombophilia screening if FH of thrombosis. Check ECG and CXR
- Start treatment for risk factors, e.g. advise to stop smoking, start antihypertensives if ↑ BP, start statin and dipyridamole S/R 200mg bd
- Refer for urgent assessment (to be seen in <1wk) and further investigation to a specialist service, e.g. TIA clinic. Specialist investigations include: CT or MRI scan to confirm diagnosis, carotid Dopplers if carotid artery territory symptoms; echocardiogram if recent MI, CCF/LVF, or murmur

Amaurosis fugax Form of TIA due to emboli passing through the retina. This causes brief loss of vision for a matter of minutes 'like a curtain'. Management is as for TIA.

Subarachnoid haemorrhage 📖 p. 560
Secondary prevention of stroke 📖 p. 564
Rehabilitation 📖 p. 204 and p. 582

Table 16.9 ABCD2 scoring system predicting future risk of stroke

ABCD2	Feature	Score
Age	<60y	0
	≥60y	1
BP	Systolic ≥140 and/or diastolic ≥90	1
Clinical features	Unilateral weakness	2
	Speech disturbance without weakness	1
	Other	0
Duration	≥1h	2
	10–59min	1
	<10min	0
Diabetes	Patient is diabetic	1
	Patient is not diabetic	0

Scoring: *High risk:* 6–7 points—8.1% 2-day risk of stroke (21% of patients)
Medium risk: 4–5 points—4.1% 2-day risk of stroke (45% of patients)
Low risk: 0–3 points—1% 2-day risk of stroke (34% of patients)

Further information
Royal College of Physicians National clinical guideline for stroke (2008) ℘ www.rcplondon.ac.uk
NICE Stroke: Diagnosis and initial management of acute stroke and TIA (2008) ℘ www.nice.org.uk

Patient information and support
Stroke Association ☎ 0303 3033 100 ℘ www.stroke.org.uk
Different Strokes ☎ 0845 130 7172 ℘ www.differentstrokes.co.uk
Speakability ☎ 0808 808 9572 ℘ www.speakability.org.uk

Management after stroke

After stroke Stroke is a family illness. 40% carers suffer psychological distress starting <6wk after discharge. Involve carers/families. Provide information/support. Address psychosocial issues and physical disability.

- Monitor and reassess frequently. Continue follow-up even when specialist services have finished. Monitor 2° prevention measures. Refer for more specialist rehabilitation if there is any deterioration in function
- Aids/appliances can help. Patients/carers may be entitled to benefits
- After stroke most patients are prescribed ≥1 drugs to ↓ risk of further stroke, but some have memory loss or problems opening containers. Provide verbal and written information about medicines and help with packaging, e.g. non-childproof tops

Screening for depression 📖 p. 199

Secondary stroke prevention Patients with a history of stroke or TIA/amaurosis fugax have a 30–43% risk of recurrent stroke within 5y. Prevention focusses on ischaemic/embolic events which account for the majority of strokes. *Preventative strategies include:*

Lifestyle advice
- Stopping smoking—📖 p. 182
- Regular exercise— 📖 p. 180
- Diet and achieving a satisfactory weight—📖 pp. 174–9
- Reducing salt intake—↓ salt of 3g/d leads to ↓ in stroke risk of 13%
- Avoiding alcohol excess—predisposes to both ischaemic and haemorrhagic stroke through action on BP—📖 pp. 184–7

Antiplatelet drugs Start patients not taking warfarin, who have had a non-haemorrhagic stroke on CT/MRI on clopidogrel 75mg od long-term[N] (aspirin 75mg od + dipyridamole S/R 200mg bd if intolerant). For patients who have had a TIA start aspirin 75mg od + dipyridamole S/R 200mg bd (dipyridamole M/R 200mg bd alone if intolerant to aspirin).

Oral anticoagulation For both 1° and 2° stroke prevention, anticoagulate with warfarin or dabigatran if there are potential causes of cardiac thromboembolism, e.g. rheumatic mitral valve disease; prosthetic heart valves; dilated cardiomyopathy; and AF associated with valvular heart disease or prosthesis. CHA2DS2-VASc score (see Table 16.10) is used to predict stroke risk and need for anticoagulation for patients with non-valvular AF.

Hypertension management 📖 p. 248
- Systolic and diastolic BP independently predict stroke. Risk escalates with increasing BP. A 5–6mmHg ↓ BP reduces risk by >30%
- After stroke (but not after TIA) defer treating hypertension until >2wk after the event as ↑ BP may be physiological response—lowering BP decreases perfusion of the brain and may be harmful

Cholesterol
- **Primary prevention** A 22% ↓ in cholesterol using a statin results in a 30%↓ in stroke in individuals with no past history of stroke/TIA. Treat if patients meet criteria for coronary prevention (📖 p. 242)
- **Secondary prevention** Treat all patients with a history of CVD with a statin regardless of baseline cholesterol. National Stroke Guidelines suggest treatment with a statin, e.g. simvastatin 40mg od, if total cholesterol is >3.5mmol/L unless contraindicated

Carotid stenosis and carotid endarterectomy Carotid endarterectomy ↓ mortality if carotid stenosis is symptomatic. Benefits ↓ as stenosis gets less—no evidence of benefit if <30% stenosis.
- **Patients without history of stroke/TIA** 2% annual risk of stroke so surgery is controversial—in general risks outweigh benefits
- **Patients with a history of stroke /TIA** Consider referral for carotid endarterectomy/carotid artery stenting if >70% carotid artery stenosis and no severe disability

Table 16.10 CHA2DS2-VASc score

	Condition	Points	Score
C	Congestive heart failure	1	0—*Low risk*—no antithrombotic therapy or aspirin 75mg od
H	Hypertension	1	
A	Age >75y	2	1—*Moderate risk*—aspirin, or oral anticoagulation depending on patient preference
A	Age 65–74y	1	
D	DM	1	
S	Female*	1	≥2—*High risk*—oral anticoagulation unless contraindicated
S	Prior stroke/TIA	2	
VASc	Vascular disease e.g. MI, peripheral arterial disease, aortic plaque	2	*Target INR for warfarin:* 2–3

* For women <65y with no other risk factors, CHA2DS2-VASc score = 0

❶ In all cases weigh benefit of treatment against potential harms. The *HAS-BLED* score may help with decision-making:
- Hypertension (uncontrolled, systolic >160mmHg)—1 point
- Abnormal liver function (cirrhosis, bilirubin >2x normal, ALT/AST/alk phos >3x normal)—1 point
- Abnormal renal function (dialysis, Cr >200micromol)—1 point
- Stroke history—1 point
- Prior major bleed or predisposition to bleeding—1 point
- Labile INR (<60% of the time in therapeutic range)—1 point
- Elderly (age ≥65y)—1 point
- Drugs predisposing to bleeding (e.g. antiplatelet agents, NSAIDs)—1 point
- Alcohol use—1 point

A score ≥3 indicates ↑ 1-year bleed risk on anticoagulation sufficient to justify caution before prescribing or more regular review

Further information
Royal College of Physicians National clinical guidelines for stroke (2012) ℘ www.rcplondon.ac.uk
NICE Clopidogrel and modified-release dipyridamole for the prevention of occlusive vascular events (2010) ℘ www.nice.org.uk

Patient information and support
Stroke Association ☏ 0303 3033 100 ℘ www.stroke.org.uk

Parkinsonism and Parkinson's disease

Parkinsonism Syndrome of:
- **Tremor** Coarse tremor, most marked at rest, 'pill-rolling'
- **Rigidity** Limbs resist passive extension throughout movement—*lead-pipe rigidity*—and juddering on passive extension of the forearm or pronation/supination—*cogwheel rigidity*
- **Difficulty in initiating movement**
- **Slowness of movement** *Mask-like* or expressionless face, ↓ blink rate, ↓ fidgeting, ↓ peristalsis
- **Abnormal gait** Small steps—*shuffling gait*—and flexed posture as if hurrying to keep up with feet—*festinant gait*
- **Micrographia** Small handwriting

Causes
- Parkinson's disease (PD)
- Other neurodegenerative diseases, e.g. Alzheimer's disease, multisystem atrophy
- Following encephalitis
- Drugs, e.g. haloperidol, chlorpromazine, metoclopramide
- Toxins, e.g. CO poisoning
- Trauma
- Normal pressure hydrocephalus

Treatment of drug-induced parkinsonism If possible, stop the implicated drug. If on an antipsychotic for schizophrenia do not stop treatment, but add an antimuscarinic (e.g. procyclidine 2.5mg tds). Consider switching to an atypical antipsychotic drug—take specialist advice.

Steele–Richardson–Olszewski syndrome Parkinsonism accompanied by absent vertical gaze and dementia. Due to progressive supranuclear palsy. *J.C. Steele, J.C. Richardson, and J. Olszewski—Canadian neurologists.*

Parkinson's disease (PD) Incurable, progressive, degenerative disease affecting the dopaminergic neurones of the substantia nigra in the brainstem, resulting in deficiency of dopamine and relative excess of acetylcholine transmitters. *Cause:* unknown. *Lifetime risk:* 1 in 40. ♂ = ♀. *Peak age at onset:* ≈65y, but 5–10% patients are diagnosed when <40y old. Prevalence ↑ with age. *J. Parkinson (1755–1824)—English physician.*

Non-motor symptoms
- **Neuropsychiatric**—apathy, anxiety/depression, visual hallucinations, psychosis, dementia, pain, olfactory disturbance
- **Sleep**—excessive daytime sleepiness, restless legs
- **Autonomic**—drooling, postural hypotension, hyperhidrosis, urinary dysfunction, dysphagia, weight↓, constipation, sexual dysfunction

Management Aims to:
- ↓ symptoms and ↑ quality of life
- ↓ rate of disease progression
- Limit side effects of treatment

Screening for depression 📖 p. 199

Referral Refer all patients to a specialist with an interest in Parkinson's disease for confirmation of diagnosis, advice on management, and to access a multidisciplinary specialist rehabilitation team.

Rehabilitation Liaise closely with the specialist rehabilitation team.
- General principles 📖 p. 204   • Specific issues 📖 p. 582

Drug treatment (*BNF* 4.9) Rarely achieves complete control of symptoms; 5–10% respond poorly. Treatment for PD should be consultant-initiated and is not started until symptoms cause significant disruption of daily activities. *Options*:

Dopamine receptor agonists (e.g. bromocriptine, pergolide). Often used alone as first-line treatment. ↑ dose gradually, according to response and tolerability. Withdraw gradually. Can also be used in association with L-dopa to ↓ off times and motor impairment.

> ⚠ Bromocriptine, pergolide, cabergoline, and lisuride have been associated with pulmonary, retroperitoneal, and pericardial fibrosis.
> - Check CXR ± spirometry, ESR, and creatinine before starting
> - Monitor for dyspnoea, persistent cough, chest pain, cardiac failure, abdominal pain, or tenderness

Levodopa (or L-dopa) Precursor of dopamine. ↑ dopamine levels within the substantia nigra. Start with low dose and ↑ in small steps—aim to keep final dose as low as possible and a compromise between ↑ mobility and dose-limiting side effects (involuntary movements, psychiatric effects). Optimum dose interval varies between individuals.
- Only effective for PD. Not effective for patients with parkinsonism due to other causes. Improves bradykinesia and rigidity > tremor
- Often given with a co-drug (carbidopa or benserazide) which prevents peripheral breakdown of levodopa to dopamine but does not cross the blood–brain barrier
- With time, there is ↓ response and troublesome side effects appear:
  - **On-off effect**—fluctuation between periods of exaggerated involuntary movements and periods of immobility
  - **End-of-dose effect** —duration of benefit after each dose reduces
  - **Abnormal involuntary movements** ↑

Other drugs
- **Monoamine oxidase B inhibition** (e.g selegiline, rasagaline). Used in severe PD in conjunction with levodopa to ↓ end-of-dose effect. Early use may postpone onset of treatment with levodopa
- **Amantadine** Improves bradykinesia, dyskinesias, tremor, and rigidity. Introduce and withdraw slowly
- **Inhibition of enzymatic breakdown of dopamine** (e.g. entacapone, tolcapone). For patients suffering from end-of-dose effect

Surgery A small proportion of carefully selected patients benefit from 'deep brain stimulation' (DBS).

Driving 📖 p. 130   Carers 📖 p. 220

Further information
NICE Parkinson's disease: diagnosis and management in primary and secondary care (2006) ℘ www.nice.org.uk

Patient advice and support
Parkinson's Disease Society ☎ 0808 800 0303 ℘ www.parkinsons.org.uk

Multiple sclerosis

Multiple sclerosis (MS) is a chronic disabling neurological disease due to an autoimmune process of unknown cause. Characterized by formation of patches of demyelination ('plaques') throughout the brain and spinal cord. There is no peripheral nerve involvement.

It is the most common neurological disorder of young adults, with a life-time risk of 1:1,000. Peak age of onset is 20–40y. ♀:♂ ≈2:1. There is a marked geographical variation—prevalence ↑ with latitude.

Presentation Depends on the area of CNS affected. Take a careful history—although a patient usually presents with a single symptom, history may reveal other episodes that have gone unheralded. Isolated neurological deficits are never diagnostic. The hallmark of MS is a series of neurological deficits distributed in time and space not attributable to other causes. Predominant areas of demyelination are optic nerve, cervical cord, and periventricular areas.

Common features

- Pain on eye movement (optic neuritis)
- Visual disturbance— ↓, blurring, or double vision
- ↓ balance and coordination
- Sensory disturbance (e.g. numbness, tingling)
- Pain (e.g. trigeminal neuralgia)
- Fatigue
- Depression
- Transverse myelitis (📖 p. 572)
- Problems with speech (e.g. slurred or slow)
- Bladder problems (e.g. frequency, urgency, incontinence)
- Constipation
- Sexual dysfunction (e.g. impotence)
- Cognitive changes (e.g. loss of concentration, memory problems)
- Dysphagia

❶ Symptoms may be worsened by heat or exercise.

Prognosis

- **Benign MS** (10%). Retrospective diagnosis. The patient has a few mild attacks and then complete recovery. There is no deterioration over time and no permanent disability
- **Relapsing-remitting MS (RRMS)** 85% patients. Episodes of sudden ↑ in neurological symptoms or development of new neurological symptoms with virtually complete recovery after 4–6wk. With time remissions become less complete and residual disability accumulates
- **Secondary progressive MS (SPMS)** After ~15y, 65% of patients with relapsing-remitting disease begin a continuous downward progression which may also include acute relapses
- **Primary progressive MS (PPMS)** 10% patients. Steady progression from the outset with increasing disability

Management If suspected, refer to neurology for confirmation of diagnosis and support from the specialist neurological rehabilitation team.

Disease-modifying drugs ↓ frequency and/or severity of relapses by ~30% and slow course of the disease. Options are β-interferon (for RRMS and SPMS), and glatiramer (for RRMS only). Prescription must be consultant-led under the NHS risk-sharing scheme—Table 16.11.

Table 16.11 Indications for β-interferon and glatiramer

	β-interferon	Glatiramer
Age	≥18y	≥18y
Contraindications	No contraindications present	No contraindications present
Walking distance	*RRMS* Can walk ≥100m without assistance *SPMS* Can walk ≥10m without assistance	*RRMS* Can walk ≥100m without assistance
Relapses	*RRMS* ≥2 clinically significant relapses in the last year *SPMS* Minimal ↑ in disability due to gradual progression and ≥2 disabling relapses in the past 2y	*RRMS* ≥2 clinically significant relapses in the last year
Stop if	• Intolerable side effects • Pregnant/planning pregnancy • ≥2 disabling relapses in <1y • Inability to walk (± assistance) persisting ≥6mo • 2° progression with observable ↑ in disability over 6mo	• Intolerable side effects • Pregnant or planning pregnancy • ≥2 disabling relapse in <1y • Inability to walk (± assistance) persisting ≥6mo • 2° progression

Natalizumab and fingolimod Approved for treatment of highly active RRMS, despite treatment with β-interferon, or rapidly evolving severe RRMS. Prescription must be consultant-led.

• **Natalizumab** Is associated with ↑ risk of opportunistic infection and progressive multifocal leucoencephalopathy (PML). If new/worsening neurological symptoms/signs refer to neurology immediately

• **Fingolimod** Is associated with macular oedema in 0.4%; routine ophthalmological review is recommended 3–4mo after initiation

Acute relapses Treat episodes causing distressing symptoms or ↑ limitation with high-dose steroids e.g. prednisolone 500mg–2g od po for 3–5d. Alternatively refer for high-dose IV steroids. Refer to specialist neurological rehabilitation if residual deficit or if frequent relapses.

Management of symptoms and disability Liaise closely with the specialist neurological rehabilitation team.

• Screening for depression 📖 p. 199
• General principles of rehabilitation 📖 p. 204
• Common neurological rehabilitation problems 📖 p. 582

Further information

NICE/RCP Diagnosis and management of multiple sclerosis in primary and secondary care (2003) 🕸 www.nice.org.uk
MS Society A guide to MS for GPs and primary care professionals (2009) 🕸 www.mssociety.org.uk

Patient advice and support

MS Society ☎ 0808 800 8000 🕸 www.mssociety.org.uk

Motor neurone disease and CJD

Motor neurone disease (MND) Is a degenerative disorder of unknown cause affecting motor neurones in the spinal cord, brainstem, and motor cortex. Prevalence in the UK ~4.5/100,000 population ♂:♀ ≈3:2. Peak age of onset ≈60y. 10% have a FH. There is *never* any sensory loss.

Patterns of disease There are 3 recognized patterns of MND:
- **Amyotrophic lateral sclerosis (ALS)** (50%). Combined LMN wasting and UMN hyperreflexia
- **Progressive muscular atrophy** (25%). Anterior horn cell lesions, affecting distal before proximal muscles. Better prognosis than ALS
- **Progressive bulbar palsy** (25%). Loss of function of brainstem motor nuclei (LMN lesions), resulting in weakness of the tongue, muscles of chewing/swallowing, and facial muscles

Clinical picture Combination of progressive upper and/or lower motor neurone signs, affecting >1 limb or a limb and the bulbar muscles. *Symptoms and signs:*

- Stumbling (spastic gait, foot drop)
- Tiredness
- Muscle wasting
- Weak grip
- Weakness of skeletal muscles
- Cramp
- Fasciculation of skeletal muscles
- Fasciculation of the tongue
- Difficulty with speech (particularly slurring, hoarseness, or nasal or quiet speech)
- Difficulty with swallowing
- Aspiration pneumonia

ⓘ MND *never* affects eye movements (cranial nerves III, IV, VI)

Management Refer to neurology for exclusion of other causes of symptoms and confirmation of diagnosis. MND is incurable and progressive. Death usually results from ventilatory failure 3–5y after diagnosis.

Drug therapy
- Riluzole (50mg bd) is the only drug treatment licensed in the UK
- Evidence suggests it extends life or time to mechanical ventilation for patients with ALS. It may also slow functional decline[N]
- It should be initiated by a specialist with experience of MND[N]
- Monitoring of liver function is essential—monthly for the first 3mo; then 3-monthly for 9mo; then annually thereafter

Support
- Involve relevant agencies early, e.g. DN, social services, carer groups, self-help groups
- Apply for all relevant benefits (📖 p. 222)
- Screen for depression (📖 p. 199)
- Discuss the future and patients' wishes for the time when they become incapacitated with patient and carer(s)
- Regular review to help overcome any new problems encountered is helpful for patients and carers

Symptom relief
- **Spasticity**—baclofen, tizanidine, botulinum toxin
- **Drooling**—propantheline 15–30mg tds po or amitriptyline 25–50mg tds
- **Dysphagia**—blend food, discuss NG tubes/PEG (📖 p. 583)
- **Depression**—common. Reassess support, consider drug treatment, and/or counselling
- **Joint pains**—analgesia
- **Respiratory failure**—discuss tracheostomy/ventilation; weigh pros and cons of prolongation of life versus prolongation of discomfort
- **Palliative care** 📖 pp. 1028–47

Creutzfeldt–Jakob disease (CJD) (human spongiform encephalopathy). Fatal, degenerative brain disease due to a rogue form of brain protein or 'prion'. *Types:*
- **Sporadic or classical** Most common form in the UK (~50 cases/y). Rare <40y. Median duration of symptoms 3–4 mo. *Cause:* unknown
- **Variant** Affects younger people than classical CJD and duration is longer, lasting a median of 14mo. *Cause:* transmitted by ingestion of nervous tissue in beef infected with bovine spongiform encephalitis or 'mad cow disease'. Compensation may be available to families
- **Iatrogenic** Cases associated with treatments using human growth hormone and human dura mater grafts. Rarely associated with corneal grafts or contaminated instruments used in surgery
- **Familial prion disease** ~20–30 families in the UK are affected with a version of CJD passed from generation to generation in an autosomal dominant pattern. Median duration of symptoms from onset is 2–5y

Presentation Long incubation (>25y in some cases). Clinical features vary according to the areas of brain most affected but are always rapidly progressive. *Common features:* personality change; psychiatric symptoms; cognitive impairment; neurological deficits (sensory and motor deficits, ataxia); myoclonic jerks, chorea, or dystonia; difficulty with communication, mobility, swallowing, and continence; coma and death.

Differential diagnosis Dementia, depression, MS, MND, SOL.

Management There is no simple diagnostic test and often families feel frustrated by early misdiagnosis. Refer to neurologist if suspected. Treatment is supportive. *Palliative care* 📖 pp. 1028–47

General principles of rehabilitation 📖 p. 204

Common neurological rehabilitation problems 📖 p. 582

Further information
NICE 🖰 www.nice.org.uk
- Riluzole for motor neurone disease (2004)
- Motor neurone disease—non-invasive ventilation (2010)

Patient advice and support
Motor Neurone Disease Association ☎ 08457 626262
🖰 www.mndassociation.org
Brain and Spine Foundation ☎ 0808 808 1000
🖰 www.brainandspine.org.uk

Spinal cord conditions

Spinal cord injury tends to affect young people, especially young men. It is devastating, and the GP and primary care team are a vital part of the ongoing support network. *Causes:* trauma (42% falls; 37% RTAs), herniated disc, transverse myelitis, tumour, abscess.

Quadriplegia and tetraplegia Caused by spinal cord injury above the first thoracic vertebra. Usually results in paralysis of all four limbs, weakened breathing, and an inability to cough and clear the chest.

Paraplegia Occurs when the level of injury is below the first thoracic nerve. Disability can vary from the impairment of leg movement to complete paralysis of the legs and abdomen up to the nipple line. Paraplegics have full use of their arms and hands.

Incomplete spinal cord injuries

- **Anterior cord syndrome** Damage is towards the front of the spinal cord, leaving the patient with loss or ↓ ability to sense pain, temperature, and touch sensations below the level of injury. Pressure and joint sensation may be preserved
- **Central cord syndrome** Damage is in the centre of the spinal cord. Typically results in loss of function in the arms, but preservation of some leg movement ± some control of bladder/bowel function
- **Posterior cord syndrome** Damage is towards the back of the spinal cord. Typically leaves patients with good muscle power, pain, and temperature sensation, but difficulty coordinating limb movements
- **Brown-Séquard syndrome** Damage is limited to one side of the spinal cord resulting in loss or ↓ movement on the injured side but preserved pain and temperature sensation, and normal movement on the uninjured side but loss or ↓ in pain and temperature sensation. *C.E. Brown-Séquard (1817–94)—French neurologist/physiologist*

Cauda equina lesion The spinal cord ends at L1/L2 at which point a bundle of nerves travels downwards through the lumbar and sacral vertebrae. Injury to these nerves causes partial or complete loss of movement and sensation. There may be some recovery of function with time.

Transverse myelitis Inflammation of the spinal cord at a single level. Symptoms develop rapidly over days/weeks and include limb weakness, sensory disturbance, bowel and bladder disturbance, back pain, and radicular pain. Recovery generally begins within 3mo but is not always complete. *Causes:*

- Idiopathic (thought to be auto-immune mechanism)
- Infection
- Vaccination
- Autoimmune disease, e.g. SLE, Sjögren's syndrome, sarcoidosis
- MS
- Malignancy
- Vascular, e.g. thrombosis of spinal arteries, vasculitis 2° to heroin abuse, spinal A-V malformation

Management Depending on severity of symptoms, admit as an acute medical emergency or refer for urgent neurological opinion.

Syringomyelia Tubular cavities (syrinxes) form close to the central canal of the spinal cord. As the syrinx expands it compresses nerves within the spinal cord. Most common in patients with previous spinal injury—although may be years before. Typically presents with wasting and weakness of hands and arms, and loss of temperature and pain sensation over trunk and arms (cape distribution). Refer to neurology.

General principles of rehabilitation 🕮 p. 204

Common neurological rehabilitation problems 🕮 p. 582

Specific problems associated with spinal cord injury

Autonomic dysreflexia (hyperreflexia) Reflex sympathetic overactivity, causing flushing and ↑ BP which may be severe. Only occurs in patients with lesions above T5/6. Usually triggered by discomfort below the level of the lesion. Presentation is with pounding headache, sweating, flushing, or mottling above the level of the lesion.

Sit the patient up and remove any obvious cause, e.g. pain, bladder distension, constipation. Give GTN spray (1–2 puff sublingual) or nifedipine 5–10mg capsule broken sublingually. If not settling, admit to hospital.

Loss of temperature control Most people with complete spinal cord injuries do not sweat below the level of the injury and many quadriplegics cannot sweat above the injury (even though they may sweat due to autonomic dysreflexia). With loss of ability to sweat or vasoconstrict, careful control of environmental conditions is essential to avoid hypothermia or overheating. In hot weather advise cooling with wet towels.

Infertility Many ♂ patients suffer infertility due to:
● Failure of ejaculation
● Retrograde ejaculation
● Thermal damage due to sitting in a wheelchair → poor-quality sperm
● Chronic infection of prostate and seminal vesicles (common)

Refer for specialist advice.

Bowel/bladder function Both bladder and bowel function are reflex actions that we learn to override as children. If the lesion is above the level of this reflex pathway (T12 for bowel and T6 for bladder function) then automatic emptying will still occur when the bladder or bowel is full—though there is no control. If the lesion is below this level there is no emptying reflex. Bladder/bowel care programmes reflect this. Useful leaflets are available from the Spinal Injuries Association.

Spasticity 🕮 p. 583	**Pressure sores** 🕮 p. 613
UTI 🕮 p. 583	**Depression** 🕮 p. 199

Patient advice and support
Spinal Injuries Association ☎ 0800 980 0501 ℘ www.spinal.co.uk
Brain and Spine Foundation ☎ 0808 808 1000 ℘ www.brainandspine.org.uk
Transverse Myelitis Society ℘ www.myelitis.org.uk
British Syringomyelia & Chiari Society
℘ www.britishsyringomyelia-chiarisociety.org

Epilepsy

Epilepsy is a group of disorders in which fits or seizures occur as a result of spontaneous abnormal electrical discharge in any part of the brain. They take many forms but usually take the same pattern on each occasion for a given individual. Prevalence 5–10/1,000. 5% of those >21y old having their first fit have cerebral pathology (10% aged 45–55y).

Epilepsy in children 📖 p. 898

Management of a fitting patient/status epilepticus 📖 p. 1070

Management after first fit 60% of adults who have one fit will never have another (90% if EEG is normal).

> ⚠ Refer *all* patients with a first suspected seizure for urgent (within 2wk) assessment by a neurologist with training and expertise in epilepsy to exclude underlying causes (e.g. tumour) and receive clear guidance on medication, work, and driving [N].

Classification of seizure types Is important, as these have implications for management and prognosis.
- **Partial seizures** The seizure is limited to one area of the brain only. Termed 'simple' if no impairment of consciousness (previously called *focal* or *Jacksonian epilepsy*) and 'complex' if consciousness is impaired (previously called *psychomotor* or *temporal lobe epilepsy*). Partial seizures may become generalized
- **Generalized seizures** Whole brain is involved. Consciousness is usually but not always impaired. 6 major types: tonic-clonic (grand mal); absence (petit mal); myoclonic; tonic; clonic; and atonic

❶ Some people have seizures that cannot be classified in this way.

Todd's palsy Focal CNS signs (e.g. hemiplegia) following an epileptic seizure. The patient seems to have had a stroke but recovers in <24h.

Causes of epilepsy in adults A cause is found in more than two-thirds of people with epilepsy. The most common causes are:
- Cerebrovascular disease
- Cerebral tumours
- Genetic, congenital, or hereditary conditions
- Drugs, alcohol, and other toxic causes
- Head trauma (including surgery)
- Post-infective causes (e.g. meningitis, encephalitis)

Assessment See Table 16.12.

Screening for depression 📖 p. 199

Long-term management of epilepsy 📖 p. 576

Epilepsy and pregnancy 📖 p. 829

Mortality Death rate is ↑ x2–3. Deaths are related to underlying condition, accidents, SUDEP, or status epilepticus.

Sudden unexplained death in epilepsy (SUDEP) Probably due to central respiratory arrest during a seizure. Minimize risk by optimizing seizure control and being aware of potential consequences of night seizures.

Table 16.12 Summary of points to cover during assessment

History	
Background	• Previous head injury • Stroke • Alcohol/drug abuse • Febrile convulsions • Meningitis or • Family history of epilepsy encephalitis
Provoking factors	• Sleep deprivation • Flashing lights • Alcohol withdrawal
Prodrome/aura	**Prodrome**—precedes fit. May be a change in mood or behaviour noticed by the patient or others **Aura**—part of the seizure that precedes other manifestations; odd sensations, e.g. déjà vu (odd feeling of having experienced that time before), strange smells, rising abdominal sensation, flashing lights
Features of the attack	**Eye witness report:** if available—colour of the patient, movement, length of fit, circumstances, after-effects **Memories of the patient:** memories of the event and/or first memories after the event, frequency of attacks, relationship to sleep, menses, etc.
Residual symptoms after the attack	• Bitten tongue • Incontinence of urine/faeces (not specific for epilepsy) • Confusion • Headache • Aching limbs or temporary weakness of limbs (Todd's palsy)
Examination	
Neurological examination	• Fever, photophobia, neck stiffness, or petechial rash? • Any residual deficit • Focal neurology • Signs of ↑ ICP (📖 p. 558)
General examination	• BP, heart sounds, heart rhythm and rate • Signs of systemic illness
Investigations (first fit only)	• ECG • Blood for U&E, Cr, eGFR, LFT, Ca²⁺, FBC, ESR/CRP

Differential diagnosis	
• Vasovagal syncope	• Normal phenomenon (e.g. déja vu)
• Psychogenic non-epileptic attacks (pseudo-seizures)	• Cardiac arrhythmias • Other cardiac disorders (e.g. aortic stenosis, HOCM)
• Tics	• TIA
• Panic attack	
• Hypoglycaemia	• Migrainous aura

Further information
NICE ℘ www.nice.org.uk
- The epilepsies: the diagnosis and management of the epilepsies in adults and children in primary and secondary care (2012)
- Referral guidelines for suspected cancer (2005)

Patient advice and support
Epilepsy Action ☎ 0808 800 5050 ℘ www.epilepsy.org.uk

Management of epilepsy

Regular GP review, at least annually, is essential.

Education Epilepsy is a diagnosis causing alarm and fear. Find out how much the patient (and family) understands about epilepsy. Acknowledge distress at diagnosis and answer their questions. Provide information on:
- What to expect—fits are controlled with drugs in 80%
- What to do during an attack
- Driving (📖 p. 130) and work—stop driving, and notify DVLA and motor insurance company. Inform employer. Do not work at heights or with/near dangerous machinery
- Avoiding risks—avoid cycling in traffic; only swim if lifeguard present
- Importance of concordance with medication
- When drug withdrawal may be considered if fit-free

Leaflets are available from Epilepsy Action. Support groups can help.

Drug therapy *BNF* 4.8.1. NICE recommends drug treatment (see Table 16.13) after the second seizure, except in specific circumstances. Drug choice is a specialist decision. ❶ Patients on anticonvulsants are entitled to free prescriptions throughout the UK.

Withdrawal of drug therapy Consider if fit-free for 2–3y. Decision to stop *must* be the patient's. Balance problems/inconvenience of drug-taking against risks of fits. Refer to neurology for supervision of drug with-drawal. If adult with grand mal epilepsy, 59% stay fit-free for 2y.

Seizure recurrence is more likely if generalized tonic-clonic seizures; myoclonic epilepsy or infantile spasms; taking >1 drug for epilepsy; ≥1 seizure after starting treatment; duration of treatment >10y; fit-free <5y.

⚠ Advise patients not to drive during withdrawal of epileptic medication or for 6mo afterwards.

Surgery Used for intractable partial seizures, hemiepilepsy, and epilepsy with focal EEG and/or radiological features.

Vagus nerve stimulation ↓ frequency of seizures for those refractory to anti-epileptic medication but not suitable for resective surgery.

Ketogenic diet Effective in some patients with refractory epilepsy—take specialist advice.

At review Review the individual's care plan. Record fits and precipitating causes; check drug concordance (frequency of repeat prescriptions) and side effects; if fit-free >2y—discuss the possibility of withdrawing medication, if appropriate. For women of reproductive age give contraception (📖 p. 756) and pre-conception advice (📖 p. 829).

Re-refer For review by a neurologist or epilepsy nurse specialist if:
- Control is poor or drugs are causing unacceptable side effects
- Seizures have continued despite medication for >2y or on two drugs
- Pointers to a previously unsuspected cause for the fits appear
- Concurrent illness (physical or psychiatric) complicates management
- For pre-conceptual advice or to discuss withdrawal of medication

Table 16.13 Commonly used drugs in epilepsy. Stress the importance of concordance. Start at a low dose, and ↑ dose until fits are controlled or side effects occur. Use monotherapy wherever possible—two drugs ↑ toxicity and side effects. Polytherapy offers no advantage over monotherapy for 90% patients. Prescribe by brand name—generic prescribing may lead to changing of brand. Changing brand carries 10% risk of worsening of seizure control.

		Ethosuximide	Sodium valproate	Carbamazepine	Lamotrigine	Clonazepam
Type of epilepsy	Absence	✓			✓	✓
	Myoclonic		✓		✓	✓
	Tonic clonic		✓¹	✓	✓	
	Partial ± 2° generalized		✓	✓	✓	
Adult starting dose		500mg od	300mg bd	100–200mg od or bd	25mg od for 2wk²	1mg nocte for 4d
Incremental dose		250mg/d at weekly intervals	200mg/d at 3-day intervals	100mg/d at weekly intervals	From starting dose to 50mg od for 2wk, then ↑ by 50mg/d at weekly intervals	↑ according to response over 2–4wk
Usual daily dose		1–1.5g od	500mg–1g bd	200–1200mg	100–200mg	4–8mg nocte
Common/important side effects		Blood dyscrasias³, nausea, sedation, vomiting, dizziness, ataxia	Pancreatitis, liver toxicity¹, blood dyscrasias³, sedation, tremor, weight ↑, hair thinning, ankle swelling	Blood dyscrasias³, rash, liver toxicity⁴, nausea, sedation, diplopia, fluid retention, dizziness, ↓ Na⁺⁵	Blood dyscrasias³, rash, fever, influenza-like symptoms, drowsiness, or worsening of seizure control	Drowsiness/fatigue, amnesia/confusion/ restlessness, muscle hypotonia, co-ordination problems, dependence, and withdrawal

1 Drug of choice for primary syndromes of generalized epilepsy.
2 Starting dose is different if used in association with other epileptics—see BNF.
3 Check FBC if bruising, mouth ulcers, or symptoms of infection (sore throat, fevers).
4 Warn about symptoms of liver disease. Check LFTS soon after starting and at review.
5 Monitor U&E at regular review.

Muscle disorders

Symptoms Muscle weakness, fatigability. Pain at rest suggests inflammation—pain on exercise, ischaemia, or metabolic myopathy.

Signs Look for associated systemic disease.
- **Myotonia**—delayed muscular relaxation after contraction, e.g. difficulty letting go after gripping something
- **Local muscular tenderness or firm muscles**—may be due to infiltration of muscle with connective tissue or fat
- **Fasciculation**—spontaneous, irregular, and brief contractions of part of a muscle; suggests LMN disease, e.g. MND
- **Lumps**—tumours are rare; lumps may be due to tendon rupture, haematoma, or herniation of muscle through fascia

Muscular dystrophies Group of genetic disorders characterized by progressive degeneration and weakness of some muscle groups.

Myotonic dystrophy (dystrophia myotonia) Autosomal dominant inheritance—abnormal DMPK gene on chromosome 19. Presents at any age. Symptoms vary from mild to severe and may include:
- **Muscle symptoms**—weakness and myotonia, particularly involves face, eyelids, jaw, neck, forearms/hands, lower legs/feet. Can affect speech and result in a lack of facial expression
- **Respiratory symptoms**—weakness of respiratory muscles → poor night-time sleep, daytime sleepiness, headaches, and difficulty waking; aspiration → recurrent chest infections
- **Eye symptoms**—cataract (may be the only problem) and ptosis
- **Reproductive problems**—infertility as a result of atrophy of the testes and problems in labour due to uterine muscle weakness
- **Learning difficulty and behavioural problems**
- **Digestive symptoms**—swallowing difficulty, abdominal pain, constipation/diarrhoea, gallstones
- **Cardiac arrhythmias**—annual ECG is advisable
- **Endocrine abnormalities**, e.g. DM
- **Anaesthetic problems**—pre-warn anaesthetist/surgeon prior to surgery

Prognosis is variable depending on severity of symptoms. Refer to confirm diagnosis and for advice on management/genetic counselling.

> *Duchenne's muscular dystrophy* Sex-linked recessive inheritance means almost always confined to boys. 30% of cases are due to spontaneous mutation. Investigation shows markedly ↑ CK (>40x normal). Presents typically at ~4y with progressively clumsy walking. Few survive to >20y old. Refer for confirmation of diagnosis and ongoing specialist support. Genetic counselling is important. *G.B.A. Duchenne (1807–75)—French neurologist.*

Patient information and support
Myotonic Dystrophy Support Group ☎ 0115 987 0080
🖰 www.myotonicdystrophysupportgroup.org
Muscular Dystrophy Campaign ☎ 0800 652 6352
🖰 www.muscular-dystrophy.org

Toxic myopathies Certain drugs can cause myopathy including:

- Alcohol
- Labetalol
- Cholesterol-lowering drugs (including statins)
- Steroids
- Chloroquine
- Zidovudine
- Vincristine
- Ciclosporin
- Cocaine
- Heroin
- PCP

Management Stop the implicated drug immediately. If symptoms do not resolve, refer for confirmation of diagnosis and management advice.

Acquired myopathy of late onset Often a manifestation of systemic disease, e.g. thyroid disease (especially hyperthyroidism), carcinoma, Cushing's disease. Investigate to find the cause. Treat the cause if found else refer for further investigation.

Polymyositis Insidious, symmetrical, proximal muscle weakness due to muscle inflammation. Dysphagia, dysphonia, and/or respiratory muscle weakness may follow. 25% have a purple rash on cheeks, eyelids, and other sun-exposed areas (*dermatomyositis*) ± nail fold erythema. CK levels are ↑. Associated with malignancy in 10% of patients >40y. Refer.

Poliomyelitis[ND]

Acute polio Spread: droplet or faecal-oral. *Incubation:* 7d. Presents with 2d flu-like prodrome then fever, tachycardia, headache, vomiting, stiff neck, and unilateral tremor ('pre-paralytic stage'). 65% who experience the pre-paralytic stage go on to develop paralysis (myalgia, LMN signs ± respiratory failure). *Management:* supportive—admit to hospital. <10% of those developing paralysis die. Permanent disability may result.

Prevention

- **1° immunization in babies and children** <10y 3 doses of the 5-part vaccine (DTaP/IPV/Hib), protecting against polio, diphtheria, whooping cough, tetanus, and *Haemophilus influenzae*, each 1mo apart—usually at 2mo, 3mo, and 4mo. If schedule is disrupted resume where stopped
- **Booster doses in children** 1 dose of 4-part vaccine (DTaP/IPV), protecting against polio, diphtheria, whooping cough, and tetanus >3y after the 1° course (usually pre-school), and another dose of 3-part vaccine (Td/IPV) against tetanus, diphtheria, and polio, 10y later (age 13–18y)
- **1° immunization in children >10y and adults** Three doses of 3-part vaccine (Td/IPV), each 1mo apart. Give booster doses after 3y and 10y
- **Booster doses for travel** Not required unless at special risk, e.g. travelling to endemic/epidemic area or healthcare workers. Boosters of Td/IPV are then given every 10y

Late effects of polio 20–30y after initial infection some patients develop new symptoms often triggered by a period of immobilization:

- ↑ muscle weakness and fatigue
- Pain in muscles and joints
- Respiratory difficulties (particularly in those who spent some time in an iron lung ventilator)—may present with symptoms relating to sleep

Once other causes are excluded, treatment is supportive.

Motor neurone disease 📖 p. 570

Myasthenia gravis/Lambert–Eaton syndrome 📖 p. 548

Other neurological syndromes

von Recklinghausen's disease (type 1 neurofibromatosis; NF1)
Autosomal dominant trait. *Criteria for diagnosis:* ≥2 of:

- ≥6 café-au-lait patches (flat, coffee-coloured patches of skin seen in first year of life, increasing in number and size with age) >5mm (pre-pubertal) or >15mm (post-pubertal)
- ≥2 neurofibromas:
  - Dermal neurofibromas—small violaceous skin nodules which appear after puberty
  - Nodular neurofibromas—subcutaneous, firm nodules arising from nerve trunks (may cause paraesthesiae if compressed) or a plexiform neurofibroma which appears as a large subcutaneous swelling
- Freckling in axilla, groin, neck base, and submammary area (women). Present by age 10y
- ≥2 Lisch nodules—nodules of the iris only visible with a slit lamp
- Distinctive bony abnormality specific to NF1, e.g. sphenoid dysplasia
- First-degree relative with NF1

Management Ongoing specialist management is essential.

Complications Affect 1 in 3 patients:

- Mild learning disability
- Short stature
- Macrocephaly
- Nerve root compression
- GI bleeding or obstruction
- Cystic bone lesion
- Scoliosis
- Pseudoarthrosis
- ↑ BP (6%)—due to renal artery stenosis or phaeochromocytoma
- Malignancy (5%)—optic glioma or sarcomatous change of neurofibroma
- Epilepsy (slight ↑)

F.D. von Recklinghausen (1833–1910)—German pathologist.

Type 2 neurofibromatosis (NF2) Much rarer than type 1. Autosomal dominant inheritance.

Diagnosis One of:

- Bilateral vestibular schwannoma (acoustic neuroma—sensorineural hearing loss, vertigo ± tinnitus)
- First-degree relative with NF2 *and either* a unilateral vestibular schwannoma *or* ≥1 neurofibroma, meningioma, glioma, schwannoma, or juvenile cataract

Management Screen at-risk patients with annual hearing tests. Once diagnosis is made, specialist neurosurgical management is needed.

Complications Schwannomas of other cranial nerves, dorsal nerve roots, or peripheral nerves; meningioma (45%); other gliomas (less common).

Ekbom's syndrome (restless legs syndrome) The patient (who is usually in bed) is seized by an irresistible desire to move his/her legs in a repetitive way accompanied by an unpleasant sensation deep in the legs. Sleep disturbance is common, as is +ve FH. *Cause:* unknown.

Management
- Exclude drug causes—common culprits: β-blockers, H_2 antagonists, neuroleptics, lithium, TCAs, anticonvulsants
- Exclude peripheral neuropathy or ischaemic rest pain
- Iron deficiency (with or without anaemia) is associated in 1 in 3 sufferers so check FBC and serum ferritin
- Also check: U&E, Cr, eGFR, fasting blood glucose, and TFTs
- Try non-drug measures first—reassurance, information, walking/ stretching, warmth, relaxation exercises, massage
- Drugs—dopamine agonists are often effective, e.g. ropinirole, pramipexole
- Refer if severe symptoms or diagnosis is in doubt

K.A. Ekbom (1907–77)—Swedish neurologist

Patient support
RLS-UK ☎ 01634 260483 ℘ www.rls-uk.org

Wernicke's encephalopathy Thiamine deficiency causing nystagmus, ophthalmoplegia, and ataxia. Other eye signs, e.g. ptosis, abnormal pupillary reactions, and altered consciousness or confusion may also occur. Consider in any patient with symptoms and a history of alcoholism.

Management Refer for confirmation of diagnosis. Meanwhile start thiamine 200–300mg od po to prevent irreversible Korsakoff's syndrome. In severe cases admit as a medical emergency. *K. Wernicke (1848–1904)—German psychiatrist.*

Korsakoff's syndrome ↓ ability to acquire new memories. May follow Wernicke's encephalopathy and is due to thiamine deficiency. Confabulation to fill gaps in memory is a feature. Refer for specialist advice on management. *S.S. Korsakoff (1853–1900)—Russian neuropsychiatrist.*

Gilles de la Tourette syndrome 📖 p. 911

Huntington's disease (chorea) Autosomal dominant trait. Testing can identify affected individuals before symptoms occur. Pre-conceptual and antenatal testing is available and should be offered to any couple with a family history on either the mother's or the father's side. Presents with movement abnormalities (e.g. hemichorea and rigidity) and dementia. Memory is relatively spared compared to cognition. Refer for expert advice. *G. Huntington (1851–1916)—US physician.*

Friedreich's ataxia The most common inherited ataxia (autosomal recessive). Prevalence—1:50,000. Presents in adolescence with progressive gait and limb ataxia, loss of proprioception, pyramidal weakness, and dysarthria. Extra-neurological involvement includes hypertrophic cardiomyopathy (most patients) and DM (10%). Treatment is supportive. Most patients become chairbound with in 15y and die in the 4th or 5th decade from cardiac or pulmonary complications. *N. Friedreich (1825–82)— German neurologist.*

Patient support
Ataxia UK ☎ 0845 644 0606 ℘ www.ataxia.org.uk

Neurological rehabilitation problems

New symptoms or limitations Consider:
- Is it due to an unrelated disease (e.g. change in bowel habit in someone who has had a stroke might indicate bowel cancer)?
- Is it due to an incidental infection (e.g. UTI, chest infection)?
- Is it due to a relapse (e.g. acute relapse in MS, TIA or further stroke in a stroke patient)?
- Is it due to a side effect of treatment (e.g. acute confusion, involuntary movements or the on-off effect in a patient with PD)?
- Is it part of a gradual progression (e.g. in MS, MND, brain tumour)?

Treat any cause of deterioration identified. If no cause is found, consider re-referring for specialist review and/or referring to the multidisciplinary rehabilitation team involved with the patient.

General principles of rehabilitation 📖 p. 204

Fatigue Consider and treat factors that might be responsible:
- Depression
- Chronic pain
- Disturbed sleep
- Poor nutrition

Action Review support, diet, and medication; encourage graded aerobic exercise; consider a trial of amantadine 200mg/d to improve symptoms[N].

Depression and anxiety Common. Diagnosis can be difficult. Standardized questionnaires, e.g. PHQ-9 (📖 p. 1001), are helpful for screening.

Action Give opportunities to talk about the impact of the illness on lifestyle. Jointly identify areas where positive changes could be made, e.g. referral to day care to widen social contact. Consider referral for counselling or to a self-help/support group. Consider antidepressant medication and/or referral to psychiatric services.

Emotionalism If the patient cries (or laughs) with minimal provocation, consider emotionalism—impairment in the control of crying. Reassure.

Sexual and personal relationships Problems are common. Useful information sheets are available at 🌐 www.outsiders.org.uk

Communication problems Speech therapy assessment is vital. Consider support via dysphasia groups and communication aids, e.g. simple pointing board (take advice from speech therapy and OT).

Poor vision Refer to an optician in the first instance. If corrected vision is still poor refer for ophthalmology review.

Respiratory infections Common. Treat with antibiotics unless in terminal stages of disease. Advise pneumococcal and influenza vaccination.

Venous thromboembolism Common but clinically apparent in <5%. Ensure adequate hydration and encourage mobility. Consider use of aspirin 75–150mg od and compression stockings if immobile. Prophylactic anticoagulation does not improve outcome.

Motor impairment Aim to maintain physical independence:
- Involve physiotherapy—often only 2–3 visits are needed
- Involve OT—a task-oriented approach is used (e.g. learning how to dress). Can also supply/advise on aids and appliances, e.g. Velcro fasteners, wheelchairs, adapted cutlery, etc
- Refer for social services OT assessment if aids, equipment, or adaptations are needed for the home
- Refer for home care services as necessary
- Give information about driving (📖 pp. 128–31) and/or employment where appropriate

Spasticity ± muscle and joint contractures Treat with physiotherapy (usually involving exercise ± splinting) ± drugs. Anti-spasticity drugs include dantrolene (25mg od), baclofen (5mg tds or rarely through a pump), and tizanidine (2mg od). Botulinum toxin can be directed at specific muscles. Refer via the specialist rehabilitation team.

Pain Most pain arises from ↓ mobility. *Other causes include:* pre-morbid disease (e.g. osteoarthritis); central pain due to neurological damage; and neuropathic pain.

Action Chronic pain, especially central pain, may respond to TCAs. Peripheral pain may respond to simple analgesia ± physiotherapy. Other options are TENS and local joint injection. A cannabinoid is now available as an oromucosal spray (Sativex®) for relief of pain/muscle spasm in MS on specialist prescription only. Refer patients with intractable pain to specialist pain clinics.

Bladder problems
- **UTI** If suspected, check urine dipstick ± send MSU for M,C&S and start antibiotics. If >3 proven UTIs in 1y refer to specialist incontinence service or urology for further assessment
- **Incontinence** 📖 pp. 450–3
- **Nocturia** Desmopressin 100–400 micrograms po or 10–40 micrograms intranasally may be helpful
- **Urgency** Modify environment, e.g. provide commode; try anticholinergic, e.g. tolterodine 2mg bd or oxybutinin 5mg tds. If not settling refer for specialist assessment

Bowel problems
- **Dysphagia** Common. Fluids are more difficult to swallow than semisolids. Formal assessment by trained staff is essential. Feeding through NG tube or percutaneous endoscopic gastrostomy (PEG) may be needed long- or short-term—in terminal disease (e.g. MND), weigh provision of nutrition against prolongation of poor-quality life
- **Constipation** Difficulty with defecation or BO <2x/wk—↑ fluid intake and ↑ fibre in diet. If no improvement, use po laxative ± regular suppositories/enemas
- **Incontinence** Exclude overflow due to constipation

Skin breakdown *Prevented by:* positioning; mobilization; good skin care; management of incontinence; pressure-relieving aids (e.g. special mattresses/cushions). Involve community nursing services.

Neurological assessment scales

A number of neurological assessment scales are in common use. Agreeing to use a formal, validated assessment scale enables comparison of observations between different team members, and also allows comparison of observations over time. Commonly used scales include:

Glasgow Coma Scale Assesses level of consciousness—📖 p. 1068

Motor scoring scale Assesses muscle power
- 0—no muscle movement
- 1—muscle flicker but no movement
- 2—moves but not against gravity
- 3—supports limb against gravity but not resistance
- 4—able to overcome mild resistance (mild weakness)
- 5—able to overcome strong resistance (normal power)

Disability severity scales Assess the impact of a particular condition on the individual. These scales are usually condition specific, e.g. the Migraine Disability Assessment Scale (MIDAS)—see Box 16.1, or Seizure Severity Questionnaire for patients with epilepsy. These scales are useful to gauge severity of symptoms and also monitor response to any treatments provided.

Daily living scales A number of scales are available that measure what the individual can do in practice. These may be:
- Non-disease specific e.g. Barthel Index, or
- Disease specific e.g. Oxford Stroke Handicap Scale

It is not really important which scale is used as long as everyone in the team uses the same scale for any given patient. Most use a graded Likert scale (e.g. 0–5) and rate activities such as:
- Mobility—walking, stairs, ability to transfer
- Personal care—dressing, washing
- Feeding—ability to prepare food, ability to feed self
- Toileting—ability to use the toilet, continence (bowels and bladder)

Quality of life scales Neurological conditions can have a profound impact on quality of life. Scales used to assess impact on quality of life may be completed by the patients themselves, or by the attending health professional. Examples include:
- **Non-disease specific scales** e.g, Euroqol EQ-5D
- **Disease specific scales**, e.g. Quality of Life in Essential Tremor (QUEST); Quality of Life in Epilepsy (QUOLIE)

Cognitive function tests e.g. The General Practitioner Assessment of Cognition (GPCOG), or 6 Cognitive Impairment Test (6CIT—📖 p. 1011).

Mental health scales, e.g.
- **Anxiety**—GAD-2 (📖 p. 993)
- **Depression**—NICE Chronic disease depression screening questions (📖 p.199); PHQ-9 (📖 p. 1001)

Box 16.1 Migraine Disability Assessment Score (MIDAS)

Used to assess the impact of migraine symptoms on lifestyle.

Instructions Please answer the following questions about ALL the headaches you have had over the last 3mo. If you did not do the activity in the last 3mo, write 0.

1. On how many days in the last 3mo did you miss work or school because of your headache?	☐ days
2. How many days in the last 3mo was your productivity at work or school ↓ by ≥½ because of your headaches? *(Do not include days you counted in question 1 where you missed work or school)*	☐ days
3. On how many days in the last 3mo did you not do household work* because of your headache?	☐ days
4. How many days in the last 3mo was your productivity in household work↓ by ≥½ because of your headaches? *(Do not include days you counted in question 3 where you did not do household work)*	☐ days
5. On how many days in the last 3mo did you miss family, social, or leisure activities because of your headaches?	☐ days
MIDAS score **TOTAL**	☐ days
A. On how many days in the last 3mo did you have a headache? *(If a headache lasted more than 1 day, count each day)*	☐ days
B. On a scale of 0–10, on average, how painful were these headaches? *(Where 0 = no pain at all, and 10 = pain as bad as can it be)*	☐

Questions A and B measure the frequency of the migraine and the severity of pain. They are not used to reach the MIDAS score but provide extra information helpful for making treatment decisions.

Interpreting the MIDAS score

I	Score: 0–5	Minimal/ infrequent disability	Tend to have little or no treatment needs. Can often manage with OTC medication. If infrequent severe attacks may require triptan
II	Score: 6–10	Mild/infrequent disability	May require medication for acute attacks, e.g. NSAID ± antiemetic or triptan
III	Score: 11–20	Moderate disability	Will need medication for acute attacks. Consider prophylaxis. Consider other causes for headaches, e.g. tension type headache
IV	Score: ≥21	Severe disability	

* Unpaid work, such as housework, shopping, and caring for children and others.

Dermatology

Skin assessment

History Use open questions at the start becoming directive when necessary—clarify, reflect, facilitate, listen. *Ask about:*

Age and gender Gives clues to likely diagnosis (see Table 17.1).

Presenting complaint Chronological account—when, where, and how the problem started. Ask directly about:
- **Skin lesions** What did the initial lesions look like? How have they evolved and extended?
- **Associated symptoms** Itching (📖 p. 594)? Sweating (📖 p. 603)? Systemic symptoms?
- **Aggravating or relieving factors**, e.g. sunlight
- **Past medical history** Similar symptoms, atopy, systemic disease, e.g. rheumatoid arthritis, coeliac disease
- **Family history** Genetic skin problems, e.g. neurofibromatosis; other family members with similar symptoms, e.g. scabies
- **Drug history** New drugs (including OTC), immunosuppressants, drug allergies
- **Occupation/hobbies** Does the problem improve when away from work/hobbies? Could the problem have been caused as a result of work/hobbies?
- **Previous treatments tried and result**

Attitudes and beliefs How does the patient see the problem? What does he/she think is wrong? How does he/she think other people view the situation? What does the patient want you to do about it?

Examination Use a systematic approach to the skin lesions:

Distribution See Figure 17.1.

Individual lesion morphology A magnifying hand lens is often helpful in looking at individual lesions. Palpation is also important to determine consistency, depth, and texture. Skin lesions—📖 p. 592.
- Are lesions monomorphic (take one form—e.g. guttate psoriasis) or pleomorphic (take many forms—e.g. chickenpox)?
- Are there 2° changes on top of primary lesions, e.g. excoriations?
- How are lesions grouped locally, i.e. ring-shaped, linear, Koebner phenomenon?

Check hair, nails, and mucous membranes Hair problems—📖 p. 602; nail changes—📖 p. 604.

Consider general examination If examination of the skin suggests systemic cause.

Action
- Summarize the history back to the patient and give an opportunity for the patient to fill in any gaps
- Draw up a problem list and outline a management plan with the patient. Further investigations and interventions are guided by the findings on history and examination—so a good history and examination is essential
- Set a review date

- Localized or generalized?
- Symmetrical? If so, are the lesions peripheral ☐ (e.g. lichen planus) or central ■ (e.g. pityriasis versicolor)?
- Do skin lesions involve the flexures ◨ (e.g. eczema) or extensor surfaces ⊞ (e.g. psoriasis)
- Are lesions limited to sun-exposed areas? 📖 p. 624
- Are lesions linear or ring-shaped? 📖 p. 592
- Is the distribution dermatomal e.g. shingles?
- Does the problem affect only one region e.g. axilla, face, groin, foot?

Figure 17.1 Assessing distribution of skin lesions

Table 17.1 Gender, age, and skin conditions

	Skin conditions that are more common
Male	Seborrhoeic dermatitis; dermatitis herpetiformis; porphyria cutanea tarda; polyarteritis nodosa; pruritus ani; tinea pedis and cruris; mycosis fungoides; squamous cell carcinoma
Female	Palmoplantar pustulosis; lichen sclerosus; lupus erythematosus; systemic sclerosis; morphoea; rosacea; dermatitis artefacta; venous ulceration; malignant melanoma
Child	Port wine stain; strawberry naevus; ichthyosis; erythropoietic porphyria; epidermolysis bullosa; atopic eczema; infantile seborrhoeic dermatitis; urticaria pigmentosa; viral infection, e.g. chickenpox, warts, molluscum contagiosum; head lice; impetigo
Adolescent	Melanocytic naevi; acne; psoriasis (particularly guttate); seborrhoeic dermatitis; pityriasis rosea; vitiligo
Early adult	Psoriasis; seborrhoeic dermatitis; lichen planus; dermatitis herpetiformis; lupus erythematosus; vitiligo; pityriasis versicolor
Middle age	Lichen planus; rosacea; pemphigus vulgaris; venous ulceration; malignant melanoma; basal cell carcinoma; mycosis fungoides; porphyria cutanea tarda
Old age	Asteatotic eczema; senile pruritus; bullous pemphigoid; venous and arterial ulcers; seborrhoeic warts; solar elastosis and keratosis; Campbell de Morgan spots; basal cell and squamous cell carcinoma; herpes zoster

Treatment of skin conditions

Skin conditions are usually treated with topical creams and lotions. Consider the vehicle as well as the active ingredient. In primary care, the choice is usually between creams or ointments.

- **Creams** Emulsions of oil and water. Well absorbed into the skin, less greasy, and easier to apply than ointments
- **Ointments** Greasy preparations suitable for chronic, dry lesions

Other alternatives include applications, gels, lotions, and pastes.

Emollients (see *BNF* 13.2.1; e.g. white soft paraffin). Useful for all dry or scaling disorders to soothe, smooth, and hydrate the skin—apply in the direction of hair growth. Effects are short-lived—advise frequent application, even after improvement occurs. Quantities to prescribe—see Table 17.2.

- Severity of the condition, patient preference, and site of application guide choice of emollient. Some ingredients rarely cause sensitization (see Box 17.1)—suspect if an eczematous reaction occurs
- Preparations such as aqueous cream and emulsifying ointment can be used as soap substitutes for hand washing and in the bath. Addition of an emollient bath oil e.g. Oilatum® or Balneum®, may also be helpful
- Avoid preparations containing an antibacterial (e.g. Dermol®), unless infection is present or a frequent complication
- Using a preparation with added urea (e.g. Balneum Plus®, Eucerin®) may improve hydration for scaling conditions or in elderly patients

Topical corticosteroids (see *BNF* 13.4)

- Used to suppress inflammatory conditions of the skin, e.g. eczema, when other measures such as emollients are ineffective used alone. Use the least potent preparation that is effective (see Table 17.3). Apply a thin layer just to affected areas >30min prior to emollients once or twice daily. Quantities to prescribe—see Table 17.2
- Creams are suitable for moist or weeping lesions, and ointments for dry, lichenified, or scaly lesions or where a more occlusive effect is wanted. Lotions may be useful when minimal application to a large or hair-bearing area is needed or for the treatment of exudative lesions
- Inclusion of urea or salicylic acid ↑ penetration of the corticosteroid

Cautions and contraindications Topical steroids:

- Are of no value in the treatment of urticaria
- Are contraindicated for rosacea and not recommended for acne
- May worsen ulcerated or secondarily infected lesions
- Should not be used indiscriminately for pruritus—they will only be of benefit if inflammation is causing the itch
- Should not be used long-term (>7–14d) on the face (and keep away from eyes) or for children. Use potent or very potent corticosteroids on the face only under specialist supervision

❶ For perioral inflammatory lesions use hydrocortisone 1% for ≤7d or, if infected (e.g. angular cheilitis), hydrocortisone + miconazole cream.

⚠ Potent topical or systemic steroids used to treat patients with psoriasis can result in rebound relapse, development of generalized pustular psoriasis, and/or local and systemic toxicity.

Table 17.2 Quantities of emollients and corticosteroids to prescribe

Area affected	Emollient*		Topical steroid**
	Cream/ointment	Lotion	
Face/neck	10–30g	100mL	15–30g
Both hands	25–50g	200mL	15–30g
Scalp	50–100g	200mL	15–30g
Both arms	100–200g	200mL	30–60g
Both legs	100–200g	200mL	100g
Trunk	400g	500mL	100g
Groins/genitalia	15–25g	100mL	15–30g

* Amounts are for an adult for 2x/d application for 1wk.

** Amounts are for an adult for once daily application for 2wk.

❶ One fingertip unit (distance from the tip of the adult index finger to the first crease) of steroid cream is sufficient to cover an area 2x the size of the flat adult palm.

Box 17.1 Ingredients that may cause skin sensitization

Beeswax
Benzyl alcohol
Butylated hydroxyanisole
Butylated hydroxytoluene
Cetostearyl alcohol (including acetyl and stearyl alcohol)
Chlorocresol
Edetic acid (EDTA)
Ethylenediamine
Fragrances
Hydroxybenzoates (parabens)
Imidurea
Isopropyl palmitate
N-(3-chloroallyl)hexaminium chloride (quaternium 15)
Polysorbates
Propylene glycol
Sodium metabisulphite
Sorbic acid
Wool fat/related substances, including lanolin

Table 17.3 Topical corticosteroid preparation potencies

Potency	Examples
Mild	Hydrocortisone 0.1–2.5%, Dioderm®, Mildison®
	• *With antimicrobials* Canesten® HC, Fucidin® H, Timodine®
	• *With crotamiton* Eurax-Hydrocortisone®
Moderate	Betnovate®-RD, Eumovate®, Synalar® 1 in 4 dilution
	• *With antimicrobials* Trimovate®
	• *With urea* Alphaderm®, Calmurid® HC
Potent	Betamethasone valerate 0.1%, Betacap®, Elocon®, Locoid®, Synalar®
	• *With antimicrobials* Aureocort®, Betnovate®-C or -N, Fucibet®
	• *With salicylic acid* Diprosalic®
Very potent	Dermovate®, Nerisone® Forte
	• *With antimicrobials* Dermovate®-NN

Changes in skin colour and eruptions

Pallor Non-specific sign which may be racial, familial, or cosmetic. Pathology suggested includes anaemia, shock, Stokes–Adams attack, vasovagal faint, myxoedema, hypopituitarism, and albinism.

Erythema 📖 p. 596　　**Hypo- and hyperpigmentation** 📖 p. 600

Linear lesions *Consider:*
- Koebner phenomenon (lesions arise in area of injury, e.g. in scratches)—occurs in psoriasis, eczema, lichen planus
- Linear urticaria
- Self-inflicted trauma—dermatitis artefacta
- Reaction to garden plants—psoralen-induced phytophotodermatitis
- Impetigo—may spread along scratch marks
- Herpes zoster—at the edge of a dermatome
- Stasis dermatitis—may follow varicose veins

Ring-shaped (annular) lesions *Consider:*
- Psoriasis
- Discoid eczema
- Urticaria
- Pityriasis rosea
- Lichen planus
- Orf
- Granuloma annulare
- Erythema multiforme
- Basal cell carcinoma
- Fungal infection, e.g. ringworm
- Erythema migrans associated with Lyme disease
- Burns (especially on a child—may be non-accidental injury)
- Cutaneous T-cell lymphoma (rare)

White patches Consider all causes of patchy hypopigmentation:
- Vitiligo
- After inflammation—cryotherapy, eczema, psoriasis, morphoea
- Pityriasis alba—white post-inflammatory patch on a child's face. No treatment needed
- Exposure to some chemicals—substituted phenols, hydroquinone
- Certain infections—pityriasis versicolor
- Tuberous sclerosis
- Halo naevus (pale area around a mole)
- Piebaldism (from birth—associated with a white forelock)
- Extensive hyperpigmentation, e.g. chloasma—patches of normal skin may appear hypopigmented

White spots Consider:
- Pustules/whiteheads, e.g. due to acne, folliculitis, or rosacea
- Molluscum contagiosum—white spots with a pearl-like appearance
- Milia—small white spots usually on upper arms/face of children; resolve spontaneously

Brown spots Consider:
- Freckles
- Moles
- Lentigos—like freckles but darker and not affected by sunlight
- Melanoma
- Café-au-lait spots— >5 associated with neurofibromatosis
- Basal cell carcinoma
- Seborrhoeic warts
- Senile keratoses
- Dermatofibroma
- Systemic disease
- Addison's disease
- Acanthosis nigrans
- Haemochromatosis

Scaling
- **Silvery scaling on the surface of red patches** Psoriasis
- **Fine scaling accompanied with rash** Pityriasis
- **Coarse, scaly skin with no rash** Ichthyosis
- **Localized, not itchy** Bowen's disease

Yellow crusting Usually due to staphylococcal infection (impetigo).

Telangiectasia Dilated distal venule/arteriole (spider naevus). *Causes:*
- **Congenital**—e.g. hereditary haemorrhagic telangiectasia
- **Venous disease in the leg**—e.g. venous stars
- **Rosacea**—facial
- **Excess oestrogen**—e.g. liver disease; the COC pill; pregnancy
- **Skin atrophy**—e.g. ageing skin, radiation dermatitis, topical steroids
- **Around BCC**

Spider naevi Small red lesions (barely visible—0.5cm diameter) in superior vena cava distribution, i.e. on the arms, neck, and chest wall. Large arteriole with numerous small vessels radiating from it giving the appearance of a spider—hence the name. Pressure applied to the central arteriole (e.g. with a pointed object) causes blanching of the whole lesion. >2 spider naevi is abnormal. *Causes:*
- **Cirrhosis**—most frequently, alcoholic
- **Oestrogen excess**—usually in association with chronic liver disease
- **Rheumatoid arthritis**—rarely
- **Viral hepatitis** (transient)
- **Pregnancy**—usually disappear in the final trimester

Blisters 📖 p. 594

Subcutaneous nodules *Consider:*
- Cysts
- Rheumatoid arthritis
- Xanthelasma
- Tumour
- Neurofibroma
- Granuloma annulare
- Furuncle
- Sarcoid
- Polyarteritis

Purpura Blue-brown discoloration of the skin due to bleeding within it. Petechiae are small dot-like purpura whilst ecchymoses are more extensive. Treat the cause. *Causes:*
- **Idiopathic**, e.g. idiopathic pigmented purpura (brownish punctate lesions on the legs)
- **Vessel wall defects** Vasculitis, paraproteinaemia, infection (e.g. meningococcal meningitis, septicaemia, glandular fever), ↑ intravascular pressure (e.g. venous disease)
- **Clotting defects** Abnormal platelet function; thrombocytopenia; anticoagulant therapy; coagulation factor deficiency
- **Defective dermal support** Dermal atrophy (e.g. ageing, steroids, disease); scurvy (vitamin C deficiency)

> ⚠ *Referral of patients with purpura*
> - Admit unwell patients with new purpura/petechiae as an emergency
> - Refer well children/young adults with unexplained petechiae immediately to be seen the same day[N]
> - For well older adults with unexplained bruising, bleeding, or purpura, check FBC, blood film, clotting screen, and ESR/viscosity/CRP[N]

Itching and blistering of the skin

Itching In any patient presenting with pruritus or itch, ask: *Are there skin lesions present?*

Skin lesions present Search for unexcoriated lesions. Investigations are not usually needed. Exceptions are patch testing for contact dermatitis and skin biopsy for dermatitis herpetiformis. *Causes:*

- Urticaria
- Contact dermatitis and allergies to food and drugs
- Prickly heat
- Skin infestations, e.g. scabies, pediculosis, insect bites
- Infections—viral, e.g. chickenpox; fungal
- Dermatitis herpetiformis
- Lichen planus
- Senile atrophy
- Psychological causes*

* excessive excoriation causes lichenification of the skin.

Skin lesions absent Large differential diagnosis. Look for pallor, jaundice, weight ↓, LN enlargement, and abdominal organomegaly. Investigate as necessary—consider urinalysis (dipstick and MSU), FBC, ESR/CRP, serum ferritin, LFTs (including alkaline phosphatase), U&E, Cr and eGFR, glucose, serum Ca^{2+}, TFTs, and CXR. If still undiagnosed—refer. *Causes:*

- Hepatic—obstructive jaundice, pregnancy
- Endocrine—DM, thyrotoxicosis, hypothyroidism, hyperparathyroidism
- Renal—chronic renal failure
- Haematological—polycythaemia vera, iron deficiency, leukaemia, Hodgkin's disease
- Malignancy—any carcinoma
- Drug allergies
- Psychological—obsessive states, schizophrenia
- Rare causes—diabetes insipidus, roundworm infection

Blisters Result from separation of skin layers. Type of blister depends on level of cleavage of the skin—subcorneal or intraepidermal blisters rupture easily, subepidermal blisters are much tougher. *Causes:*

- **Subcorneal** Pustular psoriasis (📖 p. 619), bullous impetigo (📖 p. 632)
- **Intraepidermal** Eczema (📖 pp. 606–11), HSV (📖 p. 634), VZ—chickenpox (📖 p. 652) or shingles (📖 p. 653), pemphigus, friction
- **Subepidermal** Cold or heat injury (burns—📖 p. 1114), pemphigoid, dermatitis herpetiformis, linear IgA disease
- **Other** Insect bites (may cause cleavage at any level)

Pemphigoid[G] Autoimmune disorder.

- **Bullous pemphigoid** Usually affects the elderly. An urticarial reaction may precede onset of blistering. Large, tense blisters arise on red or normal skin on the limbs, trunk, and flexures. Oral lesions in 20–30%. May be localized to one site, e.g. lower leg. *Differential diagnosis:* pemphigus, dermatitis herpetiformis, linear IgA disease
- **Cicatricial pemphigoid** Mainly affects mucous membranes in the eyes/mouth. Scarring results in visual loss. Refer to ophthalmology
- **Pemphigoid gestationis** Rare but characteristic bullous eruption associated with pregnancy. Remits after delivery but often recurs in subsequent pregnancies. 📖 p. 805

Management Refer to dermatology for skin biopsy and confirmation of diagnosis. Treatment is usually with oral steroids (prednisolone 30–60mg daily initially—reducing as symptoms improve). Other treatments include antibiotics and nicotinamide, azathioprine, or other immunosuppressants.

Prognosis Self-limiting in 50%—steroids are often stopped after ~2y.

Pemphigusᴳ Uncommon, autoimmune disorder affecting skin and mucous membranes. Affects adults (peak incidence 30–70y). *Cause:* 90% have detectable circulating autoantibodies. Associated with other auto-immune disorders, e.g. myasthenia gravis.

Presentation 50% present with oral lesions. Suspect in anyone presenting with mucocutaneous erosions/blisters. Flaccid superficial blisters then appear—sometimes months later—over scalp, face, back, chest, and flexures. As blisters are fragile they burst early and the condition may present as crusted erosions. Untreated the condition is progressive.

Management Refer to dermatology. Treatment is with high-dose systemic steroids or other immunosuppressive agents. Treatment is continued long-term although occasional remissions occur. Before treatment with steroids 75% of patients died in <4y. Now excess morbidity and mortality is due to side effects of treatment.

Dermatitis herpetiformis ♂ > ♀ (2:1). *Peak incidence:* third/fourth decade. Consists of itchy vesicular skin rash on elbows (extensor surface), knees, buttocks, and scalp, which are often broken by scratching to leave excoriations. Closely related to coeliac disease (📖 p. 412); 2–5% of patients with coeliac disease have dermatitis herpetiformis but classic symptoms of coeliac disease are uncommon. *Differential diagnosis:* scabies, eczema, linear IgA disease.

Management Refer to dermatology for skin biopsy to confirm diagnosis. Responds to withdrawal of gluten—although may take up to 1y. Controlled in the interim with dapsone or sulfapyridine.

Epidermolysis bullosa A group of genetically inherited diseases characterized by blistering on minimal trauma. Range from being mild and trivial to being incompatible with life. The most common form is *simple epidermolysis bullosa* (autosomal dominant)—blistering is caused by friction, is mild and limited to hands and feet. Patients are advised to avoid trauma.

Linear IgA disease Rare condition of blisters and urticarial lesions on the back and extensor surfaces. Refer to dermatology. Responds to dapsone.

Staphylococcal scalded skin syndrome 📖 p. 903

Further information
Electronic dermatology atlas 🖰 www.dermis.net
British Association of Dermatologists 🖰 www.bad.org.uk
• Guidelines for the management of pemphigus vulgaris (2003)
• Guidelines for the management of bullous pemphigoid (2002)

Erythema

Erythema is redness of the skin—usually due to vasodilatation. It may be localized (e.g. pregnancy—on the palms), generalized (e.g. flushing) or take the form of a red rash (e.g. drug eruption, viral exanthem).

⚠ **Erythroderma (exfoliative dermatitis)** Erythema affecting >90% skin surface. Rare, but systemic effects of skin failure are potentially fatal. ♂:♀ ≈2:1. Typical patient is middle-aged or elderly. Patchy erythema becomes universal in <48h. Accompanied by fever, shivering, and malaise. 2–6d later scaling appears. The skin is hot, red, itchy, dry, thickened, and feels tight. There may be oedema/oozing. Hair and nails may be shed. Admit as an acute medical emergency.

Causes Eczema (40%); psoriasis (25%); lymphoma (15%); drug eruption (10%); other skin disease (2%); unknown (8%).

Staphylococcal scalded skin syndrome 📖 p. 903

Erysipelas and cellulitis 📖 p. 632

Flushing Generalized erythema due to vasodilatation. Common and usually benign. Tends to affect face, neck, and upper trunk. *Cause:*
- **Physiological,** e.g. exertion, heat
- **Emotion,** e.g. anger, anxiety, embarrassment
- **Foods,** e.g. spices, chillies, alcohol
- **Endocrine,** e.g. menopause, Cushing's syndrome
- **Drugs,** e.g. opioids, tamoxifen, danazol, GnRH analogues, clomifene, nitrates, calcium channel blockers
- **Dermatological** Rosacea (unknown mechanism); contact dermatitis
- **Inflammatory** SLE; dermatomyositis
- **Infection,** e.g. slapped cheek syndrome (Fifth disease); cellulitis/erysipelas
- **Tumour** Pancreatic tumours, medullary thyroid cancer, carcinoid, phaeochromocytoma

Management Treat cause if possible (e.g. avoid alcohol, HRT). Embarrassing flushing may be helped with propranolol (e.g. 40mg od/bd) or clonidine (e.g. 50 micrograms bd). If severe and disabling and no response to conservative measures, consider referral to dermatology.

Palmar erythema Generalized reddening of the palms associated with pregnancy, liver disease, and polycythaemia.

Erythema nodosum Tender erythematous nodules 1–5cm diameter on extensor surfaces of limbs—especially shins (see Figure 17.2) ± ankle and wrist arthritis ± fever. ♀:♂ ≈3:1. Resolves in <8wk, non-scarring. No treatment needed although analgesia and mild compression may ease symptoms.

Associations ❶ 20% of cases are idiopathic with no associations.
- Streptococcal infection
- Drugs, e.g. oral contraceptives, sulfonamides
- Acute sarcoidosis
- Inflammatory bowel disease—UC, Crohn's
- Malignancy
- TB

Figure 17.2 Erythematous nodules on the shins of a patient with erythema nodosum
Reproduced from Foster, Helen, and Brogan, Paul, *Paediatric Rheumatology* (2012) with permission from Oxford University Press.

Erythema multiforme Immune-mediated disease characterized by target lesions on hands and feet (see Figure 17.3). *Causes:*
- **Idiopathic** (50%)
- **Infective** Streptococcal, HSV, hepatitis B, mycoplasma
- **Drugs** Penicillin, sulfonamide, barbiturate
- **Other** SLE, pregnancy, malignancy

Presentation Target lesions (red rings with central pale or purple area) on hands and feet. New lesions appear for 2–3wk. Frequently oral, conjunctival, and genital mucosa is affected—if severe termed *Stevens–Johnson syndrome*.

Differential diagnosis Toxic erythema, toxic epidermal necrolysis, Sweet's disease, urticaria, pemphigoid.

Management Identification and removal of the underlying cause. Mild cases resolve spontaneously and require symptomatic measures only. Admit if extensive involvement.

Figure 17.3 Typical target lesions of erythema multiforme
Reproduced from: Sladden MJ, Johnston GA (2005) Common skin infections in children: Folliculitis and herpes. *Student BMJ* **13**:265–308. Figure 2.28 with permission from BMJ Publishing.

Rosacea Relapsing-remitting chronic inflammatory facial dermatosis characterized by erythema and pustules. Most common in middle age (30–50y) and in fair-skinned people of Northern European descent. ♀ > ♂ (~3:2). No cure. *Cause:* unknown—although possible associations with the face mite *Demodex folliculorum*, *Helicobacter pylori* infection, and migraine headaches.

Presentation Earliest symptom is flushing. Erythema, telangiectasia, papules, pustules ± lymphoedema affect cheeks, nose, forehead, and chin (see Figure 17.4a). Exacerbated by sunlight and topical steroids.

Aggravating factors Sun exposure (61%); emotional stress (60%); hot weather (53%); alcohol (45%); spicy foods (43%); exercise (39%); cold weather or wind (38/36%); hot baths (37%); hot drinks (36%); cosmetics/skin care products (24%).

Complications Rhinophyma (bulbous appearance of nose—see Figure 17.4b); eye involvement—blepharitis, dry eye, and conjunctivitis.

Differential diagnosis Acne (lacks comedones and older age group); contact dermatitis, SLE, photosensitive eruptions; seborrhoeic dermatitis.

Management
- Avoid triggers
- Antibiotics—repeated treatment is usually needed over many years with prolonged courses of topical or systemic antibiotics (e.g. metronidazole 0.75% gel bd or 15% topical azelaic acid bd for 3–4mo; or lymecycline 408mg od or tetracycline 500mg bd, decreasing to 250mg od after 3wk and continuing for 4mo). Rebound may occur if antibiotics are stopped suddenly
- Refer to dermatology if rhinophyma, ocular complications, or failure to respond to treatment in general practice

Figure 17.4 Rosacea: (a) redness and pustules on nose, cheeks, and forehead and (b) rhinophyma

Reproduced from: Blount BW, Pelletier AL (2002) Rosacea: a common, yet commonly overlooked, condition. *Am Fam Physician* **66**:435–441—with permission from the American Academy of Family Physicians.

Livedo reticularis Marbled, patterned cyanosis of the skin. If not reversible by warming investigate and treat the cause. *Causes:* physiological (e.g. cold); vasculitis (e.g. SLE); hyperviscosity.

Chilblains Inflamed and painful purple pink swellings on fingers, toes, or ears. Appear in response to cold. ♀ > ♂. Advise warm housing/clothing, gloves, and woolly socks. In severe cases oral nifedipine may help.

Erythema ab igne Reticulate pigmented erythema due to heat-induced damage. Common in the elderly—especially from sitting in front of the fire or using hot water bottles to alleviate pain. In younger patients may be caused by laptop computers balanced on thighs. Explain the cause. Resolves spontaneously.

Viral rash Common, particularly in children. Appears suddenly (over hours) and is associated with symptoms of the underlying viral infection. The rash may take many forms but is usually widespread, red, maculopapular and blanches on pressure. In most cases, the underlying virus cannot be identified, but viral infections with characteristic rashes include:

- Chickenpox 📖 p. 652
- Measles 📖 p. 652
- Rubella 📖 p. 652
- Fifth disease (slapped cheek) 📖 p. 652
- Roseola infantum 📖 p. 652
- Hand, foot, and mouth 📖 p. 652

Management In all cases, no specific treatment is needed for the rash—treat the underlying viral infection symptomatically.

Rash illness in pregnancy 📖 p. 804

Lyme disease *Cause: Borrelia burgdorferi. Spread:* transmitted by ticks—usually from deer or sheep. Presents with:

- Erythema migrans (75%—see Figure 17.5)—a red macule/papule on the upper arm, leg, or trunk 7–10d after a tick bite, which expands over days/weeks to form a ring with central clearing; diameter can be up to 50cm; further smaller lesions then develop elsewhere
- Flu-like illness
- Lymphadenopathy ± splenomegaly
- Arthralgia

Symptoms are typically intermittent and changing. Complications include neurological abnormalities, aseptic meningitis, myocarditis, and arthritis.

Management Confirm diagnosis with serology. Treatment is usually with 2–3wk course of doxycycline—take microbiology advice. 🗲 Treatment with antibiotics after a tick bite but before symptoms have arisen is controversial.

Removal of ticks 📖 p. 1108

Figure 17.5 Erythema migrans following a tick bite

Pigmentation disorders

Hypopigmentation Lack of skin pigmentation. May be:
- **Generalized** Albinism; phenylketonuria; hypopituitarism
- **Patchy** Vitiligo; tuberous sclerosis; morphoea; pityriasis alba; or after inflammation (e.g. post-cryotherapy, 2° to eczema or psoriasis), infection (e.g. pityriasis versicolor), or exposure to chemicals (substituted phenols, hydroquinone)
- **Around a mole**—halo naevus

Hyperpigmentation Excess skin pigmentation. May be:
- **Genetic** Racial; freckles; neurofibromatosis; Peutz–Jegher's syndrome
- **Due to drugs** Amiodarone (blue-grey pigmentation of sun-exposed areas); psoralens; minocycline (blue-black pigmentation in scars and buccal mucosa); chloroquine (blue-grey pigmentation of face and arms); chlorpromazine (grey pigment in sun-exposed sites); cytotoxics
- **Endocrine** Addison's disease; chloasma; Cushing's syndrome
- **Nutritional** Ingestion of carrots (carotinaemia); malabsorption
- **Post-inflammatory** Varicose eczema; lichen planus; systemic sclerosis
- **Other** Benign naevi; malignant melanoma; chronic renal failure (lemon yellow); liver disease (jaundice); acanthosis nigricans

Freckles and lentigines
- **Freckles** are small, light brown macules—typically facial—which darken in the sun. They are common particularly in red heads and develop in childhood. Require no treatment
- **Lentigines** Are also brown macules but more scattered and do not darken in the sun. Most common in elderly sun-exposed skin

Chloasma Patterned macular symmetrical facial pigmentation, usually involving the forehead and/or cheeks (see Figure 17.6), ♀ >> ♂. Peak age 20–40y. Affects dark skins > fair skins.

Risk factors Pregnancy (usually fades after delivery); taking CHC or depot contraceptives (may be slow to fade when stopped); use of cosmetics, perfumes, or deodorant soap.

Management Reassurance is normally all that is needed. *Consider*:
- Stopping hormonal contraception
- Avoid irritating the skin with strong soaps/abrasive cleaners
- Vigorous photoprotection using sunscreen and hat
- 20% azelaic acid cream or 0.05% tretinoin cream may be used but requires application for >6mo to have any effect
- Rarely, patients are so worried about their appearance that camouflage cosmetics are warranted
- Laser resurfacing—mixed results—refer for expert advice

Albinism *Prevalence:* 1:20,000. Rare genetic syndrome (autosomal recessive inheritance) in which the melanocytes are unable to produce skin, hair, or eye pigment. Patients have white hair, pale skin, pink eyes, poor sight, photophobia, and nystagmus. Several different varieties exist.

Management Strict sun avoidance, sunglasses, sunscreens, refer any skin lesions for biopsy (↑ risk squamous cell carcinoma).

Figure 17.6 Chloasma of the cheek
Reproduced with permission from
🖰 www.dermnetnz.org

Figure 17.7 Vitiligo on the forearms
Reproduced with permission from
🖰 www.dermnetnz.org

Vitiligo Affects 1% of the population. ♂ = ♀. *Peak age of onset:* 10–30y. *Cause:* autoimmune; 18% have a family history. *Associations:* pernicious anaemia, Addison's and thyroid disease.

Presentation May be precipitated by injury or sunburn. Presents as smooth sharply defined white macules or patches which contain no melanocytes (see Figure 17.7). Skin appears bright white under Wood's light. Often symmetrical distribution. Hair may also be affected. *Most common sites:* hands, wrists, knees, neck, face, around eyes, and mouth.

Differential diagnosis Post-inflammatory hypopigmentation, chemical exposure.

Management Prognosis is variable—some develop a few lesions which remain static; some progress to larger depigmented areas; some repigment. There is no cure. Advise use of sunscreens for affected areas (ACBS prescription); camouflage cosmetics (refer to Changing Faces for advice on application, ACBS prescription). Consider referral to dermatology for consideration of topical steroid treatment, topical calcineurin inhibitors (tacrolimus, pimecrolimus—unlicensed), or phototherapy.

Morphoea (localized scleroderma) ♀:♂ ≈3:1. Cutaneous localized form of scleroderma. Pathologically distinct from lesions of systemic sclerosis. Internal disease is not associated. *Cause:* autoimmune but not fully understood—may follow trauma. Presents with round/oval plaques of induration and erythema which become smooth, shiny and white, with violet borders. Eventually leaving atrophic hairless pigmented patches. Affects trunk/proximal limbs. No established treatment—topical steroids are often tried. Usually resolves spontaneously in 3–5y.

Further information

British Association of Dermatologists Guidelines for the management of vitiligo (2008) 🖰 www.bad.org.uk

Patient support
Changing Faces Skin Camouflage Service
🖰 www.changingfaces.org.uk

Hair and sweat gland problems

Hair loss or alopecia May be diffuse or localized, scarring or non-scarring. Treatment is according to cause. *Differential diagnosis*:

- **Diffuse non-scarring** Male pattern baldness (responds to topical minoxidil and 1mg finasteride orally but hair loss returns as soon as stopped—neither treatment is available on NHS prescription); hypothyroidism; iron deficiency; malnutrition; hypopituitarism; hypoadrenalism; drug-induced
- **Localized non-scarring** Alopecia areata; ringworm; traumatic; hair pulling; traction; SLE; secondary syphilis
- **Scarring** Burns; radiation; shingles; tertiary syphilis; lupus erythematosus; morphoea; lichen planus

Alopecia areata[G] Common chronic inflammatory disease affecting the hair follicles ± nails (~10%). Patches of hair loss usually on the scalp (see Figure 17.8) but can affect any hair-bearing skin. 20% have a family history. Consider alternative diagnosis of tinea capitis if scales/erythema present.

Management Investigation is usually unnecessary. If mild hair loss, reassure and monitor hair loss; refer more severe cases to dermatology. Treatment options include topical/locally injected/systemic steroids ± contact immunotherapy. ~40% recover in <1y; 20% lose all scalp hair—recovery in these cases is unusual (<10%). Psychological support may be needed.

Figure 17.8 Alopecia areata

Hirsutism Excess hair in androgenic distribution (📖 p. 342)

Hypertrichosis Excess hair in non-androgenic distribution—usually face and trunk, although can be generalized. Mostly drug-induced (e.g. phenytoin, ciclosporin, minoxidil). If not, investigate to find other causes: malnutrition, anorexia nervosa, porphyria cutanea tarda, malignancy. If a cause cannot be found, treat symptomatically with electrolysis, bleaching, waxing ± depilatories.

Local hypertrichosis Can be associated with topical steroid usage, be over a melanocytic naevus, or associated with spina bifida occulta.

Hidradenitis suppuritiva Chronic inflammatory condition of sweat glands in axilla, groin, and perineum. Nodules, abscesses, cysts, and sinuses form → scarring. Treat with topical antiseptics (e.g. chlorhexidine), systemic antibiotics ± surgical drainage/excision.

Hyperhidrosis Sweating, or perspiration, is normal and essential for temperature control. The amount people sweat varies enormously. Usually sweating can be controlled with shop-bought antiperspirants and is only excessive when it cannot be controlled and interferes with the patient's quality of life. Excessive sweating may be focal or generalized.

Generalized hyperhidrosis Most likely to occur 2° to other medical conditions. Where possible treat the cause:
- **Physiological** After and during exercise; hot, humid conditions; emotional response (e.g. anxiety)
- **Infection** Can occur with any bacterial or viral infection. Consider malaria if recent history of travel
- **Non-infective** Menopause; thyrotoxicosis; phaeochromocytoma; lymphoma; leukaemia

If no cause is found, β-blockers (e.g. propranolol 40mg od/bd) or SSRIs (e.g. fluoxetine 20mg od) may be effective (unlicensed).

Focal hyperhidrosis Usually a primary condition—mainly affects the axillae, palms, soles of feet, and/or face. Affects ~5% of the population. Onset is typically in the teenage years. Distressing and socially disabling.
- Advice for patients—avoid clothing made of Lycra, nylon, and other man-made fibres, and tight clothing; wear colours that do not show the sweat, e.g. white, black; use emollient washes/moisturizers rather than soap; identify trigger factors for sweating (e.g. alcohol, crowded rooms) and avoid those situations
- Treat topically with 20% aluminium chloride (e.g. Anhydrol Forte®). Apply to clean skin at night—wash off in morning. ↓ frequency of application as symptoms subside. Treat local irritation with topical steroid, e.g. hydrocortisone 1%. Absorbent dusting powder may help axillary/plantar sweating
- Consider a trial of drug therapy with β-blockers (e.g. propranolol 40mg od/bd) or SSRIs (e.g. fluoxetine 20mg od) (both unlicensed uses)
- Refer to dermatology or vascular surgery if not responding

Secondary care treatments include:
- **Iontophoresis** For palmar/foot hyperhidrosis. A mild electric current is passed through the skin whilst immersed in a warm water bath. Multiple sessions are needed initially then treatments every 6wk–6mo
- **Botulinum toxin injections** For isolated excess sweating of the axillae/groins. ↓ sweating. Lasts 4–12mo then repeat injections are needed
- **Endoscopic transthoracic sympathectomy (ETS)** 99% effective for palmar hyperhidrosis; 80% effective for axillary hyperhidrosis; 70% effective for facial flushing, blushing, or sweating. Expect compensatory hyperhidrosis elsewhere (usually the small of the back)

Further information
British Association of Dermatologists Guidelines for the management of alopecia areata (2012) ℬ www.bad.org.uk

Patient information
Hairline International ℬ www.hairlineinternational.co.uk

Nail changes

Nail changes may be due to nail disease or indicate other dermatological or systemic disease (see Table 17.4).

Assessment

- **Take a history** Duration, initial changes, evolution of changes, other systemic or local symptoms, family history, drug and alcohol history, occupation, hobbies
- **Examine** Colour, shape, extent, and pattern of involvement; consider examination/investigation for other skin or systemic disease (guided by history and appearance of nails)

Table 17.4 Nail changes, description, and cause

Change	Description of nail	Differential diagnosis
Colour	Black transverse bands	Cytotoxic drugs
	Blue	Cyanosis
		Antimalarials
		Haematoma
	Blue-green	*Pseudomonas* infection
	Brown	Fungal infection
		Cigarette staining
		Chlorpromazine
		Gold
		Addison's disease
	Brown 'oil stain' patches	Psoriasis
	Brown longitudinal streak	Melanocytic naevus
		Malignant melanoma
		Addison's disease
	Red streaks 'splinter haemorrhages'	Infective endocarditis
		Other vasculitic disease
		Trauma
	White spots	Trauma to the nail matrix
	White transverse bands	Heavy metal poisoning
	White/brown half and half nails	Chronic renal failure
	White (leuconychia)	Hypoalbuminaemia (e.g. associated with cirrhosis)
	Yellow	Psoriasis
		Fungal infection
		Jaundice
		Tetracycline
		Yellow nail syndrome (defective lymph drainage, nails grow very slowly, may be associated with pleural effusion)

(continued)

Table 17.4 (Cont.)

Change	Description of nail	Differential diagnosis
Brittle	Nails break easily—usually at the distal end	Effect of water and detergent, iron deficiency, hypothyroidism, digital ischaemia
Clubbing ⚠ Refer any patient with unexplained clubbing for urgent CXR[N]	Loss of angle between nail fold and plate Bulbous finger tip Nail fold feels boggy	**Respiratory** bronchial carcinoma (not small cell); chronic infection; fibrosing alveolitis; asbestosis **Cardiac** SBE; congenital cyanotic heart disease **Other** inflammatory bowel disease (Crohn's > UC); thyrotoxicosis; biliary cirrhosis; congenital; AV malformation
Koilonychia	Spoon-shaped nails	Iron deficiency anaemia Lichen planus Repeated exposure to detergents
Onycholysis	Separation of the nail from the nail bed	Psoriasis Fungal infection Trauma Thyrotoxicosis Tetracyclines
Pitting	Fine or coarse pits in the nail bed	Psoriasis Eczema Alopecia areata Lichen planus
Beau's lines	Transverse grooves	Any severe illness which affects growth of the nail matrix
Ridging	Transverse	Beau's lines Eczema Psoriasis Habit tic dystrophy (thumb > other finger nails—due to habitual rubbing/picking at the cuticle) Chronic paronychia
	Longitudinal	Lichen planus Darier's disease (keratosis follicularis—genetic disorder appearing in adolescence mainly affecting skin/nails)
Nail fold telangiectasia	Dilated capillaries and erythema at the nail fold	Connective tissue disorders
Tumours of the nail fold	Benign	Viral warts Myxoid (mucus) cysts (treat with steroid injection or cryotherapy) Periungual fibroma (associated with tuberous sclerosis—appear at puberty)
	Malignant	Melanoma Squamous cell carcinoma

Atopic eczema

Affects 15–20% of schoolchildren and 2–10% of adults—usually starts <6mo of age, and by 1y 60% of those likely to develop eczema will have done so. Associated with other atopic conditions, e.g. asthma, hay fever. Remission occurs by 15y of age in 75%, although some relapse later.

Differential diagnosis Scabies; ringworm; rare syndromes, e.g. Wiskott–Aldrich syndrome; dermatitis herpetiformis.

Presentation Waxing and waning itchy condition. ❶ If no itching then unlikely to be eczema.

> *Infants* Itchy vesicular exudative eczema on face (see Figure 17.9) ± hands, often with 2° infection. May cause sleep disturbance due to itch. >½ are free of eczema by 18mo.
>
> *Children >18mo* Involves antecubital and popliteal fossae (see Figure 17.10), neck, wrists, and ankles. Lichenification, excoriation, and dry skin are common. Face may be erythematous and have typical infraorbital folds. Loss of self-esteem, behaviour, and sleep problems are common.

Adults Most commonly irritant hand dermatitis (see Figure 17.11) in a person with past history of atopic eczema—🕮 p. 609. A few continue to have generalized atopic eczema; <2% develop new eczema aged >20y. May interfere with employment/social activities. Exacerbated by stress.

Diagnosis Itchy skin *plus* ≥3 of:
- Itching in skin creases
- History of asthma or hay fever
- Onset in the first 2y of life
- Generally dry skin
- Visible flexural eczema

Assessment Ask about:
- Family (two-thirds) and personal history of atopy and eczema
- Onset and distribution of the disease
- Aggravating factors (pets, irritants, e.g. soaps/detergents, allergens)
- Sleep disturbance due to itching/rubbing
- Impact on quality of life (school work, career, social life)
- Previous treatments (including dietary restrictions), expectations of treatment and other medications being taken (e.g. steroids for asthma)

⚠ **Nipple eczema** May be Paget's disease of the breast (🕮 p. 688). Refer urgently to a breast surgeon if no response to topical treatment[N].

Complications
- **Skin thickening and scaling**
- **Bacterial infection** Secondary infection (usually with *Staph. aureus*) commonly causes exacerbations and may not be seen as obvious infection. Bacterial infection is suggested by presence of crusting or weeping or sudden deterioration of eczema
- **Viral infection** ↑ susceptibility to infection, e.g. viral warts, molluscum. *Eczema herpeticum*—propensity to develop widespread lesions with HSV and VZ; may require admission and IV aciclovir
- **Cataracts** Rarely occur in young adults with very severe eczema
- **Growth retardation** Children with severe eczema, cause unknown. A growth chart should be kept for children with chronic severe eczema

Figure 17.9 Infantile eczema on the cheeks

Figure 17.10 Childhood eczema involving both popliteal fossae

Figure 17.11 Hand (contact) dermatitis in an adult
Figures 17.9–17.11 reproduced with permission from New Zealand Dermatological Society Incorporated. Published online at ✋ www.dermnetnz.org

Management

- Education is time well spent—explain the condition and provide verbal and written information on a stepped approach to care and management of flares[N]
- Advise—loose cotton clothing; avoid wool (exacerbates eczema); avoid excessive heat; keep nails short; gloves in bed
- If a specific irritant is identified (e.g. house dust mite, pets) then avoid

Specific treatment

- **Emollients** Topical creams/ointments and bath emollients—use regularly on skin and as soap substitutes, even if skin is clear. May need to try several to find one that suits. Ideally apply 3–4x/d to moist skin. Ensure enough is supplied. Addition of an antipruritic, e.g. lauromacrogol to the emollient, may help break the scratch–itch cycle. Addition of an antiseptic to bath emollient may ↓ bacterial infection
- **Topical steroids** Prescribe the least potent strength that is effective. Use od or bd. Ointments are preferable on dry, scaly eczema; creams on wet, exudative eczema. Emollients ↓ steroid requirement
- **Antibiotics** For infected eczema—topical (alone or in combination with steroid, e.g. Fucidin® H) or oral (e.g. flucloxacillin or erythromycin 250–500mg qds for 2wk). Swab if antibiotic treatment is ineffective
- **Oral steroids** Rescue therapy while waiting for an urgent consultant opinion. Only use short courses, e.g prednisolone 20–30mg od for 5d
- **Topical immunosuppressants**, e.g. tacrolimus—on consultant advice only
- **Antihistamines** Sedative antihistamines given nocte ↓ desire to itch, e.g. promethazine, hydroxyzine
- **Bandages** Excoriated or lichenified eczema—ichthammol or zinc and calamine. Bandages can be applied at night on top of steroid ointment. Refer to dermatology
- **Wet wrapping** Used for exudative eczema—tubigrip bandage or tubular gauze soaked in emollient is applied and covered with a dry bandage. Refer to dermatology
- **Dietary manipulation** Few (<10%) benefit. Egg and milk are most commonly excluded. Refer to a dietician to avoid malnutrition

Referral *E* = Emergency admission; *U* = Urgent; *S* = Soon; *R* = Routine
- Infection with disseminated HSV (eczema herpeticum)—*E*
- Severe eczema resistant to treatment. Additional secondary care treatments include phototherapy and immunosuppressive agents—*U*
- Infection which cannot be cleared in primary care—*U*
- Severe social/psychological problems due to eczema—*S*
- Treatment requires excessive amounts of topical steroids—*S*
- Failure to control symptoms in primary care—*R*
- Patient/family might benefit from additional advice on application of treatments (e.g. bandaging techniques)—*R*
- Patch testing required if contact dermatitis suspected—*R*
- Dietary factors are suspected (refer direct to dietician)—*R*

Prurigo nodularis (nodular prurigo) Intensely itchy firm lumps 1–2cm in diameter. Cause unknown, but 80% have a history of atopy. Exclude scabies and systemic causes of itching (📖 p. 594). *Treatment:* topical steroids ± occlusion. May need sedating antihistamine for itch.

Contact dermatitis[G] Precipitated by an exogenous agent which is:
- **Irritant** (e.g. water, abrasives, chemicals, detergent), *or*
- **Allergen** (e.g. nickel—10% ♀, 1% ♂; chrome; rubber)

Clinical presentation is often indistinguishable. More common in patients with a past history of atopic eczema. In some patients contact dermatitis may be an industrial disease (📖 p. 116). *Differential diagnosis:* endogenous eczema, psoriasis, fungal infection.

Presentation Affects any part of the body but most commonly the hands—site and knowledge of occupation, hobbies, sports, etc help elucidate cause.
- **Acute** itchy erythema and skin oedema ± papules, vesicles, or blisters
- **Chronic** lichenification, scaling, and fissuring

Management
- **Identification of the allergen or irritant** Consider referral for patch testing (📖 p. 684)
- **Exclusion of the offending allergen or irritant from the environment** Although this may be impossible. There is some evidence that nickel avoidance diets can help patients with nickel sensitivity[G]. Nickel testing kits are available from dermatology departments
- **Hand care** See Table 17.5
- **Emollients** Help skin to recover—apply frequently
- **Topical steroids** Help but are secondary to avoidance measures
- **Exclude/treat secondary infection**

Table 17.5 Hand care

Hand washing	Use warm water and substitute soap with emollient, e.g. aqueous cream; dry with a clean cotton towel—avoid paper towels or drying machines
Avoidance	Avoid handling hair preparations (including shampoos), other detergents, household or industrial cleaning fluids, raw vegetables (e.g. peeling potatoes, tomato juice); fruits (e.g. peeling oranges); or raw meat
Protection	If performing any task where hands would get wet or any of the substances listed above are being handled, wear cotton gloves under PVC gloves. Wear gloves for dusty work or in the cold
Medication	Use emollients frequently throughout the day (e.g. Diprobase® cream). If necessary, apply a thin layer of steroid ointment od/bd

Further information
NICE Atopic eczema in children (2007) 🖰 www.nice.org.uk
British Association of Dermatologists 🖰 www.bad.org.uk
- Guidelines for the management of atopic eczema (2009)
- Guidelines for the management of contact dermatitis (2009)

Patient information and support
National Eczema Society ☎ 0800 089 1122 🖰 www.eczema.org

Other eczemas

Discoid (nummular) eczema
- Middle-aged/elderly patients. ♂ > ♀. Unknown cause
- **Presentation** Intensely itchy, coin-shaped lesions on limbs. Tend to be symmetrical. May be vesicular or chronic and lichenified
- **Differential diagnosis** Tinea corporis; contact dermatitis, psoriasis
- **Management** Often clears spontaneously after a few weeks but tends to recur. If treatment is needed, use a moderate or potent topical steroid. Secondary infection is common—treat with topical/systemic antibiotics. A sedating antihistamine (e.g. hydroxyzine 50mg nocte) may be useful if sleep is disturbed by itching

Venous (stasis, varicose) eczema
- Middle-aged/elderly patients. ♀ > ♂
- Associated with underlying venous disease
- **Early signs** Capillary veins and haemosiderin deposition around the ankles and over prominent varicose veins
- **Later signs** (see Figure 17.12) Eczema ± lipodermatosclerosis (fibrosis of the dermis and subcutaneous tissue) ± ulceration
- **Management** Emollients ± mild or moderate steroid ointment (avoid long-term use) and compression hosiery. Treat venous disease (📖 p. 288) or ulceration (📖 p. 612) on its own merits

Figure 17.12 Varicose eczema showing haemosiderin deposition, excoriated eczematous lesions, and lipodermatosclerosis

 Asteatotic eczema (eczema craquelé)
- **Risk factors**↑ age; overwashing; dry climate; hypothyroidism; diuretics
- **Presentation** Dry itchy eczema with fine, crazy-paving pattern of fissuring and cracking of the skin of the limbs
- **Management** Treat with emollients—occasionally a mild topical steroid is required

Pompholyx

- Sago-like intensely itchy vesicles on the sides of fingers ± palms/soles
- No associated atopic eczema or contact dermatitis
- Young adults. More common in warm weather. Frequently recurrent
- Treat with emollients and topical steroids (some need potent steroids)
- Treat any infection with oral antibiotics
- In severe cases, refer to dermatology for wet dressings

Lichen simplex chronicus Area of lichenified eczema due to repeated rubbing/scratching. May be due to habit or stress. *Treatment:* take scrapings to exclude fungal infection; topical steroids; occlusive dressing (e.g. Duoderm®) to protect skin from scratching.

Seborrhoeic dermatitis Chronic scaly eruption affecting scalp, face and/or chest. *Differential diagnosis:* psoriasis, rosacea, contact dermatitis, fungal infection. Five patterns:

- **Scalp and facial involvement** Most common in young men. Excessive dandruff, itchy scaly erythematous eruption affecting sides of the nose, eyes, ears, hairline. May be associated blepharitis
- **Petaloid** Dry, scaly eczema over the pre-sternal area
- **Pityrosporum folliculitis** Erythematous follicular eruption with papules/pustules over the back
- **Flexural** Most common in the elderly. Axillae, groins, and submammary areas. Moist intertrigo. Associated with 2° candida infection
- **Infantile** 📖 p. 903

Treatment

- **Facial, truncal, and flexural involvement** Imidazole + hydrocortisone. Pityrosporum folliculitis may respond to itraconazole 200mg od for 7d or fluconazole 50mg od for 2wk
- **Scalp lesions** Ketoconazole or coal tar shampoo. In resistant cases, apply 2% sulphur + 2% salicylic acid cream several hours before shampooing
- **Recurrence** requiring repeated treatment is common. Consider maintenance treatment with topical antifungal every other week

❶ Severe or recalcitrant seborrhoeic dermatitis is an indicator disease for HIV infection—offer HIV testing.

Dandruff Is exaggerated physiological exfoliation of fine scales from an otherwise normal scalp. More severe forms merge with seborrhoeic dermatitis and treatment is the same.

Further information

CKS Seborrhoeic dermatitis (2008) ℘ www.cks.nhs.uk
British HIV Association, BASHH and British Infection Society UK national guidelines for HIV testing (2008) ℘ www.bashh.org

Patient information and support
National Eczema Society ☎ 0800 089 1122 ℘ www.eczema.org

Ulcers

Leg ulcer Painful and debilitating condition, affecting 1% of the adult population and 3.6% of those >65y.

Cause >90% result from arterial disease, venous disease, or neuropathy. *Other causes:* trauma, obesity, immobility, vasculitis (rheumatoid arthritis, SLE, PAN), malignancy, osteomyelitis, blood dyscrasias, lymphoedema, self-inflicted.

Common sites
- **Arterial** Shin, toes, over pressure points (under heel, over malleoli)
- **Venous** Above medial or lateral malleoli of the ankle
- **Neuropathic** Sole of foot, over pressure points

History Ask about:
- Duration of ulceration
- Pain—painful, unless neuropathic when often painless
- Mobility
- Past history of ulceration, DVT, or varicose vein surgery
- History of trauma to the limb
- Systemic disease—e.g. DM, peripheral vascular disease, RA

Examination
- **Ulcer** Position; evidence of infection; surrounding callus—typical of neuropathic ulcers; evidence of tracking to involve the bones of the foot
- **Leg** Pulses; varicose veins and/or signs of venous hypertension—haemosiderin pigmentation, varicose eczema, atrophie blanche (white lacy scars), lipodermatosclerosis; sensation—↓ when peripheral neuropathy; range of joint movement

Investigation
- Bloods FBC, ESR, VDRL, blood glucose
- Ankle–brachial pressure index (📖 p. 237)
- Swab for M,C&S if any signs of cellulitis/infection
- Diabetic ulcer—if signs of infection, X-ray foot to exclude osteomyelitis

Management
- **Arterial ulcers** Refer to vascular surgery
- **Diabetic foot ulcers** Refer to a specialist diabetic foot team
- **Venous ulcers** If ABPI >0.8, can be managed in the community with graduated compression bandaging (elastic bandages applied in multiple layers over a non-adherent dressing). Change dressings 1–2x/wk. Keep skin under the bandage moist with simple emollients and treat surrounding eczema with topical steroids. Give analgesia. Encourage walking, weight ↓ if obese, and elevation of the leg when resting. 65–70% heal in <6mo. Recommend compression hosiery after healing

Referral
- **Non-healing ulcers or ulcers of uncertain cause** Dermatology
- **ABPI <0.8** Vascular surgery
- **Varicose veins** Vascular surgery—60% may benefit from vein surgery

Prevention of recurrence 5y recurrence rate is 40%—graduated compression hosiery ↓ recurrence. Below-knee class 2 stockings are adequate for most and can be prescribed with NHS prescription but are difficult to apply especially with arthritic hands. Applicators are available and can be obtained on NHS prescription, via the OT or bought from specialist disability shops.

Complications
- Infection—treat with systemic antibiotics only if rapidly advancing ulcer edge, cellulitis, or systemic symptoms
- Lymphoedema
- Contact dermatitis to topical medicaments and dressings. Consider referral for patch testing if suspected
- Malignant change—squamous cell cancer (rare). Refer for biopsy to confirm diagnosis

Pyoderma gangrenosum Uncommon cause of ulceration. Starts as a pustule/inflamed nodule that breaks down to form an ulcer that often expands rapidly and is painful (see Figure 17.13). The ulcer has a purplish margin and surrounding erythema. Usually on trunk/lower limbs. Refer to dermatology.

Causes UC (50% patients with pyoderma gangrenosum); Crohn's disease; RA; Behçet's syndrome; multiple myeloma and monoclonal gammopathy; leukaemia.

Figure 17.13 Pyoderma gangrenosum
Reproduced with permission from New Zealand Dermatological Society Incorporated.
Published online at: ℅ www.dermnetnz.org

Bed sores or pressure ulcers
- Caused by pressure necrosis of the skin. Immobile patients are at high risk—especially if frail ± incontinent
- If at risk, refer to the DN for advice on prevention of bed sores—protective mattresses and cushions, incontinence advice, guidance on positioning and movement
- Warn carers to make contact with the DN if a red patch does not improve 24h after relieving the pressure on the area. Treat aggressively and admit if not resolving

Further information
CKS Leg ulcers (2012) ℅ http://cks.nice.org.uk/leg-ulcer-venous
NICE Pressure ulcer management (2005) ℅ www.nice.org.uk

Urticaria and angio-oedema

Urticaria (hives or nettle rash) Common; affects 1 in 6 at some time. Superficial, itchy swellings of the skin or *weals* (see Figure 17.14) come and go in an attack giving the appearance of a shifting rash.

Figure 17.14 Typical urticarial lesions in a child

Angio-oedema Deeper longer-lasting swellings; painful rather than itchy. Commonly affect eyes, lips, genitalia, hands, and/or feet. May affect bowel (abdominal pain, nausea, vomiting, diarrhoea) or airway (tongue swelling, shortness of breath, wheeze). If airway compromise, consider anaphylaxis (📖 p. 1072).

Classification (see Table 17.6) Half present with urticaria alone; 1 in 10 has angio-oedema alone; the remainder have both.

Management of acute urticaria Only treat if needed:
- Try antihistamines for itch—non-sedating for daytime (e.g. cetirizine, fexofenadine) ± sedative if interferes with sleep (e.g. chlorphenamine, hydroxyzine). If one antihistamine is ineffective, try another
- Topical menthol 1% cream is an alternative/adjunct to antihistamines
- If severe, consider short-course steroids (e.g. prednisolone 40 mg od for 3–5d). If rebound symptoms after stopping, seek specialist advice

Management of chronic urticaria Check FBC, ESR, and TFTs. Assess severity and impact of symptoms. Identify potential causes. Advise to avoid non-specific aggravating factors, e.g. overheating, stress, alcohol, aspirin/codeine, and NSAIDs if aspirin-sensitive. Prescribe antihistamines for itch as for acute urticaria. If these measures do not control symptoms, refer. Other treatments are usually specialist-initiated and unlicensed. They include H_2 receptor antagonists (e.g. cimetidine, ranitidine) and anti-leukotrienes (e.g. montelukast)—response is highly variable.

Management of angio-oedema
- If anaphylaxis is suspected, give adrenaline and admit (📖 p. 1072)
- If any airway compromise, admit—even if anaphylaxis is not suspected
- Otherwise treat as for acute urticaria; monitor for airway compromise
- If not taking ACE inhibitor, refer to allergy clinic/immunology; if taking ACE inhibitor, stop—refer if symptoms continue/recur after >3mo

 Urticaria pigmentosa (cutaneous mastocytosis) Appears in infancy (usually <2wk old). Dark freckle-like lesions on the face, limbs, or trunk become urticarial when the skin is rubbed. No treatment is needed—clears spontaneously in childhood.

Table 17.6 Classification of urticaria and angio-oedema

Type	Features
Ordinary/ idiopathic	Spontaneous weals ± angio-oedema. Individual weals last 2–24h • **Acute** <6wk of continuous activity • **Chronic** ≥6wk of continuous activity—affects 1–5/1,000. May remit/relapse. Relapses are triggered by illness, stress, drugs, alcohol or hormonal changes (e.g. menstruation). 50% resolve in 3–5y; 20% persist >10y. Associated with autoimmune thyroid disease (↑ 2x); children/adolescents have ↑ prevalence of coeliac disease. Severe impact on quality of life—14% develop depression • **Episodic** (acute intermittent/recurrent) Symptoms last hours/days but recur over months/years. Treated like chronic urticaria Cause unknown. *Triggers include*: stress, overheating, drugs, alcohol, viral infections (particularly children)
Physical	Except for delayed pressure urticaria, weals last <1h. Induced by a specific physical stimulus; avoidance prevents attacks: • **Mechanical** Delayed pressure urticaria (weals appear in 2–6h and fade over 48h); symptomatic dermographism; vibratory angio-oedema • **Thermal** Cholinergic urticaria (induced by sweating); cold contact urticaria; localized heat urticaria • **Other** Aquagenic urticaria (contact with water); solar urticaria; exercise-induced anaphylaxis
Contact	Weals last <2h. Caused by allergens (e.g. nuts, shellfish, milk, eggs, penicillin, insect stings, latex) or chemicals (e.g. drugs—opioids, aspirin, NSAIDs; radio-contrast media; food additives—azo-dyes, preservatives) Refer for allergy testing if a specific allergen is suspected
Urticarial vasculitis	Individual weals last >24h; lesions are burning/painful rather than itchy and/or lesions leave scaling, bruising, purpura/petechial haemorrhages. Suspect if relentless rather than self-limiting urticaria. *Other associated features*: joint pains, fever, and/or malaise. Refer. Diagnosis is confirmed by skin biopsy. *Specialist treatment*: steroids and/or other immunosuppressive agents
Autoimmune	Urticaria, pyrexia, and malaise + disease-specific features. May be hereditary or acquired (e.g. SLE)—treat the cause
Lone angio-oedema	Swellings last <3d. *Causes*: idiopathic; drug-induced (ACE inhibitors, ARBs, NSAIDs); C_1 esterase inhibitor deficiency

C_1 esterase inhibitor deficiency (hereditary angio-oedema)
Autosomal dominant—usually presents in puberty with episodes of angio-oedema without weals. ↓ C_4 level suggests the diagnosis. Emergency treatment is with hospital admission for C_1 inhibitor concentrate infusion. Maintenance therapy (under consultant supervision with anabolic steroids or tranexamic acid) is necessary only for patients with symptomatic recurring angio-oedema or related abdominal pain.

Further information
British Association of Dermatologists Guidelines for evaluation and management of urticaria in adults and children (2007) ℬ www.bad.org.uk
BSACI Guidelines for the management of chronic urticaria and angio-oedema (2007) *Clinical and Experimental Allergy* 37:631–50.

Acne

Chronic inflammatory condition characterized by comedones, papules, pustules, cysts, and scars. Acne vulgaris is common and affects >80% teen-agers; 50% have a family history. *Peak age:* 18y; ♂ = ♀.

Cause Complex—androgen secretion results in ↑ sebum excretion; pilosebaceous duct blockage (producing comedones); colonization of the duct with *Propionibacterium acnes* bacteria and release of inflammatory mediators. Inflammatory acne is the result of the host response to the follicular *Propionibacterium acnes*.

Rarer causes

- Endocrine—PCOS, Cushing's, virilizing tumours
- Squeezing—*acne excoriée*
- Aromatic industrial chemicals—*chloracne*
- Cosmetics
- Drugs—systemic steroids, androgens, topical steroids
- Infantile—faces of male infants—cause unknown
- Physical occlusion, e.g. under a violinist's chin

Presentation Spots on face, neck ± back and chest. Examination reveals blackheads (dilated pores with black plug of keratin = comedones) and whiteheads (small cream-coloured dome-shaped papules); red pap-ules; pustules ± cysts. There may be scarring from old lesions. Burrowing abscesses and sinuses with scarring (*conglobate acne*) are seen in severe cases. Scars may become keloidal. ❶ Severity of acne (see Table 17.7) is often overestimated by the patient and minimized by the doctor.

Differential diagnosis Rosacea (📖 p. 598), bacterial folliculitis (often coexists—📖 p. 633), milia (📖 p. 621), perioral dermatitis.

Management *Aims to:*↓ number of lesions; prevent scarring; ↓ the psychological impact of the condition.

- **Misconceptions** Explain:
  - Acne is not a disease of poor hygiene. The black tip of a comedone is oxidized sebum not dirt
  - Diet is not associated with acne
  - Picking at acne does not improve it and can cause scarring
- **General measures** Wash with soap and warm (not hot or cold) water twice daily. Do not excessively scrub the skin. Use a fragrance-free water-based emollient if dry skin—avoid greasy preparations
- **Medication** (see Table 17.5) Warn patients any treatment takes weeks → months to work fully and is usually continued for months/years; reassess progress every 2–3mo and continue treatment until new lesions stop developing

Complications Acne is not a trivial disease—it can cause scars (both skin and emotional) that last a lifetime. Anxiety, social isolation, and lack of self-confidence are common—ask specifically about these factors and treat as needed.

Perioral dermatitis Papules and pustules which appear around the mouth and chin of a woman, often after use of topical steroids. Treat with oral tetracycline as for acne.

Table 17.7 Treatment of acne (see *BNF* 13.6)

Severity	Description	Management
Mild	Open and closed comedones and some papules	Topical treatment applied to the whole area (not just the spots): **Benzoyl peroxide** applied bd—start at lowest strength and build up as needed **Topical retinoids** (e.g. isotretinoin)—apply low strength preparation every 2–3 nights initially and build up strength and frequency as tolerated; warn patients to avoid the sun. Retinoids cause erythema and scaling in most patients which settles with time and acne may worsen for the first few weeks of treatment **Topical antibiotics** (e.g. clindamycin)—resistance is increasing, use only in combination with benzoyl peroxide or if benzoyl peroxide has failed. Avoid if using oral antibiotics
Moderate	More frequent papules and pustules with mild scarring	Try topical treatment first. If not working after 4–8wk, try either: **Long-term oral antibiotics** (e.g. lymecycline 408mg od or tetracycline 500mg bd) for a minimum of 8wk, or For girls, an **anti-androgen** for >6mo (e.g. cyproterone acetate in co-cyprindiol—also contraceptive) ❶ Topical benzoyl peroxide ± isotretinoin may be used simultaneously with systemic therapy
Severe	Nodular abscesses → more widespread scarring	As for moderate acne. If ineffective, or rapid relapse after antibiotics are stopped, refer to dermatology for consideration of oral retinoid treatment ⚠ Oral retinoids are teratogenic

Referral to dermatology *U* = Urgent; *S* = Soon; *R* = Routine
- Acne fulminans. Seen in adolescent males; severe acne is associated with fever, arthritis, and vasculitis—*U*
- Severe acne or painful, deep nodules or cysts and could benefit from oral isotretinoin—*S*
- Severe social/psychological sequelae—*S*
- At risk of/developing scarring despite primary care remedies—*R*
- Poor treatment response—*R*
- Suspected underlying cause for acne (e.g. PCOS—🕮 p. 725)—*R*

Further information
CKS Acne vulgaris (2013) ℘ http://cks.nice.org.uk/acne-vulgaris
Primary Care Dermatology Society Guidelines for management of acne vulgaris (2010) ℘ www.pcds.org.uk

Psoriasis

Chronic, non-infectious inflammatory skin condition. Epidermal cell prolifera-tion rate is ↑ x20 and turnover time ↓ from 28 to 4d. Affects ~2% Caucasian population (less in other races). Mean age 28y; rare <8y. ♂ = ♀. *Associations:* inflammatory bowel disease (Crohn's > UC); ↑ risk CVD (check BP, lipids; exclude DM). *Presentation:* see Table 17.8.

Cause Genetic (polygenic; 35% have a family history; if one parent affected, there is a 25% probability that a child will be affected—60% chance with two). Environmental factors trigger disease, e.g. trauma (Koebner phenomenon); infection; drugs (e.g. β-blockers, NSAIDs, lith-ium); alcohol; sunlight (aggravates psoriasis in 10%); psychological stress.

Management Explain the condition/treatment options. Discuss its chronic nature and reassure not infectious. Social/psychological problems are common. Be supportive. Advise on self-help groups.

Drug treatment (see *BNF* 13.5) Frequent emollients ±
- **Salicylic acid** ↓ surface scale. Available as Lassar's paste (apply bd) or with dithranol (Psorin®) or coal tar (e.g. Sebco®)
- **Coal tar** Anti-inflammatory + anti-scaling. The thicker the patch the stronger the preparation needed. ↓ smell by topping with emollient
- **Vitamin D analogue** (e.g. calcipotriol, tacalcitol). Plaque/scalp psoriasis—effective and no unpleasant smell or staining of clothing
- **Dithranol** Plaque psoriasis—apply to lesion only. Stains
- **Topical retinoids** (e.g. tazarotene) Mild/moderate plaque psoriasis
- **Topical steroids** (e.g. Dovobet®) Can be used on localized plaques. Less useful in widespread disease. Avoid prolonged use

❶ Plaques can become inflamed and/or aggravated on starting topical treatments, after prolonged use, or if steroids are stopped suddenly.

Referral (*E* = Emergency; *U* = Urgent; *S* = Soon; *R* = Routine)
- Generalized pustular or eythrodermic psoriasis—*E*
- Patient's psoriasis is acutely unstable—*U*
- Widespread guttate psoriasis (to benefit from early phototherapy)—*U*
- So extensive that self-management is impractical or in a sensitive area (e.g. face, hands, feet, genitalia) and symptoms are troublesome—*S*
- Severe social/psychological sequelae and/or time off work/school is interfering with employment/education—*S*
- For management of associated arthropathy (to rheumatology)—*S*
- Failure to respond to primary care management—*R*

Additional secondary care treatment options Phototherapy and PUVA; oral retinoids; cytotoxic and immunosuppressive therapy; specialist nursing services.

Further information
NICE Management of psoriasis (2012) ✆ www.bad.org.uk

Patient information and support
Psoriasis Association ✆ www.psoriasis-association.org.uk
Psoriatic Arthropathy Alliance ✆ www.paalliance.org

Table 17.8 Patterns of psoriasis

Pattern	Features
Erythroderma	📖 p. 596—admit as a medical emergency
Generalized pustular	Rare but serious. Unwell with fever and malaise. Sheets of small sterile yellowish pustules develop on an erythematous background and spread rapidly. Admit
Plaque (see Figure 17.15a)	Most common form. Well-defined disc-shaped plaques involving the knees, elbows, scalp, hair margin, or sacrum. Plaques are usually red and covered with waxy white scales which may leave bleeding points if detached. Plaques may be itchy. *Differential diagnosis:* psoriasiform drug eruption; hypertrophic lichen planus
Scalp psoriasis	Very common. May be confused with dandruff but generally better demarcated and thicker scales
Guttate (see Figure 17.15b)	Acute symmetrical raindrop lesions on trunk/limbs. Most common in adolescents/young adults—may follow streptococcal throat infection. *Differential diagnosis:* pityriasis rosea
Flexural	Affects axillae, submammary areas, and natal cleft. Plaques are smooth and often glazed. Most common in elderly patients. *Differential diagnosis:* flexural candidiasis
Nail	Nail bed is affected in 50%. Fingernails > toenails. Thimble pitting, onycholysis, and oily patches (oily brownish yellow discoloration of the nail bed—often adjacent to onycholysis). Associated with arthropathy. Treatment is difficult. *Differential diagnosis:* fungal nail infection (❶ can coexist so send clippings for mycology)
Palmoplantar pustulosis	Yellow/brown coloured sterile pustules on palms or soles
Napkin psoriasis	Well-defined eruption in nappy area of infants
Psoriatic arthropathy	~40% patients with skin changes. ♂ = ♀. See 📖 p.518

Figure 17.15 Psoriasis (a) silvery scale of plaque psoriasis and (b) widespread rash of guttate psoriasis
Reproduced with permission from ✆ www.psoriasisguide.ca

Lichen planus and keratinization disorders

Lichen planus Very itchy, polygonal, flat-topped papular lesions 2–5mm diameter, affecting flexor surfaces, palms/soles, mucous membranes (two-thirds), and genitalia in a symmetrical pattern. *Koebner phenomenon* (lesions occur in the line of damaged skin due to a scratch—see Figure 17.16a) is exhibited. Papules may have a surface network of white lines (Wickham's striae). Initially papules are red but become violaceous. Papules flatten over a few months to leave pigmentation or occasionally become hypertrophic. Two-thirds of cases occur in the 30–60y age group. ♂ = ♀. Cause unknown. *Variants*:

- **Annular** (10%). Commonly on glans penis
- **Atrophic** Rare, associated with hypertrophic lesions
- **Bullous** Blistering is rare
- **Follicular** May occur with typical lichen planus or just affect the scalp
- **Hypertrophic** Plaques may persist for years
- **Mucous membrane** (see Figure 17.16b) Alone or with skin changes

Figure 17.16 Lichen planus (a) Koebner phenomenon and (b) oral lesions
Reproduced with permission from New Zealand Dermatological Society Incorporated. Published online at: ◌ www.dermnetnz.org

Differential diagnosis Lichenoid drug eruption; psoriasis.

Complications
- Nail involvement (10%)—longitudinal pitting and grooving
- Scalp—scarring alopecia
- Malignant change ◆—it is controversial whether oral lichen planus can undergo malignant transformation. If it can, risk is low (<2% over 10y). NICE recommends patients with confirmed oral lichen planus are monitored for oral cancer as part of routine dental examination[N]

Management Emollients and moderate/high potency topical steroids provide symptomatic relief. Sedating antihistamines may be useful if sleep disturbed. Oral lesions can be treated with hydrocortisone pellets. Rarely, oral lesions are a reaction to mercury amalgam fillings—removing the fillings and replacing them with other materials may solve the problem. Refer to dermatology if:
- Diagnosis is in doubt
- Potentially scarring nail dystrophy
- Extensive involvement
- Resistant to topical treatment

Specialist treatment involves oral steroids ± PUVA.

Prognosis 50% are clear in <9mo; 15% have continuing symptoms >18mo; 20% have a further attack.

Lichen planus-like drug eruptions Recorded after treatment with:
- Thiazide diuretics
- ACE inhibitors
- Tolbutamide
- Penicillamine
- Phenothiazines
- Streptomycin
- Tetracycline
- Isoniazid
- Gold
- Quinine
- Chloroquine

Resolution after withdrawal of the drug is often slow.

Lichen sclerosus 📖 p. 731

Callosities Painless localized thickenings of the keratin layer—protective response to friction/pressure. *Management:* keratolytics, e.g. 5–10% salicylic acid ointment or 10% urea cream; attention to footwear.

Corns Painful. Develop at areas of high local pressure on the feet, e.g. where shoes press on bony protrusions. *Management:* attention to footwear, keratolytics, cushioning (e.g. corn pads). Occasionally surgery may be indicated if deformity of the foot causes recurrent corns.

Keratosis pilaris Common, sometimes inherited condition. Small horny plugs are on the upper thigh, upper arm, and face (see Figure 17.17). Associated with icthyosis vulgaris. Keratolytics, e.g. 10% urea cream improve symptoms.

Ichthyosis Inherited disorders characterized by dry scaly skin. Most common form is *ichthyosis vulgaris*: prevalence 1 in 300, autosomal dominant. Small branny scales on extensor aspects of limbs and back. Mild and often undiagnosed. *Management:* topical emollients ± bath additives. Severe cases require dermatology advice.

Keratoderma Hyperkeratosis of palms and soles. *Tylosis* is diffuse hyperkeratosis of the palms and soles. It is usually inherited (autosomal dominant) but rarely may be associated with oesophageal cancer. Acquired keratoderma occurs in women around the menopause and patients with lichen planus. Treat with keratolytics, e.g. 10% urea cream.

Milia Small white raised 1–2mm diameter spots (see Figure 17.18) resulting from small keratin-filled cysts. Usually on the face (upper cheeks and eyelids). Most common in children but can occur at any age. No treatment is required.

Figure 17.17 Keratosis pilaris   **Figure 17.18** Milia

Further information

British Society for Oral Medicine Guidelines for management of oral lichen planus (2010) ℰ www.bsom.org.uk

Primary Care Dermatology Society Pityriasis versicolor (2010) ℰ www.pcds.org.uk

Pityriasis and seborrhoeic warts

Pityriasis rosea Acute self-limiting disorder most commonly affecting teenagers and young adults. *Cause:* unknown, possibly viral. Generalized eruption is preceded by the herald patch—a single large, oval lesion 2–5cm diameter (see Figure 17.19). Several days later the rash appears consisting of many smaller lesions mainly on trunk (following the ribs giving a 'Christmas tree' pattern) but also upper arms and thighs. Lesions are oval, pink and have a delicate 'collarette' of scale. May be asymptomatic or cause mild/moderate itch. Treatment does not speed clearance. Topical steroid may relieve itch. Fades spontaneously in 4–8wk.

Herald
patch

Figure 17.19 Pityriasis rosea showing herald patch
Reproduced with permission from New Zealand Dermatological Society Incorporated. Published online at: ✍ www.dermnetnz.org

Pityriasis (tinea) versicolor Chronic, often asymptomatic, fungal infection of the skin (*Pityrosporum orbiculare*). Common in humid/tropical conditions. In the UK often affects young adults and teenagers. On untanned, white skin appears as pinkish-brown, oval, or round patches with a fine superficial scale. In tanned or darker skin patchy hypopigmentation occurs (see Figure 17.20). Involves trunk ± proximal limbs.

Management Topical imidazole antifungal (e.g. clotrimazole cream bd), or topical selenium sulfide shampoo to all affected areas at night, washed off the following morning and repeated ×2 at weekly intervals. For resistant cases, try a systemic antifungal, e.g. itraconazole 200mg od, for 1wk. Recurrences are common. Hypopigmentation may take some time to clear.

Figure 17.20 Pityriasis versicolor showing patchy hypopigmentation
Reproduced with permission from New Zealand Dermatological Society Incorporated. Published online at: ✍ www.dermnetnz.org

Pityriasis alba Finely scaled white patches on face or arms (see Figure 17.21). Affects children/young adults. Associated with atopy. Usually no treatment is required. Resolves spontaneously over months or years. If severe refer to dermatology for confirmation of diagnosis. Treatment for severe cases is with topical steroids and/or PUVA.

Figure 17.21 Pityriasis alba on a child's face
Reproduced with permission from New Zealand Dermatological Society Incorporated. Published online at: ℘ www.dermnetnz.org

Seborrhoeic wart (senile wart, basal cell papilloma) Common >60y. Often multiple—most commonly on trunk. Warty nodules, usually pigmented, 1–6cm diameter with a 'stuck-on' appearance (see Figure 17.22). Pieces of the wart can be picked off. *Cause:* unknown.

Features on dermoscopy ❶ Dermoscopy requires specialized training. Useful for distinguishing benign/malignant pigmented lesions. Typical dermoscopic features of seborrhoeic warts are:

- 'Fat fingers'
- Irregular crypts
- Fissures/ridges
- Blue-grey globules
- Light brown fingerprint-like parallel structures
- Milia-like cysts—2 types: tiny, white starry and larger, yellowish cloudy

Management Reassurance. If removal is required cryotherapy, curettage, shave biopsy, and excision biopsy are all effective.

Figure 17.22 Seborrhoeic wart with typical stuck-on appearance
Reproduced with permission from New Zealand Dermatological Society Incorporated. Published online at: ℘ www.dermnetnz.org

Further information
Primary Care Dermatology Society Pityriasis versicolor (2010)
℘ www.pcds.org.uk

Sunlight and the skin

Skin conditions worsened by sunlight HSV (cold sores); lupus erythematosus (LE); porphyria; rosacea; vitiligo.

Skin conditions improved by sunlight Acne; atopic eczema; pityriasis rosea; psoriasis (10% get worse).

Skin cancer 📖 p. 628   **Sunburn** 📖 p. 1115   **Pellagra** 📖 p. 641

Actinic (solar) keratosis (see Figure 17.23a) Single/multiple, discrete, scaly, hyperkeratotic, rough-surfaced areas over sun-exposed sites (e.g. dorsum of hands; head; neck). Occasionally occur on lower lip. More common with fairer skin types. May regress spontaneously or be pre-malignant.

Management Removal by cryotherapy, currettage, excision biopsy or topical:
- Ingenol mebutate (Picato®) gel—150 microgams/g od for 3d to scalp/ face or 500 micrograms/g od to trunk/extremities for 2d
- Fluorouracil cream (Efudix®)—apply thinly od/bd for 3–4wk
- Diclofenac gel (Solareze®)—apply thinly bd for 2–3mo
- Imiquod cream—instructions vary according to preparation.

Advise patients to wear sunblock daily; avoid sun exposure by covering up, and wear a hat with a brim. Look for other signs of sun damage/malignancy.

Complications Malignant change; cutaneous horn development (see Figure 17.23b—treat with excision or curettage; send for histology).

Figure 17.23 Actinic keratosis (a) Scalp lesions (b) Keratin horn

Solar urticaria Rare. Wheals appear within minutes of sun exposure. *Differential diagnosis:* porphyria. *Management:* sunscreens, avoidance. Refer to dermatologist if disabling.

Drug-induced photosensitivity Drugs may produce a light eruption in exposed areas, by dose-dependent or allergic mechanisms. The reaction varies according to the drug. *Common examples are:* amiodarone, chlorpropamide, furosemide, griseofulvin, phenothiazines, sulfonamides, tetracyclines, thiazides, nalidixic acid, coal tar, plant-derived psoralens.

Plant-induced photodermatitis Contact dermatitis (📖 p. 609) in light-exposed areas resulting from local sensitization of the skin by contact with psoralens from plants, e.g. carrots, celery, fennel, parsnip, common rue, giant hogweed. Oils used in perfumes derived from plants (e.g. oil of bergamot) may also contain psoralens.

Polymorphic light eruption Pruritic papules, plaques ± vesicles appear in sun-exposed areas ~24h after exposure (see Figure 17.24). Most common photodermatosis. ♀:♂ ≈2:1. *Cause:* unknown. *Management:* sunscreens and avoidance of sun exposure (sit in the shade, long sleeves, trousers, broad-brimmed hat); a short course of PUVA in the spring may help severe cases—refer to dermatology. Condition is non-scarring. *Differential diagnosis:* photoallergic contact dermatitis; drug-induced photosensitivity; lupus.

Figure 17.24 Polymorphic light eruption
Reproduced with permission from New Zealand Dermatological Society Incorporated. Published online at: ✎ www.dermnetnz.org

Actinic prurigo Rare. Starts in childhood. Papules and excoriations on sun-exposed sites. *Management:* sunscreens and avoidance. Refer to dermatology for confirmation of diagnosis and advice on further management.

Porphyria A group of rare, mostly inherited, metabolic disorders. Porphyrins are important in the manufacture of haemoglobin. Deficiency of enzymes in the porphyrin pathway results in build-up of intermediary metabolites which are toxic to the skin and nervous system. All require specialist management by either a general physician or a dermatologist. The main porphyrias are:

- **Acute intermittent porphyria** Intermittent attacks precipitated by many drugs. *Presentation:* fever, GI symptoms (vomiting, abdominal pain—can be severe); neuropsychiatric symptoms (hypotonia, paralysis, fits, impaired vision, peripheral neuritis, odd behaviour—even psychosis); *no* skin features. Urine may go deep red on standing
- **Porphyria cutanea tarda** Most common porphyria. Typically occurs in male alcoholics with liver damage. Presents with sun-induced subepidermal blisters on hands which scar. *Management:* avoidance of alcohol and aggravating drugs (e.g. oestrogens); venesection; chloroquine
- **Erythropoietic protoporphyria** Autosomal dominant; starts in childhood; red blistering eruption leaving scars on hands and nose
- **Variegate porphyria** Autosomal dominant. Common in South Africa. Skin signs are like porphyria cutanea tarda, but abdominal pain and neuropsychiatric symptoms resemble acute intermittent porphyria

Further information

British Association of Dermatologists Guidelines for the management of actinic keratoses (2007) ✎ www.bad.org.uk

Benign skin tumours

Seborrhoeic wart (senile wart, basal cell papilloma) 📖 p. 623

Chondrodermatitis nodularis 📖 p. 945   **Milia** 📖 p. 621

Naevus Benign proliferation of ≥1 normal constituent of the skin. The most common type is the melanocytic naevus or 'mole'. Most develop in childhood and adolescence. *Features:*

- **Congenital** Present at birth in 1% Caucasians (less in darker-skinned races). Usually >1cm diameter. Large ones have ↑ risk of malignancy
- **Junctional** Flat, round/oval, brown/black, 2–10mm diameter. Common sites: soles, palms, genitalia
- **Intradermal** Dome-shaped papule/nodule commonly on the face or neck. May be pigmented
- **Compound** <10mm diameter, smooth surface, variable pigmentation
- **Blue** Blue-coloured solitary naevus usually found on extremities—especially hands and feet
- **Halo** Common in children/adolescents. White halo of depigmentation surrounds the naevus which then disappears. Associated with vitiligo. New onset in adults may suggest melanoma elsewhere

Differential diagnosis Freckle, lentigo, seborrhoeic wart, haemangioma (may be pigmented), dermatofibroma, pigmented BCC, malignant melanoma.

Management Patients usually present if worried about a mole. Any change merits serious attention. *Reasons for excision biopsy:*

- Concern about malignancy (📖 p. 628)   • ↑ risk of malignant change
- Recurrent trauma/inflammation   • Cosmetic reasons

Refer for urgent dermatology assessment if malignancy is suspected. Dermoscopy features that suggest malignant melanoma—📖 p. 629

Skin tags Common. Small pedunculated polyps found in axillae, groin, neck, or on the eyelids. Reassure. Cosmetic removal can be achieved by snipping across the skin tag with scissors, cryotherapy, or diathermy.

Sebaceous cyst (epidermal cyst) Common. Round or oval, keratin-filled firm cysts, 1–3cm in diameter, within the skin. Usually a punctum is seen on the surface. Reassure. Treat any complicating bacterial infection with oral antibiotics (e.g. flucloxacillin 500mg qds). Excision is curative.

Dermatofibroma Common (♀ > ♂; young adult > elderly) and usually asymptomatic. Firm (sometimes pigmented) nodule 5–10mm in diameter, that may occur following an insect bite or minor trauma (see Figure 17.25). *Most common site:* lower legs. Treatment is with excision biopsy of symptomatic or diagnostically doubtful lesions.

Keratoacanthoma Rapidly growing nodular tumour (<2cm in diameter) of sun-exposed skin of face/arms—see Figure 17.26. A central keratin plug may fall out to leave a crater. Heals spontaneously over several months leaving a scar. *Differential diagnosis:* SCC. Treatment is with excision biopsy to exclude SCC or curettage and cautery.

Figure 17.25 Dermatofibroma

Figure 17.26 Keratoacanthoma

Keloid scar Proliferation of connective tissue presenting as firm smooth nodules/plaques in response to trauma. A scar is termed hypertrophic if changes are limited to the scar, but keloid if it extends beyond the limit of the original injury (see Figure 17.27). *Most common sites:* upper back, chest, ear lobes. More common in negroid races (2nd–4th decades).

Management Consider steroid injection into the scar. Refer to dermatologist or plastic surgeon if this is ineffective—other treatments include cryotherapy or topical silicone gel sheeting.

Pyogenic granuloma Bright red/blood-crusted nodule that bleeds easily (see Figure 17.28). Typically at the site of trauma (e.g. small cut) and enlarges rapidly over 2–3wk. Usually occurs in children/young adults. *Most common site:* finger. *Differential diagnosis:* malignant melanoma.

Management
- **Pregnant women** May disappear spontaneously after delivery
- **Other patients** Excision biopsy to exclude malignancy; topical imiquimod is an alternative if diagnosis is certain

Lipoma Common. Benign tumour of fat. Present as soft masses in the subcutaneous tissue. Often multiple. Most common on trunk, neck, and upper extremities. Removal by excision is rarely necessary.

Campbell de Morgan spot (cherry angioma) Small bright red papules on the trunk in middle-aged/elderly patients. Usually require no treatment. *Campbell de Morgan (1811–76)—English surgeon.*

Patient information

British Association of Dermatologists Patient information leaflets on: seborrhoeic warts, keratoacanthoma, dermatofibroma, pyogenic granuloma ℘ www.bad.org.uk

Figure 17.27 Keloid scar

Figure 17.28 Pyogenic granuloma

Skin cancer

⚠ **Sun safety code** 80% of skin cancer is preventable.
- Take care not to burn—protect the skin with clothing, including a shirt, trousers/skirt, hat, and ultraviolet-protective sunglasses
- Seek shade between 11 a.m. and 3 p.m
- Apply high factor sunscreen (≥SPF 30 with high UVA protection)
- Take particular care to protect children in the sun

Cutaneous malignant melanoma Every year in the UK, there are 11,900 new cases of melanoma (lifetime incidence 1 in 60) and 2,800 deaths. Incidence is rising. Particularly common in Caucasians. Frequently metastasizes and may present with metastases. *Types:*
- **Superficial spreading** 70% UK cases. ♀ > ♂. *Most common site:* lower leg in ♀ (50%); back in ♂. Macular lesion with variable pigmentation (see Figure 17.29a)
- **Nodular** (see Figure 17.29b) 20% UK cases. ♂ > ♀. Most common on trunk. Pigmented nodule grows rapidly and may ulcerate
- **Lentigo** A lentigo maligna arises in sun-damaged skin—usually on the face—and melanoma develops many years afterwards within it. Most common >60y—especially if outdoor occupation
- **Acral lentiginous** 35–60% melanoma in black-skinned populations. Affects palms, soles, and nail beds. Often detected late. Poor prognosis

Risk factors Sun exposure/sunbed use; genetic (10% have family history); multiple benign moles (>50 of >2mm diameter); congenital naevus; previous malignant melanoma; immunosuppression; fair skin type (red hair, blue eyes, and burns easily); severe sunburn in childhood/adolescence; 30% arise out of pre-existing moles, but risk of change in a benign mole (except dysplastic or congenital naevus) is small.

Assessment Encourage patients to report changes in moles early. Check the ABCDEF criteria:
- **A** Asymmetry of outline
- **C** Colour variation
- **B** Border irregularity
- **D** Diameter
- **E** Evolution—changes in size, shape, colour, and/or elevation
- **F** Funny-looking' mole—'ugly duckling' moles that stand out from the others are very discriminatory for nodular melanoma

Management Use the 7-point checklist (see Box 17.2) ± dermoscopy findings (if available) to identify changes needing referral. Refer all suspicious lesions for urgent dermatology assessment ± wide excision.

Dermoscopy ❶ Requires specialized training. Useful for distinguishing benign/malignant pigmented lesions. Use the 3-point checklist—see Box 17.3.

Specialist treatment Best chance of cure comes with complete excision. Chemotherapy/radiotherapy are of little benefit, but biological therapies (e.g. interferon, interleukin-2, ipilimumab, vemurafenib) are commonly used. A treatment vaccine is currently undergoing clinical trials.

Prognosis Relates to tumour depth at presentation. 5y survival: <0.76mm deep—95%; >4mm deep—45%; metastases—10%.

Figure 17.29 Malignant melanoma (a) superficial spreading (b) nodular

Box 17.2 The 7-point checklist for moles
Score 2 points for any major feature and 1 point for any minor feature.
Lesions scoring ≥3 points are suspicious—refer.
Major signs
- Change in size—increase in size
- Irregular colour
- Irregular shape—irregular border, asymmetry, elevation
Minor signs
- ≥7mm diameter
- Inflammation
- Oozing—including crusting/bleeding
- Change in sensation— including symptoms of minor irritation or itch

❶ One feature is enough to prompt referral if high level of suspicion.
For low-suspicion lesions, monitor for change over 8wk.

Box 17.3 The 3-point dermoscopy checklist
Each item scores 1 point—any lesion scoring 3 points warrants referral
(sensitivity 96%).
- **Asymmetry** Of colour/structure (not shape) in ≥1 perpendicular axis
- **Atypical pigment network** Irregular holes and thick lines (broadened network); streaming (irregular finger-like projections at the edge of the lesion) and pseudopods (bulbous areas of pigmentation joined to the tumour body or pigmented network at the periphery of the lesion) are also atypical
- **Blue-white structures** Blue-white veil (irregular, structureless area of confluent blue pigmentation with an overlying white 'ground-glass' haze) ± regression structures (e.g. scar-like depigmentation)

Further information
Soyer P, Angenziano G, Zalaudek I, et al. Three-point checklist of dermoscopy. *Dermatology* (2004) **208**:27–31
British Association of Dermatologists UK guidelines for the management of cutaneous melanoma (2010) ℘ www.bad.org.uk
NICE Improving outcome for people with skin tumours including melanoma: The Manual (2006) ℘ www.nice.org.uk

Squamous cell carcinoma (SCC) 20% of skin cancer in the UK. Most common >55y; ♂ > ♀. May metastasize (10%). Usually develops in sun-exposed sites, e.g. face, neck, hands. May start within an actinic (solar) keratosis (📖 p. 624) or *de novo* as a nodule which progresses to ulcerate and crust (see Figure 17.30).

Causes Chronic sun damage, X-ray exposure, chronic ulceration and scarring (aggressive SCC may develop at the edge of chronic ulcers), smoking pipes and cigars (lip lesions), industrial carcinogens (tars, oils), wart virus, immunosuppression, genetic.

Management Refer urgently to dermatology. Treated with surgical excision ± LN biopsy. Large lesions may require skin grafting. Radiotherapy is an alternative for large lesions in elderly patients.

Bowen's disease Intraepidermal SCC. Common—typically occurs on the lower leg in elderly women. Lesions are flat-edged, pink/slightly pigmented scaly plaques (<5cm diameter) and may be solitary or multiple (see Figure 17.31). *Risk factor:* exposure to arsenicals, chronic sun exposure, immunosuppression. Transformation to SCC is rare. Biopsy confirms diagnosis. Treatment is with cryotherapy, curettage, excision, or topical imiquimod/5-fluorouracil. *J.T. Bowen (1857–1941)—US dermatologist.*

Kaposi's sarcoma 📖 p. 746

Basal cell carcinoma (rodent ulcer, BCC) Most common form of skin cancer—accounts for >75% of skin cancer in the UK. Locally invasive but rarely metastasizes. Tends to occur in middle-aged/elderly patients, may be multiple and appears mainly on light-exposed areas—most commonly the face. 3 major types (see Figure 17.32—all can be pigmented):
- **Nodular** Most common. Starts as small pearly nodule ± surface telangiectasia. May necrose centrally leaving a small crusted ulcer with pearly, rolled edge
- **Superficial** ≥1 scaly erythematous plaques with pearly edges
- **Morphoeic** Waxy indurated plaque resembling a scar

Dermoscopy of pigmented BCC ❶ Requires specialized training:
- Absence of pigment network • Specks of brown/grey pigment
- Multiple blue-grey globules • Focal ulceration
- Large blue-grey ovoid nests or blotches
- Linear and arborizing (tree branch-like) telangiectasia
- Structureless or leaf-like areas towards the edge of the lesion
- Spoke wheel areas (like spokes of a wheel radiating from a central hub)

Causes Sun exposure, X-ray irradiation, chronic scarring, genetic predisposition, arsenic ingestion

Management Complete excision is the ideal. Refer routinely—if low risk to GPwSI working in a community skin cancer clinic; if uncertain or any high-risk features to dermatology. *High-risk features:*
- Site—nose/paranasal folds, scalp/temples, lips • Size >2cm
- Previously treated lesion • Immunosuppression
- Genetic disorder associated with BCC, e.g. Gorlin's syndrome

Prognosis Recurrence rate is 5% at 5y for all modalities of treatment. Development of new basal cell carcinoma at other sites is common.

Figure 17.30 Squamous cell cancer showing ulcerated nodule

Figure 17.31 Bowen's disease

Figure 17.32 Basal cell cancer. (a) Nodular BCC—pearly nodule showing surface telangiectasia. (b) Superficial BCC—scaly erythematous patch with pearly, rolled edges. (c) Morphoeic BCC (can be difficult to see)—waxy indurated plaque

Further information

British Association of Dermatologists ℗ www.bad.org.uk
- Multiprofessional guidelines for the management of the patient with primary cutaneous squamous cell carcinoma (2009)
- Guidelines for management of Bowen's disease (2006)
- Guidelines for the management of BCC (2008)

NICE Improving outcomes for people with skin tumours, including melanoma: The Manual (2006) ℗ www.nice.org.uk

Bacterial skin infection

 Impetigo Superficial skin infection due to *Staph. aureus*. Very common in childhood. A thin-walled blister ruptures easily to leave a yellow crusted lesion. May occur anywhere but most common on the face. *Differential diagnosis:* HSV, fungal infection (e.g. ringworm). Lesions spread rapidly and are contagious. Avoid spreading to other children—no sharing of towels, face flannels, etc.; some schools/nurseries/childminders prohibit attendance until lesions are cleared. Reassure that non-scarring:

- **Localized** Treat with topical antibiotics (e.g. fusidic acid cream)
- **Widespread** Treat with oral flucloxacillin or clarithromycin

Erysipelas and cellulitis Acute infection of the dermis. Often preceded by fever/'flu-like' symptoms. Usually affects face/lower leg. Appears as a painful, tender reddened area with a well-defined edge. Often the area is swollen and may blister. May be an obvious entry wound. *Differential diagnosis:* angio-oedema, contact dermatitis, gout.

Management

- **Severe infection** Admit for IV antibiotics
- **If systemically well** Mark the area before starting flucloxacillin 500mg qds or clarithromycin 500mg bd for 7–14d. Advise to seek help if infection is spreading or becoming systemically unwell
- **Facial infection** Treat with penicillin V 500mg qds (flucloxacillin 500mg qds if staphylococcal infection suspected or clarithromycin 500mg bd if penicillin-allergic). Have a low threshold for admission
- **Recurrent infections** (>2 episodes at one site). May need prophylactic long-term penicillin (e.g. penicillin V 250mg od or bd) with attention to skin care and management of any lymphoedema

Boils and carbuncles

- **Boil (furuncle)** Acute infection of a hair follicle, usually with *Staph. aureus*. A hard, tender, red nodule surrounding a hair follicle becomes larger and fluctuant after several days. Occasionally associated with fever ± malaise. Later may discharge pus and a central 'core' before healing; may leave a scar. *Predisposing factors:* usually absent—DM; HIV; obesity; blood dyscrasias; immunosuppressive drugs
- **Carbuncle** Swollen, painful area discharging pus from several points. Occurs when a group of hair follicles become deeply infected, usually with *Staph. aureus*. May be associated with fever ± malaise. *Predisposing factors:* malnutrition, cardiac failure, drug addiction, severe generalized dermatosis, prolonged steroid therapy, DM

Management

- **Non-fluctuant lesions** Apply moist heat to relieve discomfort, help localize the infection, and promote drainage
- **If fever or surrounding cellulitis or lesion is on the face** Treat with oral antibiotics, e.g. flucloxacillin 500mg qds for 7d—clarithromycin 500mg bd is an alternative if allergic to penicillin
- **If large but localized, painful, and fluctuant** Consider incision and drainage (❶ do not attempt if you are not confident). Admission may be needed if young or uncooperative child, or the boil is in a sensitive

area, e.g. genital region, face, neck, axilla, breast. Afterwards treat with oral antibiotics until inflammation resolves
- **Admit** If not settling with primary care treatment
- **If recurrent or chronic** Take swabs for culture from lesions and carrier sites (nose, axilla, and groin); treat carrier sites with topical antibiotic (e.g. Naseptin® qds for 10d). Advise improved hygiene and use of antiseptics in the bath (e.g. chlorhexidine); consider long-term antibiotics (e.g. clarithromycin 500mg od)

Folliculitis Superficial infection of the hair follicles usually caused by *Staph. aureus*. Presents as pustules in hair-bearing areas, e.g. legs, beard area. *Risk factors:* obesity, DM, occlusion from clothing, topical steroid use. *Differential diagnosis:* pityrosporum folliculitis (📖 p. 611).

Management Exclude DM; treat with topical antiseptic, or if not clearing with topical or systemic antibiotics (e.g. fusidic acid cream or oral flucloxacillin). *If recurrent or chronic:* treat as for recurrent boils.

Acute paronychia Infection of the skin and soft tissue of the proximal and lateral nail fold, most commonly caused by *Staph. aureus*. Often originates from a break in the skin or cuticle as a result of minor trauma, e.g. nail biting. Skin and soft tissue of the proximal and lateral nail fold are red, hot, and tender; nail may appear discoloured/distorted. Treat in the same way as for a boil.

Staphylococcal whitlow (felon) Infection involving the bulbous distal pulp of the finger following trauma or extension from an acute paronychia. The finger bulb is red, hot, oedematous, and usually exquisitely tender. Onset of pain is rapid and there is swelling of the entire finger pulp. *Differential diagnosis:* herpetic whitlow—📖 p. 635.

Management
- **If fluctuant** Admit for drainage and antibiotics
- **If non-fluctuant** Elevate, apply moist heat (e.g. soak in hot water), and treat with oral antibiotics; if this fails, admit for incision and drainage

Wound infection Suspect if a wound becomes painful. Look for swelling, erythema, wound tenderness ± pus. *Risk factors:*
- Malnutrition
- Carcinomatosis
- Infection near the site of incision
- DM
- Steroid therapy
- Contamination of the wound

Management If pus is present send a swab for M,C&S:
- If indurated + infection is localized to the wound suspect staphylococcus. Treat with flucloxacillin 500mg qds or clarithromycin 500mg bd
- If cellulitis around the wound suspect streptococcus. Treat with penicillin V 500mg qds or clarithromycin 500mg bd
- If foul smell, suspect anaerobes—treat with metronidazole 400mg tds

Give adequate analgesia; dress the wound frequently; review regularly; allow pus to drain. If a surgical wound, refer back to the operating surgeon if simple measures are ineffective.

⚠ **Necrotizing fasciitis** Life-threatening soft tissue infection. Usually occurs in otherwise healthy individuals after surgery/trauma (often minor). Ill-defined erythema + high fever. The wound rapidly becomes necrotic. Admit as an emergency for IV antibiotics ± surgical debridement.

Viral skin infection

Systemic viral infections 📖 p. 652   **HIV infection** 📖 p. 746

Viral warts Common and benign. Due to infection of epidermal cells with human papilloma virus (HPV). >50 types identified. The virus is transmitted by direct contact. Immunosuppressed patients are particularly vulnerable.

Genital warts 📖 p. 748

Common warts Dome-shaped papules with papilliferous surface. Usually >1. Most common on hands but may affect other areas. In children 30–50% disappear spontaneously in <6mo.

Plantar warts (verrucas) On soles of feet. Common in children. Pressure makes them grow into the dermis. Often painful. Characterized by dark punctate spots on the surface (may need to pare callus off to see). Warts group together to form mosaics.

Plane warts Smooth, flat-topped papules often slightly brown in colour. Most common on face/backs of hands. Usually >1. Manage as for common/plantar warts. Eventually resolve spontaneously. May show Koebner phenomenon.

Treatment of common, plantar, and plane warts Refer immunosuppressed patients for specialist advice. Otherwise treatment is usually unnecessary. If patients are insistent, advise over-the-counter topical salicylic acid preparations, e.g. Duofilm®, Salactol®.

HPV vaccination 📖 p. 749

Herpes simplex infection Herpes simplex virus (HSV) is transmitted by direct contact with lesions. Lesions may appear anywhere on the skin or mucosa but are most frequent around the mouth and on the lips, conjunctiva, cornea, and genitalia. Diagnosis is usually clinical.

Primary HSV stomatitis After a prodromal period (<6h) of tingling, discomfort, or itching, small tense vesicles appear on an erythematous base. These burst to form multiple, small, painful mouth ulcers. Infection may be accompanied by systemic symptoms, e.g. fever, malaise, and tender lymph nodes. ❶ May be asymptomatic and go unnoticed.

Management of 1° HSV stomatitis Give symptomatic relief—try analgesic mouthwashes, e.g. benzydamine; healing occurs in 8–12d. If seen <48h after onset prescribe oral antivirals, e.g. aciclovir 200mg 5x/d for 5d. If unable to take fluids/becoming dehydrated, admit for IV fluids.

Recurrent infection (cold sores) (See Figure 17.33) After initial infection, HSV remains dormant in the nerve ganglia. Recurrent eruptions can occur, precipitated by overexposure to sunlight, febrile illnesses, physical or emotional stress, or immunosuppression. The trigger stimulus is often unknown. Recurrent disease is generally less severe and more localized. Treat with aciclovir cream 5% 5x/d for 5d if needed (available OTC).

Figure 17.33 Cold sores

Herpetic whitlow Swollen, painful, and erythematous lesion of the distal phalanx, results from inoculation of HSV through a skin break or abrasion and is most common in health workers.

Neonatal herpes 📖 p. 748

Genital herpes 📖 p. 748

Molluscum contagiosum Most common in preschool children.
- DNA pox virus infection spread by contact—including towels. Presents as discrete pearly pink umbilicated papules, 1–3mm diameter (see Figure 17.34). If squeezed papules release a cheesy material
- Lesions are multiple and grouped—usually on the trunk, face, or neck
- Untreated lesions resolve spontaneously after 12–18mo
- In the older child, removal by expressing the contents with forceps, curettage or cryotherapy is possible but usually unnecessary

Orf Solitary, red, rapidly growing papule <1cm diameter—often on hand. Evolves into a painful purple pustule (see Figure 17.35). Patients usually have a history of close contact with sheep, e.g. vet, farmer, or cows (when termed *milker's nodule* rather than orf). *Cause*—parapox virus. *Incubation period* ~6d. Resolves spontaneously in 2–4wk. Complications include 2° infection (treat with topical/systemic antibiotics); erythema multiforme; lymphangitis.

Figure 17.34 Molluscum contagiosum
Reproduced from Lewis-Jones S (2010) *Paediatric Dermatology (Oxford Specialist Handbooks Series in Paediatrics)*. Oxford: Oxford University Press.

Figure 17.35 Orf on a thumb
Reproduced with permission from New Zealand Dermatological Society Incorporated. Published online at: 🖰 www.dermnetnz.org

Fungal infection

Table 17.9 Presentation of candidiasis

Presentation	Symptoms	Differential diagnosis
Genital infection 'Thrush' 📖 p. 737	♀ >> ♂. Itchy, sore vulvovaginitis ± white plaques on mucous membranes and cheesy discharge. Men develop a similar clinical picture	Psoriasis; lichen planus; lichen sclerosus; other causes of vaginal discharge
Intertrigo	Reddened, moist, glazed area in the submammary, inguinal, or axillary folds. In wet workers, may occur between digits. Patients may present with skin changes and/or itch	Psoriasis; tinea cruris; seborrhoeic dermatitis; bacterial skin infection
Oral	Sore mouth; poor feeding in infants. Most common in babies, patients with poor oral hygiene, or the elderly with false teeth. White plaques visible on buccal mucosa which can be wiped off ± angular stomatitis	Lichen planus; epithelial dysplasia
Nappy candidiasis	Babies in the nappy area	📖 p. 903
Chronic paronychia	Often seen in wet workers. Presents with chronic nail fold inflammation	Bacterial infection; chronic eczema
Systemic candidiasis	Occurs in immunosuppressed individuals (e.g. HIV, malignancy). Red nodules may appear on the skin	

There are two major groups of fungal skin infections seen in the UK.

Candidiasis Uniform commensal of the mouth/GI tract which causes opportunistic infection. *Risk factors:* moist, opposing skin folds; obesity; DM; neonates; pregnancy; poor hygiene; humid environment; wet work occupation; use of broad-spectrum antibiotic. Presentation—see Table 17.9.

Dermatophyte infection Tinea denotes fungal infection. Common. Affects skin, hair, or nails. Skin scrapings or nail clippings may confirm diagnosis. Presentation—see Table 17.10.

General measures for prevention of fungal infections Keep body folds separated and dry (e.g. with dusting powder) and minimize hot and humid conditions (e.g. advise open footwear).

Topical treatment of fungal infections

- **Mouth lesions** Remove tongue deposits with a toothbrush by brushing 2x/d. Treat with oral suspensions or gels (e.g. nystatin, miconazole). If false teeth advise to place imidazole gel on the teeth before insertion and sterilize overnight with dilute hypochlorite solution (e.g. Milton®)
- **Genital lesions** Imidazole cream or pessaries

- **Nail infections** If confined to the edge of 1 or 2 nails, use a lacquer or paint, e.g. amorolfine; apply 1–2x/wk after filing/cleansing for 6mo (fingernails) or 9–12mo (toenails). Avoid nail varnish/artificial nails during treatment
- **Skin lesions** Imidazole cream, spray, or powder; terbinafine cream

Systemic treatment Use for resistant, recurrent, extensive, or systemic infection, and nail or scalp infection. Warn about side effects.

- **Oral, mucocutaneous, or systemic candidiasis** Oral fluconazole 50mg od for 1–2wk—higher doses/prolonged therapy may be needed if immunosuppressed (seek specialist advice)
- **Genital candidiasis** Single oral dose of 150–200mg fluconazole
- **Tinea pedis/manuum** Oral terbinafine (250mg od for 2–6wk) or itraconazole (100mg od for 30d or 200mg bd for 7d)
- **Tinea cruris/corporis** Oral terbinafine (250mg od for 2–4wk for tinea cruris and 4wk in tinea corporis) or itraconazole (100mg od for 15d or 200mg od for 7d)
- **Nail infection** Consider if topical treatment is unsuccessful or if the proximal nail or >2 nails are involved. Confirm diagnosis with nail clipping mycology before treatment with oral terbinafine (250mg od for 6wk–3mo) or pulsed itraconazole (200mg bd for 7d, repeated after 21d, x2 for fingernail infections and x3 for toenail infections)
- **Scalp infection** If kerion (pustular boggy mass) is suspected, refer to dermatology. Otherwise, oral terbinafine (250mg od) or griseofulvin (500mg–1g od) depending on sensitivities. ⚠ Griseofulvin may be teratogenic—advise ♀ to avoid pregnancy during treatment and for 1mo afterwards and ♂ to use contraception during treatment and for 6mo afterwards

Pityriasis versicolor 📖 p. 622

Table 17.10 Dermatophyte infections

Tinea	Affects	Presentation	Differential diagnosis
Corporis 'Ringworm'	Trunk or limbs	Single/multiple plaques with scaling and erythema, especially at the edges. Lesions enlarge slowly and clear centrally (hence 'ringworm')	Discoid eczema Psoriasis Pityriasis rosea
Cruris 'Jock itch'	Groin ♂ > ♀ Common in athletes	Associated with tinea pedis. Involves upper thigh (+ scrotum rarely). Red plaque with scaling especially at the edge	Intertrigo Candidiasis Erythrasma
Pedis 'Athlete's foot'	Feet. ♂ > ♀ Young > old	Itchy, maceration between toes. *Risk factors:* swimming; occlusive footwear; hot weather	Contact dermatitis Psoriasis Pompholyx
Capitis	Hair and scalp	Defined, inflamed scaly areas ± alopecia with broken hair shafts	Alopecia areata Psoriasis Seborrhoeic eczema
Unguium	Nails— prevalence ↑ with age; rare in children. Toenails > fingernails	Begins at distal nail edge and progresses proximally to involve the whole nail. Eventually results in thickening, yellowing, and crumbling of the nail plate. Tinea pedis often coexists	Psoriasis Trauma Candidiasis

Infestations

Head lice Most common in children aged 4–11y (♀ > ♂) but may occur in anyone. Contrary to popular belief lice infest clean as often as dirty hair. Adult lice are about the size of a sesame seed, brownish grey in colour and wiggle their legs (see Figure 17.36). Only adults are contagious. Spread by close head–head contact. Lice do not jump/fly and do not remain viable away from a host.

Symptoms/signs Normally asymptomatic. Detected by contact tracing of other cases or routine inspection at home or school. Occasionally present as itchy scalp. Presence of 'nits' (eggshells—white dots attached to hair), eggs, or dead lice indicate past infection—a moving louse must be found to confirm active infection.

Detection After washing hair, apply conditioner and comb with fine-tooth detector comb (available from pharmacy). In at-risk groups e.g. schoolchildren repeat weekly. Lice are removed by the comb and seen trapped in its teeth.

Management Treat all household contacts simultaneously.

- **Prophylactic preparations** No evidence of effectiveness
- **Dimeticone** Lotion or spray. Coats lice and interferes with their water balance by preventing the excretion of water. Advise to rub into dry hair and scalp in the evening, allow to dry naturally, then shampoo off the next morning. Repeat after 7d
- **Insecticides** Effective. 4 types: malathion, phenothrin, permethrin (all available OTC, but NHS prescriptions are often sought), and carbaryl (prescription only). Malathion and phenothrin/permethrin are used as first-/second-line; carbaryl is reserved for third-line. Apply according to the manufacturer's instructions using 2 applications 7d apart. Check wet, conditioned hair with a detector comb before the first application, then every 2d until 2–3d after the second application. Supply enough for 2 applications. Shampoos are ineffective—use lotions, liquids, or cream rinses
- **Mechanical clearance** Wet-comb conditioned hair with a fine-tooth comb until all lice are removed and repeat at 3–4d intervals for 2wk. Alternative to insecticides but requires motivation
- **Other methods of treatment**, e.g. electric combs, aromatherapy (tea tree oil), herbal treatments—no evidence supporting use

❶ If pregnant/breastfeeding, treat with wet-combing or dimeticone.

Contact tracing All cases—trace close contacts over the past month and ask them to check their scalps for lice/treat as needed.

Reinfestation/resistance to treatment 3 possible reasons:

- **Reinfestation** Lice found are large adults only. Ask patient to check close contacts again. Re-treat with a different insecticide
- **Incorrect use of insecticide/mechanical clearance** Lice are at mixed stages of development. Check procedure and make sure instructions are understood. Repeat treatment with a different insecticide
- **Resistance to insecticide** Lice are seen at all stages of development. Re-treat with another product

Figure 17.36 Head lice with needle and thread to give an idea of size

Crab (pubic) lice 📖 p. 749

Scabies Extremely contagious. The scabies mite (*Sarcoptes scabei*) is ~0.5mm long and spread by direct physical contact. Average infection consists of 12 mites.

Presentation Symptoms of intense itching appear 4–6wk after infection. Examination reveals burrows (irregular, tortuous, and slightly scaly, <1cm long) on the sides of fingers, wrists, ankles, and nipples. May form rubbery nodules on genitalia. Itching results in excoriations. Untreated infection becomes chronic.

Differential diagnosis Lichen planus; dermatitis herpetiformis; papular urticaria; eczema.

Management Treat with scabicide, e.g. permethrin 5% or malathion lotion. Apply according to manufacturer's instructions. All close contacts need treatment simultaneously, which may result in all occupants of a residential home being treated. Apply to whole body including scalp, neck, face, and ears. Ensure finger/toe webs are covered, and brush lotion under the ends of finger/toenails. Reapply to whole body after 1wk and to hands alone if washed with soap <8h after application. Advise patients to launder all worn clothing and bedding after application. Itching may persist for some time after elimination of infection—use chilled crotamiton lotion and/or sedating oral antihistamines for symptomatic relief.

Complications 2° infection (treat with topical or systemic antibiotics).

Crusted 'Norwegian' scabies Affects debilitated or immunosuppressed patients There is overwhelming infection with >10,000 mites. Typically the infestation is not itchy but presents with a crusted skin rash often misdiagnosed as psoriasis. Under the microscope, crusts are seen to contain hundreds of scabies mites. Treatment is as for scabies; resistant cases can be treated with ivermectin which is available only on a named patient basis in the UK—discuss with a specialist dermatologist. ❶ People in contact with sufferers may develop a red, itchy rash themselves—treat with insecticide as for scabies.

Skin changes associated with internal conditions

Table 17.11 lists systemic internal conditions and their associated skin changes.

Table 17.11 Systemic conditions associated with skin changes

Condition	Associated skin changes
Addison's disease	Pigmentation, vitiligo
Cushing's disease	Pigmentation, hirsutism, striae, acne, truncal obesity, moon facies, buffalo hump
Diabetes mellitus	• **Diabetic dermopathy**—depressed pigmented scars on the shins • **Necrobiosis lipoidica**—shiny, atrophic yellowish-red plaques on the shins. Affects <1% diabetics but limited to those with DM or who will later develop DM • **Granuloma annulare**—palpable annular lesions on hands, feet, or face. Only rarely associated with DM. Fades spontaneously in <12mo. Differentiate from ringworm • **Xanthoma** (see *Hyperlipidaemia* below) • **Fungal infection** (🕮 p. 636) • **Vascular and neuropathic ulcers** (🕮 p. 360)
Drug eruptions	Common. Withdrawal of the offending drug usually results in clearance of the eruption in <2wk. Simple emollients ± topical steroids may ease symptoms in the interim. Occasionally patients with severe reactions may require admission for supportive treatment until effects of the drug wear off **Stevens–Johnson syndrome** (erythema multiforme—🕮 p. 597)
Hyperlipidaemia	**Xanthoma**—yellowish lipid deposits in the skin; may be eruptive (like a rash), tendinous, plane (palmar creases), tuberous (knees, elbows) **Xanthelasma**—yellowish plaques on eyelids. Not always associated with hyperlipidaemia
Inflammatory bowel disease	**Crohn's disease**—perianal abscess, sinuses, or fistulae; erythema nodosum; Sweet's disease (dark red plaques on face, arms, and legs); clubbing **Ulcerative colitis**—pyoderma gangrenosum, erythema nodosum, Sweet's disease (see *Crohn's disease*), clubbing
Liver disease	Pruritus, spider naevi, erythema, white nails, pigmentation, xanthomas (see *Hyperlipidaemia* above)
Malabsorption	Dry itchy skin, ichthyosis, eczema, oedema, dermatitis herpetiformis (associated with coeliac disease)

(continued)

Table 17.11 (Cont.)

Condition	Associated skin changes
Malignancy	**Acanthosis nigricans** Rare, epidermal thickening and pigmentation in flexures and neck. Associated with GI malignancy
	Mycosis fungoides Lymphoma that evolves in the skin. Slowly progressive becoming systemic only in terminal stages. May resemble psoriasis or eczema in early stages
	Paget's disease of the nipple—💷 p. 688
	Skin secondaries Most commonly breast, GI, ovary, lung or haematological
	Lymphoedema—💷 p. 1041

Other conditions occasionally associated with malignancy Flushing, generalized pruritus, hyperpigmentation, ichthyosis, dermatomyositis, erythroderma, hypertrichosis, pyoderma gangrenosum, superficial thrombophlebitis, tylosis

Condition	Associated skin changes
Malnutrition	**Iron deficiency** Alopecia, koilonychia, itching
	Scurvy Vitamin C deficiency—bleeding gums, woody oedema, perifollicular oedema
	Protein deficiency Pigmentation, dry skin, oedema, pale brown/orange hair
	Pellagra Nicotinic acid deficiency—photosensitive dermatitis in sun exposed areas ± dementia/diarrhoea
Neurofibromatosis	💷 p. 580
Pregnancy	Pigmentation, spider naevi, abdominal striae, pruritus, pruritic urticarial papules and plaques of pregnancy (PUPPP—1:240 pregnancies), pemphigoid gestationis (rare)
Sarcoidosis	Nodules, plaques, erythema nodosum, dactylitis, lupus pernio (dusky-red infiltrated plaques on nose ± fingers)
Thyroid disease	**Hypothyroidism**—alopecia, coarse hair, dry, puffy brownish yellow skin
	Thyrotoxicosis—pink, soft skin, hyperhydrosis, alopecia, pigmentation, onycholysis, clubbing, pretibial myxoedema (raised erythematous plaques on shins—topical steroids may help)
Tuberous sclerosis	**Adenoma sebaceum**—red/yellow fibromatous plaques—usually around nose
	Periungual fibroma—pink, fibrous projections under nailfolds
	Ash-leaf macules—white, oval macules—best seen under Wood's light
	Shagreen patches—yellowish naevi with cobblestone surface—found on the back

Chapter 18

Infectious disease

Immunization

Immunity can be induced in 2 ways

- **Active immunity** Induced using inactivated or attenuated live organisms or their products. Acts by inducing cell-mediated immunity and serum antibodies. Generally long-lasting
- **Passive immunity** Results from injection of human immunoglobulin. The protection afforded is immediate but lasts only a few weeks

Storage of vaccines Follow manufacturers' instructions. Do not store vaccines in the door of a vaccine fridge and make sure there is a maximum and minimum thermometer in the fridge. Record readings regularly and discard vaccines if not stored at the correct temperature.

Administration of vaccines Only suitably trained GPs/nurses should give immunizations. Check immunization is needed and the patient is fit. Check consent has been obtained and that immunizations are the correct ones and in date. Ensure resuscitation facilities are available. Record vaccine expiry date/batch number. Reconstitute vaccine (if necessary) and give according to manufacturer's instructions. Record date and site in the medical notes.

> **Childhood immunization** In the UK, routine vaccinations for the under 5s are usually done in the GP surgery. Routine vaccinations for older children are normally done through the school health service. Schedule for childhood immunizations—see Table 18.1.

Adult immunization

Influenza and pneumococcal vaccination Available as a Directed Enhanced Service—existing practices do not have preferred provider status. Additional payments are available through the Quality and Outcomes Framework for ensuring at-risk patients receive vaccination.

Other necessary vaccinations Can be provided as an Additional Service. Opting out incurs a 2% ↓ in global sum. A list of eligible vaccinations and terms of eligibility is available on the BMA website (℘ www.bma.org.uk). Travel vaccinations that do not fall into these criteria can be administered as a private service.

Contraindications to vaccination For specific contraindications to individual vaccinations consult the Green Book. General rules:
- **Acute illness** Delay until fully recovered. Minor ailments without fever or systemic upset are not reasons to postpone immunization
- **Severe local reaction to previous dose** Extensive area of redness/swelling that involves much of the antero-lateral surface of the thigh or a major part of the circumference of the upper arm
- **Severe generalized reaction to a previous dose** Fever ≥39.5°C <48h after vaccination; anaphylaxis, bronchospasm, laryngeal oedema, and/or generalized collapse; prolonged unresponsiveness; prolonged high-pitched or inconsolable screaming for >4h; convulsions or encephalopathy <72h after vaccination

Table 18.1 UK schedule of childhood immunization

Disease (vaccine)	Age	Comment
Tuberculosis (BCG)	High-risk neonates	1 injection
Diphtheria/tetanus/pertussis/ *Haemophilus influenzae* type b/ inactivated polio (DTaP/IPV/Hib)	2, 3, and 4mo	Primary course (3 doses, a month between each dose)
Pneumococcal conjugate vaccine (PCV)	2, 4, and 12–13mo	Primary course
Rota virus vaccine (oral Rotarix®)	2 and 3mo	Primary course
Meningococcus type C conjugate vaccine (MenC)	3 mo	1st dose
Meningococcus type C/ *Haemophilus influenzae* type b (Hib/MenC)	12–13mo	Booster dose
Measles/mumps/rubella (MMR)	12–13mo	1st dose
Influenza (Fluenz® intranasal spray)	Annually age 2–16y	1 dose per year
Diphtheria/tetanus/acellular pertussis/inactivated polio (DTP/IPV)	3y 4mo–5y (3y after completion of the 1° course)	Booster dose
Measles/mumps/rubella (MMR)	3y 4mo–5y	2nd dose
HPV vaccination	12–13y (♀ only)	3 doses over >6mo
Tetanus/low-dose diphtheria (Td/ IPV) /inactivated polio	13–14y	Booster dose
Meningococcus type C conjugate vaccine (MenC)	13–14y (or before starting higher education if no booster at 13–14y)	Booster dose

❶ Hepatitis B vaccine is also offered to neonates born to hepatitis B +ve mothers <24h after birth with booster doses at 1mo, 2mo, and 1y—🔲 p. 811

Contraindications to live vaccines (BCG; shingles; measles; mumps; oral typhoid; rubella; yellow fever). *Do not* give live vaccines:
- To pregnant women or immunocompromised patients—those on high-dose steroids for >1wk (>1mg/kg/d prednisolone for children or ≥40mg/d for adults); if haematological malignancy; if radiotherapy/ chemotherapy within 6mo; or another immunodeficiency syndrome
- <3wk after another live vaccine (but 2 live vaccines may be given together at different sites), or
- With immunoglobulin (from 3wk before to 3mo after)

❶ Patients with HIV who are not severely immunosuppressed may have live vaccine except BCG and yellow fever.

Vaccine damage payments Only payable if a patient is >60% impaired by a vaccination given within the NHS. Recipients receive a lump sum. Further information: ☎ 01772 899944 🖰 www.gov.uk.

Further information
DH The Green book: immunisation against infectious disease. 🖰 www.dh.gov.uk/greenbook
Patient information
NHS Choices 🖰 www.nhs.uk/Conditions/vaccinations

Symptoms, signs, and notification of infectious disease

Specific symptoms and signs of infection depend on the infecting organism and organs affected. For example, a chest infection will cause respiratory symptoms; a urine infection, urinary tract symptoms. Symptoms suggesting an infectious cause include:

Lymphadenopathy Palpable enlargement of the LNs.

Benign causes
- **Infective** Bacterial—pyogenic, TB, brucella; fungal; viral—EBV, CMV, HIV; toxoplasmosis; syphilis
- **Non-infective** Sarcoid, connective tissue disease (rheumatoid arthritis); skin disease (eczema, psoriasis); drugs (phenytoin); berylliosis

Malignant causes Lymphoma, CLL, ALL, metastases.

Management in adults Refer immediately for urgent investigation[N] if:
- Rapidly growing
- Non-tender, firm/hard lymph node, >3cm diameter
- Lymph nodes associated with other unexplained signs of ill health (night sweats, weight loss, persistent fever)
- Lymph nodes associated with other sinister signs, e.g. petechial rash (same day assessment), suspected head or neck tumour
- Enlarged supraclavicular nodes in the absence of local infection

Most enlarged lymph nodes are reactive lymph nodes—suggested by a short history, soft tender mobile lump, and concurrent infection. If there are no sinister features, give these 2wk to settle. If not settling, check FBC, ESR ± EBV screen. Refer lymphadenopathy >1cm diameter persisting for >6wk for urgent further investigation.

 Management in children Refer to paediatrics urgently, particularly if there is no evidence of local infection, if ≥1 of:
- Non-tender, firm/hard LN
- LN >2cm diameter
- Progressively enlarging LNs
- LNs associated with other signs of ill health (e.g. fever, weight loss)
- Enlarged axillary nodes in the absence of local infection or dermatitis
- Supraclavicular node involvement

Investigate with FBC and blood film if generalized lymphadenopathy

Table 18.2 Normal temperature as measured in different locations

Place of measurement	Normal range
Oral	35.5–37.5°C (95.9–99.5°F)
Rectal	36.6–38.0°C (97.9–100.4°F)
Axillary	34.7–37.3°C (94.5–99.1°F)
Ear	35.8–38.0°C (96.4–100.4°F)

Pyrexia/fever Oral temperature raised above 37.5°C. Normal range varies according to where measured—see Table 18.2. *Common causes:*

Infection By far, the most common cause in general practice:
- Viral infection (e.g. HIV, EBV, URTI, influenza)
- UTI
- Chest infection
- Tonsillitis
- OM
- Sinusitis
- Cholecystitis
- Cellulitis

❶ Do not forget tropical diseases, e.g. malaria in patients returning from abroad. Think of TB and SBE—especially in high-risk patients.

Cancer Lymphoma; leukaemia; solid tumours (e.g. hypernephroma).

Immunogenic causes Connective tissue disease and autoimmune disease (e.g. RA, SLE, PAN, polymyalgia rheumatica); sarcoidosis.

Thrombosis DVT; PE   *Drugs* e.g. antibiotics

Fever in children under the age of 5 📖 p. 874

Rigors Shaking episodes (sometimes violent) associated with sudden rise in fever.

Night sweats Consider TB, lymphoma, leukaemia, solid tumour (e.g. renal carcinoma), menopause, anxiety states, drug causes, e.g. opioids, SSRIs.

Pyrexia of unknown origin Defined as a fever (either intermittent or continuous) which has lasted for >3wk and for which no cause has been found. Recheck history. Re-examine carefully. Check FBC; EBV screen (depending on age of the patient); ESR; CRP; LFTs; amylase, urine (M,C&S); viral titres (including HIV); blood cultures; and CXR. If cause does not become obvious refer urgently for further investigation.

Notifiable diseases[ND] Notification of certain diseases is required under the Public Health (Control of Disease) Act 1984 and Health Protection (Notification) Regulations 2010. Notification is made to the 'proper officer of the local authority' on forms available from the HPA website (🖱 www.hpa.org.uk). *Diseases included:*

- Acute encephalitis
- Acute infectious hepatitis
- Acute meningitis
- Acute poliomyelitis
- Anthrax
- Botulism
- Brucellosis
- Cholera
- Diphtheria
- Enteric fever (typhoid / paratyphoid)
- Food poisoning
- Haemolytic uraemic syndrome
- Infectious bloody diarrhoea
- Invasive group A streptococcal disease and scarlet fever
- Legionnaire's disease
- Leprosy
- Malaria
- Measles
- Meningococcal septicaemia
- Mumps
- Plague
- Rabies
- Rubella
- SARS
- Smallpox
- Tetanus
- Tuberculosis
- Typhus
- Viral haemorrhagic fever
- Whooping cough
- Yellow fever

❶ In addition, notify other infections or contamination which could present significant risk to human health.

Illness in returning travellers

⚠ In all returned travellers who present unwell, consider imported disease *in addition* to the usual differential diagnosis. Tropical medicine is a specialized field. If unsure, seek expert advice by telephone or admit the patient.

History Ask about:

- Symptoms
- Malaria prophylaxis
- Areas travelled to (including brief stopovers)
- Health of members of the travel party
- Duration of travel
- Sexual contacts whilst abroad
- Immunizations prior to travel
- Medical treatment abroad

Examination Full examination. Particularly check for fever, jaundice, abdominal tenderness, chest signs, rashes, lymphadenopathy.

Investigations Depend on symptoms and examination findings. *Consider:* FBC, malaria testing (consult local protocols), LFTs, viral serology, blood culture, stool culture (ensure it is fresh), MSU.

Malaria[ND] 2,000 cases/y are notified in the UK. Easy to miss.

- **Symptoms** Malaria is a great mimic and can present with virtually any symptoms. Usually consists of a prodrome of headache, malaise, myalgia, and anorexia followed by recurring high fevers, rigors, and drenching sweats lasting 8–12h at a time
- **Examination** May be normal—look for anaemia, jaundice ± hepatosplenomegaly
- **Investigation** In all cases of fever in patients who have returned from a malarial endemic area—even if the plane just landed in a malarial area en route. Send a blood test for malaria daily for 3d. Tests include thick and thin film, dipstick or nucleic acid testing depending on local arrangements.
- **Management** Admit for further investigation and treatment if:
  - Very unwell
  - Unable to check a malaria test (e.g. presentation at a weekend or out of hours)
  - Malaria test +ve
  - Persistent fever despite –ve malaria test

Falciparum malaria Caused by *Plasmodium falciparum*. Accounts for ~½ UK cases—it may not present for up to 3mo after return from a malarial area. Can be fatal in <24h—especially if it occurs in pregnant women or small children (<3y). *Complications:* cerebral malaria (80% deaths); hypoglycaemia; renal failure; pulmonary oedema; splenic rupture; disseminated intravascular coagulation; death.

Benign malaria Caused by *P. vivax*, *P. ovale*, and *P. malariae*. May cause illness up to 18mo after return. All have very low mortality. Relapse may occur at intervals after initial infection as parasites lie dormant in the liver (*P. vivax* and *P. ovale*) or blood (*P. malariae*).

Typhoid[ND] **and paratyphoid**[ND] Caused by *Salmonella typhi* and *Salmonella paratyphi*; ~200 cases/y are notified in the UK.

- **Spread** By the faecal–oral route.

- **Incubation** 3d–3wk
- **Symptoms** Usually malaise, fever, headache, cough, constipation (or diarrhoea), nosebleeds, bruising, and/or abdominal pain
- **Examination** Pyrexia; relative bradycardia; rose-coloured spots on the trunk (40%); splenomegaly; CNS signs (coma, delirium, meningism)
- **Management** Admit for further investigation and antibiotics
- **Prognosis** 10% die if untreated—<0.1% if treated; 1% become chronic carriers after infection

Dengue fever Viral infection endemic in tropical and subtropical regions. ~150 cases/y are notified in the UK.
- **Spread** By the day-biting Aedes mosquito
- **Incubation** 4–7d
- **Symptoms/examination** Usually presents with a flu-like illness, sudden high fever ± red, maculopapular rash (appears 2–5d after the fever). Other symptoms—fatigue, headache, arthralgia, myalgia, nausea and vomiting, lymphadenopathy, skin hypersensitivity
- **Dengue haemorrhagic fever** Rare, severe form of dengue fever with poor prognosis. Purpuric rash appears 2–3d after onset of symptoms; minor injuries may cause bleeding; shock → death. Risk factors—previous dengue infection, age <12y, ♀, Caucasian
- **Management** Admit; treatment is supportive

Travellers' diarrhoea 50% travellers experience some diarrhoea. Most cases last 4–5d; 1–2% last >1mo. In all cases send a fresh stool sample for M,C&S at first presentation, noting on the form areas visited. Consider all the usual causes for diarrhoea (📖 p. 377) and gastroenteritis (📖 p. 410). In addition consider:

Cholera[ND] Caused by Gram –ve bacterium *Vibrio cholerae*.
- **Spread** By faecal–oral route
- **Incubation** Few hours–5d
- **Presentation** Profuse watery stool, fever, vomiting, dehydration
- **Management** Admit. Treatment is with rehydration ± antibiotics

Giardiasis ~3,800 cases/y are notified in the UK. Flagellate protozoan. Infection is suggested by an incubation period ≥2wk; watery stool with flatus ++ (explosive diarrhoea); no fever. Stool microscopy may be –ve. If suspected treat with metronidazole. Rapid response is diagnostic.

Amoebic dysentery[ND] ~100 cases/y are notified in the UK. May begin years after infection. Diarrhoea begins slowly becoming profuse and bloody ± fever ± malaise. Diagnosis is confirmed by microscopy of fresh stool. Take specialist advice on management.

Sexually transmitted infections 📖 pp. 738–49

HIV 📖 p. 746   **TB** 📖 p. 326

Hepatitis A 📖 p. 422   **Meningitis** 📖 p. 1078

Hepatitis B & C 📖 p. 742

Further information
Health Protection Agency (HPA) Topics A–Z: malaria, giardia, cholera.
🖰 www.hpa.org.uk

Infections in immunocompromised patients

Infections in patients whose host defence mechanisms are compromised range from minor to fatal. They are often caused by organisms that normally reside on body surfaces.

Opportunistic infections Infections from endogenous microflora that are non-pathogenic or from ordinarily harmless organisms. Occur if host defence mechanisms have been altered by:

- Age
- Infection
- Burns
- Neoplasms
- Metabolic disorders
- Irradiation
- Foreign bodies
- Corticosteroids
- Immunosuppressive or cytotoxic drugs
- Diagnostic or therapeutic instrumentation

The precise character of the host's altered defenses determines which organisms are likely to be involved. These organisms are often resistant to multiple antibiotics.

Organisms commonly involved

- E. coli
- CMV
- Pneumocystis
- Candida
- Herpes viruses
- Toxoplasmosis
- Mycobacteria
- Non-pathogenic streptococci
- Cryptococcal infection

Management Expert care is always required—refer promptly to the consultant responsible for the patient.

Prophylaxis

Antibiotics Used for prevention of:

- TB and meningitis in exposed patients
- Streptococcal infection in asplenic/hyposplenic patients
- Bacterial infections in granulocytopenic patients
- Pneumocystis in AIDS patients
- Recurrent UTIs

⚠ Watch for signs of superinfection with resistant organisms.

Active immunization See Table 18.3.

Passive immunization Can prevent or ameliorate herpes zoster (VZ-Ig), hepatitis A and B, measles, and cytomegalovirus infection in selected immunosuppressed patients. If a patient is in contact with any of these diseases seek advice from the consultant looking after the patient or a consultant in communicable disease control.

Immunoglobulin administration Effective for patients with hypogammaglobulinaemia. Given on a regular basis by IV infusion.

Asplenic patients All asplenic patients (or functionally asplenic patients, e.g. patients with sickle cell disease) are at ↑ risk of bacterial infection. Warn patients about severe malaria and other tropical infections when travelling abroad. Admit to hospital if infection develops despite prophylactic measures.

Ensure that asplenic patients have
- **Vaccinations** See Table 18.3
- **Prophylactic antibiotics** Oral penicillin continuously until age 16y or for 2y post-splenectomy—whichever is longer
- **Standby amoxicillin** To start if symptoms of infection begin
- **Patient-held card** Alerting health professionals to infection risk—cards and information leaflets for patients are available from
  ℜ www.orderline.dh.gov.uk ☎ 0300 123 1002

HIV 🕮 p. 746

Table 18.3 Initial immunization schedule for children and adults with immunocompromise, complement deficiency, asplenia, or splenic dysfunction

Age at presentation	Vaccination schedule
<2y	<ul><li>Routine childhood vaccination schedule (🕮 p. 645)</li><li>Further booster dose of MenACWY >1mo after the 12–13mo routine Hib/MenC and PCV13 vaccination</li><li>One further dose of Hib/MenC and PPV at >2y of age</li></ul>
2–5y	<ul><li>If already vaccinated with PCV7, vaccinate with PCV13, (2 doses > 2 months apart) and then, after ≥2mo, with PPV</li><li>If already vaccinated with PCV13, vaccinate immediately with PPV</li><li>Vaccinate immediately with Hib/MenC booster</li><li>1mo after Hib/MenC booster, vaccinate with MenACWY</li></ul>
>5y	<ul><li>Give Hib/MenC and PPV immediately</li><li>1mo after Hib/MenC and PPV, vaccinate with MenACWY</li></ul>

PCV7—pneumococcal conjugate 7-valent vaccine.
PCV13—pneumococcal conjugate 13-valent vaccine.
PPV—pneumococcal polysaccharide vaccine.
Hib/MenC—*Haemophilus influenza* b/meningitis conjugate vaccine.
MenACWY—meningitis quadrivalent (ACWY) conjugate vaccine.

❗ Start vaccinations ≥2wk before splenectomy or starting immuno-suppressive treatment.

Further information
DH The Green Book: immunization against infectious disease.
ℜ www.dh.gov.uk/greenbook

Childhood viral infections

Table 18.4 Common childhood viral infections

Condition	Duration	Main symptoms
MeaslesND	10d	**Incubation** 10–14d **Early symptoms** Fever, conjunctivitis, cough, coryza, LNs **Later symptoms** Koplik's spots (tiny white spots on bright red background found on buccal mucosa of cheeks), rash (florid maculopapular appears after 4d—becomes confluent) **Complications** Bronchopneumonia, otitis media, stomatitis, corneal ulcers, gastroenteritis, appendicitis, encephalitis (1:1,000 affected children), subacute sclerosing panencephalitis (rare)
RubellaND (German measles)	10d	**Incubation** 14–21d **Symptoms** Mild and may pass unrecognized. Fever, LNs (including suboccipital nodes), pink maculopapular rash which lasts 3d **Complications** Birth defects if infected in pregnancy; arthritis (adolescents); thrombocytopenia (rare); encephalitis (rare)
MumpsND	10d	**Incubation** 16–21d **Symptoms** Subclinical infection is common. Fever, malaise, tender enlargement of one or both parotids ± submandibular glands **Complications** Aseptic meningitis; epididymo-orchitis; pancreatitis
Chickenpox	14d	**Incubation** 10–21d (infectious 1–2d before rash appears and for 5d afterwards) **Symptoms** Rash ± fever. Spots appear in crops for 5–7d on skin and mucus membranes and progress from macule → papule → vesicle then dry and scab over **Complications** Eczema herpeticum (📖 p. 606); encephalitis (cerebellar symptoms most common); pneumonia; birth defects; neonatal infection (📖 p. 808)
Roseola infantum	4–7d	Child <2y **Symptoms** High fever, sore throat and lymphadenopathy, macular rash appears after 3–4d when fever ↓
Erythema infectiosum (Fifth disease/ slapped cheek)	4–7d	Parvovirus infection **Symptoms** Erythematous maculopapular rash starting on the face ('slapped cheeks'), reticular, 'lacy' rash on trunk and limbs, mild fever, arthralgia (rare) Contact with parvovirus in pregnancy—📖 p. 806
Hand, foot, and mouth disease	5–7d	Coxsackie virus infection **Symptoms** Oral blisters/ulcers, red-edged vesicles on hands and feet, mild fever

Management For infections listed in Table 18.4, management is supportive with paracetamol, fluids ± antibiotics for 2° infection. Teething gels may soothe mouth lesions in hand, foot, and mouth disease. Admit if any serious complications develop.

Prevention of measles, mumps, and rubella Measles, mumps, and rubella (MMR) vaccination consists of live attenuated measles, mumps, and rubella viruses. Vaccine viruses are not transmitted.

- Offer MMR to all children after their first birthday and again pre-school. Re-immunization is needed if given to children of <1y. Children with chronic illness, e.g. CF, are at particular risk from measles and should be immunized. Malaise, fever, and rash are common ~1wk after immunizations and last 2–3d. Advise on fever management. There is no link between MMR and autism or inflammatory bowel disease
- Offer children aged >18mo who have not been vaccinated (or whose vaccination status is unclear) 2 doses of MMR vaccine ≥1mo apart; if the child has received 1 dose of MMR, give a booster dose
- Offer MMR to women of childbearing age who are not immune to rubella (i.e. have not had 2 doses of MMR or are seronegative)

❶ There is no evidence that vaccination in pregnancy is harmful, but do not give to women known to be pregnant and advise women who are vaccinated to avoid pregnancy for 1mo afterwards.

Prevention of chickenpox

- Offer chickenpox (varicella) immunization (2 doses 4–8wk apart) to non-immune healthcare workers who have direct patient contact and susceptible close contacts of immunocompromised patients where continuing contact is unavoidable. Consider those with a definite history of varicella infection, immune—antibody-test others. Vaccination is contraindicated if pregnant or immunocompromised
- Non-immune immunosuppressed patients, pregnant women, or neonates (📖 p. 808) with significant exposure to chickenpox/shingles should receive zoster immunoglobulin (VZ-Ig) <3d after contact. Check antibody levels if immune status is unknown

Shingles Reactivation of latent chickenpox virus. Shingles cannot be acquired by exposure to chickenpox but contacts of patients with shingles can develop chickenpox. Infectious until all lesions have scabbed.

- **Incidence** 1 in 25. Any age—more common if immunocompromised
- **Presentation** Unilateral pain precedes a vesicular rash by 2–3 d. Crops of vesicles appear over 3–5d and are in the distribution of ≥1 adjacent dermatomes. The affected area is usually hyperaesthetic—pain may be severe. Lesions scab over and fall off in <14d
- **Management** Treat as for chickenpox. Oral antivirals (e.g. aciclovir 800mg 5x/d) are only effective if initiated <48h after onset of the rash. If immunocompromised admit for IV antivirals
- **Prevention** There is a routine shingles vaccination programme for adults aged 70y (and 79y if not previously vaccinated) in the UK

Complications Post-herpetic neuralgia; dissemination to other areas (immunosuppressed patients—admit for IV antivirals); eye involvement—refer for same day assessment to ophthalmology; Ramsay Hunt syndrome (📖 p. 538).

Streptococcal and staphylococcal infections

Streptococcal infection Several groups are pathogenic to man—A, B, C, G, D, and viridans streptococci. Presentation is varied:

- Pharyngitis
- Tonsillitis
- Wound/skin infections
- Septicaemia
- Scarlet fever

- Pneumonia
- Rheumatic fever
- Glomerulonephritis
- Neonatal sepsis
- Postpartum sepsis

- Endocarditis
- Septic arthritis
- Pneumonia
- UTI
- Dental caries

Investigation Diagnosis is usually clinical. Evidence of infection can be gained by measuring changing antibody response (ASO titres). ASO titres are ↑ in ~80% infections. Swabs are +ve if infection is on the skin or in the throat or vagina.

Treatment Most streptococci are sensitive to penicillin (e.g. penicillin V 250–500mg qds for 7–10d) although resistance is increasingly common.

Pneumococcal infection There are >85 types of S. pneumoniae. Pneumococci are carried in the noses and throats of half the population. In most people they are harmless. Spread is by droplet infection.

Presentations
- Pneumonia
- Acute otitis media
- Sinusitis

- Meningitis
- Endocarditis

- Septic arthritis (rare)
- Peritonitis (rare)

Treatment Amoxicillin 250–500mg tds for 7d (clarithromycin in allergic individuals). Resistance to penicillin in the community is still low.

Childhood vaccination Routine vaccination is offered as part of the childhood immunization programme (🔲 p. 645) using 13-valent pneumococcal conjugate vaccine (PCV) given at 2mo, 4mo, and 12–13mo of age.

Vaccination of high-risk groups A single dose of pneumococcal polysaccharide vaccine (PPV) is indicated for high-risk patients (see Box 18.1) who have not previously been vaccinated. Special rules apply to patients who are immunosuppressed or have deficient spleens (see Table 18.4, 🔲 p. 651). Booster doses are not needed except for patients with asplenia or nephrotic syndrome—when give a booster after 5–10y.

Box 18.1 High-risk patients for pneumococcal infection

Those:
- ≥65y of age
- With a cochlear implant
- With coeliac disease
- With asplenia/functional asplenia, e.g. splenectomy, sickle cell
- With immune deficiency due to disease (e.g. lymphoma, Hodgkin's disease, multiple myeloma, HIV) or treatment (e.g. chemotherapy, prolonged systemic steroids)
- With chronic heart disease, lung disease (e.g. asthma, COPD), renal disease (or nephritic syndrome), or liver disease
- With DM requiring insulin or oral hypoglycaemic drugs, *and/or*
- With CSF shunt/other conditions where leakage of CSF fluid can occur

Scarlet fever Group A haemolytic streptococcal infection. *Incubation:* 2–4d. Presents with fever, malaise, headache, tonsillitis, rash (fine punctate erythema sparing face, 'scarlet' facial flushing), and strawberry tongue (initially white turning red by third/fourth day). Treat with penicillin V 250–500mg qds for 10d (or clarithromycin if allergic). Complications include rheumatic fever (📖 p. 276) and acute glomerulonephritis.

Staphylococcal infection Usually *Staph. aureus*—occasionally *Staph. epidermidis*. Carried in the nose of ~30% of healthy adults. Antibiotic-resistant strains are common.

Presentation
- Breast abscess/mastitis
- Abscesses/furuncles/carbuncles
- Septicaemia
- Endocarditis
- Wound infection
- Osteomyelitis/septic arthritis
- Pneumonia—especially patients with COPD, influenza, or those receiving corticosteroids or immunosuppressive therapy
- Neonatal infections—usually appear <6wk after birth—pustular or bullous skin lesions on neck, axilla, or groin

Management Antibiotics (usually flucloxacillin 250–500mg qds or clarithromycin 250–500mg bd for 7–10d), abscess drainage where appropriate and general supportive measures. Where possible obtain specimens for culture before instituting or altering antibiotic regimens.

Staphylococcal scalded skin syndrome 📖 p. 903

Methicillin-resistant *Staph. aureus* (MRSA)[N] MRSA acts in the same way as any other *Staph. aureus*—it is carried harmlessly in most but occasionally causes a range of infections. It is only different because of its multiple resistance to antibiotics. Often contracted in hospital.
- ↓ tendency for multiple resistance by prudent use of antibiotics
- Wash hands thoroughly with an appropriate antibacterial preparation if they appear soiled
- If hands appear clean, wash with an alcoholic rub between each and every patient contact
- Follow local policies for management of patients who are known to be infected with or carry MRSA

Toxic shock syndrome Caused by staphylococcal exotoxin.
- **Risk factors** Tampon use; postpartum; staphylococcal wound infection; influenza; osteomyelitis; cellulitis
- **Presentation** Sudden onset of high fever, vomiting, diarrhoea, confusion, and skin rash. May progress to shock ± death
- **Management** Admit as a medical emergency—mortality 8–15%

Further information
National Electronic Library for Infection Antimicrobial resistance website 🔊 www.antibioticresistance.org.uk
Health Protection Agency (HPA) Topics A–Z: streptococcal infections, *Staphylococcus aureus*.🔊 www.hpa.org.uk
Nathwani D, Morgan M, Masterton RG, *et al.* Guidelines for UK practice for the diagnosis and management of methicillin-resistant *Staphylococcus aureus* (MRSA) infections presenting in the community. *Journal of Antimicrobial Chemotherapy* 2008; **61**(5):976–94.
🔊 http://mrsaactionuk.net/mrsaathome.html

Other bacterial infections

Haemophilus influenzae

Haemophilus influenza type b (Hib) Vaccination against Hib is routinely offered to all children (📖 p. 645) and immunocompromised patients (📖 p. 651). Prior to routine vaccination, Hib infection accounted for 60% of meningitis in children aged <5y. It was also a common cause of epiglottitis, septicaemia, and septic arthritis/osteomyelitis. Infection is now rare.

Other types Non-encapsulated *Haemophilus influenzae* (ncHi) usually causes non-invasive respiratory tract infections, e.g. OM, sinusitis. It can cause invasive disease in neonates (<1mo of age) and those with co-morbidities e.g. malignancy, immunosuppression, DM, chronic renal/liver/lung disease. Other *H. influenzae* serotypes (Hia, Hic, Hid, Hie, Hif) only rarely cause invasive disease.

Management Organisms are often penicillin-resistant. Use an alternative antibiotic e.g. clarithromycin or doxycycline. If severe infection, admit.

Clostridium infections Anaerobic, spore-forming bacilli found in dust, soil, vegetation, and GI tracts of humans and animals. 25–30 species cause disease in humans. *Presentations:*
- Food poisoning—*C. perfringens*
- Pseudomembranous colitis—overgrowth of *C. difficile* following antibiotic therapy—presents with bloody diarrhoea. Treated with vancomycin or metronidazole if toxin is isolated from stool
- Botulism—caused by a toxin released by *C. botulinum* which is ingested in contaminated food—presents with neurological symptoms and warrants immediate admission for antitoxin
- Wound infections—*C. perfringens* causes cellulitis which may → gas gangrene, septicaemia ± death—admit for IV antibiotics
- Tetanus

Tetanus (lockjaw)[ND] ~6 cases and 1 death every year in the UK. *Incubation:* 2–50d. *C. tetani* infects contaminated wounds that may be trivial, the uterus postpartum (maternal tetanus), or newborn umbilicus (tetanus neonatorum). Tetanus toxin → generalized or localized tonic spasticity ± tonic convulsions. Suspect in any patient who has not been immunized who develops muscle stiffness/spasm several days after suffering a skin wound or burn.

Management If suspected admit for specialist care. Treatment is with antitoxin, wound debridement, and general support. Effects may last several weeks. Mortality—40%.

⚠ **Tetanus-prone injuries** Any burn/wound sustained >6h before surgical treatment of that wound *or* any burn or wound that:
- Has a significant amount of dead tissue within it
- Is a puncture-type wound
- Has had contact with soil/manure likely to harbour tetanus organisms
- Is clinically infected

Prevention Tetanus vaccine:
- **Primary immunization** 3 doses of vaccine each 1mo apart. If the schedule is disrupted the course should be resumed from where it was stopped as soon as possible
- **Booster doses in children** One dose >3y after the 1° course of immunization (pre-school) and another 10y later
- **Booster doses in adults** 10y after the primary course and again 10y later. Probably gives life-long protection. If an adult has received >5 doses in total further routine boosters are not recommended
- **Open wounds** 📖 p. 1107

Diphtheria[ND] Caused by *Corynebacterium diphtheriae*. Rare in the UK since routine immunization. Spread by droplet infection or contact with articles soiled by an infected person. *Incubation:* 2–5d.

Presentation In countries where hygiene is poor cutaneous diphtheria is the predominant form. Elsewhere, characterized by an inflammatory exudate which forms a greyish membrane in the respiratory tract (may cause respiratory obstruction). *C. diphtheriae* secretes a toxin which affects myocardium, nervous and adrenal tissues.

Management Admit for antitoxin and IV antibiotics. Patients may be infectious for up to 4wk but carriers shed *C. diphtheriae* for longer.

Prevention Vaccination—given routinely in childhood in the UK (📖 p. 645). In addition give booster dose to people in contact with a patient with diphtheria or carrier, or before travel to epidemic or endemic areas.

Pseudomonas aeruginosa Common. Treatment is difficult due to multiple antibiotic resistance—if suspected, send specimen for M,C&S.
- In immunocompetent patients may cause UTI, wound infections (particularly leg ulcers—gives a characteristic greenish colouring), osteomyelitis, and skin infections (e.g. otitis externa)
- In immunocompromised patients and patients with CF, it is a common cause of pneumonia and septicaemia

Enterobacteria Examples include:
- Salmonella
- Shigella
- Escherichia
- Klebsiella
- Enterobacter
- Proteus
- Morganella
- Providencia
- Yersinia

Some are normal gut commensals. Others are pathogenic causing:
- Diarrhoea and intra-abdominal infections e.g. peritonitis, hepatobiliary
- UTI—often *E. coli*; *Proteus* species are associated with bladder stones
- Septicaemia and/or meningitis—*E. coli* is the most common cause of meningitis in neonates
- Chest infection—*Klebsiella* may cause a severe form of pneumonia
- Endocarditis—rare

Organisms are usually sensitive to trimethoprim. Severe infection requires admission to hospital for IV antibiotics.

Further information
Health Protection Agency (HPA) Topics A–Z: *Haemophilus influenza, Pseudomonas, Clostridium,* tetanus, diphtheria 🖰 www.hpa.org.uk

Haematology and immunology

Full blood count and ESR

The most commonly requested blood test is the full blood count (FBC). It gives information on:

- **Red blood cells** Haemoglobin, mean cell volume (MCV), and packed cell volume (haematocrit)
- **White blood cells** White cell count and proportion of each component—neutrophils, lymphocytes, monocytes, eosinophils, and basophils
- **Platelets** Number of platelets

❶ Reference ranges are a guide only; normal values are affected by ethnicity, age, and pregnancy. For mild abnormalities in well individuals, take laboratory advice to avoid over-investigation/referral.

Red blood cells

Mean cell volume (MCV)

- ↓ **MCV** (microcytic; <80fL). Iron deficiency anaemia. Confirm by showing that serum ferritin is ↓. *Rarer causes:* thalassaemia (suspect if MCV is 'too low' for the level of anaemia); congenital sideroblastic anaemia (very rare)
- ↑ **MCV** (macrocytic; >100fL). Vitamin B_{12}/folate deficiency; alcohol; liver disease; drugs (e.g. azathioprine, chemotherapy); haemolysis; pregnancy; hypothyroidism; marrow infiltration; myelodysplasia

Anaemia 📖 p. 662

Polycythaemia 📖 p. 679

White cells Normal white cell count is 4–11 × 10^9/L. Reasons for individual components to be ↑ or ↓ are summarized in Table 19.1.

Platelets

Thrombocytopenia ↓ platelets (<150 × 10^9/L). *Causes:*

- ↓ **production** Marrow failure; alcohol; megaloblastic anaemia
- ↓ **survival** ITP; viruses; disseminated intravascular coagulation; SLE; lymphoma; thrombotic thrombocytopenic purpura; hypersplenism; genetic disease
- **Platelet aggregation** Heparin (5% patients)
- **Drugs** e.g. omeprazole, furosemide, quinine

Thrombocythaemia (thrombocytosis) ↑ platelets (>400 × 10^9/L). *Causes:*

- **Essential thrombocytosis**
- **Reactive (2°) thrombocytosis** Due to infection, malignant disease, acute or chronic inflammatory disease, pregnancy, after splenectomy, iron deficiency, or following haemorrhage

❶ ~50% with unexplained thrombocytosis have a malignancy.

Pancytopenia Reduction in red cells, white cells, and platelets. *Causes:*

- Aplastic or megaloblastic anaemia
- Bone marrow infiltration or replacement, e.g. by lymphoma, leukaemia, myeloma, 2° carcinoma, myelofibrosis
- Hypersplenism
- Disseminated TB
- SLE
- Paroxysmal nocturnal haemoglobinuria

Erythrocyte sedimentation rate (ESR) Rate of fall of red cells in a column of blood. A measure of the acute phase response—the pathological process may be infective, immunological, malignant, ischaemic, or traumatic. Normal values ↑ with age; ♀ > ♂. ❶ ↑ in patients with severe anaemia.

Table 19.1 Differential diagnosis for white cell count changes

White cell type *Normal range (%)*	Caused of increased count	Causes of decreased count
Neutrophils *2.0–7.5 × 10⁹/L* (40–75)	• Bacterial infection • Physical injury, e.g. trauma, burns, surgery • Inflammation, e.g. PMR, RA • Myocardial infarction • Pregnancy • Malignancy—leukaemia, disseminated malignancy • Drugs, e.g. steroids	*Mild 1–2 × 10⁹/L* • Viral infections, e.g. mumps, hepatitis, influenza • Drugs, e.g. carbimazole, cytotoxics • Idiopathic/immune • Benign ethnic (Afro-Caribbean) *If <1 × 10⁹/L discuss with haematology + refer.* Warn about risks of neutropenic sepsis (🕮 p. 1025) *If <0.5 × 10⁹/L refer urgently to haematology*
Lymphocytes *1.5–4.9 × 10⁹/L* (20–45)	• Viral infection, e.g. EBV, early HIV, hepatitis, rubella • Other infections—whooping cough, toxoplasmosis • CLL and ALL ❶ Large numbers of abnormal ('atypical') lymphocytes are characteristically seen with EBV infection	• Drugs, e.g. cytotoxics, steroids • Systemic disease, e.g. influenza, SLE, uraemia • HIV infection ❶ Unless other haematological abnormalities, never needs haematology referral
Monocytes *0.2–0.8 × 10⁹/L* (2–10)	• Chronic bacterial infections (e.g. TB, SBE) • Autoimmune disorders	N/A
Eosinophils *0.04–0.44 × 10⁹/L* (1–5)	• Atopic disease, e.g. asthma (80%) • Parasitic infections (8%) • Haematological malignancy (2.5%) • Allergic/atopic skin conditions (2%) • Solid tumours (2%) • GI disease (inflammatory bowel disease; coeliac) (1.5%) • Lung disease (1%) • Connective tissue disease (0.5%)	N/A
Basophils *0.01–0.1 × 10⁹/L* (<1)	• CML /myeloproliferative disease • Hypothyroidism • Drugs, e.g. oestrogen	N/A

Anaemia: diagnosis and initial investigation

Anaemia Anaemia is a lack of sufficient red blood cells and thus haemoglobin (♂: Hb <13g/dL; ♀: Hb <12g/dL or <11g/dL first trimester and <10.5g/dL second/third trimester of pregnancy). It results if there is:

- **↓ red cell production** Defective precursor proliferation/maturation
- **↑ loss or rate of destruction** Bleeding or haemolysis
- **↓ tissue requirement for oxygen** In practice—hypothyroidism

Presentation Patients who become anaemic slowly may remain asymptomatic for a long time. As anaemia progresses pallor, exertional dyspnoea, tachycardia, palpitations, angina (especially if past history of coronary artery disease), night cramps, and cardiac bruits appear. Ultimately with severe anaemia high-output cardiac failure may develop.

❶ **Pallor** may indicate anaemia but is a very non-specific sign which may also be racial, familial, or cosmetic. *Other causes of pallor:* shock, Stokes–Adams attack, vasovagal faint, myxoedema, hypopituitarism, albinism.

Initial investigation of anaemia See Table 19.2.

Management Treat the cause—if no cause for anaemia is found, refer for specialist investigation.

Table 19.2 Investigation and differential diagnosis of anaemia

MCV	Causes	Further investigations
Low <80fL	Iron deficiency	Blood film
	Haemoglobinopathy (thalassaemia)	Reticulocyte count
	Anaemia of chronic disorder	Ferritin
		CRP/ESR/plasma viscosity
		Hb electrophoresis (if indicated)
		Rectal examination
Normal	Acute blood loss	Blood film
	Haemolysis	Reticulocyte count
	Anaemia of chronic	Hb electrophoresis (if indicated)
	disorder	Ferritin
	Uraemia	Serum B_{12}
	Haemoglobinopathy	Serum and red cell folate
	Marrow failure	Renal function
		Serum bilirubin
High >100fL	Folate and/or B_{12} deficiency	Blood film
	Alcohol	Serum B_{12}
	Liver disease	Serum and red cell folate
	Thyroid disease	Liver function
	Myelodysplasia/marrow infiltration	Thyroid function tests

Vitamin B$_{12}$ deficiency Vitamin B$_{12}$ is found in liver, kidney, fish, chicken, meats, and dairy products. Absorption takes place by active and passive mechanisms—the latter being dependent on intrinsic factor, a protein produced by gastric parietal cells.

Presentation Incidental finding of macrocytosis; symptoms/signs of anaemia; sore mouth (glossitis, mouth ulcers); neuropsychiatric problems (peripheral neuropathy, ataxia, optic atrophy, memory loss, subacute combined degeneration of the cord, rarely psychosis).

❶ B$_{12}$ levels may correlate poorly with deficiency, especially in pregnancy.

Causes of deficiency
- **Inadequate dietary intake**—e.g. vegans
- **Malabsorption**—GI disease/surgery: gastric (e.g. pernicious anaemia; gastrectomy), pancreatic (e.g. chronic pancreatitis), or ileal (e.g. coeliac disease—📖 p. 412; ileal resection)
- **Drugs**—metformin; drugs causing achlorhydria, e.g. PPIs, H$_2$ antagonists

Pernicious anaemia Autoimmune condition associated with gastric atrophy and intrinsic factor (50%)/gastric parietal cell (85%) antibodies. *Risk factors:* FH, other autoimmune disease (e.g. vitiligo, hypothyroidism), premature greying, blood groups A and HLA3. Patients have ↑ risk of stomach cancer, particularly within the first 2y of diagnosis.

Management Treat with vitamin B$_{12}$ parenterally (hydroxocobalamin IM—initially 1mg 3x/wk for 2wk then every 2–3mo). Consider oral B$_{12}$ supplements if dietary deficiency is the cause. Confirm response by repeating FBC after 8wk. Consider referral to exclude underlying GI cause.

Folate deficiency Folate is found in highest concentrations in liver and yeast but is also in spinach, other green vegetables, and nuts.

Presentation Incidental finding of macrocytosis or presents with symptoms and signs of anaemia ± polyneuropathy or dementia. Always check serum B$_{12}$ as deficiencies may coexist.

Causes of deficiency
- **Inadequate dietary intake** Common—e.g. old age, poor social conditions, malignancy, anorexia, excess alcohol (particularly spirits)
- **Malabsorption** Coeliac disease, Crohn's disease, partial gastrectomy, tropical sprue, lymphoma, diabetic enteropathy
- **Excess use** Pregnancy, lactation, prematurity, ↑ cell turnover (e.g. malignancy, haemolysis)
- **Drugs** Anticonvulsants, trimethoprim

Management In all cases, treat the cause. Supplement folate with folic acid 5mg od for 4mo. If malabsorption, may need ↑ dose to 15mg od. Treat any B$_{12}$ deficiency. For prophylaxis in chronic haemolytic states or for renal dialysis, up to 5mg od long-term is used (take specialist advice).

⚠ **Folate supplements in pregnancy** Advise women to take supplements from planning pregnancy to 12wk gestation to prevent neural tube defect. *Dose:* to prevent first occurrence—400 micrograms od; advise 5mg od to prevent recurrence, if maternal/paternal history or family history of neural tube defect, or if the mother has coeliac disease, DM, BMI >30, or is taking anticonvulsants.

Iron deficiency anaemia

Iron deficiency anaemia is the most common form of anaemia in the UK (prevalence 2–5% among adult men and post-menopausal women). RBCs are microcytic (↓ MCV) and hypochromic. Low serum ferritin and/or low transferrin saturation confirms iron deficiency. Exclude haemoglobinopathy (📖 p. 668) in those from at-risk ethnic groups or with FH.

Causes ❶ More than one cause may be present.

- **GI blood loss** Aspirin/NSAID use (10–15%); colonic carcinoma (5–10%); gastric carcinoma (5%); benign gastric ulceration (5%); angiodysplasia (5%); oesophagitis (5%); oesophageal carcinoma (1–2%)
- **Malabsorption** Coeliac disease (4–6%)—may be the presenting feature; post-gastrectomy; *H. pylori* colonization; gut resection
- **Non-GI blood loss** Menstruation (20–30%); blood donation (5%); haematuria (1%); epistaxis
- **Other** Pregnancy; lactation; premature infants; deficient diet

Management

- Investigate as shown in Figure 19.1; treat the underlying cause where possible
- Give oral iron supplements, e.g. ferrous sulfate 200mg bd—iron may cause constipation and turn stools black. If not tolerated, try a lower dose or alternative preparation, e.g. ferrous fumarate. Ascorbic acid (250–500mg bd with the iron) may enhance iron absorption
- Hb should ↑ by 1g/dL/wk—confirm response to treatment 2–3wk after starting. Continue treatment for 3mo after correction of the iron deficiency to allow replenishment of the iron stores

⚠ Asymptomatic colonic and gastric carcinoma may present with iron deficiency anaemia—seeking and excluding these conditions is a priority.

- Refer urgently for gastroscopy/specialist opinion if dyspepsia and iron deficiency anaemia[N]
- Refer urgently for suspected lower GI cancer if Hb <11g/dL in a man or <10g/dL in non-menstruating woman[N]

Failure to respond to iron supplements Consider *H. pylori* (test/treat), coeliac disease (oral iron not absorbed), continuing bleeding, non-compliance with iron, or that diagnosis is incorrect or anaemia mixed.

Follow-up Once normal, monitor Hb, MCH, and MCV every 3mo for 1y, and then annually. Give further iron supplements if Hb, MCH, or MCV fall below normal levels. Investigate further if unable to maintain Hb.

Iron deficiency without anaemia Low serum ferritin (hypoferritinaemia) is 3x as common as iron deficiency anaemia but there is a very low prevalence of GI malignancy in this group (<1% of post-menopausal women and men). Investigate as shown in Figure 19.1. Give iron supplements to replenish iron stores.

Further information
NICE Referral guidelines for suspected cancer (2005) ℘ www.nice.org.uk
British Society of Gastroenterology Guidelines for the management of iron deficiency anaemia (2011) ℘ www.bsg.org.uk

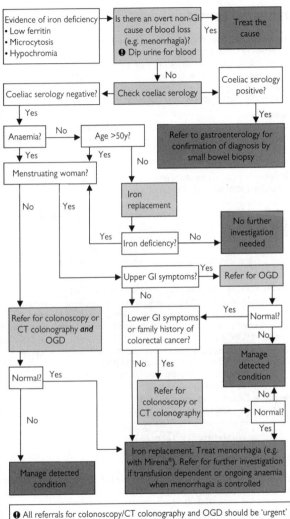

Figure 19.1 Investigation and management of iron deficiency

Other anaemias

Anaemia of chronic disease (anaemia of inflammation)
Inflammatory cytokines suppress bone marrow erythropoiesis. Usually normocytic anaemia but can be microcytic if severe. Consider:

- Leg ulcers
- Cancer
- Low eGFR contributes via low erythropoietin
- Old age
- Multi-co-morbidities.
- DM

Management

- Aim to exclude significant disorders, e.g. haematological malignancy. Suitable tests include iron (↓), transferrin (↓), ferritin (normal or ↑), LDH, serum electrophoresis, eGFR, glucose, LFTs
- Optimize management of co-morbidities

❶ Ageing is pro-inflammatory process—50% of anaemia of the elderly is unexplained after investigation.

Myelodysplastic syndrome (MDS) Common clonal, pre-leukaemia disorder affecting 1:500 >65y. Very variable severity from mild anaemia for many years to severe pancytopenia progressing to acute leukaemia within months. ❶ Isolated macrocytosis can precede anaemia for many years.

Causes Previous chemotherapy, chemical exposure, age.

Presentation Anaemia (usually macrocytic), neutropenia, thrombocytopenia, monocytosis, pancytopenia, infection, and/or bleeding. No splenomegaly or lymphadenopathy except in chronic myelomonocytic leukaemia (CMML).

Management Principally supportive—blood transfusion, erythropoietin, treat infections. Chemotherapy, e.g. azacitidine, is approved for high-risk MDS. Bone marrow transplant can be curative in young fit patients; most patients are elderly.

Prognosis Depends on cytopenias, bone marrow cytogenetics, and bone marrow blast count.

B₁₂ and folate deficiency 📖 p. 663

Haemoglobinopathy 📖 p. 668

Haemolysis Normal red cells survive 120d before being removed from the circulation—mainly by the spleen. In haemolytic anaemia red cells are destroyed faster than they are produced and anaemia develops.

Presentation May have FH. Anaemia often accompanied by jaundice due to bilirubin released when the red cells are destroyed. *FBC:* ↓ Hb; ↑ reticulocytes. Film shows polychromasia ± abnormal-shaped cells (e.g. spherocytes) or other clues as to the cause of the haemolysis (e.g. fragmented cells suggest mechanical damage). Can be exacerbated by intercurrent illness, e.g. aplastic crisis with parvovirus.

Causes See Table 19.3.

Management Refer to haematology for advice on management or if the cause is unclear. Folate supplements are usually recommended. Rarely splenectomy is needed.

Aplastic anaemia^G Bone marrow failure characterized by pancyto-penia. Rare affecting 1–2/million population. No cause is found in 70–80%. Identified causes include: genetic; drugs (inform Medicines and Healthcare products Regulatory Agency—📖 p. 146); toxins; infection.

Presentation Anaemia, thrombocytopenia (📖 p. 670), and neutropenia (recurrent infection). FBC reveals pancytopenia and lack of reticulocytes.

Management Refer urgently to haematology. Treatment is:
- **Supportive** Transfusions and antibiotics, or
- **Definitive** Aims to restore a healthy, working bone marrow. Bone marrow transplant is curative. Immunosuppressive therapy is an alternative when transplant is not an option

Further information

British Committee for Standards in Haematology
🖲 www.bcshguidelines.com
- Diagnosis and management of acquired aplastic anaemia (2009)
- Diagnosis and management of hereditary spherocytosis (2011)

Patient information and support

Aplastic Anaemia Trust 🖲 www.theaat.org.uk

Table 19.3 Causes of haemolytic anaemia

Cause	Examples
Congenital	
Membrane abnormalities	Hereditary spherocytosis or elliptocytosis
Haemoglobin abnormalities	Abnormal Hb, e.g. sickle cell anaemia—📖 p. 669
	Defective synthesis, e.g. thalassaemia—📖 p. 668
Metabolic abnormalities	Glucose-6-phosphate dehydrogenase (G6PD) or pyruvate kinase deficiency
Acquired	
Immune	Autoimmune
	● Warm, e.g. 2° to SLE, CLL, or NHL
	● Cold, e.g. 2° to EBV or mycoplasma infection
	Isoimmune (e.g. transfusion reaction; haemolytic disease of the newborn—📖 p. 820)
	Drug-induced
Hypersplenism	Malaria, lymphoma, RA, portal hypertension
Red cell fragmentation	Artificial heart valves
Activated complement	Paroxysmal nocturnal haemoglobinuria
Secondary	Renal disease, liver disease
Miscellaneous	Infections (e.g. malaria), burns, chemicals, toxins, drugs

Haemoglobinopathy

Screening

- **Pre-conceptual screening** Consider in at risk-groups and when investigating or treating infertility
- **Antenatal haemoglobinopathy screening** (📖 p. 800) Offered to all pregnant women in the UK, ideally at <10wk gestation. If the mother is a carrier, the father is offered testing ± the fetus
- **Neonatal blood spot screening** (📖 p. 851) for sickle cell disease; offered to all babies in England, Scotland, and Northern Ireland

❶ Screening results in people knowing their carrier status. Ensure results are clearly recorded in patient notes. Issue haemoglobinopathy cards to those with haemoglobinopathy and who are confirmed carriers.

Thalassaemia Autosomal recessive inherited disorder of production of α (α-thalassaemia) or β (β-thalassaemia) globin chains of haemoglobin. Many varieties are recognized, but they can classified into 2 main types:

- α° and β° thalassaemia: no gene product is produced
- α^{+} and β^{+} thalassaemia: α and β chains present but produced at ↓ rate

β-thalassaemia Common in populations from the Mediterranean; Middle East; Central, South, and South East Asia. Defective β chain production results in ↑α chain synthesis. Excess α chains precipitate in red cell precursors causing their destruction in bone marrow and spleen. This causes proliferation of marrow, bony deformity (mongoloid facies, bossing of skull, thinning of long bones), and progressive splenomegaly.

Homozygotes develop profound anaemia from 3mo of age and without repeated transfusions would die in <1y. If suspected refer urgently to paediatrics. ❶ Most infants with β° thalassaemia (β-thalassaemia major) are detected at neonatal blood-spot screening.

Specialist ongoing care is essential. Offer family members referral for genetic counselling. Children who receive transfusions grow and develop normally, but iron accumulates; chelation ↑ survival, but iron overload may cause premature death. Bone marrow transplant is curative.

α-thalassaemia Common in populations from South East Asia, Africa, and India.

- The homozygous state for α° thalassaemia is associated with fetal death at ~38wk (Barts hydrops)
- Haemoglobin H results from inheritance of α° from one parent and α^{+} from the other; patients are moderately anaemic with splenomegaly and have haemoglobin H (4 β chains combined with a haem molecule) in their red cells. Specialist management is needed

Asymptomatic patients Heterozygotes for α- or β-thalassaemia (thalassaemia trait) and homozygotes for α^{+} thalassaemia are often asymptomatic. They may have mild anaemia with hypochromic/microcytic red cells. ❶ Can be confused with iron deficiency—suspect if MCV is disproportionately low; ferritin is normal; no response to iron.

Patient information and support
UK Thalassaemia Society ☎ 020 882 0011 🖰 www.ukts.org

The sickling disorders Inherited disorder most common amongst people originating from malarial areas—Africans (1–2% newborns) and certain Mediterranean, Middle Eastern, and Indian populations. *Varieties:*

- Heterozygous state for haemoglobin S (sickle cell trait—AS)
- Homozygous state (sickle cell anaemia/disease—SS)
- Heterozygous states for haemoglobin S and haemoglobins C, D, E, or other structural variants
- Combination of haemoglobin S with any form of thalassaemia

Mechanism Haemoglobin S undergoes liquid crystal formation, as it becomes deoxygenated, causing sickling of affected blood cells. The effect of sickling is to shorten survival of red cells → haemolytic anaemia, and cause aggregation of the sickled cells, which, in turn, leads to:

- Tissue infarction—resulting in pain and/or tissue damage, e.g. stroke (10% children with sickle cell anaemia have a stroke; 5% have recurrent strokes), *and/or*
- Sequestration in the liver, spleen, or lungs—producing sudden and profound anaemia

Diagnosis FBC and film—chronic anaemia with sickling on film. Confirm diagnosis with haemoglobin electrophoresis.

Sickle cell trait Patients with <40% haemoglobin S have no symptoms, unless they are subjected to anoxia, e.g. anaesthesia.

Sickle cell anaemia Low Hb level (typically 8–9g/dL) with high reticulocyte count—although generally patients compensate well. Illness results from complications arising from acute exacerbations or 'crises' and the effects of recurrent tissue damage due to microinfarction over a long period of time. Prognosis is variable. In Africa, children usually die in <1y. In the UK, patients survive into adulthood (average survival 50y). The most common cause of death is infection.

Patients should be managed by specialist centres, aiming to prevent crises and treat complications early. There is no medication to prevent sickling. *GPs should:*

- Treat patients as if hyposplenic—give Hib, meningitis C, pneumococcal + annual influenza vaccination ± prophylactic antibiotics (📖 p. 650)
- Advise patients to avoid cold and maintain adequate hydration; warn about the dangers of anaesthetics (a Medic Alert bracelet is helpful)
- Treat infection early—be alert for aplastic crisis following parvovirus
- Give analgesia for painful crises (including opioids if needed, but avoid pethidine as may cause cerebral irritation/fits)—admit if severe
- Admit if significant crisis of any sort (e.g. stroke, dyspnoea, acute abdomen, aplastic anaemia)
- Refer for early management of long-term complications (e.g. renal failure, epilepsy)

Patient information and support
Sickle Cell Society ☎ 020 8961 7795 🖰 www.sicklecellsociety.org

Further information

British Committee for Standards in Haematology
🖰 www.bcshguide lines.com
- Significant haemoglobinopathies: guidelines for screening and diagnosis (2009)
- Management of the acute painful crisis in sickle cell disease (2003)

Bleeding and clotting disorders

Coagulation tests (sodium citrate tube; false results if under-filled)
- **Prothrombin time (PT)** Prolonged by: coumarins (e.g. warfarin); vitamin K deficiency; liver disease
- **Activated partial thromboplastin time (APTT)** ↑ in heparin treatment, haemophilia, antiphospholipid syndrome, or DIC
- **INR** Ratio of the time the sample takes to clot compared to a control

The pupuras

Vascular purpuras Result from damage to the vessel wall. Due to:
- Infection (e.g. meningococcal septicaemia, EBV)
- Immune dysfunction (e.g. Henoch–Schönlein purpura)
- Vitamin C deficiency
- Ageing (senile purpura)
- Local stasis or ↑ venous pressure (e.g. varicose veins)
- Drug reaction (e.g. steroid-induced purpura)

Thrombocytopenic purpura Purpura is related to the level of the platelet count. Bleeding is inevitable if platelet count ↓ to <5–10 x 10⁹/L.
- **Non-immune thrombocytopenic purpura** Results from conditions that damage the bone marrow, e.g. drugs (chemotherapy), aplastic anaemia (📖 p. 667), leukaemia (📖 p. 676), myeloproliferative disorders (📖 p. 678), CLL (📖 p. 678), multiple myeloma (📖 p. 674)
- **Immune thrombocytopenic purpura** Usually primary immune (ITP) but may be secondary to SLE, transfusions, or drug reactions (e.g. heparin)

Idiopathic thrombocytopenic purpura (ITP)
- **In children** Self-limiting. The child is purpuric often after a viral illness; platelet count is generally <10 x 10⁹/L, but severe bleeding is rare. Refer to paediatrics as an emergency. Usually no specific treatment is needed
- **In adults** Presentation is variable—may be acutely symptomatic (sometimes recurrent), or chronic and insidious. Presents with haemorrhage and bruising. Platelet count is ↓. Ask about drug history (particularly thiazides, quinine, or digoxin). Look for evidence of SLE or lymphoma. Examine for presence of an enlarged spleen. Refer to haematology

Impaired platelet function May occur with myeloproliferative disorder/ myelodysplasia and very high paraproteins. Causes bleeding—even if platelet count is normal.

Haemophilia 2 common forms—haemophilia A (factor VIII deficiency) and B (factor IX deficiency—Christmas disease). Sex-linked recessive disorders but 1 in 3 result from a new mutation. ♂ >> ♀. *Prevalence:* 1/10,000 (haemophilia A); 1/50,000 (haemophilia B). *Classification:*
- Carrier: ♀ heterozygotes; >25% clotting factor activity
- Mild: 5–25% clotting factor activity
- Moderate: 1–5% clotting factor activity
- Severe: 50% haemophiliacs; ≤1% clotting factor activity

Features Bleeding into joints or muscles is often delayed following trauma. If untreated, can cause permanent damage. Pressure effects occur if bleeding takes place into a confined space, e.g. intracranial bleed. Severity of bleeding is related to levels of clotting factors.

Management Follow-up should be via a specialist haemophilia centre. Pre-natal/antenatal screening is available—refer to genetics.

- **On-demand treatment** Transfusion of factor VIII or IX preparation as soon as possible after bleeding has started—most administer it to themselves; symptomatic treatment of bleeds, e.g. rest, analgesia ± physiotherapy for bleeds into muscles/joints
- **Prophylaxis** Prevents bleeds and their consequences. Agents used:
  - Tranexamic acid—prevents bleeding after minor surgical procedures for patients with mild haemophilia/carriers with symptoms
  - Desmopressin—stimulates production of factor VIII (not factor IX). Prevents/treats bleeding in mild/moderate haemophilia A
  - Factor VIII 3x/wk or factor IX 2x/wk. Given to prevent joint damage in children with severe haemophilia

Problems with treatment

- **Inhibitors** 25% of patients have antibodies to factor VIII or IX products. Treated with intravenous factor VIIa or, in children, through an immune tolerization programme
- **Infection from blood products** Not a risk with modern 'recombinant' products—historically blood products have resulted in HIV, hepatitis B and C transmission. All patients should have hepatitis B vaccination

von Willebrand's disease Autosomal dominant deficiency of vW factor. ♂ = ♀. *Prevalence:* 1% population. Most are mildly affected with easy bruising, nose bleeds, and/or menorrhagia. In severe cases bleeding may occur into joints. *FBC*—normal platelets; *clotting screen*—↑ bleeding time. Refer to haematology. Mild cases are managed with tranexamic acid, desmopressin, and/or OCP/Mirena® (for menorrhagia). In severe cases may need treatment with vW factor. *E.A. von Willebrand (1870–1939)—Finnish physician.*

Thrombophilia[G] ↑ tendency to clot. May be acquired or inherited.

Acquired 2° to obesity, immobility, pregnancy, OCP, cancer, surgery (<6wk), smoking, antiphospholipid syndrome (❶ Patients <40y with unprovoked proximal DVT/PE or <50y with ischaemic stroke should be tested for antiphospholipid antibodies). Treat the cause if possible; otherwise discuss thromboprophylaxis with the relevant specialist.

Inherited Defects in natural anticoagulants (e.g. protein S) and clotting factors (e.g. factor V Leiden). Screening in high-risk individuals (e.g. after DVT, asymptomatic relatives) does not predict thromboembolism. Refer/ discuss management with haematology if:

- Neonate/child with purpura fulminans (urgent testing)
- FH of 'high-risk thrombophilia' (protein C or S deficiency; antithrombin deficiency)
- Strong FH of unprovoked venous thrombosis (or, for ♀, oestrogen-provoked thrombosis)
- Adults that develop skin necrosis on vitamin K antagonists

Further information

British Committee for Standards in Haematology Clinical guidelines for testing for heritable thrombophilia (2010) ◌ www.bcshguidelines.com

Patient information and support

Haemophilia Society ☎ 0800 018 6068 ◌ www.haemophilia.org.uk

Anticoagulation

Indications for anticoagulation

Long term

- Prevention of recurrent VTE (including antiphospholipid syndrome and some patients with thrombophilia)
- Prevention of arterial thromboembolism in patients with cardiac disease, e.g. non-valvular AF and medium/high stroke risk; mechanical prosthetic valves; dilated cardiomyopathy

Short term

- VTE: ≥6wk after below-knee DVT; ≥3mo after proximal DVT/PE
- High-risk situations, e.g. mural thrombosis after MI; after surgery

Heparin Enhances antithrombin III activity. Sc low molecular weight heparin (LMWH) is used in the community, as it does not require daily monitoring. Indications:

- Initial treatment of VTE (whilst awaiting diagnostic testing and/or until oral anticoagulation is established)
- VTE management for cancer patients and pregnant women at high risk
- When warfarin is stopped prior to surgery
- High-risk patients on oral anticoagulants if INR is < desired range

Warfarin Antagonizes vitamin K to ↓ clotting tendency. Its effects can be reversed with vitamin K/prothrombin complex. *Target INR:*

- **Most indications:** 2.5 (range 2–3)
- **Thromboembolism on anticoagulant treatment:** 3.5 (range 3–4)
- **Prosthetic heart valves:** take specialist advice

Initiation of warfarin If no urgency for initiation (e.g. chronic AF), warfarin can be started in primary care (see Table 19.4). Check baseline FBC, clotting screen, renal and liver function. Complete a DH anticoagulant booklet for the patient to carry. Take the patient/carer through the educational points in the booklet. Ensure they understand the local monitoring system. Advise to take warfarin every evening.

Warfarin + antiplatelet therapy Except <12mo after stenting/ACS, antiplatelet agents are usually stopped if initiating warfarin. Avoid combining except on specialist advice (↑ risk of bleeding—clopidogrel > aspirin).

Monitoring See Table 19.5. After starting a new drug that may interact with warfarin, recheck INR after 5–7d.

Bleeding on warfarin

- Major bleeding—admit
- Head injury—if laceration, bruising, LOC, amnesia, persistent headache, or ↓ GCS—refer to A&E for CT scan
- Bleeding at therapeutic INR (e.g. haematuria, rectal bleeding)—investigate cause

New oral anticoagulants (e.g. dabigatran, rivaroxaban) are licensed to prevent VTE after orthopaedic surgery and for stroke prevention in patients with non-valvular AF. They have the advantage of having a fixed dose and do not require regular monitoring. However, they are not readily reversible in the community leading to concerns about bleeding.

Table 19.4 Dose regime for starting warfarin in the community

INR on day 5	Dose on days 5–7	INR on day 8	Dose from day 8	Instructions
≤1.7	5mg	≤1.7	6mg	• Give warfarin 5mg od for 4d, then check INR
		1.8–2.4	5mg	• Adjust dose as in table
		2.5–3	4mg	• Recheck INR on day 8 and adjust dose as in table
		>3	3mg for 4d	
1.8–2.2	4mg	≤1.7	5mg	• Thereafter, check INR weekly (unless 4d interval stated) and adjust dose accordingly until dose is stable in the target range
		1.8–2.4	4mg	
		2.5–3	3.5mg	
		3.1–3.5	3mg for 4d	
		>3.5	2.5mg for 4d	
2.3–2.7	3mg	≤1.7	4mg	
		1.8–2.4	3.5mg	
		2.5–3	3mg	
		3.1–3.5	2.5mg for 4d	△ **High INR**
		>3.5	2mg for 4d	INR ≥8 (lower if other risk factors for bleeding)—admit to hospital even if not bleeding
2.8–3.2	2mg	≤1.7	3mg	INR >3.7 and <8—omit warfarin 1–2d and recheck INR. Restart when INR <5 and re-titrate dose
		1.8–2.4	2.5mg	
		2.5–3	2mg	
		3.1–3.5	1.5mg for 4d	
		>3.5	1mg for 4d	
3.3–3.7	1mg	≤1.7	2mg	
		1.8–2.4	1.5mg	
		2.5–3	1mg	
		3.1–3.5	0.5mg for 4d	
		>3.5	omit for 4d	
>3.7	0mg	<2	1.5mg for 4d	
		2–2.9	1mg for 4d	
		3–3.5	0.5mg for 4d	

Reproduced with permission from *British Journal of Clinical Pharmacology* 1998 **46**:157–61.

Table 19.5 Warfarin therapy: recall periods during maintenance therapy

INR	Recall interval and action
1 high INR	Recall 7–14d. Stop treatment for 1–3d (max 1wk in prosthetic valve patients) and restart at a lower dose
	△ If INR >8 and bleeding – admit; if not bleeding, consider admission, or treat with vitamin K 2mg po or 1mg IV
1 low INR	↑ dose and recall in 7–14d
1 therapeutic INR	Recall 4wk
2 therapeutic INRs	Recall 6wk (maximum interval if prosthetic heart valve)
3 therapeutic INRs	Recall 8wk
4 therapeutic INRs	Recall 10wk
5 therapeutic INRs	Recall 12wk

△ Warfarin is a dangerous drug. In every case weigh up the pros and cons of prescribing.

Haematological malignancy

⚠ **Suspected haematological malignancy** May present with non-specific symptoms/signs. Have a high level of suspicion.

Immediate admission/ same-day referral
- FBC/blood film reported as acute leukaemia
- Suspected spinal cord compression
- Suspected renal failure due to myeloma

Urgent referral to a team specializing in blood cancers Persistent, unexplained splenomegaly.

Investigations Combinations of any of the following symptoms/signs warrant examination and further investigation with FBC, blood film, and ESR (or CRP/plasma viscosity) ± referral to a team specializing in haematological malignancy:
- Drenching night sweats and/or fever
- Weight loss
- Generalized itching—in addition check U&E, Cr, eGFR, TFTs
- Breathlessness—in addition check CXR
- Unexplained bleeding/bruising/purpura, and/or symptoms suggesting anaemia
- Recurrent infections
- Persistent bone pain—in addition check X-ray, U&E, Cr and eGFR, liver profile, bone profile, and PSA (in men)
- Alcohol-induced pain
- Abdominal pain
- Splenomegaly—refer if persistent
- Fatigue—repeat FBC, blood film, and ESR at least once if condition remains unexplained and does not improve
- Lymphadenopathy—if present ≥6wk, LNs are increasing in size, LN >2cm in size, widespread lymphadenopathy or associated weight ↓, night sweats, and/or splenomegaly, consider further investigation, discussion with specialist, and/or referral

Multiple myeloma Age usually >60y. 4,800 new cases/y in the UK and 2,600 deaths. A mutant plasma cell clone is present. The proliferating cells grow mainly in the bone marrow where they cause infiltration, localized tumours, and bone erosion. Main sites of myeloma involvement are: skull, spinal column, thoracic cage, pelvis, and proximal long bones.

Presentation
- Infection, e.g. chest infection
- Anaemia and/or bleeding
- Bone pain ± tenderness—particularly ribs, back, pelvis
- Pathological fracture
- Hypercalcaemia
- Renal failure
- Hyperviscosity syndrome (CNS features, e.g. blurred vision, altered consciousness, confusion)
- Amyloidosis (heart, tongue, carpal tunnel)

Investigation
- FBC Anaemia; *blood film*—rouleaux formation
- ESR↑↑

- *Renal function* ↑ Cr; ↓ eGFR
- *Ca²⁺* Frequently ↑
- *Serum electrophoresis* Paraprotein band
- *Urine electrophoresis* Bence Jones protein (BJP)—useful for diagnosis (❶ Occasionally may be non-secretory when BJP will be –ve)
- *Serum free light chains* (blood equivalent of Bence Jones protein)—used to measure response to treatment
- *X-ray* Erosive lesions in skull, ribs, pelvis. Fractures and vertebral collapse are common

Management Refer urgently to haematology. Specialist management depends on symptoms and whether there is tissue/organ damage.
- **Asymptomatic disease** Patients are usually monitored closely and treatment starts if symptoms or tissue/organ damage develop
- **Symptomatic disease** Treatment options include chemotherapy, steroids, biological agents (bortezomib), and/or novel agents (thalidomide, lenalidomide). Symptomatic treatment includes: thromboprophylaxis; bisphosphonates for prevention and treatment of hypercalcaemia and bone pain (bone pain may also respond to radiotherapy); dialysis for renal failure; and plasmapheresis for hyperviscosity. Intensive chemotherapy + bone marrow/stem cell transplant is offered to younger patients. Maintenance therapy is under evaluation
- **Relapsed disease** Patients who have gone into remission almost always relapse at some point. Novel/biological agents are frequently used in the treatment of relapse

Prognosis Survival is improving and ranges from weeks to many years; overall 5y survival is 37% but if <70y and fit enough to undergo intensive treatment, 5y survival is >50%.

Monoclonal gammopathy of undetermined significance (MGUS) Presence of monoclonal paraprotein band (M protein) in isolation, with no other features of myeloma or other lymphoproliferative disease. Present in 1% >50y and 5% if >80y. Usually found incidentally. Most remain stable but ~1%/y progress to myeloma or other haematological malignancy.

Management
- Exclude myeloma, other lymphoproliferative disorders, and amyloidosis; refer urgently if haematological malignancy/amyloidosis is suspected
- Refer to haematology if IgD or IgE M-protein, >15g/L IgG M-protein, or >10g/L ImA or IgM M-protein
- Monitor clinical symptoms, and check M-protein (↑ >25% should prompt re-referral), immunoglobulins, FBC, ESR, U&E, Cr, and eGFR every 3–4mo for the first year then every 6–12mo; re-refer if any significant, sustained change
- Advise patients to re-attend promptly if new symptoms (e.g. back pain, fatigue, weight ↓) develop

Further information
NICE Referral guidelines for suspected cancer (2005) ℘ www.nice.org.uk
British Committee for Standards in Haematology
℘ www.bcshguide lines.com
- Guidelines for the investigation of newly detected M-proteins and the management of MGUS (2009)
- Guidelines on the diagnosis and management of multiple myeloma (2013)

Acute leukaemia

Clonal malignant disorders (from a single cell) affecting all age groups.

Acute lymphoblastic leukaemia (ALL) Abnormal proliferation in the lymphoid progenitor cells (see Figure 19.2). Incidence is 1–4/100,000 population/y. ♂ > ♀. *Usual age range:* 2–10y, with a peak at 3–4y. Accounts for 85% of childhood leukaemia. Incidence then falls with increasing age apart from a secondary peak at ~40y.

Acute myeloid leukaemia (AML) Abnormal proliferation of a myeloid progenitor cell (see Figure 19.2). There are at least seven different subtypes. Most common leukaemia of adulthood with incidence of ~1.5/100,000 population/y. Incidence ↑ with age. Median age at presentation ~60y. ♂ = ♀. Risk factors include smoking (1:5 cases); previous chemotherapy or radiotherapy and exposure to radiation. Children with Down's syndrome are more likely to develop AML.

Presentation Short history (weeks). Symptoms/signs arise from:

Bone marrow failure Anaemia—pallor, lethargy, dyspnoea; neutropenia—infections of the mouth, throat, skin, fever; thrombocytopenia—spontaneous bruising, menorrhagia, bleeding from wounds, bleeding of gums or nosebleeds.

Organ infiltration Superficial lymphadenopathy (>50%); hepatosplenomegaly (70%); bone pain (ALL only); skin infiltration (AML only); testicular enlargement; respiratory symptoms 2° to mediastinal LNs; gum hypertrophy; unexplained irritability/behaviour change/↓ performance.

Differential diagnosis Infections, e.g. EBV; other blood conditions, e.g. aplastic anaemia, ITP, myelodysplasia; other malignancies, e.g. lymphoma, neuroblastoma, metastatic disease; rheumatoid arthritis.

Investigation
- *FBC* Normal or ↓ Hb and platelets; WCC <1 x 10⁹/L to >200 x 10⁹/L
- *Blood film* Abnormal with presence of blast cells
- *Renal function* Renal impairment if leucocyte count is very high
- *CXR* May show mediastinal mass and/or lytic bone lesions

Initial management Refer for same-day specialist opinion if:
- Abnormal blood count reported as needing urgent investigation
- Petechiae/purpura/spontaneous bleeding
- Fatigue in a previously healthy individual if accompanied by generalized lymphadenopathy and/or hepatosplenomegaly*
- Any other suspicious symptoms/signs

* Children with an abdominal mass should always be referred for same-day assessment.

Specialist management Once diagnosis is confirmed, treatment is co-ordinated in specialized centres and involves intensive supportive care, together with systemic chemotherapy and radiotherapy ± bone marrow transplant. For patients with ALL, treatment includes maintenance therapy for 2y to help maintain remission. Prognosis—see Table 19.6.

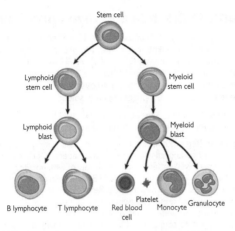

Figure 19.2 Blood cell production

Reproduced from Cancer Help UK, the patient information website of Cancer Research UK: ✆ cancerhelp.org.uk

Table 19.6 Prognosis of acute leukaemia

	Overall 5y survival
Childhood ALL	88%
Adult ALL	40% (80% achieve remission)
AML age <55y	40% (>60% for children)
AML age >55y	20%

Short-term side effects of treatment
- **Treatment side effects** Most chemotherapeutic agents have pronounced side effects, e.g. nausea, vomiting, hair loss, neuropathy
- **Immunosuppression** Any fever in a neutropenic child or adult must be taken seriously and referred immediately back to the unit in charge of care. Likewise any chickenpox contact must be referred immediately for consideration of administration of VZ-Ig, or measles contact for administration of measles Ig

Long-term side effects of treatment Heart—cardiomyopathy, arrhythmias; lung—fibrosis; endocrine system—growth delay, hypothyroidism, infertility; kidney—↓ eGFR ; secondary malignancies—may appear after many years; psychological effects.

Information and support for patients and carers
Macmillan Cancer Support ☎ 0808 808 0000 ✆ www.macmillan.org.uk
Leukaemia and Lymphoma Research ☎ 020 7405 0101
✆ www.leukaemialymphomaresearch.org.uk
CLIC and Sargent ☎ 0300 330 0803 ✆ www.clicsargent.org.uk

Chronic leukaemia and myeloproliferation

Chronic lymphocytic leukaemia (CLL) Occurs in the elderly, accounting for 40% leukaemias in that age group. Closely related to small lymphocytic lymphoma (📖 p. 681). 70–80% all diagnoses follow FBC done for another reason. Otherwise, presents with widespread painless lymphadenopathy, often noted over a period of months/years. *Examination:* check for lymphadenopathy, spleno- ± hepatomegaly.

Investigation ↑ lymphocyte count (>5 × 10⁹/L). Blood film—small lymphocytes, many of which are disrupted to form 'smear' cells.

Management Refer to haematology or discuss with a haematologist depending on age and clinical state of the patient. Once diagnosis has been confirmed, well patients with low levels of lymphocytosis are often managed in primary care with regular FBC and clinical review (at least every 6mo). Treat infections promptly. Refer for treatment if:
• Symptomatic disease (fevers, sweats, weight ↓)
• Lymphadenopathy and/or hepatosplenomegaly
• Rising lymphocyte count (↑ >50% in 2mo or doubling time of <6mo)
• Anaemia or thrombocytopenia

Specialist treatment Chemotherapy/radiotherapy. Splenectomy is indicated if massive symptomatic splenomegaly and refractory cytopenia.

❶ The term 'leukaemia' provokes fear in many. Explain the diagnosis of CLL, its benign nature in many and that prognosis can be >10y.

Chronic myeloid (granulocytic) leukaemia (CML) *Peak age:* 30–60y. Chance finding in 20%. Otherwise presents with:
• Non-specific symptoms, e.g. weight ↓, lassitude, gout, anaemia
• Splenomegaly (common)—abdominal pain, digestive symptoms, or pleuritic pain due to splenic infarction
• Bleeding (rare)—due to abnormal platelet function

Investigation *FBC:* ↑ WCC (usually >50 × 10⁹/L) ± anaemia. *Blood film:* bone marrow precursors of myeloid cells (blasts). *Cytogenetics:* Philadelphia chromosome.

Management Refer urgently to haematology. Treatment is determined by phase of the disease:
• **Chronic** (90% at diagnosis)—<10% of cells in the bone marrow are immature blasts. Treatment with tyrosine kinase inhibitors (e.g. imatinib) has dramatically improved prognosis in recent years
• **Accelerated** 10–30% of cells in the bone marrow are immature blasts. Treatment is with chemotherapy ± bone marrow/stem cell transplant, or second generation tyrosine kinase inhibitors
• **Blast** (also called acute phase, blast crisis) >30% of cells in the bone marrow are immature blasts—treated with chemotherapy

Myeloproliferative disorders Proliferation of ≥1 of the haemopoietic components of the bone marrow. Includes:
• CML
• Polycythaemia vera
• Essential thrombocythaemia
• Myelofibrosis

Erythrocytosis ↑ in the number of circulating red cells. If haematocrit is persistently ↑ for >2mo (>0.52 ♂; >0.48 ♀), investigate the cause. May be 2° (polycythaemia vera) or 2°. ❶ Hb may also appear ↑ if dehydrated (concentration effect). Secondary polycythaemia may be:

- **Appropriate** High altitude, chronic lung disease (e.g. COPD), cardiovascular disease with a right → left shunt, heavy smoking, sleep apnoea, ↑ affinity for haemoglobin (familial polycythaemia), *or*
- **Inappropriate** Caused by excess erythropoietin, e.g. 2° to hepatocellular or renal tumour, or massive uterine fibroid. May need venesection

Polycythaemia vera Also known as primary proliferative polycythaemia (PPP). Haematological malignancy resulting in overproduction of red cells. *Age range:* most >50y.

Presentation Non-specific symptoms/signs:

- Night sweats
- Dusky, cyanotic hue with red face
- Itching (especially provoked by water, e.g. after a bath)
- Splenomegaly (70%) ± hepatomegaly
- Headaches, dizziness, vertigo, and/or tinnitus
- Gout—2° to ↑ red cell turnover
- Peptic ulceration (5–10%)
- Thrombosis/haemorrhage—abnormal platelet function/hyperviscosity

Investigation Often diagnosed incidentally following FBC done for other reasons—persistently ↑ Hb + haematocrit; neutrophils and platelets may also be ↑. JAK2 mutation is +ve in >95%.

Management Refer urgently to haematology. Hb level is ↓ by regular venesection ± cytotoxics. Aspirin ↓ risk of thrombosis. Slowly progressive and survival for 10–20y is not unusual; a minority eventually transform to acute myeloid leukaemia or myelofibrosis.

Essential thrombocythaemia Patients have ↑ risk of thrombosis, but may haemorrhage due to abnormal platelet function. *FBC*—persistently ↑ platelet count >450 × 10⁹/L when reactive and other myeloproliferative causes have been excluded. Refer urgently to haematology. Treatment is with aspirin, treatment of CVD risk factors ± cytotoxics. May eventually transform to AML.

Myelofibrosis (myelosclerosis) Progressive accumulation of fibrous tissue in the bone marrow cavity, replacing normal marrow. Haemopoietic function is taken over by the spleen/liver. Patients are usually elderly and present with symptoms of anaemia, malaise, fever ± gout. The spleen is massively enlarged *FBC*—↓ Hb; *blood film*—immature erythroid cells (normoblasts) and myeloid cells (metamyelocytes/myelocytes). Red cells are teardrop-shaped. Refer urgently to haematology. Median survival is 2–3y—but many live much longer. 5–10% transform to AML.

Further information
British Committee for Standards in Haematology
℘ www.bcshguidelines.com

- Investigation and management of adults and children presenting with thrombocytosis (2010)
- Diagnosis, investigation, and management of polycythaemia/ erythrocytosis (2005)

Lymphoma

Cancer of the lymphatic system. Two main types.

Non-Hodgkin's lymphoma (NHL) Derived from malignant transformation of lymphocytes—85% B cells. Usually develops in LNs but can arise in any tissue. *Incidence:* 12,300 cases/y in the UK (4% cancers), causing 4,500 deaths/y. ♂ = ♀. 69% occur in patients >60y.

Presentation May be detected incidentally on CXR (mediastinal mass) or present with painless peripheral lymphadenopathy; abdominal mass (nodal or spleen); weight ↓; night sweats/unexplained fevers. Other symptoms are dependent on site, e.g. neurological symptoms if CNS involvement; pleural effusion; skin lesions.

Investigation FBC—may be normal if no bone marrow involvement; *monospot*—perform in all patients <30y with persistent lymphadenopathy to exclude EBV; *ESR*—usually ↑; *LFTs*—abnormal if liver involvement.

Initial management Depending on local referral pathways, consider urgent referral to oncology, haematology, or for LN biopsy if:
- Lymphadenopathy present ≥6wk
- LNs are increasing in size or LN >2cm in size
- Widespread lymphadenopathy
- Lymphadenopathy + weight ↓, night sweats, and/or splenomegaly
- Any other suspicious symptoms/signs

Specialist treatment Based on histology and stage. Treatment options include a wait-and-see approach for low-grade lymphomas; radiotherapy; chemotherapy; bone marrow transplant; monoclonal antibody therapy (rituximab); and/or immunotherapy.

Prognosis Varies widely between different types of NHL (Table 19.7) and the age of the patient. Younger, fitter patients with less widespread disease do better. Overall 51% survive 10y.

Hodgkin's lymphoma 1,900 cases/y in the UK. *Peak age ranges:* 15–35y (>50% occur <40y) and 50–70y. Derived from B lymphocytes. Two types of Hodgkin's lymphoma are recognized:
- **Classical** (95%) Reed Sternberg cells are present
- **Nodular lymphocyte predominant** (5%) 'Popcorn' cells are present

Presentation Painless lymphadenopathy (70–95% have affected cervical LNs at diagnosis), weight ↓, night sweats/unexplained fevers, pruritus. The spleen is involved in 30% → splenomegaly.

Investigation and management As for NHL.

Prognosis
- **Early stage disease** (Ann Arbor stage 1/2—affected lymph tissue is confined to 1 side of the diaphragm)—80% 10y survival
- **Late stage disease** (Ann Arbor stage 3/4—affected lymph tissue both sides of diaphragm and/or extralymphatic tissue involvement)—60% 5y survival.

T. Hodgkin (1798–1866)—*English physician/pathologist.*

Information and support

Lymphoma Association ☎ 0808 808 5555 🖰 www.lymphomas.org.uk

Table 19.7 Features of common types of *NHL*

Type	Features
High-grade NHL	
Diffuse large B cell (DLBCL)	20% of NHL (including childhood). For adults, peak age = 70y Presents with rapidly enlarging lymphadenopathy. Extranodal involvement is common. 10% have bone marrow involvement at presentation
Anaplastic large cell	Two forms. Both originate from T cells or unknown cells **Systemic form** affects children/young adults. ♂ > ♀. Usually presents at a late stage and with systemic symptoms **Cutaneous form** 5% NHL. Affects adults (peak age 61y). Presents with reddish brown skin nodules or ulceration ± regional LN involvement (25%)
Burkitt's lymphoma	Affects children—30–40% childhood lymphoma. ♂ > ♀. B-cell lymphoma. Two varieties. Endemic variety is more common in Africa and associated with EBV infection. Peak age 5–10y. Sporadic variety occurs worldwide and affects slightly older children Presents with bulky central nodal disease ± extranodal (typically abdomen), bone marrow, and/or CNS involvement
Low-grade NHL	
Follicular	Affects adults. B-cell origin. Three types divided according to the ratio of small and large cells Usually presents with disseminated disease. 50% present with bone marrow involvement. May transform to DLBCL
Small lymphocytic	4–5% NHL. Median age 60y. Clinically/morphologically identical to CLL (📖 p. 678). Distinguished by degree of lymph tissue vs. blood/bone marrow involvement Presents with diffuse lymphadenopathy and some blood/bone marrow involvement. 10–20% transform to CLL, 3% to DLBCL
Mantle cell	5% NHL. Affects adults usually >50y. ♂ > ♀ (4:1). Although classified as low grade, behaves and is treated as high-grade. Usually presents with widespread disease involving LNs, bone marrow (60–90%), peripheral blood, spleen ± gut. Poor prognosis
Marginal zone	B-cell origin. Three distinct types **Nodal** 1–3% NHL. Presents with localized lymphadenopathy **Splenic** <1% NHL. Affects adults. Presents with massive splenomegaly and blood/bone marrow involvement without lymphadenopathy **Mucosa-associated (MALT)** 10% NHL. May be associated with inflammation (e.g. *H. pylori* infection and gastric MALT; Hashimoto's thyroiditis and thyroid MALT). 70% have localized disease on presentation. Symptoms depend on the organ involved
Lymphoplasmacytic	1.5% NHL. Also called Waldenstrom's macroglobulinaemia. B-cell lymphoma. Average age at presentation is 63y Often presents late with lymphadenopathy, splenomegaly, and bone marrow involvement. May spread to the lung or GI tract. Usually associated with paraproteinaemia (IgM)

Immune deficiency syndromes

A group of diverse conditions caused by immune system defects and characterized clinically by ↑ susceptibility to infections.

⚠ Consider an immunodeficiency disorder in anyone with infections that are unusually frequent, severe, resistant, or due to unusual organisms.

History In addition to history of infection, ask about:
- Family history: immune deficiency, early death, similar disease, autoimmune illness, early malignancy
- Late separation of umbilical cord (>4wk) or shedding of primary teeth
- Failure to thrive
- Adverse reaction to immunization or viral infection
- Difficult-to-treat asthma or eczema
- Splenectomy, tonsillectomy, or adenoidectomy
- Prior prophylactic antibiotic or immunoglobulin therapy

Primary immunodeficiency As many 1° immunodeficiencies are hereditary or congenital, they appear initially in infants and children; ~80% of those affected are <20y old and, owing to X-linked inheritance ♂ >> ♀. Genetic screening is available for some conditions. Refer all suspected cases to paediatrics/immunology.

Classification >70 primary immunodeficiencies have been described. They are classified into 4 groups depending on which component of the immune system is deficient:
- B cells
- T cells
- Phagocytic cells
- Complement

Prevalence Selective IgA deficiency (usually asymptomatic) occurs in 1:400 people. All other primary immune deficiencies are rare. Excluding IgA deficiency, 50% of affected patients have B-cell deficiency; 30% T-cell deficiency; 18% phagocytic deficiencies; and 2% complement deficiency.

Presentation Table 19.8 lists some of the more common immune deficiencies. All immune deficiencies present with increased tendency to infections. Type of infection varies according to the component of the immune system involved. If suspected, refer for specialist review.

Secondary immunodeficiency Impairment of the immune system resulting from illness (including drug therapy, e.g. with cytotoxics or steroids) or removal of the spleen in a previously normal person. Often reversible if the underlying condition or illness resolves. 2° immunodeficiencies are common; most prolonged serious illness interferes with the immune system to some degree. Treat the cause.

HIV infection 📖 p. 746

Asplenia and splenectomy 📖 p. 650

Infection in the immunocompromised 📖 p. 650

Information and support for patients
Immune Deficiency Foundation ℘ www.primaryimmune.org

Table 19.8 Immune deficiency syndromes

Type	Syndrome	Clinical details
B-cell deficiency Prone to infection with Gram +ve organisms (e.g. streptococci)	Selective IgA deficiency and IgG subclass deficiencies	Variable symptoms with most only mildly affected When more severely affected, early treatment of infection may be required
	Congenital X-linked hypogammaglobulinaemia and Common variable immunodeficiency	Not inherited—cause unknown ↓ immunoglobulins Treatment is with IV immunoglobulin ↑ risk of leukaemia /lymphoma
T-cell deficiency Prone to viral, fungal, and opportunistic infections	di George's syndrome	Defect on chromosome 22 → absent/ hypoplastic thymus (and ↓ T cells), absent parathyroid glands ± cardiac and/or facial abnormalities – Mild (80%)—treated supportively – Severe—requires thymus/bone marrow transplant
	HIV	📖 p. 746
Combined B- and T-cell deficiency	Severe combined immunodeficiency	Autosomal or X-linked recessive Absence of both T-cell and B-cell immunity Presents <6mo old with frequent infections Treatment is with bone marrow transplant. Untreated most die at <1y
	Ataxia telangiectasia	Autosomal recessive Selective IgA deficiency or hypogammaglobulinaemia and T-cell dysfunction Characterized by telangiectasia, cerebellar ataxia, and recurrent chest infections Treatment is supportive ↑ risk of leukaemia /lymphoma
	Wiskott–Aldrich syndrome (partial combined immunodeficiency syndrome)	X-linked recessive ↑ IgA and IgE; normal or ↓ IgG; ↓ IgM Presents with eczema, thrombocytopenia, and recurrent infections Treatment is with bone marrow transplant—rarely survive beyond teens without ↑ risk of leukaemia /lymphoma
Phagocytic deficiency Prone to staphylococcal and Gram –ve infections	Chronic granulomatous disease	X-linked (two-thirds) or autosomal recessive Phagocyte dysfunction Usually presents <6mo of age with fungal pneumonia, lymphadenopathy, hepatosplenomegaly, and/or osteomyelitis Treatment is supportive with prophylactic antibiotics and early treatment of infections
	Agranulocytosis	Usually caused by drugs, e.g. carbimazole Absence of neutrophils Sudden onset of fever ± rigors, sore throat, mouth ulcers, headache and malaise → septicaemia If suspected check urgent FBC and/or admit

Allergies

> *'One man's meat is another man's poison.'*

Allergic diseases result from an exaggerated response of the immune system to external substances. Affects 1:6 of the British population—and is increasing. Allergic problems include:

- Asthma—□ p. 308
- Occupational asthma—□ p. 336
- Eczema—□ pp. 606–9
- Anaphylaxis—□ p. 1072
- Urticaria—□ p. 614
- Rhinitis—□ p. 942
- Conjunctivitis—□ p. 966
- Food intolerance—□ p. 685

Assessment

- Age
- Symptoms—past and present, main problem, frequency and severity, seasonal/perennial, provoking factors
- Impact on lifestyle—time off work/school, sleep
- Occupation/hobbies
- Treatment—past and present
- Home environment—pets, damp, dust, smoking
- Allergies in the past
- Family history of allergic illness
- Examination will depend on main symptoms

Investigation

IgE skin prick and serum testing Identifies IgE sensitivity to common allergens, allowing diagnosis or exclusion of atopy. Uses skin prick testing or measurement of serum IgE levels. In most places this is a 2° care procedure although it is feasible in general practice. Patients should avoid using antihistamines before skin prick testing.

Patch testing Specialist test. Identifies substances causing contact allergy. A battery of allergens on discs are applied to the skin—usually on the back—and stuck in place with tape. Skin response is then monitored.

Management

Allergen avoidance For patients with anaphylaxis, may be lifesaving:
- **Pets** Exclude the offending animal
- **Pollens** Keep windows shut (including car windows); wear glasses/sunglasses; avoid grassy spaces; fit a pollen filter on the car
- **Foods/drugs** Avoid the food/drug; avoid hidden exposure (check labels carefully); inform any school/clubs a child attends; take food with you wherever possible; record drug allergies in medical notes

House dust mite Evidence that anti-house dust mite measures are effective in the relief of asthma and eczema is weak. Measures focus on the bedroom. Advise the room should be ventilated regularly; encase mattresses, pillows, and duvets in mite-proof covers (leave in place 6mo); wash bed clothes at 60°C every 1–2wk; use a vacuum cleaner with an adequate filter; remove bedroom carpet; ↓ soft toys to a minimum and wash frequently/put in the freezer to kill house dust mites.

Medication See individual conditions.

Referral to specialist allergy clinic
- Anaphylaxis
- Food allergy
- Urticaria in which allergic aetiology is suspected
- For consideration of immunotherapy
- Occupational allergy
- If allergy diagnosis is in doubt

Bee/wasp sting allergy Accounts for ~4 deaths/y in the UK. Stings may result in a local or generalized reaction of varying severity. Treat local or mild generalized reactions with antihistamine. Supply patients with more severe reactions with an adrenaline autoinjector pen and teach them, and close contacts, to use it. If severe reaction, refer to an allergy clinic for consideration of desensitization.

Food allergy Affects 1.4% of the adult population and 5–7% of children. Types of adverse reaction to foods include:
- **IgE mediated food allergy** Acute reaction (e.g. acute peanut allergy). Symptoms include: itching, erythema, urticaria, angio-oedema, GI (e.g. vomiting, abdominal pain), sneezing, wheeze, anaphylaxis
- **Non-IgE mediated food allergy** Delayed reaction (e.g. cow's milk causing eczema). Symptoms include: erythema, itching, eczema, persistent GI symptoms (e.g. reflux, pain, loose stools, constipation)
- **Non-allergic food intolerance** May be pharmacological, e.g. tyramine in red wine/cheese, causing migraine; metabolic, e.g. lactase deficiency; or toxic, e.g. reaction to preservative rather than food
- **Food aversion** Symptoms are non-specific and unconfirmed by blinded food challenge

A limited number of foods are responsible for the majority of true food allergies: nuts (especially peanuts), wheat, eggs, fish, shellfish, cow's milk.

Management
- **IgE mediated reaction** Request skin prick testing or send blood for specific IgE testing. Advise allergen avoidance and supply an adrenaline autoinjector pen (and teach to use) if anaphylactic reaction
- **Otherwise** Try eliminating the suspected food for 2–6wk and then reintroduce. Dietician advice may be helpful

Referral Consider referral to allergy clinic or paediatrics if:
- Severe acute allergic reaction, e.g. anaphylaxis or angio-oedema
- Severe delayed reaction (e.g. severe eczema related to food)
- Confirmed IgE allergy and asthma
- Suspected multiple allergies
- Poor growth with GI symptoms
- Parental concern
- Strong suspicion of allergy despite negative tests
- No response to food avoidance

Further information
NICE Food allergy in children and young people (2011) ℘ www.nice.org.uk

Patient information and support
Allergy UK ☎ 01322 619898 ℘ www.allergyuk.org
Anaphylaxis Campaign ☎ 01252 542029 ℘ www.anaphylaxis.org.uk
Medic Alert Foundation ☎ 0800 581 420 ℘ www.medicalert.org.uk
Medi-Tag ☎ 0121 200 1616 ℘ www.medi-tag.co.uk

Breast awareness Breast awareness means knowing what your breasts look and feel like normally. Evidence suggests that there is no need to follow a specific or detailed routine such as breast self-examination, but you should be aware of any changes in your breasts.

The breast awareness 5-point code
1. Know what is normal for you
2. Know what changes to look and feel for
3. Look and feel
4. Report any changes to your GP without delay
5. Attend for routine breast screening if you are aged 50 or over

Changes to be aware of
- **Size** If one breast becomes larger or lower
- **Nipples** If a nipple becomes inverted (pulled in) or changes position or shape
- **Rashes** On or around the nipple
- **Discharge** From one or both nipples
- **Skin changes** Puckering or dimpling
- **Swelling** Under the armpit or around the collarbone (where the lymph nodes are)
- **Pain** Continuous, in one part of the breast or armpit
- **Lump or thickening** Different to the rest of the breast tissue

What should I do if I notice a change? If you do notice a change in your breasts, see your GP as soon as you can. Your GP may ask you to come back at a different time in your menstrual cycle or send you to a breast clinic for a more detailed examination.

❶ Remember that most breast changes are not cancer, even if they need follow-up treatment or further investigation.

Further information
Breast Cancer Care ✍ www.breastcancercare.org.uk
NHS Cancer Screening 'Be breast aware' leaflet and other information
✍ www.cancerscreening.org.uk/breastscreen/breastawareness.html

Breast disease

Breast symptoms

Urgent referral of patients with breast disease[N] (to be seen in <2wk) is always required for:

Lump
- Any age with a discrete, hard lump with fixation ± skin tethering
- Any age with a past history of breast cancer presenting with a further lump or other suspicious symptoms
- Asymmetrical nodularity that persists after next period (if applicable)
- Aged ≥30y with a discrete lump that persists after the next period or presents after menopause
- Aged <30y:
  - With a lump that enlarges or is fixed/hard
  - In whom there are other reasons for concern such as family history

Nipple changes
- Unilateral eczematous skin or nipple change that does not respond to topical treatment
- Nipple distortion of recent onset
- Spontaneous unilateral bloody nipple discharge

Consider a non-urgent referral if
- The woman is aged <30y and has a lump which has no suspicious features and is not enlarging
- Breast pain and no palpable abnormality, when initial treatment fails, and/or symptoms persist (use of mammography is not recommended)

⚠ In patients presenting with symptoms and/or signs suggestive of breast cancer, investigation prior to referral is not recommended.

Breast lump

History Age (malignancy is rare <30y); how and when noticed; relationship to menstrual cycle; changes in shape or size since noticed; pain; nipple discharge; skin changes; pregnancy and breastfeeding; family history; current medication (in particular contraceptive pill or HRT).

Examination With the woman seated, with arms at her sides, above her head and pressing on her hips, look at the size and shape of the breasts, skin contour, skin and nipple changes. Seat the woman at 45° supported on a couch. Ask her to place the hand on the side being examined behind her head. Ask the woman to point to or find the lump. Palpate each quadrant of the breast with a flat hand. Check the tail of the breast in the axilla. Examine both breasts. If a lump is found assess shape, size, surface, edge, consistency, mobility, and attachments. Check local LNs in axilla and supraclavicular region and for hepatomegaly.

Differential diagnosis
- Breast cancer—📖 p. 696
- Fibroadenoma— 📖 p. 692
- Breast cyst—📖 p. 692
- Duct ectasia/periductal mastitis—📖 p. 693
- Haematoma or fat necrosis—📖 p. 692
- Phyllodes tumour—📖 p. 692
- Intraductal papilloma—📖 p. 693
- Lipoma or sebaceous cyst

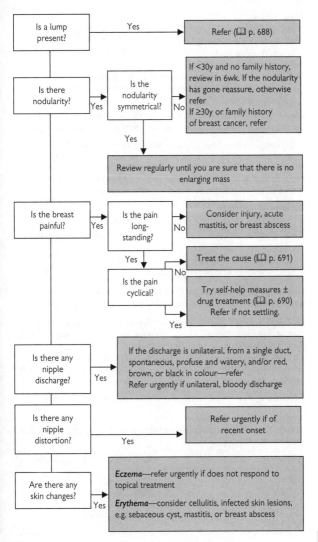

Figure 20.1 Algorithm for management of breast symptoms

Management
- **No lump** Reassure. Educate the woman about breast awareness (📖 p. 686). Consider reviewing in 6wk
- **Discrete lump** Refer
- **Asymmetrical nodularity**
  - <30y with FH of breast cancer or ≥30y—non-urgent referral
  - <30y and no family history—review in 6wk. If the nodularity has gone reassure, otherwise refer

❶ Any patient being referred with a breast lump will be concerned about the possibility of breast cancer even though most will not have cancer.

Discharge from the nipple 90% of pre-menopausal women can express milky, multiple-duct discharge. Ask about colour, quantity, and whether the discharge is unilateral/bilateral. Examine to check for lumps. Note colour/quantity of discharge and whether the discharge is coming from multiple or a single duct and is spontaneous or expressed.

Differential diagnosis
- Physiological (e.g. pregnancy)
- Duct ectasia—📖 p. 693
- Breast cancer—📖 p. 696
- Intraductal papilloma—📖 p. 693

Management
- Refer urgently if unilateral, spontaneous bloody discharge
- Refer if >50y or features suggesting pathological cause (see Table 20.1)

Breast pain or mastalgia Most common in women aged 30–50y. Use a pain chart for >2mo to distinguish cyclical from non-cyclical pain.

Cyclical breast pain Common. Two-thirds of women >35y have cyclical mastalgia which causes distress or interferes with lifestyle. Symptoms are often long-standing. *Features:*
- Usually bilateral though may not be the same intensity in both breasts
- Pain is generally felt over the lateral side of the breast, increases from mid-cycle onwards, and is relieved by menstruation

Examination may reveal tenderness ± areas of nodularity/lumpiness.

Table 20.1 Features of nipple discharge which suggest physiological or pathological cause

Physiological cause likely	Pathological cause likely—refer
Bilateral	Unilateral
Multiple ducts	Single duct
On expression only	Spontaneous
Green, milky	Red, brown, black
Stains only	Profuse and watery

Differential diagnosis

- Physiological
- Duct ectasia/periductal mastitis—📖 p. 693
- Breast cancer—📖 p. 696
- Sclerosing adenosis—📖 p. 692
- Mastitis—📖 p. 693 and p. 838
- Breast abscess—📖 p. 693
- Referred pain (e.g. cervical root pressure)

Management of mild/moderate cyclical pain 85% patients. Reassure that breast pain is a very *unusual* symptom of breast cancer. Explain the hormonal basis of symptoms. *Consider:*

- **Diet** Reducing saturated fats and caffeine may help
- **Support** Advise to wear a soft, support bra at night
- **OTC medication**—Try simple analgesia (e.g. paracetamol) and/or NSAID. Some women also find oil of evening primrose (gamolenic acid) is effective but it may take 4mo to work
- **Changing/stopping hormonal contraceptives or HRT**

Management of severe cyclical pain Defined as pain for >7d/mo for >6mo which interferes with lifestyle. Affects 15% patients. Try measures for management of mild/moderate cyclical pain first. If they fail, consider referral for specialist assessment.

Specialist treatments include: danazol, bromocriptine, tamoxifen, and LHRH analogues. Drug treatment helps ~80% of women. Treatment should be reviewed after 3–6mo and only continued if necessary. After stopping treatment, symptoms recur in about half, but are often less severe.

Non-cyclical breast pain Pain which is either continuous or intermittent but with no relationship to the menstrual cycle. Ask if the pain is localized or diffuse:

- **Well-localized/point-specific** Consider ill-fitting bras (especially underwired), breast cyst, breast abscess, mastitis, breast cancer (rarely presents with pain), chest wall causes, e.g. costochondritis
- **More generalized** Usually referred pain. Consider nerve root pain, post-herpetic neuralgia, lung disease

Management Treat the cause. If no cause can be found, refer for specialist assessment.

Eczema of the nipple Suspect underlying breast cancer. Refer for specialist assessment if no response to topical treatment—📖 p. 606.

Further information
NICE Referral guidelines for suspected cancer (2005) ✍ www.nice.org.uk

Benign breast disease

Most breast complaints are benign and have a physiological basis. Despite this, women with breast complaints tend to 'assume the worst' when a new problem is discovered. In most cases reassurance that there is nothing sinister underlying their symptoms is all that is required.

Mastalgia 📖 p. 690

Fibroadenoma An aberration of normal lobular development. Peak age 16–24y. 3 types: common, giant (>5cm diameter), and juvenile (adolescent girls). Present with a discrete, firm, non-tender, and highly mobile lump ('breast mouse'). Account for 13% of breast lumps.

Management Refer for confirmation of diagnosis—urgently if ≥30y, any personal/family history of breast cancer, or any sinister features (📖 p. 688). Diagnosis is confirmed with a combination of USS, mammography, and fine needle aspirate/core biopsy. If the lump is large (>4cm), the fibroadenoma is excised. In other groups, reassurance is usually all that is needed. 95% fibroadenomas do not enlarge after diagnosis and 25% ↓ in size or disappear with time.

❶ Fibroadenomas may calcify in older women and give a characteristic appearance in mammograms.

Sclerosing adenosis Benign condition resulting from over-proliferation of the terminal duct lobules. It can cause recurring pain and/or result in a small, firm lump in the breast. Often detected incidentally on mammography as a calcified, 'stellate' abnormality. Always refer urgently for confirmation of diagnosis. Treatment is symptomatic.

Phyllodes tumour Peak age 40–50y. 3 types—benign (most common); borderline malignant (uncommon); and malignant (rare).

Presentation and management Presents with a breast lump. Refer urgently for confirmation of diagnosis through a combination of USS, mammography, and fine needle aspirate/core biopsy. Treatment is always surgical with wide excision of the lump. Recurrence may occur.

Fat necrosis Usually history of injury ± bruising. As bruising settles, scarring results in a firm lump in the breast ± puckering of the skin. Most common in women with large breasts. Always refer urgently to a breast surgeon for triple assessment (USS, mammography + fine needle aspiration/core biopsy). Once diagnosis is confirmed, no treatment is needed. The lump often disappears spontaneously.

Breast cyst Benign and fluid-filled. Cysts may be of any size, single or multiple. Most common >35y. Usually pre-menopausal women but may occur in post-menopausal women taking HRT. Presents as a firm, rounded lump which is not fixed and not associated with skin changes/skin tethering.

First breast cyst Refer for exclusion of malignancy—urgently if ≥30y, FH of breast cancer, or other suspicious features. Diagnosis is confirmed with aspiration and/or USS and/or mammography.

Past history of breast cysts 30% of patients who have had a breast cyst develop another at a later date. If the lump is accessible, it is reasonable to attempt aspiration. There is no need to send aspirated fluid for cytology if the fluid is *not* bloodstained and lump completely resolves. Refer if the fluid aspirated is bloodstained; the lump does not disappear completely; the cyst refills; aspiration fails; or cytology reveals malignant or suspicious cells.

⚠ Do not attempt aspiration if you have not been trained to do so as there is a small but significant risk of pneumothorax.

Galactocoele Milk-containing cyst which arises during pregnancy. Refer any new lump arising in pregnancy to a breast surgeon. Repeated aspiration may be needed. Resolves spontaneously.

Duct ectasia Occurs around the menopause. Ducts become blocked and secretions behind stagnate. Presents as discharge from ≥1 duct which may be bloodstained ± breast lump ± nipple retraction ('transverse slit' appearance) ± breast pain.

Management Refer for confirmation of diagnosis—urgently if lump and/or bloodstained nipple discharge and/or nipple retraction. Usually no treatment is needed although surgery may be required to confirm diagnosis, if discharge is troublesome, or to evert the nipple.

Periductal mastitis Infected subareolar ducts. Affects younger women than duct ectasia with peak age 32y. Presents with breast tenderness ± inflammation in areolar area. May also have nipple discharge and/or retraction and/or an associated inflammatory mass/abscess.

Management Treat with antibiotics, e.g. co-amoxiclav 500/125 tds. Advise smokers that smoking can slow the healing process. If an abscess is present, refer for drainage. Refer if any residual inflammation or masses following treatment to exclude cancer. If recurrent infection, refer for consideration of surgery to remove the blocked duct.

Mastitis in lactating women 📖 p. 838

Intraductal papilloma Benign, wart-like lump that forms within a duct, just behind the areola. Perimenopausal women are more likely to have a single intraductal papilloma; younger women often have >1. May be bilateral. Presents with nipple discharge which may be bloodstained ± a subareolar lump/nodule (30%). Refer for confirmation of diagnosis—urgently if lump and/or bloodstained discharge. Usually excised.

Breast abscess Usually occurs in a lactating breast following mastitis; occasionally in a non-lactating breast in association with indrawn nipple, mammary duct ectasia, or local skin infection. Presents with gradual onset of pain in one breast segment with hot, tender swelling of the affected area.

Management Refer for surgical assessment. May be treated with repeated aspiration under ultrasound guidance or surgical incision and drainage.

Mamary duct fistula Fistula between a mammary duct and the skin. Usually a complication of a breast abscess. Refer for surgical excision.

Breast cancer screening

In the UK there has been a national screening programme for breast cancer since 1988. The aim of the programme is to detect breast cancer at an early stage in order to ↑ survival chances (stage I tumours—5y survival 84%; stage IV tumours—5y survival 18%).

Breast awareness Trials of self-examination have not ↓ mortality. Instead less formal 'Breast Awareness' is advocated—◻ p. 686.

Screening test

Women >50y Two-view mammographic screening is currently available to women aged 50–70y every 3y. This will be extended to women aged 47–73y throughout the UK by 2016. Older women can also request screening every 3y. Screening detects 85% of cancers in women aged >50y (60% of which are impalpable) and ~70–80% screening-detected cancers have good prognosis. Screening more frequently does not ↓ mortality[R]. Organization of breast cancer screening in the UK—see Figure 20.2.

High-risk women <50y Women with family history of breast cancer may be at ↑ risk of breast cancer themselves (see Figure 20.3, ◻ p. 697) and may benefit from earlier screening and/or genetic screening:

- All raised/high-risk women aged 40–49y—should be offered annual two-view mammography
- Women known to have a genetic mutation should be offered annual MRI surveillance—from 20y if TP53 mutation, and from 30y if BRCA1/2 mutation
- MRI surveillance should also be offered to women aged 30–39y with 10y risk >8%; women aged 40 –49y with 10y risk >20%; and at-risk women aged 40–49y with a dense breast pattern on mammography

Interval cancers Cancer occurring in the interval between screens. Can occur through failure to detect a cancer at screening or as a result of a new event after screening took place. In the first year after screening 20% breast cancers are interval cancers. This ↑ to ~60% in the third year.

Acceptability of screening 81% women find mammography uncomfortable, but 90% return for subsequent screens. GPs have an important role in promoting National Cancer Screening Programmes to their patients; GP endorsement ↑ uptake rates[R].

Anxiety from screening False-positive results cause anxiety as well as prompting further invasive investigations. Anxiety levels in women recalled and then found to be disease-free are higher a year after the recall appointment than in women who receive negative results at screening.

Further information

NHS Breast Screening ℘ www.cancerscreening.nhs.uk
NICE Familial breast cancer (2006) ℘ www.nice.org.uk

Information for patients ℘ www.cancerscreening.nhs.uk
- Breast screening—the facts
- Over 70? You are still entitled to breast screening

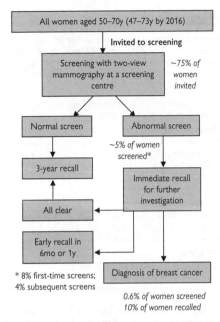

Figure 20.2 Organization of breast cancer screening in the UK

Table 20.2 Pros and cons of breast cancer screening

Benefits	Adverse effects
• Earlier diagnosis • Improved prognosis and lower mortality • Less radical and invasive treatment needed • Reassurance for those with –ve results	• Discomfort and inconvenience of screening • Radiation risks of screening (very small) • Reassurance to those women who have false –ve results • Reassurance to those who develop an interval cancer and possibly later presentation due to false sense of security • Anxiety and adverse effects of further investigation for those with false +ves • Overdiagnosis of minor abnormalities that would never develop into breast cancer • Earlier knowledge of disease and overtreatment for those who, despite early diagnosis have unchanged prognosis

Breast cancer

Breast cancer is now the most common cancer in the UK with >48,000 new diagnoses every year (including 340 new cases/y affecting men). Women have a 1 in 8 lifetime risk of developing breast cancer. Virtually all breast cancers are adenocarcinoma (85% ductal; 15% lobular).

Risk factors

Geography More common in the developed world—migrants assume the risk of the host country within two generations.

Personal characteristics
- **Age** ↑ with age—~81% of breast cancers occur in women >50y
- **Socio-economic** Higher incidence in more affluent social classes
- **Physical characteristics** Taller women have ↑ risk; women with denser breasts have 2–6x ↑ risk

Lifestyle factors
- **Obesity** ↑ risk post menopause
- **Physical activity** 30% ↓ risk if taking regular physical activity
- **High-fat diet** Probably associated with ↑ risk
- **Alcohol**↑ risk by 7%/unit consumed/d

Reproductive history
- **Early menarche or late menopause** ↑ risk
- **Pregnancy** ↑ parity results in ↓ risk (32% ↓ risk in women reporting three births compared to women reporting one); late age when first child is born ↑ risk
- **Breastfeeding** ↓ relative risk by 4.3% for each year of breastfeeding
- **Combined hormonal contraception** Slight ↑ risk (relative risk 1.24 for current users)—excess risk disappears within 10y of stopping
- **HRT** Risk ↑ by 6 cases/1,000 after 5y combined HRT use and 19 cases/1,000 after 10y use. Risk for combined oestrogen and progestogen preparations is greater than oestrogen-only preparations. HRT also ↓ sensitivity of mammography

Other past medical history
- **Past history of breast disease** Ductal or lobular carcinoma *in situ*, florid hyperplasia, and papilloma with fibrovascular core all ↑ risk
- **Ionizing radiation** Exposure ↑ risk

Family history Referral algorithm—see Figure 20.3.
- **One first-degree relative with breast cancer (mother/sister)** Risk ↑ 2x—but 95% of women with breast cancer have no family history
- **Several family members with early onset breast cancer** Refer for genetic screening—BRCA1 and BRCA2 genes account for 2–5% of all breast cancers

❶ Family relationships:
- **First-degree relative**—mother, father, sister, brother, daughter, son
- **Second-degree relative**—grandparents, grandchildren, aunt, uncle, niece, nephew, half-sister, half-brother

Breast cancer screening 📖 p. 694

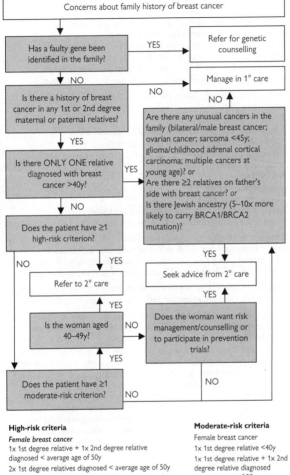

Figure 20.3 Referral of women with family history of breast cancer[N]

High-risk criteria

Female breast cancer

1x 1st degree relative + 1x 2nd degree relative diagnosed < average age of 50y

2x 1st degree relatives diagnosed < average age of 50y

1x 1st degree relative with bilateral breast cancer where first primary diagnosed at <50y

≥3x 1st/2nd degree relatives

Male breast cancer

1x 1st degree relative

Breast and ovarian cancer

1x 1st/2nd degree relative with breast cancer + another with ovarian cancer (1 must be 1st degree relative)

Moderate-risk criteria

Female breast cancer

1x 1st degree relative <40y

1x 1st degree relative + 1x 2nd degree relative diagnosed > average age of 50y

2x 1st degree relatives diagnosed > average age of 50y

Prevention Consider referral to secondary/tertiary care if family history of breast cancer (🔲 p. 697).
- Lifestyle measures—↓ alcohol intake; ↓ weight; ↑ exercise; avoid exogenous sex hormones (e.g. HRT); breastfeed
- Chemoprophylaxis—tamoxifen ↓ risk of breast cancer by 40% in high-risk women but use is limited by side effects (thromboembolism and endometrial carcinoma); other drug trials are in progress
- Prophylactic surgery—↓ risk by 90% in very high-risk women

Presentation Often found at breast screening (🔲 p. 694). Clinical presentations include:
- Breast lump (90%)
- Breast pain (21% present with painful lump; pain alone <1%)
- Nipple skin change (10%). Any red, scaly lesion or eczema around the nipple suggests Paget's disease of the breast—intraepidermal, intraductal cancer
- Family history (6%)
- Skin contour change (5%)
- Nipple discharge (3%)
- Rarely presents with distant metastases, e.g. bone pain
- In the elderly, may present with extensive local lesions

Management Refer for urgent assessment (<2wk) to a breast surgeon. Specialist investigation includes mammography, USS ± fine needle aspiration or core biopsy. If diagnosis is confirmed further investigations include tumour markers and/or CT/MRI, liver USS, and/or bone scan to evaluate spread.

Treatment Includes surgery (lumpectomy ± axillary clearance, mastectomy), endocrine therapy, radiotherapy, and/or chemotherapy.

Adjuvant endocrine therapy Oestrogen has an important role in the progression of breast cancer. Oestrogen and progesterone receptors determine the response to endocrine therapy.
- **Tamoxifen** ↑ survival of patients with oestrogen receptor +ve tumours (60% tumours) of any age but rarely causes endometrial cancer—warn patients to report any untoward vaginal bleeding. Continue tamoxifen for ≥5y— take advice from a specialist prior to stopping
- **Aromatase inhibitors,** e.g. anastrozole, letrozole, and exemestane. Block synthesis of oestrogen. Superior efficacy when compared to tamoxifen for postmenopausal women with hormone-sensitive early, breast cancer, and first choice for postmenopausal women with advanced breast cancer. Continue for ≥5y—take advice from a specialist prior to stopping
- **Trastuzumab** Monoclonal antibody directed against HER2, a receptor found in 1:5 breast cancers. Affects division and growth of breast cancer cells. Treatment option for women with early HER2 +ve cancer at high risk of recurrence and women with advanced HER2 +ve breast cancer. Administered IV every 3wk for 1y

❶ Optimum treatment regimes for breast cancer change regularly and there are regional variations. Many women will be asked to participate in clinical trials to answer important questions about best treatments.

Prognosis 73% of women diagnosed now will live 10y; 64% live ≥20y.

- Recurrence is most likely <2y after treatment—late recurrences do occur but the longer since diagnosis, the less the chance of recurrence
- Prognosis for an individual depends on age (best prognosis if 50–69y), stage of disease (see Table 20.3), grade of tumour, and oestrogen receptor status (oestrogen receptor –ve tumours have poorer prognosis)
- Women living in affluent areas have better survival rates than those in deprived areas

Psychological impact of breast cancer Depression, anxiety, marital and sexual problems are common. Be sensitive. Discuss possibilities of reconstructive surgery or breast prostheses as appropriate. Refer to the specialist breast care nurse for support and advice.

Lymphoedema 📖 p. 1041

Table 20.3 Classification of breast cancer stage

Stage	TNM equivalent	Features
In situ	Tis N0 M0	Non-invasive
I	T1 N0 M0	≤2cm diameter No LNs affected No spread beyond breast
II	T0–2 N1 M0 or T2/3 N0 M0	2–5cm diameter and/or LNs in axilla involved No evidence of spread beyond axilla
III	T0–2 N2 M0 or T3 N1/2 M0 or T4 any N M0 or Any T N3 M0 or	>5cm diameter LNs in axilla involved No evidence of spread beyond the axilla
IV	Any T/N M1	Any sized tumour LNs in axilla may be affected Distant metastases

Sentinel lymph node biopsy Prognosis and decisions about adjuvant treatment are based on knowledge of the axillary node status. The only way to assess that is to remove nodes surgically and look at them under the microscope. Axillary node clearance can result in lymphoedema and ↓ arm function. Sentinel node biopsy is the removal of the key or sentinel LN in patients undergoing surgery for early breast cancer to accurately predict the state of nodal disease in the remaining axillary LNs. Radical axillary surgery to clear the axillary nodes can then be reserved for the 20–40% with a +ve sentinel LN biopsy.

Further information
NICE Familial breast cancer (2006) ℬ www.nice.org.uk

Information and support for patients
Breakthrough breast cancer ☏ 08080 100 200 ℬ www.breakthrough.org.uk
Breast Cancer Care ☏ 0808 800 6000 ℬ www.breastcancercare.org.uk

Gynaecology

The menstrual cycle

A good working knowledge of the menstrual cycle is essential to understand its endocrine disorders and their management. One menstrual cycle lasts from the start of one period until the day before the start of the next. The average length of a cycle is 28d, but anything from 24–35d is common. The menstrual cycle is split into four (see Figure 21.1).

Follicular or proliferative phase

Hormone changes Levels of oestrogen and progesterone are low. There is ↓ negative feedback on the pituitary as a result so follicle-stimulating hormone (FSH) levels ↑. FSH stimulates follicle development in the ovary. The developing follicles then produce oestrogen.

Changes within the reproductive organs
- **Ovaries** Follicles develop. One follicle becomes dominant
- **Uterus** Lining thickens (proliferates)
- **Vagina** Tends to be drier with thicker mucus

Ovulation Occurs halfway through a cycle (~14d before the next period). The dominant follicle ruptures and an egg is released into the Fallopian tube. The follicle fills with blood after rupturing and there may be brief pain—*mittelschmerz* (reassure—no treatment needed). The egg travels along the Fallopian tube into the uterus and may be fertilized if the woman is sexually active and not using contraception.

Secretory or luteal phase

Hormone changes After ovulation, the ruptured follicle forms the corpus luteum (yellow body) and secretes progesterone and oestrogen.

Changes within the reproductive organs
- **Ovaries** Corpus luteum forms. If pregnancy does not occur the corpus luteum begins to degenerate ~4d prior to menstruation
- **Uterus** Progesterone causes the lining of the uterus to alter so that it is ready to receive a fertilized egg. The endometrium becomes oedematous, more vascular, and the glandular component becomes coiled and tortuous
- **Vagina** Mucus becomes thinner, more watery, and slippery. It becomes thicker again towards the next period as progesterone ↓
- **Other changes** Progesterone may cause 'water retention', breast tenderness, and mood changes

Periods (menstruation) With regression of the corpus luteum, oestrogen and progesterone levels ↓. This causes necrosis, bleeding, and sloughing of the endometrium, resulting in a period or menstruation. Periods begin aged 11–16y and continue until the menopause (usually 45–55y). Bleeding can last from 1–8d (average 5d) and is generally heaviest in the first 2d. Blood loss in each period is ~20–60mL (>80mL is abnormal and may lead to anaemia). Some period pain is common and normal.

Prolonged menstruation Bleeding for >5–6d/cycle. Most loss occurs in the first 3d. Long periods do not equate to ↑ menstrual loss so prolonged menstruation per se does not need investigation. Frequently goes with menorrhagia—📖 p. 708.

Menstruation | Ovulation | Menstruation

Oestrogen — FSH — Progesterone

Luteinizing hormone (LH)

FOLLICULAR PHASE — 14 — LUTEAL PHASE

0 — Days →

Figure 21.1 Hormone changes throughout the menstrual cycle

Anovulatory cycles Common around menarche, in the perimenopause, and in women with PCOS. In the absence of ovulation, there is no luteal phase of the cycle leading to variable and erratic cycle length.

Postponing menstruation
- **Combined oral contraceptive (COC) pill** Started ≥1mo before and continued throughout the time the withdrawal bleed should have occurred (2 packets back-to-back without a break). The withdrawal bleed will occur after the second packet is finished
- **Combined contraceptive patch** Can be used for 6wk without a patch-free break to postpone a period
- **Norethisterone** 5mg tds starting 3d before the anticipated onset of menstruation. Menstruation will occur 2–3d after stopping the norethisterone

Odd colour/smell of menstrual blood No known associations.

Post-coital and intermenstrual bleeding
- **Post-coital bleeding (PCB)** Non-menstrual bleeding occurring during or after sexual intercourse. Consider cervical cancer (📖 p. 726). Other possible causes include infections of the lower genital tract, cervical ectropion and polyps, trauma, and vaginal and vulval lesions
- **Intermenstrual bleeding (IMB)** Vaginal bleeding at any time during the menstrual cycle other than menstruation. May be physiological or related to use of CHC. Other causes include: endometrial polyps, uterine fibroids, endometrial hyperplasia or cancer, endometritis, and cervical, vulval or vaginal cancer

⚠ Always perform a full pelvic examination. If suggestive of cervical cancer, refer urgently (<2wk) for gynaecology opinion. Do not use cervical smears as a diagnostic test. Consider urgent referral if intermenstrual bleeding even if the cervix looks normal.

Premenstrual syndrome

Most women of reproductive age notice symptoms/bodily changes in the days/weeks leading up to their periods. These changes resolve or ↓ significantly during the period and are termed premenstrual tension (PMT), or premenstrual syndrome (PMS) if they occur on a regular basis and are severe enough to interfere with quality of life. >95% women have some symptoms but <20% seek help. Debilitating symptoms occur in 5%.

Cause Underlying mechanism is not fully understood but is thought to be due to the hormonal changes that occur after ovulation affecting neurotransmitters in the brain.

Symptoms >100 symptoms described. The most common are:
- Psychological—mood swings, nervous tension and/or irritability (when severe, termed *premenstrual dysphoric disorder*—PMDD)
- Physical—abdominal bloating, ↑ weight, breast tenderness, headache
- Behavioural—↓ visuospatial and cognitive ability, ↑ in accidents

Management Aims to alleviate symptoms. Usually symptoms return when treatment is stopped.
- Take a history of symptoms and ask the woman to keep a diary to establish cyclical nature over >2mo
- If mild/moderate symptoms—try lifestyle/dietary modification first:
  - Make allowances on days when symptoms are likely to be worst
  - Wear loose clothes if feeling bloated
  - Ensure adequate sleep and take regular exercise
  - Eat regularly—some find small, frequent meals help; avoid sweet snacks between meals; make sure diet is low in fat/salt, caffeine, and alcohol, and contains plenty of fruit/vegetables and complex carbohydrate (e.g. bread, pasta, rice, potatoes)
  - ↓ fluid intake or eat diuretic foods (e.g. strawberries, watermelon, aubergines, prunes, figs, parsley) to ease fluid retention
  - OTC remedies may help (see Table 21.1)
- Consider drug therapy or CBT (see Table 21.1) if symptoms are severe or do not respond to diet/lifestyle measures. Base choice on symptoms
- For all treatments try a 3–6mo trial. Ask women to keep a symptom diary. Be sure to follow up—as the first treatment may not work
- If symptoms are severe or primary care management is ineffective, refer to gynaecology/mental health services for specialist management

❶ Because of side effects, oestrogen patches and gonadotrophin-releasing hormone analogues are usually only used by specialists for severe or resistant PMS/PMDD.

Further information
RCOG Management of premenstrual syndrome (2007) ℳ www.rcog.org.uk

Information and support for patients and their partners
National Association for Premenstrual Syndrome ☎ 0844 815 7311
ℳ www.pms.org.uk

Table 21.1 Treatment of premenstrual tension

Treatment	Effective?	Notes
Hormonal manipulation		
COC^G	✓	First-line treatment. The RCOG recommends combined new generation pills, e.g. Yasmin® or Cilest®—given cyclically or continuously
Low-dose oestrogen^G	✓	Second-line treatment. Use 100 microgram estradiol patches. To avoid giving unopposed oestrogen, combine with dydrogesterone 10mg from day 17–28 or IUS if the uterus is intact
GnRH analogues^R	✓	Reserved for specialist care. Usually given in combination with add-on HRT
Antidepressants		
SSRIs^G	✓	↓ physical as well as psychological symptoms. First-line treatment that can be given continuously or just in the luteal phase (days 15–28)
Other drugs		
Diuretics^CE	✓	Spironolactone is effective for bloating/breast tenderness. Many women prefer 'natural' diuretics, e.g. Waterfall®, though there is no evidence of effectiveness
NSAIDs^CE	✓	Particularly helpful for premenstrual pain and to ↓ menstrual bleeding
Surgery		
Hysterectomy + oophorectomy^G	✓	Curative. Most women require HRT/testosterone replacement afterwards
Complementary therapies		
Oil of evening primrose^S	✓/✗	May help breast tenderness. Can cause fits in patients with epilepsy
Vitamin B_6^G	✓	Most studies suggest effective—advise women to take 10mg/d. High doses (>100mg/d) may cause reversible peripheral neuropathy
Chaste tree berry (*Vitex agnus-castus*)^S	✓	Evidence of effectiveness is generally positive—can cause menstrual irregularity
Magnesium supplements^G	✓	Evidence of effectiveness is generally positive. Used in the premenstrual phase
Calcium supplements^S	✓	↓ symptoms including breast tenderness and swelling, headaches, migraine, and abdominal cramps
Exercise^CE	✓	High-intensity exercise improves symptoms > low-intensity exercise
Cognitive therapy^CE	✓	Evidence that effective. Effects are smaller and slower than SSRI—but more long-lasting
Relaxation/reflexology^R	✓/✗	Conflicting evidence—can do no harm

Amenorrhoea

Oligomenorrhoea Infrequent periods (>35d between periods). Manage as for amenorrhoea.

Primary amenorrhoea No menstruation by age 16y when growth and sexual development is normal. Refer for specialist treatment. *Causes:*
- **Outflow abnormalities** Müllerian agenesis; transverse vaginal septum; androgen insensitivity (📖 p. 895), imperforate hymen
- **Ovarian disorders** PCOS; gonadal dysgenesis, e.g. Turner's syndrome—❶ gonads may have malignant potential
- **Pituitary disorders** ❶ Prolactinoma (📖 p. 370)
- **Hypothalamic disorders** Kallman's syndrome (congenital GnRH deficiency associated with anosmia)

Secondary amenorrhoea Absence of menses for ≥3mo in a previously menstruating woman. *Causes:* see Figure 21.2.

History Always consider the possibility of pregnancy.
- **Symptoms**
  - Galactorrhoea—30% prolactinomas
  - Weight change—weight ↓ may cause amenorrhoea
  - Hirsutism—may suggest PCOS or androgen-secreting tumour
  - Life crisis or upset—e.g. exams, bereavement
  - Level of exercise—high-intensity athletes, e.g. gymnasts are frequently amenorrhoeic
  - Sweats and/or flushes (suggests menopause)
  - Cyclical pain—may suggest outflow obstruction
- **Family history** Of premature menopause or late menarche
- **Drug history** Particularly contraceptives, e.g. injectable progestogens. Other drugs include: heroin, methadone, metoclopramide
- **Past history** Of chemo- or radiotherapy or gynaecological surgery

Examination
- Weight and height—common if BMI <19kg/m²
- External genitalia—structural abnormality, virilism
- Vaginal examination—including cervical smear if overdue
- Pelvic examination—ovarian masses, uterine size
- General examination—2° sexual characteristics, hirsutism, systemic disease (including visual fields/retinal examination, ? prolactinoma)

❶ For young girls, replace vaginal/pelvic examination with per-abdominal pelvic USS.

Investigation
- **Blood—** Serum prolactin; TFTs; FSH/LH ; karyotype if phenotypical abnormality; serum testosterone if LH high, hirsutism or virilism
- **USS pelvis** If structural abnormality or to confirm PCOS

Management of secondary amenorrhoea Treat the cause:
Contraception
- Injectable progestogens—stop; periods usually return within a year
- Other hormonal methods—stop; look for another cause of amenorrhoea if periods do not return in ≤3mo

If underweight Investigate and treat reasons for weight loss (e.g. anorexia). Encourage weight ↑. If no response refer to gynaecology/eating disorders clinic.

Physical exercise Explain the reason for amenorrhoea—many women refuse to cut their activity levels; consider HRT/CHC to protect bone density.

Stress Reassure. Treat any psychiatric problems—periods should return spontaneously. Set a limit for return (e.g. another 3–4mo). If periods do not return consider referral as there may be another cause.

Endocrine
- Thyroid dysfunction—treat hyper- or hypothyroidism
- Hypothalamic causes—refer to endocrinology. After 6mo amenorrhoea, there is ↑ risk of coronary heart disease and osteoporosis. Consider use of HRT or CHC
- Hyperprolactinaemia—refer to endocrinology

Gynaecological
- Premature menopause—📖 p. 711.
- PCOS—📖 p. 725

Cause not found Refer to gynaecology.

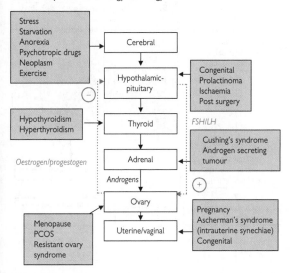

Figure 21.2 Causes of amenorrhoea

Further information
Monga A, Dobbs SP (eds) (2011) *Gynaecology by Ten Teachers.* London: Hodder Arnold. ISBN: 034098354X

Menorrhagia

Menorrhagia (heavy periods) is defined as menstrual loss ≥80mL/mo. 10% meet this criterion but 1 in 3 feel their loss is excessive. Ask about number of tampons or pads used/d, use of double protection to prevent leaks, flooding and clots to gauge bleeding. Ask how periods affect life and activities. A menstrual diary may help. *Assessment:* see Figure 21.3.

Differential diagnosis Physiological bleeding or dysfunctional uterine bleeding (50%). Exclude pregnancy. *Other causes:*

- Fibroids
- Congenital uterine abnormality, e.g. bicornuate uterus
- Pelvic infection
- Endometriosis
- Endometrial/cervical polyps
- Presence of IUCD
- Endometrial carcinoma
- Bleeding tendency
- Hormone-producing tumours

❶ Hyper- or hypothyroidism, DM, prolactin disorders, adrenal, kidney or liver disease, and some medications can also cause menstrual disturbance.

Dysfunctional uterine bleeding (DUB) Excessive menstrual loss in the absence of any detectable abnormality.

Figure 21.3 Assessment of menorrhagia in primary care

Management See Figure 21.4. *Treatment may fail if:* high blood loss; low pre-treatment loss; other uterine pathology; lack of concordance. *2° care management:* assessment of endometrium; IUS; surgery—endometrial resection and ablation, myomectomy, hysterectomy ± oophorectomy.

Heavy menstrual bleeding and no sinister pathology suspected—consider IUS (📖 p. 762). *Check:* no contraindications and ≥12mo use is anticipated

Blood flow still too great

Blood flow not ↓ to acceptable levels after >6mo use

Fit IUS—encourage women to persevere with use for >6mo

Add CHC if no contraindications

Blood flow reduced to acceptable levels

Contraindications to IUS, <12mo IUS use anticipated, or blood flow not ↓ by IUS

Requires contraception

Does not require contraception or prefers non-hormonal treatment

Try CHC (📖 p. 752). Review after 3mo

Mefenamic acid 500mg tds

or

Tranexamic acid 1g tds

Add

Continued heavy bleeding

Start on day 1 of period, and continue for days of heavy flow. Review after 3mo

Continued heavy bleeding. Try norethisterone 15mg od from day 5–26 of the menstrual cycle, or injected long-acting progestogen

Blood flow not reduced to acceptable levels after 3mo—refer

⚠ Management of very heavy bleeding
- Resuscitate as necessary—admit if shocked; IV tranexamic acid or D&C in the acute situation can ↓ haemorrhage by 75–80%.
- Reduce/stop bleeding with progestogen, e.g. norethisterone 5mg tds, for 10d. Effective in 24–48h. A lighter bleed follows on stopping. Alternatively consider tranexamic acid (1g tds for 4d) to ↓ bleeding.
- Correct anaemia and refer for gynaecology assessment.

Figure 21.4 Medical management of menorrhagia in primary care

Further information
NICE Heavy menstrual bleeding (2007) 🔗 www.nice.org.uk

The menopause

From the Greek *meno* (month) and *pausis* (halt). Menopause occurs when menstruation stops. Average age in the UK ~51y. Smoking brings it forwards by ~2y. Impact on a woman's life varies and depends on cultural, health, and social factors.

Diagnosis >12mo amenorrhoea with no other cause.

Period changes

- **Changes in menstrual pattern** Common in the years before the menopause—typically cycle shortens after 40y by up to 7–10d. Cycle then lengthens—periods may occur at 2–3mo intervals until stopping
- **Dysfunctional uterine bleeding** Common leading up to the menopause but investigate if very heavy, painful, irregular, intermenstrual, or post-coital bleeding
- **Late menstruation (>54y)** Investigate as ↑ risk of malignancy

Psychological symptoms Controversial. Some studies report depression/anxiety are more common, others find no association. Depression is multifactorial—consider social, physical, and cultural factors before resorting to HRT as a solution. Regular sustained aerobic exercise (e.g. swimming or running) ↓ psychological symptoms and insomnia.

Flushes and sweats 80% have flushes during the menopause—20% seek help. Often associated with palpitations.

Lifestyle changes Low-intensity exercise (e.g. yoga, deep breathing); cool ambient temperature; wearing natural fibres, e.g. cotton; stress ↓; avoiding trigger foods/drinks (e.g. spicy foods, caffeine, alcohol).

Drug treatments

- Hormone therapy (📖 p. 712)—effective in 80–90% of women
- Megestrol acetate (40mg od—unlicensed)—effective but carries many of the same risks as HRT—may cause vaginal bleeding on withdrawal
- SSRIs/SNRIs (e.g. venlafaxine 37.5mg bd—unlicensed)—moderately effective and may also improve mood
- Gabapentin (300mg tds—unlicensed)—↓ flushes by 45%
- Clonidine—commonly used but little evidence of effectiveness; may cause hypotension

Complementary therapies

- Black cohosh eases hot flushes—long-term effects are unknown
- Red clover may help—studies have mixed results; avoid with warfarin
- Foods containing phyto-oestrogens (e.g. soy foods) may be helpful and are unlikely to be harmful
- Natural progesterone from yams—topical preparations are ineffective
- Dong quai, evening primrose oil, vitamin E, and ginseng are no better than placebo. Avoid kava—it is linked to cases of serious liver damage

Sexual dysfunction Vaginal dryness and atrophy are common. Manage with vaginal lubricants or topical oestrogen (unless other reasons for systemic HRT). Loss of libido (especially after surgical removal of the ovaries) responds to administration of androgen (e.g. testosterone) with HRT, until libido is re-established.

Urinary problems Common—incontinence, nocturia, and urgency. Stress incontinence does not respond to HRT but topical oestrogen may improve outcome of surgery. Recurrent UTIs and incontinence in older women ↓ with use of topical vaginal oestrogen.

Ischaemic heart disease Risk is ↑ x2 after the menopause but there is no evidence to support use of HRT for 1° or 2° prevention of IHD.

Osteoporosis Consider HRT to prevent osteoporosis in premature menopause (📖 p. 511). In older women, HRT is *not* recommended as first-line treatment of osteoporosis unless there are other reasons for prescribing HRT.

Could the symptoms be due to another cause? Exclude:
• Physical illness, e.g. thyroid disease, anaemia, DM, chronic renal disease
• Side effects of medication, e.g. Ca^{2+} antagonists cause flushing
• Social problems or psychiatric illness—depression screening questionnaires can be helpful

Is the diagnosis in doubt? FSH >30iu/L on 2 occasions >1mo apart suggests the woman is postmenopausal. Check FSH:
• Following hysterectomy with conservation of ovaries
• If amenorrhoea age <45y, *or*
• If having regular bleeds due to cyclical HRT/CHC—check at the beginning of a packet (oestrogen phase) or end of the CHC-free week, respectively. CHC/HRT can ↓ FSH—to make a more accurate assessment, stop the preparation and check FSH levels 6 and 12wk after stopping

❶ It is unnecessary to check FSH in other groups >45y with amenorrhoea. FSH levels may be normal in the perimenopause.

Premature menopause Menopause in a woman <40y old. Associated with ↑ all-cause mortality and ↑ risk of osteoporosis and cardiovascular disease. *Causes:*
• Idiopathic
• Infection—TB, mumps
• Radiotherapy and/or chemotherapy
• FSH receptor abnormalities
• Surgery—bilateral oophorectomy → instant menopause; hysterectomy without oophorectomy can also induce premature ovarian failure
• Chromosome abnormalities—particularly the X chromosome
• Autoimmune endocrine disease, e.g. DM, hypothyroidism, Addison's
• Disruption of oestrogen synthesis

Management Usually HRT is recommended until the average age of menopause, i.e. 51y.

Further information
British Menopause Society ✇ www.thebms.org.uk
RCOG Alternatives to HRT for the management of symptoms of the menopause (2010) ✇ www.rcog.org.uk

Information and support for patients
Menopause Matters ✇ www.menopausematters.co.uk
The Daisy Network (premature menopause) ✇ www.daisynetwork.org.uk

Hormone replacement therapy

Short-term use of HRT is used for relief of symptoms related to oestrogen deficiency peri- and postmenopausally, e.g. flushes/sweats. Carefully balance risks against benefits for each individual.

Contraindications History of hormone-dependent cancer; thromboembolic disease (including AF); liver disease where LFTs have failed to return to normal. If past history of liver disease, gallstones, or taking liver-enzyme-inducing drugs, consider transdermal therapy.

Particular indications
- Early menopause—consider alternatives if prescribing for osteoporosis prevention alone; continue until age 51y.
- Hysterectomy before menopause even if ovaries are conserved; ~1 in 4 have early menopause.
- Second-line treatment of osteoporosis—🕮 p. 511

Choice of preparation (BNF 6.4.1.1.) Start with a low dose and provide a 3mo supply. Tablets, patches, gels, and implants are available:
- **For women without a uterus**—Give oestrogen alone, unless past history of endometriosis (endometrial foci may remain despite hysterectomy, so consider addition of a progestogen)
- **For women with an intact uterus**—Progestogen is needed for the last 12–14d of the cycle or IUS to prevent endometrial proliferation. Alternatively, use a continuous oestrogen/progestogen preparation (although not in the perimenopause or <12mo after last menstrual period)

Tibolone Oestrogenic, progestogenic, and weak androgenic action. Use in the same way as continuous combined HRT.

Topical vaginal preparations Oestrogen pessaries, creams, or rings. For vaginal dryness/atrophic vaginitis. Licence limits use 3–6mo if uterus is present although commonly used for longer. Consider prescribing a progestogen if given for longer periods or higher doses are used. Investigate abnormal bleeding.

Things to do before starting HRT

History Why does the woman want to start HRT? What are her expectations of treatment? Has she had a hysterectomy? If not, ask about bleeding pattern. Investigate abnormal bleeding prior to starting HRT.

Other points to cover
- Risk factors for osteoporosis, DVT, and CVD; FH of breast cancer
- Contraceptive requirement—HRT does not provide contraception. If <50y, CHC (🕮 p. 752) may provide contraception and alleviate menopausal symptoms
- Drug history—previous experience of HRT; levothyroxine (may need to ↑ dose of levothyroxine when start HRT—check TFTs); steroids (HRT ↓ effectiveness of steroids); anti-epileptics (↑ elimination of oestrogen)

Examination Check BP; weight; breasts (check no lumps; demonstrate breast self-examination techniques); smear is up to date; consider examination for prolapse/vaginal abnormalities if symptoms.

Starting HRT Explain the pros and cons of HRT (see Table 21.2). Support with health promotion information, e.g. about smoking cessation, breast cancer screening programme. Review after 3mo. Check BP and weight. ↑ dose if symptoms are not controlled. *Common side effects:*

- **Oestrogen-related**—Fluid retention, breast enlargement and tenderness, nausea, headaches
- **Progestogen-related**—Headache, ↑ weight, bloating, and depression (↓ by changing to a preparation with a less androgenic progestogen, e.g. dydrogesterone or medroxyprogesterone)

Bleeding Bleeding may be erratic for the first 2–3mo in patients taking cyclical HRT but should not occur after the progestogen supplement in subsequent cycles. Continuous combined preparations may cause spotting for 4–6mo; if bleeding continues >6mo, investigate to exclude endometrial abnormality and consider changing to a cyclical preparation.

Once established on HRT Review every 6–12mo and if any problems. Check BP, weight, breasts, symptoms, and bleeding pattern. Reassess risks and benefits. HRT is needed for <5y for vasomotor symptoms. When stopping, withdrawal flushes may be distressing—stop in cold weather and half the dose for 1mo first. *Reasons to stop immediately:*

- Serious neurological effects, e.g. severe headache, first fit
- Severe chest pain
- Sudden breathlessness/cough with bloodstained sputum
- Unexplained severe pain in calf
- Severe stomach pain
- Hepatitis, jaundice, liver enlargement
- BP >160mmHg systolic and/or >95mmHg diastolic
- Detection of a risk factor, e.g. DVT, stroke
- Prolonged immobility after surgery or leg injury

Table 21.2 Risks and benefits of HRT

Risks	Short-term benefits	Long-term benefits
↑ Breast cancer (RR 1.43ᵛ)	Alleviation of menopausal symptoms, e.g. flushes/ sweats/ vaginal dryness	↓ Osteoporosis
↑ DVT (RR 1.45*)		↓ Colorectal cancer
↑ Stroke (RR 1.15*)		
↑ Gallbladder disease	↓ Recurrent UTIs	
↑ Ovarian cancer if using oestrogen-only HRT for >5y		
No ↓ risk of CHD—may ↑ risk in the first year of use	❡ These figures are controversial. Subsequent studies, including long-term studies, have shown beneficial effects of HRT on symptoms, mortality, and CVD risk with no significant adverse effectsᴿ	

ᵛRelative risk in women aged 50–64y using combined HRT for 5y
*Relative risk in women aged 60–69y taking combined HRT for 5y

Further information

British Menopause Society ℘ www.thebms.org.uk
RCP (Edinburgh) Consensus conference on HRT: Final consensus statement (2003) ℘ www.rcpe.ac.uk/policy-standards/rcpe-consensus-statements
Schierbeck LL, Rejnmark L, Tofteng CL, et al. (2012) Effect of HRT on cardiovascular events in recently post menopausal women: randomized trial. *BMJ* **345**:e6409.

Information and support for women

Menopause Matters ℘ www.menopausematters.co.uk

Pelvic pain

Pelvic pain may be acute or chronic (pain for ≥6mo). *Causes:* see Table 21.3.

History Allow the woman to tell her story. Ask about:
- **Pain**—site; severity; onset (? pregnant); character/timing/pattern (e.g. relationship to menstrual cycle or sexual intercourse, exacerbating/relieving factors, effects of movement/posture); other associated features. Decide whether the cause is gynaecological—patients usually have dyspareunia and pain may be cyclical
- **Bowel (nausea and vomiting)/bladder/psychological symptoms**
- **Past history**—ectopic pregnancy, pelvic infection/surgery, other factors (be sensitive to possible history of sexual abuse or rape)

Examination Abdominal, pelvic, and vaginal examination—including rectal examination if indicated and cervical smear if overdue. Normal pelvic and vaginal examination makes a gynaecological cause unlikely.

Investigation Consider: *urine*—pregnancy test, M,C&S, dipstick for protein, RBCs, nitrites, and leucocyte esterase; *blood*—FBC, CRP, CA125; *radiology*—pelvic USS if gynaecological cause is suspected. ❶ Offer screening for STIs to all sexually active women with chronic pelvic pain.

Management of acute pelvic pain Admit if severe or if ectopic pregnancy cannot be excluded. Otherwise provide analgesia and treat the cause.

Management of chronic pelvic pain Affects 1 in 6 women in the UK. There is often >1 cause—aim to identify and address contributory factors instead of assigning a single cause.

Dyspareunia Pain on intercourse. 10% women admit sexual intercourse usually causes discomfort. It may be *superficial* (felt around the introitus) or *deep* (felt deep inside). There is a psychological element in most cases (a vicious cycle of pain leading to fear of intercourse which exacerbates symptoms). Address both physical and psychological aspects.

Superficial dyspareunia Examine if possible but do not insist. Treat cause. If no specific treatment, try lidocaine gel. *Causes:*
- **Vulval** Vulvitis—atrophic, infective (candida, HSV); dystrophy; neoplasm; lichen sclerosus; lichen planus; vulvodynia
- **Vaginal** Vaginismus; lack of lubrication; vaginitis—atrophic, infective; congenital—imperforate hymen, atresia; surgery, e.g. painful episiotomy scar; contracture—atrophy or after surgery/radiotherapy
- **Urethral** Urethritis; urethral caruncle; urethral diverticulum

Deep dyspareunia Causes: endometriosis; pelvic inflammatory disease; retroverted uterus; ovarian mass (rarely ovarian cancer); non-gynaecological causes. Examine, treat any cause found else refer for further investigation. If no cause is found or cause is untreatable, pain can be ↓ by limiting penetration. Often becomes a chronic problem.

Dysmenorrhoea (painful periods) >50% premenopausal women have some pelvic discomfort around their period; 1 in 10 find period pain significantly interferes with lifestyle.

Primary dysmenorrhoea No underlying pelvic pathology. Tends to start 6–12mo after menarche when ovulatory cycles are established. Presents with lower abdominal cramps ± backache which occur in the first 1–2d of each period. May be associated GI disturbance, e.g. diarrhoea/vomiting. Young women (<20y) with no other symptoms do not require examination unless pathology is suspected. Perform a full abdominal and pelvic examination if older woman or atypical features. Treatment is with:

- **NSAID** (e.g. mefenamic acid 500mg tds, ibuprofen 200–400mg tds)—effective in 80–90%; start when bleeding starts
- **CHC**—effective in 80–90%

❶ 10–20% do not respond—consider a missed cause.

Secondary dysmenorrhea Suggests underlying pathology. *Causes:*

- Endometriosis/adenomyosis
- Chronic pelvic infection
- IUCD/IUS
- Endometrial polyps
- Cervical stenosis
- Submucous fibroid
- History of pelvic/abdominal surgery
- Intrauterine adhesions (Asherman's syndrome)
- Psychosexual problems

Starts later than teenage years, or may present as a change in pattern, type, or intensity of usual pain. Pain can start just before the period and last throughout. Often associated with deep dyspareunia ± other symptoms, e.g. abnormal bleeding, vaginal discharge.

Assessment and management of 2° dysmenorrhoea Do an abdominal, vaginal speculum, and bimanual pelvic examination. Look for tethered/fixed uterus, uterine tenderness, masses, thickening in the posterior fornix (associated with dyspareunia and endometriosis) and/or endocervical polyps. Do a cervical smear if overdue and offer STI screen if sexually active; consider referral for pelvic USS. Treat any underlying cause, else refer for further investigation (e.g. laparoscopy, hysteroscopy).

Mittelschmerz 📖 p. 702

Table 21.3 Causes of pelvic pain

Gynaecological		Non-gynaecological	
Acute	**Chronic**	**Acute**	**Chronic**
Ectopic pregnancy	Endometriosis	Appendicitis	Irritable bowel syndrome (50%)
Pelvic inflammatory disease	Adhesions	Colitis	Interstitial cystitis
Endometriosis	Fibroids	Diverticulitis	Musculoskeletal
Torsion of fibroid	Prolapse	Cystitis	Psychological*
Dysmenorrhoea	Ovarian cyst	Renal stones	Bowel or bladder cancer
Ovarian cyst (torsion, bleeding, abscess, or rupture)	Venous congestion	Neurological	Nerve entrapment
	Pelvic inflammatory disease	Psychological	

*Psychological pain may be a consequence of and perpetuate physical pain. Diagnosis is one of exclusion.

Further information

RCOG The initial management of chronic pelvic pain (2012)
📶 www.rcog.org.uk

Endometriosis and adenomyosis

Endometriosis Presence of tissue histologically similar to endometrium outside the uterine cavity and myometrium. Most commonly found in the pelvis but can occur anywhere. Affects 10–15% of women presenting with gynaecological symptoms. Ovarian deposits may result in *chocolate cysts* or *endometriomas*.

Risk factors Heavy periods; frequent cycles. ❶ Oral contraceptives and pregnancy are protective.

Theories of pathogenesis

- **Reflux and implantation** Menstrual loss flows backwards through Fallopian tubes into the pelvis where it implants into the peritoneum and continues to grow under the influence of oestrogen
- **Transformation/induction** Peritoneal tissue transforms into endometrium under the influence of ovarian steroids or as a result of factors released when menstrual loss refluxes into the peritoneum
- **Mechanical transplantation** Endometrium transplanted from one location to another (e.g. during surgery) will grow at that new site
- **Vascular ± lymphatic spread** Thought to explain distant deposits, e.g. lungs, brain

History

- 3 cardinal symptoms: dysmenorrhoea; dyspareunia; pelvic pain (typically, varies markedly across the menstrual cycle)
- Menorrhagia   • Infertility   • Bowel/bladder symptoms

Examination Abdominal, speculum, and bimanual pelvic examination looking for pelvic tenderness, pelvic mass, and/or fixation of the uterus. Occasionally tender nodules can be felt on the utero-sacral ligaments.

Investigation Offer sexually active women a STI screen. Refer for transvaginal pelvic USS (useful to identify ovarian endometriomas but not peritoneal disease) ± to gynaecology for laparoscopy (❶ 30–50% of diagnostic laparoscopies are –ve and, if found, extent of endometriosis often does not correlate with severity of symptoms). MRI may also be useful.

Management of infertility Refer for specialist opinion—📖 p. 772
- If tubal damage—options are reconstructive surgery or IVF
- If no tubal damage—laparoscopic ablation may improve fertility

Management of pain and bleeding

- Cyclical pain and/or heavy periods—NSAID, e.g. ibuprofen 400mg tds prn from first day of period
- IUS ↓ endometriosis pain with symptom control maintained >3y; depo-medroxyprogesterone acetate injection is an alternative
- If a woman is not trying to conceive and there is no evidence of a pelvic mass, try a progestogen (e.g. norethisterone 10–15mg/d for ≥4–6mo—starting on day 5 of each cycle—if spotting occurs ↑ dose to 20–25mg/d and stop once bleeding has ceased) or continuous CHC (3 or 4 packets without a break then 7d break)
- If symptoms are not controlled—refer

Specialist treatments

- **Medical options** Include gestrinone and GnRH agonists (e.g. goserelin) ± HRT (↓ side effects and bone demineralization). Side effects can be troublesome
- **Surgical options** Include laparoscopy or laparotomy with ablation of lesions and division of dense adhesions; tubal surgery; hysterectomy. Laparoscopic ablation of mild endometriosis may ↑ fertility

❶ For all forms of specialist treatment there is a 15–20% recurrence rate. If relapse in <6mo, treatment has failed and an alternative form of treatment should be tried. If relapse in >6mo, consider the condition to have relapsed and repeat treatment.

Psychological support Many women will have had pain for years. Often there is delay in diagnosis of the cause—and, frequently, they have been told it is psychosomatic. Be sympathetic and supportive and use a cooperative strategy for management.

Adenomyosis Usually affects multiparous premenopausal women aged >35y. Caused by extension of endometrial tissue and stroma into the uterine myometrium. May coexist with endometriosis (15%) but a separate entity.

Presentation May be asymptomatic, or present with dysmenorrhoea (pain often peaks towards the end of menstruation), dyspareunia, and menorrhagia. On examination, the uterus may be symmetrically enlarged and tender.

Management No treatment needed if asymptomatic. Refer for further investigation of symptoms. MRI may confirm diagnosis but diagnosis is often only confirmed on histology after hysterectomy. Treatment is usually surgical with hysterectomy ± bilateral salpingo-oophorectomy. Medical treatment with GnRH analogues is a short-term option but symptoms return once withdrawn unless the woman has reached the menopause in the interim.

Pelvic venous congestion Chronic pelvic pain due to dilation and congestion of pelvic veins. Remains a controversial diagnosis. There is no diagnostic test; refer to exclude PID and endometriosis. Treatment is with progestogens, e.g. medroxyprogesterone 30mg od for 6mo, or GnRH analogues, e.g. goserelin 3.6mg monthly for 6mo. Symptoms often recur following treatment.

Further information

RCOG ℅ www.rcog.org.uk
- The investigation and management of endometriosis (2006)
- The initial management of chronic pelvic pain (2012)

Information and support for patients
Endometriosis UK ☎ 0808 808 2227 ℅ www.endo.org.uk
Pelvic Pain Support Network ℅ www.pelvicpain.org.uk

Prolapse

Prolapse Pelvic organs herniate into the vagina due to poor pelvic muscle tone and weakness of pelvic ligaments. Affects 12–30% of multiparous and 2% of nulliparous women. Good obstetric practice ↓ risk. Risk is ↑ by:

- Childbirth
- Menopause
- Coughing and straining
- Congenital connective tissue disorders

Terminology Named according to the organs involved:

- **Cystocoele**—bladder bulges into the vagina
- **Urethrocoele**—urethra bulges into the vagina
- **Rectocoele**—rectum bulges into the vagina
- **Enterocoele**—loops of intestine bulge into the vagina
- **Uterine**—uterus descends into the vagina

Uterine prolapse is further classified by degree. The most dependent portion of the prolapse is assessed whilst straining:

- **1st degree prolapse**—the cervix remains in the vagina
- **2nd degree prolapse**—the cervix protrudes from vagina on coughing/ straining
- **3rd degree prolapse (procidentia)**—the uterus lies outside the vagina and may ulcerate

Presentation Dragging sensation, feeling of 'something coming down', or a 'lump'. Symptoms are worse when upright, i.e. whilst awake, and exacerbated by standing for a long time, coughing, or straining.

Associated symptoms Depending on structures involved—stress incontinence (📖 p. 450), difficulty defecating, recurrent cystitis, and/or frequency of micturition. In severe cases renal failure may occur due to ureteric kinking.

Examination/investigation Check abdominal examination to exclude pelvic masses. Then in left lateral position with Sims speculum, ask the patient to bear down and watch the vaginal walls. Exclude pelvic mass by bimanual examination. Dipstick urine ± send for M,C&S.

Management Choice of treatment depends on patient preference, general health, degree of prolapse, severity of symptoms, and wish to preserve fertility and sexual activity. *Options include:*

- **Lifestyle measures** Weight ↓; smoking cessation
- **General measures** Treatment of coexisting conditions exacerbating prolapsed, e.g. chronic cough due to COPD or asthma, constipation, menopause/atrophic vaginitis
- **Physiotherapy** Pelvic floor exercises (📖 p. 841). Refer to specialist physiotherapy if simple self-help techniques fail
- **Ring pessary** Useful for those too frail for surgery, women who have symptoms but do not want surgery or as a temporary measure whilst awaiting surgery. Change pessary every 3–6mo. *Shelf pessaries* may be useful for women who cannot retain a ring pessary—consider referral
- **Surgery** Refer to gynaecology if the woman is fit for surgery and symptoms are of sufficient severity to warrant operation *and/or* she has incontinence *and/or* recurrent UTI. Surgical options include repair operations (anterior or posterior colporrhaphy), colpo-vaginal suspension, and hysterectomy (vaginal or abdominal)

Fitting a ring pessary

- Measure the approximate size required manually—the distance between posterior fornix and pubic bone can be measured roughly against the index finger
- Soften the ring in hot water and lubricate it well
- Insert the ring into the posterior fornix and tuck it above pubic bone
- Change the pessary every 3–6mo. Inspect the vagina for damage (e.g. ulceration) before inserting the new ring

Potential problems

- **Discomfort** Ring may be too big (try smaller size) or atrophic vaginitis (try topical oestrogen)
- **Infection** Remove, clear infection then try again
- **Ulceration** Remove, allow to heal, consider alternatives or reinsert when fully healed
- **Expulsion** Ring may be too small, pelvic musculature indequate, or retropubic rim unsuitable

Uterine problems

Postmenopausal bleeding (PMB) Perform a pelvic examination, including speculum examination of the cervix.

Refer urgently (to be seen in <2wk by a team specializing in gynaecological cancer):
- All women with PMB
- Endometrial thickness >4mm on USS done for another reason

Differential diagnosis Atrophic change (most common); endometrial hyperplasia; endometrial polyps; endometritis; endometrial malignancy (10% referred); cervical malignancy; fibroids; uterine sarcoma; non-genital causes (bladder and bowel).

Pelvic or abdominal mass Refer urgently for USS if abdominal/pelvic mass that is not clearly uterine fibroids and not of GI/urological origin. If USS is suggestive of cancer or urgent USS is not available, refer urgently.

Congenital abnormalities of the female genital tract
- **Duplication** Of the cervix and/or uterus; vaginal septum; bicornuate uterus (of varying degrees). Usually found incidentally. May cause problems in pregnancy/with IUD. Refer if needed
- **Imperforate hymen** May cause cryptomenorrhoea which presents as 1° amenorrhoea (📖 p. 706). Refer for surgical release if suspected
- **Ambiguous genitalia** 📖 p. 895
- **Cervical incompetence** 📖 p. 816

Uterine retroversion 20% have a retroverted, retroflexed uterus. May be difficult to palpate bimanually—push on the cervix to antevert.

Fibroids (uterine leiomyoma) Benign tumours of the smooth muscle of the myometrium affecting 1 in 5 women. Often multiple. Oestrogen-dependent so regress post-menopause. Named by location:
- Pedunculated
- Intramural (centrally in myometrium)
- Cervical
- Subserosal (bulge into peritoneum)
- Submucosal (bulge into endometrium)
- Separate from uterus, especially in broad ligament from embryonal remnants

Risk factors Nulliparity; obesity; FH of fibroids; African origin.

Presentation Usually asymptomatic. May cause:
- Pelvic pressure/discomfort and/or backache
- Menorrhagia—usually submucous fibroids distorting endometrial cavity
- Pain: torsion (pedunculated fibroid); degeneration. Red degeneration may occur in pregnancy (pain, fever, and local tenderness)
- Urinary symptoms—may press on the bladder →↑ frequency or a feeling of incomplete emptying or difficulty passing urine
- Infertility—may act as a 'natural IUCD'
- Problems in pregnancy—abnormal lie and ↑ risk of post-partum haemorrhage. Risk of miscarriage is not ↑
- Bulky uterus ± pelvic mass felt abdominally

Pelvic USS is diagnostic. Check FBC if menorrhagia. ❶ Calcified fibroids may be an incidental finding on X-ray.

Management If asymptomatic/mild symptoms—no treatment needed. Otherwise, management depends on presence of symptoms, number and location of fibroids, fertility plans, and patient's preferences:
- **Medical**—CHC or IUS ↓ menstrual loss; GnRH analogues (maximum use 6mo due to risk of osteopenia) and selective progesterone receptor modulators (e.g. asoprisnil) cause fibroid shrinkage
- **Surgical**—Uterine artery embolization; myomectomy (removal of fibroids only); hysteroscopic resection; hysterectomy

Endometrial proliferation Oestrogen causes endometrial prolife-ration; progesterone causes endometrial maturation; shedding follows withdrawal of oestrogen and progesterone. If oestrogen is given alone, the endometrium proliferates uncontrolled, resulting in irregular and heavy bleeding, polyps, and ↑ risk of endometrial carcinoma. Caused by anovulatory cycles or administration of unopposed oestrogen.

Endometrial cancer In the UK, ~7,700 women each year are diagnosed with endometrial cancer (5% of all ♀ cancers). It is predominantly a disease of postmenopausal women with 93% of cases diagnosed in women >50y (peak age 70–74y). *Risk factors:*
- Age
- Obesity
- Nulliparity
- Late menopause
- DM
- Drugs—unopposed oestrogen, tamoxifen
- Granulosa cell ovarian tumour
- FH—of breast, ovary, or colon cancer
- Previous pelvic irradiation
- Hereditary non-polyposis colorectal cancer

Risk is ↓ with current or past use of the COC pill and/or progestogens.

Presentation 15% are asymptomatic. Most present with PMB (75–80%)—any woman presenting with PMB has endometrial carcinoma until proven otherwise. Premenopausally tends to occur in overweight women and present with continual bleeding. Rarely detected on cervical smear.

Management Refer any woman with PMB to gynaecology for further investigation. Assessment comprises transvaginal USS to look at endometrial thickness ± endometrial sampling with pipelle or hysteroscopy.

Treatment TAH and BSO ± radiotherapy and/or chemotherapy depending on the likelihood of recurrence. Survival depends on the age of the patient and stage/grade of the tumour. Stage I disease—85% 5y survival; stage IV—25% 5y survival.

Endometritis Acute infection of the endometrium. Uncommon amongst premenopausal women. Usually occurs after surgery (including IUCD insertion) or childbirth. Presents with fever, lower abdominal pain, uterine tenderness, and/or purulent discharge (may be blood stained). Take high vaginal/endocervical swabs for M,C&S (including chlamydia).

Management Treat with antibiotics, e.g. doxycycline 100mg bd for 14d + metronidazole 400mg bd for 1wk or azithromycin 1g stat for chlamydia.

Pyometra is a complication (uterine cavity fills with pus)—suspect if endo-metritis fails to clear and refer to gynaecology urgently.

Further information
NICE Referral guidelines for suspected cancer (2005) www.nice.org.uk

Ovarian disease

Refer urgently to gynaecology (to be seen in <2wk) if ascites or suspected ovarian mass on abdominal/pelvic examination.[N]

Check CA125[N] (❗ particularly if >50y) if a woman reports[N]

* New IBS >50y
* Unexplained weight ↓, fatigue, or change in bowel habit
* Any of the following >12x/mo:
  * Persistent abdominal distension ('bloating')
  * Pelvic/abdominal pain
  * Feeling full ('early satiety') and/or loss of appetite
  * ↑ urinary frequency/urgency

If CA125 is ≥35iu/mL refer for USS. If suspected ovarian cancer on USS refer urgently to gynaecology (to be seen in <2wk).

If CA125 <35iu/mL consider investigating other causes of symptoms.

Causes of ↑ CA125

* 1% of healthy individuals
* Cancer—ovarian cancer (↑ in 85% with epithelial ovarian cancer); other intra-abdominal cancers
* Non-malignant conditions, e.g. endometriosis, PID, menstruation, DM, CCF, pleural effusion, liver disease, diverticulitis, appendicitis, ascites

Ovarian tumours May be solid or cystic. In ♀ of reproductive age, >80% are benign. In postmenopausal women, the proportion of malignant ovarian tumours is 50%. Classified according to tissue of origin:

* Tumours of surface epithelium—60%—see Table 21.4
* Germ cell tumours—15–25%
* Gonadal stromal tumours—5–10%
* Metastatic (from breast, stomach, colon, or genital tract)—5–10%

❗ Early tumours are often asymptomatic and may be an incidental finding on abdominal/pelvic examination or USS done for another reason.

Simple, physiological, or functional cysts Common and often incidental finding on USS in premenopausal women. May cause pain due to tension within the cyst, rupture, torsion, or bleeding into the cyst.

* **Follicular cyst** An ovarian follicle fails to rupture. Unilocular and can reach a diameter of 10cm. Usually regress during the subsequent cycle. More common in women using progesterone-only contraception
* **Luteal cyst** Forms if there is excessive bleeding into the corpus luteum. May be tender, cause abdominal pain (sometimes acute abdomen), and delay the next period

Management

* Premenopausal—check CA125 and refer to gynaecology if multilocular/solid elements; >8cm diameter; or <8cm diameter but fails to regress in <6wk. Urgent referral if CA125 ≥35iu/mL
* If postmenopausal—refer to gyanecology (urgent if CA125 ≥35iu/mL or any sinister features on USS)

Chocolate cyst/endometrioma 📖 p. 716

Table 21.4 Tumours of surface epithelium

Type of tumour	Subtype	10y survival
Serous Peak age 30–40; 20–50% of ovarian tumours; 30% bilateral	**Benign serous cystadenoma**—60% of serous tumours; 25% of all benign ovarian tumours	100%
	Borderline serous cystadenoma—10% of serous tumours	90–95%
	Malignant serous cystadenocarcinoma—35–50% of serous tumours; bilateral in 40–60%; 40–50% of all malignant ovarian tumours; 85% have spread outside the ovaries at the time of diagnosis; >50% are >15cm diameter at diagnosis	15%
Mucinous Can be very large; often multilocular; often contain viscid mucin—if burst, can cause *pseudomyxoma peritonei* (mucin -secreting cells are spread throughout the peritoneum)	**Benign mucinous cystadenoma**—peak incidence aged 30–50y; 80% of mucinous tumours; bilateral in 5–10%; 20–25% of all benign ovarian tumours	100%
	Borderline mucinous cystadenoma—10% of mucinous tumours; bilateral in 10%	90–95%
	Malignant mucinous cystadenocarcinoma—Peak age 40–70y; 10% of mucinous tumours; bilateral in 15–30%; 5–10% of all 1° ovarian cancers; average diameter at diagnosis 16cm	34%

Endometrioid—Peak age 50–60y; 30–50% bilateral; benign tumours are rare; malignant tumours account for 20–25% of all malignant ovarian neoplasms; 30% coexist with endometrial cancer; 10% coexist with endometriosis

Clear cell (mesonephroid)—5% bilateral; 5–10% of all malignant ovarian neoplasms; 25% coexist with endometriosis; associated with hypercalcaemia

Brenner (transitional cell)—Rare—2–3% of all ovarian tumours; >90% are benign. If malignant, have poor prognosis; <5% are bilateral; associated with mucinous cystadenoma and cystic teratoma in 1:10 cases

Undifferentiated carcinoma—<10% epithelial neoplasms; no histological features that characterize it

 Ovarian cysts in children Unusual. Refer any ovarian cysts >2cm found in a premenarchal child for further assessment.

Ovarian hyperstimulation Iatrogenic condition resulting from overstimulation of the ovaries in the course of infertility treatment.
- **Mild** >10% patients receiving gonadotrophin therapy. Abdominal pain/swelling ± vomiting/diarrhoea. Manage with rest and simple analgesia, e.g. ibuprofen or paracetamol prn.
- **Severe** 1% patients receiving gonadotrophin therapy. Abdominal pain/distension, vomiting/diarrhoea, ascites, pleural effusion, and/or venous thrombosis. Admit.

Further information
NICE Ovarian cancer (2011) ℘ www.nice.org.uk

Ovarian cancer and polycystic ovaries

Refer urgently to gynaecology (to be seen in <2wk)[N] if ascites or ovarian mass on abdominal/pelvic examination[N].

Check CA125 (❗ particularly if >50y) if a woman reports[N]
- New IBS >50y
- Unexplained weight ↓, fatigue, or change in bowel habit
- Any of the following >12x/mo:
  - Persistent abdominal distension ('bloating')
  - Pelvic/abdominal pain
  - Feeling full ('early satiety') and/or loss of appetite
  - ↑ urinary frequency/urgency

If CA125 is ≥35iu/mL Refer for USS. If suspected ovarian cancer on USS, refer urgently to gynaecology (to be seen in <2wk).

If CA125 <35iu/mL Consider investigating other causes of symptoms.

Epithelial ovarian cancer (EOC) 90% of ovarian cancers. 7,000 cases are diagnosed each year in the UK (2.5% of all cancers) and ovarian cancer accounts for 6% of ♀ deaths. In the UK, ~80% of patients with ovarian cancer have had symptoms for <4wk before seeing their GP.

Risk factors
- **Age** Peak age 50–70y; 85% ovarian cancers occur in ♀ >50y
- **Family history** 10% of cancers occur in women with FH. 3–4x ↑ risk if one first-degree relative with ovarian cancer—but only 40% of familial cancer is explained by known gene mutations (e.g. BRCA1/2)
- **Reproductive factors** Greater exposure to ovulation ↑ risk (e.g. infertility, nulliparity, low parity)
- **Lifestyle** ↑ risk with obesity and smoking (mucinous tumours only)
- **Other medical problems** Breast cancer aged <40y (4x ↑ risk); cervical cancer (if radiotherapy); endometriosis; benign ovarian cysts
- **Other factors** Height >1.7m; long-term perineal use of talcum powder (❡); asbestos exposure

Protective factors Pregnancy—the more pregnancies, the lower the risk; COC pill—↓ risk by 60%—protective effect is maintained >20y after the COC pill has been discontinued; breastfeeding—may ↓ risk by 20%; tubal ligation—↓ risk by 30–70%; hysterectomy—↓ risk by 50%.

Prevention Ovarian cancer fulfils some criteria for population screening. Trials are currently underway in the UK. Meanwhile, high-risk women (with ≥2 same-side family members with breast/ovarian cancer aged <50y) may be referred for specialist gynaecology and/or genetic advice ± for laparoscopic bilateral salpingo-oophorectomy.

Treatment Specialist management is with laparotomy ± adjuvant treatment with chemotherapy. *Prognosis:* stage I—92% 5y survival; stage IV (distant metastases—40% new diagnoses)—6% 5y survival.

Sex-cord stromal tumours, e.g. thecomas, fibromas, Sertoli/Leydig cell or granulosa cell tumours. Usually present early with symptoms of hormone production, e.g. precocious puberty, PMB, or virilism. Granulosa cell tumours are linked with endometrial hyperplasia/carcinoma.

Germ-cell tumours, e.g. mature teratoma (ovarian dermoid cyst), immature teratoma, dysgerminoma, endodermal sinus tumour (yolk sac tumour), mixed germ-cell tumour. Peak incidence in early 20s. Most are unilateral. Associated with ↑ AFP and ↑ β-HCG (both are used as tumour markers). Prognosis is good with the majority cured.

Polycystic ovarian syndrome (PCOS) or *Stein–Leventhal syndrome*. Up to 1 in 3 premenopausal women have polycystic ovaries on USS—1 in 3 of those women have PCOS. Cause is unknown—often there is a family history. Diagnosis requires presence of ≥2 of:

- **Oligomenorrhoea and/or anovulation**
- **Hyperandrogenism**—clinical and/or biochemical
- **Polycystic ovaries**—defined as the presence of ≥12 follicles in each ovary measuring 2–9mm in diameter and/or ovarian volume >10cm^3

Symptoms and signs May be asymptomatic or have ≥1 of:

- Menstrual irregularity—oligomenorrhoea/amenorrhoea (affects 67%— more common if BMI ≥30kg/m^2), dysfunctional uterine bleeding
- Anovulatory infertility
- Central obesity
- Acne
- Hirsutism
- Male pattern baldness

Investigations

- **USS ovaries** >12 cysts of 2–9mm in diameter (string of pearls sign)
- **Blood** ↑ testosterone (>2.5nmol/L—if >4.8 nmol/L, exclude other causes of androgen hypersecretion, e.g. tumour, Cushing's syndrome), ↓ sex hormone binding globulin (SHBG)

Complications Insulin resistance—2x ↑ incidence of DM; ↑ CVD risk— central body fat distribution, obesity, ↑ BP, ↑ triglycerides, ↓ HDL; 3x ↑ risk of stroke/TIA; ↑ endometrial cancer risk; obstructive sleep apnoea.

Management In all cases, encourage weight ↓ and exercise.

- If oligomenorrhoeic consider progestogens to induce a withdrawal bleed every 2–3mo to ↓ risk of endometrial hyperplasia
- Consider the COC pill to regulate menstruation; COC pills with anti-androgen (e.g. co-cyprindiol) may ↓ acne/hirsutism
- Consider offering annual HbA1c/FBG check—particularly if obese (BMI >30), FH of DM, or aged >40y. Screen pregnant women with PCOS for gestational DM with a GTT at <20wk gestation (📖 p. 828)
- Clomifene can be used to induce ovulation—📖 p. 772
- Metformin (unlicensed) may be helpful for insulin sensitivity and menstrual disturbance. Also used for infertility if clomifene has failed
- Hirsutism—📖 p. 342

Further information

NICE Ovarian cancer (2011) ℘ www.nice.org.uk
RCOG Long-term consequences of polycystic ovary syndrome (2007) ℘ www.rcog.org.uk

Further information and support for patients

Ovacome ☎ 0845 371 0554 ℘ www.ovacome.org.uk
CancerHelp ☎ 0808 800 4040 ℘ www.cancerhelp.org.uk
Macmillan Cancer Support ☎ 0808 808 0000 ℘ www.macmillan.org.uk
Verity Support for women with PCOS ℘ www.verity-pcos.org.uk

Conditions of the cervix

Refer urgently (to be seen in <2wk) To gynaecology:
- If clinical features of cervical cancer. Do not perform a cervical smear before referral or delay referral due to previous −ve smear
- If ascites or pelvic mass of abdominal/pelvic examination
- All patients with postmenopausal bleeding who are not taking HRT
- Patients on HRT with persistent or unexplained postmenopausal bleeding after cessation of HRT for 6wk
- All patients taking tamoxifen with postmenopausal bleeding

Consider urgent referral If persistent intermenstrual bleeding and negative pelvic examination.

Perform a full pelvic examination including speculum examination of the cervix, for patients with:
- Alterations in menstrual cycle
- Intermenstrual bleeding
- Post-coital bleeding
- Postmenopausal bleeding
- Vaginal discharge

Cervical intraepithelial neoplasia (CIN) Pre-malignant change of the cervical epithelium. The majority of these changes are found in asymptomatic women <45y (peak incidence 25–29y). CIN is a histological diagnosis resulting from biopsy—usually following an abnormal smear.
- **CIN 1** Mild/moderate dysplasia—nuclear atypia confined to basal third of the epithelium. ❶ CIN 1 may revert to normality
- **CIN 2** Nuclear atypia in basal two-thirds of the epithelium
- **CIN 3**—Severe dysplasia/carcinoma *in situ*—full thickness epithelial nuclear abnormalities

Treatment Depends on grade of histological abnormality. For women with high-grade lesions (CIN 2/3) treatment options include ablation, excision (large loop excision of the transformation zone or LLETZ, knife cone biopsy), or hysterectomy.

Cervical cancer In the UK, 3,378 women each year are diagnosed with cervical cancer (2% of all ♀ cancers). Almost exclusively occurs in women who are/have been sexually active. 2 peaks of incidence—women in their late 30s and 70s/80s. 80% are squamous cell cancer—the remainder adenocarcinoma. Incidence is dropping probably due to the cervical cancer screening programme and changes in sexual practices.

Risk factors
- Low social class
- Smoking
- Early age of 1st intercourse
- Early age of 1st pregnancy
- Multiple sexual partners
- HPV infection (types 16, 18, 31, and 33)
- History of dyskaryosis
- Method of contraception (↓ with barrier methods; ↑ if >5y COC use)
- Immunosuppression, HIV

Presentation May be found on routine cervical screening. Symptoms include post-coital, intermenstrual, postmenopausal bleeding, and/or offensive vaginal discharge. Speculum examination may reveal cervical ulceration/mass or a cervix that bleeds easily.

Management Refer urgently to gynaecology. Treatment is with surgery ± radiotherapy depending on the stage of the disease:

- **Stage 1** Microinvasive cancer (A) or cancer confined in the cervix (B). 65% women present at stage 1. 5y survival ~80–99%
- **Stage 2** Invasion into the upper third of the vagina (A) or parametria (B) but not to the pelvic side wall. 5y survival ~60–90%
- **Stage 3** Extension to the lower third of the vagina (A) or pelvic side wall (B). 5y survival ≈30–50%.
- **Stage 4** Tumour involving bladder/rectum (A) or extrapelvic spread (B). 5y survival ~20%

Prevention of cervical cancer A vaccination programme targeting girls aged 12–13y is currently underway in the UK to protect them against the strains of HPV that cause cervical cancer 📖 p. 749.

Cervical screening 📖 p. 728

Cervical erosion/ectropion Physiological. An erosion or ectropion is the area of columnar epithelium visible within the vagina when the squamo-columnar junction moves down the cervix at times of high oestrogen exposure (e.g. pregnancy, CHC, puberty). Only treat if:

- Abnormal cervical smear, *or*
- Symptoms are causing problems, e.g. post-coital or intermenstrual bleeding, or excess discharge—refer to gynaecologist for cautery. If using the CHC, consider switching to an alternative

Nabothian cysts Cervical mucus retention cysts. Usually asymptomatic—no treatment needed. Refer for cautery if troublesome discharge.

Cervicitis Presents with vaginal discharge, intermenstrual/post-coital bleeding, and/or pain. Speculum examination shows mucopurulent discharge and inflamed, friable cervix. *Causes:* Chlamydia (50%), gonococcus, and HSV. Investigate with swabs for M,C&S, and treat the cause.

Cervical polyps Develop from the endocervix and protrude into the vagina through the external os. Usually asymptomatic although there may be ↑ vaginal discharge and the lowest part of the polyp may ulcerate and bleed causing intermenstrual, postmenopausal, and/or post-coital bleeding. The vast majority are benign.

Treatment Avulsion (send for histology). Cauterize base with silver nitrate stick if possible. Frequently recur. If postmenopausal, intermenstrual, or post-coital bleeding, refer to gynaecology to exclude other pathology.

Cervical incompetence 📖 p. 816

Further information

NICE Referral guidelines for suspected cancer (2005) ℘ www.nice.org.uk

Information and support for patients

Healthtalkonline Patient experience database ℘ www.healthtalkonline.org
CancerHelp ☎ 0808 800 4040 ℘ www.cancerhelp.org.uk
Macmillan Cancer Support ☎ 0808 808 0000 ℘ www.macmillan.org.uk

Cervical cancer screening

Screening prevents ~1,000–4,000 deaths/y in the UK from squamous cell cancer of the cervix.

Taking a smear Ensure adequate training—poor smear-taking misses 20% abnormalities. Courses are available—update skills every 3y. Give all women information about the test, condition being sought, possible results of screening, and their implications.

Liquid-based cytology (LBC) Cells are collected from the cervix with a brush; the head of the brush is either broken off or rinsed into a vial containing preservative fluid before going to the laboratory for examination. LBC ↓ the number of inadequate smears taken as cervical cells can be examined even if the sample is contaminated with blood, pus, or mucus.

Timing Avoid menstruation if possible (note on the request form if unavoidable). Ideal time is mid-cycle. Routine bimanual examination is unnecessary—only do if clinically indicated (e.g. painful/heavy periods).

Screening interval See Table 21.5.

Organization of the cervical screening programme Practices undertaking cervical screening must:
- Provide information to eligible women to allow them to make an informed decision about taking part in the programme
- Perform the cervical screening test (and ensure staff are properly trained and equipped to perform the test)
- Arrange for women to be informed about the results of their tests (see Tables 21.6 and 21.7)
- Ensure that results are followed up appropriately, and
- Maintain records of tests carried out, results, and follow-up

HPV testing Infection with human papillomavirus (HPV) 16, 18, 31, and 33 is associated with CIN/cervical cancer. 99.7% of cervical cancers contain HPV DNA and women with HPV infection are 70x more likely to develop high-grade cervical abnormalities. HPV triage tests cells from LBC samples with borderline or low-grade abnormalities for high-risk HPV. Those that test −ve are returned to normal recall; those that test +ve are referred for colposcopy. HPV testing is also used as a test-of-cure after treatment for CIN.

Table 21.5 Cervical screening programmes in different parts of the UK

Nation	Age range of women screened*	Screening interval
England	25–64y	3-yearly from 25–49y 5-yearly from 50–64y
Scotland	20–60y	3-yearly
Wales	20–64y	3-yearly
Northern Ireland	25–64y	3-yearly from 25–49y 5-yearly from 50–64y

*Women older than the upper age for screening can be screened if they have never been screened previously or are under recall for previous abnormal results.

Table 21.6 Interpretation of smear results and action

Result	What does it mean?	Action
Normal	No nuclear abnormalities	Place on routine recall
Inadequate (~2% with LBC)	Insufficient/inadequate material	Repeat the smear as soon as convenient
		After three consecutive inadequate results, refer for colposcopy
Borderline or mild dyskaryosis (5–10% smears are borderline or mild)	Some nuclear abnormalities that are either inconclusive or indicative of low-grade CIN	Check HPV status If HPV –ve, return to routine 3y or 5y recall, depending on age If HPV +ve, refer for colposcopy
Moderate dyskaryosis (1% smears)	Nuclear abnormalities reflecting probable CIN 2	Refer to colposcopy
Severe dyskaryosis or worse (0.6% smears)	Nuclear abnormalities reflecting probable CIN 3	Refer to colposcopy

Other possible abnormalities seen on cervical smear
- *Dyskaryotic glandular cells*—refer for colposcopy
- *Atrophic*—common in peri-/postmenopausal women. No action
- *Endometrial cells*—may be normal if IUCD *in situ*, hormonal treatment, or first half of 28d cycle. Otherwise, discuss with laboratory. Refer if reported as abnormal
- *Inflammatory changes*—common finding. Take chlamydial, endocervical, and high vaginal swabs. Treat as necessary
- *Trichomonas, candida or changes associated with HSV infection*—treat trichomonas or candida. Discuss any new diagnosis of HSV with the patient
- *Actinomyces*—associated with IUCDs—🕮 p. 764

Table 21.7 Follow-up after colposcopy

Colposcopy result	Treatment	Follow-up
Negative (no CIN)	No	Normal recall
CIN 1	No	12mo with cytology ± colposcopy ± HPV triage (if borderline changes)
	Yes	Cytology at 6mo
CIN 2/3	Yes	If normal or borderline/mild changes— HPV testing to confirm cure; if HPV –ve return to 3y or 5y recall. If HPV +ve, repeat colposcopy
		If moderate/severe changes—repeat colposcopy

Further information
NHS Cervical Screening ℘ www.cancerscreening.nhs.uk

Information for patients
Cervical screening—the facts ℘ www.cancerscreening.nhs.uk

Vaginal and vulval problems

Refer urgently (to be seen in <2wk) to gynaecology If unexplained vulval lump or vulval bleeding due to ulceration.

Vulval pruritus/pain It is reasonable to treat in primary care. Follow-up until symptoms resolve or diagnosis is confirmed. If symptoms persist, refer—urgency depends on symptoms/concern about cancer.

Symptoms/signs
- Vaginal discharge/infection—📖 p. 736
- Vulval ulceration—genital ulcers (📖 p. 735)

Vulval itching (pruritus vulvae) Treat the cause: infection (e.g. candida, HSV, warts, threadworms, pubic lice, scabies); atrophic vulvitis; vulval dystrophy; vulval carcinoma; poor hygiene; skin conditions (e.g. eczema). ❶ Always exclude iron deficiency as a cause of itching.

Vulval lumps Common and usually benign.
- **General causes** Sebaceous cyst; varicose veins; haematoma; benign skin tumour (lipoma, papilloma, etc.); malignant skin tumour (1° or 2°)
- **Specific causes** Bartholin's gland cyst/abscess; urethral caruncle; endometriosis; carcinoma of the vulva; inguinal hernia

❶ Remember skin conditions (e.g. eczema, psoriasis) as a cause of vulval skin abnormalities.

Atrophic vaginitis Vaginal soreness, dyspareunia, and occasional spotting. The vagina looks pale and dry. Treat with topical oestrogens (usually nightly for 2wk, then 2x/wk for ≥3mo) or consider other HRT. ❶ Refer women with postmenopausal bleeding for assessment—📖 p. 721.

Vaginal cysts May arise from remnants of the mesonephric ducts (anterolaterally) or following surgery or episiotomy (posterior, lower third). Usually no treatment is needed. If symptomatic or large, refer to gynaecology for assessment ± removal.

Benign vaginal tumours Benign leiomyomas or fibromyomas are common. Refer for surgical removal.

Vaginal intraepithelial neoplasia (VAIN) Multifocal. Occurs in the upper third of the vagina—usually in association with CIN (📖 p. 726). May be asymptomatic or present with post-coital bleeding or abnormal vaginal discharge. Treatment is by local ablation.

Vaginal cancer Rare—most common >70y; 90% are squamous cell—the rest clear cell (associated with *in utero* stilboestrol), 2° tumour, or sarcoma. Presents with postmenopausal bleeding. Refer to gynaecology to be seen in <2wk. Treated with surgery (early stages) and/or radiotherapy.

Bartholin's gland swellings Painless vulval swelling due to obstruction of a Bartholin's gland duct → cyst formation. If infected, an abscess forms causing a painful, tender, red vulval lump. Cysts resolve spontaneously. Abscesses may resolve with antibiotics (if early) or discharge themselves. If not, admit for surgery (marsupialization).

Urethral caruncle Postmenopausal prolapse of the posterior urethral wall. Reddened area involving the posterior margin of the urethral opening. Usually asymptomatic—rarely bleeds or causes dyspareunia. Treat with topical oestrogen. Refer for surgery if symptoms persist.

Vulvodynia Chronic vulval pain without obvious cause. Common (4% of ♀) and may be generalized or localized. *Treatment:*

- **Topical** Avoid irritants e.g. bubblebath—use soap substitute (e.g. aqueous cream) and topical moisturizer. Lidocaine gel/cream 5% may control pain during intercourse (apply 10min before)
- **Oral** Amitriptyline (10–75mg)—start with low dose and titrate ↑ slowly; if ineffective or side effects, consider adding/substituting with pregabalin—📖 p. 218
- **Refer** If causing significant distress and not responding to treatment

Vulval dystrophy Associated with small risk of malignant change (<5%). Presents with vulval itching and/or soreness. Changes do not extend into the vagina. *Classification:*

- **Hypoplastic (lichen sclerosus)** Peak age 45–60y. Most common vulval dystrophy. 25% have a family/personal history of autoimmune disease, e.g. vitiligo, thyroid disease. Vulval skin looks atrophic ± white plaques (leukoplakia). 20% have white patches elsewhere on the body, but often these are asymptomatic
- **Hyperplasic** Usually affects postmenopausal women. There are multiple, symmetrical, thickened, hyperkeratotic lesions on the vulva

Management Treat with topical steroids—e.g. clobetasol propionate ointment od for 1mo, then alternate days for 1mo, then 2x/wk for 1mo. Refer to gynaecology/dermatology for biopsy if uncertain of diagnosis, no improvement with steroid treatment after 1mo, residual symptoms after 3mo or other lesions develop (e.g. vulval lump, other skin changes or ulceration). Symptoms may recur after treatment has stopped; retreat.

Vulval intraepithelial neoplasia (VIN) Some overlap with vulval dystrophy and may be associated with other genital tract neoplasia (e.g. CIN—📖 p. 726). Presents with abnormal vulval skin (pinky white + altered texture) ± white patches ± itch. Diagnosis is histological following skin biopsy and graded from VIN 1 (thickened epidermis—epithelial atypia in basal third only) to VIN 3 (carcinoma *in situ*/Bowen's disease with full thickness nuclear atypia). Refer patients with abnormal vulval skin (without candidal infection or other obvious cause) to gynaecology for skin biopsy. Treatment depends on site, histology, and extent.

Vulval carcinoma^G Rare—most common >70y. Most are squamous cell carcinoma; others—melanoma, basal cell carcinoma, Bartholin's gland carcinoma, and adenocarcinoma. The majority occur on the labia and spread to local LNs. Present early with chronic pruritus vulvae, vulval lump, or ulcer. Refer for confirmation of diagnosis. Treatment is surgical—5y survival rate ~95%.

Further information

NICE Referral guidelines for suspected cancer (2005) ✋ www.nice.org.uk
British Association for Sexual Health and HIV (BASHH) National guidelines on the management of vulval conditions (2007) ✋ www.bashh.org
British Association of Dermatologists Guidelines for the management of lichen sclerosus (2010) ✋ www.bad.org.uk
RCOG Vulval skin disorders (2011) ✋ www.rcog.org.uk

Information and support for patients

Vulval Pain Society ✋ www.vulvalpainsociety.org
National Lichen Sclerosus Support Group ✋ www.lichensclerosus.org

Chapter 22

Sexual health and contraception

Assessment of sexual health

Good communication skills are particularly important for clinicians when discussing sexual health problems and may improve health outcomes. Ensure a comfortable, private, and confidential environment.

General assessment Objectives are to:

- Establish a constructive relationship with the patient to enable patient and doctor to communicate effectively and serve as the basis for any subsequent therapeutic relationship
- Determine whether the patient has a sexual health problem and, if so, what that is
- Find out (where possible) what caused that problem
- Assess the patient's emotions and attitudes towards the problem. Be aware of signs of anxiety/distress. Recognize non-verbal cues
- Establish how it might be treated

History Use open questions at the start becoming directive when necessary—clarify, reflect, facilitate, listen. *Ask about:*

Presenting complaint Chronological account and concerns. If appropriate, ask about:

- Vaginal or urethral discharge
- Dysuria/other urinary symptoms
- Dyspareunia—pain on intercourse (🔲 p. 714)
- Erectile dysfunction—🔲 p. 776
- Genital skin problems—soreness, itching, ulceration, warts
- Perianal/anal symptoms
- Other symptoms, e.g. pelvic/abdominal/groin pain, deformity of the penis, haematospermia (blood in the ejaculate), retrograde ejaculation

Past medical history

- Similar symptoms—for suspected sexually transmitted infections (STIs), ask about previous STI, date of diagnosis, and treatment
- Obstetric history for women
- Urological problems and treatments or pelvic surgery
- Chronic medical problems—endocrine; cardiovascular; DM
- Medical treatment abroad—in certain countries, may be associated with ↑ HIV/hepatitis risk
- HIV testing/hepatitis B vaccination history

Drugs

- Prescription drugs, e.g. drugs associated with erectile dysfunction
- Illicit drugs—may be associated with erectile dysfunction, and history of injecting drug misuse is associated with ↑ hepatitis/HIV risk
- Allergies

Sexual history Current sexual partner (person with whom the patient had last sexual intercourse) and other recent sexual partners—if appropriate, ask about:

- Nature of relationship with partner—long-term partner; casual partner who could/could not be traced; paid-for partner
- Gender of partner

- Nature of intercourse—oral, vaginal, anal
- Contraception? Method used. Does the patient use a condom (male or female) regularly and consistently? Did it remain in place and intact?
- For women, establish date of LMP, cycle length, and regularity
- Symptoms in partner?

❶ For suspected STI, ask about all partners within the previous 3mo or incubation period of the suspected infection (if longer). If no partners are reported, note the last time the patient had sexual intercourse.

Social history
- Smoker?
- Alcohol consumption
- Travel abroad—if suspected STI, ask whether the patient had sexual intercourse abroad other than with their travelling partner, and with whom

Attitudes and beliefs
- How does the patient see the problem?
- What does he/she think is wrong?
- How does he/she think his/her partner views the situation?
- What does the patient want you to do about it?

Examination Examine the external genitalia and perianal area. Check groins for lymphadenopathy if STI is suspected. For women, perform pelvic and vaginal speculum examination. Consider digital rectal examination if indicated.

⚠ Explain the need for, and offer a suitably medically qualified chaperone for the examination of all patients. Record if a chaperone is declined.

Action
- Summarize the history back to the patient and give an opportunity for the patient to fill in any gaps
- Check that the patient has no other concerns
- Draw up a problem list and outline a management plan. Further investigations and interventions are guided by the findings on history and examination—so a good history and examination is essential
- Set a review date

Genital ulcers *Causes:* genital herpes; primary syphilis; Behçet's syndrome. If history of foreign travel, partner from abroad, or doubt about diagnosis refer to GUM clinic.

Further information
BASHH Sexual history taking (2012) ℘ www.bashh.org

Patient information about sexual health
Family Planning Association (FPA) ℘ www.fpa.org.uk
Department of Health Sexual Health Line ☎ 0800 567 123 (24h); Sexwise (for under 19s) ☎ 0800 28 29 30

Vaginal discharge

All women have some vaginal discharge. Physiological discharge varies considerably and is affected by the menstrual cycle.

- Before ovulation—mucus is clearer, wetter, stretchy, and slippery
- After ovulation—mucus is thicker and stickier

Causes of 'abnormal' discharge 5 causes account for 95% cases:

- Excessive normal secretions
- Bacterial vaginosis (BV)
- *Candida albicans*
- Cervicitis (gonococcal, chlamydial, or herpetic)
- *Trichomonas vaginalis* (TV)

Rarer causes Cervical ectropion/polyp; IUCD/IUS; chemical vaginitis (avoid perfumed or disinfectant bath additives and vaginal douches); foreign body (e.g. retained tampon—remove and treat with metronidazole 400mg tds for 7d); genital tract tumour; fistula.

History Ask about:

- **Symptoms** Vaginal discharge (itchy, offensive, colour, duration), vulval soreness and irritation, lower abdominal pain, dyspareunia, heavy periods, intermenstrual bleeding, fever, vulval pain
- **Sexual history** Recent sexual contact with new partner, multiple partners, presence of symptoms in partner, worries about STIs
- **Medical history** Pregnancy, diabetes mellitus, recent antibiotics
- **Attempts at self-medication**

Examination Always offer examination if:

- High risk for STI—age <25y; new sexual partner or >1 sexual partner in the past year; diagnosis of STI in the past 12mo
- Upper reproductive tract symptoms—abnormal bleeding (heavy, post-coital ± intermenstrual); pelvic/abdominal pain; deep dyspareunia; fever
- Pregnant, postpartum, or after miscarriage/termination
- After instrumentation (e.g. insertion of IUS/IUCD, after colposcopy)
- Recurrent infection or failed treatment
- Requesting examination/STI testing

Do an abdominal, bimanual pelvic, and vaginal speculum examination. Look for tenderness on lower abdominal or bimanual palpation, cervical erosion/contact bleeding, discharge, foreign bodies, warts, or ulcers.

Investigation Check pH of secretions with narrow-range pH paper. If >4.5, BV or TV is likely; pH is ≤4.5 with physiological discharge and candida infection. Other investigations to consider:

- High vaginal swab for M,C&S—only if symptoms/signs and/or pH consistent with specific diagnosis; the patient is pregnant, postpartum, or after miscarriage/termination; after instrumentation; or if there is recurrent infection/treatment has failed
- Endocervical swabs for gonorrhoea and chlamydia
- Viral swab if herpes is suspected (if not available, refer to GUM)
- Opportunistic cervical smear if indicated (📖 p. 728)
- Self-taken vulvovaginal swab if examination is declined

Management Treat the cause. If unclear refer to GUM or gynaecology.

Sexually transmitted infections 📖 p. 738

Bacterial vaginosis (BV) Vaginal flora is changed from *Lactobacillus* species to anaerobes. Not sexually transmitted. Affects 10–40% of premenopausal women—about half are asymptomatic. *Associated with:*
- ↑ risk of preterm delivery (and ↓ risk if treated)
- Development of PID and endometritis following abortion or birth
- Infection post-hysterectomy

Presentation Grey/white, thin, fishy-smelling, offensive discharge with no vulval soreness. On examination, the cervix looks normal; pH of secretions is >4.5. HVS for M,C&S may confirm diagnosis but treat without swab if no examination is carried out, or pH is >4.5 and typical clinical picture.

Management^G Without treatment, 50% remit spontaneously. Cure rate with all methods is ~85%. There is no benefit from treating the woman's partner. *Treatment:*
- Metronidazole 400mg bd for 5–7d or 2g single dose
- Clindamycin 2% cream 5g nocte pv for 1wk
- Recurrent infection—◆ suppressive therapy using metronidazole 400mg bd for 6d to cover each period, metronidazole 0.75% gel 2x/wk pv for 4–6mo, lactic acid gel alternate nights for >1mo, and pv probiotics are all but robust evidence of effectiveness is lacking

Candidiasis (thrush) Fungal infection—~20% of patients are asymptomatic. Predisposing factors include:

Cushing's or Addison's disease	Immunosuppression	DM
Broad-spectrum antibiotics	Steroid treatment	Pregnancy
Radiotherapy/chemotherapy	Vaginal trauma	

Presentation Well, pruritus vulvae, superficial dyspareunia, and/or thick, creamy, non-offensive discharge. *Examination:* discharge (cottage cheese) and sore vulva which may be cracked/fissured. Investigation is usually unnecessary. Confirm diagnosis if infection persists or recurs by sending a swab from the anterior fornix for M,C&S.

Management^G Only treat if symptomatic. Sexual transmission is minimal; there is no benefit from treating the partner unless overt infection:
- Try clotrimazole pessaries—cure rate ~90%
- Alternative is oral fluconazole 150mg stat, repeated after 3d if severe infection. Contraindicated in pregnancy or lactation—83% cure rate

Recurrent infection^G Advise loose, cotton underwear and avoidance of soaps, perfumes, or disinfectants in the bath. Consider vulval emollients to treat associated dermatitis. If ≥4 documented episodes (≥2 confirmed with microbiology) in a year, treat with fluconazole 150mg every 3d x3, then 150mg weekly for 6mo.

Further information

FSRH Management of vaginal discharge in non-genito-urinary medicine settings (2012) 🖰 www.fsrh.org
BASHH 🖰 www.bashh.org
- Management of bacterial vaginosis (2012)
- Management of vulvovaginal candidiasis (2007)

Sexually transmitted infection

GPs are frequently presented with symptoms/signs either presented directly or found incidentally (e.g. when doing a cervical smear) that may indicate sexually transmitted infection (STI). The easiest (and often best) option is to refer suspected cases to a genito-urinary medicine (GUM) clinic. Sometimes the patient is reluctant to go and 40% referrals never attend, so it is still necessary for GPs to know how to prevent, diagnose, and treat STI themselves.

Contact tracing Best done by GUM clinics. If a patient refuses to go, then provide him/her with a letter to give to contacts stating the disease he/she has been in contact with, treatment given, and suggesting contacts visit their local GUM clinic promptly.

Use of GUM clinics In general, refer patients:
• Who require contact tracing
• If counselling is needed, e.g. first attack of HSV, HIV
• If diagnosis is still unclear after investigation
• For confirmation of diagnosis, e.g. HSV
• If specialist treatment is required, e.g. treatment of genital warts

Prevention of STIs NICE recommends:
• Identification of high-risk patients opportunistically in general practice, e.g. at new patient checks, when attending for travel advice
• One-to-one discussions with those at ↑ risk of STIs lasting 15–20min, structured on the basis of behaviour change theories to ↓ risk-taking

High-risk groups Include patients with STIs; men who have had sex with other men; people who have come from/visited areas of high HIV prevalence; substance/alcohol misuse; early onset of sexual activity; unprotected sex; and frequent change of/multiple partners.

Young people from vulnerable groups (e.g. from disadvantaged backgrounds; in/leaving local authority care; low educational attainment). Should be offered one-to-one sessions aimed at educating them about sexual health and contraception.

Chlamydia screening A screening programme for the under 25s is currently in operation in the UK (📖 p. 740).

Vaccination A vaccine targeting the most common forms of HPV causing cervical cancer is now available in the UK. The target population is girls aged 12–14y before they become sexually active (📖 p. 749), but potentially any sexually active woman could benefit.

Prevention of HIV 📖 p. 744

Vaginal discharge 📖 p. 736

Acute pelvic inflammatory disease (PID) May be asymptomatic. Peak age 15–25y. >10% develop tubal infertility after 1 episode; 50% after 3 episodes. Risk of ectopic pregnancy ↑ x10 after a single episode. Only 70% of those with acute PID clinically have diagnosis confirmed on laparoscopy. Most cases of PID are associated with STI—usually chlamydia (50%) or gonorrhoea. In 20% no cause is found.

History

- Fever >38°C and malaise
- Acute pelvic pain (usually bilateral) and deep dyspareunia
- Dysuria
- Abnormal vaginal bleeding— heavier periods, intermenstrual and/or post-coital bleeding
- Purulent vaginal discharge

Examination Pyrexia, bilateral lower abdominal tenderness, vaginal discharge, cervical excitation, and adnexal tenderness.

Investigations Consider swabs (HVS and endocervical swab for M,C&S and chlamydia/gonorrhoea screen) and blood tests (FBC—may show leucocytosis; ↑ ESR/CRP).

Management[G] Admit if very unwell, pregnant, or if ectopic pregnancy or other acute surgical emergency cannot be excluded. *Otherwise:*

- Advise rest and sexual abstinence; provide analgesia
- Treat with ofloxacin 400mg bd and metronidazole 400mg bd for 14d; alternative is ceftriaxone 500mg IM as a single dose, followed by oral doxycycline 100mg bd and oral metronidazole 400mg bd for 14d
- If the patient has an IUCD consider removal, but only if symptoms are severe. If removed advise re alternative contraception and emergency contraception if sexual intercourse <7d ago
- Arrange contact tracing via GUM clinic
- If no improvement after 48h, admit; if slow recovery, consider referral for laparoscopy to exclude abscess formation

Chronic PID Caused by inadequately treated acute PID. Presents with pelvic pain, dysmenorrhoea, dyspareunia (1 in 5) ± menorrhagia. *Examination:* lower abdominal/pelvic tenderness, cervical excitation ± adnexal mass. Screen for chlamydia and gonorrhoea. A –ve result does not exclude diagnosis. If chronic pelvic pain with no obvious cause, refer to gynaecology. Once diagnosis is confirmed treatment options include long-term antibiotics or surgery.

Urethritis Inflammation of the male urethra. Multifactorial condition primarily sexually acquired. Mucopurulent cervicitis is the female equivalent. Characterized by discharge and/or dysuria although may be asymptomatic (found when a swab is taken following contact tracing). Treat the cause. Classified by the organisms grown:

Gonococcal urethritis N. gonorrhoeae is identified on urethral swab. Treat as for gonorrhoea (📖 p. 740).

Non-gonococcal urethritis Most common organisms identified are: chlamydia (30–50%); *Ureaplasma* (10%); *Mycoplasma genitalium* (10%); *Trichomonas vaginalis* (1–17%). In 20–30% no organism is isolated. First-line treatment is with azithromycin 1g stat. If persistent/recurrent symptoms, treat with azithromycin 500mg stat, then 250mg od for 4d and metronidazole 400mg bd for 5d.

Further information

NICE Preventing sexually transmitted infections and reducing under-18 conceptions (2007) ℘ www.nice.org.uk
BASHH ℘ www.bashh.org

- UK National Guidelines on safer sex advice (2012)
- Management of pelvic inflammatory disease (2011)
- Management of non-gonococcal urethritis (2008)

Chlamydia, gonorrhoea, and trichomonas

⚠ A single individual may have >1 STI simultaneously.

Chlamydia Major cause of pelvic pain and infertility in women.

Screening Chlamydia is a preventable cause of infertility, ectopic pregnancy, and pelvic inflammatory disease. Screening using urine testing or self-taken swabs ↓ prevalence and incidence of pelvic inflammatory disease[S]. Screening programmes aimed at young people <25y are in operation throughout the UK. Self-test kits are available through GP surgeries, sexual health/contraception clinics, and community venues (e.g. schools).

Presentation in men Usually asymptomatic. May have urethritis. Send urethral swab or first-catch urine sample for nucleic acid amplification testing (NAAT) to confirm diagnosis.

Presentation in women
- **History** >70% are asymptomatic. *Symptoms:* vaginal discharge (30%); post-coital or intermenstrual bleeding; pelvic inflammatory disease (10–30%—🕮 p. 738); dysuria
- **Examination** Mucopurulent cervicitis; hyperaemia and oedema of the cervix ± contact bleeding; tender adnexae; cervical excitation
- **Investigation** Send endocervical (if symptoms) or self-taken vulvovaginal swab (if asymptomatic) for NAAT to confirm diagnosis

❶ If ♂ or ♀ and exposed to potential infection <2wk previously, repeat test >2wk after exposure.

Management
- Doxycycline 100mg bd for 1wk or erythromycin 500mg qds for 14d; azithromycin 1g stat po is an alternative which ensures compliance
- During pregnancy/breastfeeding use erythromycin 500mg qds for 2wk
- Consider supplying home-testing kits to patients at high risk of STIs

 Presentation in neonates Conjunctivitis, pneumonia, otitis media, pharyngitis—1 in 3 affected mothers have affected babies. Seek specialist advice if suspected.

Gonorrhoea *Transmission:* ♂—1 in 5 exposures; ♀—1 in 2 exposures.

Presentation in men Depends on site of infection:
- **Urethral infection** (<10% are asymptomatic). Urethral discharge (80%); dysuria (50%) 2–5d after exposure; prostatitis; urethral stricture
- **Rectal infection** (usually asymptomatic). Anal discharge (12%); anal/perianal pain or discomfort (7%)
- **Pharyngeal infection** (>90% asymptomatic)

If asymptomatic—send first-catch urine sample for NAAT; if symptomatic send urethral ± rectal ± pharyngeal swabs (as appropriate) for NAAT and M,C&S to confirm diagnosis.

Presentation in women Infection may be asymptomatic (50%) or cause vaginal discharge (50%), lower abdominal pain; dysuria but not frequency (25%); abnormal vaginal bleeding; pelvic inflammatory disease; abscess of

Bartholin's gland; miscarriage; or preterm labour. Rectal and pharyngeal infections are usually asymptomatic.

- If asymptomatic—send self-taken vulvovaginal swab for NAAT
- If symptomatic—send endocervical swab ± rectal ± pharyngeal swab (as appropriate) for NAAT and M,C&S to confirm diagnosis

Management^G

- Ceftriaxone 500mg IM as a single dose + azithromycin 1g stat po
- Refer to GUM for contact tracing
- If persisting symptoms/signs after treatment, test for cure with swabs sent for M,C&S >72h after completion of therapy
- If asymptomatic following treatment, test for cure 2wk after treatment completion with NAAT, followed by culture if NAAT-positive
- If persistent infection, seek specialist advice

Trichomonas vaginalis (TV)

> **Presentation in neonates** Ophthalmia neonatorum. Purulent discharge from the eyes of an infant <21d old. Send swabs for NAAT and M,C&S. If confirmed, seek immediate specialist advice.

Presentation in men 15–50% are asymptomatic. *Symptoms:* dysuria, urethral discharge. Take urethral swab and first-void urine for culture.

Presentation in women 10–50% are asymptomatic. *Symptoms:*
- Vaginal discharge (25%)—mucopurulent yellow-white, smelly discharge; may be frothy
- Vulvovaginal soreness/itching • Abdominal pain • Dysuria

Examination shows typical discharge, vaginal inflammation, and strawberry cervix. Check pH of secretions with narrow-range pH paper. If pH >4.5, TV is a possibility; send HVS from the posterior fornix at the time of speculum examination for M,C&S. Sensitivity of HVS is low for TV, so if HVS is –ve, consider GUM referral for wet microscopy ± culture and contact tracing. ❶ TV may rarely be detected on cervical smear.

Management^G

- Advise patients to avoid sexual intercourse until they and their partner(s) have completed treatment and follow-up
- Metronidazole po (400mg bd for 5–7d or 2g stat)—tinidazole 2g stat is an alternative
- Consider referral to GUM clinic for contact tracing
- Resistant TV—try higher dose metronidazole: 400mg tds po + 1g od pr for 7d, or metronidazole 2g od for 3–5d. High-dose tinidazole 2g bd for 2wk ± topical vaginal tinidazole is an alternative

Further information

BASHH ℘ www.bashh.org
- Management of *Chlamydia trachomatis* genital tract infection (2006)
- UK national guideline on gonorrhoea testing (2012)
- Management of gonorrhoea in adults (2011)
- Management of *Trichomonas vaginalis* infection (2007)

National Chlamydia Screening Programme (NCSP)
℘ www.chlamydiascreening.nhs.uk

Hepatitis B and C

Hepatitis B (HBV) Common. Endemic in much of Asia and the Far East. The virus has 3 major structural antigens: surface antigen (HBsAg), core antigen (HBcAg), and e antigen (HBeAg). Spread is via infected blood, sexual intercourse, from mother to newborn baby, or via human bites. Incubation period is 6–23wk (average 17wk).

High-risk groups Patients who are/have:

- Injecting drug users
- Many sexual partners
- Adopted children from high/intermediate-risk countries
- Foster parents
- Close family contacts of a case/carrier
- Receiving regular blood/blood products and their carers
- Chronic renal/liver disease
- Prison inmates
- At risk due to occupation e.g. healthcare workers
- Staff/residents of residential accommodation for individuals with mental handicap
- Travelling to high/intermediate-risk areas
- Babies born to mothers who are chronic carriers of hepatitis B or have had acute hepatitis B in pregnancy

Presentation May be asymptomatic or present with fever, malaise, fatigue, arthralgia, urticaria, pale stools, dark urine, and/or jaundice.

Investigation LFTs (hepatic jaundice—↑ bilirubin, ↑ ALT/AST, ↑ alkaline phosphatase), hepatitis serology (see Figure 22.1).

- **HBsAg** Present from 1–6mo post-exposure. If present >6mo after the acute episode defines carrier status
- **HBeAg** Present from 6wk–3mo after acute illness. Indicates high infectivity
- **Anti-HBs** Antibodies appear >10mo after infection; imply immunity

Management In all cases advise patients to avoid alcohol. Refer for specialist advice. Treatment is supportive for acute illness. Chronic hepatitis is treated with interferon and lamivudine with varying success.

Prognosis ~85% recover fully; 10% develop carrier status; 5–10% develop chronic hepatitis—may lead to cirrhosis and/or liver carcinoma. Fulminant hepatitis and death are rare (<1%).

Prevention Advise patients re 'safe sex'. Immunize high-risk groups. Give passive immunization with human immunoglobulin to non-immune, high-risk contacts of infected patients.

❶ Hepatitis immunization of injecting drug misusers If not already infected/immune or close contact of someone already infected, use a rapid regime—immunization at 0, 7, and 21d and booster after 12mo.

Hepatitis C (HCV) Common. Spread is usually via contact with infected blood (causing post-transfusion hepatitis) but can pass from mother to baby. Not easily spread through sexual contact. In 10% no source of infection is found. Incubation is 2–25wk (mean 8wk).

Risk factors Blood transfusion; healthcare work; IV drug abuse; haemodialysis; infant of infected mother (5% risk); multiple sexual partners.

Presentation and management As for HBV. Anti-HCV antibody is detectable 3–4mo post-infection. Refer for expert advice. Avoid alcohol. 50% develop chronic infection; 5% cirrhosis; and 15% of those hepatoma.

(a) Acute hepatitis B infection with recovery

(b) Acute hepatitis B infection with progression to carrier state

Figure 22.1 Hepatitis B serology

Reproduced with permission from the US Centers for Disease Control and Prevention.

Further information
BASHH Management of viral hepatidides (2008) ℘ www.bashh.org
HPA Hepatitis A, B, and C ℘ www.hpa.org.uk
Department of Health The Green Book ℘ www.dh.gov.uk/greenbook

Information for patients
British Liver Trust ☏ 0800 652 7330 ℘ www.britishlivertrust.org.uk

HIV infection: prevention and testing

Human immunodeficiency virus (HIV) is a retrovirus infecting T-helper cells bearing the CD4 receptor. Worldwide, the HIV epidemic continues, but prophylaxis and treatment are improving prognosis in developed countries where treatment is available. It is estimated that ~1 in 3 of those infected in the UK are unaware of their diagnosis.

Transmission ~1 in 1,000 exposures. Mode of transmission may be:
- Sexual (60–70%)—heterosexual intercourse in 54%
- IV drug abuse (2%)
- Infected blood products
- Mother → child (1.5%)
- Accidental (e.g. needle stick injuries)

❶ HIV antibodies can take 3mo to develop after HIV infection, so HIV tests may miss those infected in the early stages of their disease. Consider repeating if infection may have occurred <3mo prior to testing. If in doubt, arrange a second test 3mo after the first.

Prevention of HIV infection
- Promotion of safe sex and ↓ IV drug abuse and needle sharing
- Refer to GUM for post-exposure prophylaxis if sexual contact <72h previously with an HIV-infected individual (or high-risk individual)
- Screening blood donors
- Prevention of transmission from mother to child—risk can be ↓ to <1% with antiretroviral treatment (given to the mother antenatally, during delivery, and to the neonate for first 6wk), elective Caesarean section, and advising against breastfeeding
- Trials of HIV vaccines are in advanced stages

Accidental exposure (e.g. needle stick injury). Significant exposure if:
- The source is HIV +ve
- The material is blood/another infectious body fluid (semen, amniotic fluid, genital secretions, CSF), and
- Exposure is caused by inoculation (risk of transmission 1 in 300) or by a splash onto a mucus membrane (risk of transmission 1 in 3,000)

⚠ **Immediate action** Irrigate the site of exposure with running water; establish history of HIV infection and (if possible) obtain a blood sample from the source and victim. Refer to A&E immediately for HIV post-exposure prophylaxis. Treatment is with 3 antiretroviral drugs for 4wk.

Who should be offered a test?
Universal HIV testing (offered to everyone)
- Everyone attending GUM/sexual health clinics
- Women registering for antenatal care
- Women attending for termination of pregnancy
- Everyone diagnosed with TB, hepatitis B/C, or lymphoma
- If prevalence of HIV in the local population is >2/1,000, all those registering in general practice, and all general medical admissions

High-risk patients
- If HIV is part of the differential diagnosis of the presenting condition
- If diagnosed with another STI
- Sexual partners of those known to be HIV +ve
- Men who have sex with other men and any female sexual partners

- History of injecting drug misuse
- People originating from or current/former sexual partner from a country with high HIV prevalence (>1%, e.g. sub-Saharan Africa, India)

Offer repeat testing if:
- HIV −ve, but possible exposure has occurred within the 3mo window period or since testing
- Men who have sex with men or injecting drug user—offer >1x/y
- Women who refuse an HIV test at antenatal booking—offer testing again, then a third time at 36wk

Index conditions In which HIV is part of the differential diagnosis:
- **Respiratory** TB, pneumocystis, aspergillosis, bacterial pneumonia, lung cancer
- **Neurology** cerebral toxoplasmosis; cerebral lymphoma; cryptococcal meningitis; progressive multifocal or other leucoencephalopathy; aseptic meningitis/encephalitis; cerebral abscess; SOL; Guillain–Barré syndrome; transverse myelitis; peripheral neuropathy; dementia
- **Dermatology** Kaposi's sarcoma; severe/recalcitrant seborrhoeic dermatitis or psoriasis; multidermatomal/recurrent herpes zoster
- **GI** Persistent cryptosporidiosis; chronic diarrhoea; hepatitis B/C; Salmonella, Shigella, or Campylobacter infection; oral candidiasis/hairy leukoplakia
- **Sexual health** STI; cervical cancer; CIN 2/3; VIN; seminoma
- **Haematology** Unexplained blood dyscrasia, e.g. thrombocytopenia, neutropenia, lymphopenia; unexplained lymphadenopathy; lymphoma (Hodgkin's or non-Hodgkin's); anal cancer (or intraepithelial dysplasia)
- **Ophthalmology** CMV retinitis/other infective retinal disease; unexplained retinopathy
- **Other** PUO; weight ↓; chronic parotitis/parotid cysts; head/neck cancer; mononucleosis-like syndrome (primary HIV)

Giving the result
If the result is negative Consider whether the patient needs a follow-up test in 3mo. Provide health promotion information about minimizing risk of HIV infection in future.
If the result is positive Give the result early in the consultation.
- Explain the result and its implications for the patient and their partner
- Emphasize the positive aspects of knowing the diagnosis
- Try to arrange specialist referral before the patient attends so that the patient can be given a time and date for specialist follow-up
- Give the patient time to talk through feelings and fears
- Talk about support available, e.g. friends/family; support organizations
- Provide literature about HIV and patient support organizations
- Arrange follow-up to maintain the link with primary care

Further information
BASHH ℘ www.bashh.org
- National guidelines on HIV testing (2008)
- Post-exposure prophylaxis for HIV following sexual exposure (2011)
RCOG Management of HIV in pregnancy (2010) ℘ www.rcog.org.uk

Information and support for patients with HIV and carers
NAM Aidsmap ℘ www.aidsmap.com
National AIDS Trust ℘ www.nat.org.uk
Terrence Higgins Trust ℘ www.tht.org.uk

HIV infection: clinical disease

Primary HIV Half have no symptoms. Possible symptoms:
- Mononucleosis-like picture of fever, fatigue, myalgia/arthralgia ± lymphadenopathy. Consider as a differential diagnosis of glandular fever
- Blotchy rash affecting the trunk, and orogenital/perianal ulceration
- Rarely acute neurological symptoms (aseptic meningitis, transverse myelitis, encephalitis) or diarrhoea
- FBC may show atypical lymphocytes
- Rarely, CD4 count drops acutely and conditions associated with immunosuppression, e.g. oral candidiasis or shingles, may occur

⚠ If you think a patient has primary HIV infection, seek urgent advice from a specialist. HIV tests can be negative <3mo after infection.

Progression Duration/severity of HIV infection is reflected by the CD4 count which ↓ as infection progresses. If CD4 count is <200 cells/mm³, patients have *acquired immune deficiency syndrome* (AIDS) and are at risk from opportunistic infection (e.g. pneumococcal, TB, CMV, *Pneumocystis*, toxoplasmosis, cryptosporidial diarrhoea) and AIDS-associated malignancies (e.g. Kaposi's sarcoma, lymphoma)—see Table 22.1.

Kaposi's sarcoma Purple papules or plaques on skin or mucosa of any organ. Metastasizes to lymph nodes. If suspected refer for expert help:
- **Endemic**—occurs in central Africa. Peripheral lesions, good response to chemotherapy
- **Associated with AIDS or transplant**—commonly skin or pulmonary lesions; lymphatic obstruction predisposes to cellulitis
M.K. Kaposi (1837–1902)—Hungarian dermatologist.

Management Specialist management is always needed.
Antiretroviral drugs 5 main groups:
- Entry inhibitors
- Integrase inhibitors
- Nucleoside/nucleotide reverse transcriptase inhibitors (NRTIs)
- Non-nucleoside reverse transcriptase inhibitors (NNRTIs)
- Protease inhibitors

Choice of drugs is a specialist decision. A combination is usual (highly active antiretrovirus therapy or HAART regime). Adherence to therapy is essential to avoid resistance. The aim is to ↓ viral load to an undetectable level in <6mo. Response to treatment is measured with viral load, CD4 count, and CD4 percentage. Treatment failure requires switching or increasing therapy. ❶ Do not stop or change the dose of antiretroviral drugs without taking specialist advice.

Drug interactions are common. Record antiretrovirals on GP system medication charts (even though prescriptions are usually issued by specialist centres). Check drug interactions at: 🖰 www.hiv-druginteractions.org

Prophylaxis against opportunistic infections Prophylactic antibiotics are used to prevent *Pneumocystis*, toxoplasmosis, and *Mycobacterium avium* for patients with low CD4 counts.

Psychological support Due to the stigma attached to HIV infection, patients and carers often lack the support offered by the community for most other serious illness.

Immunizations

- **Inactivated vaccines**—can be used safely; offer annual influenza vaccination, pneumococcal vaccination, hepatitis B testing and vaccination if seronegative, and hepatitis A vaccine if at risk
- **Live vaccines** (e.g oral typhoid, BCG) are generally contraindicated but give varicella (for all) and MMR (if ♀ of child-bearing age) if seronegative and CD4 count >200mm³

CVD prevention HIV is associated with ↑ risk of CVD. Check risk before, then 3–6mo after starting antiretrovirals and annually thereafter (every 5y from 40y if not taking antiretrovirals). Provide lifestyle advice (📖 p. 242), and treat hyperlipidaemia if 10y CVD risk >20%.

Sexual health Advise to use condoms with water-based lubricant for all vaginal/anal sex and condoms/dams for oral sex—even if both partners are HIV +ve (as prevents transmission of drug-resistant strains).

Contraception Efficacy of hormonal contraception is ↓ by antiretrovirals. Consider Depo-Provera® or IUS/IUCD. Advise condoms in addition to contraception. If emergency contraception is needed, first-line is an IUD; if using levonorgestrel, provide a double (3mg) dose.

Cervical screening Women with HIV have ↑ risk of HPV and cervical cancer. Annual cervical screening is recommended.

Pregnancy 📖 p. 811   **Palliative care** 📖 p. 1028

Death If HIV has contributed to death, this must be recorded on the death certificate.

Table 22.1 CD4 counts and HIV-related problems

CD4 count cells/mm³	Risk of opportunistic infection	Risk of HIV-associated tumours
>500	Minimal/none	Very small ↑ risk
200–500	Little risk unless falling rapidly, except TB	Small ↑ risk
<200	↑ risk of serious opportunistic infection, e.g. • Pneumocystis pneumonia • Toxoplasmosis • Oesophageal candidiasis	Increasing risk
<100	Additional risk of: • *Mycobacterium avium intracellulare* • Cytomegalovirus	High risk and increasingly aggressive disease

Further information

Medical Foundation for AIDS and Sexual Health HIV in primary care (2011) ℘ www.medfash.org.uk

Information and support for patients with HIV and carers

NAM Aidsmap ℘ www.aidsmap.com
National AIDS Trust ℘ www.nat.org.uk
Terrence Higgins Trust ℘ www.tht.org.uk

Other sexually transmitted infections

Genital herpes HSV is transmitted by direct contact with lesions. Lesions may appear anywhere on the skin or mucosa but are most frequent around the mouth, on the lips, conjunctiva, cornea, and genitalia.

Presentation of primary infection May be asymptomatic. If symptomatic, history and examination are diagnostic in 90% cases. Presents with multiple painful genital ulcers on a red background ± inguinal lymph nodes <1wk after sexual contact. Lesions crust over then heal. Untreated lasts 3–4wk. *Complications:* urinary retention, aseptic meningitis.

Management

- Refer to GUM if diagnosis is uncertain and for contact tracing
- Treat with aciclovir if presents within the first 5d of symptoms starting and while new lesions are still forming (↓ duration, symptoms, and complications)
- Analgesia, ice packs, and salt baths may help. 5% lidocaine ointment gives symptom relief but use with caution as may cause sensitization
- Advice—barrier methods of contraception (risk of transmission in monogamous relationships is 10%/y)
- If pregnant obtain specialist advice

Recurrent infection Reactivation of latent virus. Less severe than primary infection. Neonatal transmission rates are low (<3%)—elective Caesarean section for those with active recurrences at term is controversial. Consider suppressive therapy if ≥6 attacks/y, e.g. aciclovir 400mg bd. If breakthrough occurs, ↑ dose of antiviral, e.g. aciclovir 400mg tds.

> **Neonatal infection** Presents at age 5–21d with vesicular lesions around the presenting part or rarely systemic infection. Usually babies of women with no history of genital HSV. Refer as a paediatric emergency.

Genital warts Caused by human papillomavirus (HPV). Usually sexually transmitted, and >25% have concomitant STIs. Disease may be clinical (found on examination) or subclinical (changes associated with infection detected on smear). In women CIN (📖 p. 726) is related to infection with HPV types 16 and 18, but 90% of genital warts are caused by HPV types 6 or 11.

Presentation in women Often asymptomatic but may be associated with itching or vaginal discharge. Warts are usually seen on the vulva or introitus. Warts enlarge during pregnancy.

Presentation in men Warts are usually found on the penis or perianally.

Management of clinical warts Treatment does not eradicate the virus but removes lesions. Barrier contraception is needed for at least 3mo after the warts are gone. Treatment options in primary care:

- **Podophyllotoxin** Suitable for home treatment of unkeratinized genital warts and licensed for a 4wk course. Avoid in pregnancy. Apply 2x/d for 3d, followed by a 4d rest. This cycle is repeated 4–5x. *Side effects:* soreness/ulceration of the genital skin—advise to discontinue treatment

- **Imiquimod** Can be used at home for keratinized or non-keratinized warts. Avoid in pregnancy. Apply 3x/wk. On each occasion wash off 6–10h later. Continue for up to 16wk. Avoid unprotected intercourse after application. Can weaken latex condoms

Alternatives (usually in specialist settings)–trichloroacetic acid, excision, cryotherapy, electrosurgery.

> *Human papillomavirus (HPV) vaccination* HPV vaccines are aimed at preventing infection with strains causing cervical cancer. Currently vaccines target strains 6, 11, 16, and 18, which account for ~70% of HPV-related cancer cases and 90% of genital warts. Vaccination in the UK is targeted at girls aged 12–14y. Cervical screening in adulthood is still necessary as the vaccine does not protect against all strains causing cervical cancer.

Pubic lice Pubic (or crab) lice are similar to head lice and may be sexually transmitted. All hairy areas (including eyelashes, eyebrows, pubic and axillary hair) can be affected. Treatment options are:
- Malathion 0.5%—apply to dry hair; wash out after 12h
- Permethrin 1% cream rinse—apply to damp hair; wash out after 10min
- Phenothrin 0.2%—apply to dry hair; wash out after 2h
- Carbaryl 0.5–1% (unlicensed)—apply to dry hair; wash out after 12h
Repeat treatment after 3–7d

Scabies 📖 p. 639

Syphilis Caused by *Treponema pallidum*. Rare in the UK but incidence is increasing. *Incubation:* 9–90d. If suspected, send blood for VDRL, TPHA or treponemal antibody absorption depending on local policy. In all confirmed cases refer for specialist care. Contact tracing is essential.

4 stages
- **Primary syphilis** Chancre at the site of contact
- **Secondary syphilis** 4–8wk after chancre—systemic symptoms: fever, malaise, generalized lymphadenopathy, anal papules (conylomata lata), rash (trunk, palms, soles), buccal snail track ulcers, alopecia
- **Tertiary syphilis** 2–20y after initial infection—gummas (granulomas) in connective tissue e.g. testicular gumma
- **Quarternary syphilis** Cardiovascular or neurological complications.

Further information
BASHH 🔗 www.bashh.org
- Management of genital herpes (2007)
- Management of *Phthirus pubis* (2007)
- Management of scabies (2007)
- Management of syphilis (2008)
- Management of genital warts (2007)
Health Protection Agency (HPA) 🔗 www.hpa.org.uk

Information for patients
Family Planning Association (FPA) ☎ 0845 122 8690 (0845 122 8687 in Northern Ireland) 🔗 www.fpa.org.uk
Herpes Association ☎ 0845 123 2305 🔗 www.herpes.org.uk

Summary of contraceptive methods

80% women receive contraceptive advice and treatment through their GP. A sexually active woman has an 85% chance of becoming pregnant in <1y without contraception, and ~1 in 3 pregnancies are unplanned.

Contraceptive services Provided as an Additional Service; opting out results in a 2.4% ↓ in global sum. IUDs may be fitted as a *National Enhanced Service*; payment is available for fitting and annual review.

Choice of method See Table 22.2. *Consider:* a woman's personal preference; age; lifestyle/cultural aspects; medical history; and risk of STI. ❶ Prescriptions for contraceptives are free of charge for all women in the UK).

Before providing contraception Provide information to enable the woman to choose a method and use it effectively. Exclude pregnancy. A woman is probably not pregnant if she:
- Has been using a reliable method of contraception correctly
- Has not had unprotected sexual intercourse (UPSI) since her last period, or
- Is <7d after the start of a normal period; <4wk postpartum, <7d post-termination or miscarriage; or is fully breastfeeding, amenorrhoeic, and <6mo postpartum

❶ If in doubt, do a pregnancy test ≥3wk after the last UPSI

Emergency contraception

Copper IUCD Can be inserted ≤120h (5d) after UPSI. >99% effective. Progestogen-containing IUCDs are not suitable for this purpose.

Levonorgestrel 1.5mg po stat. Licensed ≤72h (3d) after UPSI but effective for 96h (4d). Can be used more than once if >1 episode of UPSI in a single cycle. Available OTC and on prescription. There is no evidence that treatment with levonorgestrel harms the fetus if pregnant.

Progesterone receptor modulator (ulipristal acetate 30mg stat) Can be used ≤120h (5d) after UPSI. Only use 1x/cycle.

Possible pitfalls
- **Vomiting** <3h after taking oral emergency contraception—give a replacement dose or offer a copper IUCD
- **Enzyme-inducing drugs** (e.g. anti-epileptics, St John's wort) Efficacy of oral emergency contraception may be ↓. Consider a copper IUCD or ↑ dose of levonorgestrel to 3mg (unlicensed)

All women Provide advice about ongoing contraception and prevention of STI. Advise to return if abdominal pain, next period is overdue or abnormally light/heavy, or if needs further contraceptive advice.

Sexually transmitted infections Discuss prevention of STIs with all women when providing contraception. Advise high-risk groups to use barrier methods in addition to hormonal methods of contraception.

Further information
FSRH Emergency contraception (2012) ℘ www.fsrh.org

Table 22.2 Summary of contraceptive methods

Method of contraception	% unintended pregnancies*	Advantages	Disadvantages
Sterilization (♂)	0.05 (1:2,000)	No contraindications Single procedure	Difficult to reverse Post-operative complications
Sterilization (♀)	0.5 (1:200)	No contraindications Single procedure	Requires GA and rarely results in laparotomy Post-operative complications Difficult to reverse ↑ risk ectopic pregnancy
Nexplanon® (single capsule upper arm)	0.05	Lasts 3y Immediately reversible	Needs training to insert and remove Wound infection and/or scarring Can cause irregular bleeding Progestogenic side effects
Progestogen-containing intrauterine system (IUS) (e.g. Mirena®)	0.1	Lasts 5y ↓ bleeding, ectopic pregnancy risk, dysmenorrhoea Endometrial protection	May cause erratic bleeding Progestogenic side effects Problems with insertion or retrieval
Combined contraceptive pill/patch/ring	0.3 (9)	Regular cycle and lighter periods ↓ dysmenorrhoea Cycle control	Compliance Side effects ↑ risk breast cancer, thromboembolism
Progestogen-only pill (POP)	0.3 (8)	Few side effects and contraindications	Compliance Irregular bleeding Progestogenic side effects
Intrauterine contraceptive device (IUCD)	0.6 (0.8)	Lasts ≥5y No systemic effects	Heavy periods Problems with insertion or retrieval No protection from pelvic inflammatory disease or ectopic pregnancy
Injectable progestogen (e.g. Depo-Provera®)	0.3 (3)	Avoids pill-taking ↓ bleeding and can help PMS ↓ risk of ectopic pregnancy, endometrial cancer	Menstrual irregularity Weight gain Unpredictable return of fertility ↑ risk of osteoporosis
Barrier methods (condoms, diaphragm)	2 (32)	Barrier to transmission of STIs	User-dependent Allergy
Natural methods	1 (27)	No contraindications or side effects	Teaching required High failure rate

* Failure rates stated are with perfect use. Rates in brackets are with typical use.

Combined hormonal contraception

Contraceptives containing an oestrogen and progestogen are available as:
- Combined oral contraceptive pills (COC)
- Contraceptive patches (Evra®), and
- Vaginal contraceptive rings (NuvaRing®)

COC pill Most COC come in packets of 21 pills. The woman takes the entire packet starting on the first day of her cycle and then has a 7d 'pill-free' break before starting the next packet. Pills vary by:

Oestrogen type Most COCs contain ethinylestradiol; alternatives are estradiol valerate (Qlaira®) or mestranol (Norinyl-1®).

Oestrogen content
- **Low-strength preparations** (20 microgram ethinylestradiol). Use if risk factors for circulatory disease or if oestrogenic side effects
- **Standard-strength preparations** (30–35 microgram ethinylestradiol or 50 microgram mestranol). Use for most women
- **Phased preparations** Dose of oestrogen/progestogen varies through the cycle. Try for women who have bleeding problems with monophasic products
- **Everyday (ED) preparations** Taken continuously. Can help women who find it difficult to remember to start a new packet

Progestogen type COC pills containing:
- **Levonorgestrel and norethisterone** Suitable for most women. Choose for first-time COC pill users
- **Desogestrel, norgestimate, dienogest, drosperidone, and gestodene** Consider if side effects, e.g. acne, headache, depression, weight ↑, breast symptoms, breakthrough bleeding. ❶ Desogestrel/gestodene may be associated with ↑ clotting risk
- **Cyproterone acetate** (co-cyprindiol)—Licensed for treatment of acne, not for contraception, but does provide contraception. Use for 3–4mo after resolution of symptoms. Associated with 4x ↑ risk of venous thromboembolism compared to COC containing levonorgestrel

Contraceptive patch (Evra®) 20 microgram ethinylestradiol and norelgestromin in a transdermal patch. Alternative if compliance with daily pill-taking is problematic. Apply patch on day 1 of the cycle; change patch on days 8 and 15; remove third patch on day 22 and then apply new patch after a 7d 'patch-free' interval to start the subsequent cycle.

Contraceptive vaginal ring 15 micrograms/24h ethinylestradiol and etonogestrel. Alternative low-dose preparation. Insert ring into vagina on day 1 of cycle and leave in for 3wk; remove ring on day 22; subsequent courses repeated after 7d ring-free interval.

Reasons not to prescribe combined contraception See Box 22.1.

Further information
FRSH ॐ www.fsrh.org
- Combined hormonal contraception (2012)
- UK Medical Eligibility Criteria for contraceptive use (2009)

Box 22.1 Reasons not to prescribe combined hormonal contraception*

Venous disease

- Avoid if sclerosing treatment for varicose veins or if history of current/past venous thromboembolism (VTE)
- Risk factors for VTE (use with caution if 1; avoid if >1):
  - Age ≥35y—avoid if ≥50y
  - Smoker or <1y after smoking cessation—avoid if ≥35y and if smoking ≥15 cigarettes/d
  - BMI ≥30kg/m² —avoid if BMI ≥35kg/m²
  - Family history of VTE in first-degree relative <45y—avoid if known prothrombotic coagulation abnormality, e.g. Factor V Leiden, antiphospholipid antibodies, lupus anticoagulant
  - Immobility—avoid if bed-bound or leg in plaster cast
  - History of superficial thrombophlebitis

Arterial disease

- Avoid if valvular/congenital heart disease with history of complications (e.g. pulmonary hypertension, AF, SBE) or if history of CVD including stroke/TIA, IHD, peripheral vascular disease, hypertensive retinopathy
- Risk factors for CVD (use with caution if 1; avoid if >1):
  - Age ≥35y—avoid if ≥50y
  - Smoker—avoid if smoking ≥40 cigarettes/d
  - BMI ≥30kg/m² —avoid if BMI ≥35kg/m²
  - Family history of arterial disease in first-degree relative <45y— avoid if atherogenic lipid profile
  - DM—avoid if vascular, renal, neurological, or eye complications
  - Hypertension with BP >140/90mmHg—avoid if >160/95mmHg
  - Migraine without aura—avoid if migraine with aura within 5y, attacks treated with ergot derivatives, or severe migraine lasting >72h

Liver disease Avoid if active/flare of viral hepatitis, liver tumour, or severe cirrhosis or if active gall bladder disease; seek specialist advice if history of contraceptive-associated cholestasis.

Cancer Avoid if current breast cancer; take specialist advice if no suitable alternative and past history of breast cancer, but no evidence of disease for >5y or known gene mutation for breast cancer (e.g. BRCA1).

Pregnancy-related issues Avoid if history in pregnancy of pruritus, cholestatic jaundice, chorea, or pemphigoid gestationis; or if postpartum and breastfeeding (p. 837).

Drug interactions 📖 pp. 756–7

Others Avoid if acute porphyria or haemolytic uraemic syndrome.

❶ Investigate any undiagnosed vaginal bleeding before starting combined hormonal contraception.

* Based on UK Medical Eligibility Criteria (UKMEC) 3 (theoretical or proven risks usually outweigh advantages) and 4 (unacceptable health risk) and *BNF* guidance (7.3.1).

Before starting combined contraception
- Take a history—medical, sexual health, medications, and lifestyle
- Consider asking for specialist haematology advice about thrombophilia screening if FH of DVT/PE in a first-degree relative aged <45y or multiple family members, and/or check cholesterol/triglycerides if FH of arterial disease in a first-degree relative <45y, or multiple family members
- Check BP
- Education—discuss side effects/risks of combined contraception (see Table 22.3), STIs, cervical smears, smoking, control of weight. Give both verbal and written directions on use

Starting combined contraception Contraceptive effect starts immediately if started:
- Day 1–5 of the cycle (day 1 only for estradiol valerate/dienogest pill)
- At the end of the third week postpartum
- <5d after miscarriage/TOP at <20wk gestation (day 1 only for estradiol valerate/dienogest pill)
- Changing COC pill variety or to patch or ring—start the new pill/patch/ring omitting the 7d break (or 'inactive' tablets if taking ED preparation)
- Changing from contraceptive implant, injectable progestogen, or desogestrel-only POP—start at any time until repeat injection due, implant due for removal, or last desogestrel pill taken

⚠ In all other cases and at all other times use additional contraception for the first 7d (9d if using estradiol valerate/dienogest pill).

Extended dosing^G Continuous dosing is an alternative approach to combined hormonal contraceptive administration that does not ↓ contraceptive efficacy. Several (unlicensed) regimes are in common use:
- **Short pill-free interval** Replacement of 7d break with 4d break
- **Tricycling** 3 cycles taken continuously back-to-back followed by a 7d break, i.e. 3× 21 monophasic COC, 3× rings, or 9× patches
- **Extended use** Continuous use of monophasic COC, ring, or patch until breakthrough bleeding for 3–4d, followed by a 4d or 7d break

Follow-up 3mo after starting or changing a combined contraceptive—earlier if complications. Once established, review every 6–12mo. At follow-up, assess risk factors and side effects; give health education, e.g. smoking cessation advice, benefits of long-acting reversible contraception, information about STIs; check BP.

Table 22.3 Risks and benefits of combined hormonal contraception use

Risks	Benefits
Venous thromboembolism (risk ↑ x2 but absolute risk is still very low)	Improvement in acne
Ischaemic stroke—small ↑ risk	↓ in menstrual pain and bleeding
Breast and cervical—any ↑ in risk is small and disappears <10y after combined contraception is stopped	↓ in menopausal symptoms
	↓ risk of ovarian, bowel, and endometrial cancer that persists after combined contraception has stopped
Mood changes (but no ↑ in depression)	No evidence of weight ↑

Missed doses COC pills (except Qlaira®)—see Figure 22.2; Qlaira® and contraceptive patches or rings—see *BNF* 7.3.1 and/or product literature.

⚠ **Reasons to stop CHC immediately** (pending investigation if needed):
- Sudden severe chest pain (even if not radiating to left arm)
- Sudden breathlessness (or cough with bloodstained sputum)
- Unexplained swelling or severe pain in calf of one leg
- Acute abdominal pain
- Serious neurological effects including:
  - Unusual severe, prolonged headache especially if first time or getting progressively worse
  - Sudden dysphasia, partial or complete loss of vision, disturbance of hearing, or other perceptual disorders
  - Bad fainting attack or unexplained collapse
  - First unexplained epileptic seizure
  - Weakness, motor disturbances, or numbness affecting one side or one part of body
- Hepatitis, jaundice, liver enlargement
- BP >160/95mmHg
- Prolonged immobility after surgery or leg injury
- Detection of a risk factor/contraindication (📖 p. 753)

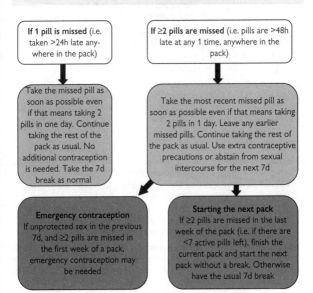

Figure 22.2 Advice for patients regarding missed COC pills

Short-term side effects Usually resolve within 2–3 cycles.

Relative oestrogen excess Breast tenderness (3.6%); nausea (1.5%); dizziness; cyclical weight ↑; bloating; vaginal discharge without infection. Use a more progestogen-dominant pill.

Relative progestogen excess Mood swings (3.9%); PMT; dry vagina; sustained weight ↑; ↓ libido; lassitude; acne. Use a more oestrogen-dominant pill.

Headache Affects 2.9% of women taking the combined contraceptive. Ask women to report ↑ in headache frequency or onset of focal symptoms when taking any combined contraceptive. If new focal symptoms, discontinue immediately and, if not typical of migraine aura and lasts >1h, admit. If headaches continue consider switching brand/alternative method of contraception.

Breakthrough bleeding Most common in the first few months of combined contraceptive use—after 6 cycles affects 1.1% women (spotting affects 3.3% women). If no vomiting/diarrhoea and no missed pills, breakthrough bleeding does not indicate ↓ efficacy. If symptoms suggest other pathology (e.g. abdominal or pelvic pain, post-coital bleeding) or breakthrough bleeding persists >3mo:

- Check compliance—any missed pills? Breakthrough bleeding may start 2–3d after a missed pill; any diarrhoea/vomiting
- Check for gynaecological causes—exclude STI (especially chlamydia); examine cervix; check smear is up to date and take smear if overdue; exclude pregnancy; consider referral for ultrasound, hysteroscopy + endometrial sampling if >45y or other risk factors for endometrial cancer

↑ oestrogen content of COC pill if on low-dose preparation. If problem persists, change progestogen. If still persists ↑ progestogen and/or try phased preparation.

Long-term risks/benefits See Table 22.3, 📖 p. 754

Acne and CHC In general acne improves when using CHC. If it fails to improve, consider switching to a brand containing a less androgenic progestogen (e.g. desogestrel, drosperidone) or one with a higher oestrogen content. Co-pyrindiol use is associated with higher risk of thromboembolism; if using for contraception as well as acne control, switch to an alternative CHC 3–4mo after symptoms have resolved.

Hepatic-enzyme-inducing drugs Combined contraceptives may interact with hepatic-enzyme-inducing drugs leading to ↓ efficacy, e.g.:

- Anti-infective agents—rifamycins (rifampicin, rifabutin), griseofulvin, antivirals (e.g. nelfinavir, nevirapine, ritonavir)
- St John's wort
- Anticonvulsants—phenytoin, carbamazepine, oxcarbazepine, phenobarbital, primidone, topiramate, modafinil

Short course (<7d) of enzyme-inducing drug Advise additional barrier contraception whilst taking the enzyme-inducing drug and for 4wk after stopping it. Omit pill/patch-free week or inactive tablets if using an 'ED' preparation.

Longer course of enzyme-inducing drug For rifampicin or rifabutin, advise alternative method of contraception, e.g. intrauterine device. For other enzyme-inducing drugs, consider ↑ the dose to ≥50 micrograms ethinylestradiol (maximum 70 micrograms) and shorten pill/patch/ring-free interval to 4d; alternatively advise another unaffected method of contraception, e.g. intrauterine device.

❶ There is no evidence that broad-spectrum antibiotics (e.g. amoxicillin) ↓ efficacy of combined contraceptives. Additional contraceptive precautions are no longer recommended.

Anticonvulsants that do not affect pill efficacy
• Sodium valproate
• Lamotrigine—but seizure frequency may ↑ when combined contraception and lamotrigine are used together and side effects of lamotrigine may be ↑ when combined contraception is stopped

Interaction with ulipristal acetate (UPA) UPA blocks the action of progesterone and so ↓ effectiveness of combined contraceptives. Advise additional contraception for 14d after using UPA when taking combined contraceptives (16d if taking estradiol valerate/dienogest pills).

Diarrhoea and vomiting Does *not* affect the contraceptive patch or ring. If a woman vomits <2h after taking a COC pill or has very severe diarrhoea, assume the COC pill has not been absorbed and treat as a missed pill (☐ p. 755).

Surgery Combined contraceptives should be discontinued and alternative contraceptive arrangements made (e.g. depo-injection, barrier methods) 4wk before major elective surgery, all surgery to the legs or surgery which involves prolonged immobilization of a lower limb. Restart the combined contraceptive on the first day of the next period occurring ≥2wk after full mobilization.

Long journeys and DVT Women taking combined contraceptives are at ↑ risk of DVT during travel involving long periods of immobility (>3h). Advise women:
• To drink plenty of non-alcoholic fluids
• To keep their legs moving whilst sitting, or walk up and down the aisle

Graduated compression hosiery is available for purchase OTC and does ↓ risk of DVT.

Further information
Family Planning Association (FPA) ☎ 0845 122 8690 (0845 122 8687 in Northern Ireland) 🖳 www.fpa.org.uk
FSRH 🖳 www.fsrh.org
• Missed pill recommendations (2011)
• Combined hormonal contraception (2012)
BNF Section 7.3.1 🖳 www.bnf.org

Progestogen-only contraceptives

Progestogen-only contraceptives thicken cervical mucus, ↓ endometrial receptivity, and inhibit ovulation. They ↓ risk of pelvic infection and can be used when oestrogen is contraindicated.

Reasons not to prescribe progestogen-only contraception

- Current breast cancer—may be used with specialist advice if disease-free for >5y and no other suitable method of contraception
- Trophoblastic disease—seek specialist advice if unsure
- Liver disease—active viral hepatitis; severe decompensated cirrhosis, or liver tumour (benign or malignant)
- If new symptoms/diagnosis of ischaemic heart disease, stroke/TIA, or migraine with aura when taking progestogen-only contraception
- Avoid if SLE with antiphospholipid antibodies (or if unknown)

❶ Investigate any undiagnosed vaginal bleeding before starting progestogen-only contraception.

Progestogen-releasing intrauterine system (Mirena®) 📖 p. 762

Progestogen-only pill (POP or 'mini-pill') (*BNF* 7.3.2.1.) Oral POPs are a suitable alternative for women for whom oestrogen-containing pills are contraindicated:

- Older women
- Heavy smokers
- Women with past history/predisposition to venous thromboembolism
- Patients with hypertension, valvular heart disease, DM, or migraine
- Breast-feeding women <6mo postpartum ❶ Delay until ≥3wk postpartum to avoid risk of heavy bleeding

Choice of POP 5 brands are currently available in the UK:

- Etynodiol 500 micrograms—Femulen®
- Norethisterone 350 micrograms—Micronor® or Noriday®
- Levonorgestrel 30 micrograms—Norgeston®
- Desogestrel 75 micrograms—Cerazette® or Nacrez®—use if compliance problems (12h window before 'missed pill'), history of ectopic pregnancy or ovarian cysts (desogestrol POPs have a stronger ovarian suppressive effect than other POPs), and/or weight >70kg

Side effects

- Higher failure rate than COC pills
- Menstrual irregularities—oligomenorrhoea, menorrhagia, amenorrhoea— examine to exclude a pathological cause ± do a pregnancy test. Menstrual irregularities tend to resolve with long-term use. If necessary, consider changing progestogen or ↑ to 2 pills/d (unlicensed)
- ↑ risk of ectopic pregnancy. If a patient presents with abdominal pain treat as an ectopic pregnancy (📖 p. 816) until proven otherwise
- *Others*—nausea and vomiting; headache; dizziness; breast discomfort; depression; skin disorders; disturbance of appetite; weight changes; changes in libido
- *Long-term*—small ↑ risk breast cancer; risk reverts to normal <10y after stopping the POP

Starting the POP
- **No previous hormonal contraception** Start on day 1–5 of the cycle—no additional contraception needed; if starting any other time, use additional contraception/abstain from sexual intercourse for 2d (9d if started after emergency contraception using ulipristal acetate)
- **Changing from COC** Start the day following completion of COC without a break (omitting 'inactive' pills if ED preparation)—no additional contraception needed
- **Changing from IUD** If POP started ≥2d before removal of copper IUD or at the time of IUS removal—no additional contraception; if started at the time of copper IUD removal, advise abstinence/barrier contraception for 7d prior to removal and for 2d afterwards
- **After childbirth** Start any time >3wk postpartum (↑ risk of bleeding earlier). Does not affect lactation. No additional contraception needed

Directions for taking the POP Take 1 tablet every day with no pill-free breaks. Take each tablet at the same time each day—if delayed >3h (>12h for desogestrel POP) treat as missed pill.

Missed pills If a pill is missed or delayed >3h (>12h for desogestrel POP), continue taking the POP at the usual time and use additional barrier methods for 2d.

⚠ Give emergency contraception if ≥1 POPs have been missed or taken >3h late (>12h late for desogestrel POP) and unprotected sexual intercourse has occurred in the 2d following this.

Diarrhoea/vomiting Continue taking the POP but use an additional barrier method during the episode and for 2d afterwards.

Interactions with other drugs Efficacy of POPs is not affected by antibacterials that do not induce liver enzymes. Efficacy is ↓ by enzyme-inducing drugs (📖 p. 756)—advise women to use an additional barrier method or alternative contraceptive method during treatment and for >4wk afterwards. Advise an alternative method of contraception if taking long-term hepatic-enzyme-inducing drugs.

Follow-up Review 3mo after starting the POP or changing from CHC—earlier if complications. Once established, review every 6–12mo—assess risk factors and side effects; give health education, e.g. smoking cessation advice, information about STIs, information about long-acting reversible contraception; check BP.

Injectable progestogens *(BNF 7.3.2.2)* Useful if oestrogen-containing preparations are contraindicated or compliance is a problem. Failure rate is <4/1,000 women over 2y.

Advantages
- Can be used to age 50y if no other risk factors for osteoporosis
- ↓ ectopic pregnancy, functional ovarian cysts, and sickle cell crises
- ↓ risk of endometrial cancer. Provides endometrial protection as part of HRT regime (unlicensed)
- May alleviate premenstrual syndrome and ↓ menorrhagia

Disadvantages
- Relatively contraindicated if DM with complications or multiple risk factors for CVD
- May ↓ bone density in first 2–3y of use. Consider DEXA scan in older women if result would influence choice
- Can mask natural menopause
- May be a delay in return of fertility of up to 1y on stopping
- Can cause menstrual disturbance—if troublesome give next injection early (8–11wk after the previous injection for Depo) or add oestrogen if no contraindications
- Other side effects, e.g. weight ↑ (up to 2–3kg), mood swings, acne

Depo-Provera® Medroxyprogesterone acetate 150mg/mL.
- Give 1× 1mL by deep IM injection into the buttock/lateral thigh or deltoid up to day 5 of the cycle. Do not rub the injection site afterwards
- If given for first time after day 5, check the woman is not pregnant and provide and advise an additional method for 7d
- Postpartum: delay until >6wk after childbirth—if not breastfeeding, first dose can be given <5d after childbirth but may cause heavy bleeding
- Repeat every 12wk. If interval is >12wk and 5d—see Table 22.4

⚠ **CSM advice about Depo-Provera®**
- In all women, weigh benefits of use for >2y against risks
- In women with risk factors for osteoporosis, consider a method of contraception other than Depo-Provera®
- In adolescents, Depo-Provera® should only be used only when other methods of contraception are inappropriate

Noristerat® Norethisterone enantate 200mg/mL. Warm first then give 1× 1mL by deep IM injection into the gluteal muscle before day 6 of the cycle or immediately after childbirth (avoid breastfeeding if baby has jaundice requiring treatment). Do not rub the injection site afterwards.
May be repeated once only after 8wk. Unlicensed if repeated further.

Interactions Effectiveness is not ↓ by antibacterials that do not induce liver enzymes. Effectiveness of Noristerat® (but not Depo-Provera®) is ↓ by enzyme-inducing drugs—advise additional contraception whilst taking these drugs and for 4wk after stopping *or* alternative method.

Progestogen implant (see *BNF* 7.3.2.2) Nexplanon® is the only implant currently available in the UK. It is a radio-opaque flexible rod (40mm × 2mm) containing 68mg of etonogestrel that is inserted subdermally into the lower surface of the upper arm on day 1–5 of the cycle. If inserted after day 5, check not pregnant and use an additional method for 7d.

Advantages Lasts 3y and, once inserted, no compliance required; can be used for women at risk of ectopic pregnancy; no effect on bone density; once removed, fertility returns immediately to normal.

Disadvantages A minor operation is needed for insertion/removal. Special training is needed, and complications of minor surgery can occur (e.g. infection, scarring). ↓ efficacy with liver enzyme-inducing drugs—advise additional method for duration of treatment and 4wk afterwards or alternative contraception if enzyme-inducing drugs are being used long-term. Cannot be used as part of a HRT regime. May cause menstrual disturbances—exclude other causes. Treat with oestrogen (Marvelon® contains the same progestogen), additional progestogen, or NSAID. Other side effects include acne, mood swings, breast tenderness, change in libido—treat symptoms as needed.

Table 22.4 Late Depo-Provera® guidelines

Timing of Depo-Provera®	Has unprotected sex occurred?	Can the injection be given?	Is emergency contraception needed?	Are condoms or abstinence advised?	Should a pregnancy test be done?
Up to 12wk and 5d since date of previous injection	N/A	Yes	No	No	No
	No	Yes	No	Yes—for the next 14d*	No
	Yes—but only in the last 3d	Yes—or give desogestrel 75 micrograms for 21d	Yes	Yes—for the next 14d*	Yes—21d later
When an injection is overdue	Yes—but only in the last 3–5d	Yes—or give desogestrel 75 micrograms for 21d	Yes—offer copper IUD	No	Yes—21d later
	Yes—>5d ago	No	No	Yes—for 21d until a pregnancy test is confirmed negative and for a further 14d* after giving Depo injection	Yes—at initial presentation and 21d later

☞ *WHO/FSRH recommendations state that injections of Depo-Provera® can be given up to 14wk and Noristerat® can be given up to 10wk after the previous injection without the need for additional barrier contraception. These guidelines also state that, when needed, additional contraception is only necessary for 7d.

Further information

NICE Long-acting reversible contraception (2005) ℅ www.nice.org.uk
FSRH ℅ www.fsrh.org
- Progestogen-only pills (2009)
- Progestogen-only injectable contraception (2009)
- Progestogen-only implants (2008)
- Nexplanon® (2010)

Patient information

Family Planning Association (FPA) ☏ 0845 122 8690 (0845 122 8687 in Northern Ireland) ℅ www.fpa.org.uk

Intrauterine devices

Intrauterine contraceptive device (IUCD) (*BNF* 7.3.4) Plastic carrier wound with copper wire/fitted with copper bands. Suitable for:

• Older parous women
• As second-line contraception in young nulliparous women, or
• For emergency contraception

Acts by inhibiting fertilization, sperm penetration of the cervical mucus, and implantation. Pregnancy rate with IUCDs containing 380mm^2 copper is <20/1,000 over 5y.

Intrauterine system (IUS) (*BNF* 7.3.2.3) The progestogen-only intrauterine system (*Mirena®*) releases levonorgestrel 20 microgram/24h directly into the uterine cavity. It acts by preventing endometrial proliferation, thickening of cervical mucus, and suppression of ovulation (some women and some cycles). Licensed uses include:

• Contraception—particularly suitable for women with heavy periods
• Primary menorrhagia—menstrual bleeding is ↓ significantly in 3–6mo
• Prevention of endometrial hyperplasia during oestrogen therapy

Emergency contraception 🔲 p. 750

Choice of devices See Table 22.5

Contraindications

IUCD only Allergy to copper; Wilson's disease; heavy/painful periods.

IUCD and IUS

• Pregnancy or <4wk postpartum
• Current or high risk of STI or pelvic inflammatory disease (includes severe immunosuppression)—a woman should not have an IUCD/IUS fitted <3mo after treatment of a pelvic infection. Following treatment of STI suitability depends on ongoing risk
• Undiagnosed uterine bleeding
• Distorted uterine cavity
• Endometrial, ovarian or cervical cancer, or trophoblastic disease
• Anticoagulation—caution—use another method if possible

Advantages

IUCD only No systemic side effects; does not mask the menopause; if fitted in a woman of >40y can remain in the uterus until menopause (unlicensed).

IUS only

• ↓ menorrhagia/dysmenorrhoea
• ↓ risk of pelvic inflammatory disease—particularly younger age groups
• ↓ risk of ectopic pregnancy compared to the IUCD
• If 45y and amenorrhoeic, can be left *in situ* for 7y for contraception (unlicensed)—change after 4y if using IUS for endometrial protection

IUCD and IUS

• Long-lasting and can be used until the menopause
• Once fitted, no compliance is needed

- Easily and immediately reversible by removal
- Can be used for women who are breastfeeding, obese, or have concurrent illness—migraine, venous thromboembolism, DM, cardiovascular disease (or ↑ risk of cardiovascular disease), or women taking long-term hepatic-enzyme-inducing drugs (e.g. anticonvulsants, antivirals)
- Can be used for HIV +ve women—but screen for STIs first and advise condom use

Disadvantages and problems

IUCD only

- **Ectopic pregnancy** Risk (0.02/100 women years) is higher than if using a hormonal contraceptive method. If pregnancy occurs, there is a 1 in 20 risk of ectopic pregnancy—consider in any woman who has IUCD and develops abdominal pain
- **↑ dysmenorrhoea/menorrhagia** Most common reason for discontinuation. Exclude infection and malposition. Exclude other gynaecological causes. Treat with NSAID or tranexamic acid or consider changing to the IUS

IUS only Progestogenic side effects:

- Changes in pattern/duration of menstrual bleeding (spotting/prolonged bleeding) are common—warn women prior to insertion. Bleeding usually becomes light/absent within 3–6mo of insertion
- Mastalgia, mood changes, change in libido—usually resolve in <6mo
- Ovarian cysts—usually resolve spontaneously; monitor with USS
- Cannot be used for emergency contraception

Table 22.5 Intrauterine devices currently available in the UK

Device	Licence	Uterine length
Flexi-T 300®	5y	>5cm
FlexiT +380®	5y	>6cm
GyneFix®	5y	Any
Load 375®	5y	>7cm
Mini TT 380 Slimline®	5y	>5cm
Multiload Cu375®	5y	6–9cm
Multi-Safe 375®	5y	6–9cm
Nova-T 380®	5y	6.5–9cm
Neo-SafeT380®	5y	6.5–9cm
T-Safe Cu380A Quickload®	10y	6.5–9cm
TT 380 Slimline®	10y	6.5–9cm
UT 380 Short or Standard®	5y	Short—5–7cm Standard—6.5–9cm
Mirena®	5y*	>6.5cm

*4y if being used for prevention of endometrial hyperplasia

IUCD and IUS

- **Fitting and removal** Requires specialist training and can be uncomfortable for the woman
- **Expulsion/malposition**—Risk of expulsion is ~1 in 20. Usually occurs <3mo after insertion—teach women to feel for threads after each period. If threads cannot be felt advise other contraception until checked by a health professional (see Figure 22.3)
- **Perforation of the uterus** Risk <1 in 1,000
- **Pelvic inflammatory disease** ↑ risk of infection <21d after insertion. Related to existing carriage of STIs. It is good practice to screen for STIs (especially chlamydia) and treat infection prior to insertion
- **Actinomyces-like organisms (ALOs) on cervical smear** Assess to exclude pelvic infection. If no signs of pelvic infection, offer choice to leave device *in situ* or change it. If symptomatic discuss antibiotic treatment with microbiology and refer to GUM/gynaecology for further management
- **Intrauterine pregnancy** Confirm intrauterine pregnancy with USS. Remove device at <12wk gestation whether or not the woman intends to continue the pregnancy. If pregnancy is >12wk or no threads are visible, refer to obstetrics/gynaecology

Insertion Special training is required. The Faculty of Sexual and Reproductive Healthcare runs a training scheme (☎ 020 7724 5669 ✍ www.fsrh.org). Accreditation must be updated every 5y. IUS/IUCDs may be inserted:

- <7d after onset of menstruation—tail end of a period is the optimum time; heaviest days of a period are best avoided
- At any other time in the cycle—if replacement of IUS/IUCD. If first device, and not in the first 7d of the cycle, ensure not pregnant and advise additional method for 7d
- Immediately after TOP/miscarriage or >4wk postpartum (unlicensed <6wk postpartum), irrespective of the mode of delivery[N]
- Always consider pre-screening for STI (especially chlamydia) ± antibiotic prophylaxis, e.g. azithromycin 1g stat, prior to insertion. Advise women to contact a doctor if any sustained pain is experienced in the first 3wk after insertion

⚠ **Cervical shock** Rare complication of IUD insertion. Presents with pallor, sweating, and bradycardia. Immediately tip the woman head down with legs raised. If symptoms/bradycardia persist, give 0.6mg atropine IV.

⚠ **Women with epilepsy** ↑ risk of seizure at the time of cervical dilation—ensure emergency drugs are available.

Follow-up Review after first period then annually. Ask about periods, pelvic pain, vaginal discharge, and discomfort to partner. Perform pelvic examination to check threads.

Figure 22.3 Missing intra-uterine device threads

Reproduced from Sadler C, White J, Everitt H, Simon C (2007) *Women's Health*, with permission from Oxford University Press.

Removal

- If pregnancy is desired—remove at any time
- If pregnancy is not desired—remove after establishing a hormonal method or use barrier methods/abstinence for ≥7d prior to removal. If urgent removal is necessary, provide emergency contraception if mid cycle and intercourse has occurred in the previous 7d (📖 p. 750)
- Menopause—remove after 1y amenorrhoea if aged >50y or after 2y amenorrhoea if aged <50y. If there is difficulty removing the device, try again after a 5d course of oestrogen (e.g. Premarin® 1.25mg od po)

Further information

FSRH Intrauterine contraception (2007) ℜ www.fsrh.org
NICE Long-acting reversible contraception (2005) ℜ www.nice.org.uk

Patient information

Family Planning Association (FPA) ☎ 0845 122 8690 (0845 122 8687 in Northern Ireland) ℜ www.fpa.org.uk

Other contraceptive methods

Sterilization There are no absolute contraindications to sterilization of men or women, provided that:

- They make the request themselves
- They are of sound mind, *and*
- They are not acting under external duress

⚠ If there is any question of a person not having the mental capacity to consent to a procedure that will permanently remove their fertility, seek advice from your medical defence organization.

Method

- **Women** Laparoscopic tubal occlusion with clips or rings (usually done under GA as a day case) or hysteroscopic sterilization with intratubal implants (usually done under LA or sedation as a day case)
- **Men** Vasectomy. Usually done under LA as a day case

Pre-referral counselling

- Alternative long-term contraceptive methods (include sterilization of partner as an alternative)
- Reversibility—sterilization is intended to be permanent; reversal is only 50–60% successful
- Failure rate—1 in 200 for ♀; 1 in 2,000 for ♂
- ↑ risk of ectopic pregnancy after tubal occlusion
- Risk of operative complications
- Effect on long-term health—no proven long-term risks
- Need for contraception before and after operation
  - *Women:* other contraception until first post-procedure period
  - *Men:* other contraception until 2 consecutive semen analyses, 2–4wk apart and ≥8wk after the procedure shows azoospermia

❶ All counselling should be supported by impartial written information.

⚠ Take additional care when counselling:

- People of <30y
- People without children
- People taking decisions during pregnancy
- People taking decisions in reaction to a loss of relationship
- People at risk of coercion by their partner, family, or health or social welfare professionals

Coitus interruptus Penis is withdrawn prior to ejaculation.

Avoidance of intercourse during times of fertility 3 methods of estimating time of ovulation are used:

- **Urine testing**—a commercial kit (Persona®) is available to buy
- **Temperature**—taken orally in the morning before drinking/getting up (thermometer is available on NHS prescription). ↑ 0.2–0.4°C indicates progesterone release from the corpus luteum. Unprotected intercourse can take place from day 3 of the ↑ until the next period
- **Mucus texture** (Billing's method). Texture of vaginal secretions is felt between finger and thumb daily. Prior to ovulation the mucus

becomes profuse and slippery, then abruptly changes to being thicker and more tacky. No unprotected intercourse from the day the mucus becomes more profuse until 3d after it becomes tacky. Patients with cycles > or <28d must vary timings

Vaginal diaphragms (*BNF* 7.3.4) Latex or silicone and flat metal spring, coiled metal rim, or arcing spring diaphragms are available. Motivation is crucial. Fitting must be performed by a doctor or nurse trained to fit diaphragms. After fitting, a woman should practise inserting, wearing, checking the diaphragm is over the cervix, and removing the diaphragm for >1wk using another form of contraception. Some vegetable/mineral oil-based lubricants (e.g. petroleum jelly (Vaseline®), baby oil) can damage caps. Water-based lubricants are safe (e.g. KY Jelly®).

❗ Spermicides (2 x 2cm strips applied to the upper surface) must always be used in combination with diaphragms and reapplied without removal if *in situ* >3h before sex takes place. The diaphragm must be left *in situ* for ≥6h (maximum 30h) after intercourse.

Follow-up Check fit and comfort after ~1wk, and discuss again the routine for use, especially the importance of spermicide. See after 3mo and then annually, but more frequently if there are difficulties, if there is a weight change of >4kg, if the woman has a baby, or after pelvic surgery. Prescribe a new diaphragm yearly.

Cervical caps (*BNF* 7.3.4) Silicone. Attach by suction. Otherwise used in the same way as a diaphragm. The inside of the cap should be filled one-third full of spermicide. Useful for women with poor muscle tone, absent retropubic ledge, or recurrent cystitis when using a diaphragm.

Spermicides to use in combination with caps or condoms (*BNF* 7.3.3) Nonoxinol '9' 2% gel (Gygel®) is the only preparation currently available in the UK.

Condoms Give protection against STIs. Male and female versions.
- A new condom should be applied for each episode of sexual intercourse (or if applied incorrectly) and only one should be used at a time; male and female condoms should not be used simultaneously
- Advise about emergency contraception in the event of an accident
- Some lubricants/topical vaginal preparations ↓ effectiveness, e.g. petroleum jelly (Vaseline®), baby oil, and oil-based vaginal/rectal preparations; water-based lubricants are safe (e.g. KY Jelly®)

Dams Are not a contraceptive but protect against STIs. Thin film that provides a barrier between the mouth/cervico-vaginal secretions or between the mouth and anus.

Further information
FSRH ℘ www.fsrh.org
- Barrier methods for contraception and STI prevention (2012)
- Sterilization (2013)

Patient information
Family Planning Association (FPA) ☎ 0845 122 8690 ℘ www.fpa.org.uk
Fertility UK ℘ www.fertilityuk.org

Teenagers and women over 40

Contraception for the under 16s

Sexual health problems One in three have sexual intercourse under the age of 16y. Those who have intercourse early are at ↑ risk of early pregnancy and STI. Worries about sexuality can add to the pressure for some. Sensitive support, clear guidance, and accurate information about contraception, sexuality, and STI are helpful. Remember to offer chlamydia screening (🔲 p. 740) to the under 25s.

Safeguarding (🔲 p. 924) ⚠ Sexual intercourse with a child under the age of 13y is rape and must be reported to the authorities.

Providing contraception to the under 16s In the UK, a doctor is allowed to give contraceptive advice and treatment to a girl aged <16y without parental consent if it is in her best interest that contraceptive advice/treatment is given and she:
- Is sufficiently mature to understand the moral, social, and emotional implications of treatment
- Cannot be persuaded to inform her parents
- Is likely to begin/continue, intercourse with or without contraception
- Is likely to suffer if no contraceptive advice or treatment is given

Confidentiality and consent 🔲 p. 50 and p. 52

Choice of contraceptive method
- **Condoms** Most commonly used contraception for adolescents. Relatively high failure rate—suggest their use in addition to another form of contraception to help prevent STIs
- **Long-acting reversible contraception (LARC)** Offer IUCD, progestogen implant, injectables, or intrauterine system to all teenagers. Provides high levels of protection against pregnancy with no need for ongoing compliance once fitted/administered. ❶ The CSM advises that medroxyprogesterone acetate (Depo-Provera®) should only be used when other methods of contraception are inappropriate as it may ↑ osteoporosis risk (use alternative if other risk factors and try not to use >2y), menstrual irregularity, and ↑ weight
- **Combined hormonal contraception** (pill, patch, or vaginal ring) Suitable method of contraception for the under 16s. Poor compliance can be a problem and leads to a relatively high failure rate
- **Progestogen-only pill** (POP) Suitable for teenagers but has the same compliance problems as combined hormonal contraception and is associated with menstrual irregularity. Useful if the teenager does not want long-acting contraception and CHC is contraindicated
- **'Morning after pill'** (levonorgestrel 1.5mg <72h or ulipristal acetate 30mg <120h after unprotected intercourse). Not suitable as regular contraception, but valuable in preventing unwanted pregnancy. Provide information on availability and make it easy for teenagers to get urgent same-day appointments to obtain a prescription

Do's and don'ts
- *Don't* insist on vaginal examination unless it is necessary
- *Do* discuss the merits of delaying sexual intercourse until older
- *Do* stress the need for protection against sexually transmitted infection

- If prescribing combined hormonal contraception for acne, dysmenorrhoea or cycle control, *do* explain its use for contraception too
- *Do* consider 'quick-starting' contraception when the young person is seen rather than waiting for the next cycle

Information and support for teenagers
Brook Advisory Service ☎ 0808 802 1234 ✆ www.brook.org.uk
Sexwise For under 19s ☎ 0800 28 29 30
Teenage Health Freak ✆ www.teenagehealthfreak.org

Contraception for women >40y

Choice of contraceptive method

- **Combined hormonal contraception** Non-smokers with no risk factors for CVD or breast cancer can use combined hormonal contraception until 50y. Consider a lower oestrogen preparation (20 micrograms ethinylestradiol). Improves menstrual and menopausal symptoms and protects bone density. Women experiencing menopausal symptoms may wish to try an extended regime (📖 p. 754)
- **Progestogen-only pill** Can be continued to 55y and can be used as the progestogen component of HRT, but three POPs daily are needed for endometrial protection (unlicensed and no data for desogestrel). Does not interfere with FSH levels
- **Injectable progestogen** Can be used up to 50y in women not at risk of osteoporosis (CSM advises benefits of using injectable medroxyprogesterone acetate for >2y should be evaluated against risks of ↓ bone density). May cause menstrual irregularity
- **Progestogen implant** Cannot be used as part of HRT regime
- **IUS** (Mirena®) Improves menorrhagia. Licensed for endometrial protection (can be used as part of an HRT regime). If 45y and amenorrhoeic, can be left *in situ* for 7y for contraception (unlicensed); change after 4y if using IUS for endometrial protection
- **IUCD** Copper intrauterine devices fitted in women >40y may remain in the uterus until post-menopause

Stopping contraception after the menopause

- **Non-hormonal methods** After 2y amenorrhoea if <50y; after 1y amenorrhoea if ≥50y
- **Combined hormonal or injectable progestogen** Use to 50y, then switch to alternative method of contraception
- **Implant, POP, or IUS** Continue to 50y; if ≥50y and amenorrhoeic, continue to 55y or check FSH—if FSH >30iu/L, repeat after 6wk and if second FSH >30iu/L stop contraception after 1y of amenorrhoea; if ≥50y and not amenorrhoeic, consider investigating abnormal bleeding and continue >55y until amenorrhoeic for 1y

Further information

Family Planning Association (FPA) ☎ 0845 122 8690 (0845 122 8687 in Northern Ireland) ✆ www.fpa.org.uk
FSRH ✆ www.fsrh.org
- Contraception for women aged over 40 years (2010)
- Contraceptive choices for young people (2010)
- UK Medical Eligibility Criteria for contraceptive use (2009)

Termination of pregnancy

The role of the GP

- The earlier in pregnancy a termination of pregnancy is performed, the lower the risk of complications. General practice is often the first stage of the referral procedure—have arrangements which minimize delay
- Termination of pregnancy (TOP), especially for 'social' reasons, is a difficult ethical area for many GPs. Whatever your views, be sympathetic and if not prepared to refer yourself, arrange for the patient to see someone who will do so as soon as possible
- Confirm pregnancy if unsure. Assess dates by bimanual palpation or arrange dating USS
- Counselling—unbiased counselling to allow a woman to reach a decision she feels is right for her—this is an important decision she will have to live with for the rest of her life. Why does she want a termination? Has she considered alternatives? Does her partner/do her parents know? What are their views?
- Ideally the woman should be given some time once she has all the information to make her decision (e.g. follow-up in a few days). Offer a let-out clause—she can always change her mind right up until the time of the procedure, and you will support her whatever decision she makes
- Consider signing form HSA1 (remember to include your qualifications)
- Discuss contraception after TOP (ideally do this before TOP so it can be started immediately after)
- Arrange follow-up after the procedure

Legal constraints The 1967 and 1990 Human Fertilization/Embryology Acts govern termination of pregnancy in the UK. Termination is allowed at <24wk gestation if termination:

- ↓ risk to the woman's life
- ↓ risk to the mother's physical/mental health (90% TOPs are carried out under this clause)
- ↓ risk to the physical/mental health of the mother's existing children
- The baby is at serious risk of being physically or mentally handicapped

There is no upper time limit if there is:

- Real risk to the mother's life
- Risk of grave, permanent injury to the mother's physical or mental health, *or*
- The baby would be born seriously physically or mentally handicapped

Terminations of pregnancy (TOPs) >24wk can only be carried out in NHS hospitals. 99% TOPs take place <20wk. Those taking place >20wk are usually performed when fetal abnormality is found on USS (or amniocentesis) or if pregnancy is concealed in the very young.

> ❶ Seek medicolegal advice from your medical indemnity organization if the patient is <16y or has a cognitive deficit that might impair ability to consent to referral and/or treatment.

Procedure

- **Medical** Oral mifepristone followed by oral and/or vaginal prostaglandin (usually misoprostol)
- **Surgical** Suction termination <15wk; dilatation and evacuation >15wk

Complications

- Infection
- Haemorrhage
- Uterine perforation
- Cervical trauma
- Failed procedure and ongoing pregnancy
- Psychological sequelae

There is no association between TOP and subsequent infertility or miscarriage/preterm delivery.

Follow-up In many areas post-procedure follow-up is undertaken by the GP. Worrying symptoms are: excessive blood loss, pain, *and/or* high temperature. Assess, consider the possibility of infection and treat if reasonably well; admit if the patient is unwell.

Check anti-D has been given if needed (📖 p. 820) and chosen method of contraception has been started.

Contraception post-termination or miscarriage <24wk

- **Combined pill/patch/ring, POP, progestogen injection/implant** Start on the day of surgical or second part of medical termination. No additional method required. If started >5d after termination (day 1 only for estradiol valerate/dienogest pill) an additional method is required for 2d (POP), 7d (combined pill/patch/ring or progestogen injection/implant) or 9d (estradiol valerate/dienogest pill)
- **IUCD or IUS** Insert at time of surgical or second part of a medical abortion. No additional method required. Otherwise delay insertion to 4wk post-abortion—use another method in the interim

Teenage pregnancy The UK has the highest teenage pregnancy rate in western Europe. Not all are unplanned. Pregnant teenagers need information and non-judgemental support to help them to reach a decision whether or not to continue with the pregnancy.

Further information

RCOG The care of women requesting induced abortion (2004) ℘ www.rcog.org.uk

Information/support for women about unplanned pregnancy

Family Planning Association (FPA) ☎ 0845 122 8690 (0845 122 8687 in Northern Ireland) ℘ www.fpa.org.uk
Marie Stopes International ☎ 0845 300 8090 ℘ www.mariestopes.org.uk
British Pregnancy Advisory Service (BPAS) ☎ 0845 730 40 30 ℘ www.bpas.org
Brook Advisory Centres (patients <25y only) ☎ 0808 802 1234 ℘ www.brook.org.uk
Antenatal results and choices (ARC) Supports parents faced with termination for fetal abnormality ☎ 0845 077 2290 ℘ www.arc-uk.org

Infertility

Failure to conceive after 1y of regular unprotected sexual intercourse in the absence of known reproductive pathology. Affects ~1 in 5 couples.

Pregnancy rates The normal rate of pregnancy in the first year is 20–25% per cycle. 84% of couples conceive after 1y of unprotected intercourse (17 in every 20 couples); 92% conceive after 2y (19 of every 20 couples); after 3y, the pregnancy rate is still ~25%/y.

Causes of infertility
- Ovulatory dysfunction ~30%
- Pelvic disease ~20%
- Male factor ~20%
- Unknown ~30%

Initial approach Most couples tend to present at about 1y. Where possible, see the couple together. This shows mutual commitment and initiates ongoing, couple-centred management.

Couple Ask about:
- **Length of time trying to conceive**
- **Frequency of and/or difficulties with sexual intercourse,** e.g. psychosexual problems, physical disability—includes excessive travelling which may limit optimal coital timing and indirectly affect fertility

Women Ask about:
- **Previous pregnancies**—children, miscarriages, same/different partner?
- **Menstrual cycle**—length of cycle (normal cycle is 21–35d duration), changes in cervical mucus through the cycle, ovulatory discomfort?
- **Past gynaecological history**—cervical smears, previous pelvic surgery, STI/pelvic inflammatory disease, PCOS
- **Past medical history**—systemic or debilitating disease, e.g. thyroid dysfunction, DM, inflammatory bowel disease, anorexia nervosa
- **Drug history**—chemotherapy, phenothiazines, cannabis, NSAIDs
- **Lifestyle**—occupation (exposure to pesticides?), smoking, alcohol, excessive exercise, stress

Men Ask about:
- **Previous children**, same/different partner?
- **PMH**—mumps, other testicular disease, STI
- **Any systemic or debilitating diseases?**
- **Drug history**—sulfasalazine, nitrofurantoin, tetracycline, cimetidine, ketoconazole, colchicine, allopurinol, α-blockers, tricyclic antidepressants, MAOI, phenothiazines, propranolol, chemotherapy, anabolic steroids, cannabis, cocaine
- **Social history**—occupation (exposure to pesticides, X-rays, solvents, paints, chemicals from smelting or welding), smoking, alcohol, excess exercise, stress, social or occupational factors which might cause testicular hyperthermia

Adverse factors Age (♀ only—fertility ↓ significantly from mid-30s), BMI <19 (♀ only) or >29 (♂ and ♀), smoking (↓ fertility by about one-third), excess alcohol (♂ only), excess caffeine (>2 cups of coffee/d—♀ only).

Examination Consider pelvic/genital examination.

GP investigations Perform investigations if no pregnancy after a year of trying to conceive—sooner if aged >35y.

Female
- Rubella status
- Chlamydia serology—indicator of possible tubal disease
- Mid-luteal progesterone—check on day 21 of the menstrual cycle for a woman with a 28d cycle; adjust timing if longer/shorter cycle. Can only be accurately interpreted after the next period as aims to 'catch' the progesterone peak 7d before the next period. Normal value (>30nmol/L) signifies ovulation
- FSH/LH—check on day 1–5 of the menstrual cycle
- Consider TFTs if symptoms/signs of thyroid disease, or prolactin if galactorrhoea or any suggestion of pituitary tumour

Male Sperm problems affect ~1 in 5 couples. Semen analysis is important even if the man already has children. If the first test is abnormal, advise loose trousers and underwear and repeat after 3mo—or as soon as possible if grossly abnormal. ❶ Abnormal sperm do not fertilize ova.

Instructions for producing a semen sample for analysis No sex for 2d beforehand and ≤7d since last sex (may affect motility). Masturbate into labelled sterile pot without use of condoms/gels. Keep the sample warm (e.g. inside pocket), and deliver to the laboratory within 2h. Handover directly to a member of laboratory staff if possible.

Referral Local protocols vary and exclusions may apply. Generally refer after 18mo of failure to conceive despite regular intercourse. Refer sooner if abnormal history, examination, or investigations, e.g.:
- **Female** age >35y; amenorrhoea/oligomenorrhoea; PCOS; previous pelvic inflammatory disease or STI
- **Male** Previous genital pathology or urogenital surgery; varicocele; significant systemic illness; persistent abnormality on semen analysis

Possible treatments GPs may need to continue to prescribe
- Clomifene—ovarian stimulation, treatment for oligospermia
- Tamoxifen—may be prescribed to women intolerant of clomifene
- Metformin—used as an adjunct to clomifene in overweight ladies with polycystic ovarian syndrome who fail to respond to clomifene alone
- Others, e.g. gonadotrophins, dopamine agonists (e.g. bromocriptine)

Counselling Consider early referral for specialist counselling. Access is through national support groups and at local specialist fertility centres. Useful contacts:
- British Infertility Counselling Association ℘ www.bica.net
- British Fertility Society ℘ www.britishfertilitysociety.org.uk

Further information

NICE Fertility: Assessment and treatment of people with fertility problems (2004) ℘ www.nice.org.uk

Advice and information for patients

Infertilitynetwork UK ☎ 0800 008 7464 ℘ www.infertilitynetworkuk.com

Sexual problems

Sexual problems may have a physical or psychological basis but *all* develop a psychological aspect in time. Both partners have a problem in ~30% cases. Be supportive—your response will determine whether the patient receives appropriate help.

Assessment

- **History of the problem** What is the problem? If new, when did it start? Why consult now? What outcome does the patient want? Is the patient complaining or is his/her partner?
- **Sexual history** Details of sex education; attitude towards sex; past history of sexual problems (or lack of problems)
- **Medical history** Chronic disease; psychiatric problems; current medication
- **Social history and recent life events**
- **Examination** Genitalia for abnormalities or tenderness—helpful but do not insist as it may scare the patient away

❶ *Always consider psychological aspects* Poor self-image; anger or resentment—relationship/financial difficulties, children, parents, work stress; ignorance or misunderstanding; shame, embarrassment, or guilt—view that sexuality is 'bad', sexual abuse; anxiety/fear about sex—fear of closeness, vulnerability, letting go, and failure.

Lack of sexual interest Usually needs specialist help. Often there are underlying psychological difficulties which may relate specifically to sex, e.g. previous child abuse, or a general psychological disorder. Women frequently lose interest around the menopause or after operations (especially mastectomy or hysterectomy) or if their partner's performance repeatedly leads to frustration (e.g. impotence). Both sexes lose interest if depressed or after traumatic events.

Vaginismus Usually apparent at vaginal examination—severe spasm of the vaginal muscles and adduction of thighs. May be detected incidentally when undertaking routine procedures, e.g. cervical smear. Try to find the root cause. *Common causes:*

- Fear of the unknown
- Local pain
- Past history of rape, abuse, or severe emotional trauma
- Defence mechanism against growing up

Management Treat any underlying medical disorder causing pain. Desensitize by encouraging the woman to examine herself, and also encourage the partner to be confident enough to insert a finger into the vagina. If no success, refer.

Orgasmic problems in women *Consider:*

Physical reasons

- Drugs—major tranquillizers, antidepressants
- Neurological disease
- Pelvic surgery—recognized complication of hysterectomy

Psychological reasons
- **Women who have never achieved an orgasm** May have psychological reasons. Give 'permission' for the woman to investigate her body's own responses further by masturbation or vibrator. When she has learned how to relax, encourage her to tell her partner and incorporate caressing into their usual lovemaking
- **Women who have lost the ability to achieve orgasm** May need specialist help, especially about current relationship or loss of self-image

Dyspareunia 📖 p. 714 **Erectile dysfunction** 📖 p. 776

Premature ejaculation Ejaculation sooner than either partner wishes. With practice men can learn to delay ejaculation. The stop/start technique may be effective: when during caressing or intercourse, a man feels he is close to climax he should stop being stimulated and relax for 30 seconds; stimulation can then recommence until he is close to climax again, when the relaxation is repeated. If this fails, the woman should squeeze the penis at the base of the glans between finger and thumb during relaxation phases. Consider referral for sex therapy if no improvement.

Delayed ejaculation May be a sign of long-standing sexual inhibition. Often patients can ejaculate by masturbation but not intravaginally. Explore anxiety and guilt feelings. Use a strategy like that for psychogenic erectile dysfunction (📖 p. 778). If that fails, refer for psychosexual counselling.

Retrograde ejaculation Semen passes into the bladder rather than the urethra—complication of TURP or bladder neck incision. May also occur as a result of spinal injury or DM. The patient can usually achieve an orgasm but there is no ejaculate or the volume of the ejaculate is ↓. Urine may be cloudy after having sex. Confirm diagnosis with urine microscopy (excess sperm in urine). Unless infertility is a problem, no treatment is required.

Haematospermia Blood in the ejaculate. Common causes include urogenital infection and minor urethral trauma, but often no cause is found. If persistent, underlying pathology is more likely. Ask about other symptoms, e.g. discharge, pain, dysuria. Examine the external genitalia and perform DRE to assess the prostate. Check MSU and semen analysis ± urethral swab (including chlamydia) if any urethral discharge/high risk of STI. Check PSA and urine cytology if patient is aged >40y. If persists and no cause is found, refer to urology.

Further information about specialist doctors/therapists
College of Sexual and Relationship Therapists
☎ 020 8543 2707 🖰 www.cosrt.org.uk
Institute of Psychosexual Medicine 🖰 www.ipm.org.uk

Information for patients
Brown P, Faulder C (1989) *Treat Yourself to Sex*. Harmondsworth: Penguin. ISBN: 0140110186.

Erectile dysfunction

50% men aged 40–70y experience inability to obtain/maintain sufficient rigidity of the penis to allow satisfactory sexual performance; 90% are too embarrassed to seek help—always ask. Incidence ↑ with age.

Organic causes (80%)

- **Cardiovascular** CHD ↑ incidence x4—more likely to have multi-vessel than single-vessel coronary artery disease; peripheral vascular disease; hypertension—incidence ↑ x2
- **DM** incidence ↑ ×3. >35% of diabetic men have erectile dysfunction. May be the presenting feature of DM
- **Neurological,** e.g. pelvic surgery, spinal injury, multiple sclerosis
- **Side effects of prescription drugs** Consider changing medication if onset of erectile dysfunction is within 2–4wk of initiation of drug therapy e.g. thiazides
- **Smoking** (incidence ↑ x2), **alcohol, or drug abuse**
- **Peyronie's disease** (📖 p. 464)
- **Testosterone deficiency or hyperprolactinaemia**

Psychogenic causes

- Performance anxiety
- Depression or stress
- Relationship failure
- Fear of intimacy

Drugs causing erectile dysfunction

- Antihypertensives
- Antidepressants (e.g. SSRIs)
- Major tranquillizers
- Anti-androgens
- Finasteride
- Cimetidine

History Ensure the presenting problem is erectile dysfunction and not other sexual difficulties; identify risk factors and distinguish psychogenic from organic causes (see Table 22.6). ❶ Many with organic erectile dysfunction develop a psychogenic component which perpetuates symptoms.

Examination and investigation

- CVD and DM—check BP, peripheral pulses, and blood for fasting lipid profile and glucose
- Psychological distress—consider depression/anxiety screening
- Testosterone insufficiency—genitals (small/absent), breasts ↑, ↓ beard (↓ frequency of shaving). If suspected, check serum testosterone, sex hormone binding globulin, free androgen index, FSH/LH ± prolactin

Table 22.6 Is erectile dysfunction organic or psychogenic?

	Psychogenic origin	Organic origin
Onset sudden or gradual?	Sudden onset	Gradual onset
Consistent loss of erections?	Inconsistent response	Consistent failure
Does the patient ever wake up with an erection?	Early-morning erections	Loss of early-morning erections
Does the patient want to have intercourse?	Relationship problems	Normal libido
Age?	Usually <60y	Usually >60y

Table 22.7 Treatment options for erectile dysfunction

Treatment	Notes
Oral drugs	
Phosphodiesterase type 5 inhibitors, e.g. sildenafil[S]	Effective for 70%. Use prn before intercourse (see Table 22.8). Only use 1x/d. Avoid if patient has unstable angina, recent stroke, or MI. *Do not* give a nitrate within 24h of use
Apomorphine	2–3mg prn 20min before sexual activity
Yohimbine[S]	Herbal remedy available OTC. 10–30mg od is effective May cause insomnia
Local drug treatments	
Intraurethral or intracavernosal alprostadil	Intraurethral preparation is effective for 40% and intracavernosal preparation for 80% patients. Used prn. Requires some manual dexterity. Takes ~10min to work. Penile pain is common. Prolonged erection and priapism results in ~1%. Advise patients to seek medical help if erection >4h
Mechanical devices	
Vacuum devices	80% effective. The penis is placed in the device and air withdrawn mechanically sucking blood into the penis. Erection is maintained by placing a constriction band around the base of the penis
Penile prosthesis	Last resort. Inflatable or rigid. Major complication is infection
Others	
Androgen supplements	Ineffective unless documented hypogonadism. Only use with specialist advice. Exclude prostatic cancer and significant CVD first, and check PSA and haematocrit at 3,6 and 12mo after initiation of treatment, then annually thereafter
Psychotherapy	Effective for some. Time-consuming and expensive but may avert the need for drugs and give permanent resolution

---

☞ Andropause/male menopause

From ~30y, testosterone levels ↓ by ~10% every decade. At the same time, sex hormone binding globulin (SHBG) level ↑, which ↓ the amount of bioavailable testosterone further. Andropause is associated with low bioavailable testosterone levels; ~30% of men in their 50s develop symptoms.

Presentation ↓ sex drive, emotional, psychological, and behavioural changes, ↓ muscle mass and muscle strength, ↑ upper and central body fat, osteoporosis and back pain, ↑ cardiovascular risk.

Management If suspected, check total testosterone and SHBG ± FSH/LH and prolactin. If hypogonadism is confirmed, refer for specialist management with testosterone replacement.

GP management Counsel the couple about the problem, its possible causes and management (see Table 22.7, 📖 p. 777, and Figure 22.4).

- Advice on lifestyle—↓ smoking and alcohol. Weight loss and ↑ exercise for obese, underactive patients improves both sexual function and cardiovascular health
- Discuss pros and cons of available drug treatment. Phosphodiesterase type 5 inhibitors (PDE5s) are the mainstays of treatment—titrate dose to effect (most people with DM need the maximum dose); warn the patient he may need 8 attempts before a satisfactory erection occurs; side effects include headache, flushing, and acid reflux
- Review progress—adjust dosage, consider other treatment options (intraurethral/intracavernosal alprostadil, vacuum devices) or treatment for psychosexual problems, and/or referral

Referral Options:

- **Urologist** If the patient has never had an erection, has a severe vascular problem, lack of success with treatment in general practice, or severe psychological distress due to erectile dysfunction
- **Endocrinologist** Hormone abnormalities (e.g. ↓ androgen, ↑ prolactin)—treatment does not always restore potency
- **Psychiatrist/psychosexual counsellor** Age <40y and no evidence of organic cause; psychosexual problem

Psychogenic erectile dysfunction Treatment in general practice is appropriate for couples who do not wish to be referred.

- See the couple together
- Recommend a manual, e.g. 'Treat Yourself to Sex' (P. Brown and C. Faulder, Penguin, 1989. ISBN: 0140110186)
- Forbid sexual intercourse
- Explain that stroking should progress slowly from non-genital to genital—if anxiety occurs, go back one step
- Progress until erection is achieved
- Give permission for intercourse (if not already achieved)
- If unsuccessful, refer to a psychosexual counsellor

⚠ All men >25y with erectile dysfunction should be screened for DM, cardiac risk factors, and signs/symptoms of vascular disease.

❶ NHS prescriptions for erectile dysfunction are available *only* for men:
- Treated for prostate cancer; with kidney failure, spinal cord injury, DM, MS, spina bifida, Parkinson's disease, polio, severe pelvic injury, or who have had radical pelvic surgery or a prostatectomy
- Already receiving drug treatment for impotence on 14.9.98
- Through specialist services for men suffering severe distress due to erectile dysfunction

Endorse NHS prescriptions with the letters 'SLS'. A consultation is currently underway to lift NHS prescribing restrictions.

Further information
British Society for Sexual Medicine Guidelines for the management of erectile dysfunction (2007) ℘ www.bssm.org.uk

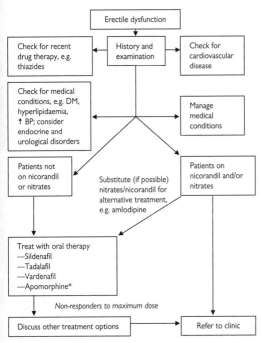

* Not as effective as PDE5 inhibitors but not contraindicated with nitrates.

Figure 22.4 Algorithm for management of erectile dysfunction

Table 22.8 PDE5 inhibitors and action times

Drug	Onset of action in min (peak action)	Duration of action in h	Doses
Sildenafil	20–30 (60)	4–6	25–50–100mg
Tadalafil	60–120 (120)	36–48	10–20mg*
Vardenafil	20–30 (60)	4–6	5–10–20mg

* For patients who anticipate sexual activity ≥2x/wk, 2.5–5mg od can be used instead.

Figure 22.4 and Table 22.8 are reproduced from British Heart Foundation Factfile: Drugs for erectile dysfunction (6/2005) available from ℘ www.bhf.org.uk

Pregnancy

Pre-conception and early pregnancy counselling

The aim of pre-pregnancy care is to give a woman enough information for her pregnancy to occur under the optimal possible circumstances. Areas to cover are:

Smoking ↓ ovulation, ↓ sperm count, ↓ sperm motility.

Once the woman is pregnant Smoking:
- ↑ miscarriage rate (x2) and risk of ectopic pregnancy
- ↑ risk of placenta praevia and placental abruption
- ↑ risk of premature rupture of membranes and preterm delivery
- ↑ risk of cleft deformities
- ↑ perinatal mortality and ↓ birth weight (by an average of ~200g)

Once the baby has delivered Smoking is associated with:
- ↑ rate of cot death
- ↑ chest infections and otitis media in children

27% of pregnant women are smoking at the time of delivery. Explain risks and advise on ways to stop—📖 p. 182.

Alcohol Fetal alcohol syndrome (growth restriction, CNS involvement, and facial deformity) is rare and tends to occur in babies of heavy drinkers—especially those who binge drink. Effects of smaller quantities of alcohol are less clear. Miscarriage rates are ↑ in moderate drinkers. Current advice is to avoid alcohol in pregnancy especially for the first 3mo. If a woman continues to drink, advise her to limit consumption to 1–2u/d.

Illicit drugs Cannabis (used by 5% mothers) is possibly associated with poorer motor skills in children and strongly linked with cigarette smoking—discourage. If taking other illicit drugs, refer for specialist care.

Diet See Box 23.1.

Folate supplementation ↓ risk of neural tube defect (open spina bifida, anencephaly, encephalocele) by 72%. For most women, recommend 0.4mg daily from when pregnancy is being planned until 13wk gestation. Recommend 5mg daily if:
- Previous child had neural tube defect
- Maternal/paternal history or family history of neural tube defect
- The mother has coeliac disease, DM, BMI >30kg/m², or is taking anticonvulsants

Only ~1 in 3 women take folic acid prior to conception. Effect of starting in early pregnancy is unevaluated. Supplements can be prescribed, are available via the Healthy Start Programme (together with vitamin C and D supplements) or are available OTC from chemists/supermarkets. Introduction of folic acid fortified flour has recently been approved.

Other supplements
- **Vitamin D** The DH recommends 10 microgram (400iu)/d but limited evidence for general use. Consider for women with poor diet or limited exposure to sunlight, those of South Asian, African, Caribbean, or Middle Eastern family origin, and those with pre-pregnancy BMI ≥30kg/m²
- **Iron** Do not routinely offer—for most, side effects outweigh benefits (📖 p. 822)

Box 23.1 Healthy eating tips for women

Eat a variety of foods including:
- Plenty of fruit and vegetables—at least five portions per day
- Plenty of starchy foods, e.g. bread, pasta, rice, or potatoes
- Protein-rich foods, e.g. lean meat, chicken, fish, eggs, beans, lentils
- Fibre, e.g. wholegrain bread, pasta or rice, fruit, and vegetables
- Dairy foods containing calcium, e.g. milk, cheese, and yoghurt

Folic acid (folate) Reduces risk of conditions, such as spina bifida. Take folic acid supplements (400 microgram) every day from stopping contraception until you are 13wk pregnant. Eat foods containing folate, e.g. green vegetables, brown rice, fortified bread, and cereals.

Iron Eat iron-rich foods, e.g. red meat, beans, lentils, green vegetables, and fortified cereals. Fruit, fruit juice, and vegetables help with iron absorption.

Food to avoid

Pâté and some unpasteurized dairy products All pâtés (including vegetable), Camembert, Brie, other ripened soft cheeses, and blue cheese—may contain *Listeria* which causes miscarriage, stillbirth, and infections in newborn babies.

Raw/undercooked meat, eggs, and ready meals Risk of food poisoning.
- Wash your hands after handling raw meat
- Keep raw meat separate from foods ready to eat
- Only eat well-cooked meat—hot right through, with no pink bits left
- Only eat eggs cooked until white and yolk are solid. Shop mayonnaise and mousses are safe but avoid home-made dishes containing raw egg
- Ensure ready meals are piping hot all the way through

Liver products and vitamin A supplements Too much vitamin A can harm a baby's development. Avoid eating liver (and liver products, e.g. pâté) and supplements containing vitamin A or fish liver oils.

Some types of fish Eat ≥2 portions of fish per week (including one of oily fish—mackerel, sardines, fresh (not canned) tuna, or trout) but:
- Avoid shark, swordfish, or marlin, and limit tuna to two steaks or four cans weekly. Mercury in these fish can harm a baby's nervous system
- Only eat 1–2 portions of oily fish per week
- Avoid raw shellfish, as they can cause food poisoning

Alcohol and caffeine Avoid alcohol. High caffeine levels can cause miscarriage or low birth weight. There is caffeine in coffee, tea, chocolate, cola, and some 'high-energy' drinks. You can drink four cups of coffee, six cups of tea, or eight cans of cola daily.

Gardening and changing cat litter
Toxoplasmosis can harm an unborn baby's nervous system and/or cause blindness. The parasite that causes it is found in meat, cat faeces, and soil. Wear gloves when gardening or changing cat litter and wash your hands afterwards.

Sexual intercourse and contraception Sexual intercourse is not known to be harmful during pregnancy. Often women contemplating pregnancy are still using contraception. Discussion about how to stop/ what to expect may be helpful (e.g. injectables, IUCD).

Exercise 📖 p. 792

Chronic disease Review of pre-existing medical conditions with referral for expert a pre-conceptual advice where necessary.
- Diabetes mellitus—refer for specialist diabetic review and change women taking sulfonylureas to metformin or insulin (📖 p. 828)
- Epilepsy—refer for specialist review of medication (📖 p. 829)
- Heart disease—refer for specialist advice if situation is not clear
- Genito-urinary disease (e.g. HIV, genital warts, bacterial vaginosis)— treat or refer for treatment/advice on mode of delivery if necessary (📖 p. 810)

Review of medication Drug handling by the body is altered during pregnancy, and drugs can cause damage to the developing fetus:
- Discontinue known teratogens prior to conception
- Advise to avoid OTC medication unless safety checked with doctor/ midwife
- Avoid prescribed medication as much as possible—few medicines have proven safety in pregnancy. If prescribing use well-known and tested drugs at the smallest possible doses, and only when benefit > risk

Problems in previous pregnancies
- Recurrent miscarriage and/or cervical incompetence (📖 p. 815)
- Congenital abnormalities/inherited disorders—pre-pregnancy counselling and detailed advice on genetic screening for high-risk pregnancies is available via regional genetics services

Rubella status Rubella in early pregnancy carries a high chance (40–70%) of deafness, blindness, cardiac abnormalities, or multiple fetal abnormalities (📖 p. 806). If rubella status is unknown, suggest it is checked. If not immune, suggest MMR immunization; avoid pregnancy for 3mo afterwards (live vaccine) and recheck immunity after 3mo.

Flu vaccination Pregnancy ↑ risk of complications and death from seasonal influenza. Offer annual flu vaccination to all pregnant women.

Work/benefits Discussion of benefits available during pregnancy (see Table 23.1) and employment law (📖 p. 792) is necessary so that women may avoid possible hazards at work, attend for antenatal care, and plan their maternity leave from early in pregnancy.

Discussion of antenatal care and screening available
- Brief discussion of antenatal screening (📖 p. 796) and antenatal care procedures (📖 p. 786) allows women to investigate their choices in pregnancy at their leisure
- Brief discussion about miscarriage and possibility of infertility allows women to be more confident about asking for help if problems with conception/early pregnancy occur

Table 23.1 Benefits available to pregnant women

Benefit	Eligibility	How to apply	Benefits gained
Statutory Maternity Pay (SMP)	• Worked for the same employer for 26wk into the 15th wk before the baby is due • Pregnant at (or have had the baby by) the 11th wk before the baby is due • Earning ≥ NI lower earnings limit in the relevant period	• Inform employer at least 28d before starting leave • Mat B1 form from midwife/GP	Paid for up to 39wk (Maternity Pay Period—MPP)—can start any time from 11th wk before the baby is due until the week of birth. • 1st 6wk—90% average earnings • 6–26wk—90% of usual earnings or £135.45/wk—whichever is lower
Maternity Allowance (MA)	• Employed/self-employed for ≥26wk in the 66wk preceding the baby's due date (test period) • Average weekly earnings of ≥£30/wk for at least 13wk of the test period • Do not qualify for SMP (e.g. changed jobs, become unemployed, self-employed)	Apply >26/40 and within 3mo of date MA due to start. Need: • Form MA1 (from Jobcentre Plus offices, employer or ℗ www.gov.uk • MATB1; and, if employed, • Form SMP1 from employer	Paid for 39wk (Maternity Allowance Period—MAP)—can start any time from 11th week before the baby until the day after birth 90% of usual earnings or £135.45/wk—whichever is lower
Sure Start Maternity Grant	• From 11wk before baby is due to <3mo after birth/adoption • Claiming Universal Credit or equivalent • No other children <16y (except if multiple pregnancy)	Form SF100 from social Jobcentre Plus offices or ℗ www.gov.uk	£500 payment

Other benefits
- **Free prescriptions/dentistry** Available to all mothers while pregnant and for 1y after the expected date of delivery. Claim if needed using form FW8
- **Universal Credit** May be available for women unable to claim SMP/MA (📖 p. 104)
- **Free milk and vitamin supplements** Women claiming Universal Credit or equivalent may be able to claim free milk and vitamin supplements if >10wk pregnant. Claim online at ℗ www.healthystart.nhs.uk or ☎ 0845 607 6823
- **Child Benefit**—📖 p. 847

Further information on maternity rights and benefits
Citizens Advice Bureau ℗ www.adviceguide.org.uk
Government website ℗ www.gov.uk

Antenatal care

Objectives of good obstetric care
- To provide a safe outcome for the mother and baby with the minimum of avoidable complications
- To make the birth experience as satisfying as possible
- To make optimal use of available resources

Pregnancy is a risky business for both mother and baby. Every year women die as a result of pregnancy—the most common causes being eclampsia, haemorrhage, pulmonary embolism, and infection.

Maternity Services Are provided by practices as an Additional Service, i.e. most practices are expected to provide routine antenatal care and postnatal care to mothers and babies from birth (or discharge from secondary care) until the 14th day after delivery, with the exception of intrapartum care and the neonatal check. Payment is included in the global sum. If a practice 'opts out' global sum is ↓ by 2.1%.

Intrapartum care Intrapartum care and neonatal checks can be provided to women by GPs at home or in GP maternity units as a *National Enhanced Service*. One payment is made for each woman who receives intrapartum care and a further payment for each neonatal check.

Definitions
- **Gravidity**—number of pregnancies a woman has had (at any stage)
- **Parity**—number of pregnancies resulting in delivery >24wk gestation (or live births <24 wk)
- **Primipara, multipara**—woman who has been delivered of a child for the first time (primipara) or second or subsequent time (multipara)

Pregnancy tests Detect urinary β-HCG. +ve from 1st day of missed period until ~20wk gestation. Remain positive for ~5d after miscarriage/termination or fetal death.

Antenatal care The first antenatal appointment should be offered as early into pregnancy as possible. Further appointments for healthy women should be offered at 16, 28, 34, 36, 38, and, if not already delivered, at 41wk. Additionally healthy nulliparous women should be offered appointments at 25, 31, and 40wk. Provide additional appointments as needed for high-risk women. See Figure 23.3 📖 p. 791.

First antenatal visit The primary function of this visit is to identify those women needing additional care. As there is so much information to be collected/discussed, consider two appointments.

History
- This pregnancy—LMP, usual cycle, fertility problems, contraception, desirability of pregnancy, any problems so far
- Estimated date of delivery (EDD)—see Figure 23.1
- Past pregnancies—outcome and complications of previous pregnancies
- Past/current medical history—illness (including psychiatric illness), drugs, allergies, varicose veins, abdominal/pelvic surgery (including female genital mutilation)

Date of first day of last menstrual period						Month →					
Day ↓	Jan	Feb	Mar	Apr	May	Jun	Jul	Aug	Sep	Oct	Nov	Dec
1	8/10	8/11	6/12	6/1	5/2	8/3	7/4	8/5	8/6	8/7	8/8	7/9
2	9/10	9/11	7/12	7/1	6/2	9/3	8/4	9/5	9/6	9/7	9/8	8/9
3	10/10	10/11	8/12	8/1	7/2	10/3	9/4	10/5	10/6	10/7	10/8	9/9
4	11/10	11/11	9/12	9/1	8/2	11/3	10/4	11/5	11/6	11/7	11/8	10/9
5	12/10	12/11	10/12	10/1	9/2	12/3	11/4	12/5	12/6	12/7	12/8	11/9
6	13/10	13/11	11/12	11/1	10/2	13/3	12/4	13/5	13/6	13/7	13/8	12/9
7	14/10	14/11	12/12	12/1	11/2	14/3	13/4	14/5	14/6	14/7	14/8	13/9
8	15/10	15/11	13/12	13/1	12/2	15/3	14/4	15/5	15/6	15/7	15/8	14/9
9	16/10	16/11	14/12	14/1	13/2	16/3	15/4	16/5	16/6	16/7	16/8	15/9
10	17/10	17/11	15/12	15/1	14/2	17/3	16/4	17/5	17/6	17/7	17/8	16/9
11	18/10	18/11	16/12	16/1	15/2	18/3	17/4	18/5	18/6	18/7	18/8	17/9
12	19/10	19/11	17/12	17/1	16/2	19/3	18/4	19/5	19/6	19/7	19/8	18/9
13	20/10	20/11	18/12	18/1	17/2	20/3	19/4	20/5	20/6	20/7	20/8	19/9
14	21/10	21/11	19/12	19/1	18/2	21/3	20/4	21/5	21/6	21/7	21/8	20/9
15	22/10	22/11	20/12	20/1	19/2	22/3	21/4	22/5	22/6	22/7	22/8	21/9
16	23/10	23/11	21/12	21/1	20/2	23/3	22/4	23/5	23/6	23/7	23/8	22/9
17	24/10	24/11	22/12	22/1	21/2	24/3	23/4	24/5	24/6	24/7	24/8	23/9
18	25/10	25/11	23/12	23/1	22/2	25/3	24/4	25/5	25/6	25/7	25/8	24/9
19	26/10	26/11	24/12	24/1	23/2	26/3	25/4	26/5	26/6	26/7	26/8	25/9
20	27/10	27/11	25/12	25/1	24/2	27/3	26/4	27/5	27/6	27/7	27/8	26/9
21	28/10	28/11	26/12	26/1	25/2	28/3	27/4	28/5	28/6	28/7	28/8	27/9
22	29/10	29/11	27/12	27/1	26/2	29/3	28/4	29/5	29/6	29/7	29/8	28/9
23	30/10	30/11	28/12	28/1	27/2	30/3	29/4	30/5	30/6	30/7	30/8	29/9
24	31/10	1/12	29/12	29/1	28/2	31/3	30/4	31/5	1/7	31/7	31/8	30/9
25	1/11	2/12	30/12	30/1	1/3	1/4	1/5	1/6	2/7	1/8	1/9	1/10
26	2/11	3/12	31/12	31/1	2/3	2/4	2/5	2/6	3/7	2/8	2/9	2/10
27	3/11	4/12	1/1	1/2	3/3	3/4	3/5	3/6	4/7	3/8	3/9	3/10
28	4/11	5/12	2/1	2/2	4/3	4/4	4/5	4/6	5/7	4/8	4/9	4/10
29	5/11		3/1	3/2	5/3	5/4	5/5	5/6	6/7	5/8	5/9	5/10
30	6/11		4/1	4/2	6/3	6/4	6/5	6/6	7/7	6/8	6/9	6/10
31	7/11		5/1		7/3		7/5	7/6		7/8		7/10

Dates are given in the format day/month

❶ As a rough guide, EDD = date of LMP + 1 year +7 days − 3 months

Figure 23.1 Expected date of delivery calculator

- Family history—↑ BP, DM, congenital/genetic abnormality, twins
- Social history—smoking, alcohol consumption, illicit drugs, support at home, work, housing, financial problems

Examination
- Check weight and calculate BMI—low BMI ↑ risk of pre-eclampsia, IUGR, and preterm delivery; high BMI is associated with pre-eclampsia
- Listen to heart and lungs; check BP, and examine abdomen
- Fetal heart with a sonic aid per abdomen from 12–14wk gestation
- Fundus can be felt per abdomen from 12wk

Investigations
- Offer early USS at 10wk–13wk 6d for dating purposes and to detect multiple pregnancy
- Offer routine anomaly scan at 18wk–20wk 6d gestation. If the placenta extends across the internal cervical os, arrange repeat USS at 32wk
- Check blood for Hb, blood group, Rhesus status, and red cell antibodies; syphilis/rubella serology, HBsAg/HIV with pre-test counselling; sickle test and/or Hb electrophoresis
- MSU for protein and bacteriuria
- Discuss and offer antenatal screening (see Figure 23.2 and 🕮 p. 796)
- Inform women <25y about chlamydia screening through the National Chlamydia Screening Programme (🕮 p. 740)

Education
- Health promotion (🕮 p. 792)
- Social security benefits (🕮 p. 785)
- Antenatal/parent craft classes
- Free prescriptions and dental care (🕮 p. 785)
- Employment rights (🕮 p. 792)
- Local services (e.g. aquanatal classes, yoga for pregnancy)
- Choice of place of delivery and options available (🕮 p. 794)
- Procedure for antenatal care—see Figure 23.3 (🕮 p. 791)
- Travel and limitations (🕮 p. 793)

Certification Supply form FW8 (application for free prescriptions and dental care) at the first antenatal appointment and form Mat B1 at 20wk.

Information
- Offer 'Screening tests and your baby' (order from 🕾 www.screening.nhs.uk/annbpublications) to all pregnant women
- Offer 'The Pregnancy Book' to all first-time pregnant women (available to download from the DH website 🕾 www.dh.gov.uk)
- Offer 'Emma's diary' to all pregnant women. Contains information and vouchers (order by e-mail: emma@emmasdiary.co.uk)

Discussion Worries about pregnancy or social situation—ask specifically about domestic violence.

Follow-up visits Ask about problems and untoward symptoms. Provide the neonatal bloodspot screening leaflet at ~28wk.

Routine checks
- BP
- Oedema
- Urine for protein
- Fundal height (from 24/25 wk)
- Fetal heart sounds (from 12–14wk)
- Fetal lie and presentation (from 36wk)

❶ Primiparous women are aware of movements from ~20wk but multiparous women often feel movements earlier.

Laboratory checks Hb and antibodies at 28wk.

Figure 23.2 NHS antenatal screening timetable

Figure 23.2 is reproduced with permission from the UK NSC antenatal and newborn screening programmes (⅋ http://cpd.screening.nhs.uk/timeline).

Women who may need additional care

- Pre-existing medical conditions, e.g. ↑ BP, cardiac, renal, endocrine, autoimmune, or haematological disorders, epilepsy, severe asthma, DM, cancer, HIV, hepatitis B, substance abuse, female genital mutilation
- Factors that make the woman vulnerable, e.g. lack of social support, domestic violence
- Age ≥40y or ≤18y
- BMI ≥30kg/m² or <18kg/m²
- Smoker
- Uterine surgery—e.g. Caesarean section, myomectomy, cone biopsy
- Previous pre-eclampsia, eclampsia, or HELLP
- Para ≥6 or ≥3 miscarriages
- Previous preterm birth, mid-trimester loss, stillbirth, or neonatal death
- Previous psychiatric illness or puerperal psychosis
- Previous baby with congenital abnormality
- Previous small-for-gestational age or large-for-gestational age baby or baby weighing <2.5kg or >4.5kg at birth
- Family history of genetic disorder

Interventions that are *not* part of routine antenatal care

- Repeated maternal weighing—only weigh if clinical management is likely to be influenced, e.g. concern about nutrition
- Breast or pelvic examination
- Iron supplementation
- Screening for chlamydia, CMV, HCV, group B streptococcus, toxoplasmosis, or bacterial vaginosis
- Screening for preterm birth by assessment of cervical length (either by USS or vaginal examination) or using fetal fibronectin
- Formal fetal movement counting
- Antenatal electronic cardiotocography
- USS >24wk
- Umbilical or uterine artery Doppler USS

Further information

NICE ぬ www.nice.org.uk

- Antenatal care: routine care for healthy pregnant women (2010)
- Improving the nutrition of pregnant and breastfeeding mothers and children in low-income households (2011)

Scientific Advisory Committee on Nutrition (SACN) The influence of maternal, fetal and child nutrition on the development of chronic disease in later life (2011) ぬ www.sacn.gov.uk

NHS Fetal Anomaly Screening Programme
ぬ www.fetalanomaly.screening.nhs.uk

Information and support for pregnant women

National Childbirth Trust (NCT) ☏ 0300 330 0700 ぬ www.nct.org.uk
Birth Choice UK ぬ www.birthchoiceuk.com
Mothers 35 plus ぬ www.mothers35plus.co.uk
Emma's Diary ぬ www.emmasdiary.co.uk
NHS Scotland ぬ www.readysteadybaby.org.uk

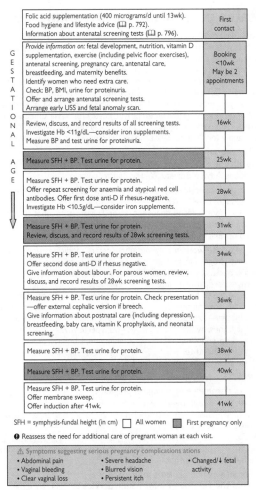

	Folic acid supplementation (400 micrograms/d until 13wk). Food hygiene and lifestyle advice (📖 p. 792). Information about antenatal screening tests (📖 p. 796).	First contact
G	*Provide information on:* fetal development, nutrition, vitamin D supplementation, exercise (including pelvic floor exercises), antenatal screening, pregnancy care, antenatal care, breastfeeding, and maternity benefits. Identify women who need extra care. *Check:* BP, BMI, urine for proteinuria. Offer and arrange antenatal screening tests. Arrange early USS and fetal anomaly scan.	Booking <10wk May be 2 appointments
E S T A T I	Review, discuss, and record results of all screening tests. Investigate Hb <11g/dL—consider iron supplements. Measure BP and test urine for proteinuria.	16wk
O N A L	Measure SFH + BP. Test urine for protein.	25wk
	Measure SFH + BP. Test urine for protein. Offer repeat screening for anaemia and atypical red cell antibodies. Offer first dose anti-D if rhesus-negative. Investigate Hb <10.5g/dL—consider iron supplements.	28wk
A G E	Measure SFH + BP. Test urine for protein. Review, discuss, and record results of 28wk screening tests.	31wk
	Measure SFH + BP. Test urine for protein. Offer second dose anti-D if rhesus negative. Give information about labour. For parous women, review, discuss, and record results of 28wk screening tests.	34wk
	Measure SFH + BP. Test urine for protein. Check presentation —offer external cephalic version if breech. Give information about postnatal care (including depression), breastfeeding, baby care, vitamin K prophylaxis, and neonatal screening.	36wk
	Measure SFH + BP. Test urine for protein.	38wk
	Measure SFH + BP. Test urine for protein.	40wk
	Measure SFH + BP. Test urine for protein. Offer membrane sweep. Offer induction after 41wk.	41wk

SFH = symphysis-fundal height (in cm) ☐ All women ▨ First pregnancy only

❶ Reassess the need for additional care of pregnant woman at each visit.

⚠ Symptoms suggesting serious pregnancy complications ations
- Abdominal pain
- Vaginal bleeding
- Clear vaginal loss
- Severe headache
- Blurred vision
- Persistent itch
- Changed/↓ fetal activity

Figure 23.3 Algorithm of antenatal care

Health promotion for pregnant women

Work For most women, work in pregnancy is safe. By law:
- Employers must assess risks to the health/safety of the pregnant woman and adjust for risks accordingly
- Women are entitled to time off work for antenatal care
- Employed women cannot work >33wk into pregnancy unless the woman's GP informs her employer that she may continue
- Employers may not require/allow return to work <2wk after childbirth
- Women who work for an employer qualify for 52wk of maternity leave. Employment rights continue throughout this period. Women can apply for flexible/part-time working hours on return to work

Further information
- **Health and Safety Executive** ℘ www.hse.gov.uk/mothers
- **Citizens Advice Bureau** ℘ www.adviceguide.org.uk

Exercise Moderate exercise is safe and healthy. Advise pelvic floor exercises (📖 p. 841). Avoid:
- Contact sports, high-impact sports, and vigorous racquet sports
- Scuba diving—possible link with fetal birth defects and may cause fetal decompression disease

Drugs Advise women to avoid unnecessary medicines (including OTC) and illicit drugs. Drugs that can be started/continued in pregnancy, if clinically necessary and benefits outweigh risks, include:

- Analgesics—paracetamol, codeine-based preparations
- Antacids and ranitidine
- Antibiotics—except tetracyclines; avoid trimethoprim in first trimester and at term
- Hormones—thyroxine, insulin
- Laxatives
- Low-dose aspirin (75mg)
- Antiemetics—cyclizine, domperidone, prochlorperazine, metoclopramide
- Antihistamines—chlorphenamine
- Antihypertensives—methyldopa, nifedipine, labetalol, doxazosin
- β-agonists—salbutamol, terbutaline
- Ipratropium
- Inhaled steroids

Drugs to discontinue or change in pregnancy
- NSAIDs—except low-dose aspirin
- Warfarin—liaise with obstetrician as may need to change to low molecular weight heparin
- Antibiotics—tetracycline, doxycycline
- Antihypertensives—ACE inhibitors, angiotensin receptor blockers
- Retinoids, e.g. isotretinoin

Further information on drugs in pregnancy
BNF and UK Teratology Information Service ☎ 0844 892 0909
℘ www.uktis.org

Complementary therapies Use as little as possible.
- **Avoid**—oil of evening primrose (possible ↑ in PROM)
- **No benefit**—raspberry leaf tea (but probably no risk either)
- **Possibly beneficial**—ginger, P6 acupressure and acupuncture for nausea and vomiting; moxibustion for breech presentation; acupuncture for backache/pelvic pain; acupuncture for insomnia
- **No/limited evidence**—St John's wort, hypnosis, aromatherapy

Smoking (📖 p. 793) Stress benefits of quitting at any stage. Halving the number of cigarettes smoked results in an average 92g ↑ in birth weight.

NHS pregnancy smoking line ☎ 0800 169 9 169

Alcohol 📖 p. 782

Diet Normal weight gain in pregnancy is 7–8kg. Do not routinely weigh unless worries about nutrition and/or weight.

Foods to avoid 📖 p. 783

Gardening and changing cat litter 📖 p. 783

Travel
- **Car** Seat belt should go above and below—*not* across—the bump
- **Air** Check specific requirements of carrier. Most airlines will not accept pregnant women >32wk (rarely, 36wk with a doctor's letter)

⚠ Travel involving long periods of immobility (>3h) is associated with ↑ risk of venous thromboembolism. Advise women to drink plenty of non-alcoholic fluids; keep their legs moving whilst sitting or walk up and down the aisle; and purchase graduated compression hosiery OTC.

Travel abroad Best time to travel is in the second trimester. Travel to high-risk areas is best postponed/cancelled. Avoid travel to places at altitudes >2,500m (↑ risk of IUGR/ pre-eclampsia).

Vaccines Assess risk/benefit ratio on an individual basis.
- **Avoid live vaccines** BCG, cholera, measles, mumps, rubella, varicella, smallpox, Japanese encephalitis. ❶ Inadvertent administration has not been shown to cause harm
- **Inactivated vaccines** Give if needed— pertussis, hepatitis A and B, meningococcal (only if significant risk of infection), inactivated polio (normally avoid), rabies, tetanus/diphtheria, yellow fever (avoid unless high risk)

❶ Pregnancy ↑ risk of complications and death from seasonal influenza. Offer annual flu vaccination to all pregnant women.

Malaria Travel to malaria areas is best avoided. If unavoidable, take precautions to avoid mosquito bites (📖 p. 172). Chloroquine and proguanil can be used in usual doses in pregnancy. Give folic acid 5mg od with proguanil. Consider mefloquine for travel to chloroquine-resistant areas. Avoid Malarone® and doxycycline.

Contaminated food/water Risk of listeriosis, toxoplasmosis, and hepatitis E. Avoid travel to hepatitis E areas—~20% death rate in the third trimester. Severe diarrhoea may be harmful to the fetus.

Insurance for travel Ensure adequate cover. Most companies insure pregnant women to 28wk, some to 32wk. In Europe, the European Health Insurance Card (EHIC) (📖 p. 45) provides free emergency medical care. It does not cover costs of transport or repatriation.

The UK has reciprocal agreements with some other countries for urgently needed medical treatment. Countries and services available are listed on the DH travel advice website (🖰 www.dh.gov.uk). Proof of British nationality or UK residence is needed.

Who should deliver where?

All those offering maternity care must give women choices about type of care, place of care and birth and the information to make those choices avoiding personal bias or preference. Who delivers where ultimately depends on the choice that the woman makes (see Table 23.2). *Options:*
• Consultant unit
• Midwife or GP/midwife unit integral with/attached to a consultant unit
• 'Isolated unit'—distant from a specialist unit and manned by midwives or midwives and GPs
• Home (~1% deliveries in the UK)

Legal position of GPs GPs are often fearful of litigation if women opt for delivery outside a specialist unit. Even women with no risk factors can run into problems—rapid intervention to save life is needed in ~5% deliveries. With midwives taking on increasing responsibility for antenatal care in the community, GP-attended home deliveries are very uncommon, and GPs perceive they lack expertise. This compounds their worry.

The legal position is that
• GPs are responsible only for their own acts or omissions
• Midwives are accountable for their own actions and decisions
• The GP only becomes responsible for a woman's care in labour when the midwife attending seeks his/her advice. The GP is then bound by terms and conditions of service to offer advice (either over the telephone or by attending), whether or not the woman had been accepted for maternity care
• If an accident occurs, the GP would be judged against standards of a colleague of similar skills and training, not a specialist obstetrician

Duties of the GP
• Provision of impartial advice about available services locally
• Discussion of the available options in a way to enable the woman to make an informed choice
• To make arrangements for provision of care

Specialist unit vs community-based care In the UK the perinatal and maternal death rates have fallen as the proportion of hospital births has risen. But this is largely due to improvements in housing, nutrition, and antenatal care rather than having babies in hospital per se. Evidence from countries where home birth is the norm suggests that birth outside the hospital setting is safe for healthy women with low-risk pregnancies.

⚠ If a woman decides to deliver away from a specialist unit, she should be informed about:
• The facilities and levels of skill and expertise available where she has chosen to deliver, and
• The facilities and specialist services that are available in a specialist unit but *not* where she has chosen to deliver

Record the discussion in her notes.

Table 23.2 Reasons why women choose home or hospital births

Home birth	Hospital birth
To avoid intervention (31%)	Safety (84%)
More in control in familiar surroundings (25%)	Previous hospital birth (6%)
Previous home birth (11%)	
More relaxed at home (10%)	
Fear of hospitals (10%)	
Continuity of care with midwife (4%)	

Advise to deliver in a consultant unit

At booking if
- Pre-existing medical disorders—epilepsy, DM, cardiac, renal, respiratory, hepatitis B, HIV, active genital herpes, IV drug abuse, history of major gynaecological surgery, or known uterine abnormality
- Familial disorder with a high risk of transmission
- ↑ BP
- Height <150cm and primigravida
- Weight at first examination <50kg or >100kg
- Past obstetric history of:
  - Perinatal death
  - Rhesus isoimmunization
  - Pre-eclampsia or eclampsia
  - Antepartum haemorrhage
  - IUGR
  - Caesarean section
  - Postpartum haemorrhage
  - Retained placenta
  - Inverted uterus
  - Shoulder dystocia

If any of the following develop during pregnancy
- Polyhydramnios
- Malpresentation
- Antepartum haemorrhage
- Prolonged pregnancy (>40wk + 10d)
- Preterm labour <37wk
- Suspected IUGR
- Pregnancy-induced ↑ BP
- Multiple pregnancy

Refer to obstetrics to discuss place of delivery if
- Primigravida <18y and >35y or ≥ para 6
- Excessive maternal weight ↑
- Failure of engagement of the head near term in a primigravida
- Past history of prolonged labour, large baby, subfertility, or cone biopsy

⚠ Other rarer medical or obstetric conditions may require specialist advice—if in doubt refer.

Further information

NICE ✆ www.nice.org.uk
- Antenatal care: routine care for healthy pregnant women (2010)
- Intrapartum care (2007)

Screening in pregnancy

Most women undergo some form of screening before/during pregnancy aiming to identify, prevent, and treat actual or potential problems (see Figure 23.2, 📖 p. 789). Offer women and their partners unbiased information verbally and in writing regarding screening and diagnostic tests, the meaning and consequences of both, what to expect in terms of results, and further options for management. The right to accept or decline should be made clear—and the decision recorded in the antenatal notes.

GPs need to be aware of techniques of prenatal diagnosis to:
- Identify all women who might benefit from genetic counselling and/or early assessment by the obstetrician, *and*
- Counsel patients about the accuracy and risk of prenatal diagnosis

Pre-pregnancy genetic screening There are many inherited diseases. Warn couples that most tests give no absolute 'yes' or 'no' but are a risk assessment. Refer couples for genetic screening before pregnancy if they want referral and have factors which put them at high risk of having a baby with a genetic disorder.

Personal or family history of genetic abnormality, e.g.:
- Cystic fibrosis
- Down's syndrome
- Sickle cell disease
- β-thalassaemia
- Haemophilia
- Fragile X syndrome
- Polycystic kidneys
- Huntington's chorea
- Duchenne and other muscular dystrophies

High risk ethnic groups, e.g.:
- Afro-Caribbean origin—sickle cell anaemia
- Indian subcontinent, Far East, southern Europe—thalassaemia
- Ashkenazi Jew—Tay–Sachs disease

❶ The Family Origin Questionnaire (available from ℳ http://sct.screening.nhs.uk) identifies those at risk of carrying a haemoglobinopathy. A blood test establishes carrier status and risk to the baby.

Older women ↑ risk of Down's syndrome (📖 p. 798).

Consanguinous couples First-degree cousins who have a baby together have an ↑ risk of congenital malformations in their offspring.

Routine antenatal screening is NOT recommended for

Vaginal/genital infections
- Bacterial vaginosis
- Chlamydia (unless <25y 📖 p. 740)
- Group B streptococcus
- Genital herpes

Other infections
- Cytomegalovirus
- Hepatitis C
- Toxoplasmosis

Genetic conditions—refer for screening only if a family member is affected:
- Cystic fibrosis
- Fragile X
- Familial dysautonomia

Others
- Thrombophilia
- Thrombocytopenia
- Preterm labour
- Domestic violence

Basic screening tests Blood and urine tests—many women are not aware these tests have been done let alone their purpose or results. Ensure women are given information about the reasons for, significance of and results of routine tests and record in the notes that permission has been given to do them. Usual tests are:

- Hb estimation (📖 p. 822)
- Antibody screen (📖 p. 820)
- Combined screen (📖 p. 798)
- Haemoglobinopathy screen (📖 p. 800)
- MSU for M,C&S (📖 p. 812)
- Hepatitis B status (📖 p. 797)
- Blood group
- Urine dipstick for proteinuria (pre-eclampsia screen 📖 p. 800)
- HIV status (📖 p. 799)
- Syphilis status (📖 p. 812)
- Rubella susceptibility

❶ Rubella immune status is not strictly a screening test for this pregnancy but does identify susceptible women (~2.5%) so that postpartum vaccination may protect *future* pregnancies.

Ultrasound scan (USS)

- **Early USS** Offer to all pregnant women at 10wk–13wk 6d for accurate gestational age assessment
- **High-resolution 'anomaly' scan** Offer at 18 wk–20wk 6d to detect fetal structural abnormalities (see Table 23.3). Detection rates vary according to the abnormality, e.g. subtle heart anomalies are less likely to be detected than gross CNS anomalies

Placenta praevia Because most low-lying placenta detected at the routine 18–20wk anomaly scan will resolve by the time the baby is born, only women with placenta praevia extending over the internal cervical os are offered another transabdominal scan at 32wk. If this is unclear, a transvaginal scan should be offered.

Table 23.3 Fetal anomalies found at the mid-pregnancy scan

Anomaly	Chance of detection at scan
Anencephaly	98%
Gastroschisis	98%
Edward's syndrome (trisomy 18)	95%
Patau's syndrome (trisomy 13)	95%
Open spina bifida	90%
Bilateral renal agenesis	84%
Exomphalos	80%
Cleft lip	75%
Diaphragmatic hernia	60%
Lethal skeletal dysplasia	60%
Serious cardiac abnormalities	50%

Further information

NICE Antenatal care: routine care for healthy pregnant women (2010) ℘ www.nice.org.uk

Chorionic villus sampling (CVS) Used to detect genetic/metabolic abnormality in high-risk pregnancies. Performed from 11wk–13wk 6d gestation. The developing placenta is sampled per abdomen with USS guidance.

- **Advantages** Undertaken earlier than amniocentesis to allow termination of affected pregnancies at an earlier stage
- **Risks** ~2–4% miscarry; limb defects (🔖)

Further information
RCOG Amniocentesis and chorionic villus sampling (2010)
🔖 www.rcog.org.uk

Amniocentesis Sampling of amniotic fluid via transabdominal needle under USS guidance >15wk gestation. Carries a 1.9% pregnancy loss risk. Amniocentesis is offered:

- If a high-risk result is obtained following first/second trimester screening for Down's syndrome
- If the woman has had a previous pregnancy affected by fetal anomaly
- If there is a strong family history of an inherited disorder

Further information
RCOG Amniocentesis and chorionic villus sampling (2010)
🔖 www.rcog.org.uk

Fetoscopy Fibreoptic visualization of the fetus. Carried out from ~18wk. Enables detection of external abnormalities, fetal blood sampling and organ biopsy. Fetal loss rate ~4%.

Down's syndrome Most common single cause of learning difficulty in children of school age. *Incidence:* 1.2/1,000 live births. Incidence ↑ with age of the mother (see Table 23.4). Screening should detect >75% of Down's syndrome pregnancies, with a screen positive rate of <3%.

Combined screening test Performed from 10wk–14wk 1d gestation. Screening test of choice, as aids early diagnosis and can be completed in one stage without the need for re-attendance. Produces a single estimate of the woman's risk of having a child with Down's syndrome using:

- **Maternal blood tests** For human chorionic gonadotrophin (HCG) and pregnancy-associated paraprotein A (PAPP-A), *and*
- **Nuchal translucency** (NT) USS measurement of the translucency of the nuchal fold in the neck of the fetus done from 11wk 2d–14wk 1d gestation

Quadruple screening test Performed from 14wk 2d–20wk; used for women who book later in pregnancy (~15%). Maternal blood is tested for alpha-fetoprotein (AFP), HCG, unconjugated estriol (uE3), and inhibin A.

Test results Are expressed as a risk assessment (e.g. 1 in 300 at term) or as a +ve or –ve result. A +ve result implies a risk >1 in 150 at term. Ensure all women with +ve results are referred promptly for counselling about further investigation (CVS/amniocentesis) and pregnancy options.

Further information
NHS Fetal Anomaly Screening Programme
🔖 http://fetalanomaly.screening.nhs.uk

Table 23.4 Levels of risk of having a Down's syndrome pregnancy in relation to a woman's age

Woman's age (y)	Risk as a ratio	
20	1:1500	⚠ The National
30	1:800	Screening Committee has recommended
35	1:270	all pregnant women, irrespective of age, should
40	1:100	be offered screening for
≥45	≥1:50	Down's syndrome

Tay–Sachs disease Genetic condition carried by 1 in 25 Ashkenazi Jews. Offer genetic screening *whether or not* there is a family history. Offer screening for other diseases commonly carried in this population (e.g. Gaucher's disease, familial dysautonomia, cystic fibrosis, Canavan's disease) *only* if there is a family history.

Antenatal HIV testing HIV testing is now offered at the booking appointment as a routine part of antenatal screening in the UK. If the woman screens negative but is at continued high risk of acquiring HIV, a repeat test may be offered later in pregnancy.

❶ If a woman screens +ve for HIV, her partner and any other children in the family should also be offered screening.

Benefits of screening Without intervention, ~25–30% babies born to mothers infected with HIV will become infected with HIV themselves. Avoidance of breastfeeding, antiretroviral therapy, and appropriate management of delivery ↓ risk of transmission to <1%.

If the screening test is declined Document refusal in the woman's notes, explore the reasons for refusal and offer screening again at 28wk.

Screening for other infections Pregnant women who are HIV +ve should be offered screening for genital infection—chlamydia, gonorrhoea, and bacterial vaginosis—done as early as possible in pregnancy and at around 28wk, as co-infection is common in certain subgroups of these women and can ↑ rate of mother-to-child transmission, as well as adversely affecting the pregnancy itself. Also check hepatitis B and C serology unless already done.

Further information
RCOG Management of HIV in pregnancy (2010) ℘ www.rcog.org.uk
British HIV Association/Children's HIV Association Management of HIV infection in pregnant women (2008) ℘ www.bhiva.org
NHS Infectious Diseases in Pregnancy Screening Programme
℘ http://infectiousdiseases.screening.nhs.uk

Chlamydia screening Is not part of routine antenatal screening, but women under the age of 25y are at high risk of chlamydia infection and may be offered screening through the National Chlamydia Screening Programme (⬜ p. 740).

Hepatitis B screening ⬜ p. 811   **Syphilis screening** ⬜ p. 812

Asymptomatic bacteriuria Detection and treatment ↓ the risk of pyelonephritis—📖 p. 812.

Haemoglobinopathy Screening for sickle cell diseases and thalassaemias should be offered to all women as early as possible in pregnancy (ideally <10wk). In both cases, women identified as being a carrier (having a trait) or having the disorder should be referred promptly for specialist counselling. Their partners should be offered screening.

Thalassaemia All women are offered FBC early in pregnancy. One of the routine FBC indices, mean cell haemoglobin (MCH) is used as a screening test for thalassaemia. If MCH is ≤27pg, a more diagnostic test using HbA2 (Hb alpha 2) chromatographic analysis is required.

Sickle cell disorders Screening policy depends on prevalence:
- **High-prevalence areas** (>1.5/10,000 pregnancies) All women are offered screening for sickle cell and other haemoglobin variants
- **Low-prevalence areas** The Family Origins Questionnaire (available from ℘ http://sct.screening.nhs.uk) is used to assess the risk of either the woman or her partner being a carrier for sickle cell and other haemoglobin variants. Those in identified high-risk groups are offered laboratory testing

Further information
NHS Sickle Cell and Thalassaemia Screening Programme
℘ http://sct.screening.nhs.uk

Anaemia 📖 p. 822   **Rhesus incompatibility** 📖 p. 820

Gestational diabetes Identify women at high risk of gestational DM at the booking appointment:
- Previous macrosomic baby (≥4.5kg)   • BMI >30kg/m^2
- DM in a first-degree relative   • Previous gestational DM
- Family origin associated with high prevalence of DM: South Asian (especially India, Pakistan, or Bangladesh); black Caribbean; Middle Eastern (especially Saudi Arabia, United Arab Emirates, Iraq, Jordan, Syria, Oman, Qatar, Kuwait, Lebanon, or Egypt)

Screening test Offer women with ≥1 risk factor screening:
- If a woman has had previous gestational DM, screen with early self-monitoring of blood glucose or offer a 2 hour 75g oral glucose tolerance test (OGTT) at 16–18wk, followed by a repeat OGTT at 28wk if the first test is normal
- For other risk factors, offer an OGTT at 24–28wk

Pre-eclampsia Check BP and urinalysis for proteinuria at each antenatal appointment to screen for pre-eclampsia (📖 p. 826).

First contact At first contact, assess the pregnant woman's level of risk for pre-eclampsia. Risk factors for developing pre-eclampsia are:
- Nulliparity or pregnancy interval of >10y   • Age ≥40y
- BMI ≥30kg/m^2 at first contact   • Multiple pregnancy
- Family (e.g. mother, sister) or past history of pre-eclampsia
- Pre-existing vascular (e.g. hypertension, DM) or renal disease

Consider ↑ frequency of BP/proteinuria monitoring in pregnancy for these women—although optimum frequency of BP checks is unclear.

⚠ Warn all pregnant women of the symptoms of advanced pre-eclampsia:
- Headache
- Problems with vision, e.g. blurring or flashing before the eyes
- Bad pain just below the ribs
- Vomiting
- Sudden swelling of face, hands, or feet

If a pregnant woman experiences any of these symptoms in pregnancy she should seek advice from a doctor or midwife as soon as possible.

Psychiatric illness At first contact, ask about:
- History of mental health problems, e.g. schizophrenia, bipolar disorder, severe depression
- Previous treatment from a specialist mental health team (including in-patient care)
- Family history of perinatal mental illness

❶ Ensure that information about any relevant history of mental illness is included in your referral letter for antenatal care.

At booking Ask:
- During the past month, have you often been bothered by feeling down, depressed, or hopeless?
- During the past month, have you often been bothered by having little interest or pleasure in doing things?
- If the woman answers 'yes' to either question, ask: is this something you feel that you need help with?

If a mental health problem is detected, further assessment (e.g. with PHQ-9—📖 p. 1001) is indicated.

Postnatal screening 📖 p. 839

Further information
NICE Antenatal and postnatal mental health (2007) ♒ www.nice.org.uk

Fetal growth and position Measure and record symphysis-fundal height (SFH) at each antenatal appointment from 24wk. Assess fetal presentation by abdominal palpation at ≥36wk. Confirm suspected fetal malpresentation by USS.

Information and support for prospective parents
Antenatal results and choices (ARC) ☏ 0845 077 2290 ♒ www.arc-uk.org
Genetic Alliance Group ☏ 020 7704 3141 ♒ www.geneticalliance.org.uk
Sickle Cell Society ☏ 020 8961 7795 ♒ www.sicklecellsociety.org
UK Thalassaemia Society ☏ 020 8882 0011 ♒ www.ukts.org
Down's Syndrome Association ☏ 0333 1212 300
♒ www.downs-syndrome.org.uk
Shine (spina bifida and hydrocephalus) ☏ 01733 555988
♒ www.shinecharity.org.uk
Tay Sachs and Allied Disease Association ☏ 01473 404 156

Common symptoms in pregnancy

Abdominal pain 📖 p. 1102

Backache Affects 60% of pregnant women—usually from the 2nd trimester onwards and worse in the evenings—may interfere with sleep/activities. Encourage light exercise (unless contraindicated, e.g. pre-eclampsia)—special land and water-based classes are run for pregnant women. Treat with simple analgesia, physiotherapy ± massage.

Bleeding 📖 p. 818

Breast soreness Most common early in pregnancy. Good support bras are essential (can be purchased from specialist clothing stores). Nipples enlarge and darken at ~12wk.

Carpal tunnel syndrome Affects ~28% pregnant women—📖 p. 486. Reassure usually resolves after pregnancy. Night splints may help. If severe consider steroid injection. Diuretics do not help. If does not resolve after pregnancy, refer for orthopaedic assessment.

Constipation Affects up to 40% of pregnant women. ↑ fluid and fibre intake. If necessary use a bulk-forming laxative, e.g. ispaghula husk. Avoid bowel stimulants as they ↑ uterine activity.

Cramp Leg cramp affects 1 in 3 in late pregnancy. Worse at night. Raising the foot of the bed by 20cm (e.g. 1–2 bricks) can help.

Fatigue
- **Early pregnancy** Almost universal symptom. Reaches peak at 12–15wk. Advise rest and adjustment of lifestyle. Reassure
- **Late pregnancy** Due to ↑ physical effort needed to do everyday tasks and sleep deprivation. Check not anaemic else reassure

Haemorrhoids Affect 8% of women in the third trimester. May be associated with itching, pain, and bleeding. Advise ↑ fibre intake. Treat prolapse with ice packs and replacement. Topical haemorrhoid applications are commonly used but lack evidence of safety or efficacy.

Headache Usually tension headache. Check BP and urine for protein to exclude pre-eclampsia (📖 p. 826). Treat with rest and analgesia. Migraine may ↑ or ↓ in pregnancy.

Heartburn Affects 70% of women in the third trimester. Reassure not harmful. Advise low-fat, bland food, small portions and frequent meals. Avoid eating late at night if worse at night, and consider raising the head of the bed (1–2 bricks under the bed). Avoid gastric irritants, e.g. caffeine. Antacid preparations, e.g. magnesium trisilicate, are helpful if lifestyle modifications are ineffective but may worsen constipation.

⚠ Pre-eclampsia can present with epigastric pain—check BP and urine for protein if epigastric/right upper quadrant pain unresponsive to simple antacids, refer for same-day assessment even if BP is normal and no/trace proteinuria (📖 p. 827).

Hypotension Common symptom of early pregnancy. Check no bleeding. Advise to avoid standing suddenly and avoid hot baths.

Insomnia Avoid drug treatment. Reassure. Relaxation techniques and mild physical exercise prior to sleep can help.

Itching/pruritus 📖 p. 805

Nausea and vomiting >80% from 4–6wk—~½ vomit. Occurs at any time of day ('morning' sickness in <20%) and made worse by odours associated with preparation/sight of food. If severe exclude multiple pregnancy, trophoblastic disease, and UTI. Symptoms usually improve by 14–16wk although persist in some.

Management Reassure—normal part of pregnancy. Adjust lifestyle, e.g. ask partner to do the shopping. Advise frequent small meals—avoid greasy/spicy foods, eat foods you can face (varies). Maintain fluid intake—small amounts frequently. Self-help measures include ginger[CE] and P6 acupressure[CE]. If severe/disabling consider antiemetics[CE], e.g. cyclizine 50mg tds. Suppositories are an effective method of administration if po route is not tolerated. If dehydrated or >2–5kg weight loss (*hyperemesis gravidarum*—1%, pregnancies) admit for rehydration.

Peripheral paraesthesia Abnormalities of sensation (e.g. tingling, pins and needles) of hands/feet are common. Reassure. Symptoms usually resolve after delivery. Carpal tunnel syndrome—📖 p. 486.

Skin changes Pigmentation (e.g. linea nigra); spider naevi; abdominal striae; chloasma/merasma; palmar erythema. *Skin rashes* 📖 p. 805.

Sweating and feeling hot Common. Check apyrexial. If apyrexial, reassure normal in pregnancy. If pyrexial, look for a source of infection.

Swelling Fluid retention affects 80%—ankles, hands/fingers, face. If severe/sudden ↑ in oedema, exclude pre-eclampsia (check BP, dipstick urine for protein).

Symphysis pubis dysfunction 3%. Symphysis separates causing discomfort/pain in lower abdomen/pelvic area radiating to lower back, upper thighs, and perineum. Pain is constant and worse on movement and resolves on rest. Treat with simple analgesia. Consider referral to physiotherapy for pelvic support belt or elbow crutches. Advise rest in a semi-recumbent position when in pain. Generally resolves after delivery but if persists refer to orthopaedics.

Urinary frequency Check MSU—UTI is common in pregnancy and associated with premature delivery—📖 p. 812.

Vaginal discharge Usually ↑ in pregnancy. Investigate if smelly, itchy, sore, or associated with dysuria.

Varicose veins Cause aching legs, fatigue, itch, and ankle/foot swelling. If ankles are swollen, exclude pre-eclampsia (check BP, dipstick urine for proteinuria). Elevate legs when sitting, provide support stockings, and encourage walking/discourage standing still. Complications include *thrombophlebitis*—treat with ice packs, elevation, support stockings, and analgesia—and DVT (📖 p. 824).

Pruritus and rashes in pregnancy

⚠ **At booking**

- Enquire if the woman has had chickenpox and/or shingles in the past. If not, advise her to make urgent contact if she develops a chickenpox-type rash or has contact with chickenpox or shingles
- Advise the woman to inform the midwife/GP urgently if she develops any rash during pregnancy or has contact with anyone who has a rash

Contact with rashes in pregnancy Many pregnant women have young children and contact with children with rashes is common. *Management—see Figure 23.4.*

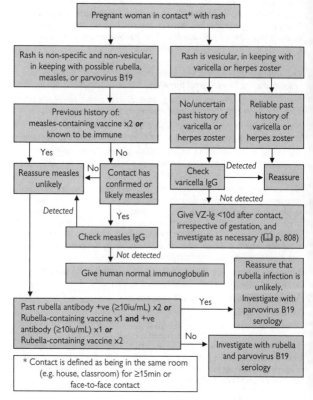

Figure 23.4 Investigation of pregnant women in contact with non-specific, non-vesicular rash, vesicular rash, or known cases of measles, rubella, parvovirus varicella, or herpes zoster

Presentation with itching If a woman presents with itching, look for a rash. If there is *no* rash consider:

Hepatic causes *Pruritus gravidarum or recurrent cholestasis of pregnancy* affects 2–20 in every 100 pregnancies and sometimes runs in families. Usually begins in the third trimester reaching a peak in the last 1mo.
- **Frank jaundice** Rare—refer urgently to an obstetrician
- **No jaundice** Check LFTs. Refer to obstetrics if abnormal. Otherwise, treat with moisturizers (e.g. Diprobase) ± oily calamine. Antihistamines do not help

Pruritus gravidarum disappears after delivery but recurs in subsequent pregnancies (40–50%) and may recur with CHC.

Other causes
- **Endocrine** DM, thyrotoxicosis, hypothyroidism—consider checking fasting blood glucose and TFTs
- **Renal** Chronic renal failure—check U&E and Cr
- **Haematological** Iron deficiency—check FBC and ferritin
- **Drug allergies**
- **Psychological** Obsessive states, schizophrenia

❶ If no cause is found and the problem persists, refer to obstetrics.

Presentation with a rash Consider:
- Common skin diseases, e.g. eczema, psoriasis, urticaria
- Skin changes specific to pregnancy
- Infectious causes:
  - Rubella
  - Parvovirus B19
  - Chickenpox/shingles
  - Measles
  - Streptococcal infection
  - Meningococcal infection
  - Enterovirus infection
  - EBV
  - CMV
  - Syphilis

Itchy rashes specific to pregnancy
- **Abdominal striae** May itch
- **Pruritic urticarial papules and plaques of pregnancy (PUPPP)** 1 in 240 pregnancies. Occurs in first/multiple pregnancies or if excessive weight ↑ in pregnancy. Intensely itchy rash usually confined to lower abdomen/buttocks. Appears at >35wk gestation. Treat with calamine and/or topical steroids. Clears spontaneously <6wk (often days) after delivery. Recurrence in subsequent pregnancies is rare
- **Pemphigoid gestationis** Rare. Starts in mid-pregnancy and appears as a generalized, intensely itchy rash. Refer for specialist management. May recur in subsequent pregnancies/with CHC
- **Impetigo herpetiformis** Rare. Starts in the third trimester. Mild itch. Systemically unwell. Refer. Remits after delivery but may recur in later pregnancies

Pregnant women with rash illness See Figure 23.5, 📖 p. 807.

Further information
Health Protection Agency (HPA) Guidance on viral rash in pregnancy (2011) ℗ www.hpa.org.uk
RCOG Obstetric cholestasis (2011) ℗ www.rcog.org.uk

Rubella and parvovirus in pregnancy

Rubella Presents with fever, LNs (including suboccipital nodes), and a pink maculopapular rash which lasts 3d. 50% of mothers infected with rubella are asymptomatic. Incubation is 14–21d and once infected, patients are infectious from 7d before the rash appears until 7d after. Asymptomatic reinfection of women who have received vaccination can also occur, so serology is essential in all pregnant rubella contacts.

Risk to the baby Abnormalities that can occur include: cataract, deafness, cerebral palsy, mental retardation, microcephaly, microphthalmia. If the mother is infected with rubella at >20wk gestation, infection does not affect the baby.

Transmission risk to the baby
- **<11wk gestation** 90% have adverse outcome
- **11–16wk gestation** 20% have adverse outcome
- **>16wk gestation** minimal risk of deafness only

Transmission risk is much lower with reinfection (<5%). There is no treatment to prevent transmission.

Management
- Contact with a non-vesicular rash or rubella— see Figure 23.4, 📖 p. 804
- Presentation with a non-specific, non-vesicular rash or suspected rubella infection—send blood for serology for rubella and parvovirus B19 (see Figure 23.6). Refer if proven infection. After further investigation and discussion of risks, women infected with rubella at <20wk may be offered termination of pregnancy

Vaccination after pregnancy Give postnatal MMR vaccination routinely to all women found not to be rubella-immune in pregnancy.

Parvovirus B19 infection Febrile illness often accompanied by tenderness of the joints/arthritis affecting hands, wrists, and knees—usually lasts 1–2wk. There may be a fine rash over the trunk and extremities. Infectious from 10d before rash appears. Incubation period 13–18d.

Parvovirus B19 in pregnancy ~50% of young women in the UK are not immune. Risk of infection in pregnancy ~1 in 400. Risk of a non-immune mother contracting the infection from a child who has Fifth disease (slapped cheek) is ~50%.

Risk to the baby If infection is at <20wk gestation, there is a 9% ↑ miscarriage rate. 3% (14–56 babies/y in the UK) develop hydrops fetalis >3wk after infection due to anaemia—½ of those babies die. There are no long-term effects from an infection which does not cause miscarriage or hydrops.

Transmission rate to the baby Depends on gestation at the time of infection. There is no treatment to prevent transmission.
- **<4wk gestation** there is no transmission
- **From 5–16wk gestation** transmission rate ~15%
- **>16wk gestation** 25–70% transmission rate (↑ with gestation)

Management
- Contact with a non-vesicular rash or parvovirus—see Figure 23.4, p. 804
- Presentation with a non-specific, non-vesicular rash or suspected parvovirus infection—send blood for serology for rubella and parvovirus B19 (see Figure 23.5). Refer if proven infection. USS surveillance is started 4wk after onset of illness or seroconversion and then every 1–2 wk until 30wk. If there are any signs of hydrops fetalis on USS, the mother is referred to a regional centre for consideration of intrauterine transfusion. Early transfusion ↑ chances of the baby's survival

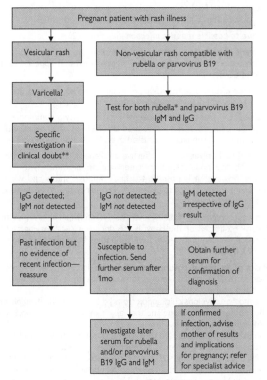

* Irrespective of past testing or immunization.
** Confirm by detection of varicella virus, antigen, or DNA in vesicle fluid.

Figure 23.5 Investigation of pregnant women with a rash illness
Reproduced in modified format with permission of the Health Protection Agency, Center for Infection, Immunisation Department: ℘ http://hpa.org.uk.

Other rash illnesses in pregnancy

Cytomegalovirus (CMV) More frequent cause of birth defect than rubella in the UK—5 in 1,000 live births—10% develop handicap. The fetus is most vulnerable when infection occurs in early pregnancy. Maternal disease may be asymptomatic or a mild flu-like illness. Occasionally there is a rash. No effective prevention strategy.

Measles Rare in the UK since introduction of routine MMR vaccination for children. Presents with coryza, lymphadenopathy, conjunctivitis, and disseminated maculopapular rash which becomes confluent. Complications include pneumonia, otitis media, and encephalitis. Infection in pregnancy can lead to intrauterine death and preterm delivery. There are no associations with congenital infection or abnormalities.

Exposure to possible measles infection See Figure 23.4, 📖 p. 804

Treatment of neonates Human normal immunoglobulin (HNIG) is given to neonates born to mothers with a measles rash that appears from 6d before to 6d after birth.

Vaccination after pregnancy Give postnatal MMR vaccination routinely to all women found not to be measles-immune in pregnancy.

Chickenpox Contact with chickenpox in pregnancy is common. People with chickenpox are infectious from 2d before the rash appears until the rash has finished cropping and crusted over. Incubation period is 14–21d.

Pre-conceptual prevention An effective chickenpox vaccine is available in the UK. There is no UK policy to screen women for immunity to varicella infection, however it is possible to check immune status and vaccinate non-immune women prior to pregnancy. Pregnancy should be avoided for 3mo after immunization.

Exposure in pregnancy If the mother has definitely had chickenpox there is no risk to herself or the baby. If she does not recall having chickenpox, check her immunity—80% have antibodies from silent infection (see Figure 23.4, 📖 p. 804).

In cases of 'at risk' exposure Arrange for VZ-Ig to be given to mother and/or baby. This can be lifesaving and significantly ↓ disease severity if given ≤10d after exposure. Babies are at risk if:
• The mother develops chickenpox from 7d before to 7d after delivery
• The mother is not immune and the baby is exposed to chickenpox <7d after birth
• The baby has been exposed to chickenpox and has potentially inadequate transfer of maternal antibodies (e.g. preterm babies <28wk, babies weighing <1,000g at birth, babies who have had blood transfusions).VZ-Ig can be given without antibody testing to these babies, but where possible, test
• Duration of protection from VZ-Ig is limited. Give a second dose if still at risk and further exposure occurs and ≥3wk since first dose. Check antibody status again before giving second dose

●⁑ Some advocate use of prophylactic aciclovir for women with significant additional risk factors, e.g. immunosuppression, smokers, women who did not receive early VZ-Ig, or those in the second half of pregnancy.

Risk to the mother Chickenpox infection complicates 2–3 in 1,000 pregnancies. Chickenpox pneumonia is more common (10%) and can be severe (1 in 1,000 mortality).

Risk to the baby Rates of transmission are higher later in pregnancy (~50% >36wk; 5–10% <28wk). Infection:

- **<20wk** Causes miscarriage. Fetal varicella syndrome affects 1–2%— segmental skin defects/scarring, limb hypoplasia ± paresis, low birth weight, microcephaly, neurological abnormalities (e.g. hypotonia, eye defects). May occur up to 28wk gestation
- **20–37wk** Intrauterine infection or death, shingles in childhood
- **1wk before–1wk after delivery** All babies should be given VZ-Ig. Onset 4d before delivery–2d after delivery carries a 20% risk of overwhelming neonatal infection—these babies should be given aciclovir in addition to VZ-Ig. Seek specialist advice

Management If clinical doubt, confirm infection by detection of varicella virus, antigen, or DNA in vesicle fluid (see Figure 23.5, 🕮 p. 807). Treat with aciclovir 800mg 5x/d po for 1wk if presents <24h after the rash appears and the mother is >20wk gestation. Monitor daily. If <28wk gestation, refer for detailed USS 5wk after infection to exclude fetal varicella syndrome.

Admit if
- Chest symptoms
- Haemorrhagic rash or bleeding
- Neurological symptoms other than headache
- Severe disease—dense rash/numerous mucosal lesions
- Significant immunosuppression, e.g. HIV +ve

Consider admission if
- Pregnancy approaching term
- Smoker
- Bad obstetric history
- Chronic lung disease
- Poor social circumstances
- Unable to monitor the woman closely, e.g homeless, traveller

Refer for urgent hospital assessment if no deterioration but:
- Fever persists, *or*
- Cropping of the rash continues >6d

❶ Warn pregnant women with chickenpox to avoid contact with anyone potentially at risk of developing severe chickenpox, especially other pregnant women or neonates.

Rash infections that cause no harm to the fetus

- Epstein–Barr virus (EBV)
- Enteroviruses—Coxsackie virus A/B; echovirus; enterovirus 68–71— cause disease, such as hand, foot, and mouth. Some enteroviruses can cause severe neonatal infection, and prophylactic immunoglobulin may be necessary—seek specialist advice

Further information
Health Protection Agency (HPA) Guidance on viral rash in pregnancy (2011) ℛ www.hpa.org.uk
RCOG Chickenpox in pregnancy (2007) ℛ www.rcog.org.uk

Other infections in pregnancy

Bacterial vaginosis Present in ~10% of pregnant women—asymptomatic in half. Associated with ↑ preterm birth (x 2). There is no screening policy in the UK, but, if detected:
• Treat with metronidazole po—400mg bd for 7d or 2g stat
• An alternative is clindamycin 2% cream 5g nocte PV for 1wk

❶ Treatment may not lower the risk to the pregnancy.

Chickenpox 📖 p. 808

Chlamydia ~1 in 20 pregnant women has chlamydia infection. During pregnancy, chlamydia infection is associated with IUGR, preterm birth, and low birthweight. It can also pass to the baby during delivery, causing eye and/or chest infections. Postpartum, chlamydia can cause womb infection. Treat if detected (📖 p. 740)—follow-up with swabs to confirm eradication. Refer any affected neonates for expert advice.

Screening As part of the National Chlamydia Screening Programme, women <25y can ask for chlamydia self-test kits at a variety of healthcare and community settings. Otherwise there is no evidence of cost-effectiveness of routine antenatal screening for STIs apart from HIV and hepatitis B.

Coughs, colds, and 'flu Little threat to the pregnancy itself. *Advise:* fluids, paracetamol, and rest. Inhaled decongestants are safe, but avoid cough linctus and OTC composite preparations. Treat any secondary infections as needed.

Cytomegalovirus (CMV) 📖 p. 808   **Enteroviruses** 📖 p. 809

Genital herpes[G] Affects ~10% of the UK population (diagnosis made in 1 in 3). Risk is greatest if the primary attack occurs at >34wk gestation. Secondary attacks are much less of a problem. Risks include:
• Passing the infection to the baby at the time of delivery
• Early labour
• IUGR (primary infection only)

❶ Elective Caesarean section is advised at term if a primary attack occurs during pregnancy at >28wk gestation. It is controversial if Caesarean section is preferable if there is an active secondary attack at the time of labour.

Gonorrhoea <1 in 1,000 pregnancies. Can pass to the baby during delivery, causing eye infections. Treat if detected—📖 p. 741. Refer affected infants urgently for expert advice. Follow-up with swabs to confirm eradication.

Group B streptococcus (GBS)[G] Bacterium carried in the vagina by >1 in 4 pregnant women (20% of non-pregnant women). Usually harmless but if transmitted to the baby during delivery can cause neonatal septicaemia, pneumonia, or meningitis.

Prevention of neonatal infection There is currently no UK screening programme to detect women carrying group B streptococcal infection during pregnancy. Treatment with IV antibiotics during labour is advised in 'high-risk' scenarios only:

• Early labour <37wk
• Prolonged (>18h) or early (<37wk) rupture of the membranes
• Group B streptococcus detected in urine in pregnancy
• If the woman has a temperature >37.8°C during labour
• If a previous baby has been affected with the condition (10x ↑ risk)

❶ If found incidentally during pregnancy (e.g. detected on a swab done for another reason), there is no evidence that treatment is effective. However antibiotics are given during labour.

Hepatitis B Prevalence of HBsAg in pregnancy is up to 1% (depending on geographical area). Women are routinely offered screening for hepatitis B infection in pregnancy. Transmission to the baby occurs during labour (up to 30% of infants of women seropositive for HBsAg and 90% of infants of women seropositive for both HBsAg and HBeAg). Infants infected are at high risk (~90%) of becoming chronic carriers and of developing chronic liver disease ± premature death.

Postnatally Refer infected women for hepatology assessment. Infected mothers should not donate their milk.

Immunization Give hepatitis B vaccine as soon as possible after birth to babies born to carrier mothers with the addition of immunoglobulin (HBIG) if the mother carries the hepatitis B e-antigen or had acute HBV infection during pregnancy. 85–95% effective in preventing neonatal hepatitis B infection. Further doses of vaccine are required at 1 and 2mo of age, and a booster dose at 1y at the same time as follow-up testing.

Hepatitis C Prevalence in pregnant women is 0.14–0.8%. Except when initial infection of the mother occurs during pregnancy (when transfer rate is much higher), transmission rate to the fetus is 5%. To date there is no evidence that HCV can be transferred to the child by breastfeeding. Infants at risk can be screened for HCV infection at 12mo (RNA screen) or 18–24mo (HCV antibody test). The majority of infants that acquire HCV infection via their mothers develop chronic hepatitis. Treatment is with interferon and achieves viral clearance rates of 40%.

HIV Prevalence of HIV among pregnant women in the UK varies from 0.04% to 0.4% depending on geographical area. Up to 50% of infants of HIV seropositive mothers are pre- or perinatally infected with HIV, accounting for 90% of HIV infections in childhood. Avoidance of breastfeeding, antiretroviral therapy, and appropriate management of delivery ↓ risk of transmission to <1%. A detailed fetal anomaly scan is important if there is first trimester exposure to antiviral treatment (including folate antagonists) as possible ↑ risk of congenital abnormality.

❶ There is a theoretical concern of mother-to-child transmission with invasive prenatal diagnosis. Take specialist advice.

Antenatal HIV testing 📖 p. 799

Fetal abnormalities include Wide set eyes, short nose, patulous lips, 'box' forehead, and growth failure. However diagnosis is usually made between 6mo and 2y of age when the child presents with lymphadenopathy, recurrent or opportunistic infections, failure to thrive, or progressive encephalopathy. Expert advice is needed throughout pregnancy and for neonatal follow-up.

Listeriosis Rare. May occur in epidemics. Infection of the mother is usually via infected food, e.g. pâté, soft cheese, milk. Detection is with blood cultures. Suspect if unexplained fever >48h, and refer for expert advice.

Maternal symptoms Fever, shivering, myalgia, headache, sore throat, cough, vomiting, diarrhoea, vaginitis.

Consequences Miscarriage (may be recurrent), stillbirth, premature labour, transmission to the fetus (in 2nd/3rd trimester). Infection in the newborn infant manifests in pneumonia ± meningitis.

Prevention See Box 23.2.

Malaria Serious complications are more common in pregnancy (cerebral malaria has 50% mortality). Suspect in any pregnant woman who has a fever and has recently visited an infected area. Seek immediate expert advice.

Measles 📖 p. 808   **Parvovirus B19** 📖 p. 806

Rubella 📖 p. 806

Syphilis Prevalence 0.07%. ~70–100% of pregnant mothers with primary, untreated syphilis transmit the disease to the fetus (1 in 3 die *in utero*). In the early latent phase, risk of transmission is ~40% and ~10–15% in the late latent phase. Neurological abnormalities as a result of congenital syphilis include encephalopathy and sensorineural deafness. Treatment ↓ risk of transmission by >98%. Refer for specialist assessment if +ve result on routine antenatal VDRL testing. ❶ +ve result is NOT specific to syphilis.

Thrush More common in pregnancy. Not harmful to the fetus. Requires treatment only if causes troublesome itching, soreness, or discharge. *Treatment:* imidazole pessaries for 1wk.

Toxoplasmosis Caused by a parasite found in raw meat and cat faeces. Up to 90% of women have not had toxoplasmosis before pregnancy and ~2 in 1,000 will catch it during pregnancy. 30–40% pass it to their fetus. Infection may result in miscarriage, stillbirth, growth problems, blindness, hydrocephalus, brain damage, epilepsy, or deafness. Risk of transmission to the fetus is related to gestation at the time of infection—third trimester ~70%; first trimester ~15%. If infection is suspected refer for specialist advice. Prevention—see Box 23.2.

Urinary tract infections 1 in 25 women develops UTI in pregnancy. If suspected, send MSU to confirm diagnosis and start antibiotics (e.g. cefalexin 250mg tds) immediately. Recurrent UTIs in pregnancy should be investigated—consider renal ultrasound >12wk after delivery.

Screening for UTI Routine screening with MSU for UTI is offered at booking. 2–5% of pregnant women have asymptomatic bacteriuria, defined as pure growth of >10^5 organisms/mL—1 in 3 will develop symptomatic infection (acute cystitis, pyelonephritis) if left untreated. Both untreated bacteriuria and frank UTI are associated with preterm delivery and IUGR. Treat for at least 1wk with suitable antibiotic (avoid trimethoprim). Check MSU following treatment to ensure infection has cleared.

Whooping cough New born babies are at particular risk of severe whooping cough infection. Pregnant women are advised to have whooping cough vaccination from 28–38wk (ideally 28–32wk) gestation to provide passive immunity for their babies.

Box 23.2 Advice for pregnant women on prevention of toxoplasmosis and listeriosis

- Only eat well-cooked meat
- Wash hands, cooking utensils, and food surfaces after preparing raw meat
- Keep raw meat and cooked foods on separate plates
- Wash all soil from fruit and vegetables before eating
- If possible get someone else to clean cat litter or use gloves and wash hands afterwards
- Use gloves when gardening and wash hands afterwards

Further information

NICE Antenatal care: routine care for healthy pregnant women (2010)
℘ www.nice.org.uk
NHS Infectious Diseases in Pregnancy Screening Programme
℘ http://infectiousdiseases.screening.nhs.uk
RCOG ℘ www.rcog.org.uk
- Management of genital herpes in pregnancy (2007)
- Prevention of early onset neonatal Group B Streptococcal disease (2012)
- Management of HIV in pregnancy (2010)
- Prevention of malaria in pregnancy (2010)
- Diagnosis and treatment of malaria in pregnancy (2010)
British HIV Association/Children's HIV Association Management of HIV infection in pregnant women (2008) ℘ www.bhiva.org

Information for patients

Department of Health Hepatitis B: how to protect your baby (2007)
℘ www.dh.gov.uk
Group B Streptococcus Support ℘ www.gbss.org.uk

Bleeding in early pregnancy

Bleeding up to 14wk into pregnancy Bleeding in early pregnancy occurs in 1 in 4 pregnancies. *Causes:*
• Bleeding in normal pregnancy—largest group
• Miscarriage
• Ectopic pregnancy
• Trophoblastic disease
• Non-obstetric conditions, e.g. friable cervix, polyp, cervical neoplasia

⚠ Any sexually active woman presenting with abdominal pain and vaginal bleeding after an interval of amenorrhoea has an ectopic pregnancy until proven otherwise.

Assessment
• Take a history of pain and bleeding—pain preceding bleeding suggests ectopic pregnancy is more likely. Have any products of conception been passed? ❶ Clots/products can be difficult to distinguish
• Check LMP and pregnancy test result (do a test if needed)
• Check pulse (>100bpm suggests shock), BP, and temperature (? toxic)
• Abdominal examination—guarding, peritonism, and/or unilateral tenderness suggest ectopic pregnancy
• Pelvic examination—with the advent of early pregnancy assessment units (EPAU), the necessity of pelvic examination is debatable. If performed, assess uterine size, cervix—is the cervix open? (A closed cervix admits only one fingertip in a multiparous woman). Is there any other cause for the bleeding?

Initial management If severe bleeding and/or pain, shocked, or toxic, admit to gynaecology as an emergency. If shocked, give 1mL Syntometrine® IM, if available, and try to gain IV access. Otherwise, refer to the EPAU to check site and viability of pregnancy with USS:
• At 5wk gestation, sac ± yolk sac is seen on scan
• At 6–7wk a fetal pole and fetal heart beat is usually seen

Blood group and rhesus status is also checked at the EPAU (📖 p. 820).

Complications of bleeding Significant sub-chorionic haematoma is associated with ↑ risk of premature rupture of membranes and IUGR—refer early for specialist antenatal care.

⚠ **Rhesus-negative women** ❶ If there is clinical doubt, give anti-D

Bleeding <12wk gestation Anti-D is not required for:
• Threatened miscarriage unless heavy or repeated bleeding and/or abdominal pain, or
• Complete miscarriage where no medical or surgical uterine evacuation

Bleeding >12wk gestation, ectopic pregnancy, and/or medical/surgical evacuation of the uterus at any gestation Give anti-D immunoglobulin (250iu IM if gestation <20wk) within 72h of bleeding— *whether or not the pregnancy is lost*—📖 p. 820.

Bleeding in early normal pregnancy Often termed *threatened miscarriage*. If fetal heart is seen on USS then there is ~97% chance of the pregnancy continuing to progress. There is no evidence that rest or abstinence from sex improves outcome.

Miscarriage Also termed spontaneous abortion. Occurs in 1 in 5 pregnancies—80% at <12wk gestation. *Risk factors:*
- Maternal age ≥35y or paternal age ≥40y
- Smoking
- BMI >29kg/m^2—if >32kg/m^2, risk is ↑ by 30%
- Excess alcohol

Causes
- Fetal abnormality (50%)
- Multiple pregnancy
- Uterine abnormality—fibroids, polyps; congenital abnormality; cervical incompetence (📖 p. 816—late second trimester miscarriages)
- Systemic disease—renal, autoimmune, or connective tissue disease— particularly SLE, PCOS, DM, systemic infection
- Drugs—cytotoxics, diethylstilbestrol
- Placental vascular abnormalities

Classification
- **Complete miscarriage** History of bleeding. No products of conception in the uterus. Provide psychological support
- **Incomplete miscarriage** Bleeding. Products of conception remain in the uterus but there is no fetal heart. Usually admitted for evacuation of retained products of conception (ERPC). Some women prefer a 'watch and wait' approach—at 3d 86% will be complete
- **Missed (or delayed) miscarriage** No bleeding. Usually discovered when no heart beat is seen on routine antenatal scan. Treatment is with ERPC. A 'watch and wait' approach is possible, but at 4wk only 66% are complete, and associated with longer bleeding

Medical management with prostaglandin analogues ± antiprogesterone priming is an alternative to ERPC and offered in some units.

❶ There is no evidence that abstinence from pregnancy for a time after miscarriage is helpful—fertility may ↑ immediately after miscarriage.

Complications
- **Early** Perforation of the uterus, retained products of conception, infection. Treat with antibiotics if infection is suspected (e.g. doxycycline 100mg od). Re-refer/readmit if shock, pain, heavy bleeding, or bleeding is not settling
- **Later** Uterine synechiae (Asherman's syndrome), cervical incompetence, psychological sequelae

Recurrent miscarriage^G ≥3 miscarriages (1–2% couples). *Check:*
- **Age**—incidence of recurrent miscarriage ↑ with age (♂ and ♀)
- **How many miscarriages**—confirmed pregnancies (not just late, heavy periods)? All with the same partner? What gestation? The more miscarriages, the lower the chance of successful pregnancy
- **Infertility treatment?** 25–30% of women who miscarry
- **Past medical history**—gynaecological problems (cervical instrumentation, PCOS); systemic disease
- **Family history**—recurrent miscarriage, thrombosis/thrombophilia

Management of recurrent miscarriage Refer for further investigation; consider checking antiphospholipid antibodies prior to referral. No cause is found in half of those referred. They have a 70% chance of successful pregnancy. Other treatable causes include:

- **Antiphospholipid antibodies** (15%). Low-dose aspirin + low molecular weight heparin from 6–34wk improves outcome
- **Inherited thrombophilia** (factor V Leiden, prothrombin gene mutation or protein S deficiency). If recurrent miscarriage >10wk, treatment with low molecular weight heparin ↑ live birth rate
- **Cervical incompetence** Diagnosis is usually made on the basis of history of suggestive symptoms in past pregnancies—≥1 late second trimester or early third trimester miscarriage (usually painless leaking of liquor or gradual painless dilatation of the cervix). Refer all women with past history for early obstetric review. Treatment is with cervical USS monitoring with cerclage if cervical length is <25mm (a stitch is placed high up around the cervix to keep it closed, e.g. Shirodkar suture. The stitch is removed at ~37wk and labour ensues rapidly if the diagnosis was correct)
- **Chromosomal abnormality in one parent** (3–5%) Refer for specialist genetics advice

Ectopic pregnancy[G] Egg implants outside the uterine cavity—95% in a Fallopian tube. Incidence ~1 in 1,000 pregnancies. *Risk factors:*

- Pelvic inflammatory disease (single episode ↑ risk x7)
- Previous ectopic (11%)
- IUD (14%)
- Infertility (15%)
- Tubal surgery
- Age >35y
- Smoking
- Multiple partners

History

- **Abdominal pain** (97%). Unilateral or bilateral, may start before bleeding; radiates to shoulder tip; ↑ on passing urine/opening bowels
- **Amenorrhoea** (75%). Peak incidence after 7wk amenorrhoea
- **Irregular vaginal bleeding** (79%). Described as 'prune juice' but may be fresh blood; usually not heavy. May pass decidual cast

Examination Shock in 15–20%; abdominal tenderness ± rebound or guarding (71%); pelvis—enlarged uterus, adnexal mass, and/or cervical excitation.

Management Admit immediately for further investigation. Resuscitate before admission as needed. Hospital management may be expectant (watch and pregnancy resolves spontaneously), medical (methotrexate), or surgical (laparotomy or laparoscopic surgery). Offer early USS in future pregnancies to confirm pregnancy is intrauterine.

Complications Death if undetected, infertility (pregnancy rate post-ectopic pregnancy is 66% with 10% having a further ectopic pregnancy).

Trophoblastic disease[G]

Hydatidiform mole Trophoblastic tumour containing 46 chromosomes (usually of paternal origin) and no fetal material. 8–20% become invasive and penetrate the uterus and/or metastasize to the lungs. Presents with:

- Bleeding in early pregnancy ± exaggerated symptoms of pregnancy
- Uterus is usually large for dates, and no fetal heart can be heard

- USS has a typical appearance; blood—↑↑ serum β-HCG
- Rarely symptoms of metastatic spread—haemoptysis, pleurisy

Refer urgently to gynaecology. If mole is confirmed, women are followed up by specialist centres. Invasive disease requires chemotherapy. Combined hormonal contraception is contraindicated until normal HCG values are obtained. Pregnancy is not advised until completion of the surveillance period—investigate with early USS and β-HCG as incidence of further molar pregnancy is ~1 in 80.

Partial mole Tumour of trophoblast containing 69 chromosomes, 1 maternal and 2 paternal sets, with some fetal tissue. A fetal heart may be seen on early USS but is absent by 8–9wk. Treat as for mole. Rarely becomes malignant (0.5%).

Choriocarcinoma Malignant trophoblastic tumour following molar (rarely normal) pregnancy. Presents with vaginal bleeding and/or metastases (shadows on CXR, dyspnoea, haemoptysis). Excellent prognosis after treatment with chemotherapy. No contraceptive restrictions after completion of therapy; pregnancy is possible >1y after treatment.

Placental site trophoblastic tumour (PSTT) Rare. Follows 3–4y after normal pregnancy. Presents with abnormal bleeding or amenorrhoea. Can present with distant metastases similarly to choriocarcinoma. Treatment is with hysterectomy ± chemotherapy. Prognosis is good.

Psychological effects of early loss of pregnancy Broach the subject with all women who have suffered early loss of pregnancy. Include the woman's partner if possible.

- Legitimize grief and acknowledge it—not all women grieve—adjust your approach accordingly; discuss worries/concerns
- Provide information about the condition which caused the loss; risk to future pregnancies (if <3 miscarriages, risk of further miscarriage is not significantly ↑; risk of further ectopic pregnancy is ~1 in 10); and self-help/support organizations, e.g. Miscarriage Association
- Warn of the anniversary phenomenon (sadness at the baby's due date or anniversary of the pregnancy loss) or sadness/jealousy on the birth of another's baby—provide ongoing support as needed
- If the woman already has young children, inform the health visitor

Further information

RCOG ℅ www.rcog.org.uk
- Management of early pregnancy loss (2006)
- Investigation and treatment of couples with recurrent miscarriage (2011)
- The management of tubal pregnancy (2004)
- Management of gestational trophoblastic disease (2010)

Patient advice and support

Miscarriage Association ☎ 01924 200799
℅ www.miscarriageassociation.org.uk
Ectopic Pregnancy Trust ☎ 020 7733 2653 ℅ www.ectopic.org
Hydatidiform Mole and Choriocarcinoma Support Service
℅ www.hmole-chorio.org.uk

Ante- and postpartum haemorrhage

Antepartum haemorrhage Any bleeding in pregnancy >24wk gestation (or the point of fetal viability) is an antepartum haemorrhage (APH). Bleeding <14wk gestation—🕮 p. 814.

Causes

Uterine
- Abruption (🕮 p. 1103)
- Placenta praevia
- Vasa praevia
- Circumvallate placenta
- Placental sinuses

Lower genital tract
- Cervical—polyp; erosion; carcinoma; cervicitis
- Vaginitis
- Vulval varicosities

⚠ *Action*
- ALWAYS admit to a specialist obstetric unit. If bleeding is severe, admit via an emergency ambulance, and whilst awaiting transport, raise legs; give O_2 via face mask; if possible, gain IV access, take blood for FBC and cross-matching, and start IV infusion
- NEVER do a vaginal examination—placenta praevia bleeds +++

Placenta praeviaᴳ Occurs when the placenta lies within the lower uterine segment. *Incidence:* 1 in 4 routine anomaly scans done at 19wk gestation show a low-lying placenta—5% stay low at 32wk <2% at term.

Associations
- ↑ with parity
- Age >35y
- Smoking
- Twins
- Preterm delivery
- Previous Caesarean section
- Endometrial damage (e.g. history of dilatation and curettage, TOP)
- Placental pathology (marginal/vellamentous cord insertions, succenturiate lobes, bipartite placenta)
- Previous placenta praevia (recurrence rate 4–8%)

Management If the placenta covers or overlaps the cervical os at routine USS at 18–20wk, follow-up USS at 32wk reveals whether the placenta is moving out of the lower segment. When the placenta remains low, management depends on whether the placenta covers the internal os (major placenta praevia) or not (minor placenta praevia). Major placenta praevia always requires delivery by Caesarean section. Normal delivery in a specialist unit may be attempted with minor placenta praevia if the placental edge is >2cm from the internal os.

❶ Women who have anterior placenta praevia on routine anomaly scanning and who have had a previous Caesarean section may have placenta accreta.

Maternal complications
- APH—typically painless bleeding >20wk with a peak incidence at 34wk
- Malpresentation—35% breech presentation or transverse lie
- Placental problems—placenta accreta and percreta especially with a history of previous Caesarean section; abruption
- Postpartum haemorrhage

Fetal complications IUGR (15%); premature delivery; death.

Primary postpartum haemorrhage (PPH) Loss of >500mL blood within 24h of delivery. Affects 1 in 100 deliveries. May occur in the community after home delivery, delivery in a community obstetric unit, or after rapid discharge from a consultant-led unit.

Causes The four Ts:
- Tone—uterine atony (90%)
- Tissue—retained products of conception
- Trauma—of the genital tract
- Thrombin—clotting disorders

Risk factors
- Age >40y
- Obesity (BMI >35kg/m²)
- Asian ethnicity
- Anaemia (Hb <9g/dL)
- Pre-eclampsia or gestational hypertension
- Past history of PPH
- Large placental site (e.g. multiple pregnancy or baby >4kg)
- Low placenta
- Abruption—known or suspected
- Prolonged labour (>12h)
- Pyrexia in labour
- Caesarean section delivery (emergency or elective)
- Operative vaginal delivery and/or mediolateral episiotomy
- Retained placenta (🕮 p. 819)

⚠ **Action**
- Call emergency ambulance for immediate transfer to hospital
- Gain IV access, take blood for FBC and cross-matching, and start IV infusion if possible
- Give ergometrine 0.5mg slowly IV if available
- Give high flow O₂ via face mask as soon as possible
- If the placenta has not been delivered attempt to deliver it by controlled cord traction
- Check for trauma and apply pressure to any visible bleeding point/ repair any visible bleeding point. Bimanual pressure on the uterus (rubbing up the fundus) may decrease immediate loss
- Some community units keep carboprost 250 micrograms for emergency use. Use if available—1mL by deep IM injection—repeat after 15min
  ❶ Contraindicated in women with asthma

Secondary PPH Excessive blood loss PV >24h after delivery. *Peak incidence:* 5–12d after delivery.

Cause Postpartum infection—sometimes associated with retained placental tissue or clot.

⚠ **Action**
- If the woman is unwell (shocked or toxic) admit to an obstetric unit for further investigation, intravenous antibiotics ± evacuation of retained products of conception
- If bleeding is slight, manage conservatively. Take a vaginal swab and start oral antibiotics—amoxicillin 500mg tds and metronidazole 400mg tds. Consider referral for USS and/or obstetric review if not settling

Further information
RCOG ⌘ www.rcog.org.uk
- Management of antepartum haemorrhage (2011)
- Management of postpartum haemorrhage (2009)
- Placenta praevia and placenta praevia accrete and vasa praevia: diagnosis and management (2011)

Haemolytic disease and rhesus isoimmunization

15% of women are RhD −ve. Development of anti-D antibodies results from fetomaternal haemorrhage (FMH) in RhD −ve women carrying a RhD +ve fetus. In later pregnancies, these antibodies cross the placenta causing rhesus haemolytic disease of the fetus which gets successively worse with each pregnancy.

All RhD −ve mothers are tested for D antibodies at booking, at 28wk, and 2-weekly thereafter. Testing is not performed once women are given anti-D prophylaxis. Anti-D titres <4u/mL (<1 in 16) are unlikely to cause serious disease. If >10u/mL, refer for specialist advice.

Effects on the fetus
- Hydrops fetalis (oedematous fetus)
- Intrauterine death

Effects on neonate
- Jaundice
- Heart failure (oedema, ascites)
- Anaemia
- Yellow vernix
- Hepatosplenomegaly
- CNS signs

❶ All neonates with haemolytic disease should be managed by specialist paediatricians. Treatment usually involves UV light for jaundice ± exchange transfusion.

Immunoprophylaxis Immunoprophylaxis for RhD −ve mothers using anti-D immunoglobulin (anti-D Ig) is given IM into the deltoid muscle as soon as possible after the sensitizing event—preferably within 72h though there is evidence of benefit up to 9d. Women already sensitized should not be given anti-D Ig.

Test for the size of fetomaternal haemorrhage In the UK, blood is taken from the mother (anticoagulated sample) as soon as possible (preferably <2h) after the sensitizing event if >20wk gestation. A Kleihauer acid elution test detects fetal haemoglobin (HbF) and identifies women with large fetomaternal haemorrhage who need additional anti-D Ig.

Other causes Anti-D antibodies are the most common cause of rhesus disease. Other causes include: Rh C, E, c, e, Kell, Kidd, and Duffy. Anti-Du antibodies are relatively common but usually harmless. Follow advice of local transfusion service about follow-up.

❶ Anti-D Ig rarely causes allergic reactions. If the woman is worried about use of blood products, an alternative approach is to check rhesus status of the father—if he is Rh −ve, then the baby is Rh −ve as well, so anti-D prophylaxis is not required.

Further information
RCOG The use of anti-D immunoglobulin for rhesus D prophylaxis (2011) ℘ www.rcog.org.uk

When should anti-D be administered?

Following spontaneous miscarriage
- ≥20wk—500iu + test the size of the fetomaternal haemorrhage
- 12–20wk gestation—250iu
- <12wk—only give anti-D if there has been an intervention (e.g. ERPC) to evacuate the uterus

Following termination of pregnancy/ectopic pregnancy
All non-sensitized RhD –ve women.

If threatened miscarriage
- All non-sensitized RhD –ve women >12wk gestation
- If bleeding continues intermittently after 12wk, give anti-D Ig 6-weekly
- <12wk gestation—only administer if bleeding is heavy, repeated, or there is associated abdominal pain (particularly if close to 12wk)

Following sensitizing events before delivery
All non-sensitized RhD –ve women after:
- Invasive prenatal diagnosis (amniocentesis, CVS, fetal blood sampling) or other intrauterine procedures
- Antepartum haemorrhage
- External cephalic version of the fetus
- Closed abdominal injury (e.g. RTA)
- Intrauterine death

<20wk—250iu; >20wk—500iu + test size of fetomaternal haemorrhage.

Routine antenatal prophylaxis
- 1–1.5% of RhD –ve women develop anti-D antibodies during pregnancy due to fetomaternal haemorrhage which is usually small and silent—most commonly in the third trimester
- Routine antenatal prophylaxis ↓ sensitization to <0.2% and should now be routine practice in the UK. Give irrespective of whether a woman has had prior anti-D prophylaxis earlier in the pregnancy
- Administration of 500iu anti-D Ig at 28wk (after blood has been taken for routine antibody screening) and 34wk gestation—or single dose of 1500iu at 28wk—↓ incidence of immunization after birth
- Women who have been given antenatal prophylaxis may still be sensitized by a large fetomaternal haemorrhage so, following any potentially sensitizing event, additional anti-D Ig should be given and a Kleihauer test performed
- Screening for anti-D antibodies after prophylaxis is uninterpretable

Postnatal prophylaxis
- 500IU–1,500iu (500iu in the UK) is given to every non-sensitized RhD –ve woman <72h after delivery of a RhD +ve infant
- >99% women have a fetomaternal haemorrhage of <4mL at delivery—a test to detect fetomaternal haemorrhage >4mL must be done so additional anti-D Ig can be given as needed
- Risk factors for high fetomaternal haemorrhage include: traumatic delivery, Caesarean section, manual removal of placenta, stillbirth and intrauterine death, abdominal trauma during the third trimester, twin pregnancy (at delivery), unexplained hydrops fetalis

A–Z of medical conditions in pregnancy

Anaemia Defined as Hb <11g/dL early in pregnancy, or <10.5g/dL after 28wk. Common in pregnancy (20%). Some ↓ in Hb is physiological due to ↑ in plasma volume, however, iron requirements ↑ x2–3 and folate ↑ x10–20 during pregnancy. Anaemia is usually due to iron deficiency. Complications include excessive fatigue and poorer fetal outcome. *Risk factors:*
• Multiple pregnancy
• Frequent pregnancies
• Haemoglobinopathy
• Starting pregnancy anaemic
• Poor diet

Screening Hb is routinely screened at booking and again at 28wk.

Management Routine use of oral iron for all pregnant women is of no proven benefit and may cause harm. Women in high risk-groups (e.g. multiple pregnancy) may routinely be given prophylaxis—follow local policies. If Hb is <11g/dL at booking or <10.5g/dL at 28wk, start iron (e.g. ferrous sulfate 200mg tds) and folate (5mg od). Repeat Hb in 2wk. If there is no response to oral iron, exclude occult infection (e.g. UTI); check haematinics; consider referral for parenteral iron.

Antiphospholipid syndrome May be primary (occurs alone) or secondary to another connective tissue disease (usually SLE). Antiphospholipid antibodies (lupus anticoagulant and/or anticardiolipin antibodies), are present together with a history of:
• Arterial or venous thrombosis, and/or
• Recurrent pregnancy loss (typically second trimester—□ p. 815)

Specialist referral is essential. Treated with low-dose aspirin + low molecular weight heparin from 6–34wk.

Asthma Affects ~5% of pregnant women.
• Generally improves with pregnancy, especially into the third trimester
• In most cases, treat asthma as usual—most drugs commonly used for treatment of asthma are safe in pregnancy ❶ Leukotriene receptor antagonists have limited safety data—seek specialist advice
• Women with poorly controlled asthma are at risk of early labour and IUGR; patients on oral steroids may need IV steroids to cover labour
• Avoid syntometrine for third stage of labour as it contains ergometrine which can cause a severe attack
• There is a tendency to worsening of asthma after delivery

Cardiac disease Risk of death is highest where pulmonary blood flow cannot be ↑, e.g. Eisenmenger's syndrome (maternal mortality 30–50%); primary pulmonary hypertension (mortality 40–50%).

Management Specialist obstetric care is needed for all patients with a pre-existing cardiac condition. Where possible refer before conception to a cardiologist for discussion of risks. Antibiotic prophylaxis for delivery may be needed for women with structural cardiac disease—seek specialist advice.

Murmurs in pregnancy Check heart sounds. Murmurs are common. Consider any heart murmurs detected during pregnancy significant and refer for further evaluation—90% will be physiological.

Depression A significant cause of maternal death.

Pre-existing depression Consider referral for pre-conceptual psychiatric advice. When antidepressants are being used, weigh up the pros and cons of discontinuing treatment during pregnancy.

Screening for depression Antenatal 📖 p. 801; postnatal 📖 p. 839

Depression in pregnancy For women with mild/moderate depression consider self-help strategies and talking therapies (e.g. counselling) first. Monitor regularly using depression questionnaires (e.g. PHQ-9—📖 p. 1001). Weigh up risks of antidepressant medication against benefits. Involve specialist mental health services early.

Postnatal depression 📖 p. 839

Diabetes 📖 p. 828 **Eclampsia** 📖 p. 1102 **Epilepsy** 📖 p. 829
HIV 📖 p. 811 **Hypertension** 📖 p. 826 **Infection** 📖 p. 810

Jaundice Any cause of jaundice may occur in pregnancy. Investigate and treat according to cause. Common causes are: viral hepatitis; gallstones; Gilbert's or Dubin Johnson syndrome.

Jaundice peculiar to pregnancy
- **Cholestasis of pregnancy/pruritus gravidarum**—📖 p. 805
- **Acute fatty degeneration of the liver** Rare. Usually >30wk gestation. The mother develops abdominal pain, jaundice, headache and vomiting. Admit for specialist care. Prognosis: ~15–20% maternal mortality; ~20% fetal mortality
- **Pre-eclampsia**—📖 p. 826
- **Severe hyperemesis** Jaundice is a complication—📖 p. 803

Pre-eclampsia 📖 p. 826

Renal disease Refer all women for specialist obstetric care.
Pre-eclampsia is more common—monitor carefully and refer early.

Renal failure If mild renal failure and no ↑ BP 96% have successful pregnancies without adverse effect. Outcomes are less good the more severe the renal failure with complications including worsening hypertension, pregnancy-related ↓ in renal function, IUGR, and preterm delivery.

Women on dialysis Conception is uncommon. High rate of miscarriage and intrauterine death. ~40–50% live birth rate. Mothers are prone to volume overload, polyhydramnios, and severe exacerbations of ↑ BP ± pre-eclampsia. Women need a 50% ↑ in duration/frequency of dialysis during pregnancy.

Renal transplant Risk of first trimester miscarriage is ↑, but pregnancies that survive are >90% successful. Immunosuppressant drugs must be continued—they are not harmful to the fetus. Pregnancy does not affect long-term survival of the transplanted kidney. Pelvic position of the transplant does not compromise vaginal delivery.

Rheumatoid arthritis (RA) Symptoms often improve during pregnancy and worsen in the puerperium. Do not use NSAIDs for joint pain >24wk gestation as can result in closure of the fetal ductus arteriosus. Paracetamol or paracetamol + codeine combinations are safe.

Disease-modifying drugs
- Sulfasalazine—folic acid supplementation is recommended
- Azathioprine—associated with IUGR
- Penicillamine—may weaken fetal collagen
- Methotrexate is contraindicated

Systemic lupus erythematosus (SLE) Exacerbations are common in pregnancy.
- **Effects on fetus** IUGR; neonatal lupus (from passively acquired maternal antibodies—usually self-limiting skin rash)
- **Effects on mother** Renal complications may worsen and be associated with ↑ BP ± pre-eclampsia; oligohydramnios; premature delivery

Management If planning pregnancy refer for review of drugs. Once pregnant refer for specialist obstetric care. Pain control—as for RA.

Immunosuppressive drugs
- Azathioprine—may cause IUGR
- Hydroxychloroquine—risk of deposits in fetal eye/ear
- Cyclophosphamide and methotrexate are contraindicated

Thyroid disease Refer for specialist obstetric advice.

Hyperthyroidism Usually Graves' disease. Severity ↓ through pregnancy. May be associated with neonatal goitre, hyper- or hypothyroidism. Continue treatment with carbimazole aiming to keep plasma T_4 at the top of the normal range. Propylthiouracil is preferred postpartum if breast-feeding, as less concentrated in breast milk.

Hypothyroidism If untreated associated with infertility, ↑ rate of miscarriage, stillbirth, and fetal abnormality. Levothyroxine dose usually needs to ↑ in pregnancy—the fetus is not affected by maternal thyroxine. Check TFTs in each trimester.

Thromboembolism[G] Most common direct cause of maternal death in the UK. Pregnancy ↑ risk of thromboembolism x10—even in very early pregnancy. *Incidence*: ~1 in 100 pregnancies (20–50% antenatal).

⚠ Suspect DVT and/or PE in any woman who is pregnant or in the puerperium who has:
- Leg pain and/or swelling
- Chest pain and/or breathlessness
- Mild unexplained fever

Management If suspected, refer as an emergency for confirmation of diagnosis and initiation of treatment. D-dimer tests are unreliable in pregnancy and should not be used.

If DVT/PE is confirmed, the woman is anticoagulated during the remainder of pregnancy and for ≥6wk postpartum (minimum 3mo total). Avoid warfarin during pregnancy—use low molecular weight heparin (LMWH) instead. Warfarin is safe postpartum and during breastfeeding.

Haematology review is usual before stopping anticoagulation. Advise women to wear graduated compression hosiery for ≥2y after DVT.

Antenatal prevention Assess risk of thrombosis:

- **High risk** Women require thromboprophylaxis with LMWH if:
  - Recurrent venous thromboembolism (VTE), or
  - Single previous VTE that is unprovoked or oestrogen-related or associated with a personal or family history of thrombophilia
- **Intermediate risk** May require thromboprophylaxis with LMWH. Seek specialist advice if:
  - Single previous VTE with no personal/family history of thrombophilia
  - Thrombophilia with no history of VTE, or
  - Pregnancy with co-morbidities (e.g. heart/lung disease, surgery, cancer, IV drug misuse, inflammatory conditions, SLE, sickle cell disease, nephrotic syndrome)
- **Lower risk** If ≥3 risk factors, consider thromboprophylaxis:
  - Age >35y
  - Obesity (BMI >30kg/m²)
  - Parity ≥3
  - Smoker
  - Gross varicose veins
  - Current systemic infection
  - Pre-eclampsia
  - Immobility (e.g. paraplegia, symphysis pubis dysfunction)
  - Long-distance travel
  - Dehydration, hyperemesis, or ovarian hyperstimulation syndrome
  - Multiple pregnancy or assisted reproduction

Postnatal prevention Assess risk of thrombosis:

- **High risk** Women require thromboprophylaxis with LMWH for 6wk postnatally if any previous VTE and required antenatal LMWH
- **Intermediate risk** Women require thromboprophylaxis with LMWH for 7d if:
  - Caesarean section in labour
  - BMI >40 kg/m²
  - Asymptomatic thrombophilia (inherited or acquired)
  - Prolonged hospital admission, or
  - Medical co-morbidities, e.g. heart/lung disease, SLE, cancer, inflammatory conditions, nephrotic syndrome, sickle cell disease, IV drug use
  - ❶ Extend the period of LMWH use if ongoing risk factors.
- **Lower risk** If ≥2 risk factors, consider thromboprophylaxis for 7d (longer if >3 risk factors):
  - Age >35y
  - Obesity (BMI >30kg/m²)
  - Parity ≥3
  - Smoker
  - Gross varicose veins
  - Current systemic infection
  - Pre-eclampsia
  - Immobility (e.g. paraplegia, symphysis pubis dysfunction)
  - Long-distance travel
  - Prolonged labour (>24h)
  - PPH >1L or blood transfusion
  - Mid-cavity rotational operative delivery
  - Elective Caesarian section
  - Any surgical procedure in the puerperium

Further information

RCOG ⌘ www.rcog.org.uk
- Reducing the risk of thrombosis and embolism during pregnancy and the puerperium (2009)
- Thromboembolic disease in pregnancy and the puerperium (2007)

NICE Antenatal and postnatal mental health (2007) ⌘ www.nice.org.uk

Hypertension in pregnancy

Chronic hypertension Hypertension present <20wk into pregnancy (or woman taking antihypertensive medication prior to pregnancy). More common in older mothers. May worsen in later pregnancy.

Management Consider changing medication (especially if taking ACE inhibitor, ARB, or chlorthiazide) to antihypertensive drugs known to be safe in pregnancy (e.g methyldopa, nifedipine, or α-blocker). Monitor BP carefully aiming to keep BP <150/100 (<140/90 if target organ damage). Pre-eclampsia is ↑ x5.

Pregnancy-induced hypertension (PIH) ↑ BP appearing >20wk into pregnancy and resolving <3mo after delivery. Affects 10% of pregnancies and risk of pre-eclampsia is ↑. Treatment is the same as for chronic hypertension. ↑ risk of developing hypertension later in life.

Pre-eclampsia (PET)[N] Affects 5–7% of primigravida and 2–3% of all pregnancies. Multisystem disease of unknown cause, developing ≥20wk into pregnancy and resolving <10d after the birth. Untreated, may progress to eclampsia—📖 p. 1102.

Risk factors for pre-eclampsia Evaluate at booking:

Moderate risk
- First pregnancy
- Age ≥40y
- Pregnancy interval >10y
- BMI ≥35kg/m² at first visit
- Family history of pre-eclampsia
- Multiple pregnancy

High risk
- Hypertensive disease during previous pregnancy
- Chronic kidney disease
- Autoimmune disease, e.g. SLE or antiphospholipid syndrome
- Type 1 or type 2 DM
- Chronic hypertension

If ≥1 high risk factor or ≥2 moderate risk factors, advise aspirin 75mg from 12wk to birth and refer <20wk for specialist obstetric care.

Criteria for diagnosis
- **BP >140/90 or >+30/+15 from booking** The earlier in pregnancy the BP rises, the more likely the pre-eclampsia will be severe
- **Proteinuria ≥0.3g/24h** Urine dipstick is a useful screening tool—if ≥1+ protein then probably significant—but ~25% false +ve rate

Interval for routine BP checks Pre-eclampsia is asymptomatic until its terminal phase, and onset may be rapid. Frequent BP screening is essential. Whenever you check BP, always check urine for protein.
- If no risk factors for pre-eclampsia—routine antenatal care
- If 1 moderate risk factor for pre-eclampsia, recheck BP at least every 3wk from 24–32wk gestation and at least every 2wk >32wk gestation
- If ≥1 high risk factor or ≥2 moderate risk factors, monitor as directed by the specialist

Thresholds for further action See Table 23.5

Risk of recurrence In subsequent pregnancy with the same partner—10–15% (usually less severe). Greater risk of ↑ BP later in life.

Eclampsia 📖 p. 1102

HELLP syndrome 📖 p. 1102

Table 23.5 Thresholds for further action

Findings		Action
New hypertension without proteinuria >20wk gestation	Diastolic BP ≥90 and <100mmHg	Refer for specialist assessment* in <48h
	Diastolic BP ≥90 and <100mmHg with significant symptoms (below)	Refer for same-day specialist assessment*
	Diastolic BP ≥100mmHg	
	Systolic BP ≥160mmHg	
New hypertension and proteinuria >20wk gestation	Diastolic BP ≥90mmHg and new proteinuria ≥1+ on dipstick	Refer for same-day specialist assessment*
	Diastolic BP ≥90mmHg and new proteinuria ≥1+ on dipstick and significant symptoms (below)	Immediate admission
	Diastolic BP ≥110mmHg and new proteinuria ≥1+ on dipstick	
	Systolic BP ≥170mmHg and new proteinuria ≥1+ on dipstick	
New proteinuria without hypertension >20wk gestation	1+ on dipstick	Repeat pre-eclampsia assessment in <1wk
	2+ on dipstick	Refer for specialist assessment* in <48h
	≥1+ on dipstick with significant symptoms (below)	Refer for same-day specialist assessment*
Maternal symptoms or fetal signs/ symptoms without new hypertension or proteinuria	Headache and/or visual disturbance with diastolic BP <90mmHg and trace or no proteinuria	Investigate cause of headache. ↓ interval to next pre-eclampsia assessment
	Epigastric pain with diastolic BP <90mmHg and trace or no proteinuria	If simple antacids are ineffective, refer for same-day specialist assessment*
	↓ fetal movements or small for gestational age infant with diastolic BP <90mmHg and trace or no proteinuria	Refer for investigation of fetal compromise. ↓ interval to next pre-eclampsia assessment

⚠ **Significant symptoms:**
- Epigastric pain
- Vomiting
- Headache
- Visual disturbance
- ↓ fetal movements
- Small for gestational age infant

* Most obstetric departments have a day case 'step-up' assessment unit.
Reproduced with permission from Action on Pre-eclampsia.

Further information
NICE Management of hypertensive disorders in pregnancy (2010) ℅ www.nice.org.uk
Action on Pre-eclampsia (APEC) PRECOG: the pre-eclampsia community guideline (2004) ℅ www.apec.org.uk

Diabetes and epilepsy in pregnancy

Pre-existing DM Affects 2–3 in 1,000 pregnancies. 95% have IDDM.

Effects on the fetus
- **In utero** Large for dates or IUGR; fetal hyperinsulinaemia; ↑ congenital abnormalities (cardiac, renal, and neural tube defects); hypoxia and intrauterine death (especially >36wk)
- **Postnatally** Hypoglycaemia; transient tachypnoea of the newborn or respiratory distress syndrome; neonatal jaundice

Effects on the mother Problems are more common if poor control.
- **In pregnancy** First trimester miscarriage; premature labour; pre-eclampsia; pyelonephritis; polyhydramnios; ↑ retinopathy
- **In labour** Fetal distress; obstruction (especially shoulder dystocia)

Management pre-pregnancy Suggest counselling via a diabetic specialist. Pay careful attention to diabetic control (aim BM 4–6mmol/L pre-meals). Advise folate supplements 5mg od until 13wk. Stop drugs contraindicated in pregnancy, e.g. ACE inhibitors, sulfonylureas.

Management during pregnancy Refer to an obstetrician early. Most women with insulin-dependent DM continue to use their pre-pregnancy insulin regime but requirements ↑ 2–3x in pregnancy. Metformin is safe in pregnancy for women with non-insulin dependent DM. USS is used to monitor fetal growth and exclude structural abnormalities. Delivery should always take place in a specialist unit with neonatal care facilities.

Retinal screening Retinopathy can worse in pregnancy. Retinal screening is important:
- At booking for all women with pre-existing DM
- At 16–20wk if any retinopathy at booking
- At 28wk for all women with pre-existing DM (not gestational DM)

Management postnatally ↓ insulin to pre-pregnancy levels (if breastfeeding may need less). Take specialist advice regarding oral hypoglycaemics and breastfeeding.

Gestational diabetes DM with onset/first recognition in pregnancy. Affects 2% of pregnancies and usually develops in the second trimester. Lower risk of congenital malformation than if pre-existing DM. Intensive management can achieve almost normal rates of macrosomia and neonatal hypoglycaemia, but there is debate whether that is necessary.

Risk factors
- Previous macrosomic baby (≥4.5kg) • BMI >30kg/m²
- DM in a first-degree relative • Previous gestational DM
- Family origin associated with high prevalence of DM: South Asian (especially Indian subcontinent); black Caribbean; Middle Eastern

Screening 📖 p. 800

Management Initially diet; some may require metformin (unlicensed) and up to 30% require insulin. Insulin is stopped immediately postpartum. Check a 6wk postpartum oral glucose tolerance test. Gestational DM usually recurs in future pregnancies; >30% develop DM in <10y.

Glycosuria in pregnancy Routine screening for glycosuria in pregnancy is not advised. Pregnant women have ↓ renal threshold and a physiologically ↑ plasma glucose level, so dipstick testing gives a high false +ve rate. If glycosuria is detected repeat the urine test—if still +ve arrange an oral glucose tolerance test.

Epilepsy in pregnancy 90% have normal pregnancies/healthy babies.

Antenatal effects on the fetus Anti-epileptic drugs including phenytoin, primidone, phenobarbital, lamotrigine, and carbamazepine, are teratogenic—especially if taken in the first trimester and if taking ≥2 drugs. Valproate is associated with the highest risk of congenital malformation and developmental delay. Topiramate is also associated with ↑ risk of cleft palate if taken in the first trimester.

Peri/postnatal effects on the fetus Haemorrhagic disease of the newborn is associated with anti-epileptic drugs—all babies should have IM vitamin K at birth; the child has ↑ risk of epilepsy.

Effects on the mother
- **In pregnancy** 10% have ↑ fit frequency. The fetus is at slightly ↑ risk of harm during a generalized tonic-clonic fit but absolute risk of harm is low. There is no evidence simple partial, complex partial, absence, or myoclonic seizures harm pregnancy in any way, unless the patient falls. Status epilepticus is associated with high infant and maternal mortality.
- **In labour/puerperium** 1–4% have fit during labour and a further 1–2% <48h after delivery

Management pre-pregnancy Discuss risks of epilepsy/anti-epileptic medication and pregnancy with all women who have epilepsy and are of childbearing age—whether or not contemplating pregnancy. Suggest referral to a neurologist for optimization of anti-epileptic drug regimes prior to pregnancy; avoid sodium valproate. Advise folic acid 5mg od from the time pregnancy is being planned until 13wk after conception.

Management during pregnancy Refer for specialist obstetric care—joint management by an obstetrician and neurologist is ideal. Anti-epileptic drug dose adjustments may be needed depending on clinical symptoms ± drug levels. Delivery should occur in a specialist centre where any fits can be managed. Encourage women to notify their pregnancy to the UK Epilepsy and Pregnancy Register (✆ www.epilepsyandpregnancy.co.uk).

Management postnatally Breastfeeding is not contraindicated if taking monotherapy, but infants should be monitored for side effects of anti-epileptic medication. If drug dose is ↑ in pregnancy, it may need to ↓ after delivery. All babies should have IM vitamin K due to ↑ risk of haemorrhage. Risk of injury to the child from maternal seizure is low. Discuss child care and minimizing risks to the child from the mother's epilepsy.

Further information
NICE ✆ www.nice.org.uk
- Diabetes in pregnancy (2008)
- The epilepsies: the diagnosis and management of the epilepsies in adults and children in primary and secondary care (2012)

Intrauterine growth and malpresentation

Intrauterine growth restriction (IUGR)[G] Babies may be small because they are premature, small for their gestation, or a combination of the two. Babies weighing <10th centile weight for their gestational age (IUGR) have different problems to premature babies.

Predisposing factors The major antenatal indicator for IUGR is low maternal weight at booking (<51kg). *Others include:*
- Multiple pregnancy
- Malformation
- Infection
- Maternal smoking
- Maternal DM
- Pre-eclampsia
- Severe maternal anaemia
- Maternal heart or renal disease
- Previous history of small baby
- Low weekly maternal weight ↑ (<0.2kg)

Antenatal detection Difficult to detect; about half are not detected until after birth. Most GPs will encounter IUGR when they do a routine antenatal check and find the symphysis-fundal height (SFH) is less than would be expected for the gestation. Other suspicious signs are oligohydramnios and poor fetal movements. Confirm suspicions with USS then seek specialist obstetric advice. Where the head circumference is relatively spared suspect placental insufficiency.

Consequences
- **Labour** More susceptible to hypoxia in labour, so require monitoring in a specialist unit where Caesarean section facilities are available and there is paediatric back-up
- **Postnatal problems** Susceptible to neonatal hypoglycaemia and jaundice. Babies <2kg may have problems with temperature regulation and require incubator facilities
- **Long-term effects** More prone in later life to cardiovascular disease and type 2 DM

Oligohydramnios Liquor volume <500mL. Rare. Associated with:
- Prolonged pregnancy
- PROM (📖 p. 832)
- Placental insufficiency
- Fetal abnormality (renal agenesis, urethral aplasia)

Confirm diagnosis with USS then refer for specialist obstetric assessment.

Large for dates Consider:
- Multiple pregnancy
- Maternal DM
- Fetal abnormality
- Polyhydramnios
- Molar pregnancy
- Large baby (>90th centile)—may have past history of large babies

Refer for USS to confirm diagnosis and exclude fetal abnormality or multiple pregnancy. Check maternal oral glucose tolerance test.

Polyhydramnios Liquor volume >2L; affects 0.15% pregnancies. *Causes*
- **Fetal abnormality,** e.g. hydrops fetalis; anencephaly (no swallowing reflex); spina bifida; oesophageal or duodenal atresia; umbilical hernia; ectopia vesicae
- **Maternal,** e.g. DM, multiple pregnancy
- **No cause found** (30–50%)

Risks Premature labour; malpresentation; cord prolapse; placental abruption; PPH.

Management Refer for USS to confirm diagnosis. Check maternal oral glucose tolerance test and refer for specialist obstetric advice.

Multiple pregnancy Detected on early antenatal USS. *Incidence:* twins—1 in 105 (1 in 3 identical); triplets—1 in 10,000. *Predisposing factors:*
- Previous twins
- Family history of non-identical twins
- Race: most common amongst African blacks; least common in Japanese
- ↑ with maternal age
- Infertility treatment—induced ovulation (e.g. clomifene); IVF and other assisted reproduction techniques

Management Refer for specialist obstetric care. Monochorionic twins are significantly higher risk than dichorionic twins. *Complications:*
- **In pregnancy** Hyperemesis; anaemia; polyhydramnios; pre-eclampsia (↑ x3); APH; placenta praevia; placental abruption
- **In labour** Malpresentation; cord prolapse; fetal distress (↑ Caesarean section rate); PPH
- **Fetus** ↑ perinatal mortality (x 5); prematurity; IUGR; malformations (↑ x2–4); twin-twin transfusion may result in 1 twin being plethoric (and jaundiced later) and the other anaemic

Breech babies[G] 3–4% babies at term. Higher incidence <37wk. Associated with ↑ risk of cerebral palsy as breech presentation is more common in premature infants and those with congenital malformation. *Risk factors:* bicornuate uterus; fibroids; placenta praevia; oligohydramnios.

Management Many turn spontaneously—especially if <36wk gestation. If a baby is found to be breech at ≥36wk gestation, confirm breech position and position of the placenta on USS and refer for specialist obstetric advice. *Specialist options:* external cephalic version (ECV); vaginal breech delivery; elective Caesarean section.

⚠ 10–15% of breech babies are discovered for the first time late in labour. If delivering at home or in a community unit, arrange transfer to a specialist unit immediately.

Follow up Congenital hip problems are more common in breech babies—refer all breech babies routinely for hip USS even if examination in the first 24h is normal.

Further information
RCOG ॐ www.rcog.org.uk
- Investigation and management of a small-for-gestational-age fetus (2002)
- Management of breech presentation (2006)

Information and support for multiple pregnancy
Twins and Multiple Births Association (TAMBA) ☏ 0800 138 0509
ॐ www.tamba.org.uk

Labour

47% of deliveries are 'normal' i.e. occur without surgical intervention, use of instruments, induction, epidural or general anaesthetic. Intrapartum care can be provided by GPs in the UK as a National Enhanced Service.

Braxton Hicks contractions Irregular tightenings of the uterus. Start ≥30wk gestation (common after 36wk). May be uncomfortable but not painful.

Premature rupture of membranes (PROM) Rupture of membranes before labour starts. Usually presents with a gush of clear fluid (± an audible pop) followed by uncontrolled leakage. If chorioamnionitis is present the woman may have abdominal pain and feel unwell. Difficult to distinguish clinically from profuse vaginal discharge or incontinence of urine. Check temperature, pulse, and BP and do a routine obstetric examination (including fetal heart). ❶ Do not perform a vaginal examination as repeated examinations can introduce infection.

Management
- **Evidence of infection**—admit for specialist obstetric care
- **<37wk gestation and suspected PROM**—admit to specialist obstetric unit for further assessment
- **≥37wk gestation**—if no signs of spontaneous labour admit for specialist obstetric assessment within 24h

Premature labour Any labour <37wk gestation. *Prevalence:* 6%—1 in 4 elective due to maternal/fetal problems. Largest contributor to neonatal morbidity/mortality in industrialized countries.

Causes of spontaneous premature labour Unknown (40%)
- Cervical incompetence
- Multiple pregnancy
- Uterine abnormality
- DM
- Pyelonephritis or other sexually transmitted or urinary infection
- Polyhydramnios
- APH

Presentation Premature rupture of membranes or contractions. If suspected admit immediately to obstetrics for further assessment.

Prolonged pregnancy/post-maturity The due date is traditionally based on pregnancy lasting 40 wk or 280d from the date of the LMP. Now most women have an early dating USS to confirm their due date. However, it is normal to deliver any time from 37–42wk. At 40wk gestation, 65% will spontaneously go into labour in the next week but 15% of women have not gone into labour by 42wk. Perinatal mortality rate is ↑ x2 from 42–43wk and x3 >43wk, so induction of labour is indicated if a pregnancy lasts >42wk.

Initial management Membrane sweep. If that is ineffective, refer for formal induction of labour (📖 p. 834). If referral is declined, ↑ antenatal monitoring to 2x weekly cardiotocography and USS (to measure maximum amniotic pool depth) as markers of fetal well-being.

Normal labour Occurs ≥37wk gestation and results in vaginal delivery of a baby in <24h. Often heralded by a 'show' consisting of mucus ± blood and/or spontaneous rupture of membranes ('waters going').

- **1st stage of labour** Time from the onset of regular contractions until the cervix is fully dilated
- **2nd stage of labour** Time from complete cervical dilatation until the baby is born. The mother has a desire to push
- **3rd stage of labour** Delivery of the placenta

Pain relief for labour Most women experience pain in labour. Strategies for pain relief include:
- **Self-help**—keep fit in pregnancy, relaxation techniques, breathing exercises, warm bath/birthing pool
- **TENS**—machines are available to hire from most obstetric units and some retail outlets
- **Entonox®**—takes 30–45s to have effect—advise women to start inhaling it as soon as the contraction starts
- **Injected opioids** (e.g. pethidine)
- **Epidural**
- **Pudendal block**—used for instrumental delivery

Advise women to discuss options with their midwife. Antenatal classes dealing with pain relief significantly ↑ a woman's confidence in managing her labour pains.

Epidural Effective method of analgesia available in most hospital units. Initiated once in established labour (cervix >3cm dilated). Regular BP, pulse, and fetal heart monitoring is required. *Particular indications:*
- Occipito-posterior position
- Breech
- Multiple pregnancy
- Pre-eclampsia
- Forceps delivery
- Maternal medical conditions, e.g. cardiac

Epidural complications during labour
- Postural hypotension
- Urinary retention
- ↑ need for instrumental delivery due to pelvic floor muscle paralysis

Epidural complications post-delivery Urinary retention, headache (especially if dural puncture).

Meconium-stained liquor Passage of fresh meconium (dark green, sticky, and lumpy) during labour may be a sign of fetal distress. Transfer immediately to a consultant unit for further evaluation.

Management Paediatrician should be present at delivery. Do not perform oropharyngeal suction if there is no evidence of fetal hypoxia.

Dystocia Difficulty in labour. May be due to problems relating to the baby, birth passage, or action of the uterus. Neonatal mortality and maternal morbidity both ↑ with duration of labour. *Possible causes:*
- Pelvic abnormality
- Shoulder dystocia (☐ p. 1104)
- Abnormal presentation
- Uterine dysfunction
- Cervical dystocia
- Cephalo-pelvic disproportion

Management If a patient in labour at home or in a community unit fails to progress as expected, admit immediately to a specialist unit for consideration of intervention to speed the labour or Caesarean section. Shoulder dystocia is an obstetric emergency—📖 p. 1104.

Induction of labour[N] Performed when it is felt the baby is better off out than in (~20% of deliveries). Only undertaken in units with facilities for continuous fetal monitoring and emergency Caesarean section.

Procedure involves Assessment of the cervix; vaginal prostaglandins; 'sweeping' of the membranes; artificial rupture of the membranes and/or IV oxytocin to maintain contractions.

Reasons for induction of labour include
• Post-maturity (most common)—offered from 41–42wk
• Premature rupture of membranes
• Intrauterine death

Assisted delivery[G] (See Table 23.5). Forceps and ventouse are used in ~11% of deliveries in the UK (range 4–25% between hospitals). Assisted delivery should only be performed with adequate analgesia (usually epidural or pudendal block) and by experienced practitioners.

Caesarean section (LSCS)[N] (See Table 23.6). Rate in England and Wales is 24.8% (range 10–65% between different hospitals). 10% are elective and usually performed at >39wk to minimize risk of respiratory complications; the other 11–12% occur after labour has started. Regional anaesthesia for LSCS is safer for mother and child than a GA.

Reasons for emergency LSCS Failure to progress (25%); presumed fetal compromise (28%); breech (14%).

Planned LSCS is indicated for
• Breech (where external cephalic version has failed)
• Multiple pregnancies where the first twin is not cephalic
• Placenta praevia or placenta accreta
• Some HIV positive women and those with primary HSV in the third trimester to ↓ virus transmission

❶ Maternal request may be an indication for LSCS; GPs should discuss risks and benefits if a request is made, and if the patient still requests a LSCS, refer for a consultant opinion.

Further information
RCOG 🔗 www.rcog.org.uk
• Preterm prelabour rupture of membranes (2010)
• Operative vaginal delivery (2011)

NICE 🔗 www.nice.org.uk
• Caesarian section guidelines (2011)
• Intrapartum care (2007—due to be updated in 2014)
• Induction of labour (2008)

Information for women
NCT Information on labour and pain relief (including epidurals) ☎ 0300 3300 770 🔗 www.nct.org.uk

Table 23.5 Forceps and ventouse

	Forceps	Ventouse
Indication	Delayed 2nd stage of labour	Delayed 2nd stage of labour
Procedure	• 'Wrigleys' forceps—for 'lift-out' deliveries • 'Neville Barnes' forceps—for high deliveries • 'Keilland's' forceps—if rotation is required	• The vacuum extraction cup is applied to the baby's head, suction is applied, and traction aids delivery • Ventouse allows rotation if the baby is malpositioned
Early complications	• Maternal trauma (episiotomy always needed) • Fetal facial bruising • Facial nerve paralysis	• 'Chignon' develops on the baby's head—resolves in ≤2d • Cephalohaematoma • Retinal haemorrhage • Neonatal jaundice (but no ↑ need for phototherapy)
Longer term complications	↑ risk of maternal faecal incontinence	
Comparison	Ventouse has ↑ failure rate compared to forceps but no ↑ CS rate. ↓ requirement for regional anaesthesia with ventouse deliveries compared to forceps deliveries Forceps result in more maternal trauma than ventouse deliveries	

Table 23.6 Comparison of Caesarean section and vaginal birth

	Complications
↑ with LSCS	*Mother—this pregnancy:* abdominal pain; bladder or ureteric injury; hysterectomy; maternal death; need for further surgery; need for admission to intensive care/high dependency unit; thromboembolism; length of hospital stay; need for readmission *Mother—future pregnancies:* not having more children; antepartum stillbirth; placenta praevia; uterine rupture *Baby:* neonatal respiratory problems
No difference	*Mother:* haemorrhage; infection; genital tract injury; faecal incontinence; back pain; dyspareunia; postnatal depression *Baby:* death (except breech); intracranial haemorrhage; brachial plexus injuries; cerebral palsy
↓ with LSCS	*Mother:* perineal pain; urinary incontinence; uterovaginal prolapse

Maternal postnatal care

Postnatal care, from hospital discharge until 14d after delivery, excluding the neonatal check, is provided as an Additional Service (maternity services) and payment is included in the global sum. 'Opting out' results in a 2.1% ↓ in global sum.

The *puerperium* is the 6wk period after delivery. Most women in the UK spend ≥6h after delivery in hospital. After discharge home, the midwife continues to visit for 2wk after the birth and then the health visitor takes over. GPs usually see the mother and baby soon after discharge and again for the 6wk postnatal check. Arrange additional reviews as needed.

The postnatal visit Discuss problems during pregnancy/delivery and postnatal contraception (see Table 23.7). Check:
- **Rhesus status** If the mother is RhD –ve and the baby RhD +ve, ensure anti-D is given <72h after delivery—📖 p. 820
- **Hb on day 5** After delivery (after the postpartum diuresis). If Hb is <10g/dL, continue iron supplements for 3mo
- **Rubella status** If non-immune, immunize as soon as possible, and ensure effective contraception for 3mo afterwards. Reassure it is safe to breastfeed after immunization
- **Temperature, pulse, and BP** ↑BP is associated with pre-eclampsia. It usually resolves <48h after delivery
- **Fundus** Day 1 = 24wk gestation size (up to umbilicus); day 5 = 16wk gestation size; by day 10, the uterus should not be palpable per abdomen. Persistent bulkiness suggests retained products of conception—refer for USS
- **Pain** Breast, abdominal, perineal, legs
- **Vaginal loss** Red, then brown, then yellowish over the first week, then serous for 3–6wk. Any fresh, red bleeding is abnormal
- **Moving about** Women should try to get mobile as soon as possible after delivery to ↓ the risk of DVT
- **Feeding** 📖 p. 870
- **Mental state** Screen for depression 4–6wk and 3–4mo postnatally (📖 p. 839)

Mother's 6wk postnatal check Discuss any problems in pregnancy or delivery. Discuss any current problems the mother has and specifically enquire about persistent vaginal loss, bladder/bowel control, and any sex-related problems. Discuss any problems with the baby—including worries about hearing/vision. Discuss feeding and contraception.

Examination/investigation
- BP and weight—if overweight discuss weight control—📖 p. 178
- Abdominal examination—uterus should not be palpable per abdomen
- Vaginal examination—only if any problems with tears/episiotomy, persistent vaginal bleeding, pain, or to perform overdue cervical smear
- Screen for depression—📖 p. 839
- Check Hb if anaemic postnatally
- Check rubella immunization has been given if not immune antenatally—if not arrange for vaccination. Check immunity 3mo after vaccination

Table 23.7 Postpartum contraception

❶ Contraception is *not* needed until 21d postpartum

Method	If not breastfeeding*:	If breastfeeding**:
COC pill/ combined patch	Start ≥3wk after delivery (patch states >28d) as ↑ risk of thromboembolism (❶ can be started immediately after miscarriage/termination) If starting on d21 (or d28 for patch) postpartum, immediate protection is provided. If starting after that time, use an additional method for 7d If PET in pregnancy—start CHC *only* when BP and biochemical abnormalities have returned to normal	Contraindicated <6wk postpartum, as it may inhibit lactation and enters breast milk in small quantities. >6wk and <6mo—use only if no other suitable method
POP	Delay until ≥3wk postpartum to avoid ↑ risk of heavy bleeding If started >3wk after delivery, start on 1st day of period for immediate protection or, if cycle is not established, use alternative protection for 1st 2d. For breastfeeding mothers, ↑ quantity of breast milk	
Injectables/ implants	Preferably delay until ≥6wk postpartum to avoid risk of heavy/ irregular bleeding. If >3wk (>4wk for implant) postpartum administer early in period or, if cycle is not re-established, check pregnancy test before administration and use additional method for 7d. If breastfeeding, delay giving injectable until ≥6wk postpartum where possible	
IUCD/IUS	Insert <48h post-delivery (but ↑ risk of expulsion) or delay until >6wk postpartum (Mirena® licence states 6wk)—take care with insertion, as the uterus may be soft and perforate easily. Use an additional method for 7d if inserted >4wk postpartum	
Cap	Refit any time from 5–6wk postpartum (even after LSCS) ❶ May require a different size postpartum	
Condoms	Useful until other methods are established and to prevent transfer of sexually transmitted diseases	
Sterilization	↑ operative and failure rate when performed at abortion or in the postpartum period Best delayed for a few months	

* Ovulation can occur within 10d of abortion and 28d of delivery.

** Advise women <6mo postpartum who are amenorrhoeic and fully breastfeeding, there is only a low chance of pregnancy (~2/1,000 women) without contraception. If any supplementary bottle feeding, baby is weaned or any vaginal bleeding (except occasional spotting) then assume the woman is fertile.

The baby's 6wk developmental check 📖 p. 852

Further information

NICE 🔊 www.nice.org.uk
- Postnatal care (2006)
- Antenatal and postnatal mental health: clinical management and service guidance (2007)

Common postnatal problems

Abdominal pain Cramping, 'period like' for the first 1–2wk after delivery, especially when breastfeeding. These are due to the uterus contracting down or involuting. Suspect infection if offensive lochia, fever, the uterus stops getting smaller day by day or is still palpable per abdomen 10d after delivery.

Breast soreness The breasts become engorged ('the milk comes in') 3–5d after the birth and may be quite painful. Support with a well-fitting maternity bra day and night. Express milk if still painful—a warm bath may help. *Other problems:*

Sore/cracked nipples Try topical remedies, e.g. Kamillosan®, and/or nipple shields. Consider advice from a breastfeeding advisor—may be a 'positioning problem'.

Skin infection Localized soreness, pain around the areola ± nipple, or in the breast after a feed—usually due to candida infection. Treat mother and baby with miconazole oral gel.

❶ Severe knife-like pain in breast during and for up to 1h after feeding suggests deeper infection—treat mother additionally with fluconazole 150mg stat and then 50mg bd for 10d (unlicensed use). Symptoms usually resolve in <3d.

Blocked duct Hard, tender lump in the breast. Advise the mother to massage that area of the breast while feeding or expressing milk.

Mastitis Tender, hot, reddened area of breast ± fever. Treat with flucloxacillin 500mg qds and NSAID, e.g. ibuprofen 400mg tds prn. Continue breastfeeding or express the milk to prevent milk stagnation if too painful for feeding.

Breast abscess Admit for incision and drainage.

Dyspareunia following perineal trauma. Almost always settles without need for surgery.

Hair loss Hair becomes thicker in pregnancy and these hairs are all shed at about the same time ~5–6mo postpartum. Reassure. Hair loss reverts to normal levels within 2–3mo. If severe, persistent, or accompanied by tiredness, consider hypothyroidism (📖 p. 840)—check TFTs.

Haemorrhoids Common and painful. *Try:*
- Local ice packs (frozen fingers of rubber gloves are the right shape)
- Topical preparations, e.g. Proctosedyl®
- Resting lying on one side
- Keeping stools soft using a stool softener
- Advising women to wash the haemorrhoids with cool water after opening bowels and gently push them through the anus (if possible)

Perineal bruising Can be very painful. Advise regular analgesia, e.g. paracetamol 1g qds ± ibuprofen 400mg tds, ice packs. Ultrasound can help—consider referral to physiotherapy.

Persistent lochia Bleeding (lochia) >6wk postpartum. Causes:

- Infection
- Retained products of conception
- Unhealed tears—cervical, vaginal or perineal
- Resumption of normal cycle
- Side effects of contraception (e.g. POP, depot injection)
- Other cervical or uterine pathology

Management

- Examine uterus per abdomen and do a bimanual vaginal examination to check involution. Perform a speculum examination and send a vaginal swab for M,C&S
- If offensive loss or systemic symptoms/signs of infection, treat with antibiotics as for endometritis (📖 p. 840). Otherwise, arrange USS
- If not settling and no cause is found, refer to gynaecology

Baby blues Very common—women become tearful and low within the 1st 10d of delivery. Be supportive. Usually resolves.

Postnatal depression Common (10–15% mothers) reaching a peak ~12wk after delivery—although symptoms are almost always present at 6wk. Often mothers do not report symptoms. NICE recommends screening all mothers for depression 4–6wk and 3–4mo postnatally by asking:

- During the past month, have you often been bothered by feeling down, depressed, or hopeless?
- During the past month, have you often been bothered by having little interest or pleasure in doing things?

If the woman answers 'yes' to either of the initial questions, ask: 'Is this something you feel you need or want help with?'

Risk factors

- Depression during pregnancy
- A bad birth experience
- Social problems (e.g. poor social support, financial problems)
- Past medical history or family history of depression or postnatal depression
- Alcohol or drug abuse

Management

- Talk through the problems. Refer to health visitor for support
- Give information, e.g. self-help groups, mother-and-baby groups
- Consider checking TFTs—especially if presenting with tiredness
- Consider referral for psychological therapies such as CBT
- Consider antidepressant medication. Of the SSRIs, sertraline 50mg od is the safest. In all cases, monitor the baby for unwanted side effects (e.g. drowsiness, respiratory depression). If not breastfeeding, fluoxetine 20mg od is the most effective antidepressant in trials
- Monitor progress using depression questionnaires, e.g. Edinburgh postnatal depression scale

⚠ Refer to the mental health team immediately if any risk of self-harm, suicide, or harm to the baby.

☙ There is evidence that oestrogen (but not progesterone) may help some women with postnatal depression[C].

Puerperal psychosis Much rarer than postnatal depression (1 in 500 births). Suspect if severe depression; high suicidal drive; mania; psychotic symptoms. In all cases seek expert help from a psychiatrist. Consider admission—under a Section if necessary. Risk of recurrence is 20%—but 50% will never be mentally ill again.

Poor abdominal and pelvic muscle tone Classes for postnatal exercise to re-tone the body are available both on dry land and in the swimming pool at most leisure centres. Pelvic floor exercises can be started <1d after delivery (see Box 23.3). Good leaflets explaining these are available from physiotherapists, local maternity units, and the NCT.

Puerperal pyrexia Temperature >38°C within 14d of delivery or miscarriage. 90% infections are in the urinary or genital tracts. Ask about:

- Urinary symptoms
- Colour and smell of lochia
- Abdominal pain
- Breast symptoms
- Any other symptoms (e.g. cough, sore throat)

Examine fully including bimanual VE and send MSU and vaginal swabs for M,C&S. *Potential obstetric causes:*

Superficial perineal infection Complicates tear or episiotomy—treat with flucloxacillin 500mg—1g qds.

Endometritis Presents with offensive lochia, lower abdominal pain, and a tender uterus. Treat with amoxicillin 500mg tds and metronidazole 400mg tds or co-amoxiclav 375mg tds. If not settling in <48h or very unwell, admit for IV antibiotics.

Mastitis See breast soreness—📖 p. 838

DVT or PE Can present with pyrexia. Refer to exclude if any leg pain/chest pain/breathlessness.

Superficial thrombophlebitis Affects 1% women. Presents with a tender (usually varicose) vein. Exclude DVT. Recovery usually occurs within a few days. Meanwhile advise the woman not to stand still and, when sitting, to elevate the leg above waist height. Support the leg, e.g. with an elasticated stocking, and try applying an ice pack to the affected area. NSAIDs, e.g. ibuprofen 400mg tds prn, may help.

Tiredness Very common in the first few months after delivery but it may be the presenting feature of postnatal depression, anaemia, or hypothyroidism. Check FBC and TFTs.

Transient autoimmune thyroiditis Up to 10% women 1–3mo after delivery. Usually presents with fatigue and lethargy.

Hypothyroidism Treat with levothyroxine for 6mo then stop for 6wk and repeat TFTs. Follow-up with annual TFTs—1 in 5 go on to develop permanent hypothyroidism.

Hyperthyroidism Refer to an endocrinologist—antithyroid treatment is not normally required but symptom control may be necessary.

Box 23.3 Pelvic floor exercises—basic techniques
- **Exercise 1** Advise the woman to pull up her pelvic muscles as if stopping herself from passing urine and hold that position for a count of 10
- **Exercise 2** Advise the woman to pull up her pelvic muscles as in exercise 1, but then relax and contract them rapidly 4 times

These exercises should be repeated as many times daily as possible long-term

Further information
NICE ℘ www.nice.org.uk
- Antenatal and postnatal mental health (2007)
- Postnatal care (2006)

General advice and support for postnatal women
Family Planning Association ☎ 0845 122 8690 ℘ www.fpa.org.uk
National Childbirth Trust (NCT) ☎ 0300 3300 770 ℘ www.nct.org.uk
NHS Direct ℘ www.nhsdirect.nhs.uk
Baby World ℘ www.babyworld.co.uk

Advice and support for women with postnatal depression
Royal College of Psychiatrists—information sheet on postnatal depression ℘ www.rcpsych.ac.uk
Association for Postnatal Illness—support and befriending by women who have suffered postnatal depression/puerperal psychosis ☎ 020 7386 0868 ℘ www.apni.org

Stillbirth and neonatal death

Stillbirth is a term applied to those babies born dead after 24wk gestation. Affects 1 in 200 pregnancies. Death may occur *in utero* or during labour. Usually presents with a lack of fetal movements and on examination no fetal heart can be detected. If suspected refer as an emergency to the nearest obstetric unit for confirmation of intrauterine death by USS.

Management In hospital mothers of babies who have died *in utero* are usually induced. Samples are routinely taken from mother and baby to try to determine cause of death.

Common causes Pre-eclampsia; IUGR; renal disease; DM; infection; malformation; post-maturity; abruption; knots in the cord. No cause is found for 1 in 5 stillbirths.

After discharge Make contact with the parents as soon as possible.

Lactation suppression Offer cabergoline 1mg as a single dose.

Registration of stillbirth A certificate of stillbirth is issued by the obstetrician which must be taken to the Registrar of deaths within 42d of the stillbirth. Parents are issued with a certificate of burial or cremation and a certificate of registration to keep. The child's name may be entered on the certificate of registration.

Funeral Parents have the option of a free hospital funeral. Burial is usually in an unmarked multiple occupancy grave. Parents may pay for a single occupancy grave or cremation. Alternatively parents may pay for a private funeral.

Benefits In the UK all maternity benefits are still payable after stillbirth— 📖 p. 785

Follow-up Is routinely arranged by the specialist obstetrician to discuss reasons for the stillbirth and implications for future pregnancies. Primary care follow-up is essential. Stillbirth is a huge burden to come to terms with. Parents do not have the regular contact with medical staff a baby brings. Ensure regular follow-up by a member of the primary care team. Broach the issues brought up by the baby's death directly. Offer an open door. Give information about support organizations, e.g. SANDS. Advise waiting 6mo–1y before embarking on another pregnancy.

Neonatal death Death of an infant <28d old. Rare in the community. In the UK, all deaths of children <18y are subject to review by the local child death review panel (📖 p. 927) and should be notified to it immediately. If the death is expected, the GP will be allowed to issue a special death certificate. If unexpected the case will be referred to the police/Coroner. Offer lactation suppression with cabergoline 250 micrograms bd for 2d, and follow-up as for stillbirth.

Further information
RCOG Late intrauterine fetal death and stillbirth (2010)
🖰 www.rcog.org.uk

Patient support and information
Stillbirth and Neonatal Death Society (SANDS) 📞 020 7436 5881
🖰 www.uk-sands.org

❗ In other sections of this book, where management differs from the norm for children, the text is highlighted in a box marked with this symbol.

Child health

Child health promotion

> 'Children are one third of our population and all our future.'
> US Select Panel for Promotion of Child Health (1981)

Patients ≤15y comprise 19% of the average practice list; under 5s see their GP more often (average 6–7x/y) and have more home visits than any other age group, except the elderly.

National Service Framework (NSF) for children Emphasizes child health promotion. It moves from rigid developmental screening to a more flexible assessment of the child within the family context. It includes:
- Immunization—📖 p. 644
- Childhood screening
- Health and development reviews—to monitor the child's development, the strengths/weaknesses of the family, and to discuss the parents' hopes and concerns, followed by early intervention as required
- Health promotion beginning antenatally and continuing to teenage years covering the full range of child health issues, e.g. diet, safety, substance abuse (drugs, smoking, and alcohol), teenage sexual health

Although most child health promotion is still carried out by the health visitor and other members of the primary healthcare team, the need for partnership with parents and involvement of other care providers (eg. schools and nurseries, social care services) is stressed.

Childhood screening The aim of screening is to discover physical, developmental, or behavioural problems as early as possible so that appropriate management can commence preventing secondary complications. There has been a move away from set times for developmental screening but the neonatal (📖 p. 848) and 6–8wk check (with emphasis on checking the eyes, heart, and hips as well as developmental milestones—📖 p. 852) are still carried out, as is a comprehensive assessment (usually by the health visitor) by 1y and again between 2–2½y.

Beyond that assessments are performed according to need. Any consultation can opportunistically be used to check immunization status, monitor development, and for health promotion. Expected developmental milestones are summarized in Table 24.2 (📖 p. 852). Liaise with the health visitor if:
- Immunizations are not up to date
- You have any worries regarding parenting abilities
- A child does not attend a primary or secondary care appointment
- You have concerns about neglect or abuse (but also see 📖 p. 924)

Neonatal bloodspot screening 📖 p. 850

Diploma in Child Health Designed to give recognition of competence in the care of children to GP vocational trainees, clinical medical officers, and trainees in specialties allied to paediatrics. Administered by the Royal College of Paediatrics and Child Health (RCPCH). Further details are available at ℘ www.rcpch.ac.uk

Health education for new parents

Reducing the risk of cot death
- Cut smoking in pregnancy
- Do not let anyone smoke in the same room as your baby
- Place your baby on his/her back to sleep
- Do not let your baby get too hot
- Do not suddenly stop using a dummy before your baby is 6mo old if your baby is used to having one
- Keep your baby's head uncovered—place your baby with his/her feet to the foot of the cot to prevent wriggling down under the covers
- It is safest for your baby to sleep in a cot in your bedroom for the first 6mo
- It is dangerous to share a bed with your baby if either parent:
  - Is a smoker—no matter where or when he/she smokes
  - Has been drinking alcohol
  - Takes medication or drugs that might make him/her drowsy
  - Feels very tired
- It is dangerous to sleep with your baby on a sofa, armchair, or settee
- If your baby is unwell, seek medical advice promptly

Protecting your baby from accidents and infections
- Keep small objects out of your baby's reach
- Stay with your baby when he/she is eating or drinking
- Make sure your baby's cot and mattress are in good condition and that the mattress fits the cot properly
- Install at least one smoke alarm
- Plan a way to escape a fire with your baby
- Never leave your baby alone in a bath or near water
- Immunize your baby
- Make sure your baby cannot reach hot drinks or the kettle or iron flex
- Only use toys suitable for your baby's age
- Never shake your baby—ask for help if crying gets too much
- Use a properly fitted baby car seat that is the right size for your baby
- Do not use a baby walker
- Wash your hands before feeding your baby and make sure your baby's bottle and teats are properly sterilized

Benefits for parents and children
- **Child benefits** Available to anyone responsible for the upbringing of a child aged <16y (those who claim and are on higher income incur an income tax charge). Claim forms are in packs given to new mothers. ☎ 0300 200 3100 ⌨ www.hmrc.gov.uk
- **Low income benefits** 📖 p. 104
- **All children <16y (18y if in full time education) and mothers <1y postpartum** and some families on low income are entitled to free prescriptions and dentistry—📖 p. 137

Further information
DH ⌨ www.dh.gov.uk
- Children's National Service Framework (2004)
- Healthy Child Programme (2009)

The neonatal check

It is essential that a full neonatal check is carried out <72h after delivery. Most neonatal checks are carried out by paediatricians in maternity units before discharge. Neonatal checks can then be provided by GMS GPs as a National Enhanced Service or by PMS GPs as part of their negotiated services if:

- The baby is discharged <24h after delivery
- The birth occurs at home or in a GP unit, or
- There is rapid discharge from obstetric unit to a peripheral unit

Parental concerns

- Discuss any worries the parent(s) might have about the child
- Review FH, pregnancy, and birth
- Arrange hepatitis B vaccination if mother is hepatitis B +ve (📖 p. 811) or BCG vaccination if in a high-risk group (📖 p. 327)

History

- **Has the baby passed urine?** For boys, is the stream good? If no urine in the 1st 24h suspect renal abnormality and admit for further investigation. If poor stream suspect posterior urethral valves, phimosis, or hypospadias
- **Has the baby passed meconium?** If no meconium in the first 24h, suspect meconium ileus and admit for further investigation

Physical examination Check the baby systematically—see Table 24.1.

Moro reflex Elicit if concerned. Support head and shoulders about 15cm from the examination couch. Suddenly allow the baby's head to drop back slightly. The response—extension of the arms followed by adduction towards the chest should be brisk and symmetrical. This reflex disappears by 6mo.

Discuss neonatal bloodspot screening 📖 p. 850

Check vitamin K has been given

- Discuss any concerns with the parent(s)
- Deficiency of vitamin K can → *haemorrhagic disease of the newborn* with potentially serious effects, including death
- All parents should be offered IM vitamin K for their baby; if IM vitamin K is declined, they should be offered oral vitamin K. ❶ One dose of oral vitamin K does not confer full protection. Formula feeds contain vitamin K supplements but breastfed babies require further doses—ensure that they get them
- Babies at high risk of bleeding (premature, low birthweight, unwell babies, and those who have undergone instrumental deliveries)—should always have IM vitamin K

Health education 📖 p. 847. Discuss:

- Feeding and nutrition
- Sleeping position
- Baby care
- Sibling management
- Crying and sleep problems
- Transport in a car

Features of common chromosomal abnormalities 📖 p. 861

Table 24.1 Check list for the neonatal examination

General appearance

Syndrome? Clusters of features, e.g. features of Down's/Turner's syndrome	Weight: small or large for gestation? Pallor, jaundice, or cyanosis ❶ Slight peripheral cyanosis is normal	Skin: birth marks; meconium staining; purpura; lanugo or evidence of post-maturity

Head and facial features

Head circumference Caput succedaneum or cephalhaematoma Fontanelles—number (if 3, ? Down's), size, and tension	Accessory auricles Ptosis Subconjunctival haemorrhage, conjunctivitis, or sticky eye? Cataract or red reflex?	Sternomastoid swelling Cleft lip Potter's facies Pierre Robin jaw (receding jaw with cleft palate)

Mouth

Cleft palate? (📖 p. 932) Tongue tie?	Profuse saliva (associated with oesophageal atresia)	Epstein's pearls

Arms and hands

Proportion of arms/fingers Oedema	Palmar creases Fingers—number, webbing, deformity	Normal movements? Erb's or Klumpke's palsy palsy (📖 p. 858)

Chest

Distortion Breast enlargement	Respiratory rate* Recession	Air entry/added breath sounds

Cardiovascular examination

Pulses (femoral/brachial)	Heart rate, rhythm, and sounds	Murmurs (📖 p. 880)

Abdomen

Umbilical infection/discharge, or hernia	Anus: patency/position	Masses**

Genitalia

♂: penis—size and shape; position of urethral orifice; testes (normal, undescended, or maldescended), hernia, or hydrocele

♀: clitoromegaly; vaginal bleeding; posterior vaginal skin tag (common)

Back, legs and feet

Sacral pit/spina bifida (📖 p. 862) Scoliosis (📖 p. 478)	Hips (📖 p. 854) Proportion of feet/legs/body	Club foot (📖 p. 497) Toes—number, webbing, deformity

CNS

Is the baby behaving normally?	Is the cry normal?	Are all 4 limbs moving equally and is the Moro reflex (if done) symmetrical?

* Respiratory rate <60 breaths/min is normal.
** Liver is usually palpable as are the lower poles of the kidneys; the spleen and bladder are never palpable.

Neonatal bloodspot screening

Neonatal bloodspot screening involves taking a blood sample obtained by pricking a baby's heel. The blood is placed on special filter paper and sent for analysis. The test is usually carried out by the midwife when the baby is 5–8d old and the result is available by 6wk.

⚠ If screening is declined, it is important to flag in the child's notes that the child has not been screened in case the child becomes ill later on.

What conditions does bloodspot testing detect? Throughout the UK babies are screened for:
- Phenylketonuria (PKU)
- Congenital hypothyroidism
- Medium chain acyl CoA dehydrogenase deficiency (MCADD)
- Cystic fibrosis (CF)
- Sickle cell disease

A pilot of screening for 5 further rare inherited metabolic disorders (maple syrup urine disease, homocystinuria, glutaric acidaemia type 1, isovaleric acidaemia, and long chain fatty acidaemia) is under evaluation.

Phenylketonuria (PKU)
- In the UK 1 in 10,000 babies has PKU (autosomal recessive trait— higher incidence in Ireland). If there is a FH, check at 48–72h of age
- Children are unable to break down phenylalanine, an amino acid present in many foods. The baby appears normal at birth but develops severe developmental delay, learning difficulty, and seizures in infancy
- The bloodspot test detects high levels of blood phenylalanine
- Treatment is with life-long dietary restriction of phenylalanine. With treatment, growth and development are normal

Congenital hypothyroidism
- In the UK, 1 in 4,000 babies is born with congenital hypothyroidism ($♀ > ♂$)
- Untreated, children with abnormally low levels of thyroid hormone fail to grow properly and have mild to severe mental disability
- The bloodspot is used to detect low levels of blood thyroxine
- Treatment with thyroxine replacement results in normal growth and development. Usually thyroxine replacement is needed lifelong

Cystic fibrosis (CF)
- In the UK, 1 in 2,500 babies is born with CF (📖 p. 330). Early treatment improves outcome and prolongs both quality and quantity of life
- Screening detects immunoreactive trypsin (IRT) which is ↑ in children with CF. If IRT is ↑, the blood is then DNA-tested for the most common gene alterations
- If a child tests +ve, it is important that parents and siblings receive genetic counselling and are offered genetic testing for the condition. If both parents are carriers of a CF gene, there is a 1 in 4 chance of any subsequent children they have together being affected
- Screening will also detect healthy carriers. This has implications not only for the child but also parents and other siblings. Ensure parents have a full explanation of results and understand their meaning

❗ Not all gene mutations are tested for. Some babies with CF will be missed by newborn screening. Continue to watch for later presentations.

Sickle cell disease

• In the UK, 1 in 2,000 babies is born with a sickle cell disorder (📖 p. 669). Infants with sickle cell disease are at risk of severe overwhelming infections and splenic sequestration crises. Early diagnosis allows prophylaxis with penicillin and vaccines, and parent training to identify children with complications and present early for treatment. This ↓ complications and deaths in young infants

• Abnormal haemoglobin is screened for using either high performance liquid chromatography (HPLC) or isoelectric focussing (IEF). If detected, a confirmatory test is performed on the original spot using a different technique from the initial screening test

• If a child tests positive, it is important that parents and siblings receive genetic counselling and are offered genetic testing for the condition

• As well as babies with sickle cell disease, this test detects babies with sickle cell trait, other heterozygous states, and other haemoglobin abnormalities (e.g. haemoglobin E, thalassaemia). Even if these have no clinical consequences for the child the current policy is to inform parents of the results. It is important that parents understand the meaning and significance of results both for the child and other family members

Medium chain acyl CoA dehydrogenase deficiency (MCADD)

• In the UK, 1 in 10,000 babies is born with MCADD (autosomal recessive trait). Infants are unable to metabolize fats effectively. If they are stressed by fasting or infection, toxic levels of fatty acids build up, causing metabolic crises, brain damage, coma, and death

• The bloodspot test detects high levels of C8 carnitine (a fatty acid of medium length). Rarely other metabolic disorders are also detected

• If a child tests +ve, parents should be offered testing for any unscreened siblings. Any subsequent babies need early screening (at 24–48h) and specialist management including regular feeding until the result is known

• Parents and siblings should be offered genetic counselling

• Treatment prevents long-term consequences, is required life-long, and involves ensuring the child does not go without food for >4–6h (longer after adolescence); has a low-fat, high-carbohydrate diet, takes L-carnitine supplements, and parents seek medical attention early if the child is unwell

Further information

UK Newborn Screening Programme Centre
🖎 www.newbornbloodspot.screening.nhs.uk

Further information for parents

UK Newborn Screening Programme Centre Leaflets about screening for parents 🖎 www.newbornbloodspot.screening.nhs.uk
National Society for Phenylketonuria (NSPKU) ☎ 030 3040 1090 🖎 www.nspku.org
Climb (Children Living with Metabolic Diseases) ☎ 0800 652 3181 🖎 www.climb.org.uk

Summary of developmental milestones

Table 24.2 Summary of developmental milestones

Development	6-week check	8 months
Gross motor	Controls head when pulled to sitting position (0–3mo) Moro reflex (0–6mo)—should be absent >6mo Holds head in line/slightly higher than body with hips semi-extended during ventral suspension (0–10wk) Lifts head momentarily when lying prone (from birth)	Bears weight on legs (3–7mo) Can be pulled to sit (14wk–6mo) Sits with support (4–6mo) Sits without support (5–8mo) Crawls (6–9mo)
Fine motor/vision	Stares (from birth) Follows horizontally to 90° (0–6wk)	Reaches out to grasp (palmar grasp) (3–6mo) Transfers and mouths (passes an object from 1 hand to the other and puts it in his mouth) (18wk–8mo) Fixes gaze on small objects (5–8mo) Follows fallen toys (4–8mo)
Hearing and speech	Responds to rattle or bell (from birth) Startle response (from birth)	Vocalizes (4–6mo) Polysyllabic babbling (6–10mo) Laughs (2–5mo) Responds to own name (4–8mo)
Social behaviour/play	Smiles (0–10wk—mean 5wk) Turns to look at observer's face (from birth)	Puts everything into mouth (4–8mo) Hand and foot regard (4–8mo) Plays peek-a-boo (5½–10mo)
⚠ Warning signs	No red reflex No visual fixation or following Failure to respond to sound Asymmetrical neonatal reflexes Excessive head lag Failure to smile	Hand preference Fisting Squint Persistence of primitive reflexes—Moro response, stepping, asymmetrical tonic neck reflex

(continued)

Table 24.2 (Contd.)

18 months	3 years	4 years
Gets to sitting position (6–11mo)	Climbs and descends stairs	Hops forward on 1 foot for 2m (3–5y)
Pulls to standing (6–10mo)	Runs (~15mo)	Stands on 1 foot for 5s (2¾–4½y)
Walks holding onto furniture (7–13mo)	Pedals tricycle (21mo–3y)	Walks heel-to-toe (3½–5¼y—backwards (4–6y)
Walks alone (10–15mo)	Jumps in 1 place (21mo–3y)	
Walks backwards (12–22mo)	Kicks a ball (15–24mo)	Bounces and catches a ball (3¼–5½y)
Climbs stairs (14–22mo)	Stands on 1 foot for 1 second (22mo–3¼y)	
Points with index finger	Picks up 'hundreds and thousands'	Copies a cross (3–4½y) and square (4–5½y)
Casts (throws) (9–15mo)	Imitates a vertical line (18–33mo)	Draws a man with 3 parts (with all features—4½–6y)
Delicate pincer grasp (10–18mo)	Copies a circle (2¼–3½y)	
Holds two bricks and bangs them together (7–13mo)	Threads beads	Recognizes colours (3–4¾y)
Scribbles (12–24mo)	Builds a tower of 8 bricks (21mo–3½y)	
Builds a tower of 3–4 bricks (16–24mo)	Matches 2 colours	
Turns to sound of name	Uses plurals (30mo–3¼y)	Speaks grammatically (2½y–4¼y)
Jabbers continually	Uses prepositions (3–4½y)	Counts to 10
Uses 'mama' and 'dada' (11–20mo—half by 15mo)	Joins words into sentences (50% by 23mo; 97% by 3y)	
Can say ≥3 words other than 'mama' and 'dada' (10–21mo)	Gives own name	
Points to eyes, nose, and mouth (14–23mo)		
Obeys simple instructions (15mo–2½y)		
Holds spoon and gets food to mouth (14mo–2½y)	Plays alone	Shares toys
Explores environment (13–20mo)	Eats with spoon and fork	Brushes teeth
Takes off shoes and socks (13–20mo)	Puts on clothes (2¼–3½y—with supervision)	Dresses without supervision (3¼–5½y)
	Washes and dries hands	Comforts friends in distress (5y)
	Separates from mother easily (2–4y)	
	Dry in the day (2–4y)	
Unable to sit, weight bear and/or stand without support	Unable to speak in simple sentences	Speech difficult to understand due to poor articulation or because of omission or substitution of consonants (confusion of 's', 'f', and 'th' disappears by 6½y)
Persistence of hand regard ± casting. No pincer grip	Unable to understand speech	
Absence of babbling or cooing; inability to understand simple commands		

Screening for hip dysplasia

Developmental dysplasia of the hip (DDH) was previously known as congenital dislocation of the hip (CDH). It ranges from dysplasia with dislocation or subluxation, through instability, to mild acetabular dysplasia with a stable hip joint. Incidence is estimated at 1–3% of newborns when all grades of severity are included, although fewer have dislocation (3 in 2,000 live births); ♀:♂≈5:1. Associated with breech presentation. Often there is a family history. 20% of cases are bilateral.

Presentation

- High-risk babies (breech presentation at 36wk even if turns prior to delivery and/or family history) are routinely screened with USS in the first 6–8 weeks of life
- Otherwise, usually detected by clinical examination as part of routine screening. Screening should take place <72h after birth and at the 6wk check. Screening tests should be taught *in vivo* by someone experienced in the technique
- Despite screening some cases slip though the net. They present as toddlers with limp/waddling gait; frequent falls; asymmetric thigh creases or limited hip abduction. Be alert for physical signs and take parental concerns seriously
- Some (particularly mild cases) go unnoticed until adulthood when they present with pain (from damage to the acetabular labrum) or premature osteoarthritis

Screening a child <3mo of age

- Screening tests should be performed in a warm room with the baby undressed and lying on a firm surface
- Flex hips and knees to 90° using one hand for each leg with thumbs on the inner side of the baby's knee and ring and little fingers behind the greater trochanters (see Figure 24.1)
- Each hip is tested separately. The examiner's hand on the opposite side from the hip being tested is used to stabilize the pelvis. Hold the thumb over the symphysis pubis and fingers under the sacrum
- Only test once as repeated testing can damage the hips

Ortolani manoeuvre Each hip is gently abducted whilst lifting the greater trochanter forward. As a dislocated hip is abducted a clunk or jumping sensation is felt. It is difficult to tell the difference between a click of a normal hip and a clunk of an abnormal one—so refer any clicky or clunky hips for further investigation (usually USS or orthopaedic review). Hip abduction of <60° in 90° of flexion is also a sensitive sign.

Barlow manoeuvre This establishes whether the hips are dislocatable. Holding the legs as described above, gently apply pressure along the line of the femur pushing it backwards out of the acetabulum. The judder of the femoral head slipping in and out of the acetabulum can be felt if the hip is dislocatable.

Figure 24.1 Screening for congenital dislocation of the hip (Ortolani test)

Examination of a child of >3mo of age

- >3mo of age, limited abduction is the most common finding in children with CDH. If the infant lies on his/her back with hips flexed at 90°, any hip which cannot abduct >75° should be viewed with suspicion
- Ortolani and Barlow tests are difficult to perform in older babies; X-ray is more useful than USS once a baby is >4.5mo old

Other signs
- Limb shortening on the affected side—compare knee levels with the child lying on his/her back and hips and knees flexed to 90°
- Asymmetry of the thighs—skin creases may asymmetric (but asymmetric in 25% of normal babies)
- Flattening of the buttock—in a prone position, the affected side may look flatter

Management Refer to an orthopaedic surgeon specializing in paediatric problems. Treatment depends on when the condition is diagnosed:
- **Young babies** Splinting in a pelvic harness to reduce and hold the hip—the hips are held in partial abduction using slings under each thigh attached to a body harness, e.g. von Rosen splint. Usually babies wear a splint for ~3mo
- **Older babies, toddlers, and adults** Surgery is required

Support for parents and children

Steps Support for patients with lower limb conditions and their families
☏ 01925 750271 🖰 www.steps-charity.org.uk

Vision and hearing screening tests

Operational senses are essential for normal development. Conditions which interfere with the senses, even if correctable, may lead to permanent impairment if not detected and treated early.

Vision screening Is carried out at the neonatal and 6wk check:
- Ask about parental worries about the child's vision
- Is there a FH of visual disorders (particularly retinoblastoma or congenital cataracts)?
- Inspect the external eye—are there any abnormalities?
- Check the red reflex in each eye (urgent referral if absent)
- Observe if the child has a fixing and following response to a bright light

A further check may be carried out by an orthoptist-led service at ~4y. Refer children for further assessment at any age where there is concern about vision on assessment or any parental concern.

> △ **Warning signs for visual problems**
> - The child does not fix on the mother's face whilst feeding by 6wk
> - In a child >6wk old, the child's eye wanders about from one side of the eye socket to the other while the child is awake and happy
> - A white spot is seen in the pupil at any age—could be cataract
> - A child holds objects close to the face whilst trying to look at them
> - A child >6mo old has a squint in one or both eyes

Tests for squint
- Sit the child on the parent's lap; stand in front of the child and shine a bright light (e.g. pen torch) at arm's length from the child
- Fix the child's head in the midline and look for the reflection of the light on the child's corneas; the reflection should be symmetrical and near the centre of the pupil (usually slightly towards the nose)
- Turn the child's head to one side keeping the eyes fixed on the light— the reflection should stay symmetrical; repeat, turning to the other side
- If reflections are not symmetrical perform a cover test

Cover test
- Sit the child comfortably on a parent's lap and shine a bright light or a place a small bright object at arm's length from the child
- Cover one eye with a card—watch for any movement of the uncovered eye to fix on the object. Then remove the card and watch the covered eye to see if it moves to fix on the object. Repeat with the other eye
- If either or both eyes move a squint is present—refer

Hearing tests All newborn babies in the UK are offered hearing tests through the neonatal hearing screening programme (NHSP):
- **Automated oto-acoustic emission (AOAE) testing** Measures integrity of the inner ear and is offered to all neonates. An earpiece is placed in the ear and quiet clicking sounds are played. In a hearing ear, the cochlea produces sounds in response to the clicks that can be analysed. Screening takes a few minutes and can be done at the bedside when the baby is asleep but responses are sometimes unclear especially if the baby is <24h old

- **Automated auditory brainstem response (AABR) testing** Assesses the entire auditory pathway and is offered to any baby not passing the AOAE test or to any baby that has a stay of >48h in a special care baby unit (in addition to AOAE testing). Sensors are placed on the head/neck and quiet clicking sounds are played through head-phones. Responses to sounds around the brain stem are analysed

⚠ **Warning signs for hearing problems**
- No startle response to loud noises at 6wk
- The child does not respond to his/her name by 8mo
- Absence of babbling or cooing by 1y
- Inability to understand simple commands by 18mo
- Inability to speak in short sentences by 2½y

When are further hearing tests necessary? Ensure referral to audiology for further assessment:
- **If the newborn hearing test indicates a problem**
- **At any age** If there is parental/professional concern; after temporal bone fracture; after bacterial meningitis/septicaemia (test hearing 4wk after discharge from hospital); after treatment with high doses of ototoxic drugs, e.g. aminoglycosides
- **At 8mo of age** If the child has FH of childhood sensorineural deafness; missed newborn hearing screen or follow-up; congenital infection (e.g. cytomegalovirus, toxoplasmosis, rubella); neurodegenerative/neurodevelopmental disorder; syndrome associated with hearing loss (e.g. Down's, Turner's); craniofacial abnormality (e.g. cleft palate); or history of severe neonatal jaundice at exchange transfusion level

Delayed speech development May be due to global or specific learning disability, deafness, or neurological problems. Parents often compare their children's development to others leading to unnecessary anxiety. The range of normal for speech development is wide:
- First words 11–20mo
- A 2y old may use anything from a few words to 2,000 words
- Children start using prepositions at any time from 3–4½y

Management If a child's speech is delayed, check other developmental milestones; examine for any neurological deficit and check hearing. Consider autism (🕮 p. 918) particularly if regression of speech. If delayed speech is the main issue, refer to speech therapy.

Further information
Royal College of Ophthalmologists Ophthalmic services for children (2009) ℘ www.rcophth.ac.uk
NHS Newborn Hearing Screening Programme ℘ www.hearing.screening.nhs.uk

Parent and child information and support
LOOK Support for families of blind or visually impaired children ☎ 0121 428 5038 ℘ www.look-uk.org
National Deaf Children's Society ☎ 0808 800 8880 ℘ www.ndcs.org.uk

Birth trauma

Head trauma

Caput succedaneum Swelling, bruising, and oedema of the presenting portion—usually scalp. Unsightly but resolves spontaneously.

Cephalhaematoma Uncommon. Haemorrhage beneath the periosteum. Unilateral and usually parietal. Presents as a lump—the size of an egg—on the baby's head. Treatment is not required, but anaemia or hyperbilirubinaemia may follow.

Depressed skull fracture Rare. Most result from forceps pressure; rarely caused by the head resting on a bony prominence *in utero*. May be associated with subdural bleeding, subarachnoid haemorrhage, or contusion/laceration of the brain itself. Seen and felt as a depression in the skull. X-ray confirms diagnosis; may need neurosurgical elevation.

Intracranial haemorrhage Rare. Suggested by lack of responsiveness, fits, respiratory distress ± shock. Admit as an emergency.

Nerve injuries

Cranial nerve trauma The facial nerve is injured most often, causing facial asymmetry especially during crying. Usually resolves spontaneously by 2–3mo of age.

Brachial plexus injury Follows stretching caused by shoulder dystocia, breech extraction, or hyperabduction of the neck in cephalic presentations. Often associated with other traumatic injuries, e.g. fractured clavicle or humerus, subluxations of the shoulder or cervical spine.
- **Partial injuries of the brachial plexus** Most recover but site and type of nerve root injury determine prognosis. If persists, refer to paediatric neurology for further investigation
  - Injuries of the upper brachial plexus (C5–6) affect muscles around the shoulder and elbow—Erb's palsy. *W.H. Erb (1840–1921)— German neurologist*
  - Injuries of the lower plexus (C7–8 and T1) affect primarily muscles of the forearm and hand—Klumpke's palsy. *A.M. Dejerine-Klumpke (1859–1927)—French neurologist*
- **Injuries of the entire brachial plexus** No movement of the arm + sensory loss. Refer immediately for neurological opinion. Prognosis for recovery is poor

Fractures

Mid-clavicular fracture Most common fracture during birth. Usually occurs due to shoulder dystocia. Most clavicular fractures are greenstick fractures and heal rapidly and uneventfully. A large callus forms at the fracture site in <1wk and remodelling is completed in <1mo. Can be associated with brachial plexus injury and/or pneumothorax.

Long bone fractures The humerus and femur may be fractured during difficult deliveries. Usually long bones heal rapidly without any residual deformity.

Cerebral palsy The term cerebral palsy identifies children with non-progressive spasticity, ataxia, or involuntary movements. It affects 0.2% of children (~1% of premature babies/babies small for dates).

Causes
- Prematurity
- *In utero* disorders
- Neonatal jaundice
- Birth trauma
- Perinatal asphyxia
- CNS trauma
- Severe systemic disease during early childhood (e.g. meningitis, sepsis)

Associated disorders
- Fits (25%)
- Squint and other visual problems
- Deafness
- Learning disability—though intelligence is often normal
- Short attention span
- Hyperactivity

Spastic syndromes 70%. Upper motor neurone involvement.
- Affects motor function and may → hemiplegia, paraplegia, quadriplegia, or diplegia
- Affected limbs are underdeveloped and have ↑ tone, weakness, and a tendency toward contractures
- A scissor's gait and toe walking are characteristic
- In mildly affected children, impairment may occur only during certain activities (e.g. running)
- With quadriplegia dysarthria is common

Athetoid/dyskinetic syndromes 20%. Basal ganglia involvement.
- Characterized by slow, writhing, involuntary movements affecting the extremities (athetoid) or proximal parts of the limbs/trunk (dystonic)
- Abrupt, jerky, distal movements (choreiform) may also occur
- Movements ↑ with emotional tension and stop during sleep
- Dysarthria is often severe

Ataxic syndromes 10%. Involvement of the cerebellum. Weakness, incoordination, and intention tremor produce unsteadiness, wide-based gait, and difficulty with rapid and fine movements.

❶ Mixed types are common.

Diagnosis Diagnosis is rarely made in infancy with certainty though often abnormalities in tone, reflexes, and posture are noted during routine developmental screening. Refer for paediatric assessment if suspected. Formal diagnosis is usually made by 2y.

Management The goal is for children to develop maximal independence within the limits of their handicap. A multidisciplinary, coordinated team approach, involving physiotherapists, occupational therapists, speech therapists, social workers, teachers, community paediatricians, and the primary healthcare team in liaison with the child and his/her parents is essential. As with all chronically disabled children, the child and parents need assistance in understanding the disability, setting realistic goals, and relieving their own feelings (📖 p. 859).

Information and support for parents
SCOPE (cerebral palsy) ☎ 0808 800 3333 🖰 www.scope.org.uk

Genetic problems

⚠ Some genetic syndromes are associated with cancer (e.g. Down's syndrome and leukaemia; neurofibromatosis and CNS tumours). Be alert to the potential significance of unexplained symptoms in this group[N].

There are 46 chromosomes—22 matching pairs with matching genes (autosomes) and one pair of sex chromosomes which may match (XX—♀) or differ (XY—♂). Genetic abnormalities are the most common cause of developmental delay. There are a huge number of genetic syndromes—many of them extremely rare. Categorize by the nature of the defect.

Chromosome number

- **Alteration in number of chromosomes** *Example:* Down's syndrome (extra chromosome 21)
- **Sex chromosome abnormalities** A sex chromosome is duplicated or deleted. *Examples:* Turner's syndrome (XO); Klinefelter's syndrome (XXY or XXYY)

Gross structural changes in chromosomes

- **Translocation** Part of one chromosome is transposed or translocated onto another. If no genetic information is lost there is no clinical effect (balanced translocation) although offspring often have problems. 6% of children with Down's syndrome have a translocation
- **Deletion** Loss of a portion of chromosome. *Example:* cri-du-chat syndrome (deletion of the short arm of chromosome 5)

Single gene abnormalities

Autosomal dominant inheritance >1,000 diseases all individually rare. Heterozygotes demonstrate the disease and 1 in 2 pregnancies of an affected individual are affected—usually ♂ = ♀. Expression of the gene may vary. *Examples:* tuberous sclerosis (📖 p. 862); Marfan's syndrome (📖 p. 283); myotonic dystrophy (📖 p. 578); neurofibromatosis (📖 p. 580).

Autosomal recessive inheritance >700 diseases that only manifest in the homozygote. Heterozygotes may be asymptomatic or show milder abnormalities. To develop severe disease, the affected gene must be inherited from both parents. The risk of an affected pregnancy is 1 in 4—usually ♂ = ♀. Affected individuals have unaffected children unless their partner is a heterozygote. *Examples:* glycogen storage diseases (📖 p. 862); PKU (📖 p. 850); sickle cell disease (📖 p. 669); thalassaemia (📖 p. 668); cystic fibrosis (📖 p. 330); MCADD (📖 p. 851).

Sex-linked disorders ~100 are recognized. Most are recessively inherited from the mother and affect only ♂ offspring. A ♂ child of a heterozygote mother has a 1 in 2 chance of developing the disease; a ♀ child has a 1 in 2 chance of carrying the disease. A ♀ child can only be fully affected by the disease if the father has the disease and the mother is a carrier when she has a 1 in 2 chance of being affected and, if not affected, will be a carrier. *Examples:* fragile X syndrome (📖 p. 863); haemophilia (📖 p. 670), red-green colour blindness (📖 p. 970), Duchenne's muscular dystrophy (📖 p. 578).

Table 24.3 Structural chromosome problems seen in general practice

Genetic problem	Features
Down's syndrome Trisomy 21 (92%) Translocation (6%) Mosaicism (2%) *Affects 1 in 1,000 live births*	*Facial abnormalities:* flat occiput, oval face (mongoloid facies), low-set eyes with prominent epicanthic folds *Other abnormalities:* single palmar crease; hypotonia; congenital heart disease Developmental delay Life expectancy is ↓, but ~½ live to 60y
Edward's syndrome Trisomy 18 *Affects 1 in 6,000 live births ♀:♂≈2:1*	*Facial abnormalities:* low-set malformed ears, receding chin, protruding eyes, cleft lip or palate *Other abnormalities:* short sternum makes the nipples appear too widely separated; fingers cannot be extended and the index finger overlaps the 3rd digit; umbilical/inguinal hernias; rocker-bottom feet; rigid baby with flexion of limbs Developmental delay Life expectancy is ~10mo
Patau's syndrome Trisomy 13 *Affects 1 in 10,000 live births*	*Facial abnormalities:* small head and eyes; cleft lip and palate *Other abnormalities:* skeletal abnormalities, e.g. flexion contractures of hands ± polydactyly with narrow fingernails; brain malformation; heart malformation; polycystic kidneys 50% die in <1mo. Usually fatal in the first year
Cri-du-chat syndrome Deletion of short arm of chromosome 5 *Affects 1 in 50,000 births*	*Facial abnormalities:* microcephaly; marked epicanthic folds; moon-shaped face; alert expression *Other abnormalities:* abnormal cry (cat-like) Developmental delay Usually fatal in the first year
Turner's syndrome XO—deletion of one X chromosome. Mosaicism may occur (XO, XX) *Affects 1 in 2,000 live female births*	Female appearance *Facial abnormalities:* ptosis, nystagmus, webbed neck *Other abnormalities:* short stature (<130cm); hyperconvex nails; wide carrying angle (cubitus valgus); inverted nipples; broad chest; coarctation of the aorta, left heart defects; lymphoedema of the legs; ovaries rudimentary or absent Lifespan is normal
Klinefelter's syndrome XXY or XXYY polysomy *Affects 1 in 1,000 live births*	Male appearance Often undetected until presentation with infertility in adult life *Clinical features:* may present in adolescence with psychopathy, ↓ libido, sparse facial hair, gynaecomastia, small firm testes *Associations:* hypothyroidism, DM, asthma *Specialist management:* androgens and plastic surgery may be useful for gynaecomastia

Polygenic inheritance Familial trends of disease are often seen but there is no simple inheritance pattern. Usually due to polygenic inheritance, i.e. the combination of genes inherited. *Examples:* neural tube defects, cleft palate; ischaemic and congential heart disease; DDH, club foot; type 1 DM; pyloric stenosis; schizophrenia.

Management of genetic disorders Depends on the specific problems of each child. A multidisciplinary approach is essential. Support the child and family. Ensure receipt of all available benefits. Tell carers about local facilities, voluntary and self-help organizations. Review regularly.

Tuberous sclerosis *Incidence:* 6/100,000. Autosomal dominant condition caused by mutations of TSC1 or TSC2 genes on chromosome 9—but two-thirds arise from new mutations. Characterized by hamartomatous lesions in the skin, nervous system, and internal organs. Usual presentation is with:
• Adenoma sebaceum (angiofibromas of the skin—seen as red-brown papules on the face—appear aged 5–10y)
• Epilepsy and developmental delay

Other features include coarsened skin over the sacrum (shagreen patch); nail fold fibromas; hypopigmented oval patches (ash leaf spots); cardiac, renal, lung, and eye abnormalities. Treatment is supportive.

Tay–Sachs disease Autosomal recessive neurodegenerative disorder caused by a mutation of the HEXA gene on chromosome 15. *Incidence:* 1 in 25 in Ashkenazi Jewish populations. 3 forms:
• **Infantile** Most common. Symptoms appear at ~6mo with relentless deterioration in neurological function until death at <4y
• **Juvenile** Symptoms appear aged 2–10y; death occurs <15y
• **Adult- or late-onset** Rare. Symptoms develop in adolescence/adulthood, e.g. unsteadiness of gait, swallowing/speech difficulty, cognitive decline, and/or psychosis. Often results in long-term disability

Antenatal screening is available (📖 p. 799)—refer if from high-risk population. Otherwise, treatment is supportive.

Glycogen storage diseases *Incidence:* ~1/25,000. Lack of ≥1 enzyme involved in glycogen synthesis or breakdown. Characterized by deposition of abnormal amounts or types of glycogen in tissues. Inheritance is autosomal recessive for all forms except type VI, which follows an X-linked inheritance. Symptoms and age of onset vary considerably:
• Predominantly liver involvement (types I, III, IV, VI) → hepatomegaly, hypoglycaemia, metabolic acidosis
• Predominantly muscle involvement (types V, VII) → weakness, lethargy, poor feeding, heart failure

Treatment involves frequent small carbohydrate meals; allopurinol (to prevent renal urate stone formation and/or gout) ± limiting anaerobic exercise. A high-protein diet is also helpful for some patients.

Neural tube defects Most neural tube defects are detected antenatally by routine antenatal USS. Inheritance is polygenic. Management is supportive. *Types of defect:*

Anencephaly Absent cerebral cortex and skull vault. Usually detected on antenatal screening. Incompatible with life—those infants born alive die within hours of birth.

Cranium defects Vary in severity from meningocele (meninges protrude through the defect) to inoperable encephalocele (brain tissue protrudes through the skull).

Spina bifida The vertebral arch is incomplete.

- **Occulta** Covered with skin and fascia. Common and usually asymptomatic though may be associated with mild gait or bladder problems
- **Cystica** Herniation of the meninges (meningocele). Uncommon but treatable usually with minor residual deficit
- **Whole cord herniation** (myelomeningocele) Is more common and often results in neurological deficit. It is associated with hydrocephalus, learning and psychological problems

⚠ *Folate supplementation* ↓ risk of neural tube defect by 72%. Supplements are available through the Healthy Start Programme, can be prescribed or bought OTC from chemists/supermarkets. Advise 0.4mg (400 microgram) od from when pregnancy is being planned to 13wk unless either parent or an existing child has a neural tube defect, or the mother has coeliac disease, DM, BMI >30kg/m², or is taking anticonvulsants—when advise 5mg od.

Fragile X syndrome Affects 1/1,250 ♂ births and 1/2,500 ♀ births. Genetic abnormality carried on the X-chromosome comprising:

- Low IQ (20–70)
- Large testes
- High forehead
- Large jaw
- Long ears
- Facial asymmetry
- Associations with ADHD, anxiety, and OCD

50% of carrier females have a normal IQ and 50% have a degree of learning disability. Consider fragile X syndrome in any child with developmental delay of unknown cause. There is some evidence that folic acid supplements ↓ hyperactive and disruptive behaviour in children with fragile X. Antenatal testing is possible for future pregnancies.

Information and support for families

Contact a Family ☎ 0808 808 3555 🖳 www.cafamily.org.uk
Genetic Alliance UK ☎ 020 7704 3141 🖳 www.geneticalliance.org.uk
Unique Rare Chromosome Disorder Support Group ☎ 01883 330766 🖳 www.rarechromo.org
Support Organisation for Trisomy (SOFT) ☎ 0333 1212 300 🖳 www.soft.org.uk
Down's Syndrome Association ☎ 0333 1212 300 🖳 www.downs-syndrome.org.uk
Turner Syndrome Support Society ☎ 0300 111 7520 🖳 www.tss.org.uk
Tuberous Sclerosis Association 🖳 www.tuberous-sclerosis.org
Cure and Action for Tay-Sachs 🖳 www.cats-foundation.org
Association for Glycogen Storage Disease (UK) 🖳 www.agsd.org.uk
Shine (Spina bifida and hydrocephalus) ☎ 01733 555988 🖳 www.shinecharity.org.uk
Fragile X Society ☎ 01371 875 100 🖳 www.fragilex.org.uk

Minor problems of neonates and small babies

See Table 24.4.

Table 24.4 Minor problems of neonates and small babies

Condition	Features	Management
Milia	Tiny pearly white papules on the nose ± palate—blocked sebaceous ducts	Disappear spontaneously—reassure
Erythema toxicum (neonatal urticaria)	Red blotches with a central, white vesicle. Each spot lasts ~24h. Spots are sterile. Baby is well	If sepsis is suspected—take a swab. Otherwise reassure—resolves spontaneously
Harlequin colour change	One side of the body flushes red whilst the other stays pale, giving a harlequin effect	A harmless vasomotor effect—reassure
Single palmar crease	Common abnormality. Associated with several genetic syndromes, e.g. Down's	Usually of no consequence unless associated with other abnormalities
Milaria (heat rash)	Itchy red rash which fades as soon as the baby is cooled (e.g. by undressing)	Reassure. Keep the baby cool if the rash appears
Peeling skin	Common among babies born after their due date	Apply olive oil, baby oil, or aqueous cream to prevent the skin cracking
Petechial or subconjunctival haemorrhage and facial cyanosis	May all occur during delivery	Resolve spontaneously—reassure. Ensure the baby has had vitamin K supplements
Swollen breasts	Due to maternal hormones. Occur in both sexes and occasionally lactate ('witche's milk')	Breast swelling usually subsides spontaneously. May become infected and require antibiotics
Sticky eye	Common. Usually due to a blocked tear duct. Swab to exclude ophthalmia neonatorum	Ophthalmia neonatorum—📖 p. 741. Blocked tear duct (📖 p. 965)—bathe with boiled water to clear when changing nappies. Avoid the use of antibiotics unless overtly infected
Sneezing	Neonates clear amniotic fluid from their noses by sneezing	Reassure

Table 24.4 (Contd.)

Condition	Features	Management
Red-stained nappy	Common in the first few days of life. Usually due to urinary urates but may be due to blood from the cord or vagina (oestrogen withdrawal bleed)	Reassure
Umbilicus	After birth, the umbilicus dries, becomes black, and separates at about 1wk of age	The umbilical stump can become infected—offensive odour, pus, periumbilical flare, malaise—requiring antibiotics If a granuloma forms at the site of separation, exclude a patent urachus (refer if present) and treat with silver nitrate cautery
Failure to regain birth weight by 2wk of age	Usually due to a feeding problem or minor intercurrent illness	Monitor weight carefully. Refer to paediatrics if no cause is apparent, or if despite treatment of the underlying cause the baby is not gaining weight
Possetting	Common The baby effortlessly brings back 5–10mL of each feed during the feed or soon after	Only of concern if the baby is otherwise unwell or failing to thrive—see gastro-oesophageal reflux If thriving, advise parents to feed the child propped up and slow down the speed at which feeds are given
Gastro-oesophageal reflux ❶ Cow's milk protein allergy (📖 p. 889) can present in a similar way	Similar to possetting, but an ↑ proportion or all of each feed is brought back May cause failure to thrive, distress ± crying More common in premature babies and those with cerebral palsy Rare complications are oesophageal stricture due to acid reflux or aspiration pneumonia	Advise parents to feed the child propped up Thickening agents (e.g. Carobel®, Nestargel®) or ready thickened feeds (e.g. SMA Staydown®) may be helpful as may Gaviscon® Infant ± ranitidine Most grow out of the condition by 12–18mo. Refer to paediatrics if failing to thrive despite simple measures, chestiness, or anaemia
Colic	Very common in newborns up to ~3mo Repeated bouts of intense, unstoppable crying The baby's body becomes tense and rigid, face goes red, and knees draw up. Often attributed to abdominal pain (although there is no objective evidence) Usually occurs in early evening Examination is normal	Cause is unknown, and symptoms resolve spontaneously with time Advise parents to try colic drops or gripe water There is no evidence that changing from cow's milk to soya-based formula is helpful Refer to paediatrics if diagnosis is in doubt, severe symptoms, other symptoms or signs (e.g. failure to thrive, severe eczema), or fails to resolve by 12wk of age
Crying	📖 p. 910	📖 p. 910

Problems of prematurity

Any baby born at <37wk gestation is considered premature. Worldwide, 11% of babies are born prematurely (7.8% in the UK). Prematurity affects all systems of the body and in general the problems are worse the more premature the baby:

- **32–36wk gestation**—premature. Generally do well—many needing only tube feeding and warmth
- **28–32wk gestation** (1–2% of births)—very preterm. In the UK, ~90% survive
- **<28wk gestation** (0.4% of births)—extremely preterm. Some babies as premature as 23–24wk gestation survive but there is a high incidence of disability

Nutrition Preterm babies <34wk suck and swallow poorly so commonly need nasogastric tube feeding. They are also at particular risk of hypoglycaemia so need frequent feeds. Breast milk—either the mother's or donated milk—is preferred, sometimes with calorie and mineral supplements. If this is not available, special low birthweight formula is used. Vitamin and iron supplements are routine until >6mo of age. Gastro-oesophageal reflux is common.

Thermoregulation Poor in preterm infants, as they have a high surface area-to-body weight ratio and little subcutaneous fat. A controlled temperature and adequate insulation with clothes and blankets, where appropriate, is important.

Respiration

- **Preterm infants >32wk gestation** May have transient tachypnoea at birth due to inability to express fluid from their lungs. Some need oxygen by headbox
- **Preterm infants <32wk gestation** There may be insufficient surfactant produced causing respiratory distress syndrome and requiring surfactant replacement and mechanical ventilation. Incidence and severity is ↓ by antenatal corticosteroids
- **Extremely premature babies** May develop chronic lung disease—defined as being ventilator- or oxygen-dependent at 36wk post-conception—due to *bronchopulmonary dysplasia*. These babies may be sent home on oxygen via nasal cannulae. They are at higher risk from respiratory infections particularly RSV. Episodes of bradycardia and apnoea are common. Have a low threshold for readmission

❶ All babies born prematurely are at ↑ risk of wheezing, asthma, and chest infections—the more premature, the greater the risk.

Prevention of RSV infection

- Take precautions to prevent exposure, e.g. avoiding busy waiting rooms in winter
- Palivizumab is a monoclonal antibody indicated for the prevention of RSV infection in infants at high risk of infection. Prescribe *only* under specialist supervision. Give the first dose before the start of the RSV season and then give monthly throughout the RSV season

Jaundice The immature liver is less able to process bilirubin so premature babies are at greater risk of developing neonatal jaundice. They are also more likely to develop kernicterus so have a lower threshold to refer for phototherapy.

Infection The immune system is poorly developed, so there is greater risk of infection. Furthermore these babies exhibit few signs, so have a low threshold to refer to paediatrics for a septic screen and antibiotics.

Anaemia Low iron stores, ↓ red cell survival, low levels of erythropoietin and repeated venepuncture lead to anaemia in premature babies. Some very premature babies may need repeated transfusion. Iron supplements are routinely given to most premature babies and should be continued until >6mo old.

Neurology Periventricular haemorrhages are common in very preterm babies. Small haemorrhages may have few consequences but more significant bleeds can lead to cystic leucomalacia, hydrocephalus, and neurodevelopmental problems—in particular cerebral palsy. Hypoxia and severe illness in the neonatal period can also lead to cerebral damage and learning disability.

Vision Retinopathy of prematurity (abnormal vascularization) may occur in very premature babies and may result in visual impairment—even blindness. All babies born at <32wk gestation or <1,501g birthweight should have ophthalmological examination prior to discharge from hospital but may need follow-up and/or laser treatment once home.

Hearing Babies requiring neonatal intensive or special care have ↑ risk of hearing problems (10–20x ↑ prevalence of significant bilateral hearing loss). They should have neonatal screening prior to discharge from hospital and appropriate follow-up.

Bonding Separation of mother and premature baby is often necessary. Poor bonding is common—and the problem is added to by fear of losing the baby. In many special care units, periods of 'kangaroo mother care' are used to improve bonding—the baby is nursed skin-to-skin attached to the mother/father's chest. Parents may be (quite understandably) very anxious when their babies first come home after a long period in special care and need more support and reassurance than other new parents.

Cot death Premature babies have ↑ risk of cot death:
- Prevention 📖 p. 847
- Management 📖 p. 926

Information and support for parents of premature babies
Bliss Support Line ☎ 0500 618 140 🖰 www.bliss.org.uk

Neonatal jaundice

Neonatal jaundice[N] In the first few days of life, most babies have ↑ serum bilirubin levels as the liver takes over the excretion of bilirubin from the placenta. Mild jaundice from age 2–6d is physiological and harmless. However, very high levels of unconjugated bilirubin are toxic, crossing the blood–brain barrier and causing encephalopathy (*kernicterus*).

High-risk babies Who require an extra visual check for jaundice in the first 48h of life include:
- Babies born at <38wk gestation
- Babies who have siblings who required phototherapy
- Babies whose mothers intend to breastfeed exclusively

Jaundice <24h after birth Any jaundice in the first 24h needs immediate referral back to hospital to exclude pathological causes (usually haemolysis or infection) and for monitoring and possible treatment.

Significant jaundice <2wk after birth May be difficult to assess (particularly in a dark-skinned baby)—examine the baby naked in natural light, check the sclera of the eyes, gums, and blanched skin. Arrange bilirubin estimation with a transcutaneous bilirubinometer (usually via midwife or paediatrics). If the bilirubin level is >250micromol/L or a reading cannot be obtained, check serum bilirubin. Refer as in Table 24.5.

Table 24.5 Bilirubin referral thresholds for babies born >38wk gestation

Age (h)	Bilirubin level (micromol/L)	Action	Bilirubin level (micromol/L)	Action
24	>100		>150	
30	>112		>162	
36	>125		>175	
42	>137		>187	
48	>150	Repeat bilirubin measurement in 6–12h	>200	Refer for investigation of underlying cause and consideration of phototherapy
54	>162		>212	
60	>175		>225	
66	>187		>237	
72	>200		>250	
78			>262	
84			>275	
90			>287	
96+			>300	

❶ Treatment thresholds differ according to gestational age at birth. Graphs for all gestational ages are available to download from: ℞ http://guidance.nice.org.uk/CG98/treatmentthresholdgraph/xls/English

Jaundice persisting >2wk (>3wk in preterm babies) Although 10% of breastfed babies are still jaundiced at 1mo of age, it is important to refer to paediatrics to exclude pathological causes, including:

- Hypothyroidism (📖 p. 850)
- Haemolysis
- Infection—particularly UTI (📖 p. 878)
- Liver disease—neonatal hepatitis or biliary atresia

Jaundice at any time If the baby is unwell, has persistently pale, chalky stools and/or dark yellow urine which stains the nappy (baby urine should be almost colourless), then refer. If conjugated bilirubin is >25micromol/L expert advice is essential.

Neonatal hepatitis Presents with persistent neonatal jaundice. Always requires specialist investigation and management. Possible causes:

- Congenital infection, e.g. HBV
- Cystic fibrosis
- Galactosaemia
- Glycogen storage diseases
- α_1-antitrypsin deficiency

Galactosaemia Inborn error of metabolism characterized by ↑ plasma galactose. Clinical manifestations depend on enzyme defect:

- **Galactokinase deficiency** Autosomal recessive inheritance. *Incidence:* 1/40,000. Presents in childhood with cataracts. Treatment involves a galactose-free diet
- **Classic galactosaemia** Autosomal recessive inheritance. *Incidence:* 1/44,000. The child appears normal at birth but becomes anorexic and jaundiced within a few days or weeks of consuming breast milk or lactose-containing formula. Vomiting, poor growth, hepatomegaly, and septicaemia are common and can be rapidly fatal. Treatment involves eliminating all sources of galactose in the diet. Long-term complications —poor growth, learning difficulty, infertility, speech and neurological abnormalities—are common

Biliary atresia *Incidence:* 1/15,000. End-stage of a sclerosing process in an initially patent biliary tree. Cause is unclear. Presents with jaundice in neonates. Prognosis has improved with laparotomy and porto-enterostomy which relieves the problem in ~50–70% of babies.

❶ Early diagnosis is particularly important so that surgery can be carried out <2mo after birth before the liver is irreversibly damaged.

Persistent physiological/breast milk jaundice Diagnosed when other causes of prolonged jaundice have been excluded. Reassure parents. Offer breastfeeding support if needed. Monitor to ensure subsides.

Further information
NICE Neonatal jaundice (2010) ℘ www.nice.org.uk

Support for parents
Children's Liver Disease Foundation ☎ 0121 212 3839
℘ www.childliverdisease.org

Feeding babies

Breastfeeding Preferred way to feed infants from birth until fully weaned or longer. However, ~1 in 3 mothers who start breastfeeding have stopped by 6wk. Most wish to continue, but problems with painful breasts/nipples, concern regarding amount of milk the baby is getting and lack of support are common reasons for stopping. Breastfeeding is something some find natural and others find difficult. Teaching mother and baby to breastfeed takes time and patience. Be supportive; ask a midwife, health visitor, or local breastfeeding advisor to help if needed.

Advantages of breast feeding

- Encourages a strong bond between mother and baby
- More convenient than bottle-feeding—the milk is ready warmed and there is no need for sterilized bottles
- Cheaper than bottle-feeding
- Protects the baby from infection
- ↓ risk of sudden infant death
- ↓ postpartum bleeding
- ↓ childhood obesity
- ↓ childhood atopy
- Possible ↓ risk of DM for baby and mother in later life
- Helps the mother ↓ weight after pregnancy
- Protects the mother against breast and ovarian cancer

Common problems with breastfeeding See Table 24.6.

Bottle-feeding

Cow's milk formula feeds Cow's milk altered to simulate the composition of human milk, with added iron and vitamins. Advise parents to choose a formula suitable for their baby and make it up exactly as the manufacturer directs. Advise parents to wash feeding bottles/teats well and sterilize them until >6mo of age. Use a cup rather than bottle >6mo.

Follow-on formula Contains more iron and casein. Not essential unless a child is not taking solids and is >6mo old. Baby milk suitable from birth can be used until a switch is made to normal cow's milk.

Unmodified cow's milk Not recommended until the baby is >1y old as less digestible and contains little iron.

Hydrolysed protein and amino acid infant formulae (e.g. Nutramigen®, Neocate®, Aptamil® pepti) are available on prescription for children with proven cow's milk protein allergy, lactose intolerance, or galactosaemia.

Soya protein-based formula Not recommended for babies <6mo of age because of concerns regarding phyto-oestrogen content. Prescribe only on consultant advice.

Healthy Start Vouchers that can be used to obtain infant formula milk, fruit, vegetables, and free vitamins are available for mothers of babies <1y and for children aged 6mo–4y from low-income households.

Further information

Drugs in Lactation Advisory Service ℘ www.ukmicentral.nhs.uk
UNICEF Baby Friendly Initiative ℘ www.babyfriendly.org.uk

Table 24.6 Common problems with breastfeeding

Problem	Possible solutions
Painful breasts and/ or nipples	Ensure correct positioning
	Treat mastitis or thrush if present
Feeding difficult despite correct positioning	Consider tongue tie. If severe, refer for frenulotomy
It is difficult to know how much milk the baby is taking at each feed	Encourage demand feeding and tell mothers to exhaust milk supply in one breast before starting the other
	Plot weight. If there are concerns about weight gain, consider other causes of failure to thrive—📖 p. 872
Breast milk does not contain all the nutrients the baby needs	Breast milk has low levels of vitamin K, D, and iron
	Ensure babies who have had oral vitamin K at birth receive additional vitamin K supplements
	Encourage weaning at 6mo
	Lactating mothers and babies from 6 months can be given vitamin D supplements if needed. Iron drops can be given to babies with low iron reserves (e.g. low birthweight, maternal anaemia)
Only the mother can feed the baby	Mothers who anticipate they will be absent from the baby for a period of time can express milk for someone else to feed to the baby in a bottle whilst they are gone. Advise mothers not to attempt this before breastfeeding is well established as the baby might find the two techniques confusing
	Two methods are commonly used:
	• Using a commercially available breast pump, or
	• By hand into a sterile bowl
	Breast milk can be frozen (special bags are available) and defrosted when required. Bottles should be sterilized and the milk warmed in the same way as for bottle-feeding
Disease can be transferred in breast milk	In general breast milk protects the baby from disease
	Some diseases can be transferred in breast milk, e.g. hepatitis B or HIV. Bottle-feeding is recommended where uncontaminated water is available
Drugs taken by the mother may have adverse effects on the baby	Mothers should take medical advice before taking any drugs (including herbal remedies). For most conditions drugs safe for use whilst breastfeeding are available
	Rarely breastfeeding is contraindicated, e.g. for women taking lithium or on chemotherapy

Sources of support for breastfeeding mothers

National Childbirth Trust (NCT) ☎ 0300 3300 700 🖰 www.nct.org.uk

La Leche League ☎ 0845 120 2918 🖰 www.laleche.org.uk

Baby Café 🖰 www.thebabycafe.org.uk

Association of Breastfeeding Mothers ☎ 0300 330 5453
🖰 www.abm.me.uk

Breastfeeding Network ☎ 0300 100 0212
🖰 www.breastfeedingnetwork.org.uk

Weaning, feeding problems, and failure to thrive

Weaning Current guidelines recommend solids should be introduced at ~6mo, although they stress individual needs of infants and choices of parents should be considered and supported. Earlier introduction of solids is linked with ↑ rates of infection and ↑ incidence of allergy and intolerance to certain foods, e.g. gluten or eggs.

Advice for parents on weaning
- Introduce solids at ~6mo of age (never <17wk)—babies are ready when they can sit up; mouth objects; are interested in food and chewing; and can reach and grab accurately
- If starting solids when the baby is <6mo old, sterilize feeding bowls/cutlery before use, and avoid egg, gluten, and fish until baby is >6mo
- Start with a few teaspoons of mashed fruit, vegetable, or cereal, and progress to home-made purées or mashed up family food without added salt/sugar. It is usual for stool to change consistency on weaning
- Babies take time to learn how to feed from a spoon and it may be messy. Wait for the baby to open his/her mouth, and allow babies to touch the food. Initially babies may only take 2–3 teaspoons/meal
- Gradually offer a wide variety of different foods and textures. Do not give raw eggs or honey to babies <1y
- Encourage 'finger foods' as soon as the baby can feed him/herself—try pieces of soft fruit, vegetable, or toast
- Continue giving the baby breast or formula milk—this is the main source of food until 1y

Feeding problems Parents commonly complain their child is not eating enough or eating the wrong foods. Look for underlying problems if the child is not growing or developing as normal.

Normal growth/development Reassure the parents that it is normal for the amount of food eaten to vary from day to day. Consider referral to the health visitor for advice/support. Advise parents to:
- Sit down for family meals wherever possible
- Restrict snacks and sugary drinks between meals
- Show little emotion when putting food in front of the child at meal times and remove the food after 15–20min without comment about what is or is not eaten; praise children when they have eaten well

Failure to thrive (faltering growth) Failure to gain weight in infancy as expected is a common problem. Usually head circumference is preserved relative to length and length relative to weight. Use UK-WHO growth charts for breastfed babies. Defined as:
- Weight consistently <3rd centile for age, or
- Progressive ↓ in weight over ≥2 major centile lines

Non-organic causes
- Lack of food due to neglect, lack of education, poverty, or famine
- Emotional problems e.g. emotional neglect, unhappy family, or other difficulties at home—this is the most common cause

Organic causes
- Chronic infection
- Heart disease
- Gastrointestinal disease, e.g. coeliac disease, chronic diarrhoea
- Metabolic disease, e.g. DM
- Respiratory disease, e.g. chronic lung disease, cystic fibrosis
- Physical feeding problems, e.g. cleft palate, pyloric stenosis

Assessment
- Ask how the child is fed—quantities, times of the day. Check formula feeds are being made up correctly
- Ask about feeding problems, e.g. regurgitation of food, vomiting
- Ask about other physical problems, e.g. breathlessness, diarrhoea
- Examine the child carefully from top to toe looking for any physical abnormalities or signs of developmental delay
- Watch the way the child interacts with you and the parent; look for evidence of neglect or maltreatment
- Look at the size of the parents—small parents have small children

Management Treat any reversible causes. Continue to measure weight, length, and head circumference regularly. Try to use the same scales on each occasion. *Refer to paediatrics:*
- If no cause for failure to thrive is found or if, despite treatment of a reversible cause, the child continues to lose or fails to gain weight
- If an abnormality requiring paediatric care is found—urgency depends on the nature of the abnormality and degree of failure to thrive

Pyloric stenosis Infantile hypertrophic pyloric stenosis usually develops in the first 3–6wk of life (rare >12wk). Failure of the pyloric sphincter to relax results in hypertrophy of the adjacent pyloric muscle. Typically affects firstborn, male infants. Pyloric stenosis runs in families and is associated with Turner's syndrome, PKU, and oesophageal atresia.

Presentation
- **Projectile vomiting** Milk—no bile. The child is still hungry after vomiting and immediately feeds again. Rarely there is haematemesis
- **Failure to thrive**
- **Dehydration and constipation** ('rabbit pellet stools')
- **Pyloric mass** (feels like an olive) is palpable in the right upper abdomen (95%)—especially if the child has just vomited
- **Visible peristalsis** In the epigastrium after a test feed

Differential diagnosis
- Possetting/reflux
- Milk allergy
- Uraemia
- Overfeeding
- Infection—especially UTI
- Adrenal insufficiency
- Gastroenteritis
- ↑ intracranial pressure
- Other causes of intestinal obstruction

Management Admit or refer urgently to paediatric surgery. After rehydration and investigation to confirm diagnosis, treatment is surgical with a Ramstedt's pyloroplasty. There are usually no long-term effects.

Information and support for parents
Birth to Five Available from ✆ www.dh.gov.uk
Parentline ✆ 0808 800 2222 ✆ www.familylives.org.uk

Fever and acute illness in the under 5s

Assessing sick children can be difficult. Infants <6mo old can be particularly difficult to assess and may deteriorate rapidly over a short period of time. Take parents concerns seriously. Physical signs are often absent or deceptive. One approach is to exclude 'alarm' symptoms and signs that might point to serious illness. In general, the younger the baby, the lower your threshold should be for seeking a paediatrician's opinion.

Remote assessment[N] Ask about the features listed in Table 24.7.
- If symptoms/signs suggesting life-threatening disease (e.g. compromised airway, breathing or circulation, or ↓ level of consciousness)—arrange for immediate hospital transfer as an emergency
- Children with any **Red** features are at high risk of serious illness. If there are no features of an immediately life-threatening illness, arrange for review by a doctor in a face-to-face setting in <2h
- **Amber** features indicate intermediate risk of serious illness. Arrange for assessment by a doctor in a face-to-face setting the same day
- Children with all **Green** features and no **Amber** or **Red** features are at low risk of serious illness and often can be managed with advice

Face-to-face assessment[N] Take a history and perform a *full* physical examination, including temperature, respiratory rate, heart rate, and capillary return. Assess for features of serious disease (see Table 24.7). Remember to check under clothing and nappies for rashes. Localizing signs may be absent (e.g. tonsillitis may cause vomiting in small children).

Further management
- If any **Red** symptoms or signs are present, refer to a paediatrician for immediate or same-day review, depending on clinical state of the child
- If any **Amber** symptoms or signs are present, and a cause is found, treat the cause. If no diagnosis is made, decide on further action based on knowledge of the family and the clinical state of the child. 3 options:
  - Advise the child's parents to call you if there is any deterioration (give advice about symptoms/signs they should watch for) or if the child fails to improve within a defined period of time
  - Arrange to review the child again within a few hours, *or*
  - Refer for paediatric review
- If all the **Green** features and no **Amber** or **Red** features are present, give advice about management at home and symptoms/signs that should prompt carers to seek further advice

 ❶ Do not prescribe antibiotics for fever of unknown cause.

Common causes of pyrexia Childhood infections are the most common cause of fever amongst children in general practice (📖 p. 876). Consider UTI if no localizing symptoms/signs. Think of TB and endocarditis—especially in high-risk patients. Do not forget tropical diseases, e.g. malaria in children returning from abroad.

Other causes of pyrexia (may present as prolonged fever) Include: malignancy (e.g. lymphoma, leukaemia), immunological causes (e.g. Still's or Kawasaki disease); drugs (e.g. antibiotics); and liver or renal disease.

Table 24.7 Traffic light system for assessment of children with fever[N]

⚠ Red—high risk symptoms/signs	Amber—intermediate risk symptoms/signs	Green—low risk symptoms/signs
Appears ill	Pallor	Normal colour of skin/lips/tongue
Colour—pale, mottled, ashen or blue	↓ response to social cues	Responds normally to social cues
No response to social cues	Wakes only with excessive stimulation	Content/smiles
Does not wake or if roused does not stay awake	↓ activity	Stays awake or awakens quickly
Weak, high-pitched or continuous cry	No smile	Strong normal cry or not crying
Grunting	Nasal flaring	Normal skin/eye turgor
Respiratory rate >60/min	↑ respiratory rate (>50/min—aged 6–12mo; >40/min aged >12mo)	Moist mucus membranes
Moderate/severe chest indrawing	Oxygen saturation ≤95% in air	None of the amber/red symptoms or signs
↓ skin turgor	Crackles in chest	
High temperature of ≥38°C aged <3mo	Tachycardia (>160bpm age <12mo; >150bpm age 12–24mo; >140bpm age 2–5y)	
Non-blanching rash	Capillary return ≥3s	
Bulging fontanelle	High temperature ≥39°C age 3–6mo	
Neck stiffness	Rigors	
Status epilepticus	Dry mucous membranes	
Focal neurological signs/seizures	Poor feeding in infants	
	↓ urine output	
	Swelling of a limb/joint	
	Non-weight bearing/not using an extremity	

Measuring temperature For infants <4wk old, measure temperature with an electronic thermometer in the axilla. For children aged ≥4wk use an electronic or chemical dot thermometer in the axilla or infrared tympanic thermometer in the ear.

Febrile convulsions 📖 p. 897

Acute illness in non-febrile children Sick children do not have to have a fever. The following are indications for referral for immediate or same-day paediatric review:
- Any symptoms or signs in the **Red** column of Table 24.7
- Persistent vomiting—more than half of the previous 3 feeds or bile stained
- Frank blood in the stools or urine
- History suggestive of apnoeic episodes

Further information

Spotting the sick child 🖰 www.spottingthesickchild.com
NICE Feverish illness in children: (2013) 🖰 www.nice.org.uk

Childhood infection

Table 24.8 A–Z of childhood infection

Infection	Page	Infection	Page
Chickenpox	📖 p. 652	Malaria	📖 p. 648
Conjunctivitis	📖 p. 966	Measles	📖 p. 652
Croup	📖 p. 937	Molluscum contagiosum	📖 p. 635
Diphtheria	📖 p. 657	Mumps	📖 p. 652
Epiglottitis	📖 p. 947	Otitis media	📖 p. 946
Erythema infectiosum	📖 p. 652	Polio	📖 p. 579
Gastroenteritis	📖 p. 410	Roseola infantum	📖 p. 652
Glandular fever	📖 p. 935	Rubella	📖 p. 652
Hand, foot, and mouth	📖 p. 652	Scabies	📖 p. 639
Head lice	📖 p. 638	Scarlet fever	📖 p. 655
Hepatitis A	📖 p. 422	Shingles	📖 p. 653
Hepatitis B/C	📖 p. 742	Sinusitis	📖 p. 942
Herpes	📖 p. 634	Skin infection	📖 p. 632
HIV	📖 p. 746	TB	📖 p. 326
Impetigo	📖 p. 632	Tonsillitis	📖 p. 934
Influenza	📖 p. 322	UTI in childhood	📖 p. 878
Kawasaki disease	📖 p. 527	Warts and verrucas	📖 p. 634
Lyme disease	📖 p. 599	Whooping cough	📖 p. 328

Viral upper respiratory tract infection (URTI) Very common. Children have >5 URTIs each year. Presents with coryza, runny eyes, and malaise. The child may also have a mild pyrexia and/or a non-specific maculopapular rash.

Management Examine to exclude tonsillitis and otitis media. If pyrexia but no other symptoms/signs, check urine to exclude UTI. Most viral URTIs settle within a few days.

Childhood pneumonia May be viral, bacterial (pneumococcal, Hib, or staphylococcal), or atypical (e.g. mycoplasma). Presents with ≥1 of:
- Fever—recurrent or persistent >38.5°C • Cough
- Chest and/or abdominal pain
- Tachypnoea, recession or other signs of respiratory difficulty
- Crepitations, ↓ breath sounds ± bronchial breathing

Management
- **Severe** If oxygen saturation <92%, cyanosis, tachypnoea (>70 breaths/min aged <1y; >50 breaths/min aged >1y), or difficulty breathing/grunting; dehydrated (or not feeding if <1y); not responding to antibiotics or the family are unable to manage—admit

- **Less severe** Manage in the community. Provide advice about management of fever and hydration. Prescribe antibiotics—amoxicillin is first-line; consider a macrolide if penicillin-allergic, mycoplasma or chlamydia is suspected as the cause of the infection or in addition to amoxicillin if first-line treatment is ineffective. Co-amoxiclav is the antibiotic of choice if pneumonia is associated with influenza. Advise parents to bring the child back for review if no better in 48h or worse in the interim

❶ Children <2y with mild symptoms of LRTI do not usually have pneumonia and may not need antibiotics. Reassess if symptoms persist.

Prevention Pneumococcal vaccination is now part of the routine childhood vaccination programme and is given at 2, 4, and 13mo.

Recurrent chest infection Consider further investigation and/or referral to look for an underlying cause if a child has a history of ≥2 probable chest infections. Possible underlying causes include:

- Asthma
- Post-infective bronchiectasis
- Oropharyngeal aspiration, e.g. due to reflux
- Congenital heart/lung defects
- Sickle cell anaemia
- Foreign body
- TB
- Cystic fibrosis
- Immune disorders, e.g. HIV, hypogammaglobulinaemia, leukaemia
- 🖝 Right middle lobe syndrome

Bronchiolitis Occurs in epidemics—usually in the winter months. Most episodes are due to respiratory syncitial virus (RSV) infection. Usually infects infants <1y old and presents with coryza ± fever progressing to irritable cough, rapid breathing ± feeding difficulty.

Examination Tachypnoea, tachycardia, widespread crepitations over the lung fields ± high-pitched wheeze.

Management Depends on severity of the symptoms.

- **Mild** Feeding well, no/mild recession, oxygen saturation >95%—advise paracetamol suspension as required and fluids. Warn carers about symptoms/signs of worsening illness
- **More severe** Lethargy, taking <½ usual feeds, dehydrated, intercostal recession ± nasal flaring, grunting, respiratory rate >70, cyanosis, oxygen saturation <95% or apnoeic episodes—admit as a paediatric emergency

High-risk infants Include:

- Premature babies
- Babies <6wk old
- Children with underlying lung disease, congenital heart disease, or immunosuppression

Have a low threshold for admission. Palivizumab, a monoclonal antibody, may be used as prophylaxis (📖 p. 866).

Prognosis Most recover fully in 10–14d. Up to half wheeze with subsequent viral URTIs.

Further information

British Thoracic Society Guidelines for the management of community acquired pneumonia in children (2011) ℛ www.brit-thoracic.org.uk

Urinary tract infection in childhood

10% girls and 3.5% boys have a urinary tract infection (UTI) in childhood—the majority in the first year of life. Amongst neonates, boys have more infections than girls. In all other age groups, ♀:♂ ≈ 10:1. 80% infections are due to *E. coli*.

Risk factors
- Poor urine flow
- History suggesting/confirmed past UTI
- Recurrent fever of unknown origin
- Antenatally diagnosed renal abnormality
- Family history of vesicoureteric reflux (VUR) or renal disease
- Constipation
- Dysfunctional voiding
- Enlarged bladder
- Abdominal mass
- Spinal lesion
- Poor growth
- High blood pressure

Consequences 5–15% develop renal scarring <2y after first infection. Infections causing renal scarring are associated with adult pyelonephritis, ↑ BP, impaired renal function, and renal failure. Prognosis is worst for children with recurrent infection, VUR, and scarring at first presentation.

Clinical presentation Depends on age and site of infection:
- **Infants and toddlers** Usually non-specific with vomiting, irritability, fever, abdominal pain, failure to thrive, and prolonged jaundice
- **Older children** Dysuria, ↑ frequency, abdominal pain, haematuria, enuresis
- **Site** Fever >38°C and/or loin pain/tenderness suggests upper UTI/acute pyelonephritis

Management[N]

Presentation with fever Suspect UTI in any child with fever >38°C with no obvious cause. Use the traffic light system (□ p. 875) to guide management. If any **Red** features, admit/refer for emergency assessment.

Urine testing Check sample if signs/symptoms of UTI, unexplained fever, or if a child fails to recover from a fever presumed due to another cause. A clean catch specimen is best. Otherwise collect using a special bag/pad.
- **If >3y**—dipstick urine. Send a sample for M,C&S if nitrite or leucocyte +ve, strong clinical suspicion of UTI, PMH of UTI, or other risk factors
- **If <3y**—dipstick urine if acutely unwell and urgent microscopy is not available. Else (and additionally) send a urine for M,C&S

Treatment of children <3y
- **With symptoms/signs of UTI**—check M,C&S and start antibiotics
- **Well with non-specific symptoms**—check M,C&S. Act on result
- **Unwell with non-specific symptoms**—check M,C&S. If urgent microscopy is not available, check urine dipstick—see Table 24.9

Treatment of children >3y Perform a urine dipstick and act on the results—see Table 24.9.

Antibiotics Trimethoprim bd for 3d for lower UTI and 7–10d for upper UTI. Review after 24–48h if not improving and send urine for M,C&S if a sample has not already been sent.

Table 24.9 Management based on urine dipstick testing[N]

Dipstick result		Management
Leukocyte esterase	Nitrite	
Positive	Positive	Start antibiotics
		If the child is <3y, or the child is unwell, or the child has a past history of urinary infection, send a sample for M,C&S
Negative	Positive	Start antibiotics; send urine for M,C&S
Positive	Negative	Send urine for M,C&S; only start antibiotics if there is strong clinical evidence for UTI or if UTI is proven on laboratory testing
Negative	Negative	Do not start treatment for UTI. Look for other possible causes of the child's symptoms
		Send urine for M,C&S if:
		• Clinical features of UTI despite dipstick results
		• The child appears unwell with no apparent cause
		• The child is <3y of age
		• The child has a past history of urine infection

Follow-up Do not check M,C&S to confirm eradication. Only start prophylactic antibiotics (trimethoprim 1–2mg/kg nocte) if >1 UTI. Treat any constipation. Advise to drink plenty of fluids.

Further investigation

Children <6mo responding to antibiotics in <48h Arrange USS ± micturating cystourethrogram (MCUG) depending on USS findings.

Children of any age with atypical infection (defined as: child very unwell, response to antibiotics took >48h, poor urine flow, abdominal/bladder mass, ↑ Cr, and/or non-*E. coli* infection). Arrange:
• Urgent USS
• DMSA scan if <3y of age, and
• MCUG if <6mo, or if <3y *and* dilation on USS, poor urine flow, non-*E. coli* infection, or FH of VUR

Children of any age with recurrent infection (defined as: ≥2 upper UTI; 1 upper UTI + ≥1 lower UTI or ≥3 lower UTI). Arrange:
• USS (urgent if <6mo old) and DMSA scan, and
• MCUG if <6mo

Balanitis 📖 p. 464

Epididymo-orchitis 📖 p. 466

Horseshoe kidney, ectopic kidney, double ureter Common malformations of the urinary tract. Usually do not affect kidney function per se but predispose to UTI. Recurrent infections may eventually cause renal damage.

Further information

NICE Urinary tract infection in children (2007) ℘ www.nice.org.uk

Congenital heart disease

Common affecting ~6 in 1,000 live births. Congenital heart disease is the major cause of heart disease in children.

Detection

Antenatal screening ~50% of severe congenital heart disease is detected *in utero* by USS. If detected during the routine 10–13wk or 18wk anomaly scan, amniocentesis is routinely offered to screen for Down's syndrome (~1 in 20 have heart disease—especially PDA, ASD, and/or VSD) and other chromosomal abnormalities.

Clinical examination Neonatal examination detects <50% of cardiac malformations not detected antenatally. The rest are detected if a murmur is found incidentally when examining the child for another reason or when the child becomes symptomatic.

Presentation

Murmur on routine examination
- **Ventriculoseptal defect (VSD)** Harsh pansystolic murmur with splitting of the 2nd heart sound
- **Atrioseptal defect (ASD)** Systolic murmur in the pulmonary area with fixed splitting of the 2nd heart sound
- **Patent ductus arteriosus (PDA)** Loud, continual 'machinery' murmur
- **Aortic stenosis** Ejection systolic murmur at the apex and left sternal edge with a soft and delayed 2nd heart sound. Slow rising pulse, ↓ BP. Rarely dizziness, faintness, or loss of consciousness on exertion
- **Pulmonary stenosis** Ejection systolic murmur with ejection click
- **Coarctation of the aorta** Ejection systolic murmur over the left side and back; absent/delayed femoral pulses and ↑ BP in upper limbs

Innocent murmurs Murmurs are a common finding in childhood particularly when examining a febrile child. The majority are not associated with heart disease—so-called 'innocent murmurs'. *Features:*
- Asymptomatic
- Soft, systolic murmur—may vary with position and does not radiate
- Normal 2nd heart sound
- No other associated signs of heart disease (normal pulses, no thrill)

Once a murmur has is known to be 'innocent', explain what that means to the parents—otherwise there may be unnecessary ongoing anxiety.

⚠ Unless the child is febrile when the murmur is heard and it disappears once afebrile, refer all children with murmurs for echo or paediatric evaluation—whether the murmur is detected at routine screening, incidentally when examining the chest for another reason, or when examined because symptomatic.

Cyanosis

- **<48h old** Likely to be due to transposition of the great arteries or severe pulmonary stenosis
- **Later presentation** Mostly due to *Tetralogy of Fallot* (see Table 24.10)

Table 24.10 Congenital cardiac abnormalities

Condition	Features
ASD	📖 p. 881
Coarctation of the aorta	📖 p. 282
Tetralogy of Fallot	Large VSD and pulmonary stenosis
	In the newborn period may present with a murmur
	Progressive cyanosis then develops over the next weeks/years ± ↓ exercise tolerance ± squatting after exercise
	Treatment is surgical
Hypoplastic left heart	Left ventricle ± mitral valve, aortic valve, and aortic arch are underdeveloped
	Presents within the 1st few days of life with heart failure
	Treatment is surgical or with heart transplant
Patent ductus arteriosus (PDA)	The ductus arteriosus fails to close after birth
	♀ > ♂. Associated with prematurity
	Symptoms depend on the size of the shunt. Presents with murmur ± failure to thrive ± heart failure
	Treatment is usually surgical closure
Transposition of the great arteries	The aorta arises from the right ventricle and the pulmonary artery from the left
	Progressive cyanosis develops within a few hours of birth
	Treatment is surgical
Valve disease	📖 p. 280
VSD	📖 p. 282

Heart failure
- Breathlessness particularly when crying/feeding
- Failure to thrive
- Sweating
- Fast respiratory and pulse rates
- Heart enlargement
- Liver enlargement
- Weight ↑ due to fluid retention

Causes of heart failure in the first week of life include:
- Left outflow obstruction
- Severe aortic stenosis
- Coarctation of the aorta
- Hypoplastic left heart

Later causes:
- Large VSD
- PDA
- Ostium primum ASD

Management In all cases, if new congenital heart disease is suspected, refer for specialist paediatric or cardiology opinion. Specialist treatment of valve lesions depends on the gradient measured across the valve. Most other congenital cardiac lesions (except some VSDs and ASDs) require surgery—staged for complex lesions.

Information and support
Children's Heart Federation 📞 0808 808 5000 🖰 www.chfed.org.uk

Diagnosis of asthma in children

Childhood asthma affects ~5% of children in the UK. Peak age of onset is 5y. 40 children/y in the UK still die from asthma.

Diagnosis Is clinical—based on recognizing a characteristic pattern of episodic symptoms in the absence of an alternative explanation. Asthma is likely if the child has >1 of the following symptoms:

- Wheeze
- Cough
- Difficulty breathing
- Chest tightness

Particularly if these symptoms:

- Are frequent and recurrent
- Occur apart from URTIs
- Are worse at night/in the early morning
- Occur in response to, or are worse after, exercise, other triggers (e.g. pets, cold/damp air) or with emotions/laughter

Other factors that ↑ the likelihood of asthma include

- Personal history of atopic disorder—probability of asthma in a child with wheeze is ↑ if: +ve skin tests, blood eosinophilia ≥4%, and/or ↑ specific IgE to cat, dog, or mite
- Family history of atopic disorder and/or asthma—the strongest association is with maternal atopy
- Widespread wheeze heard on auscultation
- History of improvement in symptoms or lung function in response to asthma therapy

Clinical features that ↓ the likelihood of asthma include

- Symptoms with colds only, with no interval symptoms— virus-associated wheeze affects up to 20% of children at some point
- Isolated cough in the absence of wheeze or difficulty breathing
- History of moist cough
- Prominent dizziness, light-headedness, peripheral tingling
- Repeatedly normal physical examination of chest when symptomatic
- Normal PEFR or spirometry when symptomatic
- No response to a trial of asthma therapy
- Clinical features pointing to an alternative diagnosis

Further action Based on history and examination, decide how likely the probability of asthma is:

High probability Start a trial of treatment (📖 p. 884). Review and assess response. Reserve further testing for those with a poor response.

Intermediate probability In some children (particularly if <5y) there are not enough features to make a firm diagnosis of asthma, but no features suggesting an alternative diagnosis. There are three possible approaches to reaching a diagnosis:

- **Watchful waiting with review** If mild, intermittent wheeze and/or symptoms that occur only with viral URTIs
- **Trial of treatment with review** Bronchodilators and/or corticosteroids. Choice depends on frequency and severity of symptoms.
  - If a treatment is beneficial, a diagnosis of asthma is probable. Find the minimum effective dose of therapy. At a later point consider a trial of reduction/withdrawal of therapy

- If it is unclear if a child has improved, try withdrawing the treatment. If treatment is not beneficial, consider further testing and/or referral
- **Spirometry** Possible >5y. ❶ Normal spirometry/PEFR testing, if performed when the child is asymptomatic, does not exclude asthma.
  - If evidence of airway obstruction, assess change in FEV_1 in response to bronchodilator and/or reponse to treatment. ↑ in FEV_1 of >12% from baseline and/or beneficial treatment trial supports a diagnosis of asthma. Otherwise consider further testing and/or referral
  - If no evidence of airways obstruction—consider testing for atopic status, bronchodilator reversibility when symptomatic (using home PEFR) and/or bronchial hyper-responsiveness (e.g. exercise challenge in those with symptoms brought on by exercise). Consider specialist referral

If low probability of asthma Consider more detailed investigation and/or specialist referral.

❶ Do a CXR if severe disease or clinical suggestion of another condition.

Reasons for referral *E* = Emergency; *U* = Urgent; *S* = Soon; *R* = Routine
- Severe exacerbation of asthma or severe URTI—*E*
- Unexpected clinical findings, e.g. focal signs, abnormal voice or cry, dysphagia, inspiratory stridor—*E/U*
- Persistent wet or productive cough—*U/S*
- Failure to thrive—*U/S*
- Diagnosis unclear or in doubt—*U/S/R*
- Failure to respond to conventional treatment (particularly inhaled corticosteroids >400 micrograms/d or frequent use of steroid tablets)—*S*
- Excessive vomiting or possetting—*S/R*
- Symptoms present from birth or perinatal lung problem—*S/R*
- Family history of unusual chest disease—*R*
- Nasal polyps—*R*
- Parental anxiety or need for reassurance—*R*

❶ This is only a rough guide; urgency of referral will depend on the clinical state of the child.

Differential diagnosis See Table 24.11, 📖 p. 886

Prognostic factors
- The earlier the onset of wheeze, the better the prognosis—most children presenting at <2y become asymptomatic by mid-childhood
- Male gender—risk factor for asthma in pre-pubertal children—but boys are more likely to 'grow out' of asthma during adolescence
- Coexistent atopy—risk factor for persistence of wheeze
- Frequent/severe episodes of wheezing in childhood—associated with recurrent wheeze that persists into adolescence

Further information
British Thoracic Society/SIGN British guideline on the management of asthma (2011) ℘ www.sign.ac.uk

Information and support for parents and patients
Asthma UK ☏ 0800 1216244 ℘ www.asthma.org.uk

Management of asthma in children

Symptoms/signs of a severe asthma attack in children >2y

- Oxygen saturation <92%
- PEFR 33–50% best/predicted (>5y)
- Too breathless to talk
- ↑ heart rate (>140bpm age 2–5y; >125 bpm >5y)
- ↑ respiratory rate (>40 breaths/min age 2–5y; >30 breaths/min >5y)
- Use of accessory neck muscles

Life-threatening signs in children >2y Oxygen saturation <92% plus ≥1 of:

- PEFR <33% best/predicted (>5y)
- Silent chest (inaudible wheeze)
- Poor respiratory effort
- Agitation
- Cyanosis
- Altered consciousness

Symptoms/signs of a significant asthma attack if <2y

- Oxygen saturation of <92%
- Marked respiratory distress
- Cyanosis
- Too breathless to feed

Life-threatening features

- Episodes of apnoea
- Poor respiratory effort
- Bradycardia

Management of an acute asthma attack 🕮 p. 1095

Aims of treatment

- To minimize symptoms and impact on lifestyle (e.g. absence from school; limitations to physical ability)
- To minimize the need for reliever medication
- To prevent severe attacks/exacerbations

GP services and self-management 🕮 p. 310. For children ensure that the following are checked and recorded at least annually:

- Symptom score, e.g. Children's Asthma Control Test (from 4–11y), Asthma Control Questionnaire (>5y)
- Exacerbations, oral steroid use, and time off school/nursery due to asthma since last check
- Inhaler technique and medication adherence (prescription frequency)
- Personalized asthma self-management action plan
- Exposure to tobacco smoke (e.g. parental smoking)
- Growth—height and weight centile

Drug therapy Use a stepwise approach (see Figure 24.2 and Figure 24.3, 🕮 p. 887). Start at a step appropriate to the initial severity of symptoms. Aim to achieve control of the condition and then ↓ by stepping down.

Exacerbations Treat exacerbations early. A rescue course of prednisolone (30–40mg/d if aged >5y or 20mg/d if aged 2–5y) for 3–14d may be needed at any step and any time. Alternatively, leukotriene antagonists can be used for children with episodic asthma—start at the onset of asthma/coryzal symptoms and continue for 7d.

Short-acting β_2 **agonists** (🕮 p. 306) (e.g. salbutamol). Work more quickly and/or with fewer side effects than alternatives. Use prn unless shown to benefit from regular dosing. Using ≥2 canisters/mo or >10–12 puffs/d is a marker of poorly controlled asthma.

Figure 24.2 Summary of stepwise management in children aged <5y
Reproduced in modified format with permission from the British Thoracic Society and SIGN.

Inhaled corticosteroids (📖 p. 306) Most effective preventer. May be beneficial even for children with mild asthma. Consider if:
- Exacerbations of asthma needing oral corticosteroids in the last 2y
- Using inhaled β_2-agonists ≥3x/wk
- Symptomatic ≥3x/wk or ≥1 night/wk

Oral steroids 📖 p. 306

Add-on therapy Before initiating a new drug, check compliance, inhaler technique, and eliminate trigger factors.
- **Inhaled long-acting β_2 agonists** (📖 p. 306) (e.g. salmeterol). Are first-choice add-on therapy for children aged >5y to improve lung function and symptoms. Do not use without inhaled steroid—use of combination inhalers is recommended. Stop if of no benefit
- **Leukotriene receptor antagonists** (e.g. montelukast). May ↓ symptoms and exacerbations and ↑ lung function. First-choice add-on therapy for children <5y
- **Theophylline or β_2-agonist slow-release tablets** May ↓ symptoms and ↑ lung function but side effects are common

Stepping down Review and consider stepping down at intervals ≥3mo. Maintain on the lowest dose of inhaled steroid controlling symptoms. When reducing steroids, cut dose by 25–50% each time. Children with milder asthma and a clear seasonal pattern can step down more quickly in their good season.

Selection of inhaler device If possible use a metred-dose inhaler. Inadequate technique may be mistaken for drug failure. Emphasize patients must inhale slowly and hold their breath for 10s after inhalation. Demonstrate inhaler technique before prescribing and check at follow-ups. Spacers or breath-activated devices are useful for children who find activation difficult and essential for children <5y. Dry powder inhalers are an alternative for older children.

Expected PEFR in children 📖 p. 304

Allergen avoidance 📖 p. 311

Complementary therapy 📖 p. 312

Asthma in adolescents Common but may be under-diagnosed due to under-reporting of symptoms, so specifically ask about symptoms:
• Breathlessness/wheezing with exercise is common; if due to asthma, it should respond to pre-treatment with a β_2-agonist
• Depression/anxiety may make asthma symptoms more prominent
• Advice about risks of smoking/passive smoking is very important
• Inhaler preference is important in ensuring good treatment adherence
• Complementary or alternative medicine use is common and may be linked with adherence to prescribed medication
• Discuss career choice and highlight occupations that may ↑ symptoms

Table 24.11 Differential diagnosis of wheezing in children

Clinical clue	Possible diagnosis
Perinatal and family history	
Symptoms present from birth or perinatal lung problem	CF, chronic lung disease, ciliary dyskinesia, developmental anomaly
Family history of unusual chest disease	CF, developmental anomaly, neuromuscular disorder
Severe upper respiratory tract disease	Defect of host defence
Symptoms and signs	
Persistent wet cough	CF, recurrent aspiration, host defence disorder
Excessive vomiting or possetting	Reflux ± aspiration
Dysphagia	Swallowing problems ± aspiration
Abnormal voice or cry	Laryngeal problem
Focal signs in the chest	Developmental disease, post-viral syndrome, bronchiectasis, TB
Inspiratory stridor as well as wheeze	Central airways or laryngeal disorder
Failure to thrive	CF, host defence defect, gastro-oesophageal reflux
Investigations	
Focal or persistent radiological changes	Developmental disorder, post-infective disorder, recurrent aspiration, inhaled foreign body, bronchiectasis, TB

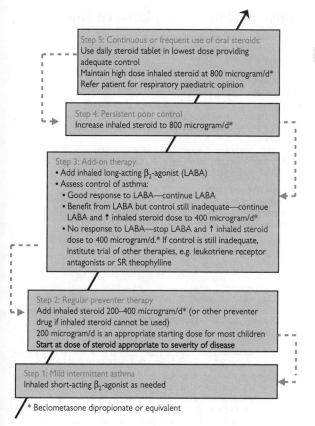

Step 5: Continuous or frequent use of oral steroids:
Use daily steroid tablet in lowest dose providing adequate control
Maintain high dose inhaled steroid at 800 microgram/d*
Refer patient for respiratory paediatric opinion

Step 4: Persistent poor control
Increase inhaled steroid to 800 microgram/d*

Step 3: Add-on therapy
• Add inhaled long-acting β₂-agonist (LABA)
• Assess control of asthma:
  • Good response to LABA—continue LABA
  • Benefit from LABA but control still inadequate—continue LABA and ↑ inhaled steroid dose to 400 microgram/d*
  • No response to LABA—stop LABA and ↑ inhaled steroid dose to 400 microgram/d.* If control is still inadequate, institute trial of other therapies, e.g. leukotriene receptor antagonists or SR theophylline

Step 2: Regular preventer therapy
Add inhaled steroid 200–400 microgram/d* (or other preventer drug if inhaled steroid cannot be used)
200 microgram/d is an appropriate starting dose for most children
Start at dose of steroid appropriate to severity of disease

Step 1: Mild intermittent asthma
Inhaled short-acting β₂-agonist as needed

* Beclometasone dipropionate or equivalent

Figure 24.3 Summary of stepwise management in children aged 5–12y
All doses given refer to beclometasone dipropionate (BDP) administered via metred dose inhaler. For other drugs/formulations, adjust dose accordingly (see *BNF* Section 3)
Reproduced in modified format with permission from the British Thoracic Society and SIGN.

Further information
British Thoracic Society/SIGN British guideline on the management of asthma (2011) ↗ www.sign.ac.uk

Patient information and support
Asthma UK ☎ 0800 1216244 ↗ www.asthma.org.uk

Constipation and malabsorption

Constipation[N] Frequent complaint amongst all age groups of children. Take a careful history—diagnose constipation if ≥2 of:
- Abnormal stool pattern:
  - <3 stool per wk (except breastfed babies >6wk)
  - Hard, large or rabbit-dropping stool
  - Overflow soiling (children >1y)
- Symptoms associated with defaecation:
  - Distress on stooling or anal pain
  - Bleeding associated with hard stool
  - Straining
  - Poor appetite or abdominal pain that improves after stool passed
  - Posture indicating retaining stool (straight legs, back arch, tiptoe)
- History of previous constipation or anal fissure

Serious underlying causes
- Hirschsprung's disease
- Coeliac disease
- Hypothyroidism
- Anorectal abnormalities
- Neurological conditions
- Abdominal tumours

Management Refer for specialist assessment if any red flag symptoms/signs suggesting a serious underlying cause:
- Delay in passing meconium or constipation since birth
- Abnormal appearance, position or patency of the anus
- Ribbon-like stool
- New leg weakness, deformity (e.g talipes), or neuromuscular signs
- Asymmetrical gluteal muscles, sacral naevus, sinus or pit, or scoliosis
- Abdominal distension with vomiting or gross distension

If there is faltering growth, check coeliac serology and TFTs.

Treatment of idiopathic constipation Diagnose if serious underlying causes have been excluded. Use a macrogol as first-line laxative adjusting dose according to response. Add a stimulant laxative if ineffective. If macrogols are not tolerated use a stimulant ± alternative softener. Continue medication for several weeks after regular bowel habit has been established. In addition to medication, advise about balanced diet and adequate fluid intake. Refer for specialist assessment if not responding to treatment in ≤3mo (≤1mo if <1y old).

Diarrhoea and vomiting 📖 p. 376

Malabsorption In all cases refer for investigation and treatment of the cause. Usually presents with:
- Chronic diarrhoea
- Failure to thrive or weight ↓
- Steatorrhoea, and/or
- Iron or other nutrient deficiency

Causes in children
- **Common** Cow's milk intolerance (cow's milk protein allergy, or lactose intolerance); coeliac disease
- **Rarer** Cystic fibrosis; chronic infection (e.g. giardiasis); inflammatory bowel disease

Cow's milk protein allergy Affects ~3% of children. Mainly occurs in bottle-fed infants <6mo old but affects 0.5% of purely breastfed babies as cow's milk protein from the mother's diet is secreted in breast milk.

Presentation May be family history. Often affects >1 body system:
- **Gastrointestinal symptoms** (50–60%). Diarrhoea (occasionally with blood); colic; less commonly constipation
- **Skin symptoms** (50–70%). Urticaria; eczema
- **Respiratory and other symptoms** (20–30%). Wheeze; rhinitis; conjunctivitis

Diagnosis Often clinical—try withdrawing cow's milk. If this resolves symptoms and they return with reintroduction then cow's milk protein allergy is likely. Skin prick/RAST tests have high false +ve and –ve results.

Treatment
- Eliminate cow's milk—usually by replacing cow's milk formula with hydrolysed protein milk formula (e.g. Nutramigen®)
- 10% of babies are also intolerant to hydrolysed protein formula and require amino acid formula (e.g. Neocate®)
- Advise parents that solids should be dairy-free
- Most children grow out of cow's milk protein intolerance and can be challenged with foods containing milk from 12mo

Lactose intolerance Rare in infancy; more common in childhood.

Presentation in infancy Severe symptoms of abdominal distension, diarrhoea (explosive and watery) ± vomiting and failure to thrive. Stools test +ve for reducing sugars. Treatment is with a lactose-free diet.

Presentation in later childhood (>2y) Due to lactase deficiency.
- Common—incidence is very variable depending on place of origin—but for people of European origin ~10–15% (higher if of Asian origin)
- Symptoms tend to be milder with abdominal pain and/or distension ± diarrhoea and/or vomiting appearing at any time from 2y of age to adulthood. Symptoms improve when milk products are removed from the diet. Tolerance of milk products is variable—cheese and yoghurt are better tolerated as lactose is hydrolysed by bacteria

 Soya milk does not contain lactose. Milk from other animals (e.g. goat's milk) does contain lactose. Soya milk contains phyto-oestrogens and has high glucose content, do not use if <6mo of age or long-term except with specialist advice.

Cow's milk intolerance following gastroenteritis Temporary cow's milk intolerance is common after a bout of gastroenteritis in children and can result in continuing diarhhoea (>2wk). Try excluding cow's milk from the diet. If symptoms improve, wait until all symptoms have gone and then reintroduce cow's milk. If symptoms do not improve, refer for further investigation.

Further information
NICE Constipation in children and young people (2010) ℠ www.nice.org.uk

Gut atresia, hernias, and intussusception

Oesophageal atresia 📖 p. 385

Duodenal atresia Usually associated with other abnormalities—particularly Down's syndrome. If not detected on antenatal USS, presents postnatally with bile-stained vomiting. AXR reveals a 'double bubble' with air in stomach and first part of duodenum but none beyond. Requires surgical correction.

Anorectal atresia (imperforate anus) 1 in 4,000 live births. Usually the baby fails to pass meconium and no anus is visible. There is often a fistula to the urethra (boys) or vagina (girls). Treatment is surgical. In the period after surgery, anal dilation is vital to prevent stricture and starts 2wk post-op. It requires use of graded dilators by the baby's parents for several months. Faecal incontinence may be a problem but can usually be managed using a combination of dietary manipulation, enemas, and drug treatment.

Umbilical hernia Common. Due to a defect in the umbilical ring when the cord separates. More common in people of black ethnic origin and associated with certain syndromes (e.g. trisomy 13 and 18). Usually resolves spontaneously. Strangulation is rare. Refer for surgery if an umbilical hernia persists until >2y of age.

Inguinal hernia
- **Non-acute** History of intermittent groin ± scrotal swelling—the spermatic cord may be thickened on the affected side. Refer to paediatric surgery for repair (herniotomy)
- **Acute** Sudden appearance of an irreducible groin or scrotal swelling—necessitates emergency admission for reduction and repair

Diaphragmatic hernia *Incidence:* 1 in 2,500 live births. A defect in one hemidiaphragm allows the bowel to herniate into the chest cavity → pulmonary hypoplasia *in utero* or lung compression postnatally. Detected antenatally on USS or postnatally when the child develops respiratory distress soon after birth—CXR confirms diagnosis. Corrective surgery is associated with high mortality but once successfully repaired the child usually has no further difficulties.

Exomphalos and gastroschisis
- **Exomphalos** Complete return of the gut into the abdominal cavity fails to occur during intrauterine life. At birth there is a swelling at the umbilicus, consisting of gut covered by a membrane
- **Gastroschisis** There is a defect in the abdominal wall through which exposed gut prolapses

Exomphalos and gastroschisis are usually detected antenatally at routine USS. Delivery then takes place at a specialist centre where surgical repair can be undertaken soon after birth. Once repaired prognosis is good.

Intussusception The invagination of one part of the bowel into the lumen of the immediately adjoining bowel. It is the most common cause of intestinal obstruction in young children and usually occurs in previously healthy children. *Incidence:* 2 in 1,000 live births. *Peak age:* 5–18mo ♂:♀ ≈2:1.

Associations
- Seasonal variation suggests an underlying viral cause—rota- and adenoviruses have both been implicated
- Intestinal polyps
- Meckel's diverticulum
- Henoch–Schönlein purpura

Types
- **Ileo-ileal** Ileum invaginates into adjacent ileum
- **Ileo-colic** Most common type—an ileo-ileal intussusception extends through the ileo-caecal valve
- **Ileo-caecal** The apex of the intussusception is the ileo-caecal valve
- **Colo-colic** Colon invaginates into adjacent colon—may be secondary to bowel tumour

Presentation Very variable. Always have a high index of suspicion.
- Abdominal colic—paroxysms of pain during which the child draws up his/her legs—the child often screams with the pain and becomes pale. Episodes usually are 10–15min apart and last 2–3min but become more frequent with time
- Vomiting—early symptom
- Rectal bleeding—passage of blood ('redcurrant jelly stool') or slime per rectum is a late sign
- Sausage-shaped mass in the abdomen—usually in the right upper quadrant—though not always present

⚠ The child becomes rapidly worse if not treated early, becoming toxic and developing an obstructive picture with distended abdomen ± faeculent vomiting.

Differential diagnosis Other causes of bowel obstruction; gastroenteritis; constipation; haemolytic uraemic syndrome.

Management Admit as an acute surgical emergency. Untreated intussusception is usually fatal. Treatment is with reduction by air or barium enema, or surgery.

Growth disorders

Take every opportunity to weigh and measure every child. Plot height, weight (and head circumference if <1y) on centile charts. Always correct the age of the child for prematurity at birth.

Failure to thrive 📖 p. 872   **Obesity** 📖 p. 178

Calculating expected height Small parents have small children and tall parents have tall children—always calculate expected height of the child before deciding the child has short stature or excessive height.

> Expected height = (mother's height + father's height) ÷ 2
> *Then:* add 6cm for a boy or subtract 6cm for a girl.

❶ 3% of 'normal' children fall under the 3rd and 3% above the 97th centile.

Short stature Height <3rd centile. Mainly healthy children (80%) but may indicate physical or emotional problems—especially if both parents have heights >3rd centile or serial measurements show growth has fallen below that expected from the centile chart. *Causes:*

- **Genetic** Achondroplastic dwarfism; familial short stature; Turner's syndrome; familial growth delay (children have delayed pubertal growth spurt but eventually reach normal height)
- **Physical** Low birthweight conditions; endocrine causes, e.g. growth hormone deficiency, hypopituitarism, hypothyroidism, DM; chronic illness, e.g. severe asthma, heart disease, chronic infection
- **Non-organic** Poor nutrition; emotional neglect; eating disorders

Assessment

- Ask how the child eats and about problems with feeding the child— appetite, food fads, special diets, quantities/times, snacks, etc.
- Ask about other physical problems, e.g. breathlessness, diarrhoea
- Examine the child carefully from top to toe looking for any physical abnormalities or signs of developmental delay
- Watch the way the child interacts with you and the parent. Look for evidence of neglect or maltreatment
- Look to see how large the parents are—2 small parents will probably have a small child

Management Treat reversible causes. Continue to measure height and weight regularly. Refer to paediatrics if no cause for short stature, or an abnormality requiring specialist care, is found, or if, despite treatment of a reversible cause, the child fails to grow along his/her growth curve.

Pituitary dwarfism ↓ function of the anterior pituitary gland, causing short stature or failure to thrive. Skeletal maturation, assessed by bone age, is usually >2y behind chronologic age. *Causes:*

- Idiopathic
- Genetic
- Midline defect, e.g. cleft palate
- Pituitary tumour, e.g. craniopharyngioma

Management Specialist management is essential. Treatment is with growth hormone ± cortisol, thyroid hormone, and/or gonadal sex steroids.
❶ Growth hormone treatment ↑ risk of slipped femoral epiphysis.

Excessive height Most children with height >97th centile come from tall families. Pathological causes of excess height are rare and include pituitary adenoma (gigantism), thyrotoxicosis, precocious puberty, Marfan's syndrome, and homocystinuria. Refer if a child is much taller than predicted height or deviates from his/her growth curve.

Head growth At birth, head circumference is 32–37cm (term infant); the anterior fontanelle measures 2.5 x 2.5cm, becoming smaller until it closes any time from 6mo–18mo. Most head growth occurs in infancy. Consider referring children with head circumference <3rd or >97th centile.

- **Microcephaly** 1 in 1,000 births. Small head out of proportion with the size of the body. Associated with developmental delay. *Causes:* genetic, intrauterine infection (e.g. rubella, CMV), chromosome abnormality, fetal alcohol syndrome, hypoxia
- **Macrocephaly** Large head circumference. *Causes:*
  - *Hydrocephalus* —suspect if head circumference deviates from the normal curve or if there are signs of ↑ intracranial pressure—refer
  - *Megalencephaly* —usually benign and familial—rarely associated developmental delay
- **Asymmetrical skull** *Causes:* postural effects, e.g. children who always sleep on one side (reassure–usually resolves with time); craniosynostosis (premature fusion of skull sutures—if suspected refer for prompt neurosurgical opinion)

Disorders of puberty

Delayed puberty Affects ~2%. No pubertal changes by 13y in girls or 14y in boys, or no progression of puberty over 2y. May be constitutional (>50% boys) or pathological (80% girls). In all cases, refer to a paediatrician for further assessment. *Pathological causes:*

- Failure of the ovaries/testes (1° or hypergonadotrophic hypogonadism)
- Failure of stimulation of normal gonads to produce sex hormones (2° or hypogonadotrophic hypogonadism)

Precocious puberty Puberty before the normal age for the population (in the UK: <8y for girls; <9y for boys). Affects 4–5% girls. ♀:♂≈ 5:1. In all cases, refer for further investigation. *Types:*

- **Central or true precocious puberty** (80%). Premature activation of the hypothalamic–pituitary–gonadal axis. No pathological cause is found in 50–60% ♂ and 90% ♀. There may be a family history
- **Pseudo-precocious puberty** (20%). ↑ level of sex hormones in the absence of excess FSH or LH. There is usually a pathological cause

Other problems of puberty

- **Asymmetric breast growth in girls** Almost universal. Reassure that usually evens out by the time of full maturation
- **Gynaecomastia in boys** ~50% during puberty. Small, firm lump under one/both nipples. Reassure. Usually resolves without treatment
- **Primary amenorrhoea (without delayed puberty)** 📖 p. 706
- **Premature pubarche (or adrenarche)** Early appearance of pubic ± axillary hair and body odour, without other signs of precocious puberty. If no other abnormalities of androgen excess, reassure

Information and support for children and parents
Child Growth Foundation ☎ 020 8995 0257
🖰 www.childgrowthfoundation.org

Other childhood endocrine problems

Diabetes mellitus 📖 p. 344   **Addison's disease** 📖 p. 368

Congenital goitre Enlarged thyroid gland present at birth ± hypo- or hyperthyroidism. Hypothyroid babies are treated with thyroxine; if there is tracheal compression or hyperthyroidism treatment is surgical.

Hypothyroidism

Neonatal (congenital) hypothyroidism 📖 p. 850

Juvenile (acquired) hypothyroidism Usually due to autoimmune thyroiditis (Hashimoto's thyroiditis). Often insidious onset with ↑ weight, constipation, dry or coarse hair, and sallow, cool, or mottled coarse skin. In children there may also be growth retardation, delayed skeletal maturation ± delayed puberty. TFTs confirm diagnosis. Refer to paediatrics for specialist management. Treatment is with thyroxine replacement.

Hyperthyroidism

Neonatal hyperthyroidism Rare but potentially life-threatening. Occurs in infants of mothers with current or prior Graves' disease due to passage of autoantibodies across the placenta. *Presentation:*

* Feeding problems
* ↑ BP
* Irritability
* Tachycardia
* Exophthalmos
* Goitre
* Frontal bossing
* Microcephaly
* Failure to thrive
* Vomiting
* Diarrhoea

Refer for specialist management. Affected infants generally recover in <4mo. Long-term consequences include premature fusion of the cranial sutures (craniosynostosis) and developmental delay.

Juvenile hyperthyroidism Usually Graves' disease (📖 p. 364).

Features due to hyperthyroidism	*Eye features*
* Weight ↓	* Double vision
* Tremor	* Eye discomfort ± protrusion
* Palpitations (may have AF)	(exophthalmos and proptosis)
* Hyperactivity	* Lid lag
* Diffuse goitre ± thyroid bruit	* Ophthalmoplegia

TFTs confirm diagnosis. Refer for specialist management. Treatment is with antithyroid medication. Spontaneous resolution in <2y is the norm.

Congenital adrenal hyperplasia (CAH) Also known as *adrenogenital syndrome* or *adrenal virilism*. Autosomal recessive trait due to absence or deficiency of any of the enzymes needed for synthesis of cortisol. Each enzyme block causes a characteristic deficiency. 2 patterns:

* Androgens accumulate causing virilization of an affected female fetus
* Androgen synthesis is impaired causing inadequate virilization of an affected male fetus (much rarer)

Presentation and management Ambiguity of the external genitalia. Less severe forms may go unnoticed until puberty. There may be a family history of CAH, ambiguous genitalia, or neonatal death. Rarely presents with Addisonian crisis. Refer for specialist management. Treatment is usually with glucocorticoid ± mineralocorticoid replacement.

Male hypogonadism ↓ function of the testes. 3 types:
- **Primary** Damage to the Leydig cells impairs androgen (testosterone) secretion, e.g. Klinefelter's syndrome, anorchia (absent testes)
- **Secondary (hypogonadotrophic)** Disorders of the hypothalamus or pituitary impair gonadotrophin secretion which may result in impotency and/or infertility. e.g. panhypopituitarism
- **Resistance to androgen action** Presentation depends on age of onset:
  - *In utero* —ambiguity of genitalia or female appearance, small penis, incomplete testicular descent
  - *In childhood* —delayed or impaired puberty, impaired development of male sexual characteristics ± gynaecomastia
  - *In adulthood* —↓ libido, impotence, loss of muscle power, testicular atrophy, fine wrinkling of the skin around eyes and lips, sparse body hair, osteopeonia, gynaecomastia

Management Refer for specialist investigation. Treatment depends on the nature of the deficiency.

Androgen insensitivity syndrome (AIS) X-linked genetic disorder affecting 1 in 62,000 male births. Abnormalities within androgen receptors result in the individual being genotypically male (46XY) but phenotypically female. External genitalia are female in complete AIS (CAIS), but are often ambiguous in partial AIS (PAIS). The testes fail to descend and are usually found in the groin—rarely within the abdomen. At puberty, breast development occurs and female contours form, but there is little or no pubic or axillary hair. Patients often present with primary amenorrhoea.

Management As diagnosis is often made in teenage years, young people with CAIS have usually been treated as female since birth. Specialist support is always required. Testes are usually removed as they have malignant potential, and oestrogens given to complete secondary sexual development.

Dealing with sexual ambiguity detected at the neonatal or 6-week check
- Be honest—do not guess the gender of the child
- Explain that there are rare conditions where girls may be virilized or boys undermasculinized, causing girls to look like boys and vice versa
- Arrange paediatric assessment as soon as possible for further investigations, gender assignment, and ongoing management

Funny turns and febrile convulsions

Funny turns Small children are often brought to the GP by their parents because they have had a funny turn. The major questions are: was the episode a fit? If so, what caused it? If not, then is there another serious underlying cause, e.g. heart disease?

History A good history from a witness is essential. Ask:
- When did the attack happen and where?
- Were there any precipitating events or warning signs, e.g. viral illness; fever; strong emotions (was the child angry or upset?); head injury?
- What happened? Did the child lose consciousness? Jerk his limbs? If so, was the jerking generalized or restricted to one area of the body? What did the child look like during the attack, e.g. colour, floppiness? Did anything else happen during the attack, e.g. tongue biting?
- How long did the attack last?
- What happened after the attack? Was the child conscious straight away? Was there disorientation or drowsiness?

Also check
- General history—is the child well? Does the child have any ongoing medical problems? Past medical history—serious illness, neurological and/or developmental problems, heart problems.
- Birth history—problems in pregnancy, birth trauma
- Family history—epilepsy

Examination Full general/neurological examination; developmental milestones. Plot head circumference/weight on centile chart.

Differential diagnosis Epileptic attacks—febrile convulsion or childhood epilepsy (🕮 p. 898); non-epileptic attacks.

Non-epileptic attacks Usually self-limiting and harmless. Frightening for parents/carers, so education about likely duration and cause of attacks and reassurance the child will come to no harm are important.

Simple blue breath-holding attacks Onset usually >6mo of age. Common. Provoked by frustration or upset. *Signs:* +ve Valsalva manoeuvre, cyanosis, stiffening, and coma. No treatment needed—spontaneous recovery. Most children 'grow out' of the attacks by 3y.

White reflex asystolic (anoxic) attacks Most common from 6mo—2y. Usually triggered by minor injury or anxiety. *Signs:* vagal asystole, pallor, rapid coma, stiffening, upward eye movement ± urinary incontinence. No treatment needed—spontaneous recovery.

Reflex syncope or vasovagal attacks ('faints') 🕮 p. 551

Others causes are rare in children but include
- Cardiac arrhythmias—refer if recurrent loss of consciousness or collapse on exertion for paediatric cardiology assessment
- Hyperventilation
- Benign monoclonus of infancy
- Benign paroxysmal vertigo
- Sleep phenomena
- Hypoglycaemia
- Fictitious or induced illness

Febrile convulsions Epileptic seizures provoked by fever in otherwise normal children. *Prevalence:* 3–5% of children aged 6mo–5y (peak age 18mo). There is often a family history. Seizures are usually brief (<5min) and generalized. *Causes (in order of decreasing frequency):* viral infections; otitis media; tonsillitis; UTI; gastroenteritis; LRTI; meningitis; post-immunization.

Management of the fitting child 📖 p. 1070

Further management Most children do not require admission. Check temperature, assess respiratory/heart rate, capillary return, and level of consciousness. Examine for a source of infection. If there is no obvious cause and not being admitted, check an MSU.

> ⚠ Complex convulsions are more likely to be provoked by a serious condition. Suspect serious pathology if a child has:
> • Had a prolonged (>10min) or focal febrile convulsion, *or*
> • Not recovered within an hour of a febrile convulsion

Admit if
• Complex seizure, the child was drowsy before the seizure, is irritable, systemically unwell or 'toxic', and/or the cause of the fever is unclear
• Symptoms/signs of meningitis (📖 p. 1078); petechial rash; recent or current treatment with antibiotics (may mask symptoms/signs of meningitis); or aged <18mo (meningitis may have non-specific signs)
• The cause of the fever requires hospital management in its own right
• Early review by a doctor is not possible, inadequate home circumstances, or the carer is anxious or unable to cope

For children not being admitted Reassure parents/carers that febrile convulsions do not harm the child. Antipyretics (e.g. paracetamol) do not prevent convulsions but are useful for symptom control. Advise parents to seek urgent medical help if the child deteriorates in any way, develops a non-blanching rash, fits again, or they are worried. Arrange early review (in <24h). Recommend that immunization schedules are completed.

Consider outpatient referral if
• Diagnosis of febrile convulsion is in doubt
• Febrile convulsions have been frequent, severe, and/or complex, and prophylactic treatment (with buccal midazolam, rectal diazepam or continuous anticonvulsants) might be indicated
• The child is at ↑ risk of epilepsy, e.g. coexistent neurological or developmental conditions; history of epilepsy in a first-degree relative
• Parents/carers are anxious despite reassurance or request referral

Prognosis Febrile convulsions recur in subsequent febrile illness in ~30% of children. 1% of children having a febrile convulsion go on to develop epilepsy (compared to 0.4% of children who do not).

Further information

NICE The epilepsies: the diagnosis and management of the epilepsies in adults and children in primary and secondary care (2012) 🖰 www.nice.org.uk

Childhood epilepsy

Childhood epilepsy is a susceptibility to continuing seizures. Prevalence ↑ with age from ~4 in 1,000 children at 7y to ~5 in 1,000 children at 16y. 60% of adult epilepsy starts in childhood.

Risk factors Neurological abnormalities or developmental delay; family history; past history of febrile convulsions—1% develop epilepsy.

Diagnosis Seizures, faints, and funny turns can be difficult to distinguish and diagnose (📖 p. 896). A reliable eye witness account is the key.

⚠ Refer to a specialist paediatrician with training and expertise in epilepsy for diagnosis. All children who have had a first non-febrile seizure should be seen in <2wk[N].

Management of the fitting patient 📖 p. 1070

Long-term management of epilepsy 📖 p. 576

Epileptic syndromes In children, epilepsy is considered in terms of the 'epileptic syndrome'. Identifying a syndrome enables predictions about cause, severity, and prognosis. Epileptic syndromes are characterized by a set pattern of seizure type(s) ± other features: physical appearance; age at onset; family history; associated learning disability and/or developmental delay; associated neurological findings; and EEG (should be undertaken in any child with a history of ≥2 epileptic seizures).

❶ It is not possible to identify a syndrome in 30%—and symptoms/signs may take months to evolve until diagnosis can be made in others.

Benign rolandic epilepsy Also known as *childhood epilepsy with centrotemporal spikes*. 15–20% of childhood epilepsy. Starts in children aged 2–12y (peak age 7–10y)—usually stops by 13y. Frequently, there is a family history. Clonic, partial sensorimotor attacks affect the face, tongue, pharynx, hand, and arm. Most common on falling asleep (>½ have seizures only during sleep) or soon after waking. Secondary generalization to tonic-clonic seizures may occur. EEG is characteristic. Use of drug treatment depends on frequency and severity of seizures.

Juvenile myoclonic epilepsy (JME) 4–12% of childhood epilepsy. Age of onset 5–24y (peak age 10–16y). 50% have FH of epilepsy. Presents with sudden, brief, bilaterally symmetrical and synchronous involuntary muscle contractions. Upper body > lower body. May cause the patient to throw objects or fall. Consciousness is often maintained. Frequently occurs soon after waking. Triggers may include light (50%), tiredness, or emotion. Generalized tonic-clonic seizures—often starting with a series of myoclonic jerks—appear <4y after onset of myoclonic seizures in ~90%. Absence seizures also occur in 15–30%. EEG is characteristic.

Management and prognosis Usually treated with sodium valproate—fits may not be well controlled with medication. JME does not remit spontaneously. Lifelong medication is needed—relapse rate is ~90% on withdrawal of anti-epileptic medication.

Absence seizures (petit mal) 10–12% of childhood epilepsy. Age of onset 4–10y (peak age 5–7y); ♀ > ♂; ~15% have a family history. The child stops what he is doing and may stare into middle space for a period of seconds (mean 4–20s). Can occur 50–100x/d. Deterioration in school performance may be the first sign. Separating absence attacks from day-dreaming can be difficult. EEG is characteristic.

Management and prognosis 80% become seizure-free with sodium valproate. ~15% go on to develop JME. ~10% (without other adverse factors) have absence or tonic-clonic seizures in adult life.

Localization-related epilepsies Up to 30% of childhood epilepsy. Focal (partial) seizures that may be *symptomatic* (known underlying cause) or *cryptogenic* (cause not found). Clinical features, disabilities, and prognosis depend on cause and location of the brain abnormality.

Infantile spasms (West's syndrome) Starts in the first year of life (*peak age:* 4mo). Runs of tonic spasms—usually flexion spasms ('salaam' spasms)—occur every 5–10s. Characteristic EEG. Associated with loss of vision and social interaction. Treatment is with steroids and anti-epileptics (usually vigabatrin). Poor prognosis—30–50% have cerebral palsy; 85% have a cognitive disability; 20% death rate.

Sturge–Weber syndrome Unilateral capillary naevus (port wine stain)—usually over the forehead/eyelid; epilepsy (90%); developmental delay (50%); hemiparesis and/or homonymous hemianopia (30%) and glaucoma in the affected eye. Treatment is supportive.

Lennox–Gastaut syndrome Severe, early onset form of epilepsy (starts aged 2–6y) with multiple seizure types and typical EEG. Often resistant to treatment.

Particular problems to look for in children with epilepsy

- **Developmental problems**—25% have special educational needs; >20% have moderate/severe learning disability. Specific cognitive disability (e.g. with reading or arithmetic) may have a serious impact on a child's education if not recognized
- **Social stigmatization** (perceived or experienced) is common. Children may have problems making friends because they are not allowed to do everything other children do or have funny turns and are considered 'odd'. Psychosocial problems include lack of confidence, poor self-esteem, behavioural problems (e.g. conduct disorder, school refusal), dependence on others, anxiety, and depression
- **Adverse effects of anti-epileptic drugs**—for girls discuss the risk to unborn child and interactions with contraception
- **Physical trauma**—may occur as a result of having a seizure

Further information

NICE ℘ www.nice.org.uk
- The epilepsies: the diagnosis and management of the epilepsies in adults and children in primary and secondary care (2012)
- Referral guidelines for suspected cancer (2005)

Information and support for children and parents
Epilepsy Action ☎ 0808 800 5050 ℘ www.epilepsy.org.uk

Arthritis in children

Joint and limb pains are common in children. Arthritis is rare.

Presentation of arthritis in children

Older children Usually present with well-localized joint pains ± hot, tender, swollen joints.

Babies and young children May present with immobility of a joint or a limp, but the diagnosis can be extremely difficult.

Differential diagnosis of joint pains in children
* Juvenile idiopathic arthritis (JIA—incidence 1 in 10,000)
* Infections, e.g. TB, rubella, Lyme disease
* Rheumatic fever
* Henoch–Schönlein purpura
* Traumatic arthritis
* Hypermobility syndrome
* Leukaemia, lymphoma, or bone malignancy
* Sickle cell disease
* SLE and connective tissue disorders
* Transient synovitis of the hip (irritable hip)
* Septic arthritis
* Perthes' disease
* Slipped femoral epiphysis

Septic arthritis 📖 p. 521

Types of childhood arthritis See Table 24.12.

Management of children with arthritis
* If suspected, refer urgently to paediatrics for confirmation of diagnosis
* Once confirmed, ensure the child is referred to a specialist paediatric rheumatology unit to avoid long-term disability. These units have multidisciplinary facilities for rehabilitation, education, and surgical intervention (if necessary) and support both the family and the child
* NSAIDs and paracetamol help pain and stiffness, but corticosteroids and immunosuppressants (e.g. methotrexate) are often required for systemic disease. Monoclonal antibody therapy may be used if first-line disease-modifying agents are ineffective
* Ensure families apply for any benefits that might be available to them
* Tell families about self-help and support groups
* Support families in any applications made to adapt the home or school environment for the child's condition

Information and support for parents and children
Arthritis Research UK ☎ 0300 790 0400 ⌨ www.arthritisresearchuk.org
Children's Chronic Arthritis Association ☎ 01905 745 595
⌨ www.ccaa.org.uk

Table 24.12 Childhood arthritis

Type of arthritis	Features
Oligoarthritis or pauciarticular onset arthritis	
Persistent:	Most common form of JIA (50–60%) but still rare
	Peak age: 3y. ♀ >> ♂
	Affects ≤4 joints—especially wrists, knees, and ankles. Often asymmetrical
	Associated with uveitis (often with +ve anti-nuclear antibody) which requires regular screening by slit lamp examination—rarely causes blindness
	Generally prognosis is good, with remission in 4–5y
Extended:	Chronic arthritis with an oligoarticular onset of the disease, which progresses to involve >4 joints. Joints tend to be stiff rather than hot and swollen
Still's disease* **(Systemic onset JIA)**	10% of JIA—only 1 in 3 have arthritis at the onset of the disease
	Affects boys and girls equally up to 5y—then girls are more commonly affected
	Presentation:
	• Fever—high, swinging, early evening temperature for >2wk
	• Rash—pink maculopapular rash with fever
	• Musculoskeletal pain—arthralgia, arthritis, myalgia
	• Generalized lymphadenopathy
	• Hepatosplenomegaly
	• Pericarditis ± pleurisy (uncommon)
	Investigations: blood—↑ ESR/CRP; FBC—↑ neutrophils, ↑ platelets. Autoantibodies are –ve
	⚠ *Differential diagnosis:* malignancy—particularly leukaemia or neuroblastoma; infection
Polyarticular onset JIA	Starts with or without a preceding systemic illness at any age >1y. Usually occurs in teenagers producing widespread joint destruction
	There is symmetrical arthritis of hands, wrists, PIP joints ± DIP joints
	Rheumatoid factor is usually –ve (+ve in 3%—often teenage girls)
Enthesis-related JIA	Affects teenage and younger boys, often producing an asymmetrical arthritis of lower limb joints and tendon insertions. Heel pain and soft tissue swelling are common
	Associated with HLA-B27 and acute anterior uveitis
	Represents the childhood equivalent of adult ankylosing spondylitis. ~60% of childhood sufferers develop ankylosing spondylitis later in life
Juvenile psoriatic arthritis	Polyarthritis affecting large and small joints, including fingers and toes. The arthritis can be very erosive
	Psoriasis may be present in the child or a first-degree relative (📖 p. 618)

**G.F. Still (1868–1941)—English paediatrician.*

Paediatric dermatology

Birthmarks

Strawberry naevus (capillary haemangioma)
- Not usually present at birth
- Occurs anywhere on the skin surface
- Starts as a small, red patch, then grows rapidly over a few months into a bright red vascular lump
- After initial growth, the naevus stays the same size for 6–12mo, then involutes and disappears by 5–7y
- No treatment is needed. Parents may need considerable reassurance
- If interfering with feeding, breathing, or vision—refer for treatment with intralesional steroids or laser

Port wine stain (naevus flammeus)
- Present at birth
- Irregular red/purple macule which often affects one side of the face
- Permanent—may become darker and lumpy in middle age
- May be associated with other abnormalities, e.g. intracranial vascular malformation (Sturge–Weber syndrome—📖 p. 899)

Salmon patch (stork mark)
- The most common vascular naevus (~50% neonates)
- Small, telangiectatic lesion forming a pink macule—most commonly at the nape of the neck or on the upper face
- Facial lesions resolve spontaneously—those on the neck may persist. No treatment is needed

Mongolian blue spot
- Bluish discoloration of the skin, usually over buttocks and lower back in dark-skinned babies
- Of no clinical significance but may occasionally be mistaken for bruising and non-accidental injury
- Usually disappears by 1y

Congenital melanocytic naevi ~1.5% of neonates.
- Noted at birth as raised nodules or plaques of black or brown
- May be hairy, irregular, and single or multiple
- Classified by size: <1.5cm—small; 1.5–20cm—medium; >20cm—large
- There is a risk of malignant change to melanoma—the larger the naevus the greater the risk
- Laser therapy can improve cosmetic appearance

Nappy rash Most common type of nappy eruption. Usually seen in young infants—rare >12mo. An irritant dermatitis due to skin contact with urine or faeces.

Presentation Glazed erythema in the napkin area, sparing skinfolds. Secondary bacterial or fungal infection is common.

Differential diagnosis
- Seborrhoeic eczema
- Candidiasis
- Napkin psoriasis

Management
- Advise parents to keep the nappy area dry
- Give baby as much time as possible with the nappy off
- Apply moisturiser as soap substitute
- Apply a barrier cream between nappy changes—although this may interfere with the action of some modern nappies
- Topical treatment with an antifungal combined with hydrocortisone is effective if the nappy rash is not clearing

Infantile seborrhoeic eczema
- Starts in the first few weeks of life
- Affects body folds—axilla, groins, behind ears, neck ± face and scalp (*'cradle cap'*). Flexural lesions present as moist, shiny, well-demarcated scaly erythema. On the scalp, neck, and behind the ears, a yellowish crust is usual
- Treat flexural lesions with emollients and 1% hydrocortisone ointment, or with clotrimazole and hydrocortisone cream
- Scalp lesions respond to OTC cradle cap creams

Candidiasis Often complicates nappy rash or infantile seborrhoeic eczema. Erythema, scaling, and pustules involve the flexures. There may be associated satellite lesions. Treatment is with a topical antifungal, e.g. clotrimazole.

Juvenile plantar dermatosis Presents with red, dry, fissured and glazed skin principally over the forefeet. Sometimes involves the whole sole. Usually starts in primary school years and resolves spontaneously in mid-teens. Due to wearing socks and/or shoes made from synthetic materials. Emollients help but topical steroids are ineffective. Advise cotton socks and leather shoes.

Accessory nipples Commonly seen on the milk line in both male and female infants. Usually small and inconspicuous. No treatment is required.

Staphylococcal scalded skin syndrome Rare but serious skin infection seen in infants/young children. Caused by staphylococcal infection releasing epidermolytic toxin causing widespread erythema/blistering. The epidermis shears off giving the appearance of scalded skin. Admit as a paediatric emergency for IV antibiotics and supportive treatment. ❶ Can also affect immunosuppressed adults.

Acne 📖 p. 616
Psoriasis 📖 p. 618
Atopic eczema 📖 p. 606
Scabies 📖 p. 639
Head lice 📖 p. 638
Urticaria 📖 p. 614
Impetigo 📖 p. 632
Warts 📖 p. 634
Molluscum contagiosum 📖 p. 635

Further information
Electronic dermatology atlas 🖱 www.dermis.net

Diagnosis of cancer in children

Every year in the UK, 1,550 children are diagnosed with and 260 children die from cancer. The most common type of childhood cancer is acute leukaemia (1 in 3) followed by brain tumour (1 in 4). Risk of developing cancer for an individual child is ~1:500. 5y survival is 78%; of those that survive 5y, 10% die as a result of tumour recurrence or treatment effects.

Diagnosis of childhood malignancy is a particular challenge in primary care. GPs rarely see children with cancer, and the cancers that children get are often unfamiliar to them. Always have a high index of suspicion and if in doubt refer for a specialist opinion. Referrals should be made to a paediatrician or specialist in children's cancer.

❶ Some congenital/genetic syndromes may be associated with ↑ risk of childhood cancer (e.g. Down's syndrome—leukaemia; neurofibromatosis and tuberous sclerosis—CNS tumours).

Abdominal distension[N] If persistent or progressive, examine the abdomen:
- If a mass is found, refer immediately
- If the child is uncooperative and abdominal examination is not possible, or if examination is difficult, consider referral for urgent abdominal USS

Unexplained or persistent back pain[N] Examine the child and check FBC and blood film. Consider X-ray and/or discussion with a paediatrician. If no cause is found, refer urgently.

Admission or referral to be seen the same day[N] Any child with:
- Hepatosplenomegaly
- Unexplained petechiae
- Unexplained urinary retention
- ↓ conscious level
- Headache and vomiting that cause early morning waking or occur on waking, as these are classic signs of ↑ intracranial pressure ❶ <1% of patients presenting with headache have a brain tumour
- Children <2y with new-onset seizures (excluding febrile convulsion); bulging fontanelle; extensor attacks; and/or persistent vomiting
- FBC suggesting malignancy
- Mediastinal, hilar, or thoracic mass on CXR

Referral to be seen the same day or within 2wk[N] Any child with:
- New-onset seizures
- Cranial nerve abnormalities
- Visual disturbances
- Leg weakness—refer immediately if gait abnormalities or motor or sensory signs
- Other motor/sensory signs
- Abdominal mass
- Skin nodules in a baby that could be metastatic neuroblastoma
- Proptosis
- Shortness of breath—particularly if not responding to bronchodilators

Urgent referral to be seen in <2wk[N] Refer:
- When a child presents several times (≥3x) with the same problem, but with no clear diagnosis
- If white papillary reflex (leukocoria)
- If aged ≥2y with persistent headache where you cannot carry out an adequate neurological examination in primary care
- If aged <2y with:
  - Abnormal ↑ in head size
  - Arrest/regression of motor development and/or altered behaviour
  - Abnormal eye movements and/or lack of visual following
  - Poor feeding/failure to thrive
  - New squint/change in visual acuity
- If unexplained mass at any site that has ≥1 of the following features— the mass is:
  - Deep to the fascia
  - Non-tender
  - Progressively enlarging
  - Associated with a regional lymph node that is enlarging
  - >2cm in diameter
- If lymphadenopathy with ≥1 of the following features (particularly if no evidence of local infection and/or associated with general ill health, fever or weight loss):
  - Non-tender, firm, or hard lymph nodes
  - Lymph nodes >2cm in size
  - Lymph nodes progressively enlarging
  - Any axillary nodes (in the absence of local infection or dermatitis)
  - Any supraclavicular nodes
- If unexplained haematuria
- If persistent localized bone pain/swelling and X-ray suggesting cancer
- If unexplained deteriorating school performance or developmental milestones, or unexplained behavioural and/or mood changes
- If rest pain or unexplained limp—consider X-ray and/or discussion with a paediatrician before, or as well as, referral
- If family history of retinoblastoma and/or visual problems

Investigations[N] Check FBC and blood film if:
- Pallor and/or fatigue
- Unexplained irritability
- Unexplained fever
- Persistent or recurrent URTIs
- Generalized lymphadenopathy
- Persistent or unexplained bone pain (additionally, consider X-ray)
- Unexplained bruising

❶ If the FBC and blood film indicate leukaemia, admit or make a referral for the child to be assessed by a paediatrician the same day.

Consider referral[N] When there is persistent parental anxiety, even when a benign cause is considered most likely.

Further information
NICE Referral guidelines for suspected cancer (2005) ℘ www.nice.org.uk

Specific childhood cancers

Acute leukaemia 📖 p. 676   **Brain tumour** 📖 p. 558

Lymphoma 📖 p. 680   **Sarcoma** 📖 p. 505

Gonadal tumours

- Testicular tumours 📖 p. 468
- Ovarian tumours 📖 p. 725

Neuroblastoma Tumour derived from neural crest tissue. 90 cases/y are reported in Great Britain—6% of all paediatric tumours. Neuroblastoma tends to affect children <4y old (50% <2y; 90% <9y). *Sites:* adrenal medulla—50%; abdominal sympathetic ganglia—25%; chest—20%; pelvis—5%; neck—5%.

Presentation Variable and often non-specific—depends on site of the tumour and extent of metastases. ~½ present with metastatic disease.

- **General effects** Pallor, fever, anorexia and weight ↓, failure to thrive, diarrhoea, irritability, flushing, ataxia
- **Local effects of tumour** Abdominal mass (or thoracic mass on CXR); local spread may cause paraplegia or cauda equina syndrome. Infants <6mo may have rapidly progressive intra-abdominal disease
- **Effects of metastases** Lymphatic and haematogenous spread, particularly to liver, lungs, and bone, is common. Associated symptoms:
  - Bone pain ± pathological fracture
  - Breathlessness
  - Periorbital bruising (looks like a black eye), proptosis, or Horner's syndrome
  - Firm skin nodules (usually babies—'blueberry muffin appearance')

Investigate with a FBC If persistent or unexplained bone pain (X-ray is also needed); pallor or fatigue; unexplained irritability; unexplained fever; persistent or recurrent URTI; generalized lymphadenopathy; and/or unexplained bruising.

If neuroblastoma is suspected Carry out an abdominal examination (and/or urgent USS), and consider CXR and FBC. If any mass is found, refer urgently.

Specialist management Treatment is with surgery, chemotherapy, and/or radiotherapy. Early stage disease has a 95% 5y survival; late stage disease has 20% 5y survival. Children with extra-abdominal tumours and those who are <1y at diagnosis have better prognosis.

Wilms' nephroblastoma 80 cases/y in Great Britain. Kidney tumour composed of primitive renal tissue; L > R; bilateral in 10%. Usually affects children <5y old (peak age: 2–3y). ♂ > ♀. 10% occur in children with rare syndromes, e.g. Beckwith–Wiedemann syndrome, aniridia, or hemihypertrophy. A few cases are familial.

Presentation

- **General effects** Fever, anorexia and weight ↓, anaemia
- **Local effects of tumour** Unilateral abdominal mass ± pain ± unexplained haematuria
- **Effects of metastases** 10% have metastases to liver, lungs, or bone (rare) at presentation. May present with symptoms/signs of metastases

Management If a child presents with abdominal distension, examine the abdomen. *Refer if:* intrabdominal mass (immediate) or unexplained haematuria (urgent). Treatment is with surgery ± chemotherapy ± radiotherapy. 5y survival is 85% (higher for early stage tumours).

Retinoblastoma Rare tumour of the eye. 40 cases/y in Great Britain. 40% are <1y old at diagnosis; 95% are <5y old. May be familial (10%—dominant inheritance) when the tumour is usually bilateral; genetic testing is available. May be detected as a white pupillary reflex seen at developmental screening. Alternatively may present with squint or inflammation of the eye. Refer suspected cases to ophthalmology urgently.

Specialist treatment Depends on size and location of tumour, whether unilateral or bilateral, and whether family history. Options include thermotherapy, brachytherapy, chemotherapy, or surgery. 5y survival is 99%.

Ongoing care When a diagnosis of cancer is made, most children embark on an intensive regime of treatment. They are referred to tertiary paediatric oncology units that share care with local hospitals and have direct access to advice/admission via those units. Outreach nurses provide support in the community (e.g. administration of IV drugs via Hickman lines) to maintain as normal a lifestyle as possible.

⚠ Immunosuppression can be a major problem. Any febrile episode in a neutropenic child requires immediate referral to a specialist unit. Chickenpox can be particularly serious—seek specialist advice from the treating unit if the patient is in contact with any other child with chickenpox.

The GP's role Treatment for childhood cancer is increasingly successful with cure rates of >80% for many forms of cancer. The role of the GP is important even if it is peripheral. Keep in touch with the family and up to date with what is going on. Provide support to the child and other family members. Give advice on benefits or local services that might be useful. Ensure prescriptions are supplied promptly.

Palliative care Sadly, despite treatment, some children progress to the terminal stages of their cancer. General principles of palliative care apply (📖 pp. 1028–47) but the emotional traumas are often much greater. If possible engage specialist palliative care services early. Try to maintain continuity of care with as few professionals involved as possible. Provide ongoing support to family members after the child has died.

Further information

NICE Referral guidelines for suspected cancer (2005) ℘ www.nice.org.uk

Information and support for patients and their carers

Children with Cancer UK ☎ 020 7404 0808
℘ www.childrenwithcancer.org.uk
CLIC and Sargent ☎ 0300 330 0803 ℘ www.clicsargent.org.uk
Neuroblastoma Society ☎ 020 8940 4353 ℘ www.nsoc.co.uk
Childhood Eye Cancer Trust (CHECT) ☎ 020 7377 5578
℘ www.chect.org.uk
Together for Short Lives (Hospices and Palliative Care) ☎ 0808 8088 100 ℘ www.togetherforshortlives.org.uk

Behaviour problems

GPs are commonly asked to 'sort out' behaviour problems of children by parents at their wits' ends. 2–10% of all children are said to have behaviour problems depending on how problems are defined and measured.

Differentiation between normal behaviour and behavioural problems can be difficult—especially if you do not know the child or family well. A significant problem is more likely:
• When the behaviour is frequent and chronic
• When >1 problem behaviour occurs, *and*
• If behaviour interferes with social and cognitive functioning

There is no right or wrong way to deal with these problems and the approach outlined in Figure 24.4 is just one way to tackle them.

Managing the problem For simple problems, parental education, reassurance, and a few specific suggestions tailored to the situation are often sufficient. Follow-up is important to ensure that the problem is resolving. If simple measures are not succeeding within 3–4mo, consider referral to other agencies, e.g. health visitor, school nurse, child and adolescent mental health team. Specific behavioural techniques include:

Behaviour modification Behaviour modification is a learning process requiring care givers to set consistent rules and limits. Parents should try to minimize anger when enforcing rules and ↑ +ve contact with the child.

Discipline Ineffective discipline may result in inappropriate behaviour. Scolding or physical punishment may briefly control a child's behaviour if used sparingly but may ↓ the child's sense of security and self-esteem. Threats to leave or send the child away are damaging. *Options:*
• **+ve reinforcement for appropriate behaviour** This is a powerful tool for controlling a child's behaviour with no adverse effects
• **Time-out procedure** The child must sit alone in a dull place for a brief period. Time-outs are a learning process for the child and are best used for controlling a single inappropriate behaviour or a few at one time

Breaking vicious circle patterns The child's behaviour (be it normal for that developmental stage or abnormal) evokes a response in the parent or carer which provokes the child to behave in that manner further—thus generating another response from the parent. Try to identify vicious circle patterns and suggest alternative parental responses which make the behaviour futile.

Sleep problems 📖 p. 912   **Toilet training** 📖 p. 914

Parent information and support

Green C (2006) *New toddler taming: A parents guide to the first four years.* London: Vermilion. ISBN: 0091902584

Green C (2000) *Beyond toddlerdom: Every parent's guide to the 5–10s.* London: Vermilion. ISBN: 0091816246

Parentline 📞 0808 800 2222 🖰 www.familylives.org.uk

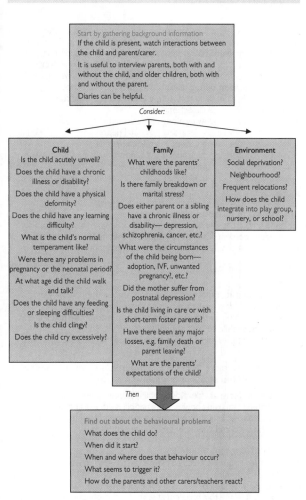

Start by gathering background information
If the child is present, watch interactions between the child and parent/carer.

It is useful to interview parents, both with and without the child, and older children, both with and without the parent.

Diaries can be helpful.

Consider:

Child

Is the child acutely unwell?

Does the child have a chronic illness or disability?

Does the child have a physical deformity?

Does the child have any learning difficulty?

What is the child's normal temperament like?

Were there any problems in pregnancy or the neonatal period?

At what age did the child walk and talk?

Does the child have any feeding or sleeping difficulties?

Is the child clingy?

Does the child cry excessively?

Family

What were the parents' childhoods like?

Is there family breakdown or marital stress?

Does either parent or a sibling have a chronic illness or disability— depression, schizophrenia, cancer, etc.?

What were the circumstances of the child being born— adoption, IVF, unwanted pregnancy?, etc.?

Did the mother suffer from postnatal depression?

Is the child living in care or with short-term foster parents?

Have there been any major losses, e.g. family death or parent leaving?

What are the parents' expectations of the child?

Environment

Social deprivation?

Neighbourhood?

Frequent relocations?

How does the child integrate into play group, nursery, or school?

Then

Find out about the behavioural problems
What does the child do?

When did it start?

When and where does that behaviour occur?

What seems to trigger it?

How do the parents and other carers/teachers react?

Figure 24.4 Assessment of childhood behaviour problems

Information and support for children
Childline 24h confidential counselling service ☎ 0800 1111
🖰 www.childline.org.uk

Excessive crying Babies vary considerably in the amount they cry and ease with which they are soothed. Likewise parents vary in their ability to tolerate a crying baby. Babies cry for many reasons—discomfort, hunger, loneliness, separation, boredom, etc. If a baby is crying excessively:
- Take a history from the parent—when does the baby cry, can he/she be consoled, what do the parents do when the baby cries
- Examine fully from head to toe to exclude causes of discomfort, e.g. nappy rash, otitis media, eczema
- Check the baby is growing along his/her centile line
- Consider family stress (including postnatal depression—📖 p. 839) as a reason why the parent cannot tolerate the crying
- Treat any underlying cause found and support the family. Information about behavioural techniques used to manage babies that cry excessively is available from Cry-sis ☎ 08451 228 669 🖱 www.cry-sis.org.uk

Feeding problems 📖 p. 872

Rhythmic behaviour Head rocking or banging, thumb sucking, self-stimulation, baby behaviour, and many other variants all occur during normal development. They usually appear if the child is tired, uncertain, or anxious. Reassure parents. Most resolve spontaneously.

Fears and phobias

Fears
- Fears of the dark, monsters, and spiders are common in 3–4y olds
- Fears of injury and death are more common in older children
- Statements made by the parents in anger or jest may be taken literally by preschool children and can be disturbing
- Frightening stories, films, or TV programmes may be upsetting and intensify fears

Phobias Phobias cause persistent, unrealistic, yet intense anxiety in reaction to external situations or stimuli.

Management Normal developmental stage-related fears must be differentiated from true phobias. If the phobia is intense and interferes with the child's activity, or if the child does not respond to simple reassurance, refer to the child and adolescent mental health team.

School refusal and truancy

Children <10y Younger children may refuse to go to school or recurrently complain of abdominal pain, nausea, or other symptoms that justify staying home. Usually school refusal is a form of separation anxiety, although occasionally it is due to a problem at school, e.g. problems interacting with the teacher or friends or bullying. Advise parents to consult the school—a star chart with a star from the teacher for each morning the child goes to school without a fuss may help. Relapses can occur if the child is absent or after holidays.

Older children School refusal is a more difficult problem. Speak to parents and child together and separately. Try to ascertain if there is a genuine reason why the child avoids school. Liaise with the school. If not succeeding, refer to the child and adolescent mental health team.

Conduct disorders Poor behavior, e.g. aggression, destructive tendencies, and antisocial behaviour are common complaints. Tolerance varies from family to family. Try simple strategies such as rewarding good behaviour and ignoring poor behaviour ± 'time-out' strategies (younger children—📖 p. 911). If not succeeding, refer to the child and adolescent mental health team.

Childhood depression 📖 p. 921

Hyperactivity 📖 p. 916

Tics Sudden, rapid, repetitive non-rhythmic motor movements of no apparent purpose. Commonly involve facial grimacing, head movements or shoulder movements. Average age of onset ≈5y. Tics are present at some point in ~4% of children. Often a family history is present. Tics come and go and vary in intensity and frequency. They are often precipitated by stress. Most disappear during adolescence but in 20% they persist into adulthood.

Gilles de la Tourette syndrome ♂:♀ ≈3:1. Characterized by multiple motor tics and irrepressible verbal outbursts—sometimes obscene. There may also be repetitive blinking, nodding, gesturing, echoing of speech, and/or stuttering. Usually begins in childhood. Associated with obsessive–compulsive disorder and ADHD. Probable genetic aetiology.

Management Spontaneous remissions do occur. Clonidine or antipsychotic medication may help if severely affected (usually specialist initiated). Treat any associated obsessive–compulsive disorder (📖 p. 996) or ADHD (📖 p. 917). *G. Gilles de la Tourette (1857–1904)—French neurologist.*

⚠ **Behavioural problems and maltreatment**[N] Consider maltreatment (📖 p. 924) if there is behavioural change inconsistent with age/development that is not explained by a medical condition (e.g. ADHD, autism) or stressful situation (e.g. parental separation). In particular, suspect maltreatment if:
- A child repeatedly scavenges, steals, hoards, or hides food, or
- There is precocious or coercive sexualized behaviour

Refugee children Many child refugees have traumatic backgrounds. Approach children with sensitivity and consider involving specialist child mental health and specialist refugee support services early.

Further information
NICE When to suspect child maltreatment (2009) ℰ www.nice.org.uk

Parent information and support
Parentline ☏ 0808 800 2222 ℰ www.familylives.org.uk
Cry-sis Support for families with crying and sleepless babies ☏ 08451 228 669 ℰ www.cry-sis.org.uk

Child information and support
Childline 24h confidential counselling service ☏ 0800 1111 ℰ www.childline.org

Sleep problems

Sleeping patterns and habits of children vary considerably and should only be regarded as problems when they are presented as such by the family. First, take a careful history. Ask about:

- **Medical problems,** e.g. night cough related to asthma, itching from eczema, obstructive sleep apnoea. Treat appropriately
- **Physical problems,** e.g. hunger or cold
- **Night terrors**
- **The sleep pattern**—usually ≥1 of:
  • Difficulty settling
  • Waking during the night
  • Waking early in the morning
- **The amount of daytime sleep**

General advice In all cases it is helpful to recommend a regular calming bedtime routine (e.g. bath, story, cuddle, bed) and minimal fuss when a child does wake at night, e.g. try to settle back to sleep without taking out of cot, not rewarding waking with games, snacks, etc.

Resistance to going to bed The baby/child who cries incessantly when put to bed is a common problem with a peak age of 1–2y. The child cries when left alone or climbs out of bed and seeks the parents. *Causes include:*

- Separation anxiety
- Increasing attempts by the child to control his/her environment
- Long naps late in the afternoon
- Rough, overstimulating play before bedtime
- A disturbed parent–child relationship and/or tension in the home

Management Letting the child stay up, staying in the room and comforting the child or punishing the child are all ineffective. Options include:

- **Leaving the child to cry** This often does work and the crying diminishes after a few nights but it is very hard for parents to do and can be impossible if they are in shared accommodation
- **Controlled crying** The child is left to cry for a set length of time, e.g. 2–10min, before the parent returns to settle him/her again with minimum fuss and then leaves. Length of time before returning is gradually ↑. Easier for parents than leaving the child to cry and still effective
- **Staying with the child until he/she sleeps but gradually withdrawing proximity,** e.g. sit on bed with child, after a few nights sit next to bed, then nearer door, etc. until the child learns to go to sleep alone; this method is gentler than the above but may take longer

Waking during the night Occurs in half of all children aged 6–12mo and is related to separation anxiety. In older children, episodes often follow a stressful event (e.g. moving home, illness).

Management Allowing the child to sleep with the parents, playing, feeding, or punishing the child usually prolong the problem.

- Try the methods used for resistance to going to bed—but advise parents to always check to see that the child is not ill/needing a clean nappy, etc. before being left to cry

- Scheduled waking where a child is woken 15–60min before the time he/she usually wakes and then resettled has also been shown to improve night waking
- If a child wakes early, another strategy is to make toys or books accessible. The child may then amuse him-/herself for a period of time without disturbing his/her parents. Some 2–3y olds wander around without waking the parents—fitting a stair gate across the child's bedroom door prevents the child coming to any harm doing this
- Use of sedatives, e.g. promethazine (for children >2y), is often discouraged but can be useful particularly when parents feel desperate. Only use as a short-term measure

Nightmares Occur during rapid eye movement (REM) sleep. Nightmares can be caused by frightening experiences (e.g. scary stories, television violence), particularly in 3–4y olds. The child usually becomes fully awake and can vividly recall the details of the nightmare. An occasional nightmare is normal, but persistent or frequent nightmares warrant evaluation by an expert.

Sleepwalking (somnambulism) Involves walking clumsily, usually avoiding objects. The child appears confused but not frightened. 15% of children aged 5–12y have sleepwalked one or more times. It is most common amongst school-aged boys and may be triggered by a stressful event.

- Advise parents/carers not to try to wake the child
- If the child is in danger, gently steer him/her away from any harm
- If the child sleepwalks frequently, consider taking action to prevent the child coming to any harm whilst sleepwalking, e.g. stair gate across bedroom door
- If the sleepwalks occur repeatedly at the same time, waking the child ~15min before the predicted time can break the cycle

Night terror Sudden awakening with inconsolable panic and screaming. Usually occurs in the first 1–3h of sleep. Episodes last seconds → minutes. *Features:*

- Blank or confused stares
- Incomplete arousal with poor responsiveness to people
- Amnesia for the episode

Night terrors are most common in children aged 3–8y and require no treatment apart from simple reassurance. Advise parents not to wake the child as this ↑ the disturbance. If frequent consider waking the child before episodes occur and keeping the child awake for a few minutes to break the cycle. If the terrors persist beyond 8y, consider a diagnosis of temporal lobe epilepsy.

Parent information and support
Parentline ☎ 0808 800 2222 ⌖ www.familylives.org.uk
Cry-sis Support for families with crying and sleepless babies
☎ 08451 228 669 ⌖ www.cry-sis.org.uk

Toilet training

Most children can do without nappies by day from 2–3y and by night from 2–5y. How to approach toilet training will vary from child to child.

General rules

- **Wait until the child is ready** This usually means that the child can indicate to the parent that he/she is going to the toilet and has shown an interest in using the potty or toilet. It is helpful to have a potty or child's toilet seat to put on the normal toilet for the child to become familiar with before starting toilet training
- **Pick a good time** When the child can have a few days at home without nappies in an environment where accidents do not matter. Make sure the child has plenty of spare clothes available
- **Keep the potty handy or stay within easy reach of the toilet** If a child says he/she wishes to go, sit the child immediately on the toilet. Reward any result with praise. Do not punish the child for accidents— advise the parent to ask the child to help clear up any mess and reinforce that it would be better to use the potty/toilet next time
- **Until the child (and parent) are confident in the child's ability to use the toilet continue using nappies when out and at night.** Take the child to the toilet at night before bedtime. When dry nappies are consistently noted in the mornings, try the child without nappies at night—a plastic sheet on the mattress is a good idea. Even when a child has been dry day and night for some time, accidents are common if the child is tired, unwell, or unsettled (whether excited or unhappy)

❶ If the child does not succeed within a few days, either try training pants or revert to nappies and try again at a later date.

Nocturnal enuresis[N] Involuntary voiding of urine during sleep on >2 nights/wk. Affects 8% of children aged 4½y and 1.5% at 9y. ♂ > ♀. Tends to run in families. Distressing for child and parents with effects on emotional and social well-being. Cause is not fully understood:

- 1–2% have an underlying physical abnormality—usually UTI, constipation, or DM (rarely congenital anomalies, diabetes insipidus, or pelvic mass). Exclude with history and examination—consider urinalysis if recent onset, daytime symptoms, or symptoms/signs of ill health
- Occasionally caused by emotional distress or recent illness—consider if the child has been dry for 6mo prior to onset. Explore possible triggers that may need treating. Consider maltreatment, particularly if parents blame/punish the child despite advice that it is not the child's fault

Management See Table 24.13. Often resolves with time.

Further information
NICE Nocturnal enuresis: the management of bedwetting in children and young people. (2010) ℘ www.nice.org.uk

Information for parents of children with enuresis
ERIC (enuresis resource and information) ☎ 0845 370 8008
℘ www.eric.org.uk

Table 24.13 Management of enuresis

Method	Features
Advice and information	Reassure parents and children that enuresis is not the child's fault. In particular, advise:
	• That punitive measures should not be taken
	• On ways to limit the impact of bedwetting, e.g. bed protection
	• On regular toileting 4–7x/d and before bed
	• On appropriate fluid intake (1–1.4L/d in a child aged 4–8y)
	• To avoid caffeine
	• About self-help organizations/sources of support, e.g. ERIC
Reward systems	For example, star chart
	Use for agreed behaviour (e.g. going to the toilet before bed) rather than a dry night
Lifting and waking	Useful short-term measure but will not promote long-term dryness. However, young people who have not responded to treatment may find self-waking with an alarm clock useful
Enuresis alarms	An alarm is triggered to wake the child when urine makes contact with a sensor. With time the child wakes in response to bladder contractions rather than the alarm
Refer to school nurse or paediatric enuresis clinic	First-line treatment when advice/rewards fail. Usually some effect in <4wk but may take months until the child is completely dry at night. Continue until 2wk of dry nights—restart if relapse
Desmopressin	Synthetic version of antidiuretic hormone. Taken at night
Usually specialist initiated	Side effects include headache, nausea, nasal congestion, nosebleed, sore throat, cough, flushing, and mild abdominal cramps
	❶ There is a risk of water overload—advise only one mug of fluid from 1h before desmopressin dose to 8h afterwards
	Used when alarm is unsuccessful or unsuitable or in combination with an alarm. If effective continue for 3mo, then withdraw to assess whether still needed
Anticholinergics/ imipramine	Specialist initiation only for children who have not responded to other treatments

Encopresis Most children are continent of faeces by 2½–3y. Faecal soiling after this age usually occurs during the day. If:
• Bowel control, but the child passes stool in unacceptable places, the cause is usually emotional. Expert help from child and adolescent mental health services is needed—refer. Consider maltreatment (📖 p. 924)
• A firm stool is passed occasionally in the toilet but usually in the pants, developmental delay (either mental or social) is likely. Try a firm, consistent training programme
• Soft stool oozes out, causing constant soiling, consider overflow incontinence secondary to constipation (📖 p. 888)

Poor progress at school

~20% of school-aged children require special educational services at some point in their schooling. ♂: ♀ ≈5:1. Consider:
- Is a child's physical illness affecting school work, e.g. asthma, eczema?
- Is medication affecting academic performance (e.g. anticonvulsants)?
- Is the family stable or is there family upset?
- Does another family member have a chronic/life-threatening illness?
- Is the child's home environment conducive to doing school work?
- Is this school refusal?
- Is the child happy at school?
- Is there a problem with vision or hearing?
- Is the child of normal intelligence?
- Does the child interact socially with adults and other children?
- Have developmental milestones been met?
- Does the child have specific difficulty with certain aspects of his school work, e.g. mathematics, reading, writing?

Severe learning difficulty 📖 p. 919

Specific learning disorders

Dyslexia and dyscalculia Difficulty in information learning/processing. Intelligence is often normal/high and the child appears bright and alert. There may be a family history.
- **Dyslexia** Difficulty with letters/words, resulting in problems with reading, writing, and spelling. Affects up to 10% of the population. ♂ > ♀
- **Dyscalculia** The core problem is difficulty handling numbers and mathematical concepts. Less common than dyslexia

There is considerable overlap between dyslexia, dyscalculia, and also dyspraxia. If suspected liaise with the child's school. Formal testing by an educational psychologist can confirm the diagnosis. Specialized educational assistance and support are helpful.

Dyspraxia (developmental coordination disorder) Difficulty affecting movement/coordination. Affects 2–6% of the population; ♂ > ♀ Intelligence is often normal/high. Features are variable but include:
- Clumsiness
- Poor posture
- Awkward gait
- Reading and writing difficulties
- Difficulty holding a pen or pencil properly
- Poor short-term memory
- Poor body awareness
- Confusion about which hand to use
- Difficulties throwing/catching balls
- Poor sense of direction
- Difficulty hopping, skipping, and/or riding a bike
- Slow to learn to dress and feed

Diagnosis involves specialist community paediatric multidisciplinary assessment. Treatment is supportive.

Speech and language delay 📖 p. 857

Hyperactivity Difficult to define as claims a child is hyperactive often reflect the tolerance level of the person complaining. Active children with shorter-than-average attention spans create management problems.

Hyperactivity may have an underlying cause (e.g. an emotional disorder, CNS dysfunction, a genetic component) or may be an exaggeration of normal temperament. Often it is stage-related—support until that stage has passed. Simple behaviour management techniques help (📖 p. 908).

Attention deficit hyperactivity disorder (ADHD)[N]

- Common neurodevelopmental disorder interfering with normal social functioning, learning, and development
- Aetiology is probably multifactorial with overstimulation, family environment, and genetic factors all contributing
- Affects up to 9% of the school age population in the UK; ♂:♀ ≈ 6:1
- Other emotional, behavioural, and learning problems may coexist
- Long-term ADHD is associated with low academic achievement, substance misuse, unemployment, and antisocial tendencies

Presentation ❶ Many of these behaviours are seen in normal children.
- **Inattention** Poor attention to detail and organization of tasks; appears not to listen; easily distracted; forgetful; lack of concentration
- **Impulsivity** Lack of social awareness; shouts out answers to questions; difficulty waiting (unable to take turns or wait in a queue); excessive talking—interrupts others; lack of social awareness
- **Hyperactivity** Fidgets; inappropriate running/climbing/leaving seat

Assess duration of symptoms, how much functioning is impaired, and whether problems occur in different settings/areas of functioning—a report from school can be useful. ❶ Diagnosis of ADHD should only be made by a specialist.

Differential diagnosis
- Learning disability
- Hearing problems
- Epilepsy
- Autistic disorder
- Thyroid disease
- Drug ingestion
- Psychological problems (depression, emotional trauma, e.g. divorce)

Management
- **Mild/moderate impairment** Watchful waiting to see if problems persist, or refer for parent training/education
- **Persistent problems/severe impairment** Refer to community paediatrics or the child and adolescent mental health team for formal diagnosis. Specialist treatment includes behavioural therapy ± drug therapy (e.g. methylphenidate)
- **In all cases** Self-help and local support groups can be helpful

Autistic spectrum disorder 📖 p. 918

Further information
NICE Attention deficit hyperactivity disorder (2008) ℘ www.nice.org.uk

Information and support for parents and children
British Dyslexia Association ☎ 0845 251 9002 ℘ www.bdadyslexia.org.uk
Dyspraxia Foundation ☎ 01462 454 986
℘ www.dyspraxiafoundation.org.uk
National Attention Deficit Disorder Information and Support Service (ADDISS) ☎ 020 8952 2800 ℘ www.addiss.co.uk
Independent Panel for Special Education Advice (IPSEA)
☎ 0800 018 4016 ℘ www.ipsea.org.uk

Autism and severe learning difficulty

Autistic spectrum disorders[N] Impair social interaction and communication and affect ~1% of the population; ♂ > ♀ (≈4:1). *Risk factors:*

- Family history (including family history of psychosis)
- Premature birth (<35wk)
- CNS malfunction/dysfunction
- Valproate in pregnancy
- Intellectual disability
- Genetic disorders, e.g. Down's syndrome, fragile X, tuberous sclerosis, muscular dystrophy, neurofibromatosis

Features of autism Triad of features present in the first 3y of life and not attributable to another disorder (e.g. language delay):

- Impaired reciprocal social interaction (A symptoms)
- Impaired imagination associated with abnormal verbal and non-verbal communication (B symptoms)
- Restricted repertoires of activities and interests (C symptoms)

Features of Asperger's syndrome Impaired reciprocal interaction and stereotyped behaviour but without delay in speech or cognitive development. Better prognosis than autism.

Diagnosis Not apparent at birth; usually detected from 18mo–3y when failure of social interaction and lack of speech becomes apparent. Asperger's syndrome may present later. GPs play a vital role in detection. Consider the possibility of autistic spectrum disorder if concerns about development/behaviour are raised—but be aware of other explanations. Look for specific abnormalities of:

- **Spoken language,** e.g. ↓/absent, monotone, repetitive, only about own interests, rude/inappropriate, one way rather than conversation
- **Responding to others,** e.g. ↓ responsiveness, misunderstanding of others' intentions, −ve response to requests of others
- **Interacting with others,** e.g. ↓ awareness or ↓ tolerance of others entering personal space, plays alone, unaware of socially expected behaviour, difficulty making friends, lack of enjoyment
- **Eye contact/gestures,** e.g. ↓ eye contact, inappropriate/absent gestures/facial expressions
- **Ideas and imagination,** e.g. lack of imagination/creativity, failure to appreciate social niceties
- **Unusual or restricted interests,** e.g. dislike of change, over-reaction to stimuli, lack of flexibility, overfocussed/unusual interests
- **Rigid and repetitive behaviours,** e.g. repetitive stereotyped movements/play, strict adherence to rules
- **Other features,** e.g. unusual profile of skills/deficits, immature social/emotional skills, lack of common sense, excessive trust

Refer to or discuss with the local autism or community paediatric team if there are concerns. ❶ Diagnosis of autistic spectrum disorder should only be made by a specialist.

Checklists (e.g. the Checklist for Autism in Toddlers or CHAT—🖰 www.nas.org.uk) may be useful to assess toddlers with problems with social interaction or language delay but should not be used to make or exclude a diagnosis.

Management Life-long conditions; often severely disabling requiring a lot of support from community services. Most interventions are behavioural and delivered in an educational setting. Medication may be used for specific issues, e.g melatonin for sleep problems. Be approachable, willing to listen, and an advocate for the family. Give information about self help and signpost to support organizations and benefits (📖 p. 922).

Severe learning difficulty (mental handicap) May exist alone or with other disabilities. Often noted by a parent first—take any concerns seriously. Causes are varied—many are rare. Divide into:

- **Congenital** Genetic (e.g. Down's syndrome, fragile X); metabolic (e.g. congenital hypothyroidism); others (e.g. rubella in pregnancy)
- **Acquired,** e.g. trauma, meningitis, birth injury

Outlook

- **IQ 50–70** 80% of people with learning disability. Most lead an independent life and require just special attention to their schooling
- **IQ 35–49** Special schooling or extra support within mainstream schooling, and supervision may be needed
- **IQ <35**—severe learning difficulty. Limited social activity and speech may be impaired. Special schooling and medical services are needed

Management Refer to paediatrics/genetics to ensure no treatable cause is missed. *Then:*

- **Communicate with carers** Explain referrals; test results and their implications; the local system and who is responsible for what. Find out about the condition (as far as possible) and tell the carers where to get more information. Ensure carers receive information about benefits and housing/schooling options available
- **Refer to other community services,** e.g. paediatrician; severe learning disability service. Ensure follow-up happens and assist with assessment of special needs for schooling, housing, and employment. Provide ongoing prescriptions where appropriate
- **Manage medical problems not related to disability**
- **Promote concordance** With long-term therapy ± education or rehabilitation programmes
- **Reproduction** Offer family planning, pre-conceptual counselling, and/ or antenatal diagnosis for parents and patients with severe learning difficulty reaching reproductive age

The chronically disabled child 📖 p. 922

Further information

NICE Autism: recognition, referral, and diagnosis of children and young people on the autism spectrum (2011) ℳ www.nice.org.uk

Information and support for parents and children
National Autistic Society of the UK (NAS) ☎ 0808 800 4104
ℳ www.nas.org.uk
MENCAP ☎ 0808 808 1111 ℳ www.mencap.org.uk
Independent Panel for Special Education Advice (IPSEA) ☎ 0800 018 4016
ℳ www.ipsea.org.uk

Adolescence

Changes of adolescence start gradually—from ~10y for girls and ~12y for boys—and are complete by the age of ~17y. Adolescence is characterized by rapid physical development and emotional change. Adjusting to these changes causes problems:

- **Concerns about appearance** Some become very concerned about their appearance. They need reassurance, especially if not growing or maturing as quickly as their friends
- **Clothes/style** Are important to express solidarity with friends and declare independence
- **Hormonal changes** Lead to body shape, voice, hair, and skin changes, body hair growth, and menstruation. Adjustment can be difficult
- **Acne** May need treatment—especially if scarring
- **Dieting and consumption of junk food** Are common. Rarely, eating disorders develop

Consent 📖 p. 52   **Confidentiality** 📖 p. 50

School problems
- **School refusal** 📖 p. 910
- **Truancy** Usually children who are unhappy at home and frustrated at school. They spend their days with others who feel the same
- **Poor school work** Emotional problems, e.g. worry about problems at home, often affect school work and make it difficult to concentrate; pressure to do well/pass exams may be counterproductive. Exams are important, but advise parents not to let them dominate life or cause unhappiness

Maltreatment 📖 p. 924

Behaviour problems It is normal for teenagers and their parents to complain about each other's behaviour and disagree frequently. Parents often feel they have lost control over their child. Adolescents resent parental restrictions on their freedom—but still want parental guidance. Advise parents to lay down sensible ground rules and stick to them. Evidence suggests children are at greater risk of getting into trouble if their parents do not know where they are—advise teenagers to let their parents know where they are going and parents to ask.

Sexual problems and contraception 📖 p. 768

Trouble with the law ♂ > ♀. Most young people do not break the law—when they do, it usually only happens once. Repeated offending may reflect family culture or may result from unhappiness—always ask about emotional feelings when an adolescent is repeatedly getting into trouble.

Drugs, solvents, and alcohol Most teenagers never use drugs or inhale solvents, and of those that do, most never get beyond the experimenting stage. Alcohol is the most common drug causing problems for adolescents but consider the possibility of any form of drug use (📖 p. 188) when parents notice serious, sudden changes in behaviour.

Emotional problems Teenage unhappiness is common and does not necessarily indicate depression (~½ 14y olds feel miserable; ¼ are self-deprecatory; 8% have suicidal thoughts). However, emotional disorders are often not recognized, even by family and friends. Over-eating, excessive sleepiness, promiscuity, and a persistent over-concern with appearance may be signs of emotional distress. More obviously, phobias and panic attacks appear.

Rarely, changes in behaviour and mood can mark the beginning of more serious mental health disorders. Bipolar disorder and schizophrenia, as well as more common disorders such as anxiety, may emerge during adolescent years. Refer for mental health assessment if concerned.

Distinguishing normal adolescent behaviour from mental illness Teenage behavioural problems may be signs of mental illness if:
● They go on for more than a few weeks
● They do not vary, e.g. persistently low mood in all circumstances
● They are severe, e.g. self-harming behaviour, violence
● There is a significant impact on relationships, school performance, and/or usual activities

Childhood depression[N] Response to childhood stress. Distinguish from depressive symptoms occurring as part of other emotional or conduct disorders. Most common in adolescence ($♀ > ♂$).

Diagnosis Difficult, especially among adolescents. Adolescents often do not communicate well with their parents and have little contact with health professionals—resulting in late diagnosis.

Presenting features
● Unhappiness and/or tearfulness, apathy, boredom, ↓ ability to enjoy life
● Antisocial behaviour—$♂ > ♀$—especially after bereavement
● ↓ school performance—may admit to poor concentration
● Separation anxiety reappearing in adolescence
● Frequent unexplained illness or undue worries about health
● Self-harm
● Bipolar depressive disorder is rare before puberty, and mania must be present to make a diagnosis

Management Unless a mild episode related to a single precipitating event and no other risk factors for depression, refer for specialist advice. Specialist treatment includes counselling, family therapy, CBT, and drug therapy (❶ With the exception of fluoxetine, risks of treatment with SSRIs outweigh benefits in children).

Disorders of puberty 📖 p. 893

Eating disorders 📖 p. 1014

Further information
NICE Depression in children and young people (2005) ℅ www.nice.org.uk

Information and support for parents and children
Parentline ☎ 0808 800 2222 ℅ www.familylives.org.uk
Childline ☎ 0800 1111 ℅ www.childline.org.uk
Brook Advisory Service ☎ 0808 802 1234 ℅ www.brook.org.uk
Sexwise For under 19s ☎ 0800 28 29 30

The chronically disabled child

Chronic disability due to a wide variety of causes affects ~10% of children in the UK.

Effects on the child Vary from child to child, depending on the nature of the disability, personality of the child, and support the child has at home and in the community. Common problems include:

- Physical discomfort—both due to the disability and to painful or embarrassing treatments
- Alterations in the normal pattern of growth and development and/or physical differences may lead to social isolation and ↓ motivation
- Frequent hospitalizations and outpatient visits prevent the child integrating into school or ongoing community activities
- Dependence—the disability may prevent the child reaching his/her own goals and achieving his/her own independence. Many children also realize the additional burden they cause their parents and carers

Effects on the family Vary from family to family depending on financial and/or social support, relationship between parents and other siblings, and many other factors. Stress may cause family break-up, especially when other marital and intra-family problems exist. Common problems:

- Grieving for the loss of the 'ideal child'—conditions that affect the appearance of the child particularly affect attachment between parents and child. The grief might take the form of shock, denial, anger, sadness, depression, guilt, or anxiety and may occur any time in the child's development
- Neglected siblings
- Inconsistent discipline—due to demands placed on the family and sympathy for the child—resulting in behaviour problems
- Marginalization of one parent—one parent tends to take on the bulk of the caring activities. There is a danger the other parent starts to feel inadequate and isolated with respect to the care of the child
- Major expense and time commitment—frequently one parent has to give up work to look after a disabled child resulting not only in loss of income, but loss of that parent's independence and opportunities for the future
- Social isolation
- Confusion over the health, benefits, and social services available

Care coordination Inconsistent policies and funding, inadequate access to facilities (including physical barriers to access), and poor communication and coordination between the healthcare, educational, and community support systems → misery for children with disability and their families. Without coordination of services, care is crisis-oriented.

Care coordination requires knowledge about the child's condition, the family, and the community in which they function. In all cases *someone* should be designated responsible for coordinating care—the best person to do that will vary according to circumstances. Regardless of who assists in coordination of services, the family and child must be partners in the process.

Rehabilitation The general principles of rehabilitation for adult patients apply to children too—📖 p. 204 and p. 282

Role of the GP

- The GP of any patient with a chronic illness in the community is a team member and may be the key worker who coordinates care
- The GP provides continuity of care, particularly when the child is under the care of several different secondary care teams, or during the transition from child to adolescent or adult services
- Maintain an open door policy and encourage children and carers to seek help for problems early
- Be flexible with appointments to avoid long waits and allow carers and other family members to attend to their own health needs
- Try to become familiar with a child's disease, even if it is rare. It is impossible to plan care without knowledge of course and prognosis, and an easy way to lose a child's confidence if you appear ignorant of their condition
- If progress is slower than expected or stalls, consider other medical problems (e.g. anaemia, infection), behavioural problems, and communication problems (e.g. poor vision/hearing)
- Remember that children with disability are at ↑ risk of maltreatment and that symptoms/signs of maltreatment may be difficult to distinguish from the effects of the child's underlying problem
- Information alone can improve outcome

Support for carers 📖 p. 220

Information for parents and children

Benefits information ✆ www.gov.uk

Contact a Family Support and information for families with disabled children (any disability) ☎ 0808 808 3555 ✆ www.cafamily.org.uk

Whizz-Kidz Mobility for non-mobile disabled children ☎ 020 7233 6600 ✆ www.whizz-kidz.org.uk

Tourism for all Holidays for families with a disabled child
☎ 0845 124 9971 ✆ www.tourismforall.org.uk

Safeguarding children

Children may be mistreated if harm is inflicted upon them or if a responsible person fails to prevent them from coming to harm. In the UK, there are ~50,500 children on child protection registers or the subject of child protection plans. Classification—see Table 24.14.

Table 24.14 Classification of child abuse: >1 type may occur concurrently

PHYSICAL Hitting, shaking, throwing, burning, suffocating, poisoning, including fabricated or induced illness	EMOTIONAL The child is made to feel worthless, afraid, unloved, or inadequate. Includes age-inappropriate expectations and witnessing domestic violence
NEGLECT Failure to meet the child's basic needs (including medical needs); allowing the child to be exposed to danger	SEXUAL Forcing/enticing a child to participate in sexual activities—physical contact or production of pornographic material

Circumcision of female children or forced marriage <16y
Both illegal in the UK. Children may be taken abroad to be circumcised/married. If you suspect that this might be going to happen to any patient, inform social services and/or the police immediately.

Risk factors ❶ Any child may be a victim of maltreatment.

Parent/carer factors
- Mental illness/learning disability
- Substance/alcohol abuse
- Being abused themselves
- Ongoing physical illness
- Parental conflict/domestic violence/divorce
- Unemployment/poor living conditions

Child factors
- History of sibling abuse
- Learning/behaviour/physical problems
- Unplanned pregnancy/premature birth
- Poor attachment to parents/carers
- Environment high in criticism
- 'Looked after' children (those under the guardianship of the state, e.g. those in local authority or foster care)

Presentation *Always have a high index of suspicion.*

Suspect maltreatment if
- The child discloses it
- Story is inconsistent with injuries (⚠ bruising, bleeding, fractures, or other injuries in children not independently mobile are suspicious)
- Characteristic injuries—marks consistent with cigarette burns; scalds (especially if symmetrical or doughnut-shaped on buttocks); finger mark or bite mark bruises; perineal bruising or anogenital injury; linear marks consistent with whipping; buckle or belt marks
- Late presentation or lack of concern about injury/illness
- Behaviour of the child is suggestive, e.g. withdrawn, 'frozen watchfulness', sexually precocious behaviour, abnormal interaction between child and parents, unwilling to speak about the injury
- STI or pregnancy in any child <13y (consider if the child is older)
- The child is persistently smelly/dirty and/or inadequate home environment (including food and hygiene)

Consider maltreatment within your differential diagnosis if
- Encopresis, enuresis, or daytime incontinence of urine (📖 p. 914)
- Failure to thrive (📖 p. 872)
- Severe or persistent infestations (e.g. scabies, head lice), oral injuries, or urinary/anogenital symptoms without adequate explanation
- Failure to attend healthcare appointments and/or poor concordance with treatment plans for significant medical conditions
- Unusual/frequent presentation to healthcare professionals
- Injury as a result of inadequate supervision
- Behavioural problems (📖 p. 908)
- Inappropriate dress (e.g. underdressed in cold weather)

⚠ **Immediate action**[N] Do *not* ask leading questions.
- **Listen and observe** Record the history given, any report of maltreatment, the child's appearance and behaviour, any physical signs, and interaction between the child and parent/carer
- **Seek an explanation** From the accompanying adult and (if possible) the child. Record the explanations given. An inadequate explanation is implausible, inadequate, inconsistent (over time or between the child and parent/carer), or based on cultural practice (does not justify harm)
- **Make a decision** If child maltreatment is likely, a possibility or can be excluded

Further action Welfare of the child is *paramount*.

Share your concerns and plans For further action with parents and child *unless* you believe doing so will ↑ risk to child. Record any discussions, referrals, and actions taken.

If child maltreatment is a possibility Check the child's/other family members' records for worrying features; consider asking other practice members if they have concerns; and do ≥1 of the following:
- Seek further information from other agencies (e.g. school, social services) or other health professionals (e.g. health visitor, specialists involved with care)
- Discuss concerns with a more experienced colleague, e.g. practice safeguarding lead, locality named professional for safeguarding, or senior paediatrician
- Arrange to review the child at a date appropriate to concern— follow-up if the appointment is cancelled or is not kept

❶ At any stage your level of concern may change and lead you to exclude or suspect maltreatment.

If you suspect that child maltreatment is likely Refer to children's social care following local child protection procedures. Follow-up telephone referrals in writing in <24h. Urgency of action taken depends on the nature of the suspected maltreatment.

Responding to child protection enquiries Under Section 47 of the Children Act (1989), GPs have a legal obligation to share relevant information whether or not they have consent of the parents.

Further information

GMC Protecting children and young people (2012) ℅ www.gmc-uk.org
NICE When to suspect child maltreatment (2009) ℅ www.nice.org.uk

Child death

Sudden infant death syndrome (cot death) ~1 in 2,000 babies/y are found unexpectedly dead in the first year of life in the UK. These deaths are most common in winter months and at night (midnight–9 a.m.). An identifiable cause for the death can be found for 37%—the rest remain unexplained ('*cot deaths*'). Theories include cardiac arrhythmia and apnoeic attacks. *Peak age:* 1–4mo; ♂ > ♀.

Risk factors for cot death
- Baby sleeping face down
- Smoking (mother and other family members)
- Overheating
- Minor intercurrent illness
- Twin or multiple pregnancy
- Low birth weight
- Social disadvantage
- Young mother
- Large numbers of siblings

Reducing the risk of cot death 📖 p. 847

Management if you are the first person contacted
- Check an ambulance is on its way and go immediately to the scene. Start resuscitation, unless clearly inappropriate. Continue until the baby gets to hospital
- If it is clear the baby is dead and cannot be resuscitated, inform the parents sympathetically. Contact the police/Coroner and the designated paediatrician for unexpected death in childhood. Arrange for the baby to be taken to A&E, not to a mortuary
- Take a brief history. Record the circumstances of death immediately (e.g. position when found, bedding, vomit). Listen to the parents. Mention the baby by name and do not be afraid to express your sorrow
- If the baby is a twin, the surviving twin is at ↑ risk of cot death and should be admitted to hospital for observation

Management if you learn that a baby has died
- Provide information as requested to the rapid response team, and attend the initial case discussion if possible
- Consider taking part in the scene of death visit to support parents

Follow-up
- Review within a few days. There may be some anger directed towards you as often babies have been seen in general practice within a few days or weeks of the death. Do not be defensive or become angry
- Discuss suppression of lactation if breastfeeding (📖 p. 842)
- Advise parents about likely grief reactions—guilt, anger, ↓ appetite, sleeplessness, hearing the baby cry. Do not forget siblings—they can be deeply affected too. Continue regular review as long as needed and wanted. Be sensitive to anniversaries. Watch for psychiatric illness
- Ensure parents have received written information about cot death including details of self-help organizations and helplines. Consider referral for counselling—ideal timing for referral varies
- Refer for specialist obstetric assessment early in the next pregnancy and make sure parents are put in touch with the Care of Next Infant (CONI) scheme. Discuss the use of apnoea alarms

Death of a child in other circumstances Death of a child is always difficult. Accidents are the most common cause of death followed by death from childhood cancer. Principles of management used for cot death can be applied.

Child death review
- All deaths of children <18y (excluding stillbirths) are subject to review by a local child death review panel and should be notified to it
- Unexpected deaths are investigated by a rapid response team, involving police, a senior paediatrician, and other professionals as appropriate
- This rapid response team notifies and gathers information from other professionals involved with the child, including the GP, carries out an initial case discussion, arranges a visit to the scene of death, and then arranges post-mortem informed by the investigation
- Further case discussions take place following post-mortem. The GP should be invited and sent a report. An appropriate professional is identified to inform the parents of the findings
- The panel arranges support for the parents throughout this procedure—regard this as additional to GP support

Apnoea alarms Commonly issued to or purchased by parents if they are worried about the risk of cot death. An apnoea alarm cannot be useful unless parents are taught basic life support to a proficient standard. An alarm should not be supplied without this training. There is no evidence that apnoea alarms prevent cot deaths.

Near-miss cot deaths Parents may rush a child to A&E or the GP after an episode of pallor ± floppiness. Parents may have attempted mouth-to-mouth resuscitation before the baby starts to respond to them, or may have simply touched the baby or lifted the baby up and received a response. Usually there are no residual symptoms or signs.

Management Difficult. Parents may have misinterpreted normal irregularities in sleep or the child might be unwell and have a physical cause for symptoms, e.g. early stages of a viral infection. Usually parents are very anxious by the time you see the child. Take a careful history and examine the child from top to toe. Treat any cause of symptoms found. Be as reassuring as possible and play down anxieties.

⚠ If the child has any risk factors for cot death, there is a clear history of apnoea, the child comes from a difficult social background, or parents are unable to cope following the episode—admit the child for observation and further assessment.

Information and parent support
Lullaby Trust ☎ 0808 802 6868 (bereavement support); 0808 802 6869 (information and support) ℘ www.lullabytrust.org.uk
Child Bereavement Charity ☎ 01494 568900
℘ www.childbereavement.org.uk
Child Death Helpline ☎ 0800 282 986 ℘ www.childdeathhelpline.org.uk

Ear, nose, and throat

The mouth

⚠ **Oral surgery referral**[N]

Urgent referral To exclude malignancy, ALL:

- Mouth ulcers persisting for >3wk
- Lumps in the mouth persisting >3wk
- Red or white patches in the mouth—including suspected lichen planus—that are painful, swollen, or bleeding

❶ For patients with persistent symptoms/signs related to the oral cavity, in whom a definitive diagnosis of a benign lesion cannot be made, refer or follow up until the symptoms and signs disappear. If the symptoms/signs have not disappeared in ≤6wk, make an urgent referral.

Non-urgent referral Patients with unexplained red and/or white patches of the oral mucosa that are not painful, swollen, or bleeding—including suspected lichen planus.

Dry mouth *Causes:* anxiety, drugs or Sjögren's syndrome. Look for cause, and rectify if possible. Prescribe artificial saliva, e.g. Glandosane®.

Sore mouth Treat the cause. *Consider:*

- Oral thrush
- Aphthous ulcers
- HSV
- Dry mouth
- Trauma (e.g. burn)
- Side effects of chemo- or radiotherapy
- Anaemia
- Hand, foot, and mouth disease (child)
- Gingivitis

Mouth ulcers Treat the cause. *Consider:*

- Aphthous ulcers
- Trauma, e.g. sharp tooth, false teeth
- Crohn's disease/UC
- Coeliac disease
- Drugs, e.g. steroids, gold
- Reiter's disease
- Behçet's disease
- HSV
- Herpes zoster
- Vincent's angina
- Erythema multiforme
- Self-inflicted, e.g. burns

Leukoplakia Thick whitish, grey patch usually on the inside of the cheek, the tongue, or gum. It is the mouth's reaction to chronic irritation of the mucous membranes. ♂ > ♀. Common in patients who smoke, patients with ill-fitting dentures, and patients who habitually chew on their cheek. Usually benign but may be an early sign of oral cancer. NICE recommends referral to oral surgery to exclude malignancy in *all* cases[N].

Erythroplakia Reddened area that results when the lining of the mouth thins. The area appears red because the underlying capillaries are more visible. Erythroplakia is a much more ominous predictor of oral cancer than leukoplakia. NICE recommends referral to oral surgery to exclude malignancy in *all* cases[N].

Tongue problems

- **Blue tongue** Central cyanosis—📖 p. 232
- **Dry and furred tongue** Suggests dehydration
- **Geographic tongue** Irregular smoother redder patches that change position over time on the dorsum of the tongue. Due to papillae loss. Asymptomatic or causes soreness. Rarely due to vitamin B_{12} deficiency
- **Large tongue** Consider acromegaly, amyloidosis, myxoedema

- **Smooth tongue** Iron, riboflavin, nicotinic acid, B_{12} or folate deficiency; idiopathic—usually elderly; antibiotic use
- **Sore tongue** Glossitis of anaemia; Crohn's disease; coeliac disease; carcinoma of the tongue; psychogenic causes
- **Strawberry tongue** Yellowish white tongue coating with the dark red papillae of the tongue projecting through. Associated with scarlet fever although also present in Kawasaki's disease
- **Ulcer** Assume any non-healing ulcer is due to carcinoma of the tongue until proven otherwise. Refer for biopsy to an oral surgeon. Treatment is with surgery or laser ablation ± radiotherapy

Halitosis Common after sleep. *Short-term halitosis* is associated with acute illness, e.g. tonsillitis, appendicitis (foetor oris), gastroenteritis, diabetic ketoacidosis.

Chronic halitosis Is usually caused by bacterial putrefaction of food debris and dental plaque and is related to poor oral hygiene. Associated with gingivitis ± periodontitis. Smoking, alcohol, isosorbide dinitrate, and disulfiram exacerbate the problem. Rarely caused by metabolic disorders, e.g. trimethylaminuria (TMAU or fish odour syndrome).

Management Examine the mouth and recommend a dental check. Advise oral hygiene, e.g. regular brushing of teeth/tongue, dental flossing; smoking cessation; diet advice—avoid garlic, onions, curries; treat any local infection, e.g. gingivitis; mouthwashes, e.g. 0.2% aqueous chlorhexidine gluconate help ↓ dental plaque. Refer if causing distress.

Aphthous ulcers Painful white ulcers. Common, affecting ~20%. Usually idiopathic but may be associated with poor health, stress, Crohn's, coeliac, and Behçet's disease. Most are short-lived. Large ulcers (up to 2cm diameter) can take ~6wk to heal. Most resolve spontaneously. Topical therapies are effective, e.g. hydrocortisone lozenges qds (dissolve in contact with the ulcer). If ulcers are recurrent, check FBC, iron, and folate levels. Refer any ulcer not significantly improving >3wk after presentation to exclude malignancy, or if recurrent ulcers cause distress.

Oral cancer >6,200 new cases/y in the UK. Incidence is increasing. Usually squamous cell carcinoma. ♂ > ♀. Major risk factors are smoking and high alcohol consumption. Lip cancer has good prognosis (>90% 5y survival), but overall survival is poor (51% 2y survival) mainly due to poor public awareness/late presentation. Usually presents with leukoplakia (white patch), erythroplakia (red patch), or non-healing ulcer (>3wk).

Management Refer suspicious lesions to oral surgery for biopsy.

Lichen planus 📖 p. 620	**Erythema multiforme** 📖 p. 597
Oral thrush 📖 p. 636	**Behçet's disease** 📖 p. 519
Herpes simplex virus (HSV) infection (cold sores) 📖 p. 634	

Further information
NICE Referral guidelines for suspected cancer (2005) ℘ www.nice.org.uk

Support and information for patients
Mouth Cancer Foundation ☎ 01924 950 950
℘ www.mouthcancerfoundation.org

Dental and jaw problems

Gums

- **Bleeding gums** Consider periodontal disease (most common cause); pregnancy; leukaemia; bleeding disorders; scurvy
- **Hypertrophied gums** Associated with phenytoin use
- **Blue line** Along the margin of the teeth—suggests lead poisoning
- **Gum inflammation** Gingivitis—consider immunodeficiency; vitamin C deficiency; DM, leukaemia; drugs; e.g. phenytoin, nifedipine, ciclosporin

Vincent's angina Pharyngeal infection with ulcerative gingivitis. *Management:* penicillin V 250mg qds po + metronidazole 400mg tds po. *J.H. Vincent (1862–1950)—French bacteriologist.*

Periodontal disease Disease of the periodontal ligament caused by bacterial plaque and exacerbated by smoking and DM. Occurs in the normal population >30y. Leads to gingivitis, dental abscesses, and tooth loss. Encourage patients to register with a dentist[N]—regular dental care helps prevent dental emergencies and periodontal disease. Patients experiencing difficulty finding an NHS dentist should telephone their local Primary Care Organization and ask to be found a dentist.

⚠ Refer urgently to a dentist if unexplained tooth mobility for >3wk[N].

Toothache Pain/excessive sensitivity to temperature may be a problem with exposed dentine or pulp infection—advise to see a dentist.

Dental abscess Facial swelling and pain related to bacterial infection. Refer to a dentist. Prescribe analgesia if there will be a delay.

Complications of tooth extraction

- **Haemorrhage** Apply pressure by placing wet gauze over socket and get patient to bite hard for 15min—refer to dentist if not stopping
- **Painful socket and bad taste in mouth** Infection—refer to a dentist. Give analgesia if delay is likely

Loss of tooth through trauma 📖 p. 1108

 Cleft lip and palate *Incidence:* 1:600 live births—half have other abnormalities too (e.g. hypoplastic mandible). Often—though not always—detected at routine antenatal USS. The cleft may be unilateral or bilateral and involve lip and/or palate. Cleft lips are usually repaired in the first few days of life; cleft palates at ~3mo depending on the weight of the baby.

Problems associated with cleft lip and/or palate
- Feeding difficulties with associated poor weight gain
- Aspiration pneumonia
- Hearing problems—particularly glue ear. In some areas children with cleft palate are routinely given grommets at ~18mo. Treat otitis media promptly. Audiology review is important
- Speech problems—refer for speech therapy
- Dental problems—universal with cleft palate. Orthodontic treatment is always required

Temporomandibular joint (TMJ) dysfunction Common disorder affecting ~70% of the population—only 5% seek treatment. Typically presents in early adulthood. ♂:♀ ≈ 1:4. Aetiology is complex—malocclusion and trauma play a part and are exacerbated by psychogenic factors.

Assessment Take a careful history noting pain—duration, location, and nature; precipitating/relieving factors; joint noises; restricted jaw function, e.g. locking, poor bite; and non-specific symptoms, e.g. headache, earache, and tinnitus. Examine the head and neck, including the TMJ and mandibular movement. Exclude other disease. Do not X-ray as this yields little useful information—CT/MRI may be ordered by specialists.

Patterns of disease There are 3 patterns of disease:
- **Myofacial pain and dysfunction** Due to clenching/teeth grinding. Pain is usually worse in the morning. Stress, anxiety, and depression are key features. Poor sleep is common. May have diffuse muscle tenderness
- **Internal derangement** The articular disc is in an abnormal position and causes restriction of mandibular movement. Pain is usually continuous and exacerbated by jaw movement
- **Osteoarthrosis** Degeneration of the joint seen on older patients. Crepitus and sounds from the joint occur on jaw movement

Management Reassure and explain the benign nature of the disorder. Suggest simple analgesia, e.g. paracetamol ± ibuprofen. Resting the jaw and avoiding stress may help. Refer those with ongoing problems to oral surgery.

Specialist treatment A bite appliance to wear at night helps 70%. Physiotherapy, behavioural therapy, and exercises also help. Drug treatments include NSAIDs, antidepressants, opioids, and muscle relaxants. Surgery is occasionally necessary if medical treatment fails.

Dislocated jaw 📖 p. 1113   **Fractured mandible** 📖 p. 1113

Information and support
British Association of Oral and Maxillofacial Surgeons Salivary gland disorders; temporomandibular joint disorders ℬ www.baoms.org.uk
Cleft Lip and Palate Association (CLAPA) ℂ 020 7833 4883
ℬ www.clapa.com

Sore throat

Each GP sees ~120 patients with sore throat every year—mostly children and young adults. 70% sore throats are viral in origin—the rest bacterial (mostly Group A β-haemolytic streptococci).

Clinical picture Pain on swallowing; fever; headache; tonsillar exudates; nausea and vomiting; and/or abdominal pain (especially in children due to abdominal lymphadenopathy).

❶ Viral and bacterial infections are indistinguishable clinically but association with coryza and cough may point to a viral aetiology.

Differential diagnosis Glandular fever especially in young adults, with persistent sore throat.

Investigation Not usually undertaken.
- Throat swabs cannot distinguish commensal organisms from clinical infection (40% carry Group A β-haemolytic streptococci), are expensive and do not give instant results so are rarely used
- Rapid antigen tests give immediate results but have low sensitivity limiting usefulness

Management 90% recover in <1wk without treatment. Complications are rare. Advise analgesia and antipyretics (e.g. paracetamol and/or ibuprofen),↑ fluid intake, and salt water gargles.

Use of antibiotics Antibiotic prescription can probably be avoided in most patients, but educating patients about the reasons for not prescribing is vital to maintain a good doctor–patient relationship.
- **Benefits** Antibiotics give a modest benefit in symptom relief (8h less symptoms) and may confer slight protection against some complications (e.g. quinsy, otitis media). There is no evidence antibiotics protect against rheumatic fever or acute glomerulonephritis
- **Risks** Possibility of side effects with antibiotic use; ↑ in community antibiotic resistance; 'medicalizing' a self-limiting condition—prescribing ↑ faith in antibiotics encouraging re-attendance with sore throat

Most patients should be given simple advice and/or a 'delayed prescription' (phenoxymethylpenicillin or erythromycin qds)—for patients to collect if no better in 2–3d (70% do not collect the script). Avoid amoxicillin as this causes a rash in those with glandular fever.

Reasons to give antibiotics immediately[N]
- Acute sore throat where ≥3 Centor criteria are present: tonsillar exudate, tender anterior cervical lymphadenopathy/lymphadenitis, history of fever, and absence of cough
- Patient is systemically very unwell
- Symptoms and signs suggestive of serious illness and/or complications (e.g. peritonsillar abscess, peritonsillar cellulitis)
- High risk of serious complications because of pre-existing co-morbidity, e.g. significant heart, lung, renal, liver, or neuromuscular disease, immunosuppression, cystic fibrosis, and young children born prematurely

Complications of sore throat All rare:

- **Quinsy (peritonsillar abscess)** Usually occurs in adults. *Signs:* unilateral peritonsillar swelling, difficulty swallowing (even saliva), and trismus (difficulty opening jaw). Refer for IV antibiotics ± incision and drainage
- **Retropharyngeal abscess** Occurs in children. *Signs:* inability to swallow, fever. Refer for IV antibiotics ± incision and drainage
- **Rheumatic fever** 📖 p. 276   • **Glomerulonephritis** 📖 p. 442

Indications for referral to ENT

Urgent referral Any unexplained sore throat for >1mo[N].

Referral for tonsillectomy[G]

- **Recurrent acute tonsillitis** Young children have a lot of throat infections, and most will 'grow out' of the problem without the need for surgery. Tonsillectomy is only considered if children miss a lot of school, e.g. >5 attacks/y for 2y causing school absence
- **Airway obstruction** Very large tonsils causing sleep apnoea
- **Chronic tonsillitis** >3mo + halitosis
- **Recurrent quinsy**
- **Unilateral tonsillar enlargement** To exclude malignancy.

⚠ Tonsillectomy carries a small risk of severe haemorrhage. Readmit any patient with bleeding post-operatively for observation.

Glandular fever (infectious mononucleosis) Consider in teenagers or young adults presenting with sore throat lasting >1wk. Caused by Epstein–Barr virus (EBV). Spread by droplet infection and direct contact ('kissing disease') and has a 4–14d incubation period. Presents with sore throat, malaise, fatigue, lymphadenopathy, enlarged spleen, palatal petechiae, and/or rash (10–20%). Send blood for FBC (atypical lymphocytes) and glandular fever antibodies (Monospot or Paul Bunnell).

Management Advise rest, fluids, and regular paracetamol, avoid alcohol. Try salt water gargles or aspirin gargles (only if >16y). Consider a short course of prednisolone for severe symptoms. Treat 2° infection with antibiotics. Counsel re the possibility of prolonged symptoms (up to several months). ⚠ Do not prescribe amoxicillin as it causes a rash.

Complications 2° infections; rash with amoxicillin; hepatitis; jaundice; pneumonitis; neurological disturbances (rare).

Tonsillar tumour Most often elderly. *Signs:* unilateral tonsillar swelling, dysphagia, sore throat, earache. Refer for excision biopsy.

⚠ Refer any unexplained, sore throat present for >1mo for urgent ENT assessment[N].

Further information

NICE 🖱 www.nice.org.uk
- Respiratory tract infections: antibiotic prescribing (2008)
- Referral guidelines for suspected cancer (2005)

Information for patients

Patient UK Information leaflets on sore throat. URTI, tonsillitis, tonsils and adenoids, and glandular fever 🖱 www.patient.co.uk

Hoarseness and stridor

Hoarseness Change in quality of the voice affecting pitch, volume, or resonance. Occurs when vocal cord function is affected by a change in the cords, a neurological or muscular problem. *Causes:*

- **Local causes** URTI (most common); laryngitis; trauma (shouting, coughing, vomiting, instrumentation); carcinoma; hypothyroidism; acromegaly
- **Neurological problems** Laryngeal nerve palsy; motor neurone disease; myasthenia gravis; multiple sclerosis
- **Muscular problems** Muscular dystrophy
- **Functional problems**

Assessment Weight ↓, dysphagia, or neck lumps add to suspicions of malignancy. Check TFTs in those with weight gain. Indirect laryngoscopy with a mirror can be difficult and give a poor view. ENT departments have thin fibreoptic scopes for direct visualization in outpatients.

⚠ *Refer urgently for chest X-ray (CXR)*[N] If hoarseness persisting >3wk—particularly smokers >50y and heavy drinkers.

If there is a POSITIVE finding on CXR Refer urgently to a team specializing in the management of lung cancer.

If there is a NEGATIVE finding on CXR Refer urgently to a team specializing in the management of head and neck cancer.

Laryngitis Hoarseness, malaise ± fever and/or pain on using voice. Usually viral and self-limiting (1–2wk) but occasionally 2° bacterial infection occurs.

Management Advise patients to rest voice, take OTC analgesia, e.g. paracetamol and/or ibuprofen, try steam inhalations. Consider antibiotics if bacterial infection is suspected (e.g. phenoxymethylpenicillin 250mg qds for 1wk).

Vocal cord nodules Can cause hoarseness. Usually precipitated by overuse of the voice—typically in singers. They can be visualized at laryngoscopy. Initial treatment is resting the voice but sometimes nodules have to be removed surgically.

Functional disorders Hysterical paralysis of the vocal cord adductors due to psychological stress. Can cause the voice to ↓ to a whisper or be lost completely. More common amongst young women.

Management Refer for laryngoscopy to exclude organic cause. Speech therapy and psychological support may help.

Laryngeal carcinoma ♂ > ♀. Smoking is the main risk factor. The first sign is usually hoarseness, followed by stridor, dysphagia, and pain,

Management Refer urgently to ENT if suspected. Diagnosis is confirmed with laryngoscopy and biopsy. Treatment is with surgery ± radiotherapy. Early tumours confined to the vocal cord have 80–90% 5y survival.

Post-laryngectomy problems After laryngectomy patients have a permanent tracheostomy and require practical and psychological support. *Problems include:*

- Excessive secretions
- Recurrent pneumonia
- Stenosis of the tracheostomy site—refer to ENT/oral surgery if severe
- Communication difficulties—ensure referred to speech therapy
- Maintenance of adequate diet—refer to dietician if not maintaining weight and recurrence of tumour has been excluded

Stridor Noise created on inspiration due to narrowing of the larynx or trachea—much more common in children than adults. Treat the cause.

> ⚠ *Signs of severe airway narrowing*
> - Distress
> - ↑ respiratory rate
> - Pallor and cyanosis
> - Use of accessory muscles and tracheal tug

Causes Congenital abnormalities of the larynx; epiglottis; croup (laryngotracheobronchitis); inhaled foreign body; trauma; laryngeal paralysis.

 Laryngomalacia (congenital laryngeal stridor) Common among small babies. Due to floppy aryatic folds and the small size of the airway. Stridor becomes more noticeable during sleep, excitement, crying, and with concurrent URTIs. Normally resolves without treatment. Parental concern may necessitate referral.

Croup Common viral infection occurring in epidemics in autumn and spring. Starts with mild fever and runny nose. In younger children (<4y), oedema and secretions in the larynx and trachea result in a barking cough and inspiratory stridor. The cough typically starts at night and is exacerbated by crying and parental anxiety. Some children have recurrent attacks associated with viral URTI.

Management Steam helps. There is also evidence that steroids can be helpful—give oral dexamethasone 0.15mg/kg or prednisolone 1–2mg/kg. Admit as a paediatric emergency if there is intercostal recession, cyanosis, or the child's carers are unable to cope.

Acute epiglottitis in children Bacterial infection causing a swollen epiglottis. Can potentially obstruct the airway. Much rarer since introduction of routine *Haemophilus influenza* type b (Hib) immunization. Consider if stridor, drooling, fever, and upright 'leaning forward' posture.

⚠ If suspected do not examine the child's throat as this can precipitate complete obstruction.

Management Refer urgently but try to maintain a calm atmosphere to avoid distressing the child. Examination will be undertaken in hospital with full resuscitation facilities on hand. *Treatment:* IV antibiotics.

Adult epiglottitis Much less common than childhood epiglottitis and less likely to cause complete airway obstruction. Refer for IV antibiotics.

Inhaled foreign body Refer to ENT for assessment.

Neck lumps and salivary gland problems

Neck lumps are common and can be the first sign of serious underlying pathology. Accurate assessment is important to differentiate harmless lumps from those needing further investigation and treatment. Ask about local symptoms in the head/neck and systemic symptoms (e.g. fever, anorexia, weight ↓). Differential diagnosis—see Figure 25.1.

⚠ **Refer urgently to ENT**[N]
- Any unexplained lump in the neck of recent onset
- Any previously undiagnosed lump that has changed over 3–6wk.

Lymphadenopathy Most enlarged LNs are reactive LNs—suggested by a short history, soft tender mobile lump, and concurrent infection.

⚠ **Check FBC, blood film + ESR (or CRP/viscosity)** And consider further investigation, discussion with a specialist, and/or referral if[N]:
- Lymphadenopathy present ≥6wk
- LNs are increasing in size
- Associated weight ↓, night sweats, and/or splenomegaly
- LN >2cm in size
- Widespread lymphadenopathy

Causes of lymphadenopathy
- **Benign infective** Viral infection, e.g. EBV, CMV, adenovirus, HIV; bacterial infection, e.g. streptococcal sore throat, TB; toxoplasmosis; syphilis
- **Benign non-infective** Sarcoid; connective tissue disease (e.g. RA); skin disease (e.g. eczema, psoriasis); drugs (e.g. phenytoin)
- **Malignant** Lymphoma, CLL, ALL, metastases—head and neck cancer may present with enlarged cervical LNs

Branchial cyst Arises from embryonic remnants of the second branchial cleft in the neck. Most common in young adults. Presents as a smooth swelling in front of the anterior border of the sternomastoid at the junction of its upper and middle thirds—often during a viral URTI. Position is characteristic. *Examination:* fluctuant lump that does not move on swallowing. Treatment is by excision—refer to ENT.

Thyroglossal cyst The thyroid gland develops from the lower portion of the thyroglossal duct. If a portion of this duct remains patent it can form a thyroglossal cyst. Usually presents in young adults (peak age 15–30y) with either a painless, smooth, cystic midline swelling between the isthmus of the thyroid gland and the hyoid cartilage or just above the hyoid cartilage or, if the cyst is inflamed, a painful, tender lump with localized swelling. *Examination:* the cyst rises as the patient sticks out his tongue. Refer to ENT for excision.

Salivary gland strictures and stones
- **Salivary stones** 80% of calculi are seen in the submandibular duct system. Less frequently they occur in the parotid duct system and rarely in other salivary glands
- **Strictures** of the salivary gland duct occur as a complication of a pre-existing calculus, due to mucus plugs or following trauma to the duct wall (e.g. cheek biting)

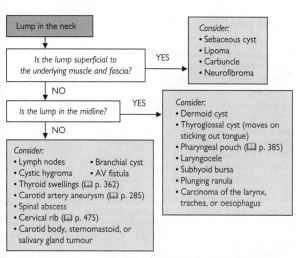

Figure 25.1 Differential diagnosis of neck lumps

Presentation Pain and swelling on eating due to obstruction of saliva flow. The gland may appear normal or be tender and swollen. Sometimes stones can be visualized at the salivary duct orifice or felt on bimanual palpation. Both stones and strictures predispose to infection in the gland.

Management Refer to ENT/oral surgery for confirmation of diagnosis—stones are seen on plain X-rays or sialography. Some stones pass spontaneously but most require surgical removal—the whole gland may be removed to prevent recurrent problems. Strictures can often be dilated.

Acute parotiditis Unilateral parotid swelling and pain caused by bacterial infection. Predisposing factors include DM, immunosuppression/compromise, local fibrosis following radiotherapy, and autoimmune destruction (e.g. Sjögren's). Precipitating factors include surgery, dehydration, salivary stones/strictures, and poor oral hygiene. Treat with antibiotics (e.g. amoxicillin 500mg tds for 1wk) and rehydration. If not settling consider abscess formation—refer to ENT/oral surgery for drainage.

Mumps 📖 p. 652

Salivary gland tumours Present with a lump/swelling in a salivary gland—80% in the parotid gland. Treated with surgery ± radiotherapy.

⚠ Refer urgently to ENT/oral surgery if unexplained swelling in the parotid or submandibular gland for >1mo[N]. Refer sooner if pain, rapid growth, hard fixed mass, weight ↓, or facial nerve palsy.

Further information
NICE Referral guidelines for suspected cancer (2005) ॐ www.nice.org.uk

Nasal problems

Anosmia

Bilateral anosmia More common than unilateral. *Causes:*
- **Local causes** URTI, rhinitis, enlarged turbinates, nasal polyps
- **Central causes** CNS tumours, after head injury, meningitis, hydrocephalus, Kallman's syndrome

Unilateral anosmia One-sided loss of the sense of smell. *Causes:* head injury, frontal lobe lesion.

Taste disturbance Taste of food is often dependent on smell. Any cause of anosmia can also result in taste disturbance. Other causes of taste disturbance include:
- Drugs—taste disturbance is a side effect of ACE inhibitors
- Glossopharyngeal nerve palsy—taste loss on posterior third of the tongue
- Facial nerve palsy (📖 p. 537)
- Chronic adrenal insufficiency—↑ sensitivity to taste
- Malignancy—taste sensations, e.g. metallic taste with pancreatic cancer

Nasal discharge
- **Clear discharge** May be physiological (e.g. due to cold air), due to allergy (e.g. hay fever), or viral (e.g. URTI)
- **Clear fluid after trauma** Can indicate CSF leak
- **Green discharge** Indicates active bacterial infection
- **Yellow discharge** May indicate viral/bacterial infection or allergy
- **Persistent blood stained discharge** ⚠ Tumour of the nose or post-nasal sinus until proven otherwise—refer urgently to ENT

❶ The term *rhinorrhoea* is also used to mean nasal discharge. The term *coryza* is usually applied to watery discharge from nasal mucus membranes that occurs when a patient has a viral infection.

CSF rhinorrhoea Clear fluid dripping from the nose after trauma can indicate a fracture of the roof of the ethmoid labyrinth and CSF leak. Fluid tests +ve for glucose. It suggests significant trauma—consider referral for head injury assessment. Spontaneous healing of the CSF leak is the norm but if it persists refer to neurosurgery for dural closure.

Nasal obstruction Common symptom experienced occasionally by many. Usually obstruction is bilateral. ⚠ Assume persistent unilateral blockage is neoplastic until proven otherwise—refer urgently to ENT.

Causes of nasal obstruction
- **Mucosal swelling** Coryza, rhinitis (📖 p. 942), iatrogenic, nasal polyps
- **Septal deviation** Trauma, congenital, e.g. 2° to cleft lip
- **Other** Tumour, enlarged adenoids, foreign body (📖 p. 1108)

Deviated nasal septum Common in adults—usually 2° to injury. May be associated with external deformity. Nasal blockage is unilateral. Treat mucosal swelling due to rhinitis first as that may be sufficient to control symptoms. If unsuccessful, refer for surgery (submucous resection).

Septal haematoma May occur after injury and causes nasal blockage. Presents as a bilateral soft bulging of the septum. Refer urgently to ENT for evacuation to prevent cartilage destruction.

Septal perforation Can cause bleeding, crusting, and discomfort. *Causes:* trauma, nose picking, cocaine use, post-operative, malignancy. Refer if suspicion of malignancy, otherwise treat symptomatically (e.g. vaseline or naseptin for crusting)—surgical closure is often not successful.

Post-nasal drip Draining of nasal secretions down the back of the throat. Treat as for chronic sinusitis (📖 p. 942). *Symptoms include:*
• Feeling of mucus in the back of the throat
• Chronic cough—usually worse in the morning and improves in the day
• Morning sore throat
• Nasty taste in the mouth/bad breath

Causes URTI, sinusitis, allergic and/or vasomotor rhinitis, nasal polyps, deviated nasal septum.

Nasal polyps Most common in ♂ aged >40y—associated with asthma, allergic rhinitis, and chronic sinusitis. Consider CF in children <16y. *Symptoms:* nasal blockage; watery discharge; post-nasal drip; change in voice; loss of smell; taste disturbance.

Signs Polyps are smooth and pale, usually bilateral, and commonly arise from the middle meatus and middle turbinates. They may completely block the nasal passage. They can be confused with enlarged inferior turbinates but are more mobile and lack sensation.

Management Try medical treatment—steroid nasal drops (e.g. fluticasone nasal drops od) until polyps shrink (maximum 1mo), and then steroid nasal spray to ↓ recurrence. Swab and give antibiotics if purulent nasal discharge. Refer for consideration of polypectomy if medical treatment fails. ❶ Polyps often recur after surgery.

⚠ Refer unilateral polyps with an unusual or irregular appearance especially if ulcerating and/or bleeding, for exclusion of malignancy.

Nose bleed/epistaxis 📖 p. 1074 **Nasal foreign body** 📖 p. 1108

Snoring and sleep apnoea 📖 p. 338

Fractured nose Undisplaced nasal fractures usually heal without intervention. X-ray is unhelpful. Give adequate analgesia. Advise that bruising may be extensive and the nose will feel blocked for 1–2wk.

Associated injuries Consider assessment for head injury (📖 p. 1112). Always look for associated fractures of the zygoma/maxillary bones ('step' deformity in the orbit, dental malocclusion, difficulty opening the jaw, diplopia). Refer urgently to the maxillofacial surgeons if present.

Assessment for permanent deformity Can be difficult at the time of the injury due to soft tissue swelling—reassess 7–10d after injury. Refer promptly any patient with significant deformity or if the patient is unhappy with the appearance of the nose to ENT. Reduction should take place <3wk after fracture. Deviation of the nasal septum may not be correctable at the time of manipulation and, if symptomatic, will need a later submucous resection.

Sinusitis and rhinitis

Acute sinusitis Infection of ≥ 1 paranasal sinus (maxillary, frontal, ethmoid, or sphenoid). Usually follows URTI—10% are due to tooth infection. Presents with frontal headache/facial pain (may be difficult to distinguish from toothache)—typically worse on movement/bending ± purulent nasal discharge ± fever.

Management[N] Most sinusitis resolves spontaneously in 7–10d. Advise analgesia (paracetamol ± ibuprofen) and fluids for all patients. Steam inhalation may also help. *Treatment options:*
- Decongestants—little evidence of effectiveness
- Steroid nasal sprays (e.g. beclometasone 2 puffs to each nostril bd)
- Antibiotics (e.g. amoxicillin 500mg tds)—reserve for patients with frontal sinusitis, severe symptoms, symptoms persisting >2.5wk, or at high risk of serious complications (e.g. CF, immunosuppression)

Chronic/recurrent sinusitis >3mo of symptoms or >3 episodes of sinusitis in any year. Presents with post-nasal drip; frontal headache/facial pain; and/or blocked nose. Associated with nasal polyps (📖 p. 941) and vasomotor rhinitis. Treat as for acute sinusitis. Refer to ENT if symptoms are interfering with life—surgery may help.

Rhinitis Inflammation of the nasal mucosa. Affects >1:5 people. May be allergic (most children; 1:3 adults) or non-allergic (e.g. *vasomotor*—triggered by physical/chemical agents such as cold air, tobacco, or perfumes; *drug-induced*). If allergic cause is suspected, ask about potential allergens: pollen, animals, fungi/moulds, occupational allergens (e.g. flour, latex).

Symptoms Nasal discharge, itching, sneezing ± nasal blockage/congestion. Symptoms may be seasonal (only certain times of the year) or perennial (all year); intermittent (<4d/wk or <4wk at a time) or persistent. Make an assessment of severity. Patients have moderate/severe symptoms if ≥1 of: troublesome symptoms; abnormal sleep; impairment of daily activities/sport/leisure; problems at work/school. If symptoms are intrusive and difficult to control, refer for allergy testing.

Signs Swollen inferior turbinates; ↓ nasal airway; pale or mauve mucosa; nasal discharge; 'allergic crease' on bridge of nose from persistent rubbing (young sufferers with allergic rhinitis).

Management of allergic rhinitis General measures include ↓ in allergen exposure; nasal douching with saline nose drops ± steam inhalation. Drug treatment—see Table 25.2.

Desensitization 50—70% success rate. Risk of anaphylaxis is high so provision is limited to specialist centres—refer via an allergy clinic.

Table 25.1 Predominant pollen types at different times of year in the UK

Jan	Feb	Mar	Apr	May	Jun	Jul	Aug	Sep	Oct	Nov	Dec
Alder Hazel		Elm Willow Ash	Silver birch (25%)	Oak	Weed pollen						
				Grass pollen (60%)				Fungal spores			

Table 25.2 Drug treatment of allergic rhinitis (*BNF* 12.2.1 and 12.2.2)

Category	Notes
Nasal steroids	Effective if applied properly and can be used safely long-term
	Take several days to work—try for >2wk before abandoning. Often started at high dose—when symptoms are controlled, dose is ↓ to the minimum that maintains symptom control
	Choose preparations with minimal systemic absorption if using >1mo (e.g. fluticasone, mometasone). If nasal irritation, sore throat, or nosebleeds switch to a preparation without benzalkonium chloride preservative, e.g. Flixonase Nasules® or Rhinocort®
Oral steroids	Only rarely needed. *Consider for:* severe nasal obstruction; short-term rescue medication for uncontrolled symptoms; or control of symptoms for important social/work events (e.g. examinations)
	Use 20–30mg prednisolone po for 5–7d in combination with nasal steroids. Injected preparations are not recommended
Oral antihistamines	Choose a non-sedative antihistamine, e.g. loratadine 10mg od. May be used alone or in combination with nasal steroids. Improve associated symptoms (e.g. conjunctivitis) as well as nasal symptoms
Topical antihistamines	e.g. Azelastine nasal drops—useful as a rescue therapy
	Faster acting than oral antihistamines—onset of action is in <15min
Leukotriene receptor antagonists	e.g. Montelukast 10mg od
	As effective as antihistamines. Useful for patients with concurrent asthma. Combination with antihistamines does not ↑ efficacy
Topical/oral decongestants	e.g. Ephedrine nasal drops tds/qds
	Effective (drops >> oral preparations) in reducing nasal congestion
	Discourage use of nasal drops for >10d as vasoconstriction → mucosal damage → worsening of nasal congestion—a vicious cycle termed *rhinitis medicamentosa*. Not caused by oral preparations
Topical anticholinergics	e.g. Ipratropium bromide nasal spray tds—↓ rhinorrhoea but no effect on other nasal symptoms
Topical chromones	e.g. Sodium cromoglicate or nedocromil sodium nasal spray—less effective than nasal steroids but may be useful for children or pregnant women wishing to avoid steroids

Non-allergic rhinitis Treat as for allergic rhinitis—treatment is often less successful.

Hay fever Rhinitis and/or conjunctivitis and/or wheeze due to an allergic reaction to pollen. Occurs at different times in the year depending on which pollen is involved (see Table 25.1).

Management When the pollen count is high—keep windows shut (including car windows—consider pollen filter for the car); wear glasses/sunglasses; avoid grassy spaces. Treat as for allergic rhinitis. Topical chromone eye drops (e.g. nedocromil) may help eye symptoms.

Further information
British Society for Allergy and Clinical Immunology (BSACI) Guidelines for the management of allergic and non-allergic rhinitis (2008). See ℅ www.bsaci.org

Earache and external ear problems

Earache Ear pain is a common presenting symptom. Think of:

- **Local causes** *Outer ear:* otitis externa; furunculosis; impacted wax; pinna pain (perichondritis); malignant disease of the ear. *Middle ear:* otitis media; barotrauma; myringitis; mastoiditis
- **Referred pain** Trigeminal nerve (dental abscess/caries, impacted molar teeth, TMJ dysfunction); facial nerve (HSV infection, Ramsay Hunt syndrome); vagus nerve (tumours of the piriform fossa, larynx, or post-cricoid area); glossopharyngeal nerve (tonsillitis/quinsy/post-op tonsillectomy, tumour of the base of the tongue or tonsil, neuralgia); cervical nerves C2/3 (cervical sponylosis)

△ Refer urgently to ENT if unilateral unexplained pain in the head/neck area for >4wk, associated with otalgia (earache) but normal otoscopy[N].

Myringitis Inflammation of the tympanic membrane. Myringitis bullosa describes painful vesicles on the tympanic membrane associated with mycoplasma or viral URTIs. A similar picture occurs with Ramsay Hunt *syndrome* (🕮 p. 538).

Discharge from the ear Otorrhoea is discharge from the ear. Major causes are: otitis externa; otitis media; and cholesteatoma.

❶ Always exclude a perforated drum in discharging ears—beware of cholesteatoma. If you cannot visualize the drum—review the patient. Clear fluid leaking from an ear after head injury may suggest a CSF leak. Fluid tests +ve for glucose. This implies a head injury with force—refer to A&E for further assessment.

Otitis externa Inflammation ± infection of the external ear canal. Common—affecting ~10% at some time. Adults > children. Associated with eczema of the ear canal. *Risk factors include:* swimming, humid environment, narrow ear canal, hearing aid use, and mechanical trauma (e.g. cleaning ears out with cotton buds or after syringing).

Acute otitis externa <6wk duration. Presents with ear pain (often severe), discharge (may be offensive), and hearing loss ± lymphadenopathy behind/ in front of the ear. If the ear canal is not obscured by debris/discharge, it appears red, swollen, and inflamed. Moving the pinna may be painful.
❶ Acute episodes have a tendency to recur.

△ Diabetics and immunosuppressed patients can develop a severe necrotizing form of otitis externa—refer to ENT early.

Chronic otitis externa (>3mo duration) Ongoing discharge from the ear ± hearing loss. Causes canal stenosis and permanent hearing ↓.

Management Although very common, can be difficult to treat. Take a swab if any discharge.

- Advise analgesia, e.g. paracetamol ± ibuprofen
- Prescribe ear drops—options are: aluminium acetate drops (as effective as antibiotics); and antibiotic and/or steroid drops (e.g. Locorten-Vioform®)
  ☛ If you cannot see the eardrum to ensure that it is intact, use of potentially ototoxic gentamicin ear drops is controversial

- Adding oral antibiotics (e.g. flucloxacillin/erythromycin qds) does not improve outcome[CE]—only use if treatment with drops alone has failed or administration of ear drops may be ineffective, e.g. debris within the canal, very swollen canal, uncooperative child

❶ Skin of the pinna adjacent to the ear canal is often affected by eczema. Treat with topical corticosteroid cream/ointment—avoid prolonged use.

If no response after 1wk, Try alternative ear drop, e.g. Otosporin® (contains neomycin, hydrocortisone, and an antifungal—polymyxin B) ± oral antibiotics. If swab result is available, prescribe based on the result. Consider gentle syringing to remove infected material. Refer to ENT for aural toilet/advice on further management if no response.

Furunculosis Boil in the ear canal. Presents with severe ear pain—may be exacerbated by moving the tragus or opening the jaw. Exclude DM.
- If no surrounding cellulitis—advise OTC analgesia and application of hot compresses; most will settle. If not settling, prescribe topical antibiotics and steroid drops, e.g. Gentisone HC®, 3 drops qds for 1wk
- If surrounding cellulitis—prescribe flucloxacillin 250–500mg qds for 7d
- Refer to ENT for incision and drainage if not settling

Foreign bodies in the ear 📖 p. 1108

Ear wax Normal. Becomes a problem only if causes deafness, pain, or other ear-related symptoms. Factors preventing normal extrusion of wax from the ear (e.g. wearing a hearing aid, using cotton buds to clean ears) ↑ the chance of ear wax accumulating.

Ear syringing Indicated if impacted wax causes loss of hearing, discomfort, or tinnitus. Avoid syringing if there is deafness in the other ear or a history of perforation of the eardrum (including grommet), previous mastoid operation, or chronic middle ear disease (e.g. chronic suppurative otitis media, cholesteatoma). If ear syringing is contraindicated, refer to ENT for removal under direct vision, e.g. with microsuction.

Perichondritis of the pinna Infection of the pinna due to ear piercing or laceration. If not treated quickly can result in destruction of cartilage and 'cauliflower ear'. *Pseudomonas* is a common infecting organism so treat with oral ciprofloxacin 500–750mg bd. If not settling, refer as an emergency to A&E.

Chondrodermatitis nodularis helicis (CNH) Caused by pressure on the ear (e.g. against pillow at night, tight headwear). Tender lump often with overlying scaling/ulceration on the outer helix of the pinna. Tender to lie on and painful in the cold. Advise relief of pressure ± topical steroid/antibiotic cream. If this fails, cryotherapy or surgical excision is effective. *Differential diagnosis:* SCC, BCC, gouty tophus.

Haematoma of the pinna 📖 p. 1113

Accessory auricle *Incidence:* 1.5:100 live births. Small skin lesion consisting of skin ± cartilage in front of the ear. No treatment is necessary but accessory auricles are often removed for cosmetic reasons.

Bat ears Common congenital abnormality. A fold of the pinna is absent. The child is noted to have protruding ears. Runs in families. Referral for surgery is indicated if the condition is causing psychosocial problems.

Otitis media

Acute suppurative otitis media (OM) Common, acute inflammation of the middle ear. Parental smoking ↑ children's risk of OM—encourage parents to stop smoking. Caused by viral/bacterial infection.

Presentation Ear pain—usually unilateral ± fever/systemic upset. Ear discharge may be associated with relief of pain if there is a spontaneous perforation of the eardrum. *Examination:* red, bulging drum. If perforation has occurred the external canal may be filled with pus obscuring the drum. ❶ If you can't see the drum, review the patient after treatment.

Management^N

- In 80%, symptoms resolve in ≤4d without treatment. Advise fluids and paracetamol and/or ibuprofen for analgesia and fever control. Symptoms resolve 24h earlier with antibiotics but antibiotics carry the risk of side effects and use ↑ community antibiotic resistance. Consider using a 'delayed' approach—prescribing if symptoms are no better in 4d
- Consider prescribing immediately (e.g. amoxicillin tds) for children with bilateral OM or acute OM with otorrhoea
- Prescribe immediately if very systemically unwell or at high risk of serious complications because of pre-existing co-morbidity, e.g. significant heart, lung, renal, liver, or neuromuscular disease, immunosuppression, CF, young children born prematurely
- If recurrent attacks (>4 episodes in 6mo) or if acute perforation does not heal in <1mo—refer to ENT

Chronic suppurative otitis media Persistent drainage (>1mo) from the ear associated with tympanic membrane perforation and conductive hearing loss. Not usually painful.

- **Central perforation** 'Safe disease'. Treat as for otitis externa (📖 p. 944). Refer to ENT if there is persistent discharge, deafness, vertigo, or earache. Surgery to close the drum may help
- **Attic or marginal perforation** 'Unsafe disease'. May indicate *cholesteatoma*. Refer to ENT for further assessment

Serous/secretory otitis media (glue ear) Non-infected fluid accumulates in the middle ear due to dysfunction/obstruction of the Eustachian tube, e.g. 2° to throat or ear infection, or tonsillar hyperplasia. Most common cause of hearing loss in childhood. More common in children with Down's syndrome or cleft lip/palate. *Symptoms:* deafness ± earache, difficulties with speech/language, ± behavioural problems. *Signs:* dull, concave drum with visible peripheral vessels ± fluid level and/or air bubbles behind the drum.

 Management in children Untreated, 75% have no symptoms in <3mo; 5% have bilateral hearing loss persisting >12mo. Glue ear resolves as the child grows older—treatment is aimed at ↓ impact of symptoms until natural resolution. If not resolving, refer to community audiology/ENT depending on local policy. Specialist treatment options include watchful waiting or grommet insertion.

Grommets Air-conducting tubes inserted through the eardrum to drain the middle ear. Most are extruded spontaneously <9mo after insertion. May need reinsertion if deafness recurs. Patients can swim/bathe but should avoid diving. If discharge from the ear, treat with antibiotic/steroid ear drops ± aural toilet (see Otitis externa—📖 p. 944).

Management in adults Uncommon in adults—usually follows URTI and spontaneously resolves in <6wk. If not resolving or no history of preceding URTI, refer to ENT to exclude post-nasal space tumour.

Mastoiditis Rare complication of acute OM—infection spreads to the mastoid. *Symptoms:* persistent, throbbing earache; creamy, profuse ear discharge; increasing conductive deafness; fever and general malaise. *Signs:* tenderness ± swelling over the mastoid; ear may stick out; drum is red/bulging or perforated—if the eardrum is normal, it is not mastoiditis. Refer to ENT as an emergency. Treatment is with IV antibiotics.

Cholesteatoma Skin or stratified squamous epithelium growing in the middle ear. Thought to result from formation of a *retraction pocket* in the pars flaccida of the eardrum. Local expansion as the drum desquamates can damage adjacent structures (e.g. facial nerve; semicircular canals—resulting in vertigo). If infected there is an offensive discharge from the ear. *Signs:* perforation of the pars flaccida of the drum with pearly white discharge within it and conductive deafness. Refer to ENT. Treatment is with suction to clear out the cholesteatoma and/or surgery. Following surgery, the ear should be dry and trouble-free—if not, refer back to ENT. Life-long follow-up is required as cholesteatoma recurs.

Tympanosclerosis Thickening and calcification of the tympanic membrane as a result of scarring from recurrent ear infections or after grommet insertion. Usually asymptomatic. No action is needed.

Barotrauma Due to changes in atmospheric pressure (e.g. air travel, diving) in those with poor Eustachian tube function. Presents with a sensation of pressure/pain in one/both ears, hearing loss ± vertigo. There is fluid behind the drum (or perforated drum), haemorrhagic areas in the drum ± conductive hearing ↓. Usually resolves spontaneously in 2–3wk. If perforation has not healed in <1mo refer to ENT.

Prevention Valsalva manoeuvre, yawning, or sucking boiled sweets during flight—particularly during take-off/landing—encourages the Eustachian tube to open to allow pressure to equalize. Decongestants may help, e.g. pseudoephedrine 120mg 30min prior to flight. Patients with otitis media should not fly.

Further information

NICE Respiratory tract infections: antibiotic prescribing (2008) ℛ www.nice.org.uk

SIGN Diagnosis and management of childhood acute otitis media in primary care (2003) ℛ www.sign.ac.uk

Clinical Evidence Williamson I *Otitis media with effusion* (2004) ℛ www.clinicalevidence.com

Deafness

Congenital deafness Usually detected on neonatal screening (📖 p. 856). *Causes:*
- Genetic (50%)
- Intrauterine infection, e.g. rubella
- Drugs given in pregnancy, e.g. streptomycin
- Birth asphyxia
- Meningitis
- Severe neonatal jaundice

Childhood-onset deafness Temporary deafness is common due to middle ear infections but permanent deafness rare (1–2:1,000). ↓ hearing is often noticed by parents or teachers—take concerns seriously and refer for assessment. Deafness causes long-term speech, language ± behavioural problems and early intervention makes a difference.

Management History, examination, assess development (including speech and language), consider referral for audiology or to ENT. *Causes:*
- **If no earache** Bilateral glue ear (📖 p. 946); impacted wax; hereditary cause; sequel of meningitis, head injury, or birth complications
- **If earache** Acute otitis media (📖 p. 946); impacted wax

Adult-onset deafness Common and debilitating, leading to isolation and depression. Presentation tends to be late. *Causes:* See Table 25.3.

Presentation Usually hearing loss develops insidiously with increasing problems understanding others when there is background noise. Tinnitus may be the presenting problem.

Useful screening questions
- Do other people mumble a lot?
- Do you find yourself frequently saying 'pardon'?
- Does the family say the TV is too loud?
- Do you miss hearing the doorbell or 'phone?
- Do you occasionally get the wrong end of the stick in a conversation?

Management Examine the drum; exclude wax; consider post-nasal space tumour. If no self-limiting cause is found, refer for a hearing test to quantify hearing loss and assess suitability for hearing aid.

⚠ *Refer to ENT if:*
- Conductive deafness of unknown cause
- Sudden deafness if no wax visible
- Asymmetrical deafness—refer urgently to ENT[N] to exclude rare, dangerous diagnoses, e.g. acoustic neuroma, cholesteatoma

Benefits for deaf people 📖 p. 222

Presbyacusis Very common. Causes bilateral symmetrical sensorineural deafness in the over 50s. Deafness is gradual in onset. High frequencies are more severely affected, so speech discrimination—particularly of high-pitched voices—is lost first. Examination is normal. Refer for an audiogram to confirm diagnosis and then for a hearing aid if appropriate.

Otosclerosis Bilateral conductive deafness due to adherence of the stapes footplate to the bone around the oval window. May be FH (50%). If deteriorates in pregnancy, avoid prescribing combined contraceptives. Refer to ENT for assessment to replace the stapes with an implant.

Table 25.3 Causes of adult deafness

Conductive deafness	Sensorineural deafness
Impacted wax (📖 p. 945)	Presbyacusis
Debris/foreign body in the ear canal	Infections (measles, meningitis)
Perforation of the eardrum	Ménière's disease (📖 p. 951)
Middle ear effusion (glue ear)	Drugs, e.g. aminoglycosides, furosemide
Otosclerosis	Acoustic neuroma
	Noise-induced deafness

Noise-induced deafness Caused by exposure to noise >85dB. May occur in work or non-work settings (e.g. firearm sports). Immediate indications are ringing in the ears/muffling of hearing after exposure. Refer to audiology. Avoid further excessive noise exposure. Hearing aids may help. If employment-related, may be eligible for compensation (📖 p. 116; war veterans—📖 p. 223). Employees should be protected from noise and provided with ear protection if working in noisy environments.

Acoustic neuroma Slow-growing neurofibroma arising from the acoustic nerve. *Symptoms:* unilateral sensorineural deafness, tinnitus ± facial palsy. *Management:* refer to ENT. Treatment is surgical.

⚠ Refer urgently to ENT to exclude acoustic neuroma if unilateral or asymmetrical sensorineural deafness[N].

Hearing aids Can help anyone with reduced hearing, but they never restore perfect hearing. Aids may be:
- **Body-worn, behind-the-ear, or in-the-ear**
- **Analogue or digital** Most traditional aids are analogue aids and amplify all sounds, including background noise. Digital aids can be programmed to filter out background noise and customized to the individual's pattern of hearing loss; whistle less; and can have different settings for different sound environments, e.g. TV, crowded rooms
- **Bone conduction aids** For those with conductive hearing loss or if unable to wear conventional aids due to surgery/malformation
- **CROS/BiCROS aids** For those with unilateral complete deafness. CROS hearing aids pick up sound from the side with no hearing and feed it to the better ear. BiCROS aids amplify sound from both sides and feed it into the ear that has some hearing

Cochlear implants Benefit patients of any age with profound bilateral sensorineural hearing loss. 2 components—one external (worn behind the ear) and the other internal (surgically implanted). Intense speech therapy is needed for several years to interpret signals from the implant.

Information and support for deaf patients and their carers
National Deaf Children's Society ☎ 0808 800 8880 🖥 www.ndcs.org.uk
Action on Hearing Loss ☎ 0808 808 0123 *Text phone:* 0808 808 9000 🖥 www.actiononhearingloss.org.uk
British Deaf Association ☎ 0207 697 4140 🖥 www.bda.org.uk
Hearing Concern LINK ☎ 0300 111 1113 🖥 www.hearinglink.org

Tinnitus and vertigo

Dizziness and giddiness 📖 p. 549

Tinnitus Ringing or buzzing heard in the ears or head. Occasional tinnitus is common (15% of population) but 2% are severely affected. Patients with tinnitus that interferes with daily life and sleep are prone to depression. *Cause:* often unknown. May accompany hearing loss or be due to noise exposure, head injury, Ménière's, anaemia, ↑ BP, or drugs (loop diuretics, tricyclics, aminoglycosides, aspirin, NSAIDs).

Management Reassure patients that there is no sinister cause. Refer to audiology for a hearing aid if there is deafness. Drugs are not helpful but look for and treat associated depression. Psychological support is important—consider referral to a hearing therapist and/or support group (e.g. Tinnitus Association). Masking with background music/radio or an aid that produces white noise (available via ENT) can help. Surgical sectioning of the cochlear nerve is a last resort → deafness.

Indications for referral to ENT
- **Objective tinnitus**—noise can be heard by an observer; rare and may be due to vascular malformations or TMJ problems
- **Unilateral tinnitus**—especially if associated with deafness; refer to exclude acoustic neuroma

Vertigo An illusion that the surroundings are spinning. Ask about duration and frequency, associated nausea, deafness and tinnitus, and recent viral symptoms. *Causes:*
- **Episodic vertigo lasting a few seconds or minutes** Commonly due to benign positional vertigo
- **Episodic vertigo lasting minutes to hours** Consider Ménière's disease
- **Prolonged vertigo (>24h)** Peripheral lesion, e.g. viral labyrinthitis or trauma, or a central lesion (usually associated with other signs), e.g. multiple sclerosis, stroke, tumour

Examination
- Look for neurological signs especially cerebellar signs, cranial nerve lesions, and Romberg's sign
- Assess BP, nystagmus, eardrums, and hearing
- Hallpike manoeuvre:
  - Move the patient quickly from a sitting position to a lying supine position with head turned to one side and extended over the end of the bed—look for nystagmus and ask about vertigo
  - Repeat with the head turned to the other side

Nystagmus Involuntary, oscillatory eye movements—can be congenital or due to labyrinthine or visual system problems. Refer all cases for assessment, unless associated with self-limiting labyrinthitis.

⚠ Sudden attacks of vertigo can be dangerous. Consider risks of swimming, dangerous machinery, and ladders. Advise patients to stop driving and inform the DVLA—if group 1 licence can resume once symptoms are controlled; group 2 licences are restored if symptom-free >1y.

Benign positional vertigo Recurrent attacks of sudden-onset vertigo, lasting only a few seconds or minutes. Occur with sudden changes in posture. Common after head injury or viral illness. Possibly caused by otoliths in the labyrinth. Diagnosis is based on history and a +ve Hallpike test. Normal tympanic membrane.

Management Usually self-limiting (few weeks)—although may continue intermittently for years. Reassure. Labyrinthine sedatives are not helpful. Teach the patient to minimize symptoms by sitting and lying in stages. Habituation may occur by maintaining the trigger position until vertigo settles. If not settling, perform or refer to ENT for Epley's manoeuvre[C] (rapid repositioning of head to move otoliths out of the labyrinth) and/or refer to physiotherapy for exercises/vestibular rehabilitation.

Viral labyrnthitis Usually follows a viral URTI.
- **Symptoms and signs** Sudden onset of vertigo, prostration, nausea and vomiting, no associated loss of hearing, normal tympanic membrane
- **Treatment** Labyrinthine sedatives, e.g. cyclizine or prochlorperazine
- **Natural history** Usually resolves in 2–3wk—if persists >6wk refer

Ménière's syndrome Overdiagnosed in patients with recurrent vertigo and deafness. It is a complex of symptoms including clustering of attacks of vertigo and nausea, tinnitus, a sense of fullness in the ear, and sensorineural deafness which may be progressive. *Aetiology:* idiopathic dilation of endolymphatic spaces.

Management
- Refer all suspected cases to ENT or neurology to confirm diagnosis
- Provide information and advise about support organizations
- Treat acute attacks with labyrinthine sedatives, e.g. cyclizine or prochlorperazine. Consider buccal/rectal routes of administration if vomiting. Do not use long-term
- Encourage patients to mobilize after an acute attack
- Betahistine taken regularly may help in some patients, as may thiazide diuretics, a low-salt diet, vestibular rehabilitation, tinnitus maskers, and/ or hearing aids
- There is some indication that stress may precipitate attacks
- Look out for and treat concurrent anxiety and depression

 Vertebro-basilar insufficiency Common in *older patients.* *History of dizziness* on extension and rotation of the neck. Normal tympanic membranes. May have associated cervical spondylosis and neck pain. Provide lifestyle advice. ✒ Some advocate use of a cervical collar.

Labyrinthectomy is a last resort and can help vertigo but results in deafness on that side. *P. Ménière, (1799–1862)—French ENT surgeon.*

Information and support for patients
Action for Hearing Loss ☎ 0808 808 0123 ✆ www.rnid.org.uk
British Tinnitus Association ☎ 0800 018 0527 ✆ www.tinnitus.org.uk
Ménière's Society ☎ 0845 120 2975 ✆ www.menieres.co.uk

Ophthalmology

'The eye is the window of the mind'
Richard II, William Shakespeare (1564–1616)

❶ Community-based optometrists are a valuable resource available to GPs to help differentiate eye conditions and refine referral pathways. Getting an optometrist's opinion can also assist in setting the appropriate priority level for referral or prevent unnecessary referrals.

Assessment of the eye

History Ask about pain, redness, watering, change in appearance of the eye, altered vision, and if the problem is unilateral or bilateral. Distinguish between blurred and double vision. Enquire about trauma, previous similar episodes, systemic illness, and eye disease in the family. If using medication, take a drug history (including eye drops).

Visual acuity Test and record the central (macular) vision of each eye separately for near and distance vision with glasses on. Cover the non-test eye carefully. On a full-size Snellen chart, line '6' can be read by the normal eye at 6m (see Figure 26.3—🕮 p. 957). If unable to read the 6/9 line, use a pinhole to improve refraction. Near vision can be checked using a near-vision testing card (see Figure 26.2—🕮 p. 956) or newspaper.

Examination

- The eyelids should be symmetrical. Check the skin around the lids, the position, eyelashes of, and any inflammation, crusting, or swelling of the lid or lid margin
- Use a bright light to examine the eye surface—it should be bright and shiny. Use a fluorescein stain if any indication of corneal damage
- Note any redness—if most marked around the lid lining and periphery of the eye conjunctivitis is likely, whereas a duskier redness around the margin of the cornea (ciliary congestion) suggests disease of the cornea, iris, or deeper parts of the eye (uvea)

Examining the ocular media Takes practice. Darken the room and ensure you have good batteries in your ophthalmoscope.
- Check the red reflex (opacities within the eye appear as a shadow)
- Examine the disc—place your hand on the patient's forehead and support the lid with your thumb; use your right eye for the patient's right eye and vice versa, Look for the shape, colour and size of the cup
- Follow each of the 4 main vessels to the periphery
- Examine the macula by asking the patient to look directly at the light
- Examine the peripheral retina by asking the patient to look up, down

❶ Dilating the pupils with a short-acting mydriatic (e.g. 0.5–1% tropicamide) makes examination much easier, but warn patients they may have temporarily blurred vision and should not drive home.

Visual fields Test peripheral vision by sitting in front of the patient and comparing their visual field to your own (1 eye at a time)—the most basic test is to check the patient can see hand movement in each of the 4 quadrants. Refer for formal tests. Visual field defects— 🕮 p. 971.

Eye movements If the patient complains of double vision, move an object to the nine positions of gaze (see Figure 26.1). Ask the patient to tell you in which direction the double vision increases.

Pupils Should be round, central, of equal size, and respond equally to light and accommodation *Pupil abnormalities*:
- **Horner's syndrome** 🕮 p. 300
- **Fixed dilated pupil** *Causes:* trauma (e.g. blow to the iris), mydriatic drops, acute glaucoma, third nerve palsy

- **Afferent pupillary defect** Pupils are the same size but there is a ↓ in constriction response to light in the affected eye. Shine a bright light in the better eye for 3s, then move it rapidly to the affected eye. If the afferent pathway is ↓, the first pupil movement is dilation not constriction. *Causes:* optic neuritis, retinal disease
- **Argyll Robertson pupil** Bilateral small irregular pupils with no light response. Occurs in patients with DM or neurosyphilis. *D. Argyll Robertson (1837–1909)—Scottish ophthalmologist*
- **Holmes–Adie pupil** Accommodation is partially paralysed, causing blurring of near vision, slight pupil dilation, and a very slow pupil response to light and accommodation (minutes). Occurs unilaterally in young adults and is not associated with serious neurological disease. *G.M. Holmes (1876–1965)—Irish neurologist; W.J. Adie (1886–1935)—British neurologist*

Referral See Table 26.1

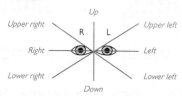

Figure 26.1 The nine positions of gaze (straight ahead is one position)

Table 26.1 Eye referrals

Emergency (direct to A&E or emergency eye clinic)	Sudden loss of vision Acute glaucoma Perforating injury, intraocular foreign body Chemical burns Retinal detachment Corneal ulcer Sudden onset of diplopia or squint + pain Temporal arteritis with visual symptoms—📖 p. 524
Same-day (<24h)	Hyphema or vitreous haemorrhage Orbital fracture Sudden onset of ocular inflammation e.g. iritis or ophthalmic herpes zoster Corneal foreign bodies or abrasions
Urgent (<2wk)	Central visual loss Sinister 'floaters' Flashing lights without a field defect Chronic glaucoma with pressure >35mmHg
Routine	Gradual loss of vision Chronic glaucoma (unless pressure >35mmHg) Chronic red eye conditions Painless diplopia or squint Chalazion/stye/cyst Ptosis

N.48

She waved

N.36

Faces the sun

N.24

Painting the rainbow

N.18

Life was like a flying dogfish

N.14

Quietly a storm drove purple ducks
across the road. The chimney top

N.12

Glowed in the dusk and my sister let her
biscuit fall through ashes. September was

N.10

In drizzling mood when hedgehogs threw
pinecones in the dark. Squirrels played classical
music.

N.8

We won a feather duster by encouraging Jessica to bake an
enormous apple pie and pirouette between the tables.

N.6

Queuing had never appealed to the young porcupines but swimming held great drama for
the blue and pink ostrich.

N.5

Delight was exceeding the pleasures of everyday ambulation and breaking the pattern of a melancholy
existence to see the trees.

Figure 26.2 Near-vision testing card—reading types are read at 30cm with
reading glasses if used

Reproduced from Collier J, Longmore M, Amarakone K (2013) *Oxford Handbook of Clinical Specialties*, with permission from Oxford University Press.

H

T

O Y

H U V

A T Y M

X O W U H

Y U V T X O

A W I U H V T

❶ These Snellen charts are for illustration purposes only. Lines on a full-sized chart are read from a distance of 6m with distance glasses if worn. Read from the top of the chart to the bottom. *Interpretation:*

Able to read	6	Normal vision	6/6
down to the	9	Can see at 6m what a normal person can see at 9m	6/9
line labelled:	12	Can see at 6m what a normal person can see at 12m	6/12
	18	Can see at 6m what a normal person can see at 18m	6/18
	36	Can see at 6m what a normal person can see at 36m	6/36
	60	Can see at 6m what a normal person can see at 60m	6/60
Counts fingers		Counts fingers held at 0.5m distance	CF
Hand movement		Perceives hand moving at 0.25m distance	HM
Perceives light		Can see a torchlight when shone into the eye	PL
No perceived light		Blind	No PL

Figure 26.3 Snellen charts

Reproduced from Collier J, Longmore M, Amarakone K (2013) *Oxford Handbook of Clinical Specialties*, with permission from Oxford University Press.

Eye trauma

In all cases

- Take a careful history; establish the nature of the trauma (i.e. what hit the eye and with what force?)
- Measure acuity and examine both eyes carefully recording your findings
- If the patient is unable to open the injured eye, try to instill local anaesthetic drops and then examine—if unable to do so, refer to eye casualty for assessment
- Encourage accident prevention, e.g. wearing protective goggles

Corneal abrasion

- Take a careful history to exclude high-speed particles, (e.g. from strimmer) that could cause penetrating injury
- Abrasions may cause severe pain—if so apply a few drops of local anaesthetic (e.g. proxymetacaine 0.5%) before examining
- Use fluorescein stain, with cobalt blue light illumination to detect abrasion—stains green (see Figure 26.4)
- If the abrasion is vertical, ensure no foreign body is left in the eye by everting the upper lid
- Abrasions normally heal in <48h; advise chloramphenicol 0.5% eye drops qds until healing is complete
- Eye padding is not needed except to protect the eye after a local anaesthetic

Superficial foreign bodies Cause discomfort, a 'foreign body sensation', and watering. They can be difficult to see so examine very carefully (see Figure 26.5), including everting the eyelids. The foreign body sensation may come from an abrasion.

Management

- If metal or a penetrating injury is suspected, refer to eye casualty
- Superficial foreign bodies can be removed with a corner of clean card after instilling local anaesthetic. If that fails or if you are not confident, refer to eye casualty
- After removal, treat with topical antibiotics, e.g. chloramphenicol 0.5% drops 2-hourly for 3d, then qds for 4d
- If left >12h, a rust ring may form around a metal foreign body—refer to eye casualty for removal

Arc eye Due to corneal epithelial damage as a result of exposure to UV light. Seen in welders, sunbed users, skiers, mountaineers, and sailors who do not use adequate eye protection. Symptoms include severe eye pain, watering, and blepharospasm a few hours after exposure.

Management Pad the eye and give analgesics and cyclopentolate 1% eye drops bd (causes pupil dilation). Recovery should occur in <24h—if not refer. Advise on suitable protective wear for future exposure.

Blunt injury Caused by fists, squash balls, etc. The result may be anything from a 'black eye' to globe rupture. Globe rupture is usually obvious with a wound and severely ↓ vision. More minor injuries include subconjunctival haemorrhage (📖 p. 967) or corneal abrasion.

Refer urgently if
- Visual acuity is affected
- Lacerated conjunctiva
- Double vision
- *Hyphaema*—blood in the anterior chamber
- Unable to see posterior limit of a subconjunctival haemorrhage—may indicate orbital fracture
- Persistent pupil dilation—usually recovers spontaneously but may indicate a torn iris
- Any signs of retinal damage (oedema, choroidal rupture), *or*
- You cannot assess the eye, e.g. if lid swelling/pain prevents examination

'Blow out' fracture of the orbit Uncommon fracture due to blunt trauma to the eye (e.g. squash ball injury). Can present with blurred or double vision and pain on moving the eye. *Signs:* enophthalmos (often masked by swelling), infraorbital nerve loss, and inability to look upwards due to trapping of inferior rectus muscle. Refer for X-ray and assessment of eye trauma via A&E.

Penetrating wounds Refer urgently to eye casualty if penetrating injury is a possibility, i.e. history of flying object or working with hammers, drills, lathes, or chisels where a metal fragment may fly off. X-ray/CT scan can confirm diagnosis and help locate the foreign body. *Symptoms/signs:*
- Wound may be tiny
- Eye is painful and waters
- Vision may initially be normal, or may be very poor, depending on the size of the foreign body
- Photophobia, hyphaema, and/or pupil distortion

⚠ **Do not remove large foreign bodies (dart or knife)** Support the object with padding whilst transferring the patient supine to eye casualty or A&E. Cover the other eye to prevent damage from conjugate movement.

Chemical burns Can cause great damage—particularly alkali injuries. Use topical anaesthetic (e.g. proxymetacaine 0.5%) before examining. Hold the lids open, brush out any powder, and irrigate with large amounts (1–2L) of clean saline or water immediately. Do not try to neutralize the acid or alkali. Refer urgently to eye casualty.

Figure 26.4 Corneal abrasion, stained with fluorescein, appears green

Figure 26.5 Corneal foreign body

Eye pain, papilloedema, and orbital disease

Eye pain *Consider:*

- **Painful conditions** Corneal foreign body, keratitis, iritis, scleritis, acute glaucoma, ophthalmic shingles, arc eye
- **Gritty eye discomfort** Conjunctivitis, entropion, trichiasis, dry eye, episcleritis
- **Pain on moving the eye** Optic neuritis
- **Referred pain** Tension type headache, migraine, refractive error, trigeminal neuralgia, ophthalmic shingles, giant cell arteritis, ocular muscle imbalance, ↑ ICP
- **Photophobia** Painful vision in normal light. 1 of the 3 principal features of meningism associated with meningitis; discomfort in the light can also be due to eye disease, e.g. conjunctivitis, and migraine

Papilloedema (see Figure 26.6). *Causes:*

- Intracranial SOL
- Encephalitis
- SAH
- Benign intracranial hypertension
- Malignant hypertension
- Optic neurtitis
- Disc infiltration, e.g. leukaemia
- Ischaemic optic neuropathy
- Retinal venous obstruction
- Metabolic causes, e.g. hypocalcaemia

> ⚠ Refer suspected papilloedema for same-day specialist medical opinion.

Swelling around the eyes Oedema around the eyes gives the face a bloated appearance. Swollen eyelids may partially close the eyes. In severe cases the whole face becomes oedematous. Associated with nephrotic syndrome, allergic reactions (e.g. pollen, dust, or insect bites), angio-oedema, and periorbital cellulitis.

Exophthalmos The eyes protrude from the orbit and thus have a staring appearance. Stand at the same level as the patient and look at the patient's eyes. There should be no white of the sclera visible below the iris. If the eye is pushed forward, as in exophthalmos, white sclera is seen below the iris and the patient can look upwards without moving his/her eye-brows (distinguishes from lid retraction).

- **Bilateral** Caused by Graves' disease (📖 p. 364)
- **Unilateral** Caused by Graves' disease (📖 p. 364), orbital disease (e.g. tumours, cellulitis); vascular disease, e.g. cavernous sinus thrombosis, carotid-cavernous fistula; sinus disease (e.g. tumour)

> **Microphthalmios** 1:1,000 live births. Small eyes. Associated with Down's syndrome and other genetic abnormalities.

Orbital inflammation

Preseptal cellulitis Infections of the upper lid may cause significant swelling and redness around the eye. Typically affects children following mild trauma. The eye is unaffected—infection is localized to skin and superficial tissues. Treat as localized cellulitis with oral antibiotics (e.g. flucloxacillin). Monitor carefully as can progress to orbital cellulitis.

Orbital cellulitis Typically due to spread of infection from the paranasal sinuses. Usually presents with pain, double/blurred vision, and general malaise. *Signs:* fever, eyelid swelling, proptosis, and inability to move the eye. Severe cases can lead to septicaemia, meningitis, and cavernous sinus thromboses. If suspected, refer immediately to ophthalmology for IV antibiotics/surgical drainage.

Orbital tumours The eye is in a confined space within the orbit. Any ↑ in mass pushes the eye forwards. *Symptoms/signs:*

- Unilateral proptosis is tumour until proven otherwise
- Orbital pain—especially in rapidly growing malignant tumours
- Lid swelling/distortion
- Limitation of eye movements ± diplopia
- ↓ visual acuity if involvement of optic nerve, retina, or vascular supply

⚠ If suspected—refer for urgent ophthalmology opinion.

Tumours may be

- **Primary** Benign or malignant—any orbital structure may be involved, e.g. lacrimal gland (carcinoma or adenoma); retina (retinoblastoma in children, melanoma); optic nerve (neurofibroma, astrocytoma, meningioma); lymphoid tissue (lymphoma); connective tissue (rhabdomyosarcoma—rapid growing, causing proptosis, ocular inflammation, and poor vision due to optic nerve involvement)
- **Due to spread from adjacent structures,** e.g. post-nasal space tumour
- **Due to blood-borne metastases,** e.g. breast, leukaemia, neuroblastoma, Ewing's sarcoma

Information for patients and carers
Eye Care Trust ⌖ www.eyecaretrust.org.uk
Micro- and Anophthalmic Children's Society (MACS) ☎ 0800 169 8088
⌖ www.macs.org.uk

Macula

Normal optic disc

Retinal blood vessels

Acute papilloedema: disc margins are absent

Figure 26.6 The normal retina (left) and papilloedema (right)

Lid disease

Ingrowing lashes (trichiasis) Causes an irritable foreign body feeling in the eye ± recurrent infection. In severe cases, the ingrowing lashes may damage the cornea. Refer to ophthalmology.

Loss of eyelashes (madarosis) Usually due to blepharitis (📖 p. 964), in which case the condition is bilateral and associated with other symptoms/signs of blepharitis. Other causes include plucking/rubbing (may be unilateral or bilateral), alopecia areata, and discoid lupus (scarring madarosis). Sometimes no cause is found. Treat the cause if possible.

Depigmentation of the eyelashes (poliosis) Vitiligo can affect the eyelids. There is usually a family history. Associated with other autoimmune disease (e.g. thyroid disease) and Vogt–Koyanagi–Harada syndrome (a rare disorder of ocular depigmentation associated with chorioretinal disease, anterior uveitis ± tinnitus and meningism).

Entropion In-turning of the eyelids due to degenerative changes or secondary to scarring. Most commonly affects the lower lid. ↑ with age (rare <40y). The eyelashes rub on the cornea and irritate the eye. Taping the lower lid to the cheek can give temporary relief. If left untreated, can cause corneal vascularization, ulceration, and infection. Refer for rapid surgical correction.

Ectropion Turning out of the lower eyelid. Causes eye irritation and watering. Most common in the elderly or those with facial nerve palsy (📖 p. 538). Refer for surgery.

Ptosis From the Greek meaning 'to fall', ptosis describes drooping of the upper eyelid. When the normal eye is looking straight forwards, the margin of the upper lid is situated ~2mm above the pupil. Ask the patient to look downwards as far as possible and then upwards as far as possible. The lid margin should move >8mm. The lid margin moves <4mm in patients with severe ptosis. Treat the cause where possible. To determine the cause, look at the pupil:
- **Dilated pupil** Oculomotor nerve palsy—refer urgently to neurology
- **Constricted pupil** Horner's syndrome
- **Normal pupil** Old age, congenital, myasthenia gravis, muscular dystrophy, myopathy, botulism

 Congenital ptosis Unilateral/bilateral weakness of the levator muscle. Children may compensate by tilting their heads upwards to see better. ~50% have associated superior rectus muscle weakness. Refer for surgical correction if obstructing vision as may cause amblyopia.

Neurological causes of ptosis
- **Oculomotor (3rd nerve palsy)** Often ptosis is complete if the pupil is dilated. Refer urgently to neurology to exclude cerebral haemorrhage or tumour[N]
- **Horner's syndrome** 📖 p. 300
- **Tabes dorsalis** 2° to syphilis

Muscular and mechanical causes of ptosis
- **Senile** Most common cause of ptosis—due to age-related changes in the levator muscle. Refer if causing problems
- **Myasthenia gravis** 📖 p. 963
- **Muscular dystrophy,** e.g. myotonic or oculopharyngeal dystrophy
- **Myopathy,** e.g. Graves' disease
- **Mechanical** Swelling of the eyelid due to allergy or mass effect of tumour

Causes of localized eyelid swelling
- Stye
- Papilloma
- Chalazion
- Xanthelasma
- Sebaceous cyst
- Marginal cyst of Zeis/Moll
- Dermoid cyst—usually upper inner and outer angles of the orbit
- BCC (rodent ulcer)—usually at the lid margin
- Lacrimal gland and lacrimal sac disorders (📖 p. 965)

Stye Common eyelid infection. 2 forms:

External stye (hordeolum externum) Most common form of stye. Infection of a lash follicle or associated gland of Moll (sweat gland) or Zeis (sebum gland) usually by *Staphylococcus aureus*. Confined to the skin and always points outwards. Treat with hot compresses and oral or topical antibiotics (e.g. chloramphenicol ointment)

Internal stye (hordeolum internum) Abscess of a meibomian gland. Often causes less swelling than external stye. May point inwards onto the conjunctiva (seen as red patch with yellow centre before it bursts) or outwards through the skin. Treat in the same way as external stye with hot compresses and oral or topical antibiotics.

Marginal cyst of Zeis or Moll Non-infected swellings of the glands of Zeis/Moll. No treatment needed unless troublesome when refer.

Chalazion/Meibomian cyst Following an internal stye, the Meibomian gland may become blocked forming a cyst. Cysts may resolve spontaneously but often become infected (treat with topical antibiotics) and/or chronic. If recurrent infection or chronic cyst refer to ophthalmology for incision and curettage. ❶ Refer early if <7y as large cysts can affect refraction and generate amblyopia.

Squamous cell papilloma Benign skin tumour—which may form a horn-like lesion. Refer for excision/curettage.

Blepharitis 📖 p. 964   **Xanthelasma** 📖 p. 233

Basal cell carcinoma (rodent ulcer, BCC) 📖 p. 630

Further information
NICE Referral guidelines for suspected cancer (2005) ℅ www.nice.org.uk

Information for patients
Eye Care Trust Patient information on eyelid and tear gland disorders
℅ www.eyecaretrust.org.uk
Patient.co.uk Patient information on stye and chalazion
℅ www.patient.co.uk

Blepharitis and tear duct problems

Blepharitis Chronic, low-grade, inflammation of meibomian glands and lid margins. Presents with long history of irritable, burning, dry, red eyes. Eyelids have red margins ± scales on the eyelashes (see Figure 26.7). On elevation of the upper lid, look for inflamed meibomian glands. Associated with dry eyes, internal stye (📖 p. 963), and ingrowing eyelashes.

Differential diagnosis Lid papilloma and warts can become inflamed and mimic blepharitis.

Management Prolonged treatment over 2–3mo with regular eye care 3x/wk is needed. Warn patients to persevere as there may be no improvement for up to 2wk:

1. **Warmth** Apply a facial sauna, microwaveable EyeBag® or hot, moist flannel to the eyes for 5–10min. This is to open the skin pores and meibomian glands. The face should be red after heating.
2. **Massage** Press on the eyelids with a cotton bud to release the meibomian gland secretions—these are seen as thin curly lines. Pressure should not be too light, nor firm enough to cause discomfort.
3. **Clean** With the eyes gently closed, use diluted tea-tree oil baby shampoo (10 parts water to 1 part baby shampoo) on a cotton bud to rub along the eyelashes for 15–20s, top and bottom. Clean any remaining shampoo from the lids with a clean facecloth using clear, warm water. Alternatives to baby shampoo include bicarbonate of soda solution or sterile, impregnated Lid-Care® wipes.

After an initial treatment period, it is often necessary to continue to use warm compresses and lid scrubs from time to time to keep the lid scales under control. Treat dry eye symptoms with preservative-free tear supplements, e.g. Liquifilm Tears®.

Exacerbations Treat with topical antibiotics (place a 1cm strip of fucithalmic or chloramphenicol ointment onto a clean finger and rub it into the base of the eyelashes). Oral antibiotics (e.g. doxycycline 50mg od) for 3mo may be useful for patients not responding to lid care and topical antibiotics. Topical steroid drops or ointment may sometimes be useful but use only on specialist advice.

Figure 26.7 Scaling on the eyelashes in blepharitis

Dry eye syndrome (keratoconjunctivitis sicca) Tear secretion ↓ with age. Dry eyes cause eye irritation and redness which is often worse in centrally heated buildings. The eye feels gritty, vision is occasionally blurred, and there is reflex watering of the eye in severe cases. Commonly associated with blepharitis.

Causes ↓ tear production (e.g. age, Sjögren's syndrome); ↑ evaporation of tears (e.g. exposure keratitis).

Management
- Treat with artificial tears, e.g. Viscotears®, Hylo-Care® Liquifilm Tears®. If one preparation does not work, try another. Always use preservative-free drops—hypersensitivity can be a problem with prolonged use
- Treat any associated lid disease, e.g. blepharitis
- If simple medication fails try combined short- and long-acting drops, e.g. Liquifilm Tears® tds and Celluvisc® tds
- Refer to ophthalmology if continuing symptoms despite treatment

❶ Longer acting drops, (e.g. Celluvisc®, Viscotears®) blur vision for a time. Short-acting drops (e.g. Liquifilm Tears®) only give relief for ~30min and may need very frequent application.

Watering eyes (epiphora) Due to overproduction of tears or out-flow obstruction. Caused by corneal irritation (e.g. blepharitis, dry eyes, corneal abrasion, foreign body, conjunctivitis, entropion), iritis, acute glaucoma, ectropion, blocked tear duct.

Acute dacryocystitis Acute infection of the tear sac, can spread to surrounding tissues. Treat immediately with antibiotics, e.g. flucloxacillin. Abscess can form—if it does surgical drainage is required so refer.

Chronic dacryocystitis Seen in the middle-aged and elderly. Presents with a watery eye which discharges mucus regularly. The eye does not look inflamed. Refer for syringing of the lacrimal system or surgery.

Infantile dacryocystitis (blocked tear duct) Delay in canalization/obstruction of the lacrimal duct causing persistent watering or sticky eyes in 20% babies. Vision is normal and there is no conjunctival inflammation. If the lower lid conjunctiva is reddened, swab to exclude chlamydia (☐ p. 740).

Management Advise parents to bathe the lids with cooled boiled water. Avoid antibiotic eye drops unless there is clear infection. Spontaneous resolution is the norm. 4% fail to clear by 1y—refer to a paediatric ophthalmologist. Treatment is by probing the duct to clear it.

Information for patients
Eye Care Trust Patient information on blepharitis, eyelid, and tear gland disorders ℰ www.eye-care.org.uk
Patient.co.uk Patient information on blepharitis, dry eyes, watery eyes, and blocked lacrimal duct in children ℰ www.patient.co.uk

The red eye and conjunctivitis

⚠ **'Red flag' signs of a potentially dangerous red eye**
- ↓ visual acuity
- Pain deep in the eye—not surface irritation as with conjunctivitis
- Absent or sluggish pupil response
- Corneal damage on fluorescein staining
- History of trauma

Refer the patient to be seen by a specialist the same day.

Differential diagnosis Think systematically about the structures within the eye to come to a differential diagnosis—see Table 26.2.

Conjunctivitis Inflammation of the conjunctiva is the most common eye problem seen in general practice (see Figure 26.8)—1 in 8 children have an episode of acute infective conjunctivitis every year. Presents with unlateral/bilateral red eye with surface irritation; eye discharge (clear, mucoid, or muco-purulent); sticking of the eyelids, especially on waking; no change in visual acuity. Examination may reveal enlarged papillae under the upper eyelid and/or pre-auricular lymph node enlargement.

Bacterial or viral conjunctivitis Clinically difficult to distinguish—doctors get it right only ~50% of the time. Both present with acute red eye—usually starting in one eye and often spreading to involve both, together with watery/purulent discharge. The eyes are often crusted ± stuck together on waking. Visual acuity is not impaired. Both may occur in association with viral URTI.

Management of acute infective conjunctivitis
- Usually self-limiting condition; 65% settle in 2–5d without treatment; advise patients to bathe the affected eye(s) with boiled, cooled water morning and night, avoid contact lens use, and use simple hygiene measures (e.g. hand washing and not using shared towels)
- If symptoms are not improving in 3–5d, review the diagnosis and consider treatment with topical chloramphenicol qds for 5d
  ❶ Chloramphenicol is available OTC.

⚠ Advise patients to seek medical advice if: ↓ visual acuity, eye becomes painful rather than sore/gritty, significant photophobia, eyelid swelling, or symptoms are not improving in 5d.

Allergic conjunctivitis Bilateral symptoms appear seasonally (e.g. hay fever) or on contact with an allergen (e.g. animal fur). Presents with red, watery, itchy eyes ± photophobia ± family/personal history of atopy. *Signs:* follicles in the lower tarsal conjunctiva and 'cobblestones' under the upper lid.

Management of allergic conjunctivitis Treat with topical or systemic antihistamines (e.g. sodium cromoglicate, nedocromil, or olopatadine eye drops). Avoid topical steroids due to long-term complications (cataract, glaucoma, fungal infection). Consider cold compress and washout with cold water during acute exacerbations. Refer if symptoms are persistent despite treatment, or if vision is affected.

Table 26.2 Differential diagnosis of red eye

Structure	Condition	
Inflammation of the orbit	• Thyroid eye disease/exomphalos (📖 p. 365)	• Tumour (📖 p. 961) • Orbital cellulitis (📖 p. 961)
Lid disease	• Stye (📖 p. 963) • Chalazion (📖 p. 963)	• Blepharitis (📖 p. 964) • Allergic eye disease
Scleral inflammation	• Scleritis/episcleritis (📖 p. 969) • Post-operative inflammation	
Conjunctival disease	• Viral infection • Bacterial infection • Chlamydial infection	• Allergy • Subconjunctival haemorrhage
Corneal disease	• Foreign body/trauma (📖 p. 958) • Corneal ulceration (📖 p. 968) • Ophthalmic shingles (📖 p. 969)	• Corneal abrasion (📖 p. 958) • Dry eye (📖 p. 965) • Arc eye (📖 p. 958)
Uveal/iris inflammation	• Anterior uveitis (📖 p. 959) • Posterior uveitis/toxoplasma	
Other causes of red eye	• Acute glaucoma (📖 p. 977) • Post-operative endophthalmitis (📖 p. 979)	

Ophthalmia neonatorum 📖 p. 741

Herpes simplex keratoconjunctivitis 📖 p. 968

Subconjunctival haemorrhage Spontaneous painless localized haemorrhage under the conjunctiva (see Figure 26.9). Common in the elderly. Looks alarming but generally painless (may cause some aching of the eye). Clears spontaneously in 1–2wk but may recur. *Associations:* ↑ BP, clotting disorders, leukaemia, ↑ venous pressure. Check BP. If severe/recurrent, check FBC and clotting screen.

❶ Consider referral if follows trauma—especially if the posterior edge of the haemorrhage cannot be seen (may be associated with orbital haematoma, penetrating injury, or orbital fracture).

Pterygium 📖 p. 968

Figure 26.8 Acute infective conjunctivitis

Figure 26.9 Subconjunctival haemorrhage

Corneal, sclera, and uveal disease

Corneal abrasions 📖 p. 958   **Arc eye** 📖 p. 958

Superficial foreign bodies 📖 p. 958   **Corneal arcus** 📖 p. 233

Pterygium Common (see Figure 26.10). Found particularly in people who work outdoors in hot, dusty climates. Creamy coloured raised triangular plaque on the conjunctiva on either side of the cornea—nasal side > temporal side. No need to treat unless encroaching over the pupil and causing visual loss → refer for surgical excision—recurrence is possible. ⓘ Differential diagnosis is carcinoma *in situ*—if any atypical features, refer for excision biopsy.

Figure 26.10 Pterygium

Corneal vascularization Growth of blood vessels onto the cornea. Occurs in patients with severe lid disease, rosacea, or due to excessive contact lens wear. If a contact lens wearer, advise to remove contact lenses for at least 2mo. Refer to ophthalmology for specialist management to prevent long-term damage.

Keratitis, keratoconjunctivitis, and corneal ulceration

• Keratitis is inflammation of the cornea
• Keratoconjunctivitis is inflammation of the conjunctiva and cornea

Presentation Presents with a very painful eye, blurred vision, photophobia, and profuse watering. On examination there is ↓ visual acuity, circumcorneal injection (blood vessel dilatation concentrated around the limbus), conjunctivitis (particularly the quadrant most associated with the injury/infection) ± a creamy white, disc-shaped lesion on the central or inferior cornea. The pupil may be small due to reflex miosis. Corneal ulcers stain green with fluorescein—use a bright light with a blue filter to see them.

Causes Bacterial—2° to trauma, foreign body, dry eyes, entropion, blepharitis; viral—herpes simplex, herpes zoster, or adenovirus; fungal; protozoal—history of foreign travel/contact lens wear; non-infective, e.g. 2° to autoimmune disease or trauma.

Management Treatment depends on cause. Delay in treatment may result in loss of sight so refer for same-day ophthalmology assessment.

Herpes simplex infection and dendritic ulcer HSV keratitis is common and can be recurrent in the same eye with the virus lying dormant within the trigeminal nerve between attacks. Presents with acute keratitis or keratoconjunctivitis. Occasionally may present as an irritable eye with little discomfort. Examination and fluorescein staining reveal a characteristic corneal ulcer with a delicate branching pattern (dendritic ulcer). Refer for urgent (same-day) ophthalmology opinion. Treatment is with 3% aciclovir ointment 5x/d continued for 3d after healing.

⚠ There is a danger of massive amoebic ulceration and blindness if steroid eye drops are administered to patients with dendritic ulcer.

Ophthalmic shingles Zoster in the ophthalmic branch of the oculomotor (3rd) nerve. Pain, tingling, or numbness around the eye precedes a blistering rash and inflammation. In 50% the eye is affected with conjunctivitis, scleritis, episcleritis, keratitis, iritis, visual loss, and/or oculomotor nerve palsy. Nose tip involvement makes eye involvement likely (nerve supply is the same as the globe). Prescribe oral aciclovir (800mg 5x/d) and refer immediately. The cornea may become anaesthetic/scarred and require grafting.

Episcleritis The episclera is the thin layer of vascular tissue overlying the sclera. Episcleritis is unilateral in two-thirds of cases. It presents with diffuse inflammation of the eye with minimal tenderness and no discharge. Try treatment with an NSAID (e.g. ibuprofen 400mg tds or ketorolac 0.5% eye drops qds). If NSAID is ineffective, refer to ophthalmology for consideration of treatment with steroids.

Scleritis Inflammation of the sclera. Can be unilateral or bilateral. ♀ > ♂. *Peak age:* 40–60y. Affects the anterior or posterior segment and may be diffuse, nodular, or necrotizing. Presents with painful, red eye. Vision may be blurred due to corneal, iris, or posterior segment involvement, and visual acuity ↓. The eye is tender to touch and may have a deep purple hue. Look for scleral nodules. There may be accompanying uveitis and keratitis.

Associations In ~50%, associated with systemic illness, e.g. herpes zoster, rheumatoid arthritis, systemic lupus erythematosus, polyarteritis nodosa, Wegener's granulomatosis, trauma, infection, or surgery.

Management Refer urgently to ophthalmology. Treated with steroids. Complications include cataract, glaucoma, and retinal detachment.

Iritis (anterior uveitis) Most common in young/middle-aged adults. Acute onset of pain, photo-phobia, blurred vision and ↓ visual acuity, watering, circumcorneal redness, small or irregular pupil ± keratitic precipitates on the posterior surface of the cornea ± *hypopyon* (anterior chamber pus, causing a white 'fluid level' line). Pain ↑ as eyes converge and pupils constrict. May be secondary to corneal graft rejection or eye infections, e.g. toxoplasmosis, herpes virus keratitis. In 30% associated with seronegative arthropathies, e.g. ankylosing spondylitis.

Management Refer urgently to ophthalmology. Complications include posterior synechiae (irregular pupil shape), glaucoma, and cataract. Relapses are common.

Visual field loss and blindness

Visual field loss Not all patients who have a visual field loss are aware of it. ❶ If you suspect visual field loss, refer to a community optometrist or ophthalmology for formal field testing. *Causes:* see Figure 26.11.

Blindness Is defined as inability to perform any work for which eyesight is essential (not the total absence of sight). In practice this means <3/60 vision (may be >3/60 if patient has severe visual field defect, e.g. glaucoma). 157,000 people are registered blind in England.

Partial sightedness Does not have a standard definition but usually implies vision in the range 3/60—6/60; 155,000 people are registered partially sighted in England.

Major causes of blindness in the UK
- **Elderly** Macular degeneration; glaucoma
- **Younger patients** Diabetic retinopathy; uveitis; inherited retinal disease; retinovascular disease

❶ Worldwide, cataract, glaucoma, and chlamydial infection causing trachoma are common causes.

Registration of blindness and partial sight Voluntary in England. Refer patients for low vision assessment. Application is made by a consultant ophthalmologist to social services.

Support Many patients benefit from links with national support organizations that provide information, and active local organizations who support the blind and partially sighted with drivers and guides.

Driving 📖 p. 129

Colour blindness

Congenital colour blindness Inherited as a sex-linked characteristic. ♂:♀ ≈20:1. The Ishihara test consists of series of cards with a number in coloured dots against a contrasting background of more coloured dots. Coloured dots are paired to detect different patterns of colour blindness. Lack of red/green discrimination is most common. Colour blindness prohibits certain types of employment (e.g. airline pilot).

Impaired colour recognition Occurs later in life. Red is the most common colour affected. May be an early sign of an optic nerve disorder. Patients complain of colour looking 'washed out' (desaturated) in one eye compared to the other—refer.

Information and support for patients and carers

Royal National Institute for the Blind Information and talking book service ☎ 0303 123 9999 🖰 www.rnib.org.uk
Partially Sighted Society ☎ 0844 477 4966 🖰 www.partsight.org.uk
LOOK (for families of blind/visually impaired children) ☎ 0121 428 5038 🖰 www.look-uk.org
National Blind Children's Society ☎ 0800 781 14444 🖰 www.nbcs.org.uk

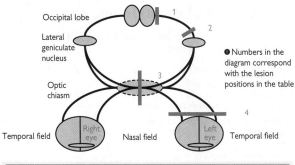

Defect (lesion position)	Description and causes
Bilateral homonymous hemianopia (1)	Normal eyes; normal pupillary responses; no conscious vision (cortical blindness) *Cause:* bilateral damage to the visual cortex—usually CVA
Homonymous hemianopia (1)	Half the visual field is affected symmetrically in both eyes. Macular fibres may be preserved (macular sparing) if the posterior cerebral artery is functional. *Cause:* strokes involving the middle cerebral artery
Quadrantanopia (2)	Loss of a homonymous (symmetrical) quadrant of vision indicates temporal lobe disease with superior defect and parietal lobe disease with inferior loss. *Causes:* vascular events, tumours, trauma
Bitemporal hemianopia (3)	The temporal side of the visual field is affected in both eyes. If one nerve is completely affected, a junctional scotoma results. *Causes:* compressive chiasmal lesions, e.g. pituitary tumour, craniopharyngioma, or meningioma
Altitudinal defect (4)	Field defect respecting the horizontal. *Cause:* optic nerve disease, e.g. optic neuropathy, optic neuritis
Enlarged blind spot (4)	Blind spot is enlarged if the optic disc is enlarged. *Causes:* papilloedema, disc inflammation, infiltration with lymphoma
Central scotoma (4)	Loss of central vision with normal visual field around it. May be unilateral or bilateral • **Bilateral causes** toxic (e.g. tobacco), B_{12} deficiency, MS, age-related macular degeneration, inherited • **Unilateral causes** glioma of optic nerve, vascular lesion
Tunnel vision	Loss of peripheral vision in all directions. *Causes:* glaucoma, retinitis pigmentosa, retinal detachment, functional visual loss (visual fields having no anatomical correspondence)
Loss of vision from one eye	Due to lesions of the retina or optic nerve anterior to the optic chiasm. *Causes:* retinal detachment, retinal vein occlusion, optic neuropathy, infiltration of the nerve, demyelination, compression of the nerve

Figure 26.11 Visual field loss, position of lesion, and causes

Sudden loss of vision in one eye

⚠ Always refer as an emergency to ophthalmology—unless you are certain it is migraine or stroke.

Causes of sudden loss of vision covered elsewhere

- Acute glaucoma (📖 p. 977)
- Migraine (📖 p. 554)
- Stroke/amaurosis fugax (📖 p. 562)
- Temporal arteritis (📖 p. 524)
- Wet AMD (rapid rather than sudden loss of vision— 📖 p. 974)

Retinal vein occlusion Incidence ↑ with age. More common than arterial occlusion. *Presents with:*

- Sudden loss of vision in one eye—typically on waking (branch retinal vein occlusion causes partial visual loss) ± afferent pupil defect
- Fundus like 'a stormy sunset'—scattered haemorrhages, engorged veins, disc swelling ± cotton wool spots
- ~90d after retinal vein occlusion, the eye may become painful due to neovascular glaucoma

Causes

- Glaucoma
- ↑ BP
- Hypercholesterolaemia
- Arteriosclerosis
- Polycythaemia
- ↑ homocysteine

Management Refer as an emergency to ophthalmology. Laser treatment may prevent neovascular glaucoma and vitreous haemorrhage due to retinal neovascularization. Macular oedema may be helped by intraocular steroids or intraocular anti-vascular endothelial growth factor medication (e.g. bevacizumab or ranibizumab).

Retinal artery occlusion Usually due to thromboembolism. Sudden visual loss in one eye (counting fingers or light perception) and afferent pupil defect. The retina appears white ± cherry red spot at the macula. A retinal embolus may be visible. Exclude temporal arteritis (📖 p. 524).

⚠ *If the patient presents <1h after onset* Applying then releasing firm eyeball pressure can sometimes dislodge an embolus into one of the smaller branches and thus preserve some vision.

Management Refer as an emergency to ophthalmology. There is no reliable treatment. Optic atrophy and blindness is the usual outcome. Treat any risk factors for atherosclerosis or embolism, i.e. ↑ BP, hyperlipidaemia, smoking, DM, carotid/cardiac disease.

Vitreous haemorrhage Presents with sudden ↓ in vision, loss of red reflex, and difficulty visualizing the retina. *Risk factors:* DM with new vessel formation, bleeding disorders, retinal tear/detachment, central retinal vein occlusion, trauma, head injury, tumour. Refer urgently to ophthalmology. Treatment is with vitrectomy and repair of retinal damage with laser- or cryotherapy.

Retinal detachment Affects 1:7,000 people each year. *Presents with:*

- Painless loss of vision—'like a curtain' coming across the vision
- Rate of detachment can vary. Upper retinal detachments tend to occur more quickly—causing loss of lower part of vision

- 50% have premonitory symptoms—flashing lights or floaters before eyes due to abnormal retinal stimulation prior to the detachment
- If the macula is detached central vision is lost and may not completely recover—even after retinal reattachment
- Examination reveals visual field loss (± central visual loss), afferent pupil defect, and a grey retina which may balloon forwards

Causes
- Idiopathic
- Trauma
- DM
- After cataract surgery
- Myopia
- Retinopathy of prematurity
- Inherited eye disease

Management Refer urgently for treatment to secure the retina.

Floaters Small dark spots in the visual field usually caused by opacities in the vitreous. Floaters continue to move when the eye comes to rest. *Risk factors:* myopia, cataract operation, trauma. Usually harmless and may settle with time but patients may benefit from vitrectomy if floaters are interfering with vision (e.g. preventing reading).

⚠ Sudden showers of floaters in one eye ± flashing lights can indicate retinal detachment which may be difficult to see on examination. Floaters associated with eye pain/inflammation may indicate posterior uveitis.

General rules for referral
- If long-standing floaters/flashes, then no need for referral
- If symptoms are of recent onset (<6wk) and no other symptoms, refer urgently to ophthalmology outpatients
- If symptoms are of recent onset (<6wk) and associated with any visual field loss, ↓ acuity, or pain/inflammation of the eye, refer as an ophthalmology emergency

Optic neuritis Disc swelling due to inflammation or demyelination. Presents with rapid visual loss (hours to days) and ↓ colour vision (red desaturation); discomfort on eye movements; temporary worsening of symptoms when hot; optic disc swelling. Refer urgently to ophthalmology for confirmation of diagnosis. Steroids may help in severe cases. Visual loss usually stabilizes after week 2 and recovers over 6wk.

Causes Multiple sclerosis (1:4 patients with MS present with optic neuritis—□ p. 568); DM; viral infections, e.g. influenza, measles, chickenpox; familial, e.g. Leber's disease.

Anterior ischaemic optic neuropathy (ANION) Occurs when the short ciliary arteries are damaged. 2 forms:
- **Arteritic** Due to arterial inflammation (e.g. temporal arteritis, SLE)
- **Non-arteritic** Results from arterial emboli

Presentation Central vision drops suddenly and irreversibly. Examination reveals a complete or altitudinal visual field defect. The disc appears swollen and pale ± haemorrhages. May be accompanied by symptoms of the underlying condition (e.g. temporal arteritis—□ p. 524).

Management Refer as an ophthalmology emergency. Treatment depends on cause.

Gradual loss of vision

Causes of gradual loss of vision covered elsewhere

- Chronic glaucoma (📖 p. 976)
- Cataract (📖 p. 978)
- Diabetic retinopathy (📖 p. 352)

Age-related macular degeneration (AMD) Most common cause of blindness in the UK—2% of people >65y old are blind in one or both eyes due to AMD. Always a bilateral disease but one eye is usually more severely affected than the other. *Risk factors:* ↑ age, +ve family history, smoking, ↑ BP.

Presentation Difficult to detect in primary care. Signs are often minimal. *Symptoms:*

- In all cases, there is deterioration/distortion of central vision—affects reading/face recognition first—worse with changes in lighting
- A dark patch that rapidly fades may be noticed on waking—can be interpreted as 'seeing a shadowy figure' and be very frightening
- With severe visual loss patients may see visual hallucinations—usually of faces or stars. These can also be very frightening

Dry (geographic) AMD All patients start with this form of AMD. Caused by atrophy of the neuroretina. The cells of the macula break down, resulting in drusen formation (yellowish lipid deposits). As number/size of drusen ↑, central vision ↓.

Wet AMD Accounts for 50% of blindness due to AMD. In some patients with dry AMD, drusen lifts the retinal pigment epithelium away from its blood supply. New blood vessels grow from the choroid and may bleed forming scars → irreversible loss of central vision.

Management If progressive loss of vision, refer to ophthalmology for confirmation of diagnosis—urgently if recent onset or rapid ↓ in vision. For those with dry AMD and loss of vision, treatment with AREDS2 food supplement (containing omega-3 fatty acids, antioxidants, and zinc) ↓ progression by 25%[R]. Treatment of other coexisting conditions (e.g. cataract and glaucoma) can also help. Provision of visual aids, registration of blindness and social support are important.

Aflibercept Is a monoclonal antibody to the vascular growth factor that stimulates new vessel growth. It is approved as an effective treatment by NICE for the treatment of patients with active wet AMD and visual symptoms. It is only administered in secondary care settings. Injections are given into the eye 1x/mo for 3mo with further injections thereafter, titrated against disease activation. Ranibizumab and bevacizumab are alternatives.

Central serous retinopathy (CSR) Typically occurs in hypermetropic middle-aged patients. Vision is blurred and distorted particularly for reading. The cause is a serous leakage of fluid from abnormal choroidal vessels. The condition is generally self-limiting but can be bilateral and chronic. Refer to ophthalmology for photodynamic therapy.

Macular hole Typically ♀ in mid-60s. Presents with gradual central visual loss/distortion and colour loss. If it occurs in the non-dominant eye, the patient may be relatively asymptomatic. Refer to ophthalmology. Vision takes 4–12mo to recover following treatment.

Macular dystrophies Several inherited retinal diseases (e.g. Best's disease; Stargardt's macular dystrophy; Bull's eye maculopathy) present with progressive loss of central vision either in early adulthood or aged 40–60y. Ask if there is a history of visual loss in a family.

Retinitis pigmentosa Familial disorder resulting in retinal degeneration. Usually first noticed in adolescence and progresses to blindness. 2 forms exist—the autosomal dominant form is more common than the autosomal recessive form and milder.
- **Symptoms** Night blindness, loss of visual field, difficulty in light adaptation, gradual loss of central vision
- **Signs** Black pigment flecks in the retina, optic atrophy, attenuated blood vessels

Epiretinal membrane Presents with distortion and blurred central vision, particularly for near vision. Associated with previous peripheral vascular disease, retinal detachment/break, branch retinal vein occlusion, uveitis, trauma, or tumour. Refer to ophthalmology for vitrectomy and membrane peel.

Optic atrophy Signs: gradual visual loss; pale optic disc. Causes: glaucoma, MS, ischaemia (e.g. retinal artery occlusion), retinal damage (choroiditis, retinitis pigmentosa), toxic (tobacco amblyopia, methanol, arsenic, quinine). Refer for confirmation of diagnosis to ophthalmology or neurology.

Compressive lesions of the optic pathway (e.g. meningioma, glioma, abscess, arteriovenous malformation). Can cause visual field defects—type depends on the site of the lesion—🔲 p. 971

Uveal and retinal tumours

Melanoma Most common tumour affecting the eye. Usually detected during routine examination by an optometrist. Other presentations include gradual central visual loss and/or retinal detachment. Can affect the iris, ciliary body, or choroids. Refer for urgent ophthalmology opinion.

Secondaries Metastasis to the eye can occur from tumours of the breast, lung, or kidney. Appear as pale elevations of the choroid. Symptoms are variable but include visual loss and retinal detachment. Refer urgently for confirmation of diagnosis.

Retinoblastoma 🔲 p. 907

Further information

NICE Macular degeneration (age-related)—ranibizumab and pegaptanib (2008) ℅ www.nice.org.uk
AREDS2 Research Group. (2013) Lutein + zeaxanthin and omega-3 fatty acids for age-related macular Degeneration. The Age-Related Eye Disease Study 2 (AREDS2) randomized clinical trial. *JAMA* **309**:2005–15.

Information and support for patients

Macular Disease Society ☎ 0300 3030 111 ℅ www.maculardisease.org
RP Fighting Blindness ☎ 0845 123 2354 ℅ www.rpfightingblindness.org.uk

Glaucoma

Chronic simple glaucoma (open-angle) (COAG) Common. Affects ~2% of all >40y olds. Accounts for ~1:4 ophthalmology outpatient appointments and 10% of new blindness registrations.

Risk factors

- ↑ intraocular pressure (IOP) >21mmHg—the major risk factor—but 30% of newly diagnosed glaucoma patients have 'normal' pressure
- Family history (↑ risk x10)
- Abnormal BP (↑ in elderly)
- ↑ age
- Myopia
- Black race
- ↑ plasma viscosity

❶ Steroid use (systemic or topical in or close to the eye) can cause ↑ intraocular pressure.

Presentation May be detected during routine optometrist examination or through routine screening for diabetics or patients with family history. Otherwise patients present late as glaucoma is asymptomatic and visual acuity is preserved until visual fields are severely impaired. *Signs:* optic nerve damage (glaucomatous disc cupping), visual field loss (sausage-shaped blind spots), and ↑ intraocular pressure.

Variants

- **Ocular hypertension** ↑ intraocular pressure with no field loss
- **Normal tension glaucoma** Field loss, disc cupping but normal intraocular pressure

Management Advise all patients >40y to have regular optometry check-ups. Those with a family history of glaucoma should have biannual checks of their intraocular pressures (*tonometry*) and annual visual field checks at an optician from 40y of age. Refer patients with ↑ pressures, or in whom you notice (or are doubtful about) disc cupping to ophthalmology for assessment. Patients with ↑ intraocular pressure must be followed up life-long. Aim is to ↓ intraocular pressure to slow disease progression (even with 'normal' pressures).

Medical treatment

- Topical prostaglandin analogue (e.g. latanoprost od in the evening)— ↑ outflow of aqueous
- Topical β-blocker (e.g. timolol 0.25% bd)—↓ aqueous secretion. Caution in patients with asthma or heart failure. Often combined with a topical prostaglandin analogue. *Side effects:* allergy and dry eyes
- Topical carbonic anhydrase inhibitor (e.g. dorzolamide tds, or bd if in combination with a β-blocker)—↓ aqueous secretion. *Side effects:* blurred vision, tiredness, dyspepsia
- Topical α-agonist (e.g. brimonidine bd)—↓ aqueous secretion and ↑ outflow. *Side effects:* local reactions, headache, dry mouth, tiredness

Surgery Trabeculectomy is considered when the 'target' intraocular pressure is not met with medical treatment (especially in patients <50y). *Side effects:* failure, worsening cataract.

Acute angle closure glaucoma (AACG) Uncommon. Affects 0.1% of patients >40y—typically elderly, long-sighted women with early cataract. Closed-angle glaucoma may present in one of 3 ways:

• **Latent** Usually picked up when screening the opposite eye after an episode of acute/subacute glaucoma. The patient is asymptomatic and IOP normal, but the anterior chamber is shallow with a narrow angle.

• **Subacute** Episodic haloes around bright lights, impaired vision ± frontal headache/eye pain. Attacks are precipitated by the pupil dilating, e.g. at night or entering a darkened room, and relieved by sleep or entering a brighter environment. Examination between attacks is normal but during an attack, the pupil is semi-dilated and cornea slightly clouded. Patients with subacute glaucoma are at risk of an acute attack

• **Acute** Blockage of aqueous drainage from the anterior chamber causes a sudden ↑ in IOP from 15–20 to 60–70mmHg. There may be a history of previous subacute attacks. The patient complains of eye pain with acute loss of vision in 1 eye ± abdominal pain/nausea/vomiting

Examination Vision ↓; cornea looks hazy (due to oedema); pupil is fixed and dilated (often slightly oval in shape with long axis vertical); circumcorneal redness; eyeball feels hard (due to ↑ pressure); poor fundal view ± cataract.

Management Refer acute or subacute glaucoma as an emergency to ophthalmology. Specialist treatment is with miosis to open drainage channels (e.g. pilocarpine 4% drops) and acetazolamide ± apraclonidine and/or latanoprost drops to ↓ aqueous production. Surgery or laser treatment (peripheral iridotomy) to allow free aqueous circulation is undertaken once intraocular pressure has been ↓. Patient may need prophylactic surgery on the contralateral eye to prevent AACG in that eye too. AACG may damage the trabecular meshwork and patients are at risk of developing chronic glaucoma following an attack. Regular check-ups are necessary.

Neovascular or secondary glaucoma May occur in patients with diabetic retinopathy, central or branch retinal vein obstruction, or ocular ischaemia. Blood vessels grow across the iris and the iridiocorneal angle, preventing fluid drainage. Pressures can be very high (40–70mmHg) and the patient may suffer pain from corneal oedema. Treatment is surgical and, in severe cases, if the eye is blind, it is removed.

Congenital glaucoma 1:10,000 live births. ♂ > ♀. Usually bilateral. Presents with irritation of the eye (watering, rubbing), photophobia, large eyes with large, fixed pupils ± cloudy cornea. Refer urgently for paediatric ophthalmic opinion. Surgery is needed to prevent blindness.

Further information
NICE Diagnosis and management of chronic open-angle glaucoma and ocular hypertension (2009) ℰ www.nice.org.uk

Information and support for patients
International Glaucoma Association ☎ 01233 648170
ℰ www.glaucoma-association.com

Cataract

Lens opacity is found in 75% >65y olds. Most do not need treatment.

Risk factors for cataract

- Old age
- DM
- +ve family history
- Prolonged steroid treatment
- ↑ BP
- Excessive alcohol
- Smoking
- Prenatal rubella/toxoplasma (congenital cataract)
- Hypocalcaemia
- Eye trauma
- Radiation exposure

Presentation

In adults

- Blurred vision and gradual loss of vision
- Dazzles and haloes around objects—especially in sunlight
- Frequent spectacle changes due to changing refractive index

❶ Unilateral cataract may not be noticed by the patient—but loss of binocular vision affects judgement of distance.

 In children Cataracts present with squint, white pupil, nystagmus, amblyopia, or loss of binocular vision. May be hereditary or associated with Down's syndrome, galactosaemia, or congenital rubella.

Signs A shadow in the red reflex/absent red reflex; difficulty visualizing the fundus.

Types of cataract

- Congenital cataract—localized and usually polar
- Nuclear cataracts—central; most common in old age
- Cortical lens opacities
- Subcapsular cataracts—usually linked to old age or steroid use.
- Dot cataracts—common in DM
- Traumatic cataract
- Mature cataract (see Figure 26.12)

Figure 26.12 Mature cataract

Management of adult cataract Check fasting blood glucose to exclude DM. Advise patients to have their visual acuity checked regularly. Refer to ophthalmology if ↓ sight (or any other symptom) interferes with social functioning, driving, or independence.

Surgical treatment Removal of the natural lens ± posterior chamber lens implantation. Usually done as a day case procedure under LA. Healing takes 2–6wk depending on the technique used. 75–95% without other ocular pathology have 6/12 vision or better 3mo post-op. Patients require testing for new spectacles 6wk post-op to allow refractive changes to settle.

Complications of cataract surgery
- Intraocular infection (endophthalmitis)—rare (0.1%); presents with pain and blurred vision ± red eye ± tenderness. Refer back to the operating surgeon urgently—antibiotics injected within 2–3h can preserve vision. Delayed referral (>12h) will lead to blindness
- Posterior capsule rupture
- Broken or protruding sutures—cause sensation of a foreign body on the cornea or pain—may need to be removed
- Vitreous haemorrhage
- Glaucoma
- Posterior capsule opacification (5–30% <5y post-op) symptoms are similar to the original cataract; treatment is with laser therapy to create a hole in the capsule

 Management of childhood cataract Refer immediately to ophthalmology.

Information for patients
Eye Care Trust ✆ www.eye-care.org.uk
Royal College of Ophthalmologists ✆ www.rcophth.ac.uk
Moorfields Eye Hospital ✆ www.moorfields.nhs.uk/EyeHealth

Refractive errors and squint

Glasses check Look through the patient's glasses:
• If image is magnified (prescription '+')—the patient is long-sighted
• If image is reduced (prescription '−')—the patient is short-sighted

Amblyopia (lazy eye) Poor vision in the absence of ocular or visual pathway disorder. Squint, ptosis, cataract, unequal refractive errors, or astigmatism can cause the image from one eye to be disregarded. If this persists >7–8y of age, it becomes irreversible. Treatment is with glasses ± patching, and squint surgery if necessary.

Refraction errors

Hypermetropia (long sight) Most common refractive error. Common in infants and lessens with age. Distant objects focus behind the retina. Ciliary muscle contraction (to make the lens more convex) is needed to focus the image. This can lead to convergent squint, eye tiredness, and headache. Convex lenses are used for correction.

Myopia (short sight) Distant objects focus in front of the retina. There is often a +ve FH. Concave lenses are used to correct the defect. Contact lenses may be necessary in high myopia (>−8 diopters). Myopia is unusual <6y old and tends to worsen until the late teens. Regular (6-monthly) eye checks are needed to ensure correct lenses are prescribed. In adults increasing myopia can indicate developing cataracts. High myopia (8–20 diopters) predisposes to retinal detachment—these patients should have an annual eye examination (more frequent if floaters).

Astigmatism Curvature across the cornea or lens differs in the vertical/ horizontal planes. Objects are distorted longitudinally or vertically. Lenses can be used to correct this defect.

Presbyopia Age-related loss of accommodation. The lens becomes less easy to deform from 45–65y. Focussing on close objects (accommodation) is more difficult and glasses may be needed for near-work (e.g. reading).

Refractive procedures Increasingly being undertaken as an alternative to spectacles. *LASIK (Laser Assisted In Situ Keratomileusis)* is a combination of surgery and laser therapy. It can be used for higher degrees of refractive error and astigmatism. Complications are rare.

Non-paralytic squint Abnormality of coordinated eye movement; 3% of children have a congenital squint. Due to an imbalance in the muscles of the eye; there is full range of eye movement in both eyes and no double vision. Note the light reflexes from different parts of the cornea—they should be symmetrical. If not, there is a squint. Squint may be convergent (esotropia) or divergent (exotropia). Esotropia (see Figure 26.13) is most common and often associated with long-sightedness.

Predisposing factors Family history of squint, high refractive errors, neurological disease (e.g. cerebral palsy), cataract, Down's syndrome, Turner's syndrome, retinoblastoma, optic atrophy, craniofacial anomalies, retinal disease.

Childhood screening for squint 📖 p. 856

Figure 26.13 Esotropic squint

Management Refer to ophthalmology. Without treatment, children with squint risk developing amblyopia, failure of binocular vision, and long-term visual problems. Visual maturity occurs at 7–8y. Eye patching, correction of refractive errors (spectacles), and realignment surgery can improve sight up to this age.

Paralytic squint Caused by damage to the extraocular muscles or the nerves supplying them. Usually acquired and caused by cranial nerve palsy. Results in diplopia—maximal when looking in the direction requiring the action of the paralysed muscle. The image from the eye that is not moving correctly is peripheral to the image from the normal eye. Refer for urgent neurology/ophthalmology opinion[N]. Once sinister causes have been excluded, management involves treatment of the underlying condition ± patching and/or prism spectacles ± surgery.

Pseudosquint

- **Wide epicanthic folds** Give the appearance of a squint—corneal reflections are symmetrical.
- **Intermittent deviation of the eyes in neonates** Common. Check red reflex is present. Normally settles by 3mo—squint after this time is significant. Refer.

Gaze palsy Inability to perform coordinated movements of the 2 eyes together in the same direction. In all cases, refer to neurology—treatment depends on cause (see Table 26.3).

- Horizontal gaze palsy—loss of conjugate eye movements to one side
- Vertical gaze palsy—loss of conjugate eye movements upwards

Table 26.3 Ocular nerve palsies

Nerve	Effect of paralysis	Causes of nerve palsy
3rd Oculomotor nerve	Ptosis and ophthalmoplegia—eye looks down and out. Surgical causes are also associated with pain, proptosis, and pupil dilation	*Surgical:* berry aneurysm (posterior communicating artery); cavernous sinus lesions. *Medical:* microvascular disease e.g. DM
4th Trochlear nerve	Superior obique muscle is paralysed. Causes diplopia and torticollis. The eye cannot look down and inwards	Trauma (30%), DM (30%), idiopathic
6th Abducens nerve	Lateral rectus paralysed. Causes diplopia. The eye is turned in and cannot move laterally from the midline	Tumour, trauma to the base of the skull, vascular

Contact lenses and drugs for the eye

Contact lenses 20% are worn because they are more suitable for the eye condition than spectacles, 80% for cosmetic/convenience reasons. Some are worn just to change eye colour. Contact lenses are used in high myopia or hypermetropia, presbyopia, and after cataract removal because thick spectacle lenses cause visual field distortion. They are also useful when the cornea has been damaged, e.g. after ulceration or trauma and in keratoconus (a rare corneal degenerative disease).

Types of lens Hard, gas-permeable (larger hard lenses are designed to allow air to reach the cornea), and soft lenses are available. Some soft lenses are 'daily disposable' or 'monthly disposable'. Hard and gas-permeable lenses can correct for minor astigmatism; normal soft lenses cannot as the lens is too flexible. A high astigmatism requires spectacles or a special (toric) soft lens (delicate and needs careful cleaning). Patients with poor tear secretion do not tolerate contact lenses well.

Care of lenses Careful cleaning of the lenses and contact lens container is vital—particular solutions are used for each type of lens, and these should not be interchanged. Contact lenses can be stained by fluorescein or rifampicin—ask before prescribing.

Complications
- Eye infection
- Corneal abrasion or vascularization (painful, watery eye after lens removal)
- Sensitization to cleaning agents (redness, stinging, swollen eyelids)
- Giant papillary conjunctivitis
- Losing the lens within the eye
- Keratitis
- Acanthamoeba infection

Drugs and the eye Many eye complaints can be treated with topical medication.
- Ointments last longer in the eye than drops but can cause blurring of vision—they are better used at night
- Antibiotics should generally be given as drops, enabling clearance through the nasolacrimal system. In severe infections 2-hourly drops should be used, reducing to qds after 48 h
- Antibiotic preparations (e.g. chloramphenicol, fusidic acid) can potentially become contaminated with bacteria so should be changed regularly

Mydriatics (e.g. tropicamide, cyclopentolate) dilate the pupil and cause cycloplegia thus causing blurred vision. They are used to dilate the pupil for examination and to prevent adhesions to the lens in iritis. They can precipitate acute closed-angle glaucoma in susceptible patients.

Miotics (e.g. pilocarpine) constrict the pupil and ↑ aqueous drainage. They are used in glaucoma. They can cause systemic side effects, e.g. sweating, ↑ BP, pulmonary oedema.

Local anaesthetic drops (e.g. oxybuprocaine, proxymetacaine) can help examination of painful eyes and foreign body removal. Protect the eye with an eye pad until the anaesthetic has worn off to prevent corneal damage (corneal reflex is suppressed).

Steroid eye drops are used in scleritis, episcleritis, iritis. Prescribe only after slit lamp examination and on the advice of an ophthalmologist. Can cause severe eye damage if used when a dendritic ulcer is present. Long-term use may cause glaucoma, thinning of the cornea/sclera and may facilitate fungal infection.

β-blocking drops (e.g. timolol, betaxolol) are used in glaucoma. Beware of systemic side effects—bronchospasm, bradycardia.

α₂ receptor agonists (e.g. brimonidine) are used in glaucoma. May cause dry mouth, headache, fatigue.

Prostaglandin analogues (e.g. latanoprost, bimatoprost) used in glaucoma. May cause lash growth and ocular inflammation.

Mental health

Mental health assessment

Assessing a patient with mental health problems in primary care can be challenging. Aims (may need >1 appointment to achieve):

- Establish a constructive relationship to enable effective two-way communication and serve as the basis for subsequent encounters
- Assess the patient's emotions and attitudes
- Perform an assessment of the patient's risk to self and/or others
- Determine if the patient has a mental disorder and, if so, which
- Find out (where possible) what caused the mental disorder
- Explore how best it might be treated

Psychiatric history

Informants GPs may be approached by concerned relatives/friends. Talk to them (be careful to maintain confidentiality); establish concerns/circumstances, relevant past history, and outline the patient's pre-morbid personality.

The consultation Try to review old notes *before* seeing the patient. Use open questions at the start, becoming directive when necessary—clarify, reflect, facilitate, listen. Be open and ready to ask about suicide, sex, drugs, etc. Ask about:

- **Presenting complaint**—chronological account, past history of similar symptoms. Ask directly about thoughts of suicide and self-harm
- **Family history**—psychiatric illness, recent loss or serious illness of a family member, bereavement, depression, suicide or attempted suicide, psychosis, alcoholism, drug use
- **Personal history**—abuse (as a child, domestic violence), substance misuse, serious illness (including past psychiatric history and major physical illness), recent significant events (e.g. childbirth, house move)
- **Attitudes and beliefs**—how does the patient see him/herself? What does he/she think is wrong? How does he/she think other people view the situation? What does the patient want you to do about it?
- **Occupation**—unemployed? Happy in job?
- **Home situation**—housing, relationships, social support, debt etc.

Mental state examination *Check:*

- Appearance and behaviour—signs of self-neglect or malnutrition, eye contact, rapport, movements, agitation, or aggression
- Speech—spontaneity, volume, tone, rate, amount, continuity (flight of ideas, loosening of associations)
- Mood—depressed or elevated. Consider screening for depression, e.g. screening questions for patients with chronic disease (🕮 p. 199), screening questions for pregnant or post-natal women (🕮 p. 839), PHQ-9 (🕮 p. 1001)
- Thinking—form, content, flow, possession
- Perception—illusions, hallucinations, pseudohallucinations
- Cognition—cognitive screen, e.g. 6CIT (🕮 p. 1011)
- Insight—patient's understanding of his/her illness, its effects, and need for treatment

Action

- Summarize the history back to the patient and give an opportunity for him/her to fill in any gaps or clarify any points
- Draw up a problem list and management plan with the patient
- Set a review date

High-risk groups for psychiatric illness

Women

- More vulnerable to depression and eating disorders
- During pregnancy and in the post-partum period
- When looking after children <5y old, especially lone parents who also go out to work
- When subjected to domestic violence
- During the menopause

Men More at risk of suicide.

People with long-term physical health problems e.g.

- Diabetes
- Heart disease
- Chronic disabling lung disease
- Cancers
- Dementia
- Disabling neurological disorders: stroke, PD, MS, MND

Substance abusers Drug abuse; alcoholism.

People suffering adverse life events

- Bereavement
- Relationship break-up
- Unemployment
- Financial problems

Minority ethnic groups More likely to suffer mental health problems due to social and economic deprivation, isolation from their usual culture, racism, and past exposure to war or torture (>50% of refugees have mental disorders).

Carers All carers are at risk of depression (~40% of carers of stroke victims are depressed). This starts early after the onset of care-giving. It is good practice to:

- Identify all carers and mark their records
- Check carers' mental and physical health annually
- Inform carers that they are entitled to a needs assessment
- Ask patients if you can share information with their carers
- Inform carers about support groups and carer centres

Residents of care homes and nursing homes 50% have depression.

Mental health symptoms and signs

Acute confusion 📖 p. 1010   Anxiety 📖 p. 992

Depression 📖 p. 1000

Abnormal beliefs Decide whether a belief is normal in the context of the patient. If not, decide if the belief is a:
- **Delusion,** i.e. a belief that does not seem to have a rational basis and which is not amenable to argument, *or*
- **Overvalued idea,** i.e. belief that is odd but understandable, given the patient's background

Compulsions Forced behaviours, repeated despite inappropriateness or unreasonableness, and associated discomfort in response to an obsession. Can be disabling, e.g. repeated hand washing hundreds of times a day. Obsessive–compulsive disorder—📖 p. 996

Abnormal perceptions *Consider:*
- **Illusion** Misinterpretation of information, e.g. seeing a coat on a hanger and interpreting it as a person. Can happen if ↓ level of conscsciousness or occasionally if visual impairment—particularly AMD
- **Hallucination**
- **Pseudohallucination** Vivid perception which is recognized as not being real, e.g. delirium tremens
- **Depersonalization** Feeling of being unreal—like an actor playing yourself. Associated with a wide range of mental illness, e.g. depression, schizophrenia
- **Derealization** Feeling of everything around you being unreal—like in a dream. Often linked to depersonalization

Hallucinations Sensory experiences in the absence of external stimuli. May be visual, auditory, gustatory, olfactory, or tactile.
- **Visual/tactile/auditory hallucinations** Suggest mental illness
  - Visual and tactile hallucinations suggest organic disorder, e.g. dementia, acute delirium, metabolic encephalopathy, drug abuse
  - Auditory hallucinations suggest psychosis
- Hallucinations experienced when the patient is falling asleep (**hypnagogic hallucination**) or waking up (**hypnapompic hallucination**) are features of narcolepsy
- **Olfactory and gustatory hallucinations** Often occur together. May be suggestive of psychosis but also occur with temporal lobe epilepsy and olfactory bulb tumours

Thought disorders Consider disorders of:

Content
- **Ideas of reference** Patients feel they are noticed by everyone around them/stand out from the crowd; media content, e.g. television or radio, refers to the patient; or that others are talking/thinking about the patient. Becomes a delusion of reference when insight is lost. Associated with schizophrenia, depressive states, and acute and chronic cognitive impairment
- **Delusions**

Flow
- **Flight of ideas** Leaps from idea to idea. There is always some association between ideas but may seem odd, e.g. rhymes. Associated with manic illness
- **Perseveration** Persistence of a verbal or other behaviour beyond what is apparently intended, expected, or needed. Associated with dementia and brain damage, e.g. cerebral palsy, CVA
- **Loosening of association** Series of thoughts appear only distantly (or loosely) related to one another or completely unrelated. Associated with schizophrenia
- **Thought block** Abrupt and complete interruption in the stream of thought leaving a blank mind. Associated with schizophrenia

Form
- **Preoccupation** The patient thinks about a topic frequently but can terminate the thoughts voluntarily. Common symptom, e.g. in anxiety states. Ask about preoccupation with suicide in depressed patients
- **Obsession** Thought or image repeated in spite of its inappropriateness or intrusiveness and associated discomfort. The thought and efforts to stop it ↑ anxiety and can be disabling

Possession
- **Thought insertion** Thoughts do not belong to the patient but have been planted there by someone else. One of the first-rank symptoms of schizophrenia
- **Thought withdrawal** Opposite of thought insertion. The patient perceives a thought is missing and has been removed by someone else. A first-rank symptom of schizophrenia
- **Thought broadcasting** The patient believes his/her thoughts can be heard by other people—either directly or via the newspapers, radio, etc. Associated with schizophrenia

Delusions Beliefs held unshakably despite available counter-evidence and which are unexpected in view of circumstances and background. The belief is usually (but not always) false.
- **Primary delusions** Belief arrives in the head fully formed, e.g. thought insertion; strongly suggestive of schizophrenia
- **Secondary delusions** Belief arises on the basis of experience, e.g. someone who has lost their job several times through no fault of their own may believe they are unemployable

Paranoid delusions Delusions (usually primary) which concern the relationship between the patient and other people. Associated with schizophrenia, depressive states, and acute and chronic cognitive impairment.
- **Delusions of persecution** Most common type of paranoid delusion. Belief that a person or an organization is intentionally harassing or inflicting harm upon the patient. Associated with schizophrenia, depressive states, and acute and chronic cognitive impairment
- **Delusions of grandeur** Beliefs of possessing exaggerated power, importance, knowledge, or ability. Associated with mania and schizophrenia

Psychological therapies

In the UK, the Improving Access to Psychological Therapies (IAPT) programme in England and similar programmes in other areas of the UK have
dramatically ↑ access to psychological therapies. These may be used alone
or in combination with drug therapies.

Who should be referred? Consider referral for patients with:
- Stress
- Grief reactions
- Eating disorders
- Body dysmorphic disorder
- Medically unexplained symptoms
- Depression
- Phobias
- Somatization
- Obsessive–compulsive disorder
- Anxiety
- Panic disorder
- Personality disorders
- Post-traumatic stress disorder

Problem-solving therapy (PST) Can be an effective tool for use
in the GP surgery[M]. Involves drawing up a list of problems and generating
and agreeing solutions, broken down into steps, for patients to work on as
homework between sessions—📖 p. 1003

Cognitive behaviour therapy (CBT)
- **Behavioural therapies** Aim to change behaviour. Usually the therapist
  uses a system of graded exposure (systematic desensitization),
  combined with teaching a method of anxiety reduction.
- **Cognitive therapy** Focusses on people's thoughts and the reasoning
  behind their assumptions on the basis that incorrect assumptions (that
  are often unconscious) → abnormal reactions which then reinforce
  these assumptions further (a vicious cycle)

The patient learns to recognize negative or unhelpful thinking patterns.
By enabling the patient to be more aware of this and teaching ways that
the patient can challenge cognitive errors, more helpful thinking styles can
result. Patients must then practice re-evaluating their thoughts and associated behaviours. At least as effective as drug treatment[M].

Individual non-facilitated self-help

Computerized CBT (CCBT) Particularly useful for patients with mild
symptoms or who do not wish to be referred to specialist psychological
therapy services.
- Free online interactive CCBT, e.g:
  - Living Life to the Full ♒ www.livinglifetothefull.com
  - The Mood Gym and e-Couch ♒ www.moodgym.anu.edu.au/welcome
- Other computerized CBT, e.g. Beating the Blues. A fee is payable, but
  some PCOs have purchased this program for use by patients free of
  charge in GP surgeries ♒ www.beatingtheblues.co.uk

Bibliotherapy For patients who are not computer-literate, self-help books
based on CBT techniques are an alternative, e.g.:
- **Gilbert P** (2000) *Overcoming Depression*. London: Constable &
  Robinson. ISBN: 1841191256
- **Burns D** (2000) *Feeling Good: The New Mood Therapy*. London: Harper
  Collins. ISBN: 9780380810338

Guided self-help Based on a CBT approach and available through psychological therapy services. Helpful for patients with mild symptoms. Uses books/printed materials under the supervision of a trained facilitator who introduces, monitors, then reviews the outcome of each treatment. Usually there is minimal contact with the facilitator (<3h).

Mindfulness-based cognitive therapy Skills training programme designed to enable patients to prevent the recurrence of depression; ↓ relapse by >50% in the first year after treatment. 8wk group programme aimed at patients who have ≥3 depression relapses, with 4 further follow-up sessions in the year following therapy.

Behavioural activation Therapist and patient work together, with the aim of identifying effects that the patient's behaviour might have on symptoms, mood, and problems. Then they address any problematic behaviours. Techniques may include reducing avoidance, activity scheduling, graded exposure, and initiating positively reinforced behaviours.

Interpersonal therapy (IPT) Individual or group therapy concentrating on the difficulties that arise in maintaining relationships with others. Focusses on current, not past, relationships and works on the premise that if interpersonal conflicts are resolved, both relationships and mood will improve. Useful for patients who can identify relationship difficulties.

Psychoeducational groups Group therapy can be used to explore depression or chronic physical health conditions, e.g. diabetes. Run by trained practitioners, they also involve the element of peer support.

Applied relaxation Group or individual therapy that teaches patients to relax quickly in different situations. Establishes the cues that herald feelings of anxiety and helps the patient to relax when those cues are felt. Effective treatment for anxiety states[M].

Counselling Usually reflective listening to encourage patients to think about and try to resolve their own difficulties. There is little evidence of beneficial effects or cost-effectiveness[N], but if there is a specific, identifiable cause for the patient's symptoms, counselling directed at the cause may be helpful, e.g.:

• Relationship breakdown—counselling is available through organizations, such as RELATE (🖰 www.relate.org.uk)
• Bereavement—counselling is available via organizations, such as CRUSE (📞 0870 167 1677; 🖰 www.cruse.org.uk)
• Debt—counselling is available from the Citizens Advice Bureau, National Debtline (📞 0808 808 4000), or the Consumer Credit Counselling Service Debt Remedy website (🖰 www.stepchange.org)

Further information

NICE 🖰 www.nice.org.uk
• Depression (2009)
• Generalised anxiety disorder and panic disorder in adults (2011)
• Common mental health disorders (2011)

SIGN Non-pharmaceutical management of depression in adults: a national clinical guideline (2010). 🖰 www.sign.ac.uk

Anxiety

Anxiety is only considered abnormal when it occurs in the absence of a stressful trigger, impairs physical, occupational, or social functioning, and/ or is excessively severe or prolonged. Features include:

Psychological symptoms	*Physical symptoms*	
• Fearful anticipation	• Dry mouth	• Paraesthesiae
• Irritability	• Tremor	• Tinnitus
• Sensitivity to noise	• Dizziness	• Headache
• Restlessness	• Epigastric discomfort	
• Poor concentration	• Difficulty swallowing	
• Worrying thoughts	• Frequent/loose motions/flatulence	
• Insomnia and/or nightmares	• Chest discomfort/constriction	
• Depression	• Difficulty breathing/hyperventilation	
• Obsessions	• Palpitations/awareness of missed beats	
• Depersonalization	• Frequency/urgency of micturition	
• Fear of losing control/dying	• Sexual dysfunction	
	• Menstrual problems	

Generalized anxiety disorder (GAD) Long-term condition, fluctuating in severity and nature, often beginning in adolescence. Lifetime prevalence ~5%. Key features are excessive, difficult-to-control worry about a number of events/activities occurring on most days for ≥6mo. Consider if history of anxiety/worry or if frequent attender with chronic physical health problem or no physical health problem but needing reassurance about somatic symptoms or repeated worrying about a wide range of different issues.

Associations

* Anxiety is often accompanied by depression (🔲 p. 1000) and may be a feature of early schizophrenia
* Other conditions which can cause anxiety and/or mimic symptoms of anxiety include drug/alcohol use or withdrawal, caffeine abuse, thyrotoxicosis, hypoglycaemia, temporal lobe epilepsy, phaeochromocytoma

Assessment Check TFTs. Use GAD-2 score (see Box 27.1) for screening:

* **If score ≥3**, consider anxiety disorder
* **If score <3** but you suspect anxiety is a factor, ask '*Do you find yourself avoiding places or activities and does this cause you problems?*'—if the answer is yes, consider anxiety disorder.

Management

* Avoid caffeine, excess alcohol, and illicit drugs
* Use a stepped treatment approach (see Figure 27.1)[N]
* Provide information about self-help organizations/support groups
* Try to identify causes of anxiety
* Consider using an anxiety scale (e.g. Hamilton Anxiety Scale) to record baseline morbidity and progress at follow-up

Psychological therapies 🔲 p. 990

* **Low intensity**—individual non-facilitated self-help; individual guided self-help; psychoeducational groups
* **High intensity**—CBT or applied relaxation

Ongoing symptoms

Step 4: offer referral for specialist treatment

Step 3: offer-high intensity psychological intervention and/or drug treatment

Step 2: offer low-intensity psychological interventions

Step 1: identification and assessment, education, and active monitoring

❶ Offer the least obtrusive, most effective treatment first

Figure 27.1 Stepwise approach to GAD management

Drug treatment

- SSRIs (e.g. sertraline 50–150mg od)—warn patients medication may take >1wk to work and of possible side effects (short-term ↑ in anxiety; GI symptoms). If >60y or other risk factors for GI bleeding, consider co-prescribing a PPI
- Follow-up every 2–4wk in the first 3mo then every 3mo
- If drug treatment is effective, continue for >1y
- If no benefit, consider alternative SSRI/SNRI or adding a psychological therapy; pregabalin is an option if unable to tolerate SSRI/SNRI. Do not offer antipsychotic medication
- Avoid benzodiazepines except for acute crises; restrict use to <4wk

⚠ Patients <30y may have ↑ suicidal thoughts when they start an SSRI/SNRI—warn about this risk and follow-up <1wk after starting medication and then weekly for 1mo to monitor suicide/self-harm risk.

Refer to specialist mental health services if severe anxiety with marked functional impairment plus:

- Risk of self-harm/suicide, or
- Significant co-morbidity (e.g. substance misuse, personality disorder or complex physical health problems), or
- Self-neglect, or
- Inadequate response to step 3 interventions

Box 27.1 GAD-2 short screening tool

Over the last 2wk, how often have you been bothered by any of the following problems?	Not at all	Several days	> half the days	Nearly every day
1. Feeling nervous, anxious, or on edge	0	1	2	3
2. Not being able to stop or control worrying	0	1	2	3

GAD-2 was developed by Spitzer RL, Williams BW, Kroenke K et al. with an educational grant from Pfizer Inc.

Panic disorder Panic attacks are very common, but panic disorder is uncommon: lifetime prevalence—1% of ♂; 3% of ♀.
- **Panic attack** Period of intense fear with characteristic symptoms. Can be spontaneous or situational
- **Panic disorder** Chronic disorder; recurrent panic attacks associated with persistent fear of having (or the consequences of) another attack

Symptoms Anxiety builds up quickly and unexpectedly without a recognizable trigger and patients often describe an intense feeling of apprehension or impending disaster. Common associated symptoms:
- Shortness of breath/smothering sensations
- Choking
- Palpitations and ↑ heart rate
- Chest discomfort or pain
- Sweating
- Dizziness, unsteady feelings, or faintness
- Nausea or abdominal pain
- Depersonalization/derealization
- Numbness or tingling sensations
- Flushes or chills
- Trembling or shaking
- Fear of dying
- Fear of doing something crazy or uncontrolled

Examination Obvious distress; sweating; tachycardia; hyperventilation. ↑ BP is common and usually settles. Otherwise examination is normal.

Associations Depression (56%); GAD; agoraphobia; substance misuse; suicide (↑ risk).

Differential diagnosis Alcohol withdrawal; drug misuse/withdrawal, other psychiatric disorders (e.g. psychosis); hyperthyroidism; temporal lobe epilepsy; cardiac arrhythmia; labyrinthitis; hypoglycaemia; hyperparathyroidism; phaeochromocytoma (very rare).

Management of acute panic attack 📖 p. 1120

Management of panic disorder Use a stepped treatment approach:
- **Step 1** Recognition and diagnosis. Educate about the condition, signpost to support in the community, and discuss treatment options. Commence active monitoring. Avoid alcohol, illicit drugs, and caffeine
- **Step 2** Treatment in primary care—offer (in order of effectiveness) psychological therapy (CBT), drug treatment or self-help (bibliotherapy or CCBT). Choice depends on severity of symptoms, co-morbidities and patient preference
- **Step 3** Consideration of alternative treatment—if one step 2 treatment is ineffective, change to or add another
- **Step 4** Offer referral for specialist treatment if ≥2 primary care treatments have failed

Drug treatment ❶ Do not use benzodiazepines for treatment of patients with panic disorder—associated with poorer long-term outcome.
- Offer SSRI, e.g. paroxetine, citalopram. Warn about possible transient ↑ in anxiety on starting treatment. Minimize initial side effects by starting at low dose and ↑ slowly. Review in <2wk and at 4, 6, and 12wk
- If SSRI is not suitable or ineffective, offer a TCA (e.g. imipramine, clomipramine) or non-drug treatment
- If effective, continue for ≥6mo, reviewing every 8–12wk
- Minimize discontinuation symptoms by tapering dose over time

Phobias As GAD but limited to certain situations. 2 main features:
- **Avoidance** Of the circumstances that provoke anxiety
- **Anticipatory anxiety** If there is a prospect of meeting that situation

Simple phobia Inappropriate anxiety in the presence of ≥1 object/situation, e.g. flying, enclosed spaces, spiders. Common in early life; most adult phobias are a continuation of childhood phobias. *Lifetime prevalence:* 4% ♂; 13% ♀.

Management Treatment is only needed if symptoms are frequent, intrusive, or prevent necessary activities. Exposure therapy is effective. Obtain through psychological therapy services or through the private sector, e.g. British Airways' 'fear of flying' course.

Social phobia Intense/persistent fear of being scrutinized or negatively evaluated by others leads to fear and avoidance of social situations (e.g. using a telephone, speaking in front of a group). Significantly disabling; not just shyness. May be generalized (person fears most social situations) or specific (related to certain activities only).

Management
- **Drug therapy** SSRIs—continue ≥12mo or long-term if symptoms remain unresolved, there is a co-morbid condition (e.g. depression, GAD, panic attacks), a history of relapse, or early onset
- **Psychological therapies** CBT (cognitive restructuring) ± exposure

Agoraphobia Onset is often aged 20–40y with an initial panic attack. Subsequently, panic attacks, fear of fainting and/or loss of control are experienced in crowds, away from home, or in situations from which escape is difficult. Avoidance results in patients remaining within their homes where they know symptoms will not occur. Other symptoms include depression, depersonalization, and obsessional thoughts.

Management Difficult to manage in general practice. Diagnosis is often delayed as patients will not come to the surgery and ongoing management complicated by refusal to be referred to psychiatric services. Prognosis is best when there is good marital/social support. *Options:*
- **Behaviour therapy,** e.g. exposure, coping with panic attacks. Home visits may be required but should be resisted as part of therapy
- **Drug treatment** SSRIs (citalopram and paroxetine are licensed); MAOIs; TCAs (imipramine and clomipramine are commonly used). Relapse rate is high. Benzodiazepines can be used if frequent panic attacks, particularly if initiating other treatment but beware of dependence

Further reading
NICE ℵ www.nice.org.uk
- Generalized anxiety disorder and panic disorder in adults (2011)
- Common mental health disorders (2011)

Patient information and support
Triumph over phobia (TOP) UK ☎ 0845 600 9601 ℵ www.topuk.org
Anxiety Care ℵ www.anxietycare.org.uk
No More Panic ℵ www.nomorepanic.co.uk

Other anxiety-type disorders

Stress 📖 p. 998   **Post-traumatic stress disorder** 📖 p. 998

Mixed anxiety and depression Combinations of anxiety and depression are common—particularly amongst women. Prevalence ~10%. When anxiety and depression occur together symptoms are more severe; there is ↑ functional impairment; illness is more chronic/persistent; and there is poorer response to treatment. Treat as for anxiety and/or depression, depending on the predominating features. Refer for psychiatric assessment if management strategies are not working.

Obsessive–compulsive disorder (OCD) Recurrent obsessive thoughts and compulsive acts. Lifetime prevalence ~2% although minor obsessional symptoms are more common. ♂:♀≈ 2:3. Tends to present in young adults. Patients may have symptoms for years before seeking help as they know that their thoughts/actions are irrational and are embarrassed to tell anyone. Relatives may highlight the problem.

Features
- **Obsessional thinking** Recurrent persistent thoughts, impulses, and images causing anxiety or distress
- **Compulsive behaviour** Repetitive behaviours, rituals, or mental acts done to prevent or ↓ anxiety
- **Other features** Indecisiveness and inability to take action, anxiety, depression, and depersonalization

Screening questions[N]
- Do you wash or clean a lot?
- Do you check things a lot?
- Is there any thought that keeps bothering you that you would like to get rid of but can't?
- Do your daily activities take a long time to finish?
- Are you concerned about orderliness or symmetry?
- Do these problems trouble you?

Management in adults
- **Mild functional impairment** Offer short CBT (<10h), including exposure-response prevention (ERP) or group therapy
- **Moderate functional impairment** Offer more intensive CBT (>10h) or drug therapy (SSRI, e.g. fluoxetine 20–40mg od)
- **Severe functional impairment** Offer psychological therapy + drug treatment. If inadequate response at 12wk, offer a different SSRI or clomipramine. Refer if symptoms persist

---

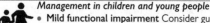

Management in children and young people
- **Mild functional impairment** Consider guided self-help. Include support and help for family and carers
- **Moderate/severe functional impairment** Offer CBT including ERP adapted to patient's age in a group or individual setting. Refer if symptoms do not improve. Drug therapy should only be initiated in secondary care

Body dysmorphic disorder (BDD) Preoccupation with an imagined defect in appearance or markedly excessive concern over a slight physical anomaly. *Prevalence:* 0.5–0.7%.

Features Time-consuming behaviours, e.g. mirror gazing, comparing self to others, camouflage, reassurance seeking, and skin picking.

Screening questions[N]
- Do you worry about the way you look and wish you could think about it less?
- What specific concerns do you have about your appearance?
- On a typical day, how many hours a day is it on your mind (>1h excessive)?
- What effect does it have on your life?
- Does it make it hard to do your work or be with friends?

Management As for OCD, however all children/young people should be offered CBT.

Somatization Physical symptoms in response to emotional distress. Characterized by an excessive preoccupation with bodily sensations combined with a fear of physical illness. Common feature of depression, anxiety, schizophrenia, and substance use.

Medically unexplained symptoms 🔲 p. 200

Somatization disorder Chronic condition. History of numerous unsubstantiated physical complaints. Starts at <30y and often persists many years. ♀:♂ ≈10:1; lifetime prevalence 0.1–0.2% though mild symptoms are much more common. Presents with:
- >2y history of multiple symptoms with no physical explanation
- Refusal to be reassured that there is no explanation for the symptoms
- Impaired social/family functioning due to these symptoms and/or associated behaviour

Management of somatization disorder
- Reattribution involves acknowledging/taking symptoms seriously, offering necessary examination and investigations, asking about psychosocial problems, and explaining the link between symptoms and stress
- Treat co-morbid psychiatric problems (e.g. depression, anxiety, panic)
- Beware of risks of drug interaction—self-medication with multiple OTC (or even prescription) drugs is common
- Beware of side effects of medication—these patients do not tolerate prescribed drugs well and have a heightened awareness of side effects
- Refer to the specialist mental health team if risk of suicide, marked functional impairment, impulsive or antisocial behaviour

Further information
NICE Obsessive–compulsive disorder: core interventions in the treatment of obsessive–compulsive disorder and body dysmorphic disorder (2005) ℰ www.nice.org.uk

Patient information and support
OCD Action ☏ 0845 390 6232 ℰ www.ocdaction.org.uk

Chronic stress

We all suffer from stress and, most of the time, the pressures of everyday life are a motivating force. A problem only arises when those pressures exceed the individual's ability to cope with them.

Causes of stress Virtually anything we do can cause stress. The most common causes of stress-related morbidity in the UK are:
- Work problems
- Family problems
- Financial problems
- Legal problems
- Exam stress

The stress epidemic 10.8 million working days are lost each year in the UK due to stress (11% of all sickness absence). The Health and Safety Executive estimates ~0.4 million people in the UK are experiencing work-related stress at a level they believe is making them ill; up to 5 million people feel 'very' or 'extremely' stressed by their work; and work-related stress costs society >£4 billion every year. Occupational stress is most likely to affect those working in the health, social work, and education sectors.

Presentation Most patients do not consult their GP with stress, unless they feel it is affecting their health. Common symptoms include:
- Mood swings
- Anxiety
- Depression
- Low self-esteem
- Poor concentration and/or memory
- Fatigue and/or lethargy
- Poor or ↑ appetite
- ↑ smoking, alcohol, and/or caffeine consumption
- Sleep disturbance
- Headaches
- Loss of libido
- Menstrual abnormalities
- Dry mouth
- Other unexplained aches/pains, e.g. muscular pains, chest pains
- Worsening of pre-existing conditions, e.g. irritable bowel syndrome, eczema, asthma, psoriasis, migraine

The GP's role is to identify stress as a cause of presenting symptoms; educate patients about stress and links between symptoms and stress; identify sources of stress; provide support and self-management strategies (see Box 27.2); treat medical problems arising out of stress e.g. depression; and provide certification if stress is so great that unable to work.

Post-traumatic stress disorder (PTSD) May occur in 25–30% of those who have experienced/witnessed traumatic events, e.g. major accident, fire, assault, military combat. It can affect people of all ages.

Symptoms Most develop symptoms immediately after the event but it is common for sufferers not to present until months/years afterwards. In ~15%, onset of symptoms is delayed. 65% experience chronic symptoms:
- **Intrusive recollections** Thoughts; nightmares; flashbacks
- **Avoidant behaviour** Of people, places, situations, or circumstances resembling/associated with the event; refusal to talk/think about the event; excessive rumination about questions about the event (e.g. why me? How could it have been prevented?)
- ↑ **arousal** ↑ anxiety/irritability, insomnia, ↓ concentration, ↑ vigilance
- **Numbing of emotions** Inability to experience feelings; feelings of detachment; giving up previous activities; amnesia for parts of the event

Associations Depression, anxiety; drug/alcohol abuse and dependence.

Management Treat any other associated psychiatric illness.

- **Watchful waiting** If mild symptoms have been present <4wk. Be supportive and listen. Arrange follow up in <1mo
- **Trauma-focussed psychological treatment** CBT and/or eye movement desensitization and reprocessing (EMDR). Refer if severe symptoms <4wk or ongoing intrusive symptoms >4wk after trauma
- **Drug treatment** (e.g. paroxetine, mirtazapine) Not first-line treatment. Reserve for those refusing or with continuing symptoms despite psychological therapy

❶ Debriefing after traumatic events is unhelpful.

The stressed GP 📖 p. 8

Box 27.2 Self-help stress management strategies

10 tips for chronic stress relief

- Ensure you get enough sleep and rest—avoid using sleeping tablets to achieve this (see Insomnia—📖 p.194)
- Look after yourself and your own health, e.g. don't skip meals, sit down to eat, take time out to spend time with family and friends, make time for hobbies and relaxation, do not ignore health worries
- Avoid using nicotine, alcohol, or caffeine as a means of stress relief
- Work off stress with physical exercise—↓ levels of adrenaline released and ↑ release of natural endorphins which → a sense of well-being and enhanced sleep
- Try relaxation techniques
- Avoid interpersonal conflicts—try to agree more and be more tolerant
- Learn to accept what you can't change
- Learn to say 'no'
- Manage your time better—prioritize and delegate; create time buffers to deal with unexpected overruns and emergencies
- Try to sort out the cause of the stress, e.g. talk to line manager at work, arrange marriage or debt counselling, arrange more childcare

Time management made easy This technique aims to transform an overwhelming volume of work into a series of manageable tasks.

- Make a list of all the things you need to do
- List them in order of genuine importance
- Note whether you really need to do the task, what you need to do personally, and what can be delegated to others
- Note a timescale in which each task needs to be done, e.g. immediately, within a day, within a week, within a month, etc.

Further information

Health and Safety Executive (HSE) 🖰 www.hse.gov.uk/stress

NICE Post-traumatic stress disorder (PTSD): the management of PTSD in adults and children in primary, secondary, and community care (2005) 🖰 www.nice.org.uk

Patient advice and support

Stress Management Society ☎ 0844 357 8629 🖰 www.stress.org.uk

International Stress Management Association (UK) 🖰 www.isma.org.uk

Depression

2.3 million people suffer from depression in UK at any time. ♂:♀ ≈1:2.

Recognition ~30–50% cases are not detected, although most are mild cases, more likely to resolve spontaneously. Diagnosis of mental illness is stigmatizing. This can lead to 'collusion' between patient and doctor during consultation to avoid diagnosis, doing little to tackle the problem.

Screening questions for depression[N] If +ve response to either question, investigate further, e.g with PHQ-9 (Figure 27.2).

- During the last month, have you often been bothered by feeling down, depressed, or hopeless?
- During the last month, have you often been bothered by having little interest or pleasure in doing things?

Causes and co-morbidity Associated with:
- **Psychiatric disorders,** e.g. anxiety, alcohol abuse, substance abuse, eating disorders
- **Physical disorders,** e.g. PD, MS, dementia, thyroid disorders, Addison's disease, hypercalcaemia, RA, SLE, cancer, HIV and other chronic infections, cardio- and cerebrovascular disease, learning disability
- **Drugs causing symptoms of depression** β-blockers, anticonvulsants, Ca^{2+} channel blockers, corticosteroids, oral contraceptives, antipsychotic drugs, drugs used for PD (e.g. levodopa)

Biopsychosocial assessment (BPA) Discuss:
- Current symptoms (nature, onset, duration, severity)
- PH of depression and/or mood elevation (? bipolar disorder)
- FH of mental illness
- Quality of relationships
- Living conditions—social support
- Employment/financial worries
- Alcohol/substance misuse
- Suicidal ideation
- Treatment options
- Past experience of/response to treatments

In addition consider discussing:
- Co-morbid mental/physical health problems
- Awareness of sources of help
- The patient's views about the cause of his/her symptoms
- Need for follow-up

Symptoms Present >50% of the time in the past 2wk. Two key features:
- Depressed mood, *and/or*
- ↓ interest or pleasure, which must be disabling to the patient

Other symptoms:
- Change in appetite/weight
- Insomnia or hypersomnia
- Fatigue or loss of energy
- Poor concentration
- Poor appetite or overeating
- Insomnia or hypersomnia
- Low energy or fatigue
- Low self-esteem
- Psychomotor agitation/retardation
- Sense of worthlessness or guilt
- Recurrent thoughts of death/suicide
- Feelings of hopelessness
- Poor concentration or difficulty making decisions

❶ Sleep disturbance and fatigue have high predictive value for depression and should prompt enquiry about other symptoms.

Name:			Date:		
Over the last 2 weeks, how often have you been bothered by any of the following problems? (use ✓ to indicate your answer)		Not at all	Several days	More than half the days	Nearly every day
1.	Little interest or pleasure in doing things	0	1	2	3
2.	Feeling down, depressed, or hopeless	0	1	2	3
3.	Trouble falling or staying asleep, or sleeping too much	0	1	2	3
4.	Feeling tired or having little energy	0	1	2	3
5.	Poor appetite or overeating	0	1	2	3
6.	Feeling bad about yourself— or that you are a failure or have let yourself or your family down	0	1	2	3
7.	Trouble concentrating on things, such as reading the newspaper or watching television	0	1	2	3
8.	Moving or speaking so slowly that other people could have noticed. Or the opposite—being so fidgety or restless that you have been moving around a lot more than usual	0	1	2	3
9.	Thoughts that you would be better off dead, or of hurting yourself in some way	0	1	2	3
	Add columns:				
				Total:	
10.	If you ticked off any problems, how difficult have these problems made it for you to do your work, take care of things at home, or get along with other people?	Not difficult at all			
		Somewhat difficult			
		Very difficult			
		Extremely difficult			

Figure 27.2 The Patient Health Questionnaire (PHQ-9)
The Patient Health Questionnaire (PHQ-9) is reproduced with permission of Pfizer Inc.

Examination
- **General appearance** Self-neglect, smell of alcohol, weight ↓
- **Assessment of mood** Looks depressed and/or tired, speech monotone or monosyllabic, avoids eye contact, tearful, anxious or jumpy/fidgety, feeling of distance, poor concentration, etc.
- **Psychotic symptoms** Hallucinations, delusions, etc. (🕮 p. 1006)

Assessing severity of depression Can be done using a depression symptom count or patient self-complete measure, such as the PHQ-9.
- **Subthreshold depressive symptoms** Fewer than 5 symptoms of depression (PHQ-9 of <5)
- **Mild depression** ≥5 symptoms of depression that result in only mild functional impairment (PHQ-9 of 5–9)
- **Moderate depression** Symptoms or functional impairment are between 'mild' and 'severe' (PHQ-9 of 10–14 indicates moderate depression; PHQ-9 of 15–19 indicates moderately severe depression)
- **Severe depression** Most symptoms and the symptoms markedly interfere with functioning ± psychotic symptoms (PHQ-9 ≥20)

Assessment of suicidal intent ❶ Always ask patients directly about suicidal ideas and intent (🕮 p. 1118). *Risk factors for suicide:*
- ♂ > ♀
- Age 40–60y
- Living alone
- Divorced > widowed > single > married
- Unemployment
- Chronic physical illness
- Past psychiatric history
- Recent admission to psychiatric hospital
- History of suicide attempt/self-harm
- Alcohol/drug misuse
- Family history of suicide

Cultural considerations Some cultures have no terms for depression. Patients may present with physical symptoms (somatization) or use less familiar 'cultural-specific' terms to describe depressive symptoms, e.g. 'sorrow in my heart'.

Management of depression[N] Use a stepped care approach starting at the step most appropriate for the patient.

Step 1 All patients—assess severity. Provide education about depression and information about support available to both the patient and carers/family members as appropriate. Discuss treatment options.

If sleep is a problem Discuss sleep hygiene (🕮 p. 194): establish regular sleep/wake times; avoid excess eating, smoking, or alcohol before sleep; create a proper environment for sleep; take regular exercise.

Subthreshold or mild depression Active monitoring—watchful waiting for <2wk to see if spontaneous recovery occurs. Simple problem-solving strategies may be useful in the GP surgery (see Figure 27.3).

Step 2 Persistent subthreshold or mild/moderate depression.
- **Low-intensity psychosocial interventions** (🕮 p. 990) Individual guided self-help; CCBT; structured group exercise programme (e.g. exercise prescription)
- **Group-based peer support** For people with a shared chronic physical health problem

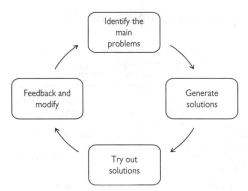

Figure 27.3 Simple problem solving strategy to use in the surgery

- **Drug treatment** Do not use routinely for subthreshold/mild depression—consider if: past history of moderate/severe depression; subthreshold symptoms that have been present >2y; subthreshold/mild depression that persists after other interventions

Step 3 Moderate/severe depression or mild/subthreshold depression that has not responded to treatment.

- **High-intensity psychological interventions** (🕮 p. 990) Individual or group-based CBT, interpersonal therapy, behavioural activation, behavioural couples therapy (if relationship difficulties)
- **Drug treatment** Usually SSRI
- **Combined treatments** Antidepressant medication + high-intensity psychological intervention (CBT or interpersonal therapy)
- **Collaborative care** For people with physical health problems. Case management supervised by a mental health professional providing education + psychological/pharmacological treatments with follow-up

Step 4 Referral to psychiatry *U* = Urgent; *S* = Soon; *R* = Routine
- High suicide risk—*U*
- Severe self-neglect—*U*
- Depression complicated by psychotic symptoms—*U*
- Depression complicated by significant psychiatric co-morbidity or psychosocial factors—*R/S*
- Inadequate response to multiple treatments—*R*

Safety-netting Follow-up if patients do not attend appointments. Give patient ± family/carers clear advice on what to do if the patient's mood deteriorates and how to access urgent support, both in and out of hours.

Further reading

NICE 🖰 www.nice.org.uk
- Depression (2009)
- Depression in adults with a chronic physical health problem (2009)

Patient information and support

Depression Alliance ☏ 0845 123 2320 🖰 www.depressionalliance.org
Samaritans ☏ 08457 909 090 🖰 www.samaritans.org

Drugs for treating depression

(BNF 4.3)

When should antidepressants be started? Consider for:
- Patients with moderate/severe depression ± psychological therapy
- Dysthymia (subthreshold depressive symptoms lasting >2y)
- Mild depression if other treatment strategies have failed—📖 p. 998

What should I tell the patient? Giving patients information ↑ compliance. When starting antidepressant drugs explain:
- The reasons for prescribing
- Timescale of action—unlikely to have any effect for 2wk; effects build up to maximum effect at 4–6wk, and
- Likely side effects including possible exacerbation of anxiety in the first 2wk of treatment

Which drugs are available? The major groups are:

Selective serotonin re-uptake inhibitors (SSRIs) (e.g. fluoxetine 20mg od; citalopram 20–40mg od; sertraline 50–150mg od). Usually first choice as less likely to be discontinued due to side effects and safer in overdose. Warn of possible short-term ↑ in anxiety/agitation when starting medication and advise patients to stop if significant. GI side effects, including dyspepsia are common. Consider co-prescribing a PPI for stomach protection if >60y or other risk factors for GI bleeding.

 Only fluoxetine has been shown to be of benefit for the treatment of depression in children—📖 p. 921.

 Elderly people—particularly those taking SSRIs—are prone to hyponatraemia when taking antidepressants.

Serotonin and noradrenaline re-uptake inhibitors (SNRIs) (e.g. venlafaxine 37.5mg bd, duloxetine 60mg od). Avoid if uncontrolled hypertension. Venlafaxine is also contraindicated if high risk of arrhythmia.

Tricyclic and related anti-depressants (TCAs) (e.g. lofepramine 70mg od/bd/tds; trazodone 150–300mg daily). Titrate dose up from low dose until the patient feels the drug is helping *or* until side effects intrude[S]. Common side effects include drowsiness, dry mouth, blurred vision, constipation, urinary retention, and sweating. Use with caution for patients with CVD because of risk of arrhythmia, patients with prostatic hypertrophy (↑ risk of retention), and patients with raised intraocular pressures (↑ risk of acute glaucoma).

Mirtazapine 15–45mg nocte. Presynaptic α2-adrenoreceptor antagonist. ↑ central noradrenergic and serotonergic neurotransmission. Causes sedation during initial treatment and may also cause weight ↑.

Reboxetine 4–6mg bd. Selective inhibitor of noradrenaline re-uptake. Not recommended for elderly patients.

- Genetic—people with a diagnosis of psychosis are more likely to suffer from DM and/or CVD even after exclusion of other risk factors
- Social exclusion—↓ attendance at chronic disease management clinics, ↓ participation in screening programmes

Annual reviews in primary care All patients with confirmed non-organic psychotic illness require long-term follow-up in primary care.
- **Regular reviews** Case registers help ensure regular reviews take place. Check a written care plan has been drawn up by the psychiatric service involved. Follow-up if a patient does not attend for review
- **Check mental health** Assess symptoms; compliance with medication; efficacy of treatment; medication side effects; risks of suicide
- **Check physical health** Annual screening and review of smoking, exercise, BMI (and/or waist circumference), BP, FBG or HbA1c, FBC, renal and liver function, lipids, prolactin (if taking anti-psychotic medication), TFTs (if taking lithium)
- **Education** Involve family if possible—information about psychotic illness and treatment (reinforce compliance), early signs of relapse, where to access help, benefits of ↓ smoking, exercise, healthy diet, weight control, sensible drinking, and avoidance of illicit drugs, e.g. cannabis/amphetamines, which exacerbate symptoms and ↑ risk of relapse
- **Help with lifestyle change,** e.g. referral to smoking cessation clinic, dietician or weight management programme; exercise prescription
- **Social support** Assistance may be needed with: carer support, finances, housing, employment, structured daily activity, transport, social network. Those who can help include: social services, community mental health team, housing officer, disability support workers

Driving and psychotic illness Advise patients to inform the DVLA. Driving should cease during the acute illness (all vehicles) and until stable with insight for ≥3y (LGV/PCV drivers)—📖 p. 131

> **Emergency management of severe psychosis**
> - Severe crises that endanger the individual or others are difficult to manage in primary care. Treatment in hospital may be required
> - If unwilling to accept voluntary admission, use compulsory admission under the Mental Health Act (📖 p. 1122)
> - Sedation whilst awaiting admission may be required—try oral medication first, e.g. lorazepam 1–2mg or chlorpromazine 50–100mg po; if oral medication is refused and severe agitation, consider lorazepam 1–2mg IM or chlorpromazine 50mg IM (↓ dose for elderly patients and avoid if the patient is epileptic, has been drinking, or taking barbiturates)

Further information
IRIS Initiative 🖱 www.iris-initiative.org.uk
- GP guidance: emerging psychosis and young people (2010)
- GP guidance: physical health issues of emerging psychosis (2010)

Patient information and support
Royal College of Psychiatrists Patient information leaflets 🖱 www.rcpsych.ac.uk
MIND ☎ 0300 123 3393 🖱 www.mind.org.uk

Schizophrenia and mania

Management of first presentation If psychotic illness is suspected, ask yourself whether the patient is a risk to self/others
- If a risk, request emergency specialist assessment and/or acute admission voluntarily or under the Mental Health Act (🔲 p. 122)
- If no immediate risk refer through the local rapid-access early intervention in psychosis service (🔲 p. 1006)

Physical health problems of people with psychosis 🔲 p. 1006

Driving and psychosis 🔲 p. 131

Schizophrenia Is a frightening and disabling condition in which the sufferer is unable to distinguish his internal from the outside world. Lifetime prevalence ≈1%. Peak age of onset—♂ (15–25y); ♀ (25–35y).

First rank symptoms Reliable markers in ~70% of patients. ≥1 symptom is suggestive of schizophrenia:

- Auditory hallucinations in the form of a commentary
- Hearing thoughts spoken aloud
- Hearing voices referring to the patient, made in the 3rd person
- Somatic hallucinations
- Thought broadcasting
- Thought withdrawal, insertion, and interruption
- Delusional perception
- Feelings or actions experienced as made or influenced by external agents (passivity feelings)

First presentation of schizophrenia Typically a young person <35y with +ve symptoms (delusions, hallucinations, and/or thought disorder). The patient may lack insight, so the initial approach may come from a relative/friend. See the patient.
- Ask about physical and psychological symptoms—in particular thoughts and perceptions
- Assess the patient's behaviour and appearance. Look for evidence of self-care, loss of affect, poverty of thought, and social withdrawal
- Try to elicit any history of drug abuse
- Ask friends, neighbours, or relatives present to tell you about the patient's behaviour

Differential diagnosis Illicit drugs, temporal lobe epilepsy, delirium, dementia, affective disorder, personality disorder.

Chronic schizophrenia Characterized by thought disorder and −ve symptoms (poverty of thought, apathy, inactivity, lack of volition, social withdrawal, and loss of affect). Aim to treat the disease, prevent relapse, and improve quality of life.

Antipsychotic medication Initiate only under specialist supervision. Safety concerns include:

- Weight ↑
- Insulin resistance/diabetes
- Dyslipidaemia
- Cardiovascular disease
- Prolonged Q-T syndrome
- Extrapyramidal syndrome

❶ All patients taking antipsychotic agents should have annual review of BMI, BP, FBG/HbA1c, lipids, FBC, U&E and eGFR, LFTs, and prolactin.

Regular primary care review 🔲 p. 1007

Mania and hypomania Most of us experience ups and downs in our mood according to the circumstances we find ourselves in.

Mania Is characterized by a persistently high or euphoric mood out of keeping with circumstances. Other signs include:

Hypomania Is a less severe form of mania.

- ↑ pressure of speech
- ↑ energy and activity
- ↑ appetite
- ↑ sexual desire
- ↑ pain threshold

- ↓ desire/need for sleep
- ↓ insight
- Grandiose delusions
- Hallucinations
- Labile mood

- Over-assertiveness
- Spending sprees
- Disinhibition
- Self-important ideas
- Poor concentration

Differential diagnosis Hypoglycaemia; alcohol or drug abuse; prescribed drug side effects (e.g. steroids); temporal lobe epilepsy; frontal lobe dysfunction (e.g. due to tumour or stroke); thyrotoxicosis.

Regular primary care review 📖 p. 1007

Drug treatment (*BNF* 4.2.3)
- Lithium is the drug of choice—initiate only under specialist supervision
- Check levels weekly until the dose is constant for 4wk, then monthly for 6mo. Then, as long as the dose is constant, check levels every 3mo
- If levels are slowly rising, suspect nephrotoxicity
- Check plasma creatinine, eGFR, and TFTs every 6mo
- Avoid changing proprietary brands as bioavailability varies
- *Toxicity:* blurred vision, diarrhoea/vomiting, ↓ K⁺, drowsiness, ataxia, coarse tremor, dysarthria, hyperextension, fits, psychosis, coma, shock
- *Alternative drugs:* sodium valproate; carbamazepine

Bipolar disorder or manic depression Consists of episodes when the patient has mania (bipolar I) or hypomania (bipolar II) against a background of depression. Lifetime prevalence ~1%. ♂:♀ ≈1:1. Peak incidence is in late teens and early 20s—90% develop the disorder before 30y. Management is as for mania.

Referral to the specialist mental health team *U* = Urgent; *S* = Soon; *R* = Routine.
- ↑ in risk to self or others—*U*
- Poor response to treatment/persistent symptoms—*U/S/R*
- Significant side effects of medication—*R*
- Problems with adherence to treatment regime—*S/R*
- Suspected co-morbid substance misuse—*R*
- Patient new to your practice—*R*

Further information
NICE 🖰 www.nice.org.uk
- Schizophrenia (2009)
- Bipolar disorder (2006)

Patient information and support
MIND ☎ 0300 123 3393 🖰 www.mind.org.uk
Rethink ☎ 0300 5000 927 🖰 www.rethink.org
Manic Depression Fellowship ☎ 0808 802 1983 🖰 www.mdf.org.uk

Acute delirium

Common condition seen in general practice—particularly amongst elderly patients. May occur *de novo* or be superimposed upon chronic confusion of dementia (📖 p. 1012) causing sudden worsening of cognition.

Presentation
- Global cognitive deficit with onset over hours/days
- Fluctuating conscious level—typically worse at night/late afternoon
- Impaired memory—on recovery amnesia of the events is usual
- Disorientation in time and place
- Odd behaviour—may be underactive, drowsy, and/or withdrawn *or* hyperactive and agitated
- Disordered thinking—often slow and muddled ± delusions (e.g. accuse relatives of taking things)
- Disturbed perceptions—hallucinations (particularly visual) are common
- Mood swings

Examination Can be difficult. If possible, do a thorough general physical examination to exclude treatable causes.

Possible causes
- **Infection** Particularly UTI, pneumonia; rarely, encephalitis/meningitis
- **Drugs** Opioids, sedatives, levodopa, anticonvulsants, recreational drugs
- **Metabolic** Hypoglycaemia, hyponatraemia, uraemia, liver failure, hypercalcaemia, other electrolyte imbalance (rarer)
- **Alcohol or drug withdrawal**
- **Hypoxia,** e.g. pneumonia, exacerbation of COPD, cardiac failure
- **Cardiovascular** MI, stroke, TIA
- **Intracranial lesion** Space-occupying lesion, ↑ ICP, head injury (especially subdural haematoma)
- **Thyroid disease**
- **Carcinomatosis**
- **Epilepsy** Temporal lobe epilepsy, postictal state.
- **Nutritional deficiency** B_{12}, thiamine, or nicotinic acid deficiency

Differential diagnosis
- Deafness—may appear confused
- Dementia—longer history and lack of fluctuations in conscious level; in practice may be difficult to distinguish especially if you come across a patient who is alone and can give no history
- Primary mental illness, e.g. schizophrenia (📖 p. 1008); mania (📖 p. 1009); anxiety state (📖 p. 992)

Management Is aimed at treating all remediable causes.

Admit to hospital or refer to intermediate care if:
- The patient lives alone
- The patient will be left unsupervised for any duration of time
- If carers (or residential home) are unprepared/unable to continue looking after the patient, *and/or*
- If history and examination have indicated a cause requiring acute hospital treatment

Possible investigations to consider in the community
- Cognitive function test, e.g. 6CIT (see Table 27.1)
- Urine—dipstick for glucose, ketones, blood, protein, nitrates, and leucocyte esterase; send for M,C&S
- Check finger-prick capillary glucose to exclude hypoglycaemia
- Blood—FBC, ESR, U&E, eGFR, LFTs, Ca²⁺, TFTs
- ECG
- CXR

Management at home
- Acute confusion is frightening for carers—reassure and support them
- Treat the cause, e.g. antibiotics for UTI or chest infection
- Try to avoid sedation as this can make confusion worse. Where unavoidable use lorazepam 0.5–1mg po/IM prn
- Involve district nursing services and/or intermediate care services, e.g. to provide incontinence aids, nursing care, additional support
- If the cause does not become clear despite investigation or the patient fails to improve with treatment admit for further investigation and assessment

Assessment of capacity to make decisions 📖 p. 122

Table 27.1 The 6 Cognitive Impairment Test (6CIT)

	Question	Response	Score
1.	*What year is it?*	Correct: 0; Incorrect: 4	
2.	*What month is it?*	Correct: 0; Incorrect: 3	
Remember the following address: e.g. John Brown, 42, West Street, Bedford			
3.	*What time is it (to the nearest hour)?*	Correct: 0; Incorrect: 3	
4.	*Count backwards from 20 to1*	Correct: 0; 1 error: 2; >1 error: 4	
5.	*Months of the year backwards*	Correct: 0; 1 error: 2; >1 error: 4	
6.	*Repeat the memory phrase*	Correct: 0; 1 error: 2; 2 errors: 4; 3 errors: 6; 4 errors: 8; All incorrect: 10	
	Total		

Instructions on scoring Ring the appropriate score results for each question; add up the scores to produce a result out of 28.

Score

- 0–7   Not significant
- 8–9   Probably significant—refer; possible dementia
- 10–28   Significant—refer; likely dementia

Dementia

Generalized impairment of intellect, memory, and personality, with no impairment of consciousness. Prevalence ↑ with age (rare <60y; 5% >65y; 20% >80y). *Common causes:* Alzheimer's disease (60%); vascular (multi-infarct) dementia; dementia with Lewy bodies.

Presentation Patients may be aware of 'being a bit forgetful' but usually relatives complain about their behaviour. Early symptoms are loss of short-term memory and inability to perform normally simple tasks. Alternatively patients present later with failure to cope at home or self-neglect occasionally leading to crisis. To diagnose dementia there must be a clear history of progressive impairment of memory and cognition ± personality change. Always assess level of support in the home, housing, and ability to cope (both patient and carers). Review medications to identify any that might impair cognition.

Examination Check general appearance—look for self-neglect, malnutrition, abuse; screen for cognitive deficit, e.g. with 6CIT (🔲 p. 1011).

Investigation Aimed at detecting treatable causes: check FBC, U&E, eGFR, LFTs, Ca^{2+}, TFTs, glucose, B_{12}, folate. Consider: MSU, CXR, ECG.

Differential diagnosis
- Acute delirium—🔲 p. 1010   • Depression—🔲 p. 1000
- Communication difficulties—deafness, dysphasia, or language difficulties

Prevention[N]
- 2° prevention: review and treat vascular risk factors
- Offer referral to genetic counselling to those thought to have a genetic cause for their dementia, and refer unaffected relatives

General management
- **Refer** All patients should be referred to the mental health services for the elderly or a memory assessment clinic for formal diagnosis, exclusion of treatable causes, ongoing specialist support and assessment, and care planning. Refer to a social worker for community support
- **Apply principles of rehabilitation** (🔲 p. 204; 🔲 p. 582)
- **Support carers** (🔲 p. 220). Advise re benefits (🔲 p. 222), self-help groups, respite care. Warn that dementia is progressive and prepare carers for a time when the patient does not recognize them
- **Discuss whilst sufferer still has capacity** Along with carers, the use of advanced statements, lasting power of attorney (🔲 p. 122), advanced decisions to refuse treatment, and preferred place of care plans
- **Treat concurrent problems** (e.g. UTI, chest infection, anaemia, pain) They make dementia worse. Consider possible side effects of medication. ❶ 40% have concurrent depression
- **Management of memory loss** Notebook to record 'tasks must do'; electronic prompts on mobile phone; medication dispensers

Management of behavioural (non-cognitive) symptoms
- Maintain a constant environment if possible

- Safety—arrange for door catches to prevent wandering, and take up loose carpets to prevent falls; consider fire and electrical safety
- Avoid sedatives wherever possible as may worsen confusion—if needed use very low dose and review regularly

⚠ *Antipsychotic drugs for patients with dementia*[N] Do not use antipsychotics for mild to moderate non-cognitive symptoms because of the risk of severe adverse reaction, CVA (2x risk), and death. Consider in severe agitation only if:
- Risks and benefits have been assessed and discussed
- Patient is carefully monitored for changes in cognition
- Co-morbid conditions, such as depression, have been considered
- Dose is started low and titrated upwards
- Treatment is time-limited and regularly reviewed

Driving and dementia Inform the DVLA. Licensing depends on clinical condition.

Assessment of capacity to make decisions 📖 p. 122

Alzheimer's dementia Most common form of dementia. *Cause:* unknown—defective genes found on chromosomes 14, 19, and 21. *Risk factors:* FH, Down's syndrome (onset at ~30y), late onset depression, hypothyroidism, history of head injury. Presents with steady ↓ in memory and cognition. *Onset:* any age—normally >40y. ♀:♂ ≈0.7.

Drug management of cognitive symptoms Specialist-initiated—refer. Preferred drug varies according to severity of cognitive deficit:
- **Mild/moderate** Anticholinesterase inhibitors (e.g. donepezil, galantamine, rivastigmine) ↓ rate of decline.
- **Moderate/severe** Memantine ↓ clinical/cognitive decline

Alois Alzheimer (1864–1915)—German neuropathologist/psychiatrist.

Vascular (multi-infarct) dementia Multiple lacunar infarcts or larger strokes cause generalized intellectual impairment. Tends to occur in a stepwise progression with each subsequent infarct. The final picture is one of dementia, pseudobulbar palsy, and shuffling gait with small steps. Treatment is as for secondary prevention of TIA/stroke—📖 p. 564

Lewy body dementia Fluctuating but persistent cognitive impairment, parkinsonism, and hallucinations. No specific treatment. Avoid antipsychotics as they can be fatal. Use benzodiazepines if tranquillization is necessary. *Friedrich H. Lewy (1885–1950)—German neurologist.*

Pick's dementia Dementia characterized by personality change associated with frontal lobe signs such as gross tactlessness. Lack of restraint may lead to stealing, practical jokes, and unusual sexual adventures. Treatment is supportive. *Arnold Pick (1851–1924)—Czech neurologist/psychiatrist.*

Further information

NICE Dementia (2006 with 2011 update) 🖱 www.nice.org.uk

Patient information and support

Alzheimer's Society ☎ 0300 222 1122 🖱 www.alzheimers.org.uk
Benefits enquiry line ☎ 08457 123 456
Carers UK ☎ 0808 808 7777 🖱 www.carersuk.org

Eating disorders

Identification of and screening for eating disorders Target groups for screening include:
- Young women with low BMI compared with age norms
- Patients consulting with weight concerns who are not overweight
- Women with menstrual disturbances or amenorrhoea
- Patients with GI symptoms
- Patients with symptoms/signs of starvation—sensitivity to cold, delayed gastric emptying, constipation, ↓ BP, bradycardia, hypothermia
- Patients with physical signs of repeated vomiting—pitted teeth ± dental caries, general weakness, cardiac arrhythmias, renal damage, ↑ risk of UTI, epileptic fits, ↓ K⁺
- Children with poor growth
- Young people with type 1 DM and poor treatment adherence

Screen target populations with simple screening questions[N]
- Do you worry excessively about your weight?
- Do you think you have an eating problem?

△ Patients who are pregnant or have DM are at particular risk of complications if they have eating disorders. Refer early for specialist support and ensure everyone involved in care is aware of the eating disorder.

Anorexia nervosa Prevalence 0.02–0.04%. ♀ >> ♂. Usually begins in adolescence. Peak prevalence at 16–17y. *Features:*
- Refusal to keep body weight >85% of that expected (BMI <17.5kg/m²)
- Intense fear of gaining weight, though underweight
- Disturbed experience of body weight or shape or undue influence of shape on self-image
- Amenorrhoea in women for ≥3mo and ↓ sexual interest

Patients tend to have a set daily calorific intake, e.g. 600–1,000 calories, and may employ strategies, e.g. bingeing and vomiting, purging, or excessive exercise to try to lose weight. Depression and social withdrawal are common as are symptoms 2° to starvation.

Management[N]
- Give ongoing support and information
- Check electrolytes
- Refer to a specialist eating disorders clinic (if available) or the mental health team. Treatment involves family therapy for adolescents, psychotherapy, and possible admission for refeeding

Follow-up Patients with enduring anorexia nervosa not under 2° care follow-up should be offered an annual physical and mental health check.

△ Many patients with anorexia nervosa have compromised cardiac function. Avoid prescribing drugs which adversely affect cardiac function (e.g. antipsychotics, TCAs, macrolide antibiotics, some antihistamines). If prescribing is essential then follow up with ECG monitoring.

Bulimia nervosa Prevalence 1–2%. Mainly ♀ aged 16–40y. *Features:*
- Recurrent episodes of binge eating, far beyond normally accepted amounts of food
- Inappropriate compensatory behaviour to prevent weight ↑, e.g. vomiting; use of laxatives, diuretics, and/or appetite suppressants. Bulimics can be subdivided into those that purge and those that just use fasting and exercise to control their weight
- Self-image unduly influenced by body shape (see Anorexia nervosa)
- Normal menses and normal weight. If low BMI classified as anorexia

Management
- Give ongoing support and information
- Check electrolytes
- First-line treatment:
  - Evidence-based self-help programme, e.g. Overcoming Bulimia—available from ℘ www.overcomingbulimiaonline.com
  - Antidepressant medication—fluoxetine 60mg od is the drug of choice
- If unsuccessful, refer to a specialist eating disorders clinic (if available) or the mental health team. CBT may help

Advice for patients purging
- **Vomiting** Advise patients to avoid brushing their teeth after vomiting, rinse with a non-acid mouthwash after vomiting, and ↓ acid oral environment (e.g. by limiting acid foods)
- **Laxatives** Where laxative abuse is present, advise patients to gradually ↓ laxative intake. Laxative abuse does not significantly ↓ calorie absorption

Binge eating disorder A pattern of consumption of large amounts of food, even when a patient is not hungry. Common. Usually associated with obsessive feelings about food and body image, feelings of guilt/disgust about the amounts consumed, and/or a feeling of lack of control.

Management
- Give ongoing support and information
- Provide an evidence-based self-help programme as a first step and/or antidepressant medication (SSRI is the drug group of choice)
- If unsuccessful refer for specialist help. CBT might be helpful
- In all cases, provide concurrent advice and support to tackle any co-morbid obesity (📖 p. 178)

Body dysmorphic disorder 📖 p. 997

Further information
NICE Core interventions in the treatment and management of anorexia nervosa, bulimia nervosa, and related eating disorders (2004) ℘ www.nice.org.uk

Patient support and information
Beating Eating Disorders (BEAT) ☎ 0845 634 1414 (adults) ☎ 0845 634 7650 (youths) ℘ www.b-eat.co.uk

Other psychological conditions

Seasonal affective disorder (SAD) 'Winter blues'—recurrent disorder involving 'seasonal' episodes of depression, usually in the winter months. Affects ~2% adults. ♀:♂ ≈2:1. Peak incidence in third decade.

Symptoms Depression + ↑ sleep, ↑ food intake (with carbohydrate craving), and weight ↑. 30% experience elatory mood swings in summer.

Management SSRIs (particularly sertraline); phototherapy (30–90min/d in the early morning—effects should be seen within 3wk). Light boxes can be borrowed from psychiatry departments, hired, or bought (contact SAD Association for more information ℬ www.sada.org.uk).

Borderline personality disorder Patients may prefer 'emotional instability disorder'. Affects ~1% of the population. ♀ > ♂ *Features:*
- Pervasive and maladaptive patterns of behaviour, thinking, and control of emotions
- Significant instability of personal relationships, self-image, and mood
- Impulsive behaviour
- Tendency towards suicidal thoughts/self-harm
- Possible transient psychotic symptoms

Recognition Consider if repeated self-harm, persistent risk-taking, or marked emotional instability. If suspected, refer for specialist assessment.

Crisis management[N]
- Assess current risk to self/others—if a risk, request emergency specialist assessment and/or acute admission voluntarily or under the Mental Health Act (📖 p. 1122)
- Ask about past episodes and management strategies that worked
- Help to identify manageable changes that might enable the patient to deal with current problems
- Offer follow-up and contact the patient if the appointment is not kept
- Refer for specialist care if risk/distress continues to ↑

Specialist treatment of personality disorder
- Intensive structured psychological therapy, e.g. STEPPS programme
- Drugs—SSRIs are used for impulsive behaviour; low-dose antipsychotics for paranoid ideas; mood stabilizers for emotional instability. ❶ Be careful taking over prescribing from specialist care—there are no drugs licensed for use for borderline personality disorder and evidence of efficacy is poor

⚠ Risk of overdose is ↑ amongst patients with personality disorder.

Factitious disorder (Munchausen syndrome) Intentional feigning of physical/psychological symptoms to assume the sick role (± hospital admission). Can be difficult to detect. Differs from *malingering* as there is no external reward (e.g. financial). *Common presentations*
- **Physical** Dermatitis artefacta, PUO, bruising disorders, brittle DM, diarrhoea of unknown cause; neurological symptoms, e.g. pseudoparalysis or pseudofits (neurologica diabolica); abdominal pain (laparotomophilia migrans); chest pain (cardiopathia fantastica)

- **Psychological** Feigned psychosis, fictitious bereavement, fictitious overdose

Management Exclude any other basis for presenting pathology. Explain findings to the patient exploring possible causes. Assess psychological and social difficulties. Consider referral to specialist mental health services. *Baron H.K.F.F. von Munchausen (1720–1797)—German traveller/soldier.*

Munchausen's syndrome by proxy Caregiver—typically a mother with child—seeks repeated medical investigations and needless treatment for the person he/she is caring for. The child or person being cared for may actually be harmed by the carer to achieve these aims. Commonly reported symptoms include: neurological symptoms, bleeding, rashes.

Management Often difficult to detect and even harder to prove. A form of abuse that must be taken seriously and handled with care (🕮 p. 924). Involve all relevant agencies early (e.g. social services, paediatrics).

Malingering Intentional production or feigning of physical or psychological symptoms to assume the sick role for a known external purpose. Malingering is not considered a mental illness or psychopathology, although it can occur in the context of other mental illnesses. Forms:
- **Pure malingering** The individual falsifies all symptoms
- **Partial malingering** The individual has symptoms but exaggerates the impact they have upon daily functioning
- **Simulation** The individual acts out symptoms of a specific disability
- **False attribution** The individual has valid symptoms but is dishonest as to the source of the problems, e.g. attributing neck pain to an RTA to obtain compensation

Differential diagnosis True medical or psychiatric illness yet to be diagnosed; factitious disorder; somatization disorder

Common motivating factors
- Avoidance of work and/or other responsibility
- Litigation to obtain money
- Obtaining narcotics
- Avoidance of/release from jail
- Need for attention

Management Difficult. As doctors, we tend to believe our patients.
- Exclude causes for symptoms through careful history/examination
- Avoid prescribing drugs and unnecessary referrals as these might perpetuate symptoms
- Avoid certifying the patient as unfit to work or to perform activities— if the patient is unhappy about this, suggest a second opinion
- Tactfully explain your findings and conclusions to the patient and explore the reasons for the behaviour
- Provide support to find more appropriate ways to solve problems

Further information

NICE Borderline personality disorder (2009) ℘ www.nice.org.uk

Patient/relative information and support

Emergence ℘ www.emergenceplus.org.uk
Borderline Personality Disorder (BPD) central ℘ www.bpdcentral.com
Self Injury and Related Issues (SIARI) ℘ www.siari.co.uk

Cancer and palliative care

Principles of cancer care

If cancer is suspected, comprehensive assessment of patient and disease is needed before treatment decisions are made. Treatment can be:

- **Radical** Curative intent—surgery and/or drug/radiotherapy
- **Adjuvant** Given after surgery when micrometastatic disease is suspected—decision to proceed is based on the likelihood of relapse
- **Neoadjuvant** Given prior to definitive treatment to make treatment easier and more likely to succeed
- **Palliative** When cure is not possible and symptom management is the priority—📖 p. 1028

Assessment of the tumour

- **Histological nature of the tumour** Tissue of origin; cancer type (e.g. adenocarcinoma, squamous cell cancer); degree of differentiation; and tumour grade. High-grade, poorly differentiated tumours tend to have a poorer outcome than low-grade, well-differentiated tumours
- **Biological behaviour of the tumour** Tumour markers produced by cancers may be a useful adjunct to histological classification and staging and can be used to influence and monitor efficacy of treatment—see Table 28.1. ❶ Tumour markers can be ↑ in non-malignant conditions
- **Anatomical extent of the tumour** Determined through clinical, radiological, biochemical, and surgical assessment. Routine blood tests (e.g. LFTs, bone profile) may also indicate the presence of metastases

Cancer staging Staging allows the plan of treatment to be made.

TMN classification Widely used classification of tumours. Exact criteria for staging depend on the primary organ site:

- **T** Primary tumour—graded T_1–T_4 with increasing size of primary
- **N** Regional lymph nodes—advancing nodal disease is graded N_0–N_3
- **M** Presence (M_1) or absence (M_0) of metastases

Stage grouping

- **Stage 1** Clinical examination reveals a tumour confined to the primary organ. The lesion tends to be operable and completely resectable
- **Stage 2** Clinical examination shows evidence of local spread into surrounding tissue and first draining LNs. The lesion is operable and resectable but there is a higher risk of further spread of disease
- **Stage 3** Clinical examination reveals extensive primary tumour with fixation to deeper structures and local invasion. The lesion may not be operable and may require a combination of treatment modalities
- **Stage 4** Evidence of distant metastases beyond the site of origin. The primary site may be surgically inoperable

Other factors

- **Patient's performance status** The Eastern Cooperative Oncology Group (ECOG) Performance Status Scale is widely used (see Table 28.2). Patients with ECOG score >2 are usually deemed unsuitable for most chemotherapy interventions
- **Mortality, morbidity, and efficacy of the procedure**
- **Patient preferences**

Table 28.1 Tumour markers and associated conditions

Tumour marker	Associated conditions	
	Malignant conditions	*Non-malignant conditions*
CEA	GI tract cancers (particularly colorectal cancer)	Cirrhosis Pancreatitis Smoking
CA 19–9	Colorectal cancer Pancreatic cancer	Cholestasis
CA 125	Ovarian cancer Breast cancer Hepatocellular cancer	Cirrhosis Pregnancy Peritonitis Endometriosis
αFP	Hepatocellular cancer Germ cell cancers (not pure seminoma)	Liver disease—hepatitis/cirrhosis Pregnancy Open neural tube defects
HCG	Germ cell cancers Choriocarcinoma and hydatidiform mole	Pregnancy
PSA	Prostate cancer	BPH Prostatitis Prostate instrumentation Acute urinary retention Physical exercise Old age

Table 28.2 ECOG Performance Status Scale

Classification	Description
ECOG 0	Fully active; able to carry on all activities without restriction
ECOG 1	Restricted in physically strenuous activity but ambulatory and able to carry out work of a light or sedentary nature
ECOG 2	Ambulatory and capable of all self-care; confined to bed or chair 50% of waking hours
ECOG 3	Capable of only limited self care; confined to bed or chair 50% or more of waking hours
ECOG 4	Completely disabled; cannot carry out any self-care; totally confined to bed or chair

The GP's role Treatment for cancer is increasingly successful but also increasingly complex. Treatment of cancer is largely a specialist activity, but the role of the GP is important at this time, even if mainly supportive.
- Keep in touch with the family and up to date with treatment—provide support (e.g. advice on benefits/local services), preventive care (e.g. flu vaccination for patients and/or carers), and general medical care
- Liaise with the secondary care teams involved, and provide continuity if care is passed from one specialist team to another
- If the patient does not survive, provide ongoing support to the family

Surgery for cancer

Surgery has 3 main roles in cancer management:

Diagnosis and staging Advances in imaging and laparoscopic techniques have ↓ the number of patients requiring open surgery to confirm a cancer diagnosis. Surgical staging remains important in:

- Breast cancer—'sentinel' axillary node biopsy is needed to accurately predict the state of nodal disease
- Ovarian cancer—tumour deposits on the peritoneal surface are poorly visualized with conventional imaging. Direct visualization is required using laparotomy or laparoscopy
- Certain abdominal malignancies—laparoscopic assessment of extent and spread of tumour may be performed prior to resection

Curative surgery

Non-metastatic disease Surgery with curative intent is dependent on complete resection of the tumour with a margin of normal tissue. Local control of tumours with a propensity to spread to lymph nodes may be improved with resection of the draining group of nodes, e.g. vulval tumours. However, even if the tumour was completely resected, surgery can still fail to cure either as a result of:

- Development of metastatic disease as a result of the presence of micrometastatic deposits unidentifiable at the time of surgery
- Development of local relapse as a result of inadequate margins. Surgical margins can be limited by patient-related factors (e.g. only a partial lobectomy may be possible in patients with lung cancer because of poor underlying respiratory function) or by tumour-related margins (e.g. invasion of the tumour to a vital structure such as the aorta)

Metastatic disease Surgery may be curative in a limited number of tumours with metastases. However, this is much less common, requires careful patient selection, and is best performed by a specialist team. Circumstances in which curative surgery may be offered include:

- Isolated metastases from breast cancer with a long disease-free interval
- Liver metastases from colorectal cancer
- Pulmonary metastases from osteosarcoma or soft tissue sarcoma

Palliative surgery Surgery can be effective in achieving good symptom control in the palliative setting, but decision to proceed must be carefully considered particularly as patients may have limited life expectancy, poor performance status, and rapid tumour progression. Ideally such decisions should be multidisciplinary and involve surgeons specialized in oncology and experienced in palliative management (see Table 28.3).

Table 28.3 Situations in which palliative surgery should be considered

Situation	Comments
Cancers causing obstructive symptoms e.g. bowel, ovary, ureter, bronchus ❶ Most malignancy-associated bowel obstructions are functional, not anatomical	Surgery to relieve the obstruction may be warranted even if the underlying disease is incurable with locally advanced disease or distant metastases **Bowel obstruction** this occurs most commonly in patients with colonic or ovarian cancer **Oesophageal or bronchial obstruction** laser therapy of an intraluminal mass may restore the lumen **Obstructive hydronephrosis** nephrostomy or ureteric catheters may relieve the obstruction **Placement of a stent** may help relieve the symptoms of dysphagia, dyspnoea, jaundice, and large bowel obstruction
Fistulae	Fistulae, often arising as a result of pelvic tumours or as a side effect of radiotherapy, can be associated with distressing malodours and excessive discharge Surgery may provide excellent palliation but may not be useful in those with multiple sites of fistulae or rapidly advancing intra-abdominal disease where life expectancy is limited
Jaundice	*Radiological and/or endoscopic stent placement:* can relieve obstructive jaundice secondary to extrinsic pressure from lymph nodes on the biliary system or intrinsic pressure from cholangiocarcinoma or pancreatic carcinoma **Complications** infection or blockage necessitate replacement **Surgical relief** by choledochoenterostomy; avoids the problems associated with stents and may be indicated in a small minority with excellent performance status and slowly growing disease
Spinal cord compression and brain tumours	Urgent referral for neurological assessment for decompressive surgery or vertebroplasty is indicated for confirmed spinal disease or operable brain tumours
Gastrointestinal bleeding	A wide range of endoscopic techniques have been developed to stop bleeding from benign and malignant causes, including sclerotherapy with adrenaline, laser coagulation, and radiological embolization These techniques may avoid the need for major surgery in patients who have a limited life expectancy
Bone metastases	Prophylactic fixation of a long bone may reduce either pain and/or the risk of pathological fracture in patients with: • Lesions in weight-bearing bones • Destruction of >50% of the cortex • Pain on weight-bearing • Lytic lesions In all cases fixation should be followed by radiotherapy to control growth and promote healing
Pain	If the expected morbidity of the procedure is low, surgical debulking of large, slowly growing tumours can reduce pain. Neurosurgical approaches such as cordotomy are only rarely considered

Chemotherapy

Chemotherapy is the use of chemical agents in the cure or palliation of malignant disease.

Drug groups Include:
- Antibiotics, e.g. bleomycin
- Alkylating agents, e.g. busulfan
- Antimetabolites, e.g. methotrexate, 5-fluorouracil
- Alkaloids, e.g. vincristine
- Platinum derivatives—DNA intercalating agents, e.g. cisplatin
- Enzymes, e.g. asparaginase
- Hormones, e.g. sex hormones, corticosteroids
- Biological agents, e.g. interferon, monoclonal antibodies (e.g. rituximab)
- Others, e.g. hydroxycarbamide, retinoids

These agents work in a variety of ways to inhibit tumour growth and/or cause tumour cell damage. Normal cells may be damaged at the same time as tumour cells, resulting in the high levels of toxicity experienced by patients.

Choice of agent Depends on known activity of the agent, cost, and patient factors. It is a specialist decision.

Types of tumour Response to chemotherapy depends on type and grade of tumour being treated. Broadly tumours can be divided into:
- **Those likely to respond** Leukaemia, lymphoma (Hodgkin's and intermediate-/high-grade non-Hodgkin's), testicular tumours, small cell lung cancer, embryonal tumours, choriocarcinoma, ovarian cancer, sarcoma, breast cancer, prostate cancer
- **Those that may respond** Low-grade non-Hodgkin's lymphoma, GI cancer, brain/CNS tumours, melanoma, bladder and uterine cancer
- **Those unlikely to respond** Non-small cell lung, renal, pancreatic, head and neck, cervical, and liver cancer

Combination chemotherapy Often different chemotherapeutic agents are combined to ↑ their chances of effect. Agents acting in different ways may potentiate each others' actions, and using combinations reduces the risk of resistance (if one agent does not have any effect, another may). Choosing agents with different side effect profiles reduces cumulative toxic effects.

Intermittent chemotherapy Particularly useful for cytotoxic drugs. Intermittent treatment exploits the difference in recovery rates between normal and malignant tissues. Gaps between cycles of treatment allow normal tissue (particularly the immune system) to recover, but the malignant tissue does not recover to such a large extent (see Figure 28.1). The population of malignant cells diminishes relative to the normal cells with each cycle.

Adjuvant chemotherapy Given to prevent relapse after primary treatment of a non-metastatic tumour for which relapse rate is known to be high. An example is adjuvant chemotherapy for breast cancer.

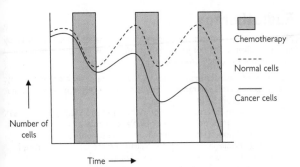

Figure 28.1 Action of cytotoxic chemotherapy on normal and cancer cell populations

Neutropenic sepsis Neutropenic sepsis is defined as fever of ≥38.0°C for ≥2h when the neutrophil count is <1.0 × 10⁹/L. *Causes:*
- Chemotherapy (most common cause)
- Radiotherapy—if large volumes of bone marrow are irradiated, e.g. pelvic radiotherapy
- Malignant infiltration of the bone marrow, e.g. prostate/breast cancer

Risks of neutropenia Bacterial and fungal infection. Risk of infection ↑ sharply as neutrophil counts fall to <1.0 × 10⁹/L, with greatest risk at counts <0.1 × 10⁹/L. Neutropenia for >5d is a further risk factor. Usually patients are most at risk in the nadir period from 1wk after therapy.

Presentation and primary care management Symptoms/signs may be minimal—have a high index of suspicion. Neutropenic, septic patients can deteriorate rapidly and become hypotensive or moribund within hours. Early referral for investigation and specialist management is critical.
- If a high-risk patient complains of chills, fever, rigors, sore throat, or generalized aches, check an urgent FBC
- Mouth ulcers and ↑ fatigue can be signs of neutropenia

⚠ Development of fever in a patient with neutropenia is a medical emergency caused by infection until proven otherwise.

Information for patients about side effects of chemotherapy
Chemocare ✍ www.chemocare.com
Cancer Research UK ☎ 0808 800 4040 ✍ www.cancerhelp.org.uk
Macmillan Cancer Support ☎ 0808 808 0000 ✍ www.macmillan.org.uk

Radiotherapy

Mechanism of action Ionizing radiation damages cells. Radiotherapy aims to deliver a dose of irradiation to an area which allows normal tissues, but not the cancer, to recover from the damage.

Delivery of radiotherapy May be used alone or with chemotherapy. Once maximum dose of radiotherapy has been received by any area, that area cannot usually be irradiated again

- **External beam** External source of ionizing radiation (e.g. gamma rays) is aimed at a target point in the body. Patients may be immobilized, e.g. with boards/moulds, to ensure delivery of treatment to the correct place. Can be single dose (e.g. for palliative reasons) or fractionated into several doses spread over weeks. Fractionation ↑ effect
- **Brachytherapy** Delivery of radiation by placing a radioactive source within or close to the malignancy, e.g. caesium-137 in the uterus

Side effects Skin reactions—see Table 28.4; non-skin reactions—see Table 28.5.

Table 28.4 Managing post-radiotherapy skin reactions

RTOG score*	Description	Skin appearance	Treatment
0	Normal	Normal	Aqueous cream bd to delay onset of reaction
1	Faint erythema	Skin slightly pink or red	Aqueous cream tds or prn
2A	Tender or bright erythema (dry desquamation)	Skin red, dry and scaly— some itch and tingling	Frequent aqueous cream (qds or prn) Diprobase® cream or soft white paraffin (avoid excess build-up) Hydrocortisone cream may be used sparingly on itchy areas. Review use after 7d—discontinue if the skin breaks
2B	Patchy moist desquamation, oedema	Skin inflamed with patches of epidermis broken down and moist	Apply hydrogel dressings to moist areas with appropriate 2° dressing, eg surgipad or foam dressing Apply aqueous cream to other parts of the field
3	Confluent moist desquamation	Epidermis blisters and sloughs; underlying dermis is exposed and sore. Oozing of serous fluid	Apply hydrogel or foam dressing suitable for the amount of exudate Review frequently Swab and treat with oral antibiotics (e.g. flucloxacillin 500mg qds) if any signs of infection
Post-radio-therapy			Reaction may continue for several weeks post-treatment. Continue with use of aqueous creams until skin returns to normal If RTOG 2B/3 apply principles of moist wound healing as in 2B and 3 above or (if patient is not allergic to silicone) a silicone dressing If infection is suspected apply silver-impregnated dressings or silver sulfadiazine cream (Flamazine®)

*RTOG stands for Radiotherapy and Oncology Group.

Treatment may be

- **Curative,** e.g. childhood tumours, lymphoma, seminoma, head/neck tumours, bladder cancer, squamous/basal cell skin cancer
- **Adjuvant** Pre-operatively to ↓ size/extent of otherwise inoperable tumours or post-operatively to treat microscopic foci remaining after tumour removal (e.g. in treatment of breast cancer)
- **Palliative** For control of distressing symptoms. Only symptomatic sites of disease are targeted, e.g. bone metastases, haemorrhage; obstruction of a viscus; neurological complications; fungating tumours

Table 28.5 Non-skin side effects of radiotherapy

Side effect	Description/action
Sore mouth/ throat	Associated with radiotherapy to the head/neck. Advise patients to visit the dentist prior to treatment; avoid smoking, alcohol, and spicy foods; rest voice when radiotherapy reaction becomes established
	Consider treatment with: normal saline/bicarbonate mouthwashes; antiseptic mouthwashes (e.g. chlorhexidine—though alcohol may sting); soluble aspirin (can be gargled) or paracetamol; benzydamine mouthwash; topical local anaesthetics; topical steroids; coating agents (e.g. sucralfate). If insufficient fluid/food intake, consider nutritional support via NG tube and/or referral for gastrostomy (if weight loss >10%)
Dysphagia	May result from thoracic radiotherapy. Avoid smoking, spirits, and spicy food. Consider treatment with: antacid; sucralfate; soluble paracetamol or aspirin; NSAID po/PR
Nausea and vomiting	Radiotherapy to the abdomen often causes nausea as a result of serotonin release. Consider prophylactic antiemetic therapy with a serotonin inhibitor, e.g. ondansetron
Diarrhoea	Frequently accompanies abdominal/pelvic radiotherapy *Management:* dietary modification (e.g. ↓ dietary fibre) may help. Supply with loperamide—4mg initial dose then 2mg every 2h until symptoms settle (4mg every 4h at night). *Proctitis:* may accompany rectal/prostatic irradiation. Treat with rectal steroids
Pneumonitis	Acute pneumonitis can develop 1–3mo after treatment and is associated with a fever, dry cough, and breathlessness. *Differential diagnosis:* pneumonia. CXR—shows lung infiltration confined within the treatment volume
	Management: steroids—start with 40mg od prednisolone and reduce over a period of weeks as improvement occurs ❶ Pulmonary fibrosis may occur >12mo after treatment
Cerebral oedema	Can occur after cranial irradiation. Steroid dose is ↓ after completion of radiotherapy. Consider ↑ dose again
Memory loss	Depending on the parts of the cranium irradiated, both long- and short-term memory problems can occur after cranial irradiation. Treatment is supportive; some recovery may occur
Somnolence syndrome	Occurs within a few weeks of brain irradiation. *Presents with:* nausea/ vomiting; anorexia; dysarthria; ataxia; profound lethargy
	Treatment is supportive. Recovery may occur spontaneously

Palliative care in general practice

'Any man's death diminishes me because I am involved in mankind'
Devotions Meditation 17, John Donne (1572–1631)

⚠ Death is the natural end to life—not a failure of medicine.

Palliative care starts when the emphasis changes from curing disease and prolonging life to relieving symptoms and maintaining well-being or 'quality of life'. On average, GPs have 1–2 patients with terminal disease at any time and can get more personally involved with them than other patients.

End-of-life care (EOLC) 75% of deaths are 'predictable' and follow a period of chronic illness where end-of-life care (for those likely to die in <12mo) would be appropriate.

Problems arising are a complex mix of physical, psychological, social, cultural, and spiritual factors involving both patients and carers. To respond adequately good lines of communication and close multidisciplinary teamwork is needed. Local palliative care teams are invaluable sources of advice and support and frequently produce booklets with advice on aspects of palliative care for GPs.

Symptom control must be tailored to the needs of the individual. A few basic rules apply:
- Carefully diagnose the cause of the symptom
- Explain the symptom to the patient
- Discuss treatment options
- Set realistic goals
- Anticipate likely problems
- Review regularly

Identification It may be difficult to identify when patients are nearing end of life, particularly for non-cancer illness (see Figure 28.2). This can lead to access to EOLC not being offered at all or being offered late.

Advanced care planning The 2008 National End-of-life Care Strategy recommends assessment of people identified as approaching the end of life and agreement with them about how to meet their preferences using advanced care planning with regular review. This may include:
- Symptom control
- Discussion about preferences for care including 'do not attempt to resuscitate' directives (📖 p. 1052)
- Advance directives to withhold treatment (📖 p. 123)
- Discussion about preferred place of death—60–67% of people would prefer to die at home; currently 53% die in hospital but 40% have no medical necessity to die there

Communication about EOLC People are more likely to talk about end of life with their GP than any other professional, but only 33% of GPs are confident to initiate a discussion with a patient about end-of-life issues. Specific training ↑ confidence.

Preferred priorities for care (PPC) The PPC document is a tool for discussion and recording of EOLC wishes. It is available to download from the NHS EOLC website.

The Gold Standards Framework Aims to improve quality of palliative care provided by the primary care team by improving the practice-based organization of care of dying patients. The Framework focusses on: optimizing continuity of care, teamwork, advanced planning (including out-of-hours), symptom control, and patient, carer, and staff support. Evaluation data show the framework ↑ the proportion of patients dying in their preferred place and improves quality of care as perceived by the practitioners involved.

Liverpool Care Pathway Is a model of 'best practice' to improve care of the dying in the last hours/days of life. It covers physical, psychological, social, and spiritual aspects of care and widely used in the community, both in care homes and in private residences. Over recent years the Liverpool Care Pathway has gained a controversial reputation as a 'pathway to death' but, if used correctly, with full consultation with all medical staff and family members/carers involved, it still has a very important place in managing the final days/hours of a patient's life.

Further information

NHS National End-of-Life Care Programme
℠ www.endoflifecareforadults.nhs.uk
Dying Mattters ℠ www.dyingmatters.org
NHS End-of-Life Care Programme Preferred Priorities for Care ℠ www. endoflifecareforadults.nhs.uk/tools/core-tools/preferredprioritiesforcare
Gold Standards Framework ℠ www.goldstandardsframework.org.uk
Liverpool Care Pathway ℠ www.mcpcil.org.uk/liverpool-care-pathway
Help the Hospices Directory of hospice and palliative care services in the UK ℠ www.helpthehospices.org.uk/hospiceinformation

Patient advice and support
Macmillan Cancer Support ☏ 0808 808 0000 ℠ www.macmillan.org.uk

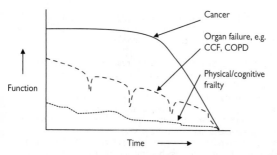

Figure 28.2 Trajectories of decline at the end of life

Pain and general debility

Pain control Pain control is the cornerstone of palliative care. Cancer pain is multifactorial—be aware of physical and psychological factors.

Principles of pain control 📖 p. 212

Pain-relieving drugs 📖 p. 214

Management of specific types of pain Table 28.6

Weakness, fatigue, and drowsiness Almost a universal symptom.

Reversible causes
- Drugs—opioids, benzodiazepines, steroids (proximal muscle weakness), diuretics (dehydration and biochemical abnormalities), antihypertensives (postural hypotension)
- Emotional problems—depression, anxiety, fear, apathy
- Biochemical abnormalities—hypercalcaemia, DM, electrolyte disturbance, uraemia, liver disease, thyroid dysfunction
- Anaemia   • Infection
- Poor nutrition   • Prolonged bed rest
- Raised intracranial pressure (drowsiness only)

Management Treat reversible causes. Provide advice on modification of lifestyle. If drowsiness/fatigue persist consider a trial of dexamethasone 4mg/d or antidepressant. Although steroids make muscle wasting worse, in the short term they may improve general fatigue and well-being. Provide psychological support to patients and carers. Consider referral to physiotherapy; review aids and appliances; review home layout (possibly with referral to OT); and/or review home care arrangements.

Hypercalcaemia Occurs with 10% malignant tumours—particularly myeloma (>30%) and breast cancer (40%).

Presentation and differential diagnosis 📖 p. 366

⚠ Always suspect hypercalcaemia if someone is iller than expected for no obvious reason. Untreated hypercalcaemia can be fatal.

Management Depending on the general state of the patient, make a decision whether to treat the hypercalcaemia or not. If a decision is made *not* to treat, provide symptom control and do not check the serum calcium again. If you decide to treat:
- **Asymptomatic patient with corrected calcium <3mmol/L** Monitor
- **Symptomatic and/or corrected calcium >3mmol/L** Arrange treatment with IV fluids and bisphosphonates via oncologist/ palliative care team immediately. Check serum calcium 7–10d post-treatment. 20% do not respond, and there is no benefit from re-treating with the same bisphosphonate. Zoledronic acid, although more expensive than pamidronate, works for ~2x as long (6wk). Consider maintenance with regular IV bisphosphonate. Many initially responsive to bisphosphonates become unresponsive with time; monthly sc denosumab is an option for those with persistent/relapsed hypercalcaemia of malignancy

Table 28.6 Management of specific types of pain

Type of pain	Management
Bone pain	• Try NSAIDs and/or strong opioids • Consider referral for palliative radiotherapy, strontium treatment (prostate cancer), or IV bisphosphonates (↓ pain in myeloma, breast and prostate cancer) • Refer to orthopaedics if any lytic metastases at risk of fracture for consideration of pinning
Abdominal pain	• **Constipation** is the most common cause; 🕮 p. 1035 • **Colic** try loperamide 2–4mg qds or hyoscine hydrobromide 300 micrograms tds s/ling. Hyoscine butylbromide (Buscopan®) 20–60mg/24h can also be given via syringe driver • **Liver capsule pain** dexamethasone 4–8mg/d. Titrate dose to the minimum that controls pain. Alternatively try NSAID + PPI cover • **Gastric distension** may be helped by an antacid ± an anti-foaming agent (e.g. Asilone®). Alternatively a prokinetic may help, e.g. metoclopramide or domperidone 10mg tds before meals • **Upper GI tumour** often neuropathic element of pain; coeliac plexus block may help; refer to the palliative care team • **Consider drug causes** NSAIDs are a common iatrogenic cause • **Acute/subacute obstruction** 🕮 p. 1033
Neuropathic pain (pain associated with altered sensation)	• Often burning/shooting pain; usually only partially responsive to opioids—titrate to the maximum tolerated dose of opioid • If inadequate add a neuropathic agent, e.g. amitriptyline 10–25mg nocte, increasing as needed every 2wk to 75–150mg. Alternatives include gabapentin, pregabalin, duloxetine, and clonazepam • If pain is due to nerve compression resulting from tumour, dexamethasone 4–8mg od may help • *Other options:* TENS; nerve block; topical lidocaine patches; specialist treatment options, e.g. ketamine (seek expert advice)
Rectal pain	• Topical drugs, e.g. rectal steroids • Tricyclic antidepressants, e.g. amitriptyline 10–100mg nocte • Anal spasms—glyceryl trinitrate ointment 0.1–0.2% bd • Referral for local radiotherapy
Muscle pain	• Paracetamol and/or NSAIDs • Muscle relaxants, e.g. diazepam 5–10mg od, baclofen 5–10mg tds dantrolene 25mg od, increasing at weekly intervals to 75mg tds • Physiotherapy, aromatherapy, relaxation, heat pads
Bladder pain/ spasm	• Treat reversible causes. ↑ fluids. Toilet regularly • Try oxybutynin 5mg tds, tolterodine 2mg bd, propiverine 15mg od/ bd/tds, or trospium 20mg bd • Amitriptyline 10–75mg nocte is often effective • If catheterized—try instilling 20mL of intravesical bupivacaine 0.25% for 15min tds or oxybutynin 5mL in 30mL od/bd/tds • NSAIDs can also be useful • Steroids, e.g. dexamethasone 4–8mg od may ↓ tumour related bladder inflammation • In the terminal situation hyoscine butylbromide 60–120mg/24h or glycopyrronium 0.4–0.8mg/24h sc can be helpful
Pain of short duration	For example, dressing changes—try a short-acting opioid e.g. fentanyl citrate 200 micrograms lozenge sucked for 15min prior to the procedure or a breakthrough dose of oral morphine 20min prior to the procedure

Anorexia, nausea, and vomiting

Anorexia Treat nausea, mouth problems, pain, and other symptoms.
↓ psychological distress and treat depression. Advise small, appetizing
meals frequently in comfortable surroundings.

Drugs that may be helpful
- Alcohol pre-meals
- Metoclopramide or domperidone 10mg tds pre-meals—to prevent
  feeling of satiety caused by gastric stasis
- Dexamethasone 2–4mg od or prednisolone 15–30mg od for
  short-term appetite enhancement

General principles of management of nausea and vomiting
- **Assess** Try to identify likely cause—see Table 28.7
- **Review medication** Could medication be the cause? Which
  anti-emetics have been used before and how effective were they?
- **Try non-drug measures**
- **Choose an antiemetic** If cause can be identified, choose an antiemetic
  appropriate for the cause (see Table 28.7). Use the antiemetic ladder
  (see Figure 28.3). Administer antiemetics regularly rather than prn and
  choose an appropriate route of administration
- **Review frequently**—Is the antiemetic effective? Has the underlying
  cause of the nausea/vomiting resolved? Avoid changing antiemetic
  before it has been given an adequate trial at maximum dose

❶ If there is >1 cause for nausea/vomiting, you may need >1 drug.

Route of administration
- For prophylaxis of nausea and vomiting—use po medication
- For established nausea or vomiting—consider a parenteral route e.g. syringe
  driver (📖 p. 1046)—persistent nausea may ↓ gastric emptying and drug
  absorption. Once symptoms are controlled consider reverting to a po route

Non-drug measures Do not forget non-drug measures to ↓ nausea:
- Avoidance of food smells and unpleasant odours
- Relaxation/diversion/anxiety management
- Acupressure/acupuncture

Figure 28.3 The antiemetic ladder

Table 28.7 Causes of vomiting and choice of antiemetic

Mechanism of vomiting	Antiemetic
Drug/toxin-induced or metabolic, e.g. hypercalcaemia	Haloperidol (1.5–5mg nocte)
	Levomepromazine (5mg stat or 6.25mg nocte)
	If persistent nausea due to opioids, consider changing opioid
Chemotherapy/radiotherapy	Granisetron (1mg bd) or ondansetron (8mg bd po or 16mg od PR)—chemotherapy- or radiotherapy-induced vomiting
	Haloperidol 1.5–5mg nocte—radiotherapy-induced vomiting
	Dexamethasone 4–8mg daily po/sc—often given as part of a chemotherapy regime
	Metoclopramide 20mg tds
↑ intracranial pressure	Dexamethasone 4–16mg/d
	Cyclizine 50mg bd/tds (or 150mg/d via syringe driver)
Anxiety, fear, or pain	Benzodiazepines, e.g. diazepam 2–10mg/d or midazolam sc
	Cyclizine 50mg bd/tds
	Levomepromazine 6–25mg/d
Motion/position	Cyclizine 50mg tds po/sc/IM
	Hyoscine po (300 micrograms tds) or transdermally (1mg/72h)
	Prochlorperazine po (5mg qds) or buccal (3–6mg bd)
Gastric stasis*	Domperidone 10mg tds or metoclopramide 10mg tds (particularly if multifactorial with gastric stasis and a central component)
Gastric irritation	Stop the irritant if possible, e.g. stop NSAIDs
	Proton pump inhibitors, e.g. lansoprazole 30mg od or omeprazole 20mg od
	Antacids
	Misoprostol 200 micrograms bd—if caused by NSAIDs
Constipation	Laxatives/suppositories/enemas
Intestinal obstruction	Refer for surgery if appropriate
	Cyclizine, haloperidol, or levomepromazine
	Dexamethasone 4–8 mg/d—antiemetic and ↓ obstruction
	If vomiting cannot be controlled consider referral for venting gastrostomy or antisecretory agents (e.g. octreotide)
Cough-induced	📖 p. 1038
Unknown cause	Cyclizine 50mg tds or 150mg/d via syringe driver
	Levomepromazine 6–25mg/d
	Dexamethasone 4–8mg daily po/sc
	Metoclopramide 10–20 mg tds/qds po

* Vomits of undigested food without nausea soon after eating.

❗ Drugs with antimuscarinic effects (e.g. cyclizine) antagonize prokinetic drugs (e.g. metoclopramide)—if possible, do not use concurrently.

Other GI problems

Mouth problems Review medication making the mouth sore or dry. Refer to the DN for advice on mouth care (e.g. use a toothbrush to keep the tongue clean). Consider mouthwashes, e.g. saline, Oraldene®, chlorhexidine, benzydamine (for pain). Try ¼–½ ascorbic acid 1g effervescent tablet/d— place on tongue and allow to dissolve.

Specific measures
- Oral thrush—treat with fluconazole 50mg od for 7d and soak dentures in sodium hypochlorite fluid for ≥12h to prevent reinfection
- Painful mouth—benzydamine mouthwash ± lidocaine spray
- Ulcers or painful areas—hydrocortisone pellets topically qds after eating and nocte
- Oral cancer pain—topical NSAIDs, e.g. soluble aspirin or diclofenac
- Chemotherapy-induced ulcers— sucralfate suspension
- Dry mouth—review medication that might be causing dry mouth, e.g. antidepressants, opioids. Try salivary stimulants, e.g. iced water, pineapple chunks, chewing gum, boiled sweets, or mints. Consider saliva substitutes, e.g. Glandosane® spray
- Radiotherapy-induced dryness—pilocarpine
- Excessive salivation—amitriptyline 10–100mg nocte, hyoscine, or glycopyrronium via syringe driver

Dysphagia May be due to physical obstruction (by tumour bulk) or functional obstruction (neurological deficit).
- Treat the cause if possible, e.g. celestin tube for oesophageal tumour
- If the patient is hungry and wishes to be fed consider referral for a percutaneous endoscopic gastrostomy (PEG)
- If the patient does not wish to have a PEG ask whether he/she would like subcutaneous fluids and treat symptomatically with mouth care, anxiolytics, analgesia, and sedation

Hiccup A distressing symptom. Treatment is often unsatisfactory.
- **General measures** Rebreathing with a paper bag; pharyngeal stimulation by drinking cold water or taking a teaspoon of granulated sugar
- **Peripheral hiccups** Irritation of the phrenic nerve or diaphragm—try metoclopramide (10mg tds), antacids containing simeticone (e.g. Asilone®), dexamethasone (4–12mg/d), or ranitidine (150mg bd)
- **Central hiccups** Due to medullary stimulation, e.g. ↑ ICP, uraemia—try chlorpromazine (10–25mg tds/qds), dexamethasone (4–12mg/d), nifedipine (10mg tds), or baclofen (5mg bd)

Ascites Free fluid in the peritoneal cavity. Common with ovarian cancer (50% patients). Presents with abdominal distension. *Signs:* shifting dullness to percussion ± fluid thrill. Depending on clinical state consider referring for radio- or chemotherapy if appropriate.

Symptom control
- Give analgesia for discomfort
- Refer for paracentesis and/or peritoneovenous shunt
- Try diuretics—furosemide 20–40mg od and/or spironolactone 100–400mg od. May take a week to produce maximal effect.
  - ❶ Monitor albumin level—if low, diuretics make ascites worse

- Dexamethasone 2–4mg daily may help—discontinue if not effective
- 'Squashed stomach syndrome'—try prokinetics, e.g. domperidone or metoclopramide 10mg tds

Constipation Passage of hard stools less frequently than the patient's own normal pattern. It is a very common symptom. Occult presentations are common in the very elderly and frail and include:

- Confusion
- Abdominal pain
- Loss of appetite
- Urinary retention
- Overflow diarrhoea
- Nausea/vomiting

⚠ Constipation can herald spinal cord compression (🔲 p. 478). If suspected, do a full neurological examination.

Management Pre-empt constipation by putting everyone at risk (e.g. patients on opioids) on regular aperients. Treat reversible causes, e.g. give analgesia if pain on defecation, alter diet (e.g. add prunes), ↑ fluid intake.

- Treat with regular stool softener (e.g. lactulose, macrogol) ± regular bowel stimulant (e.g. senna) or a combination drug (e.g. co-danthrusate). Titrate dose against response
- If that is ineffective consider adding rectal measures. If soft stools and lax rectum—try bisacodyl suppositories (❗ must come into direct contact with rectum); if hard stools—try glycerin suppositories; insert into the faeces, and allow to dissolve
- If still not cleared refer to the district nurse for lubricant ± stimulant enema (usually acts in ~20min). Once cleared leave on a regular aperient, with instructions to ↑ aperients if constipation recurs

Gut fistulae Connections from the gut to other organs—commonly skin, bladder, or vagina. Bowel fistulae are characterized by air passing through the fistula channel. If well enough for surgery, refer to a surgeon. If not fit for surgery consider referring to palliative care for octreotide.

Diarrhoea Clarify what the patient/carer means by diarrhoea. Less common than constipation but can be distressing for the patient and difficult for the carer—especially if incontinence results.

Management
- ↑ fluid intake—small amounts of clear fluids frequently
- Screen for infection (including pseudomembranous colitis if diarrhoea after a course of antibiotics) and treat if necessary
- Ensure no overflow diarrhoea 2° to constipation; no excessive/erratic laxative use; and no other medication is causing diarrhoea
- Consider giving aspirin (300–600mg tds)—↓ intestinal electrolyte and water secretion caused by prostaglandins. May particularly help with radiation induced diarrhoea
- Consider ondansetron 4mg tds for radiotherapy-induced diarrhoea
- Consider giving pancreatic enzyme supplements, e.g. Creon® 25,000 tds prior to meals if fat malabsorption (e.g. 2° to pancreatic carcinoma)
- Otherwise treat symptomatically with codeine phosphate 30–60mg qds or loperamide 2mg tds/qds
- Refer to palliative care if unable to control symptoms

Skin, neurological, and orthopaedic problems

Bed sores Due to pressure necrosis of the skin. Immobile patients are at high risk—especially if frail ± incontinent. Likely sites of pressure damage—shoulder blades, elbows, spine, buttocks, knees, ankles, and heels. Bed sores heal slowly in terminally ill patients and are a source of discomfort and stress for both patients and carers (who often feel guilty that a pressure sore is a mark of poor care).

• If at risk refer to the DN or palliative care nursing team for advice on prevention of bed sores—protective mattresses and cushions, incontinence advice, advice on positioning and movement
• Warn carers to make contact with the DN or palliative care nursing team if a red patch does not improve 24h after relieving the pressure on the area
• Treat any sores that develop aggressively and admit if not resolving

Wound care Large wounds can have major impact on quality of life. Patients with advanced disease have major risk factors for development and poor healing of wounds—immobility, poor nutrition, skin infiltration ± breakdown due to malignancy. Skin infiltration causing ulceration or fungating wounds can be particularly distressing.

Management The primary aim is comfort. Healing is a secondary aim and may be impossible. Always involve the DN and/or specialist palliative care nursing team early. Many hospitals also have wound care specialist nurses who are valuable sources of advice.

Specific management problems See Table 28.8.

Raised intracranial pressure Occurs with 1° or 2° brain tumours. Characterized by
• Headache—worse on lying
• Vomiting
• Confusion
• Diplopia
• Convulsions
• Papilloedema

Management
• Unless a terminal event, refer urgently to neurosurgery for assessment. Options include insertion of a shunt or cranial radiotherapy
• If no further active treatment is appropriate start symptomatic treatment—raise the head of the bed, start dexamethasone 16mg/d (stop if no response in 1wk), analgesia

Spinal cord compression 📖 p. 478

Bone fractures Common in advanced cancer due to osteoporosis, trauma as a result of falls, or metastases. Have a low index of suspicion if a new bony pain develops. Treat with analgesia. Unless in a very terminal state, confirm the fracture on X-ray and refer to orthopaedics or radiotherapy urgently for consideration of fixation (long bones, wrist, neck of femur) and/or radiotherapy (rib fractures, vertebral fractures).

 In the elderly, fracture of a long bone can present as acute confusion.

Table 28.8 Common wound management problems

Problem	Management
Pain	Exclude infection; ensure the dressing is comfortable; limit frequency of dressing changes
	Ensure adequate background analgesia; consider additional analgesia for dressing changes and/or topical opioids on the dressing
Excessive exudate	Use high absorbency dressings with further packing on top ± plastic pads to protect clothing
	Change the top layer of the dressing as often as needed but avoid frequent changes of the dressing placed directly on the wound
	Protect the surrounding skin with a barrier cream/spray
Necrotic tissue	Use desloughing agents
	Referral for surgical debridement may be necessary
Bleeding	Prevent bleeding during dressing changes by:
	• Avoiding frequent dressing changes
	• Using non-adherent dressings or dressings which liquefy and can be washed off (e.g. Sorbsan®) *and*
	• Irrigating the wound with saline to remove dressings
	If there is surface bleeding—put pressure on the wound; if pressure is not working try:
	• Kaltostat®
	• Adrenaline—1mg/mL (or 1:1,000) on a gauze pad, or
	• Sucralfate liquid—place on a non-adherent dressing and apply firmly to the bleeding area
	Consider referral for radiotherapy or palliative surgery (e.g. cautery)
Odour	Treat with systemic and/or topical metronidazole
	Charcoal dressings can be helpful
	Seal the wound, e.g. with additional layer of cling film dressing
	Try disguising the smell with deodorizers (e.g. Nilodor®) used sparingly on top of the dressing—short-term measure. Long-term, the deodorant smell often becomes associated with the smell of the wound for the patient
Infection	Usually chronic and localized
	Irrigate the wound with warm saline or under running water in the shower/bath
	If the surrounding skin is inflamed—swab the wound and send for M,C&S then start oral antibiotics, e.g. flucloxacillin 250–500mg qds or erythromycin 250–500mg qds. Alter antibiotics depending on sensitivities of the organisms grown

Respiratory problems

Cough Troublesome symptom. Prolonged bouts of coughing are exhausting and frightening—especially if associated with breathlessness and/or haemoptysis.

Haemoptysis 🔲 p. 297

Breathlessness Affects 70% of terminally ill patients. It is usually multifactorial. Breathlessness always has a psychological element—being short of breath is frightening. Causes—see Figure 28.4.

Management of cough and breathlessness

General non-drug measures

- Generally reassure. Explain reasons for breathlessness/cough and adaptations to lifestyle that might help, e.g. sitting up straight
- Breathing exercises can help—refer to physiotherapy
- Exclude treatable causes (see Box 28.1 and Figure 28.4)
- Steam inhalations/nebulized saline can help with tenacious secretions
- Try a stream of air over the face if the patient is breathless, e.g. fan, open window

General drug measures

- Try simple linctus 5–10mL prn for cough
- Oral or subcutaneous opioids to ↓ the subjective sensation of breathlessness—start with 2.5mg morphine sulfate solution 4-hourly and titrate upwards. Opioids may also help with cough—try pholcodine 10mL tds or morphine sulfate solution as for breathlessness. If already on opioids, ↑ dose by 25%. Titrate dose until symptoms are controlled or side effects
- Try benzodiazepines—2–5mg diazepam od/bd for associated anxiety + lorazepam 1–2mg s/ling prn in between. Diazepam acts as a central cough suppressant—try 2–10mg tds for cough
- Oxygen has a variable effect and is worth a try, although a hand-held battery fan or electric fan may be just as effective
- Hyoscine 400–600 micrograms 4–8-hourly (or 0.6–2.4mg/24h via syringe driver) and/or ipratropium inhalers/nebulized ipratropium ↓ secretions

Specific measures

- **Chest infection** Treat with nebulized saline to make secretions less viscous ± antibiotics (if not considered a terminal event)
- **Post-nasal drip** Steam inhalations, steroid nasal spray or drops ± antibiotics
- **Laryngeal irritation** Try inhaled steroids, e.g. Clenil® 100 micrograms/ actuation 2 puffs bd
- **Bronchospasm** Try bronchodilators ± inhaled or oral steroids. ❶ Salbutamol may help cough even in the absence of wheeze
- **Gastric reflux** Try antacids containing simeticone (e.g. Asilone®)
- **Lung cancer** Try inhaled sodium cromoglicate 10mg qds; local anaesthesia using nebulized bupivacaine or lidocaine can be helpful— refer for specialist advice (avoid eating/drinking for 1h afterwards to avoid aspiration). Palliative radiotherapy or chemotherapy can also relieve cough in patients with lung cancer—refer

Stridor Coarse wheezing sound that results from the obstruction of a major airway, e.g. larynx.

Management

- Corticosteroids (e.g. dexamethasone 16mg/d) can give relief
- Consider referral for radiotherapy or endoscopic insertion of a stent if appropriate
- If a terminal event—sedate with high doses of midazolam (10–40mg repeated prn)

Box 28.1 Reversible causes of cough

- Infection
- Malignant bronchial obstruction/lung metastases
- Bronchospasm
- Gastro-oesophageal reflux
- Aspiration
- Drug-induced, e.g. ACE inhibitors
- Treatment-related, e.g. total body irradiation
- Heart failure
- Secretions
- Pharyngeal candidiasis

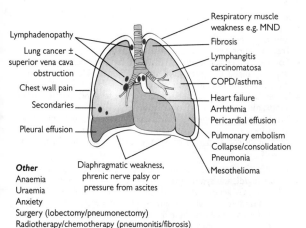

Other
Anaemia
Uraemia
Anxiety
Surgery (lobectomy/pneumonectomy)
Radiotherapy/chemotherapy (pneumonitis/fibrosis)

Figure 28.4 Causes of breathlessness

Reproduced from: Lynch J, Simon C (2007) *Respiratory Problems*, with permission from Oxford University Press.

Haematological and vascular problems

Bleeding/haemorrhage In all patients likely to bleed (e.g. in end-stage leukaemia) pre-warn carers and give them a strategy.

Severe, life-threatening bleed Make a decision whether the cause of the bleed is treatable or a terminal event. This is best done in advance but bleeding cannot always be predicted.
• **Severe bleed—active treatment**—🕮 p. 1075
• **Severe bleed—no active treatment:**
  • Stay with the patient
  • Give sedative medication, e.g. midazolam 20–40mg sc/IV or lorazepam 1–2mg s/ling. If in pain, consider sc opioid
  • Support carers, as big bleeds are extremely distressing

Non-life-threatening bleed: first aid measures
• In all cases: reassure; monitor frequently
• Surface bleeding—pressure on wound; if pressure is not working, try Kaltostat® or adrenaline (1mg/mL or 1:1,000) on a gauze pad
• Nosebleeds—nasal packing or cautery

Non-life-threatening bleed: follow-up treatment Follow-up is directed at cause if appropriate:
• Anticoagulants—check INR
• Treat infection that might exacerbate a bleed
• Consider ↓ bleeding tendency with tranexamic acid 500mg qds
• Upper GI bleeding—stop NSAIDs, start PPI in double standard dose and consider referral for gastroscopy
• Lower GI bleeding—consider rectal steroids to ↓ inflammation or oral tranexamic acid ± referral for colonoscopy
• Radiotherapy—consider referral if haemoptysis, cutaneous bleeding, or haematuria
• Referral for chemotherapy or palliative surgery, e.g. cautery, are also options

Anaemia Do not check for anaemia if no intention to transfuse.
• **If Hb <10g/dL and symptomatic** Treat any reversible cause (e.g. iron deficiency, GI bleeding 2° to NSAIDs). Consider transfusion
• **If transfused** Record whether any benefit is derived (as if not, further transfusions are futile) and the duration of benefit (if <3wk—repeat transfusions are impractical). Monitor for return of symptoms; repeat FBC and arrange repeat transfusion as needed

Superior vena cava (SVC) obstruction Due to infiltration of the vessel wall, clot within the superior vena cava or extrinsic pressure. 75% are due to 1° lung cancer (3% of patients with lung cancer have SVC obstruction). Lymphoma and clotting associated with long central lines are the other major causes.

Presentation
• Shortness of breath/stridor
• Headache worse on stooping ± visual disturbances ± dizziness and collapse

- Swelling of the face—particularly around the eyes, neck, hands and arms, and/or injected cornea
- *Examination:* look for non-pulsatile distension of neck veins and dilated collateral veins (seen as small dilated veins over the anterior chest wall below the clavicles) in which blood courses downwards

Management

- Treat breathlessness (opioids—5mg morphine sulfate solution 4-hourly ± benzodiazepine, depending on the level of anxiety)
- Start corticosteroid (dexamethasone 16mg/d)
- Refer urgently for oncology opinion. Palliative radiotherapy has a response rate of 70%. Stenting ± thrombolysis is also an option

Lymphoedema Due to obstruction of lymphatic drainage, resulting in oedema with high protein content. Affects ≥1 limbs ± adjacent trunk. If left untreated, lymphoedema becomes increasingly resistant to treatment due to chronic inflammation and subcutaneous fibrosis. Cellulitis causes rapid ↑ in swelling. *Causes:*

- Axillary, groin, or intrapelvic tumour
- Axillary or groin surgery (including biopsy)
- Post-operative infection/radiotherapy

Presentation

- Swollen limb ± pitting
- Impaired limb mobility and function
- Discomfort/pain related to tissue swelling and/or shoulder strain
- Neuralgia pain—especially when axillary nodes are involved
- Psychological distress

Management See Table 28.9

Table 28.9 Management of lymphoedema

Avoid injury to limb	In at-risk patients (e.g. patients who have had breast cancer with axillary clearance) or those with lymphoedema, injury to the limb may precipitate or worsen lymphoedema. Do not take blood from the limb or use it for IV access or vaccination
Skin hygiene	Skin care with moisturizers e.g. Diprobase®, Emulsiderm®
	Topical treatment of fungal infection
	Systemic treatment of bacterial infection
External support	Intensive—with compression bandages
	Maintenance—with lymphoedema sleeve (contact breast care specialist nurse for more information on obtaining sleeves)
Exercise	Gentle daily exercise of affected limb gradually increasing range of movement
	❶ Must wear a sleeve/bandages when doing exercises
Massage	Very gentle fingertip massage in the line of drainage of lymphatics
Diuretics	If the condition has developed or deteriorated since prescription of corticosteroid or NSAID or if there venous component, consider a trial of diuretics
	Otherwise diuretics are of no benefit

Problems with mental well-being

Anxiety All patients with terminal disease are anxious at times for a variety of reasons, including fear of uncontrolled symptoms and of being left alone to die. When anxiety starts interfering with quality of life, intervention is justified.

Management: non-drug measures Often all that is needed:
- Acknowledgement of the patient's anxiety
- Full explanation of questions + written information as needed
- Support—self-help groups, day care, patient groups, specialist home nurses (e.g. Macmillan nurses)
- Relaxation training and training in breathing control
- Physical therapies, e.g. aromatherapy, art therapy, exercise

Management: drug measures
- **Acute anxiety** Try lorazepam 1–2mg s/ling prn or diazepam 2–10mg prn
- **Chronic anxiety** Try an antidepressant, e.g. fluoxetine 20mg od. Alternatives include regular diazepam e.g. 5–10mg od/bd, haloperidol 1–3mg bd/tds, or β-blockers, e.g. propranolol 40mg od–tds—watch for postural hypotension

If anxiety is not responding to simple measures, seek specialist help from either the psychiatric or palliative care team.

Depression A terminal diagnosis commonly makes patients sad. 10–20% of terminally ill patients develop clinical depression but in practice it is often difficult to decide whether a patient is depressed or just appropriately sad about his/her diagnosis and its implications. Many symptoms of terminal disease (e.g. poor appetite) are also symptoms of depression so screening questionnaires for depression are often unhelpful. If in doubt, a trial of antidepressants can help.

Assessment of suicide risk Ask about suicidal ideas and plans in a sensitive but probing way. It is a common misconception that asking about suicide can plant the idea into a patient's head and make suicide more likely. Evidence is to the contrary.

Management: non-drug measures
- Support, e.g. day and/or respite care; carers group; specialist nurse support (e.g. Macmillan nurse; CPN); ↑ help in the home
- Relaxation—often ↑ the patient's feeling of control over the situation
- Explanation—of worries/problems/concerns about the future
- Physical activity—exercise; writing

Management: drug measures
- Consider starting an antidepressant—📖 p. 1004
- All antidepressants take ~2wk to work
- If immediate effect is required consider using flupentixol 1mg od (beware as can cause psychomotor agitation)

If not responding or suicidal refer for psychiatric opinion.

Terminal anguish and spiritual distress Characterized by over-whelming distress. Often related to unresolved conflict, guilt, fears, or loss of control.

Anxiety can be increased if
- Patients are unaware of the diagnosis but feel people are lying to them
- They have certain symptoms, such as breathlessness, haemorrhage, or constant nausea or diarrhoea
- Weak religious conviction—convinced believers and convinced non-believers have less anxiety
- There are young dependant children or other dependant relatives
- Patients have unfinished business to attend to, such as legal affairs

Action Listening can itself be therapeutic. Talk to the patient, if possible, about dying and try to break down fears into component parts. Address fears that can be dealt with. As a last resort, and after discussion with the patient (where possible) and/or relatives, consider sedation.

Confusion 📖 p. 1010

Insomnia 📖 p. 194

The last 48 hours

It is notoriously difficult to predict when death will occur. Symptoms and signs of death approaching include:

- Day-by-day deterioration
- Difficulty swallowing medicines
- Gaunt appearance
- ↓ intake of food and fluids
- Profound weakness—needs assistance with all care; may be bed-bound
- Drowsy or ↓ cognition—often unable to cooperate with carers

Goals of treatment in the last 48h

- Ensure patients are comfortable—physically, emotionally, and spiritually. Consider using the Liverpool Care Pathway (📖 p. 1029)
- Make the end of life peaceful and dignified—what is dignified for one patient may not be for another; ask
- Support patients and carers so that the experience of death for those left behind is as positive as it can be

Patients' wishes Dying is a unique and special event for each individual. Helping to explore a patient's wishes about death and dying should not be a discussion left to the last 24h.

Advance directives/lasting power of attorney 📖 pp. 122–3

Out-of-hours providers Alert out-of-hours providers if a patient is dying at home. This will ensure appropriate response to calls and avoid unnecessary and unwanted admissions. Consider a 'just-in-case' box to leave at the patient's home containing drugs that might be needed should the patient deteriorate outside normal working hours.

Different cultures Different religious and cultural groups have different approaches to the dying process. Be sensitive to cultural and religious beliefs. Never assume; if in doubt ask a family member.

Assessment of patient needs Ask which problems are causing the patient/carers most concern and address those concerns where possible. Patients often under-report symptoms.

Physical examination Keep examination to a minimum to avoid unnecessary interference. Check sites of discomfort/pain suggested by history or non-verbal cues; mouth; bladder and bowel.

Psychological assessment Find out what the patient wants to know. Gently assessing how patients feel about their disease and situation can shed light on their needs and distress.

Investigations Any investigation at the end of life should have a clear and justifiable purpose (e.g. excluding a reversible condition where treatment would make the patient more comfortable). The need for investigations in the terminal stage of illness is minimal.

Review of medication Comfort is the priority. Stop all unnecessary medication.

Symptom control Dying patients tolerate symptoms very poorly because of their weakness. Nursing care is the mainstay of treatment, GPs do have a role:

- Ensure new problems do not develop, e.g. use of appropriate mattresses and measures to prevent bed sores
- Treat specific symptoms, e.g. dry mouth

- Think ahead—discuss treatment options that might be available later, e.g. use of a syringe driver, buccal, PR, or transcutaneous preparations to deliver medication when/if the oral route is no longer possible; use of strong analgesia which may also have a sedative effect
- Ensure there is a clear management plan agreed between the medical and nursing team and the patient/family members. Anticipate probable needs of the patient so that immediate response can be made when the time comes—define clearly what should be done in the event of a symptom arising/worsening; ensure drugs or equipment that may be needed are in the home; inform the out-of-hours service

Excessive respiratory secretion (death rattle) Noisy, moist breathing. Can be distressing for relatives. Reassure that the patient is not suffering or choking. Try repositioning and/or tipping the bed head down (if possible) to ↓ noise. Treat prophylactically—it is easier to prevent than remove accumulated secretions. *Suitable drugs:*
- Glycopyrronium—non-sedative; give 200 micrograms sc stat and review after 1h. If effective, give 200 micrograms every 4h sc or 0.6–1.2mg/24h via syringe driver
- Hyoscine hydrobromide—sedative in high doses; give 400 micrograms sc stat and review response after 30min. If effective, give 400–600 micrograms 4–8 hourly or 0.6–2.4mg/24h via syringe driver. If the patient is conscious and respiratory secretions are not too distressing, it may be more appropriate to use a transdermal patch (Scopoderm® 1.5mg over 3d) or sublingual tablets (Kwells®). Dry mouth is a side effect.

Terminal breathlessness Distressing symptom for patients/carers. Support carers in attendance and explain management:
- Diamorphine or morphine: dose depends on whether the patient is being converted from oral morphine (or an alternative opioid). If no previous opioid, start diamorphine 5mg/24h sc. If previously on oral morphine, divide the total 24h dose by 3 to obtain the 24h sc dose of diamorphine or by 2 to obtain the 24h sc dose of morphine. ↑ dose slowly as needed
- Midazolam 5–10mg/24h sc
- If sticky secretions—try nebulized saline ± physiotherapy

Terminal restlessness *Causes:*
- **Pain/discomfort** Urinary retention, constipation, pain which the patient cannot tell you about, excess secretions in throat
- **Opioid toxicity** Causes myoclonic jerking. The dose of morphine may need to be ↓ if a patient becomes uraemic
- **Biochemical causes**—↑ Ca^{2+}, uraemia—❶ if it has been decided not to treat abnormalities do not check for them
- **Psychological/spiritual distress**.

Management Treat reversible causes, e.g. catheterization for retention, hyoscine to dry up secretions. If still restless, treat with a sedative. This does not shorten life but makes the patient/relatives more comfortable. *Suitable drugs:* haloperidol 1–3mg tds po; chlorpromazine 25–50mg tds po; diazepam 2–10mg tds po, midazolam (10–100mg/24h via syringe driver or 5mg stat), or levomepromazine (50–150mg/24h via syringe driver or 6.25mg stat).

Terminal anguish and spiritual distress 📖 p. 1043

Syringe drivers

Syringe drivers are used to aid drug delivery when the oral route is no longer feasible. Indications include:
- Intractable vomiting
- Severe dysphagia
- Patient too weak to swallow
- ↓ conscious level
- Poor gut absorption (rare)
- Poor patient compliance

Types of syringe driver In recent years, many PCOs, hospitals, and hospices have been changing their syringe drivers from the traditionally used blue or green Graseby drivers, which are being phased out. Newer devices with additional safety and monitoring features (e.g. McKinley T34 or Alaris) are now in common use. It is important to find out which devices are used in your locality and how they work.

⚠ Incorrect use of syringe drivers is a common cause of drug errors. Each PCO should use just one type of syringe driver to ↓ risks of errors.

Drugs that can be used in syringe drivers See Table 28.10.

General principles Draw up the prescribed 24h medication. The diluent of choice in most cases is water for injection but 0.9% sodium chloride should be used if using levomepromazine, diclofenac, octreotide or ondansetron; cyclizine should not be diluted with saline. Then set the rate on the syringe driver.
❶ Local policies may differ. Hands-on training is essential.

Mixing drugs in syringe drivers Provided there is evidence of compatibility, drugs can be mixed in syringe drivers. Diamorphine or morphine can be mixed with:
- Cyclizine
- Hyoscine hydrobromide
- Hyoscine butylbromide
- Midazolam
- Ondansetron
- Dexamethasone (<4mg/24h)
- Levomepromazine
- Haloperidol
- Metoclopramide
- Glycopyrronium

If combining 2 or 3 drugs in a syringe driver, a larger volume of diluent may be needed (e.g. 20 or 30mL syringe). If >3 drugs are needed in 1 syringe driver, reassess treatment aims.

Common problems with syringe drivers
- **If the syringe driver runs too slowly** Check it is switched on; check the battery; check the cannula is not blocked
- **If the syringe driver runs too quickly** Check the rate setting
- **Injection site reaction** If there is pain or inflammation, change the injection site

Further information
Sdrivers—Drug Compatibility Database ℘ www.pallcare.info
Palliative Care Adult Network Guidelines ℘ http://book.pallcare.info/

Table 28.10 Drugs that can be used in syringe drivers

Indication	Drugs
Nausea and vomiting	Haloperidol 2.5–10mg/24h
	Levomepromazine 5–200mg/24h (causes sedation in 50%)
	Cyclizine 150mg/24h (may precipitate if mixed with other drugs)
	Metoclopramide 30–100mg/24h
	Octreotide 300–600 micrograms/24h (consultant supervision)
Respiratory secretions	Hyoscine hydrobromide 0.6–2.4mg/24h
	Glycopyrronium 0.6–1.2mg/24h
Restlessness and confusion	Haloperidol 5–15mg/24h
	Levomepromazine 50–200mg/24h
	Midazolam 20–100mg/24h (and fitting)
Pain control	Diamorphine ⅓–½ dose oral morphine/24h
	Morphine ½–⅔ dose of oral morphine/24h
	Oxycodone ½ dose oral oxycodone/24h

❶ Subcutaneous infusion solution should be monitored regularly, both to check for precipitation (and discoloration) and to ensure the infusion is running at the correct rate.

Emergencies in general practice

Emergency patient encounters

Emergency calls Nearly all requests for emergency care are made by telephone. General rules:

- **Train surgery staff** to handle distressed callers, recognize serious problems, and act appropriately when such calls are received
- **Where possible use a single number for patients to access help** If using an answering machine, ensure the message is easily heard and contains clear instructions. Worried patients find it difficult to cope with complicated telephone referral systems or messages
- **Appear helpful** rather than defensive from the outset. Keep calm and friendly—even in the event of provocation. Worried callers often appear abrupt or demanding
- **Record** the time of the call, date, patient's name, address and a contact telephone number, brief details of the problem, and action taken (even if calls are being recorded)
- **Collect only information you need to decide what action is necessary** If the patient needs to be seen, collect enough information to decide where and how quickly the patient should be seen, and whether extra equipment or help is needed
- **If giving advice** make it simple and in language the patient can understand. Repeat to make sure it has been understood. Consider asking the patient/carer to repeat what you have told them. Always tell callers to ring back if symptoms change or they have further worries
- **If a visit is indicated** ensure the address is right and ask for directions if you are not sure where to go. Try to give a rough arrival time
- **In some cases** (e.g. major trauma, large GI bleeds, suspected MI, burns, overdoses) call for an emergency ambulance at once
- **If a call seems inappropriate** consider the reason for it—e.g. depression might provoke recurrent calls for minor ailments

⚠ If in doubt—see the patient.

Emergency home visits

- Try to stick to the problem you have been called about
- Take a concise history and examine as appropriate
- Make a decision on management and explain it to the patient and any carers in clear and concise terms that they can understand. Repeat advice several times ± write it down
- Record history, examination, management suggested, and advice given for the patient's notes
- Always invite the patient and carers to ring you again should symptoms change, the situation deteriorate, or further worries appear
- For inappropriate calls, take time to educate the patient and/or carers about self-management and use of emergency GP visiting services
- Always consider hidden reasons for seemingly unnecessary visits

Being prepared

- Ensure that you have a reliable car with a full tank of fuel
- Have a good street map of the area ± Ordinance Survey map ± an electronic in-car navigation system

- Carry a large, strong torch in the car
- Carry a mobile telephone to enable you to call for help as needed
- Check your drug box is fully stocked and all items are in date
- Check all equipment carried is operational, and carry spare batteries
- Carry a list of emergency telephone numbers
- Know which chemists have extended opening hours and/or carry the chemist's rota

Safety and security

- In all cases ensure someone else knows where you are going, when to expect you back, and what to do if you do not return on time
- If going to a call you are worried about either take someone with you to sit in the car or call the police to meet you there before going in
- If you reach a call and find you are uncomfortable, make sure you can get out. Note the layout of the property and make sure you have a clear route to the door
- Set up your mobile phone to call the police or your base at a single touch of a button. Consider carrying an attack alarm
- If possible have separate bags for drugs and consultation equipment; leave the drug box locked out of sight in the boot of the car when doing a visit

Referral letters Good communication is essential when referring patients to other doctors and agencies, especially in emergency situations. Ensure all referral letters include:
- Address of the referrer (including telephone number if possible)
- Name and address of registered GP if not the referrer
- Date of referral
- Name, address, and date of birth of the patient (and any other identifiers available, e.g. hospital or NHS number)
- Name of the person to whom the patient is being referred (or department if not a named individual)
- Presenting condition—history, examination, investigations already performed with results, treatments already tried with outcomes
- Relevant past medical history and family history
- Current medication and any intolerances/allergies known
- Reason for referral (what you want the recipient of the letter to do) e.g. to investigate symptoms, to reassure parents
- Any other relevant information, e.g. social circumstances
- Signature (and name in legible format) of referrer

❶ Consider using carbonized paper to keep copies of emergency referral letters.

The doctor's bag 📖 p. 100

Managing a resuscitation attempt outside hospital

⚠ Ventricular fibrillation complicating acute MI is the most common cause of cardiac arrest that members of the primary healthcare team will encounter. Success is greatest when the event is witnessed and attempted defibrillation is performed with the minimum of delay.

Resuscitation equipment See Table 29.1.
- Resuscitation equipment is used relatively infrequently. Staff must know where to find equipment at the time it is needed and should be trained to use the equipment to a level appropriate to the individual's expected role
- Each practice should have a named individual with responsibility for checking the state of readiness of all resuscitation drugs and equipment on a regular basis, ideally once a week. In common with drugs, disposable items like the adhesive electrodes have a finite shelf life and will require replacement from time to time if unused

Training Training and practice are necessary to acquire skills in resuscitation techniques. Resuscitation skills decline rapidly and updates and retraining using manikins are necessary every 6–12mo to maintain adequate skill levels. Level of resuscitation skill needed by different members of the primary healthcare team differs according to the individual's role:
- All those in direct contact with patients should be trained in basic life support and related resuscitation skills such as the recovery position
- Doctors, nurses, and other paramedical workers such as physiotherapists should also be able to use an automatic external defibrillator (AED) effectively. Other personnel (e.g. receptionists) may also be trained to use an AED

⚠ It is unacceptable for patients who sustain a cardiopulmonary arrest to await the arrival of the ambulance service before basic resuscitation is performed and a defibrillator is available.

Performance management Accurate records of all resuscitation attempts and electronic data stored by most AEDs during a resuscitation attempt should be kept for audit, training, and medicolegal reasons. The responsibility for this rests with the most senior member of the practice team involved. Process and outcome of all resuscitation attempts should be audited—both at practice and PCO level—to allow deficiencies to be addressed and examples of good practice to be shared.

Ethical issues
- It is essential to identify individuals in whom cardiopulmonary arrest is a terminal event and where resuscitation is inappropriate
- Overall responsibility for a 'Do not attempt to resuscitate (DNAR)' decision rests with the clinician in charge of the patient's care
- Seek opinions of other members of the medical and nursing team, the patient, and any relatives in reaching a DNAR decision

- Record the DNAR decision in the patient notes, the reasons for that decision, and what the relatives have been told; provide a copy of the DNAR form for the patient/carers to keep in the home
- Ensure that all members of the team involved with the patient's care are aware of the decision and have it recorded in their notes too.
  ❶ Remember to send a notification to the local ambulance service and OOH provider
- Review the decision not to attempt resuscitation regularly in the light of the patient's condition

Further information

Resuscitation Council (UK) Cardiopulmonary resuscitation guidance for clinical practice and training in primary care (2001) ℘ www.resus.org.uk
BMA, RCN and Resuscitation Council (UK) Decisions relating to cardio-pulmonary resuscitation (2007) ℘ www.resus.org.uk

Table 29.1 Resuscitation equipment needed

Equipment	Notes
Defibrillator with electrodes and razor	An automated external defibrillator should be available wherever and whenever sick patients are seen
	Regular maintenance is needed even if the machine is not used
	After the machine is used the manufacturer's instructions should be followed to return it to a state of readiness with minimum delay
Pocket mask with one-way valve	All personnel should be trained to use one
Oro-pharyngeal airway	Suitable for use by those appropriately trained. Keep a range of sizes available
Oxygen and mask with reservoir bag	Should be available wherever possible. Oxygen cylinders need regular maintenance-follow national safety standards
Suction	Simple, mechanical, portable, handheld suction devices are recommended
Drugs	Epinephrine/adrenaline—1mg IV.
	Amiodarone—300mg IV—for VF resistant to defibrillation
	Naloxone—for suspected cases of respiratory arrest due to opioid overdose
	⚠ There is no evidence for the use of alkalizing agents, atropine, buffers, or calcium salts before hospitalization
	Drugs should be given by the intravenous route, preferably through a catheter placed in a large vein, for example in the antecubital fossa, and flushed in with a bolus of IV fluid
	If IV access cannot be obtained, give drugs via the intraosseous route (IO). In a child, if IV/IO access is not available and cannot easily be obtained, but a tracheal tube is in place, consider giving adrenaline (100 microgram/kg) via the tracheal tube
Other	Saline flush, gloves, syringes and needles, IV cannulae, IV fluids, sharps box, scissors, tape

Adult basic life support

Basic paediatric life support 📖 p. 1060

Adult basic adult life support (ABLS) Is a holding operation—sustaining life until help arrives. BLS should be started as soon as the arrest is detected—outcome is less good the longer the delay (see Figure 29.1).
1. **D**anger Ensure safety of rescuer and patient
2. **R**esponse Check the patient for any response
- Is he **A**lert? Yes/No
- Does he respond to **V**ocal stimuli? Yes/No
- Does he respond to a **P**ainful stimulus (pinching the lower part of the nasal septum)? Yes/No
- Is the patient **U**nconscious? Yes/No

If he responds by answering or moving Do not move the patient unless in danger. Get help. Reassess regularly.

If he does not respond Shout for help; turn the patient onto his back.

3. **A**irway Open the airway—place one hand on the patient's forehead and tilt his head back. With fingertips under the point of the patient's chin, lift the chin to open the airway.

⚠ Try to avoid head tilt if trauma to the neck is suspected

4. **B**reathing With airway open, look, listen, and feel for breathing for no more than 10s—look for chest movement, listen at the victim's mouth for breath sounds, feel for air on your cheek.

If breathing normally Turn the patient into the recovery position (📖 p. 1071), get help, and check for continued breathing.

If not breathing or only making occasional gasps/weak attempts at breathing: get help then start chest compressions.

❶ In the first few minutes after cardiac arrest, a victim may be barely breathing or taking infrequent, noisy, gasps. Do not confuse this with normal breathing. If you have any doubt whether breathing is normal, act as if it is *not* normal.

5. **C**irculation Start chest compressions if not breathing:
- Kneel by the side of the victim and place the heel of one hand in the centre of the victim's chest. Place the heel of your other hand on top of the first hand. Interlock the fingers of your hands and ensure that pressure is not applied over the victim's ribs. Do not apply any pressure over the upper abdomen or the bottom end of the bony sternum
- Position yourself vertically above the victim's chest and, with arms straight, press down on the sternum 5–6cm
- After each compression, release all the pressure on the chest without losing contact between your hands and the sternum. Compression and release should take an equal amount of time
- Repeat at a rate of ~100–120x/min

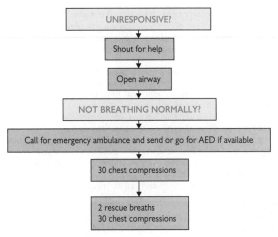

Figure 29.1 Adult basic life support (ABLS) algorithm

Figure 29.2 Automated external defibrillator (AED) algorithm

Figures 29.1 and 29.2 are reproduced with permission from the Resuscitation guidelines (2010)
℗ www.resus.org.uk

6. Combine chest compression with rescue breaths

- After 30 compressions open the airway using head tilt and chin lift
- Pinch the soft part of the victim's nose closed, using the index finger and thumb of your hand on his forehead. Allow the victim's mouth to open, but maintain chin lift
- Give a rescue breath—take a normal breath and place your lips around the victim's mouth (mouth-to-nose technique is an alternative) making sure that you have a good seal. Blow steadily into his mouth for ~1s whilst watching for the chest to rise
- Maintaining head tilt and chin lift; take your mouth away from the victim and watch for the chest to fall as air comes out
- Take another normal breath and blow into the victim's mouth again to give a total of 2 effective rescue breaths. Then return your hands without delay to the correct position on the sternum and give a further 30 chest compressions
- Continue chest compressions and rescue breaths in a ratio of 30:2

If rescue breaths do not make the chest rise

- Check the victim's mouth, and remove any visible obstruction
- Recheck that there is adequate head tilt and chin lift
- Don't attempt >2 breaths each time before returning to chest compressions

❶ **Chest-compression-only CPR** If you are unable or unwilling to give rescue breaths, give continuous chest compressions only at a rate of 100–120/min.

⚠ Only stop to recheck the victim if the patient shows signs of regaining consciousness (e.g. coughs, opens eyes, moves purposefully) AND starts to breath normally; otherwise resuscitation should not be interrupted.

Use of automated external defibrillators (AEDs) in adults Programme AEDs to deliver a single shock followed by a pause of 2min for the immediate resumption of CPR.

If a patient arrests Unless an AED is immediately available, start CPR according to the guidelines for basic life support.

As soon as the AED arrives. See Figure 29.2.

- Switch on the AED and attach the electrode pads. If >1 rescuer is present, continue CPR whilst this is done. (Some AEDs automatically switch on when the AED lid is opened)
  - Place one AED pad to the right of the sternum below the clavicle
  - Place the other pad in the mid-axillary line with its long axis vertical
- Follow the voice/visual prompts. Ensure nobody touches the victim whilst the AED is analysing the rhythm

If a shock is indicated Ensure that nobody touches the victim. Push the shock button as directed (fully automatic AEDs deliver the shock automatically). Immediately resume CPR and continue to follow the prompts.

If no shock is indicated Immediately resume CPR and continue to follow the prompts.

Use of AEDs in children 📖 p. 1062

When to go for assistance It is vital for rescuers to get assistance as quickly as possible. If you are the only rescuer, go for assistance before starting CPR.

When >1 rescuer is available
- One should start resuscitation while another rescuer goes for assistance
- Another should take over CPR every 2min to prevent fatigue. Ensure minimum of delay during changeover of rescuers

Duration of resuscitation Continue resuscitation until:
- Further qualified help arrives from the emergency medical services
- The victim starts breathing normally, *and/or*
- You become exhausted

Pad position for external defibrillators Place 1 pad to the right of the sternum below the clavicle. Place the other pad vertically in the mid-axillary line approximately level with the V6 ECG electrode position or female breast (although clear of any breast tissue).

Advising about CPR over the telephone If you receive a phone call for advice about an <u>adult</u> who has collapsed and is not breathing, call for emergency ambulance support. Advise the person with the patient to perform compression-only CPR. This is easier to describe, more acceptable to the general public, and more effective than traditional compression/ventilation CPR. ❶ Children need compressions and ventilation.

Management after successful treatment of cardiac arrest
- Turn into the recovery position (📖 p. 1071)
- Give oxygen aiming to keep oxygen saturation at 94–98%
- Transfer to hospital as soon as possible by emergency ambulance

Further information
Resuscitation Council (UK) Resuscitation guidelines (2010)
🖥 www.resus.org.uk

Adult advanced life support

See Figure 29.3. Advanced life support has 3 basic stages:
- Revive the patient using basic life support (📖 p. 1054). Basic life support should be started if there is any delay in obtaining a defibrillator but must not delay shock delivery
- Restore spontaneous cardiac output, using an automated external defibrillator (📖 p. 1056) or manual defibrillator
- Review possible causes for cardiac arrest and take action as needed

Precordial thump Appropriate *only* if the arrest is witnessed and a defibrillator is not to hand—may dislodge a pulmonary embolus or 'jerk' the heart back into sinus rhythm. Use the ulnar edge of a tightly clenched fist, and deliver a sharp impact to the lower half of the sternum from a height of ~20cm then immediately retract the fist.

VF/VT arrest
- Attempt defibrillation (1 shock 150–200J biphasic or 360J monophasic)
- Immediately resume chest compressions (30:2) without reassessing rhythm or feeling for the pulse. Continue CPR for 2min then pause briefly to check the monitor
- If VT/VF persists give a 2nd shock (150–360J biphasic or 360J monophasic); continue CPR for 2min then pause briefly to check the monitor
- If VT/VF persists give a 3rd shock (150–360J biphasic or 360J monophasic), then continue CPR for 2min
- After the 3rd shock (and whilst continuing CPR) administer adrenaline (epinephrine) 1mg IV and amiodarone 300mg IV (lidocaine 1mg/kg is an alternative if amiodarone is not available). Give drugs IO if IV access cannot be obtained
- Repeat 2min CPR, rhythm check, defibrillation sequence while VT/VF persists
- Give adrenaline (epinephrine) 1mg IV immediately before alternate shocks (i.e. approximately every 3–5min)

Non-VT/VF arrest
- Start CPR 30:2. Without stopping CPR, check that the leads are attached correctly
- Give adrenaline (epinephrine) 1mg IV as soon as IV access is achieved
- Continue CPR 30:2 until the airway is secured, then continue chest compression without pausing during ventilation
- Recheck the rhythm after 2min and proceed accordingly—if VT/VF change to VF/VT arrest (shockable rhythm) algorithm
- Give adrenaline (epinephrine) 1mg IV every 3–5min (alternate loops)

Fine VF Fine VF difficult to distinguish from asystole is very unlikely to be shocked successfully into a perfusing rhythm. Continuing good-quality CPR may improve the amplitude and frequency of the VF and improve the chance of successful defibrillation to a perfusing rhythm.

Organized electrical activity If organized electrical activity is seen during the brief pause in compressions, check for a pulse.
- If a pulse is present, start post-resuscitation care (📖 p. 1057)
- If no pulse, continue CPR and follow the non-shockable algorithm

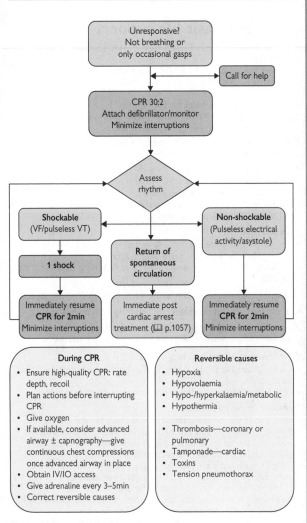

Figure 29.3 Adult advanced life support algorithm

Reproduced with permission from Resuscitation guidelines (2010) ℗ www.resus.org.uk

Further information
Resuscitation Council (UK) Resuscitation guidelines (2010) ·
℗ www.resus.org.uk

Paediatric basic life support

Basic paediatric life support (see Figure 29.4) is a holding operation until help arrives.

1. **Danger** Ensure safety of rescuer and patient
2. **Response** Check the child for any response
- Is he **Alert**?
- Does he respond to **Vocal** stimuli?
- Does he respond to **Painful** stimuli (pinch lower part of nasal septum)?
- Is he **Unconscious**?

If he responds by answering or moving Do not move the child unless in danger. Get help. Reassess regularly.

If he does not respond Shout for help. Assess airway.

3. **Airway** Open the airway. Do not move the child from the position in which you found him unless you have to:
- Gently tilt the head back—with your hand on the child's forehead
- Lift the chin—with your fingertips under the point of the child's chin

If unsuccessful
- Try jaw thrust—place the first 2 fingers of each hand behind each side of the child's jaw bone, and push the jaw forward
- Try lifting the chin or jaw thrust after carefully turning the child onto his back

⚠ Avoid head tilt as much as possible if trauma to the neck is suspected

4. **Breathing** Look, listen, and feel for breathing (maximum 10s)

If breathing normally Turn the child carefully into the recovery position (📖 p. 1071) if unconscious, and check for continued breathing.

If not breathing or not breathing normally:
- Carefully turn the child onto his back and remove any obvious airway obstruction
- Give 5 initial rescue breaths—note any gag or cough response

Technique for rescue breaths
- Ensure head tilt (neutral position for children <1y) and chin lift
- If age ≥1y, pinch the soft part of the child's nose closed with the index finger and thumb of the hand which is on his forehead. Open the child's mouth a little, but maintain the chin upwards
- Take a breath and place your lips around the child's mouth (mouth and nose if <1y*), ensuring you have a good seal. Blow steadily into the child's airway over ~1–1.5s, watching for the chest to rise
- Maintaining head tilt and chin lift, take your mouth away and watch for the chest to fall as air comes out
- Take another breath and repeat this sequence 5 times

❶ If you have difficulty achieving an effective breath, consider airway obstruction—📖 p. 1086.

---

* If the nose and mouth cannot both be covered, place your lips around the mouth alone as for an older child, or nose alone (close the child's lips to prevent air escape).

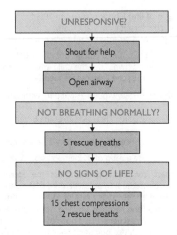

If lone rescuer, after 1 minute call for help then continue

Figure 29.4 Paediatric basic life support (PBLS) algorithm

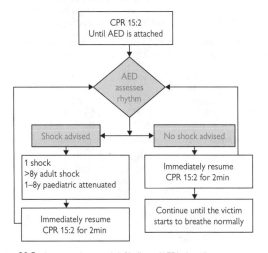

Figure 29.5 Automated external defibrillator (AED) algorithm

Figure 29.4 and Figure 29.5 are reproduced with permission from Resuscitation guidelines (2010)
🔗 www.resus.org.uk

5. **Circulation (signs of life)** Check (maximum 10s) for:
- Any movement, coughing, or normal breathing (not agonal gasps)
- Pulse—child ≥1y carotid pulse; child <1y brachial pulse

If circulation is present Continue rescue breathing until the child starts breathing effectively on his own. Turn the child into the recovery position (📖 p. 1071) if unconscious, and reassess frequently.

If circulation is absent Or slow pulse (<60bpm) with poor perfusion or you are not sure:
- Give 15 chest compressions. Then give 2 rescue breaths, followed by 15 further chest compressions
- Continue the cycle of 2 breaths followed by 15 chest compressions

❶ Lone rescuers may use a ratio of 30 compressions:2 rescue breaths.

Technique for chest compressions Compress the sternum 1 finger's breadth above the xiphisternum by at least a third of the depth of the chest. Release the pressure then repeat at a rate of ~100–120 compressions/min.
- **Children <1y with a lone rescuer** Use the tips of 2 fingers
- **Children <1y with ≥2 rescuers** Place both thumbs flat on the lower third of the sternum with tips pointing towards the child's head and encircle the lower part of the child's ribcage with the tips of the fingers supporting the infant's back. Press down with both thumbs
- **Children >1y** Place the heel of 1 hand over the lower half of the sternum. Lift the fingers. Position yourself vertically above the chest with arm straight, and push downwards. For larger children use both hands with fingers interlocked to achieve satisfactory compressions

⚠ Stop to recheck for signs of a circulation only if the child moves or takes a spontaneous breath—otherwise continue uninterrupted.

Use of automated external defibrillators (AEDs) in children
- **Children >8y** Use the standard adult AED (see Figure 29.5)
- **Children <8y** Paediatric pads or a paediatric mode should be used if available—if not, use the adult AED as it is. ❶ Shockable rhythm is rare in children <1y, but if present benefits of AED use outweigh risks

If a patient arrests Start CPR according to the guidelines for PBLS.

As soon as the AED arrives follow Figure 29.5
- Switch on the AED and attach the electrode pads. If >1 rescuer is present, continue CPR whilst this is done. (Some AEDs automatically switch on when the AED lid is opened)
  - Place one AED pad to the right of the sternum below the clavicle.
  - Place the other pad in the mid-axillary line with its long axis vertical
- Follow the voice/visual prompts. Ensure nobody touches the victim whilst the AED is analysing the rhythm

If a shock is indicated Ensure nobody touches the victim. Push the shock button as directed (fully automatic AEDs deliver the shock automatically). Immediately resume CPR and continue to follow the prompts.

If no shock is indicated Immediately resume CPR and continue to follow the prompts.

When to go for assistance It is vital for rescuers to get assistance as quickly as possible when a child collapses.

When >1 rescuer is available One should start resuscitation while another rescuer goes for assistance.

Lone rescuer Perform resuscitation for 1 minute before going for assistance (and consider taking a young child/infant with you to minimize interruption in CPR). The only exception to this is a witnessed sudden collapse—as in this case cardiac arrest is likely to be due to arrhythmia and the child may need defibrillation so seek help immediately

Duration of resuscitation Continue resuscitation until:
- Child shows signs of life (spontaneous respiration, pulse, movement)
- Further qualified help arrives from emergency medical services
- You become exhausted

Cervical spine injury
- If spinal cord injury is suspected (e.g. if the victim has sustained a fall, been struck on the head or neck, or has been rescued after diving into shallow water) take particular care during handling and resuscitation to maintain alignment of the head, neck, and chest in the neutral position
- A spinal board and/or cervical collar should be used if available

Advising about CPR over the telephone If you receive a phone call for advice about a *child* who has collapsed and is not breathing, call for emergency ambulance support. Advise the person with the patient to perform compression and ventilation CPR. ❗ For adults advise compression-only CPR.

Management after successful treatment of cardiac arrest
- Turn into the recovery position (📖 p. 1071)
- Give oxygen, aiming to keep oxygen saturation at 94–98%
- Transfer to hospital as soon as possible by emergency ambulance

Resuscitation of the newborn 📖 p. 1066

Further information
Resuscitation Council (UK) Resuscitation guidelines (2010)
🖰 www.resus.org.uk

Paediatric advanced life support

See Figure 29.6. Cardiac arrest in children is rare. Except where there is underlying heart disease, it is usually a consequence of respiratory arrest which results in asystole or pulseless electrical activity and has poor prognosis. Good airway management and providing high-flow oxygen for very sick children is therefore important in preventing cardiac arrest.

Basic paediatric life support Follow the algorithm in Figure 29.4.

Unable to ventilate? Consider foreign body in the airway and initiate airway obstruction sequence—📖 p. 1086

Checking the pulse
- **Child** Feel the carotid pulse in the neck
- **Infant** Feel the brachial pulse on the inner aspect of the upper arm

Once the airway is protected By tracheal intubation, continue chest compression without pausing for ventilation. Provide ventilation at a rate of 10–12/min and compression at 100–120/min. When circulation is restored, ventilate the child at a rate of 12–20 breaths/min.

Adrenaline (epinephrine) dose
- IV or intraosseous (IO) access—10 micrograms/kg adrenaline (0.1mL/kg of 1:10,000 solution). Give as soon as possible if non-shockable rhythm
- If circulatory access is not present and cannot be quickly obtained, but the child has a tracheal tube in place, consider giving adrenaline 100 micrograms/kg via the tracheal tube (1mL/kg of 1:10,000 or 0.1mL/kg of 1:1,000 solution). This is the least satisfactory route of administration

⚠ Do not give 1:1,000 adrenaline IV or IO.

VF/pulseless VT Less common in paediatric life support.
- Defibrillation:
  - Give 1 shock of 4J/kg, or
  - If using an AED for a child of <8y, deliver a paediatric attenuated adult shock energy
  - If using an AED for a child >8y, use the adult shock energy
- For VF/pulseless VT persisting after the 3rd shock, resume chest compressions and give adrenaline 10 micrograms/kg and amiodarone 5mg/kg
- Continue 2min cycles of CPR and shocks. Give adrenaline in alternate cycles and amiodarone one further time after the fifth shock

Magnesium Magnesium treatment is indicated in children with documented hypomagnesaemia or with polymorphic VT ('torsade de pointes'), regardless of cause. Give IV magnesium sulfate over several minutes at a dose of 25–50mg/kg (to a maximum of 2g).

Intravenous fluids In situations where the cardiac arrest has resulted from circulatory failure, a standard (20mL/kg) bolus of crystalloid fluid should be given if there is no response to the initial dose of adrenaline.

Further information
Resuscitation Council (UK) Resuscitation guidelines (2010)
🖰 www.resus.org.uk

During CPR

- Ensure high-quality CPR: rate depth, recoil
- Plan actions before interrupting CPR
- Give oxygen
- Obtain IV/IO access
- Give adrenaline every 3–5min
- If available, consider advanced airway ± capnography—give continuous chest compressions once advanced airway in place
- Correct reversible causes

Reversible causes

- Hypoxia
- Hypovolaemia
- Hypo-/hyperkalaemia/metabolic
- Hypothermia

- Thrombosis—coronary or pulmonary
- Tamponade—cardiac
- Toxins
- Tension pneumothorax

Estimating the weight of a child for drug/fluid doses

- Use a recent weight from the parent-held child record if available
- Otherwise for children >1y, weight (in kg) ≈ 2x (age + 4)

Figure 29.6 Paediatric advanced life support (PALS) algorithm
Figure 29.6 is reproduced with permission from Resuscitation guidelines (2010)
🔊 www. resus.org.uk

Resuscitation of the newborn

Follow the algorithm in Figure 29.7.

Rapid assessment of the infant at birth Start the clock. Assess colour, tone, breathing, heart rate.

A healthy baby
- Born blue
- Good tone
- Cries seconds after delivery
- Good heart rate (120–150bpm)
- Rapidly becomes pink during the first 90s

An ill baby
- Born pale
- Poor tone/floppy
- Slow/very slow heart rate (<100bpm)
- Not breathing/inadequate breathing by 90–120s

Clamping the cord 1min after delivery for newborns not requiring resuscitation. If resuscitation is needed, delay until the baby is breathing.

Heart rate and pulse oximetry Heart rate is best judged by listening with a stethoscope—in many cases it can also be felt by palpating the umbilical cord. If available and the infant needs resuscitation, use pulse oximetry to measure pre-ductal oxygen saturation and heart rate. Place sensor on the right hand/wrist. In healthy term babies, oxygen saturation ↑ from 60% soon after birth to 90% at 10min.

Airway Open the airway by placing the head in a neutral position (neck neither extended nor flexed). If the occiput is prominent and the neck tends to flex, place a support under the shoulders—but do not overextend the neck. If the baby is floppy, apply jaw thrust or chin lift as needed.

Breathing Inflation breaths are breaths with pressures of ~30cm of water for 2–3s. Use air rather than oxygen.

If heart rate ↑ You have successfully inflated the chest. If the baby does not start breathing alone, continue to provide regular breaths at a rate of ~30–40 breaths/min until the baby starts to breathe alone.

If heart rate does not ↑ Either you have not inflated the chest or the baby needs more help. If the chest does not move, consider:
- Is the baby's head in the neutral position? Do you need jaw thrust?
- Do you need a longer inflation time?
- Do you need a second person's help with the airway?
- Is there obstruction, e.g. meconium (laryngoscope and suction)?
- What about an oropharyngeal (Guedel) airway?

Chest compressions Only commence after inflation of the lungs.
- Grip the chest in both hands so that the thumbs of both hands can press on the sternum at a point just below an imaginary line joining the nipples and with the fingers over the spine at the back
- Compress the chest quickly—↓ the AP diameter of the chest by at least a third with each compression. Ratio of compressions to inflations is 3:1

Drug support For a few babies inflation of the lungs and effective chest compression are not sufficient to produce effective circulation. IV or intra-osseous drugs may be helpful.

Figure 29.7 Newborn life support algorithm
Reproduced with permission from the Resuscitation guidelines (2010) ℗ www.resus.org.uk

Drug doses
- **Adrenaline (epinephrine)** 10 microgram/kg (0.1mL/kg of 1:10,000 solution), increasing to 30 microgram/kg (0.3mL/kg of 1:10,000 solution) if ineffective
- **Sodium bicarbonate** 1–2mmol/kg (2–4mL 4.2% bicarbonate solution)
- **Glucose** 250mg/kg (2.5mL/kg of 10% glucose)
- **For emergency volume replacement** (e.g. history of a bleed)—use 10mL/kg 0.9% saline given over 10–20s. Repeat if needed

Further information
Resuscitation Council (UK) Resuscitation guidelines (2010)
℗ www.resus.org.uk

Coma

Patients in coma/pre-coma nearly always require emergency admission.

When you receive the call for assistance
- Advise the attendant (unless history of possible spinal injury) to turn the patient onto his/her side
- Call an ambulance to meet you at the scene

On reaching the patient
- Assess the need for basic life support:
  - Airway patent?
  - Breathing satisfactory?
  - Circulation adequate?
- Turn into the recovery position (📖 p. 1071) if no contraindications, e.g. spinal injury
- Call for ambulance support if you have not already done so
- Ensure the patient is warm
- Try to establish a diagnosis (see Figure 29.8)

As soon as possible
- Insert an airway
- Give oxygen
- Establish IV access
- Transfer to hospital—unless the condition has resolved, e.g. hypoglycaemia, fit

Possible causes
- **Drugs** Sedatives or hypnotics, opioids, alcohol, solvents, carbon monoxide poisoning
- **Vascular** Stroke, low cardiac output, e.g. post-MI, ruptured AAA
- **CNS** Fit or post-ictal state; hydrocephalus (e.g. blocked shunt); cerebral oedema (e.g. meningitis, SAH, head injury); concussion; extradural or subdural haematoma
- **Metabolic** Hypo- or hyperglycaemia; hypothermia; hypopituitarism
- **Infection** Meningitis or septicaemia, pneumonia

Assessment and management See Figure 29.8.

Table 29.2 The Glasgow Coma Scale

Eye opening	Spontaneous	4	To pain	2
	To voice	3	None	1
Best verbal response	Oriented	5	Incomprehensible	2
	Confused	4	None	1
	Inappropriate words	3		
Best motor response	Obeys command	6	Flexion	3
	Localizes pain	5	Extension	2
	Withdraw	4	None	1

Total score = Eye opening + Best verbal + Best motor response scores

Examine

A **Airway**—does the patient have a patent airway? Consider turning into the recovery position to keep the airway clear if unconscious but has circulation and is breathing (📖 p.1071)

B **Breathing**—is the patient breathing? What is the respiratory rate? What is the oxygen saturation (if pulse oximeter available)? Consider giving oxygen (if peripheral oxygen saturation is ≤94%)

C **Circulation**—BP and pulse rate; haemorrhage control if bleeding

D **Disability**—level of consciousness (e.g. Glasgow Coma Scale)

E **Exposure**—look for clues to underlying cause e.g. signs of injury, smell of alcohol, rashes, pinpoint pupils/needle marks on limbs, temperature

Ask any attendants about
• Onset of symptoms /collapse
• Previous medical history
• Current medication
• Injury
• Social circumstances

Look for clues at the scene e.g. suicide notes, repeat prescription forms, Medic Alert bracelets.

Give 1mg IM glucagon (or 0.5mg if weight <25kg) or 50–250ml 10% glucose in 50ml aliquots (2–5ml/kg 10% glucose if child <12y)

May need to repeat glucagon after 20min

Follow with carbohydrate if good response—📖 p.1100

Check BM —— BM <2.5

—— BM >7

BM normal

Is opioid overdose suspected?   Yes

No

Consider hyperglycaemic states (📖 p.1100) Admit for further investigation

Adult or child >12y—give naloxone 0.4–2mg IV every 2–3min to a maximum of 10mg

Child 1mo–12y—give naloxone 10 microgram/kg. If no response give 100 microgram/kg

Repeat doses may be required

Is meningococcal disease suspected?

Yes   No

Give IV/IM benzylpenicillin immediately while awaiting transport unless previous anaphylactic reaction. *Dose:*
Adult or child >10y—1.2g
Child 1–9y—600mg
Infant <1y—300mg

ADMIT

Figure 29.8 Assessment and management of the unconscious patient

The fitting patient

Epilepsy Children—📖 p. 898   **Febrile convulsions** 📖 p. 897
Adults—📖 p. 574

Status epilepticus If >1 seizure without the patient regaining consciousness *or* fitting continues >5min despite medication.

When the call for assistance is received Instruct the attendant:
- To stay with the fitting patient
- To move anything from the vicinity that might cause injury
- To turn the patient onto his/her side

⚠ **Management of a major fit or status epilepticus**
- Ensure that the airway is clear
- Turn the patient into the recovery position (see Figure 29.9)
- Prevent onlookers from restraining the fitting patient
- Do not give drugs for the first 5min—many fits stop spontaneously
- After 5min treat with:

Midazolam buccal liquid	*or*	**Rectal diazepam**	
>10y 10mg	6mo–1y 2.5mg	Elderly 10mg	1mo–2y 5mg
5–10y 7.5mg	<6mo 300	>10y 10–20mg	Neonate 1.25–2.5mg
1–5y 5mg	microgram/kg	2–10y 5–10mg	

Alternatively, if IV access is established and resuscitation facilities are available, treat with IV lorazepam (adult and child ≥12y—4mg; child <12y—100 microgram/kg—maximum 4mg)
- If the fit continues >5min after medication administration, call for an emergency ambulance
- Drugs can be repeated ×1 after 10–15min; consider checking finger prick blood glucose if prolonged fit

Admit any patient with a fit immediately if
- Possibility that 2° to other illness, e.g. meningitis, subdural haematoma
- Recovery after the fit is incomplete (other than feeling sleepy)
- Status epilepticus (even if fits are controlled)

Follow-up Refer for urgent specialist assessment (to be seen in <2wk):
- Any adult who has a first fit
- Any child who has a first fit not related to fever

Delirium tremens (DTs) Major alcohol withdrawal symptoms usually occur 2–3d after an alcoholic has stopped drinking. *Features:*
- **General** Fever, tachycardia, ↑ BP, ↑ respiratory rate
- **Psychiatric** Visual/tactile hallucinations, acute delirium, apprehension
- **Neurological** Tremor, fits, fluctuating level of consciousness

⚠ **Action** DTs have 15% mortality—always admit as an emergency.

Further information
NICE ◌ www.nice.org.uk
- The epilepsies: the diagnosis and management of the epilepsies in adults and children in primary and secondary care (2012)
- Referral guidelines for suspected cancer (2005)

Figure 29.9 The recovery position. When a patient is unconscious but has circulation and is breathing, it is important to:

- Maintain a good airway
- Ensure the tongue does not cause obstruction
- Minimize the risk of inhalation of gastric contents

For this reason the victim should be placed in the recovery position. This allows the tongue to fall forward, keeping the airway clear.

Putting a patient into the recovery position

- Remove the patient's glasses
- Kneel beside the patient and make sure that both legs are straight (A)
- Place the arm nearest to you out at right angles to the body, elbow bent with the hand palm uppermost (A)
- Bring the far arm across the chest, and hold the back of the hand against the patient's cheek nearest to you (B)
- With your other hand, grasp the far leg just above the knee and pull it up, keeping the foot on the ground (B)
- Keeping the patient's hand pressed against his cheek, pull on the leg to roll the patient towards you onto his side (C)
- Adjust the upper leg so that both the hip and knee are bent at right angles (D)
- Tilt the head back to make sure the airway remains open (D)
- Adjust the hand under the cheek, if necessary, to keep the head tilted
- Check breathing regularly

⚠ Monitor the peripheral circulation of the lower arm. If the patient has to be kept in the recovery position for >30min, turn the patient onto the opposite side.

The unconscious child The child should be in as near a true lateral position as possible with his mouth dependent to allow free drainage of fluid. The position should be stable. In an infant this may require the support of a small pillow or rolled-up blanket placed behind the infant's back to maintain the position.

Cervical spine injury If spinal cord injury is suspected (for example, if the victim has sustained a fall, been struck on the head or neck, or has been rescued after diving into shallow water) take particular care during handling and resuscitation to maintain alignment of the head, neck, and chest in the neutral position. A spinal board and/or cervical collar should be used if available.

Anaphylaxis

Severe systemic allergic reaction that is life-threatening. *Common causes:*

- **Foods** Nuts, milk, fruit, fish and shellfish, eggs, pulses (beans, peas)
- **Drugs** Antibiotics, aspirin and other NSAIDs, opioids
- **Insect stings** Wasp or bee   • **Latex**

Features Often history of anaphylaxis/severe allergic reaction. Anaphylaxis is likely when *all* of the following are met:

- **Sudden onset/rapid progression** Of symptoms over minutes
- **Life-threatening:**
  - Airway problems—difficulty breathing/swallowing; feeling that throat is closing; hoarseness; stridor, *and/or*
  - Breathing problems—↑ respiratory rate; wheeze; shortness of breath; oxygen saturation <92%; cyanosis (late sign); confusion due to anoxia; respiratory arrest, *and/or*
  - Circulation problems—shock (pallor, clammy, tachycardia—bradycardia is a late feature); ↓ BP; faintness/dizziness; collapse; agitation/confusion; loss of consciousness. May cause myocardial ischaemia and ECG changes even if normal coronary arteries
- **Skin and/or mucosal changes** Flushing, erythema, urticaria, and/or angioedema, rhinitis and/or conjunctivitis—subtle/absent in 1 in 5

  ❶ Skin or mucosal changes alone are *not* a sign of an anaphylactic reaction, although they may develop into one.

Other symptoms Abdominal symptoms, e.g. abdominal pain, vomiting or incontinence; anxiety ± sense of impending doom.

Differential diagnosis

- **Life-threatening** Severe asthma; septic shock
- **Non-life-threatening** Simple faint; hyperventilation/panic attack; breath-holding attacks in small children; lone urticaria/angio-oedema

Action If suspected when the initial call comes in, request an emergency ambulance immediately. Ask if the patient has had a similar event before. If so, does he/she have an adrenaline auto-injector device? If yes, advise immediate use. Then visit—on attendance, follow the algorithm in Figure 29.10. Patients with airway/breathing problems may prefer to sit up; if low blood pressure, lie flat (on left side if pregnant) with legs elevated; if unconscious and breathing, place in the recovery position (📖 p. 1071).

Follow-up Warn patients or parents of the possibility of recurrence. Advise sufferers to wear a device (e.g. Medic-Alert bracelet) that will inform bystanders or medical staff should a future attack occur. Refer all patients after their first anaphylactic attack to a specialist allergy clinic. Consider supplying sufferers (or parents) with an adrenaline auto-injector device (e.g. EpiPen®) which can be used to administer IM adrenaline (epinephrine) immediately should symptoms recur. If you supply an auto-injector device, teach anyone likely to need to use it how to operate the device. IM adrenaline is very safe.

Further information

Resuscitation Council UK Emergency medical treatment of anaphylactic reactions for first medical responders (2008) ℘ www.resus.org.uk

Anaphylactic reaction?

Check:
Airway	Breathing
Circulation	Disability (e.g. confusion, coma)

Exposure (e.g. skin changes, facial or lip swelling, wheezing/stridor)

Diagnosis—look for:
- Acute onset of illness, *and*
- Life-threatening airway changes—swelling, hoarseness, stridor, *and/or*
- Life-threatening breathing changes—rapid breathing, wheeze, fatigue, cyanosis, oxygen saturation <92%, confusion, *and/or*
- Life-threatening circulation problems—pale, clammy, low BP, faintness, drowsy/coma, *and usually*
- Skin changes

Call for help
Lie the patient flat
Raise the patient's legs

Give adrenaline (epinephrine) 1:1,000 solution
>12y: 0.5mL (500 micrograms) IM
6–12y: 0.3mL (300 micrograms) IM
<6y: 0.15mL (150 micrograms) IM

If skills and equipment are available

Establish an airway
Monitor
- Pulse oximetry
- ECG
- BP

Give as soon as possible:
High-flow oxygen (>10L/min)
IV fluid challenge:
Adult: 500mL—1L
Child: crystalloid 20mL/kg
Repeat as needed
Repeat IV colloid if this might be the cause of anaphylaxis

Give after initial resuscitation:
Antihistamine (chlorphenamine)—
IM or slow IV:
>12y: 10mg
6–12y: 5mg
6mo–6y: 2.5mg
<6mo: 250 micrograms/kg
Hydrocortisone — IM or slow IV:
>12y: 200mg
6–12y: 100mg
6mo–6y: 50mg
<6mo: 25mg

Figure 29.10 Emergency treatment of anaphylaxis[G]

Information and support for patients
Allergy UK ☎ 01322 619898 🖳 www.allergyuk.org
Anaphylaxis Campaign ☎ 01252 542029 🖳 www.anaphylaxis.org.uk
Medic-Alert Foundation Supply Medic-Alert bracelets. ☎ 0800 581 420
🖳 www.medicalert.org.uk

Shock

Shock is due to inadequate blood flow to the peripheral circulation. It results in ↓ BP (± tachycardia), peripheral cyanosis, and ↓ urinary output.

Anaphylactic shock 📖 p. 1072

Septic shock 📖 p. 1078

Cardiogenic shock (e.g. due to MI, arrhythmia, tamponade). *Signs:*
- Hypotension—systolic BP <80–90mmHg
- Pulse rate may be normal, ↑, or ↓
- Severe breathlessness ± cyanosis

Action
- Sit the patient up if possible. Call for ambulance assistance
- Gain IV access. Treat underlying cause, e.g. atropine for bradycardia; diamorphine, furosemide, and GTN spray (if tolerated) for acute LVF
- If available give 100% oxygen—unless COPD when 24%

Hypovolaemic shock Usually due to haemorrhage. *Signs:*
- **Initially** Tachycardia (pulse >100bpm), pallor, sweating ± restlessness
- **Later** Decompensation—sudden fall in pulse rate and BP. Young people may decompensate very rapidly—if tachycardic treat as a medical emergency—speed could be lifesaving

Gastrointestinal bleeding 📖 p. 1076   **Lacerations** 📖 p. 1074

Very heavy menstrual bleeding 📖 p. 709

Ruptured abdominal aortic aneurysm (AAA) In the community, death rate from ruptured AAA is ~90% (80% before reaching hospital and 10% during surgery). Consider ruptured AAA in any patient with ↓ BP and atypical abdominal symptoms (especially if pulsatile abdominal mass).

⚠ In a patient with a known AAA, abdominal pain represents a ruptured AAA unless proven otherwise.

Dissecting thoracic aneurysm
- Typically presents with sudden tearing chest pain radiating to the back
- Consider if ↓ BP and chest pain (especially if pain radiates to the back)
- As dissection progresses, branches of the aorta are sequentially occluded causing: hemiplegia (carotid artery); unequal pulses and BP in the 2 arms (subclavian artery); paraplegia (spinal arteries); acute renal failure (renal arteries); aortic incompetence (proximal extension) and MI (cardiac arteries)

Action for ruptured AAA or dissecting thoracic aneurysm
- Lie the patient down flat, and raise legs above waist height
- Call for emergency ambulance assistance
- Gain IV access and (if possible) take blood for FBC and cross-matching—try to insert 2 large-bore cannulae
- If available, start IV fluids. Give rapidly over 10–15min
- If available, give 100% oxygen—unless COPD when give 24%

Nosebleed/epistaxis Usually due to ruptured blood vessels on the nasal septum. *Causes:*

- **Young** Nose picking, coryza, allergic rhinitis, blood dyscrasias
- **Elderly** Degenerative arterial disease, ↑ BP, nose picking, coryza, allergic rhinitis, medication (anticoagulants or aspirin), blood dyscrasias, telangiectasia, tumour. Often no cause is found

Manage as in Figure 29.11. Recurrent minor nosebleeds—refer to ENT.

Figure 29.11 Acute management of nosebleed in the community

Bleeding in terminally ill patients Bleeding can be a terminal event in patients with cancer. Where possible, make a decision in advance about whether to treat severe bleeding and prepare carers.

- **If a decision is made to treat** Treat as for hypovolaemic shock, and admit to hospital as an emergency. ❶ If bleeding from a lung tumour, protect the airway and lie the patient on the side of the tumour
- **If a decision is made not to treat** Stay with the patient, and give sedative medication (e.g. midazolam 20–40mg sc or IV or diazepam 10–20mg PR ± analgesia). Support the carers

Other rarer causes of shock Admit as medical emergencies:
- **Neurogenic** Due to cerebral trauma or haemorrhage, e.g. head injury, subarachnoid haemorrhage
- **Poisoning**   • **Liver failure**

Gastrointestinal bleeding

Take all gastrointestinal (GI) bleeds seriously; 7% of patients admitted to hospital with acute GI bleeding die.

Causes of GI bleeding

Upper GI bleed
- Peptic ulcer
- Gastritis
- Mallory–Weiss tear
- Oesophagitis
- Oesophageal or gastric cancer
- Oesophageal varices
- Drugs—steroids, anticoagulants, NSAIDs
- Angiodysplasia
- Haemangioma
- Bleeding disorders
- Swallowed blood from nosebleed

Lower GI bleed
- Diverticulitis
- Colitis—infectious or inflammatory
- Large bowel tumour or polyp
- Haemorrhoids
- Anal fissure
- Angiodysplasia (A-V malformations are common)
- Haemangioma
- Bleeding disorders
- Blood from upper GI bleed

Risk factors

Upper GI bleed
- History of alcohol abuse
- History of chronic liver disease
- History of NSAID use
- History of oral steroid use

Lower GI bleed
- Change in bowel habit
- History of diverticulitis
- History of UC

All GI bleeds
- Anticoagulant use
- Serious medical conditions (e.g. cardiovascular/respiratory/renal disease)
- Recent tiredness (? due to anaemia)

Presentation

Upper GI bleeding Typical presentation:
- Haematemesis—vomiting of blood
- Melaena—passage of black, offensive, tarry stool, consisting of digested blood per rectum. Always indicates a significant bleed. ❶ Iron tablets may cause black stools

Lower GI bleeding Passage of fresh blood per rectum. Brisk bleeding is a medical emergency but often patients complain of small amounts of bleeding related to passage of stool. Mixed blood and stool implies bleeding proximal to the sigmoid colon; blood around the stool implies a more distal bleed; blood on the toilet paper or in the pan not mixed with stool is often from anal bleeding due to haemorrhoids or an anal fissure.

❶ Very heavy upper GI bleeds can present with fresh red bleeding PR.

Other features That may be present and indicate a significant bleed (may precede bleeding):
- Faintness or dizziness, especially on standing
- Patient feels cold or clammy
- Collapse ± cardiac arrest

Examination
- Colour—pallor, peripheral cyanosis
- BP, pulse, and JVP—tachycardia, ↓ BP/JVP, and/or postural drop
- Depending on clinical state, perform abdominal ± rectal examination
- If history is suggestive of haemorrhoids/anal fissure, check anus
- Examine any vomitus/stool

Action

- When a call for help is received—arrange immediate emergency transfer of the patient to hospital if a significant acute GI bleed is suspected
- Arrange to see the patient if diagnosis from history or severity of bleed is unclear
- Regard as an emergency until proved otherwise

On assessment Briefly assess the severity of the bleed from history and examination. If a significant GI bleed is suspected:
- Lie the patient flat and lift legs higher than body (e.g. feet on a pillow)
- Insert a large-bore IV cannula—the opportunity may be lost by the time the ambulance crew arrives. If possible take a sample for FBC and cross-match on insertion
- If available, give oxygen
- If available, start IV fluids
- Transfer as rapidly as possible to hospital

Follow up for patients with less severe bleeds Except for patients with haemorrhoids/anal fissure, all patients presenting with GI bleeding, even if the bleeding does not cause any circulatory compromise, require further investigation to establish the cause of the bleeding. Refer urgently to a lower GI team if:
- ≥60y with rectal bleeding persisting ≥6wk without anal symptoms—even without change in bowel habit
- ≥40y with a combination of rectal bleeding persisting ≥6wk, combined with a change in bowel habit towards looser stools/↑ stool frequency

Coffee-ground vomit Vomiting of altered blood—looks like coffee granules. Implies upper GI bleeding—although less severe than fresh red blood. History and examination is as for acute GI bleed. Always admit to hospital for further assessment.

Management in terminally ill patients If a terminally ill patient has a severe, life-threatening bleed, make a decision whether the cause of the bleed is treatable or a terminal event. This is best done in advance, but bleeding cannot always be predicted.

If active treatment is indicated Treat as for acute GI bleeding.

If no active treatment is indicated
- Stay with the patient
- Give sedative medication, e.g. midazolam 20–40mg sc or IV or diazepam 10–20mg PR ± analgesia
- Support carers, as big bleeds are extremely distressing

❶ Unless a patient is very near to death, admit all palliative patients with non-life-threatening GI bleeds related to their underlying condition. Palliative treatment options include laser treatment and arterial embolization—both can be performed on frail patients.

Meningitis and encephalitis[ND]

Meningitis and encephalitis present in similar fashion. Usually rapid onset (<48h). Typical symptoms may be preceded with a prodrome of fever, vomiting, malaise, poor feeding, and lethargy which is often indistinguishable from a viral infection. Particularly significant early signs include:

- Severe leg pain—so bad that the child cannot stand/walk
- Cold hands or feet when the child is running a fever
- Pale skin ± blueness around the lips

Typical symptoms/signs

Meningism
- Headache
- Photophobia
- Stiff neck—cannot put chin on chest
- Kernig's sign +ve—with hips fully flexed, resists passive knee extension

↑ intracranial pressure
- Drowsiness
- Irritability
- ↓ pulse rate
- ↓ consciousness
- Fits
- ↑ BP
- Abnormal tone/ posturing
- Vomiting
- Bulging fontanelle (baby)
- Focal neurological signs

Septicaemia/septic shock
- Fever
- Peripheral shutdown—cool peripheries, mottled skin, cyanosis, capillary refill time >2s
- Arthritis
- Hypotension
- Peripheral oxygen saturation of ≤95%
- Tachycardia
- ± rash—petechiae suggest meningococcus
- Tachypnoea

⚠ Small children or immunocompromised patients may not present with typical signs. Go on gut feeling.

⚠ **Action**

- Call an emergency ambulance and get the patient to hospital as soon as possible
- If shocked, lie the patient flat and raise legs above waist height
- If symptoms/signs of meningococcal disease, give IV/IM benzylpenicillin immediately while awaiting transport. *Dose:*
  - Adult or Child ≥10y—1.2g
  - Child 1–9y—600mg
  - Infant <1y—300mg
- DO NOT delay transfer to hospital to give antibiotics
- Withhold penicillin ONLY if there is a clear history of anaphylaxis in response to a previous dose (a rash following penicillin is not a contraindication). Cefotaxime is an alternative (adult or child >12y— 1g; child <12y—50mg/kg)
- For meningitis without signs of meningococcal disease, only give penicillin if urgent transfer to hospital is not possible
- If possible gain IV access whilst awaiting the ambulance and take blood for cultures. Consider starting IV fluids/plasma expander. Give 10mL/kg rapidly over 10–15min
- If available give 100% oxygen

Contact tracing/prophylaxis for meningococcal disease

- Meningitis and acute encephalitis are notifiable diseases
- Contact tracing is undertaken by the local public health department
- For a single case, only close contacts ('kissing contacts'), e.g. people living in the same household, require prophylactic antibiotics and vaccination

Prophylactic antibiotics

- **Ciprofloxacin** 500mg as a single dose (age 5–12y—250mg; <5y—30mg/kg—maximum 125mg), *or*
- **Rifampicin** 600mg bd for 2d (child 10mg/kg for 2d unless <1y when dose is 5mg/kg bd for 2d). Rifampicin colours urine red

Vaccination Offer close contacts vaccination appropriate to the serotype of the confirmed case.

Late-onset effects Be alert for:

- Hearing loss (formal audiology testing should be organized by the treating hospital)
- Ongoing neurological problems, e.g fits, hemiparesis
- Orthopaedic problems, e.g bone and joint damage, leading to poor limb growth
- Psychosocial effects, e.g learning disability, behavioural difficulties

Meningitis vaccination

- **Group C strains** responsible for 40% of meningococcal disease
- **Group B strains** responsible for most of the rest
- **Group A strains** common in other parts of the world; rare in the UK

Meningitis B vaccination (Bexsero) In the UK, currently only available privately but not through the NHS. Protects against 88% of meningitis B strains. A booster dose is needed after >1mo (>2mo if aged >2y but <11y); children <2y require 3 doses >1mo apart.

Meningococcal A&C vaccine No protection against group B strain. Immunize individuals travelling abroad to high-risk areas with the Meningococcal A&C vaccine, even if they have received the Meningitis C conjugate vaccine beforehand.

Meningitis C conjugate vaccine

- For infants, doses are given at 3mo and 12–13mo as part of the routine childhood vaccination programme
- A booster dose is given at 13–14y (or before starting higher education if no booster at 13–14y)
- Vaccine may be given to HIV +ve patients
- A gap of 6mo is recommended between a dose of the Meningococcal A&C vaccine, usually given for travel purposes, and Meningitis C conjugate vaccine
- Do not use Meningitis C conjugate vaccine for travel purposes as the greatest risk is from group A infection

Further information

NICE Bacterial meningitis and meningococcal septicaemia (2010)
℘ www.nice.org.uk

Telephone helplines for families

Meningitis Research Foundation ☎ 080 8800 3344 ℘ www.meningitis.org
Meningitis Trust ☎ 0808 80 10 338 ℘ www.meningitis-trust.org

Chest pain and palpitations

Chest pain Common symptom.

⚠ Always think—could this be an acute coronary syndrome (ACS), PE, dissecting aneurysm, or pericariditis?

On receiving the call for assistance Ask:
- Nature and location of the pain
- Duration of the pain
- Other associated symptoms—sweating, nausea, shortness of breath, palpitations
- Past medical history (particularly heart disease, high cholesterol)
- Family history (particularly heart disease)
- Smoker?

Action
- Consider differential diagnosis (see Table 29.3)
- If ACS is suspected call for ambulance assistance before (or instead of) visiting
- Otherwise visit (or arrange surgery appointment), assess, and treat according to cause

History Ask about:
- Site and nature of pain. Any history of trauma?
- Duration
- Associated symptoms (e.g. breathlessness, nausea)
- Provoking and relieving factors
- PMH, FH (e.g. heart disease), drug history, smoking history

Examination
- Check BP in both arms
- General appearance—distress, sweating, pallor
- JVP and carotid pulse
- Respiratory rate
- Apex beat
- Heart sounds
- Lung fields
- Local tenderness
- Pain on movement of chest
- Skin rashes
- Swelling or tenderness of legs (? DVT)

Investigations ECG and CXR may be helpful.

Palpitations The uncomfortable awareness of heart beat. Can be physiological (e.g. after exercise, at times of stress) or signify arrhythmia. Can cause a feeling of faintness or even collapse (e.g. Stokes–Adams attack, due to AV block). Ask the patient to tap out the rhythm.
- **Bradycardia** 📖 p. 272
- **Occasional missed beat** Suggests ventricular ectopics—📖 p. 268
- **Tachycardia** 📖 p. 268

Table 29.3 Causes of acute chest pain

Diagnosis	Features
Acute coronary syndrome (📖 p. 1082)	Band-like chest pain around the chest or central chest pressure/dull ache ± radiation to shoulders, arms (L > R), neck, and/or jaw Often associated with nausea, sweating, and/or shortness of breath
Pericarditis (📖 p. 277)	Sharp, constant sternal pain relieved by sitting forward May radiate to left shoulder ± arm or into the abdomen Worse lying on the left side and on inspiration, swallowing, and coughing
Dissecting thoracic aneurysm (📖 p. 1074)	Typically presents with sudden tearing chest pain radiating to the back Consider in any patient with chest pain (especially if radiates through to the back) and ↓ BP
PE (📖 p. 1090)	Acute dyspnoea, sharp chest pain (worse on inspiration), haemoptysis, and/or syncope. Tachycardic and mild pyrexia
Pleurisy	Sharp, localized chest pain, worse on inspiration May be associated with symptoms and signs of a chest infection
Pneumothorax (📖 p. 1090)	Sudden onset of pleuritic chest pain or ↑ breathlessness ± pallor and tachycardia
Oesophageal spasm, oesophagitis	Central chest pain. May be associated with acid reflux (although not always) May be described as burning but often indistinguishable from cardiac pain May respond to antacids
Musculoskeletal pain	Localized pain—worse on movement May be a history of injury
Shingles	Intense, often sharp, unilateral pain Responds poorly to analgesia May be present several days before rash appears
Costochondritis	Inflammation of the costochondral junctions – tenderness over the costochondral junction and pain in the affected area on springing the chest wall
Bornholm's disease	Unilateral chest and/or abdominal pain, rhinitis. Coxsackie virus infection. Treat with simple analgesia
Idiopathic chest pain	No cause apparent. Common Affects young people > elderly people. ♀ > ♂

⚠ If a patient is acutely unwell with chest pain and the cause is not clear, err on the side of caution and admit for further assessment.

Acute coronary syndrome

The term acute coronary syndrome (ACS) covers:
- **Myocardial infarction** Both ST segment elevation MI (STEMI) and non-ST segment elevation MI (NSTEMI), and
- **Unstable angina**

Initial primary care management is the same for STEMI, NSTEMI, and unstable angina.

Presentation May be new onset or a rapid deterioration in stable angina. Presenting features include:
- Sustained central chest pain (>15min)—typically described as central crushing/pressure, band-like pain
- Pain radiating to the arms, jaw, back, or upper abdomen (may be the only symptom)
- Symptoms resulting from sympathetic autonomic stimulation, e.g. nausea, vomiting, sweating
- Symptoms relating to shock, e.g. breathlessness, hypotension, collapse

Other factors to consider
- Does the patient have risk factors for cardiac disease?
- Has the patient had previous investigations for chest pain? If so, what investigations were done, when, and what were the results?
- Does the patient have a history of ischaemic heart disease? If so, what is the current treatment and what has been tried in the past?

⚠ Diagnosis of acute coronary syndrome (ACS) is sometimes difficult (e.g. patients with DM may have silent MI): have a high index of suspicion.

Examination Pulse, BP, JVP, heart sounds, chest (? pulmonary oedema).

ECG Do not do an ECG if it delays transfer of the patient to hospital. Normal ECG does not exclude ACS. If an ECG is done, fax it to the receiving hospital. ECG changes—see Table 29.4.

Action

When the call for assistance is made If ACS is suspected, arrange immediate transfer to hospital. For reperfusion interventions (thrombolysis or percutaneous coronary intervention) to be effective, they must be carried out as soon as possible after the onset of pain. Seeing the patient before arranging transfer introduces unnecessary delays.

If possible attend the patient once the ambulance has been called:
- Give pain relief with either sublingual GTN or IV/IM opioid (e.g. morphine 5–10mg—half dose if elderly/frail) or both
- Give aspirin 300mg po (unless contraindicated)
- Consider giving IV/IM antiemetic (e.g. metoclopramide 10mg)
- Measure oxygen saturation with pulse oximeter—only give oxygen if saturations are <94%. Aim for saturations of 94–98% (88–92% if known COPD and at risk of CO_2 retention)
- If bradycardia, consider giving atropine 500 micrograms IV and further doses of 500 micrograms if needed to a maximum of 3mg

❗ To avoid inadvertent replication of medication when the patient reaches hospital, record all drugs that have been given (name of the drug, dose and route of administration, time administered). Send this information to hospital with the patient.

Table 29.4 Features of STEMI, NSTEMI, and unstable angina

	STEMI	NSTEMI	Unstable angina
Chest pain present?	Yes	Yes	Yes
ECG changes	ST elevation (≥1mm in ≥2 adjacent limb leads or ≥2mm in ≥2 adjacent anterior chest leads) or New LBBB	Normal or Signs of myocardial ischaemia: • ST segment depression • T wave inversion/ flattening	Normal or Signs of myocardial ischaemia: • ST segment depression • T wave inversion/ flattening
Troponin levels*	Raised	Raised	Normal

* Usually done in hospital. Indicates myocardial muscle necrosis. Becomes +ve 3–6h after onset of pain and may remain +ve for 7–14d.

Thrombolysis in general practice May be appropriate in places where transfer to hospital takes >30min. Special training and equipment are needed.

Late calls If the patient is seen pain-free after an acute episode.

Admit as an emergency if the patient
- Has signs of complications that require emergency admission (e.g. pulmonary oedema)
- Is seen <12h after the acute episode and the ECG is abnormal or ECG is unavailable

Arrange same day specialist assessment if the patient
- Is seen <12h after the acute episode, is well and ECG is normal
- Is seen 12–72h after the acute episode and there are no reasons for immediate emergency admission

If the patient is seen >72h after an acute episode and is well Assess clinically, perform ECG, and arrange blood test for troponin. Refer to cardiology for routine follow-up/more urgently, depending on the clinical situation. For patients with new-onset chest pain, most areas run rapid access chest pain clinics.

In the interim, start regular aspirin; supply with GTN spray, and warn to call for assistance (by calling ambulance and/or emergency GP) if chest pain lasts >15min despite GTN spray.

Further information
NICE Chest pain of recent onset (2011) ℘ www.nice.org.uk

The choking adult

⚠ If blockage of the airway is only partial, the victim will usually be able to dislodge the foreign body by coughing. If obstruction is complete, urgent intervention is required to prevent asphyxia (see Figure 29.12).

Is foreign body airways obstruction (FBAO) likely?
- Sudden onset of respiratory distress whilst eating?
- Is the victim clutching his neck?

Is the patient coughing effectively?

Signs of an effective cough include
- In response to the question 'Are you choking?' the victim answers and says 'Yes'
- Fully responsive—able to speak, cough, and breathe
▶▶ Encourage the victim to cough, and monitor.

Signs of an ineffective cough include
- In response to the question 'Are you choking?' the victim either responds by nodding or is unable to respond
- Breathing sounds wheezy
- Unable to breathe
- Attempts at coughing are silent
- Unconscious
▶▶ Call for assistance (e.g. dial 999) and assess conscious level.

If victim IS conscious but has absent/ineffective coughing
- Give up to 5 back blows as needed
- If back blows do not relieve the obstruction, give up to 5 abdominal thrusts as needed

Following back blows or abdominal thrusts Reassess:
- **If the object has not been expelled and the victim is still conscious** Continue the sequence of back blows and abdominal thrusts
- **If the object is expelled successfully** Assess clinical condition (including abdominal examination if abdominal thrusts used). If there is any suspicion part of the object is still in the respiratory tract or there are any intra-abdominal injuries as a result of abdominal thrusts, refer to A&E for assessment

If the victim becomes UNCONSCIOUS
- Support the victim carefully to the ground
- Immediately call an ambulance
- Begin CPR (📖 p. 1054), with 30 chest compressions at a rate of 100–120/min—even if carotid pulse is present

Foreign body in the throat Occurs after eating—fish bone or food bolus are most common. Can cause severe discomfort, distress, and inability to swallow saliva.

Management Refer immediately to A&E or ENT for investigation (lateral neck X-ray ± laryngoscopy). Most fish bones have passed and the discomfort comes from mucosal trauma. Food boluses often pass spontaneously (especially if the patient is given a smooth muscle relaxant) but occasionally need removal under GA.

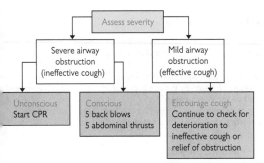

Figure 29.12 Algorithm for the management of choking in adults

Figure 29.12 is reproduced with permission from the Resuscitation guidelines (2010) ℰ www.resus.org.uk

Back blows for adults
- Stand to the side and slightly behind the victim
- Support the chest with 1 hand and lean the victim well forwards so that when the obstructing object is dislodged it comes out of the mouth
- Give up to 5 sharp blows between the shoulder blades with the heel of the other hand

Abdominal thrusts for adults
- Stand behind the victim and put both arms around the upper part of the abdomen
- Lean the victim forwards
- Clench your fist and place it between the umbilicus and bottom end of the sternum
- Grasp this hand with your other hand and pull sharply inwards and upwards. Repeat up to 5 times as needed

Further information
Resuscitation Council (UK) Resuscitation guidelines (2010)
ℰ www.resus.org.uk

The choking child

⚠ If the child is breathing spontaneously, encourage his own efforts to clear the obstruction. ONLY intervene if ineffective (see Figure 29.13).

Is foreign body airways obstruction (FBAO) likely? Look for:
- Sudden onset of respiratory distress in a previously well child—often witnessed by the child's carer
- Respiratory distress associated with coughing, gagging, or stridor
- Recent history of playing with or eating small objects

Is the child coughing effectively?

Signs of an effective cough include
- Fully responsive—crying or verbal response to questions
- Loud cough and able to take a breath before coughing
- ▶▶ Encourage the child to cough and monitor.

Signs of an ineffective cough include
- Unable to vocalize
- Quiet or silent cough
- Unable to breathe ± cyanosis
- Decreasing level of consciousness
- ▶▶ Call for assistance (e.g. dial 999), and assess conscious level.

If the child IS conscious but has absent/ineffective coughing Give up to 5 back blows as needed. If back blows do not relieve the obstruction, give up to 5 chest thrusts (infants <1y) *or* up to 5 abdominal thrusts (children ≥1y) as needed. Then reassess:
- **If the object has *not* been expelled and the victim is still conscious** Continue the sequence of back blows and chest (for infant) or abdominal (for children) thrusts. ❶ Do not leave the child
- **If the object is expelled successfully** Assess clinical condition (including abdominal examination if abdominal thrusts used). If there is any suspicion part of the object is still in the respiratory tract or there are any intra-abdominal injuries as a result of abdominal thrusts, refer to A&E

If the child is UNCONSCIOUS ❶ Do not leave the child.
- Place on a firm, flat surface—call out/send for help if not arrived
- Open the mouth and look for any obvious object. If one is seen, make an attempt to remove it with a single finger sweep
- Open the airway and attempt 5 rescue breaths. Assess effectiveness of each breath—if a breath does not make the chest rise, reposition the head before making the next attempt
- If there is no response to the rescue breaths, proceed immediately to chest compression—regardless of whether the breaths were successful. Follow the PBLS sequence (📖 p. 1060) for 1min before summoning help if not already there

If it appears the obstruction has been relieved Open and check the airway. Deliver rescue breaths if the child is not breathing. If the child regains consciousness and is breathing effectively, place him in a safe side-lying (recovery) position, and monitor breathing and conscious level whilst awaiting the arrival of the emergency services.

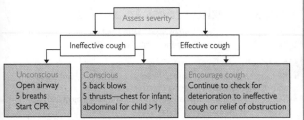

Figure 29.13 Algorithm for management of paediatric foreign body airway obstruction (PFBAO)

Figure 29.13 is reproduced with permission from the Resuscitation guidelines (2010) ℘ www.resus.org.uk

Back blows for small children/infants
- Place the child in a head-downwards, prone position (e.g. across your lap). Support the head if needed by holding the jaw
- Deliver a smart blow with the heel of one hand to the middle of the back between the shoulder blades. Repeat up to 5 times as needed

Back blows for older children
- Support the child in a forward-leaning position
- Deliver a smart blow with the heel of one hand to the middle of the back between the shoulder blades from behind. Repeat up to 5 times as needed

Chest thrusts for infants <1y
- Turn the child into a supine position with head down (e.g. by holding the child's occiput and laying the child along your arm, supported on your thigh)
- Deliver 5 sharp chest thrusts (like chest compressions but slower rate ~20/min) to a point 1 finger's breadth above the xiphisternum

Abdominal thrusts for children ≥1y
- Stand behind the child (kneel if small child). Place your arms under the child's arms and encircle his torso
- Clench your fist and place it between the umbilicus and xiphisternum
- Grasp your clenched hand with your other hand and pull sharply inwards and upwards. Repeat up to 5 times as needed

❶ Ensure that pressure is not applied to the xiphoid process or the lower rib cage as this may cause abdominal trauma.

Further information
Resuscitation Council (UK) Resuscitation guidelines (2010)
℘ www.resus.org.uk

Acute breathlessness in adults

Attend as soon as possible after receiving the call for help. If there is likely to be any delay, call for emergency ambulance assistance.

On arrival
- Be calm and reassuring—breathlessness is frightening and panic only adds to the sensation of being breathless
- Direct history and examination to finding the cause as quickly as possible—treat according to the cause
- If no cause can be found—do not delay—admit to hospital as an acute medical emergency

Causes See Table 29.5.

Acute left ventricular failure (acute LVF) Severe acute breathlessness due to pulmonary oedema. Urgent action is needed to save life.

Presenting features
- Sudden acute breathlessness
- Fatigue
- Cough ± haemoptysis (usually pink and frothy)
- Tends to occur at night
- Some relief gained from sitting/standing

Signs
- Dyspnoea
- Tachycardia—gallop rhythm may be present
- Coarse wet-sounding crackles at both bases
- Ankle/sacral oedema if right heart failure also present
- ± hypotension

Action
- If severe call for emergency ambulance support
- Sit the patient up
- Be reassuring—it is very frightening to be very short of breath
- Give oxygen if available—aim for peripheral oxygen saturations of 94–98% (if history of COPD give 24% oxygen and aim for saturations of 88–92%)
- Give IV furosemide 20–50mg slowly (or bumetanide 1–2mg)
- Give IV morphine 5–10mg or diamorphine 2.5–5mg over 5min
- Give metoclopramide 10mg IV (can be mixed with morphine/diamorphine)
- Give GTN spray 2 puffs sublingually

Admission Depends on severity and cause of attack, response to treatment, and social support. *Always admit if:*
- Alone at home
- Inadequate social support
- Suspected cause of acute LVF warrants admission (e.g. acute MI)
- Very breathless and no improvement over 30min with treatment at home
- Hypotension or arrhythmia

Table 29.5 Causes of acute breathlessness

Diagnosis	Features
Asthma 📖 p. 1092	Breathlessness and wheeze. Usually in association with a past history of asthma, though can present de novo *Signs of a severe attack include:* inability to speak in sentences, tachycardia, pulsus paradoxus, ↑ respiratory rate, use of accessory muscles of respiration, drowsiness or exhaustion
Anaphylaxis 📖 p. 1072	One or both of: • Respiratory difficulty, e.g. wheeze, stridor • Hypotension *Other features may include:* erythema, angio-oedema, generalized pruritus and/or itching of the palate and/or external auditory meatus, rhinitis, nausea ± vomiting, palpitations, urticaria, conjunctivitis, sense of impending doom
Acute left ventricular failure	**Symptoms** Sudden acute breath-lessness Fatigue Cough ± haemoptysis Tends to occur at night Some relief from sitting/standing	**Signs** Dyspnoea Tachycardia ± gallop rhythm Coarse crackles at both bases Ankle/sacral oedema if right heart failure also present ± hypotension
Arrhythmia 📖 p. 268–73	Usually palpitations (although not always) associated with chest pain, collapse or funny turns, sweating, breathlessness, and/or hyperventilation. May be a PMH/FH of similar symptoms or thyroid disease
PE 📖 p. 1090	Acute dyspnoea, sharp chest pain (worse on inspiration), haemoptysis, and/or syncope. Tachycardic and mild pyrexia
Acute exacerbation of COPD 📖 p. 318	Worsening of previously stable COPD. Presents with ≥1 of: ↑ dyspnoea ↓ exercise tolerance ↑ fatigue ↑ fluid retention ↑ wheeze Chest tightness ↑ cough ↑ sputum purulence ↑ sputum volume Upper airways symptoms, e.g. cold, sore throat New-onset cyanosis Acute confusion
Pneumonia 📖 p. 324	Breathlessness, cough, fever, sputum, ± sharp, localized chest pain, worse on inspiration
Pneumothorax 📖 p. 1090	Sudden onset of pleuritic chest pain or ↑ breathlessness ± pallor and tachycardia
Choking 📖 p. 1084	Think of aspirated foreign bodies in any history of sudden onset of stridor or symptoms of respiratory distress
SVC obstruction 📖 p. 1040	Acute breathlessness, headache worse on stooping, swelling of the face and/or neck with fixed elevation of JVP—admit for assessment
Air hunger due to shock 📖 p. 1074	Inadequate blood flow to the peripheral circulation—usually associated with ↓ BP (± tachycardia) and peripheral cyanosis
Hyperventilation 📖 p. 1120	Breathlessness associated with fear, terror, and a sense of impending doom

Pulmonary embolism and pneumothorax

Pulmonary embolism Venous thrombi—usually from a deep vein thrombosis in the leg—pass into the pulmonary circulation and block blood flow to the lungs. Without treatment 20% with proximal deep vein thrombosis develop pulmonary embolus (PE). PE is listed as a cause of death on 12,000–13,000 death certificates every year in the UK.

Risk factors

- Immobility—long flight or bus journey, post-op, plaster cast
- Smoking
- Combined hormonal contraception
- Pregnancy or puerperium
- Malignancy
- Past history or family history of DVT, PE, or clotting tendency

Symptoms Acute dyspnoea, pleuritic chest pain, haemoptysis, syncope. Large clots can be rapidly fatal.

Signs

- Hypotension
- Tachycardia
- Cyanosis
- ↑ JVP
- Tachypnoea
- Pleural rub

Look for a source of emboli—although DVT may not be clinically obvious.

⚠ Have a high level of suspicion. Patients may have minimal symptoms/ signs apart from some pleuritic pain and dyspnoea. PE in the community can be linked with surgical procedures done 2–3wk previously.

Differential diagnosis

- Pneumonia and pleurisy
- Acute coronary syndrome
- Other causes of acute breathlessness—acute LVF, asthma, exacerbation of COPD, pneumothorax, shock (e.g. due to anaphylaxis), arrhythmia, hyperventilation
- Other causes of acute chest pain—aortic dissection, rib fracture, musculoskeletal chest pain, pericarditis, oesophageal spasm, shingles

Immediate action If suspected, give oxygen as soon as possible (aim to keep SpO$_2$ at 94–98%) and admit as an acute medical emergency.

Further management In all cases of proven PE, anticoagulation is started in hospital or by a hospital-at-home service before discharge to general practice. Warfarin should be continued for ≥3mo. Aim to keep the INR ~2.5 (range 2–3).

Spontaneous pneumothorax Risk factors:
- Previous pneumothorax
- Smoking
- Ascent in an aeroplane
- Diving

Cause
- **In patients <40y** Usually due to rupture of a pleural bleb. The typical patient is tall, thin, and male ($\male:\female \approx 6:1$)
- **Patients >40y** Usually due to COPD (70–80%)
- **Rarer causes** Asthma, pneumonia, TB, lung cancer, pulmonary fibrosis

Presentation Sudden onset of pleuritic chest pain or ↑ breathlessness ± pallor and tachycardia. Look for resonant percussion note, ↓ or absent breath sounds—signs may be absent if the pneumothorax is small.

Management
- Refer for same-day CXR
- If pneumothorax is confirmed, seek specialist advice about further management
- Small pneumothoraces usually resolve spontaneously (50% collapse takes ~40d to resorb)—monitor until completely resolved
- Larger pneumothoraces may require admission for aspiration or a chest drain
- Smoking cessation ↓ risk of recurrence

Traumatic pneumothorax Trauma may not initially be obvious—ask about injections around the chest area, e.g. acupuncture (to neck and shoulders as well as chest); aspiration of breast lump, etc. Presentation and management is as for spontaneous pneumothorax.

Tension pneumothorax Complication of traumatic pneumothorax; rare after spontaneous pneumothorax. A valvular mechanism develops—air is sucked into the pleural space during inspiration but cannot be expelled during expiration. The pressure within the pleural space ↑ and the lung deflates further; the mediastinum shifts to the opposite side of the chest, and venous return ↓. Can be rapidly fatal.

Clinical features
- Agitated and distressed patient, often with a history of chest trauma
- Tachycardia
- Sweating
- Signs of a large pneumothorax—↓ breath sounds and ↓ chest movement on the affected side
- Mediastinal shift—trachea deviated away from the side of the pneumothorax

Action If tension pneumothorax is suspected:
- Sit the patient upright if possible
- Insert a large-bore cannula through the 2nd intercostal space of the chest wall in the mid-clavicular line on the side of the pneumothorax to relieve the pressure in the pleural space
- Transfer as an emergency to hospital

Acute asthma in adults

Many deaths from asthma are preventable. Delay can be fatal. Factors leading to poor outcome include:
- Doctors failing to assess severity by objective measurement
- Patients or relatives failing to appreciate severity
- Underuse of corticosteroids

⚠ Regard each emergency asthma consultation as acute severe asthma until proven otherwise.

Risk factors for developing fatal or near-fatal asthma

A combination of severe asthma recognized by ≥1 of
- Previous near-fatal asthma
- Previous admission for asthma—especially if within 1y
- Requiring ≥3 classes of asthma medication
- Heavy use of β_2-agonist
- Repeated attendances at A&E for asthma care—especially if within 1y
- Brittle asthma

and adverse behavioural or psychosocial features recognized by ≥1 of
- Non-compliance with treatment or monitoring
- Failure to attend appointments
- Self-discharge from hospital
- Psychosis, depression, other psychiatric illness, or deliberate self-harm
- Current or recent major tranquillizer use
- Denial
- Alcohol or drug misuse
- Obesity
- Learning difficulties
- Employment/income problems
- Social isolation
- Childhood abuse
- Severe marital/legal/domestic stress

Assess and record
- Peak expiratory flow rate (PEFR)
- Symptoms and response to self-treatment
- Heart and respiratory rates
- Oxygen saturation by pulse oximetry (if available)

⚠ Patients with severe or life-threatening attacks may not be distressed and may not have all the characteristic abnormalities of severe asthma. The presence of any should alert the doctor.

Levels of severity of acute asthma exacerbations

Moderate asthma exacerbation
- Increasing symptoms
- PEFR >50 to 75% predicted
- No features of acute severe asthma

Acute severe asthma Any one of:
- PEFR 33–50% best or predicted
- Respiratory rate ≥25 breaths/min
- Heart rate ≥110/min
- Inability to complete sentences in 1 breath

Life-threatening asthma Any 1 of the following with severe asthma:
- PEFR <33% best/predicted
- O_2 saturation <92%
- Silent chest
- Cyanosis
- Feeble respiratory effort
- Bradycardia
- Dysrhythmia
- Hypotension
- Exhaustion
- Confusion
- Coma

Near-fatal asthma Respiratory acidosis and/or requiring mechanical ventilation with ↑ inflation pressures.

Brittle asthma
- **Type 1** Wide PEFR variability (>40% diurnal variation for >50% of the time for a period of >150d) despite intense therapy
- **Type 2** Sudden severe attacks on a background of apparently well-controlled asthma

Management See Figure 29.14, 🕮 p. 1094

Admit to hospital if
- Life-threatening features
- Features of acute severe asthma present after initial treatment
- Previous near-fatal asthma

Lower threshold for admission if
- Afternoon or evening attack
- Recent nocturnal symptoms or hospital admission
- Previous severe attacks
- Patient unable to assess own condition
- Concern over social circumstances

If admitting the patient to hospital
- Stay with the patient until the ambulance arrives
- Send written assessment and referral details to the hospital
- Give β_2 bronchodilator via an oxygen-driven nebulizer in the ambulance

Follow-up after treatment or discharge from hospital
- GP review within 48h
- Monitor symptoms and PEFR
- Check inhaler technique
- Written asthma action plan
- Modify treatment according to guidelines for chronic persistent asthma
- Address potentially preventable contributors to admission

Further information
BTS/SIGN British guideline on the management of asthma (2011 with 2012 update) ✆ www.sign.ac.uk

Moderate asthma	Acute severe asthma	Life-threatening asthma
INITIAL ASSESSMENT		
PEFR >50% to 75% best or predicted	PEFR 33–50% best or predicted	PEFR <33% best or predicted
FURTHER ASSESSMENT		
SpO_2 ≥92% Speech normal Respiration <25 breaths/min Pulse <110 beats/min	SpO_2 ≥92% Cannot complete sentences Respiration ≥25 breaths/min Pulse ≥110 beats/min	SpO_2 <92% Silent chest, cyanosis, or poor respiratory effort Arrhythmia or hypotension Exhaustion, altered consciousness
MANAGEMENT		
Treat at home or in the surgery *and* ASSESS RESPONSE TO TREATMENT	Consider admission	Arrange immediate admission
TREATMENT		
β_2 bronchodilator: Via spacer—give 4 puffs initially (1 puff and 5 tidal breaths through spacer x4) and a further 2 puffs every 2min according to response to a maximum of 10 puffs or Nebulizer (preferably oxygen-driven) — 5mg salbutamol or 10mg terbutaline **Steroid** — prednisolone 40–50mg po **If good response to initial treatment** (symptoms improved, respiration and pulse settling, and PEFR >50%) continue or step up usual treatment and continue prednisolone for 5d	**Oxygen** (if available) to maintain SpO_2 94–98% β_2 bronchodilator: Nebulizer (preferably oxygen-driven)—5mg salbutamol or 10mg terbutaline or Via spacer—give 4 puffs initially and a further 2 puffs every 2min according to response to a maximum of 10 puffs **Steroid**—prednisolone 40–50mg po or hydrocortisone 100mg IV **If no response in acute severe asthma—ADMIT**	**Oxygen** (if available) to maintain SpO_2 94–98% β_2 bronchodilator and ipratropium: Nebulizer (preferably oxygen-driven) — 5mg salbutamol or 10mg terbutaline, and 0.5mg ipratropium or Via spacer — give 4 puffs initially and a further 2 puffs every 2min according to response to a maximum of 10 puffs **Steroid** — prednisolone 40–50mg po or hydrocortisone 100mg IV **ADMIT**

Figure 29.14 Management of acute severe asthma in adults

Figure 29.14 is modified from the British guideline on the management of asthma (2011) with permission from SIGN/British Thoracic Society.

Acute asthma in children

Assess and record
- Pulse rate—increasing heart rate generally reflects ↑ severity
- Respiratory rate and breathlessness
- Use of accessory muscles—best noted by palpation of neck muscles
- Amount of wheezing
- Degree of agitation and conscious level

Levels of severity
Child >5y See Figure 29.15, 📖 p. 1096
Child 2–5y See Figure 29.16, 📖 p. 1097

Child <2y Assessment of children <2y can be difficult.
- **Moderate asthma**
  - SpO_2 ≥92%
  - Audible wheezing
  - Using accessory muscles
  - Still feeding
- **Severe asthma**
  - SpO_2 <92%
  - Cyanosis
  - Marked respiratory distress
  - Too breathless to feed
- **Life-threatening asthma**
  - Apnoea
  - Bradycardia
  - Poor respiratory effort

⚠ If a patient has signs and symptoms across categories, always treat according to the most severe features.

Management
Child >5y See Figure 29.15, 📖 p. 1096
Child 2–5y See Figure 29.16, 📖 p. 1097

Child <2y Intermittent wheezing attacks are usually in response to viral infection, and response to bronchodilators is inconsistent.
- **If mild/moderate wheeze**
  - A trial of bronchodilators can be considered if symptoms are of concern—use a metered dose inhaler and spacer with a face mask
  - If no response consider alternative diagnosis (aspiration pneumonitis, pneumonia, bronchiolitis, tracheomalacia, CF, congenital anomaly) and/or admit
- **If severe wheezing** Admit to hospital
- **If any life-threatening features** Admit immediately as a blue light emergency

Follow-up after treatment or discharge from hospital
- GP review within 1wk
- Monitor symptoms, PEFR, and check inhaler technique
- Written asthma action plan
- Modify treatment according to guidelines for chronic persistent asthma
- Address potentially preventable contributors to admission

ASSESS ASTHMA SEVERITY		
Moderate exacerbation	**Severe exacerbation**	**Life-threatening asthma**
SpO$_2$ ≥92% PEFR ≥50% best or predicted Able to talk Heart rate ≤125/min Respiratory rate ≤30/min	SpO$_2$ <92% PEFR 33–50% best or predicted Too breathless to talk Heart rate >125/min Respiratory rate >30/min Use of accessory neck muscles	SpO$_2$ <92% plus any of: PEFR <33% best or predicted Silent chest Poor respiratory effort Agitation Altered consciousness Cyanosis
β$_2$-agonist 2–10 puffs via spacer (2 puffs every 2min according to response up to a maximum of 10 puffs) **Steroid**—consider soluble prednisolone 30–40mg po	**Oxygen** via face mask **β$_2$-agonist** 2–10 puffs via spacer (2 puffs every 2min according to response up to a maximum of 10 puffs) or Nebulized salbutamol 2.5–5mg or terbutaline 5–10mg **Steroid**—soluble prednisolone 30–40mg po Assess response to treatment 15min after β$_2$-agonist	**Oxygen** via face mask **Nebulize:** • Salbutamol 5mg or terbutaline 10mg + • Ipratropium 0.25mg **Steroid**—soluble prednisolone 30–40mg po or IV hydrocortisone 100mg
IF POOR RESPONSE ARRANGE ADMISSION	**IF POOR RESPONSE REPEAT β$_2$-AGONIST AND ARRANGE ADMISSION**	**REPEAT β$_2$ AGONIST VIA OXYGEN-DRIVEN NEBULIZER WHILST ARRANGING IMMEDIATE HOSPITAL ADMISSION**
GOOD RESPONSE Continue β$_2$-agonist via spacer or nebulizer as needed (maximum every 4h) If symptoms are not controlled repeat β$_2$-agonist and refer to hospital Continue prednisolone for up to 3d Arrange follow-up clinic visit	**POOR RESPONSE** Stay with the patient until the ambulance arrives Send written assessment and referral details Repeat β$_2$-agonist via oxygen-driven nebulizer in the ambulance	

Figure 29.15 Management of acute asthma in children aged >5y

Figures 29.15 and 29.16 are modified from the British guideline on the management of asthma (2011) with permission from SIGN/British Thoracic Society

⚠ *Lower threshold for admission if*
- Attack in late afternoon or at night
- Recent hospital admission or previous severe attack
- Concern over social circumstances or ability to cope at home

ASSESS ASTHMA SEVERITY		
Moderate exacerbation	**Severe exacerbation**	**Life-threatening asthma**
SpO$_2$ ≥92% Able to talk Heart rate ≤140/min Respiratory rate ≤40/min	SpO$_2$ <92% Too breathless to talk Heart rate >140/min Respiratory rate >40/min Use of accessory neck muscles	SpO$_2$ <92% plus any of: Silent chest Poor respiratory effort Agitation Altered consciousness Cyanosis
β$_2$-agonist 2–10 puffs via spacer ± face mask (2 puffs every 2min according to response up to a maximum of 10 puffs) **Steroid**—consider soluble prednisolone 20mg po	**Oxygen** via face mask **β$_2$-agonist** 2–10 puffs via spacer ± face mask (2 puffs every 2min according to response up to a maximum of 10 puffs) or Nebulized salbutamol 2.5mg or terbutaline 5mg **Steroid**—soluble prednisolone 20mg po Assess response to treatment 15min after β$_2$-agonist	**Oxygen** via face mask **Nebulize:** • Salbutamol 2.5mg or terbutaline 5mg + • Ipratropium 0.25mg **Steroid**—soluble prednisolone 20mg po or IV hydrocortisone 50mg
IF POOR RESPONSE ARRANGE ADMISSION	**IF POOR RESPONSE REPEAT β$_2$-AGONIST AND ARRANGE ADMISSION**	**REPEAT β$_2$-AGONIST VIA OXYGEN-DRIVEN NEBULIZER WHILST ARRANGING IMMEDIATE HOSPITAL ADMISSION**

GOOD RESPONSE	**POOR RESPONSE**
Continue β$_2$ agonist via spacer or nebulizer as needed (maximum every 4h) If symptoms are not controlled, repeat β$_2$ agonist and refer to hospital Continue prednisolone for up to 3d Arrange follow-up clinic visit	Stay with the patient until the ambulance arrives Send written assessment and referral details Repeat β$_2$-agonist via oxygen-driven nebulizer in the ambulance

Figure 29.16 Management of acute asthma in children aged 2–5y

⚠ *Lower threshold for admission if*
• Attack in late afternoon or at night
• Recent hospital admission or previous severe attack
• Concern over social circumstances or ability to cope at home

Further information

BTS/SIGN British guideline on the management of asthma (2011 with 2012 update) ℘ www.sign.ac.uk

Acute abdominal pain

❶ Signs may be masked in elderly patients or those on corticosteroids. Small children with abdominal pain are difficult to assess.

History Consider:
- **S**ite of pain—see Figure 29.17
- **O**nset: how long? How did it start? Change over time?
- **C**haracter of pain: type of pain—burning, shooting, stabbing, dull etc.
- **R**adiation
- **A**ssociated symptoms, e.g nausea, vomiting, diarrhoea
- **T**iming/pattern, e.g. constant, colicky, relationship to food
- **E**xacerbating and relieving factors, including previous treatments tried and results
- **S**everity

Examination
- Temperature
- Pulse
- BP
- Jaundice
- Anaemia
- Site of pain (see Figure 29.17)
- Guarding/rebound tenderness
- Rectal/vaginal examination as necessary

Management Treat the cause (see Table 29.6)—if unsure admit as a surgical emergency to hospital. If possible, give analgesia prior to transfer to hospital.

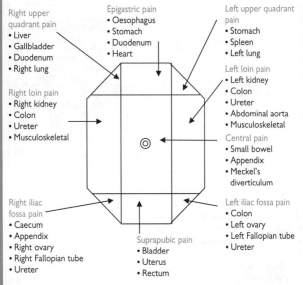

Right upper quadrant pain
- Liver
- Gallbladder
- Duodenum
- Right lung

Epigastric pain
- Oesophagus
- Stomach
- Duodenum
- Heart

Left upper quadrant pain
- Stomach
- Spleen
- Left lung

Right loin pain
- Right kidney
- Colon
- Ureter
- Musculoskeletal

Left loin pain
- Left kidney
- Colon
- Ureter
- Abdominal aorta
- Musculoskeletal

Central pain
- Small bowel
- Appendix
- Meckel's diverticulum

Right iliac fossa pain
- Caecum
- Appendix
- Right ovary
- Right Fallopian tube
- Ureter

Suprapubic pain
- Bladder
- Uterus
- Rectum

Left iliac fossa pain
- Colon
- Left ovary
- Left Fallopian tube
- Ureter

Figure 29.17 Site of abdominal pain gives important clues about the organ involved

Table 29.6 Differential diagnosis of acute abdominal pain

Renal and gynaecological causes

Renal colic	p. 444	Dysmenorrhoea	p. 714
UTI/pyelonephritis	p. 448	Endometriosis	p. 716
Hydronephrosis	p. 454	Pelvic inflammatory disease	p. 738
Henoch–Schönlein purpura	p. 526	Ovarian torsion/bleed/ rupture	
Ectopic pregnancy	p. 816	Gynaecological malignancy	

GI causes

Irritable bowel syndrome	p. 418	Perforated bowel	
Constipation	p. 378	Appendicitis	p. 394
Diverticular disease	p. 401	Meckel's diverticulum	p. 395
Gallbladder disease	p. 428	Pancreatitis	p. 430
Liver disease		Bowel obstruction	p. 400
Inflammatory bowel disease	p. 414	Intussusception	p. 895
Gastroenteritis	p. 410	Strangulated hernia	p. 392
Gastritis	p. 387	Volvulus	p. 400
Peptic ulcer	p. 388	GI malignancy	

Other causes

Spinal arthritis	p. 476	Mesenteric adenitis	p. 394
Muscular pain		Acute coronary syndrome	p. 1082
Heart failure	p. 262	Pneumonia	p. 324
Sickle cell crisis	p. 669	Subphrenic abscess	p. 394
Ruptured spleen		DM—ketoacidosis	p. 1100
Torsion of the testis	p. 466	Porphyria	p. 625
Leaking/ruptured AAA	p. 1074	Addison's disease	p. 368
Shingles/post-herpetic neuralgia	p. 653	Lead poisoning	

Acute abdominal pain in pregnancy p. 1102

Ruptured spleen May occur immediately following trauma or present days/weeks later. Diseased spleens (e.g. glandular fever, malaria, leukaemia) rupture more easily.

Presentation
- History of abdominal trauma
- Blood loss: tachycardia, ↓ BP ± postural drop, pallor
- Peritoneal irritation: guarding, abdominal rigidity, shoulder tip pain
- Paralytic ileus: abdominal distension, lack of bowel sounds

⚠ *Action* If suspected, admit as a blue light surgical emergency.

Endocrine emergencies

Hypoglycaemia Known diabetic on oral/insulin therapy. Short history. May present with coma, fits or odd/violent behaviour, tachycardia ± ↑ BP. There may or may not have been warning signs/symptoms—sweating, hunger, tremor. ❶ Younger children may present atypically with behavioural changes or headache.

Investigation Blood sugar (on blood testing strip) <2.5mmol/L.

⚠ **Action**
- If conscious give simple carbohydrate, e.g. 3 glucose tablets, 100mL of milk or a sugar-containing soft drink, e.g. Lucozade®, 5 sweets (e.g. Jelly Babies®), or GlucoGel®
- If unable to take oral carbohydrate—give IM glucagon 1mg (children <25kg—0.5mg)—takes ≤5min to act—may have poor effect if the patient is starved or drunk—*or* IV glucose (adult: 50–250mL of 10% solution in 50mL aliquots; child: 2–5mL/kg of 10% solution)
- Once the patient has regained consciousness supplement with simple carbohydrate as for the conscious patient and, as symptoms improve give complex carbohydrate, e.g. biscuits
- Repeat glucose testing in <15min then monitor hourly blood sugars over the next 4 hours and 4-hourly for the following 24h
- Maintain a high glucose intake for several hours if the patient has a severe episode of hypoglycaemia due to a sulfonylurea
- Review reasons for the hypoglycaemia

Hyperglycaemic ketoacidotic coma Usually occurs in patients with type 1 DM but may rarely occur in patients with type 2 DM. May be the way in which DM presents (i.e. can occur in young patients not known to be diabetic). Presents with a 2–3d history of deterioration often precipitated by infection. Typically the patient is dehydrated with Kussmaul breathing (deep sighing breaths), ketotic (fruity) smelling breath, shock (↓ BP and postural drop, tachycardia) ± coma. ⚠ Can present with vomiting and abdominal pain mimicking acute abdomen—always check for ketotic breath and Kussmaul breathing.

Investigation BM is usually >20mmol/L and urine (if available) tests +ve for ketones.

⚠ **Action** Arrange to admit as an emergency to hospital. If shocked/coma—lie flat, elevate feet, and resuscitate:
- Airway—check airway is clear
- Breathing—give O_2 if available to maintain SpO_2 at 94–98%
- Circulation—gain IV access if possible and give 1L (child: 10mL/kg) 0.9% saline rapidly. Repeat up to 3x as needed

Hyperosmolar hyperglycaemic state Also known as hyperglycaemic hyperosmolar non-ketotic coma (HONK). Predominantly occurs in patients with type 2 DM (very rarely type 1 DM). Presents with <1wk history of deterioration, ↓ level of consciousness, dehydration ++, ↓ BP with postural drop. Often precipitated by other illness, e.g. infection, MI. May be a presenting feature of type 2 DM. Blood sugar (on blood testing strip) is >35mmol/L.

⚠ **Action** Admit immediately to hospital.

Myxoedema coma

Typical presentation

- >65y old
- History of thyroid surgery/ radioactive iodine
- May be precipitated by MI, stroke, infection, or trauma
- Looks hypothyroid
- Hypothermia
- Hyporeflexia
- Heart failure
- Cyanosis
- Bradycardia
- Coma
- Seizures

Investigation Finger prick blood glucose may be ↓.

⚠ Action

- Keep warm
- Treat heart failure with diuretics ± opioids and nitrates—📖 p. 1088
- Admit as an emergency to hospital

Hyperthyroid crisis (thyrotoxic storm)

Risk factors

- Recent thyroid surgery/history of radioactive iodine
- Infection
- Trauma
- MI

Presentation

- Fever
- Agitation and/or confusion
- Coma
- Tachycardia/AF
- Diarrhoea and vomiting
- Acute abdomen
- May have goitre ± thyroid bruit

⚠ Action Admit as an emergency to hospital.

Hypoadrenal (Addisonian) crisis May occur in patients on long-term steroids (treatment or replacement) if the steroids are stopped suddenly or not ↑ during intercurrent illness *or* may be a presenting feature of congenital adrenal hyperplasia or Addison's disease. Presents with vomiting, hypotension, and shock.

Management Give IM or IV hydrocortisone:

- Adults and children >12y: **100mg**
- Children 1mo–12y: **2–4mg/kg**

Admit to hospital for further management.

Prevention of Addisonian crises

- Warn all patients taking long-term steroids not to stop their steroids abruptly and to tell any doctor treating them about their condition
- Advise patients to carry a steroid card or Addison's disease self-help group emergency card, and wear a Medic-Alert bracelet or similar in case of emergency
- Double dose of steroid prior to dental treatment or if intercurrent illness (e.g. URTI)
- If vomiting, replace oral steroid with IM hydrocortisone

Obstetric emergencies

Resuscitation of the newborn 📖 p. 1066

Eclampsia Occurs when a pregnant woman has a fit as a result of pre-eclampsia. Usually BP is very high and, if the baby is not yet born, it becomes distressed. There is a serious risk of stroke in the mother. Women with pre-eclampsia have a 2% chance of eclamptic seizure. 44% occur after the baby is born—usually <24h after delivery. Give buccal midazolam (10mg) or PR diazepam (10–20mg) or IV lorazepam (4mg) and admit as an acute 'blue light' emergency.

HELLP syndrome Occurs in pregnancy or <48h after delivery. Associated with severe pre-eclampsia.
- **H**aemolysis
- **E**levated **L**iver enzymes
- **L**ow **P**latelets

Signs Hypertension (80%); right upper quadrant pain (90%); nausea and vomiting (50%); oedema.

Management Admit for obstetric assessment.

Obstetric shock *Causes:*
- Haemorrhage—APH (📖 p. 818); placental abruption (remember— bleeding may be internal and not seen per vaginum); PPH (📖 p. 819)
- Ruptured uterus
- Inverted uterus
- Pulmonary embolus
- Anaphylaxis (usually drugs)
- Amniotic fluid embolism
- Broad ligament haematoma
- Septicaemia

⚠ Action
- Call for help
- Arrange immediate admission to the nearest specialist obstetric unit (or A&E, if necessary)
- Gain IV access and start IV fluids; give O₂ via face mask (if available)
- Treat the cause if apparent

Fetal distress Signifies hypoxia. *Signs:*
- Passage of meconium during labour
- Fetal tachycardia (>160bpm at term)
- Fetal bradycardia (<100bpm, seek urgent obstetric assistance)

⚠ Action
- Give the mother oxygen via a face mask and turn her onto her side
- Transfer immediately to a specialist obstetric unit for further assessment ± delivery

Acute abdominal pain in pregnancy Non-obstetric causes of abdominal pain may be forgotten or signs may be less well localized than in the non-pregnant patient (📖 p. 1098).

Appendicitis Mortality is higher in pregnancy and perforation more common (15–20%). Fetal mortality is 5–10% for simple appendicitis but rises to 30% when there is perforation. Due to the pregnancy, the appendix is displaced and pain is often felt in the paraumbilical region or subcostally. Admit immediately if suspected.

Cholecystitis Pregnancy encourages gallstone formation. Symptoms include RUQ pain, nausea, and vomiting. Diagnosis can be confirmed on USS. Treatment is the same as outside pregnancy aiming for interval cholecystectomy after birth.

Fibroids Torsion or red degeneration. Fibroids ↑ in size in pregnancy. They may twist if pedunculated. Red degeneration occurs usually after 20wk and may occur until the puerperium. It presents as abdominal pain ± localized tenderness ± vomiting and low-grade fever. Confirm diagnosis with USS. Treatment is with rest and analgesia. Pain resolves within 1wk.

Ovarian cysts Torsion or rupture of a cyst may both cause abdominal pain as may bleeding into a cyst. USS can confirm the presence of a cyst. Management depends on the nature of the cyst and the severity of the pain. Admit for assessment.

If <20wk gestation, also consider
- Miscarriage 📖 p. 815
- Ectopic pregnancy 📖 p. 816

If >20wk gestation, also consider
- Labour 📖 p. 832
- Pubic symphysis dehiscence 📖 p. 803
- Placental abruption
- Uterine rupture
- Haematoma of the rectus abdominis Rarely bleeding into the rectus sheath and haematoma formation occurs spontaneously or after coughing in late pregnancy. May cause swelling and abdominal tenderness. USS can be helpful. If unsure of diagnosis admit to exclude acute surgical or obstetric cause of pain

Uterine rupture Rare in the UK. Associated with maternal mortality of 5% and fetal mortality of 30%. 70% are due to dehiscence of Caesarean section scars. Rupture occurs most commonly during labour but occasionally in the 3rd trimester or after an otherwise normal delivery.

Presentation Pain is variable but usually severe, bursting, constant lower abdominal pain ± heavy vaginal bleeding. Generally associated with profound shock in the mother and fetal distress. If in labour, the presenting part may disappear from the pelvis ± contractions stop.

⚠ **Action** Admit as an acute emergency to a specialist obstetric unit.

Placental abruption (abruptio placentae) Part of the placenta becomes detached from the uterus. Consequences depend on the degree of separation and the amount of blood loss.

Presentation
- Typically constant pain—may be felt in the back if posterior placenta
- Woody hard, tender uterus
- Shock ± PV bleeding
- Fetal heart absent or signs of fetal distress (fetal tachycardia or bradycardia)

⚠ **Action** If suspected admit as an acute emergency to the nearest specialist obstetric unit.

Shoulder dystocia Affects <1% deliveries but is a life-threatening emergency. Occurs when the anterior shoulder impacts upon the symphysis pubis after the head has delivered and prevents the rest of the baby following. Most cases of shoulder dystocia are unanticipated.

Clues
- Prolonged 1st or 2nd stage of labour
- 'Head bobbing'—the head consistently descends then returns to its original position during a contraction or pushing in the 2nd stage

❶ If shoulder dystocia occurs in the community there is usually not time to transfer a woman to a specialist unit.

⚠ *Action* Call for help. Consider episiotomy. Then try any of these procedures (no particular order):
- Roll the mother onto hands and knees and try delivering posterior shoulder first
- Flex and abduct the mother's legs up to her abdomen (upside down squatting position)—try delivery again
- Deliver the posterior arm—put a hand in the vagina in front of the baby—ensure the posterior elbow is flexed in front of the body and pull to deliver the forearm. The anterior shoulder usually follows
- External pressure—ask an assistant to apply suprapubic pressure with the heel of the hand—a rocking movement can help
- Adduction of the most accessible (preferably anterior) shoulder. Simultaneously put pressure on the posterior clavicle to turn the baby. If unsuccessful continue rotation through 180 degrees and try again

Cord prolapse The cord passes through the os in front of the presenting part of the baby. If the presenting part squashes the cord, umbilical blood flow is restricted causing fetal hypoxia and distress (fetal mortality 10–17%).

Risk factors
- Malpresentation—breech/ transverse/oblique
- Cephalo-pelvic disproportion
- Multiple pregnancy
- Preterm rupture of membranes
- Polyhydramnios
- Pelvic tumours

⚠ *Action*
- Minimize handling of the cord to prevent spasm
- Try to keep the cord within the vagina
- Call for help

Aim to prevent presenting part from occluding the cord. Try:
- Displacing the presenting part upwards with the examining hand
- Get patient into knee/elbow position—head down
- If possible, drop the head end of the bed
- Fill the bladder with 500–750mL normal saline via a catheter and clamp the catheter

Admit as an emergency to the nearest specialist obstetric unit—usually treated with emergency Caesarean section.

Retained placenta The 3rd stage of labour is complete in <10min in 97% of labours. If the placenta has not been delivered in <30min (to allow for cervical spasm), it will probably not deliver spontaneously.

⚠ **Action**
• Avoid excessive cord traction
• Check the placenta is not in the vagina—remove if it is
• Check the uterus

If the uterus is well contracted Cervical spasm is probably trapping an otherwise separated placenta—wait for cervix to relax to enable removal of the placenta.

If the uterus is bulky The placenta may have failed to separate. Try:
• Rubbing up a contraction
• Putting the baby to the breast (stimulates uterine contraction)
• Giving a further dose of syntometrine
• If the placenta will still not deliver, admit as emergency for manual removal

Uterine inversion Rare.

⚠ **Action** Do not remove the placenta if attached until the uterus is replaced. If noted early, try to replace the uterus. Otherwise admit as an emergency. The mother may become profoundly shocked so set up an IV infusion before transfer if possible, and give O_2 via a face mask.

Broad ligament haematoma Presents in a recently delivered woman as obstetric shock without excessive PV bleeding. Examination reveals pain and tenderness on the affected side. The uterus is deviated from that side.

⚠ **Action** Admit as an acute emergency to the nearest specialist obstetric unit.

Amniotic fluid embolism Very rare. Mortality ~80%. Presents with shock, cyanosis, and dyspnoea. May occur at the height of a contraction.

⚠ **If suspected**
• Call for help
• Resuscitate—Airway; Breathing; Circulation
• Transfer as an emergency to the nearest A&E or obstetric unit

Accidents and injuries

Road accidents Doctors are not legally obliged to attend an accident they happen to pass—but most feel morally obliged to do so.

Immediate action
- Assess the scene
- Ensure that emergency services have been called
- Take steps to ensure your own safety and that of others, e.g. park your vehicle defensively; wear a reflective jacket if available; turn on hazard lights; use warning triangles
- Ensure all vehicle ignitions are turned off
- Triage casualties into priority groups—decide who to attend first
- Forbid smoking

Immediate treatment
- Check the need for basic resuscitation:
  - Airway patent?
  - Breathing adequate?
  - Circulation intact?
- Resuscitate as necessary (📖 p. 1054 or inside back cover)
- Control any haemorrhage with elevation and pressure
- DO NOT attempt to move anyone who potentially could have a back or neck injury until skilled personnel and equipment are available
- Do not give anything by mouth
- Use coats and rugs to keep victims warm
- If available give analgesia (e.g. opioids—but not if significant head injury or risk of intraperitoneal injury; Entonox®—from ambulance)
- If shocked set up IV fluids if available
- Take directions from the paramedics—they are almost certainly more experienced than you in these situations

Medicolegal issues
- Ensure your medico-legal insurance covers emergency treatments
- Keep full records of events, action taken, drugs administered, origin of drugs, batch numbers, and expiry dates
- A GP can charge a fee to the victims for any assistance given

Road safety Road accidents are responsible for 30–40% of all fatal accidents. *Prevention:*
- Wear seat belts and appropriate protective clothing (e.g. helmet if riding a pedal or motorcycle)
- Avoid alcohol/other drugs that hamper performance when driving
- Supervise children close to roads; teach them the Green Cross code
- Keep speed down
- Keep vehicles well maintained
- When cycling, use cycle tracks if available
- Do not drive if tired or ill
- Ensure that children are properly strapped in

Burns and scalds 📖 p. 1114

Head and facial injury 📖 p. 1112

Poisoning and overdose 📖 p. 1116

Muscle injuries/sprains 📖 p. 502

Drowning 📖 p. 1126

Fractures 📖 p. 1110

Whiplash 📖 p. 475

Figure 29.18 Who should have tetanus vaccination?

The content of the figure is as follows:

OPEN WOUND

Tetanus-prone injuries
- Wounds/burns that require surgical intervention that is delayed for >6h
- Wounds/burns that show a significant degree of devitalized tissue or a puncture-type injury, particularly where there has been contact with soil/manure.
- Wounds containing foreign bodies
- Compound fractures.
- Wounds/burns in patients who have systemic sepsis.

High risk Heavy contamination with material likely to contain tetanus spores and/or extensive devitalized tissue.

Fully immunized (i.e. ≥5 doses of vaccine at appropriate intervals), or primary immunization complete and boosters up to date but incomplete
→ No vaccination needed—give human tetanus immunoglobulin if high-risk, tetanus-prone wound

Not immunized, immunization status unknown, primary immunization incomplete or boosters not up to date
→ Give an immediate dose of tetanus vaccine and further doses as needed to complete the recommended schedule. Give human tetanus immunoglobulin at a different site if tetanus-prone wound

Schedule
Primary immunization 3 doses with 1mo between each (i.e. 2nd dose 1mo after 1st dose and 3rd dose 1mo after 2nd dose)
Booster doses 1 booster dose 5y after primary immunization (3y if child <10y) and a 2nd booster dose 10y after the first booster dose

Haematoma Subungual—📖 p. 487; pinna—📖 p. 1113

Wounds Most patients with significant lacerations present directly to A&E. If a patient presents to general practice, perform immediate care (elevate bleeding limb and apply pressure to arrest bleeding). Advise nil by mouth and transfer to A&E.

Minor lacerations
- Ensure no foreign body is in the wound—if in doubt refer for X-ray/surgical exploration (especially important if injury was with glass)
- Wash wound and clean away debris and any necrotic material
- Check there is no damage to underlying nerves, tendons, bone, or blood supply before dressing or closing a wound
- Aim to oppose the skin edges without tension to allow healing
- Do not attempt to close a wound if you are not confident that you can achieve an adequate result
- Always refer cuts through the lip margin to A&E; consider referral to A&E for any facial wounds and wounds in children
- Check tetanus status (see Figure 29.18)
- In assault cases take particular care to document all injuries carefully, e.g. with photographs, drawings, and measurements of wounds
- Consider non-accidental injury in children—📖 p. 924

Closing the wound Options:
- **Skin closure strips** Use for small cuts in non-hairy skin not under tension or in addition to sutures for larger wounds
- **Skin 'glue' (e.g. Histoacryl®)** Quick (takes 30s to set) and can be used on hairy skin such as the scalp
- **Suturing** Undertake training before attempting suturing.
  - Infiltrate wound edges with 1% lidocaine (maximum 2mg/kg)
  - Addition of adrenaline (epinephrine) can help haemostasis but must not be used on digits or extremities, as necrosis can occur
  - Take care to oppose edges accurately—start interrupted sutures in the middle of the wound
  - Use appropriate suture (e.g. adult face 5–0 monofilament nylon remove after 5d; limbs or trunk 3–0 nylon—remove after 1–2wk)

> **Pretibial lacerations** The shin has poor blood supply especially in the elderly. Flap wounds are common, may heal poorly ± break down to form ulcers. *Management:* wash wound. Carefully realign the flap; secure with skin closure strips without tension, and bandage. Advise elevation of the leg. Review regularly to check healing.

Airgun pellets Common. Refer for X-ray. Can be difficult to remove—leave in place if not in a harmful position. If in a joint, refer for removal.

Fish hooks Infiltrate with lidocaine. Push the hook forwards through the skin until the barb is exposed. Cut the barb off and then ease the hook back through the skin the same way it entered.

Knocked-out teeth Ask the patient to suck tooth clean, reinsert, or store in milk or saliva and send to a dentist.

Coin and other foreign body ingestion Most coins will pass through the gut without any problems. If asymptomatic, they can be left to take their course (advise checking stools to ensure passed). If symptomatic refer for X-ray and consideration for endoscopic removal. If there is any indication of aspiration refer urgently.

Foreign bodies in the ear Most common in children. Try to remove under direct vision with forceps but avoid pushing objects deeper into the canal and causing damage. Do not poke around with forceps in an uncooperative child. Removal under GA may be needed. Insects can be drowned in oil and syringed out.

Foreign bodies in the nose Common in young children. Any child with smelly discharge from one nostril has a foreign body in the nose until proven otherwise—refer for exploration under GA. Do not try to remove yourself unless the object is very superficial and the child cooperative. You might push the object further in and cause trauma.

Removal of ticks Use a commercially available tick remover when possible. If a tick remover is not available, grip the tick as close as possible to the skin with a pair of tweezers, and firmly pull the tick out of the skin.

Animal bites ~200,000 people are bitten by dogs each year in the UK. Animal bites are contaminated and wound infection is common. Clean with soap and water. Check tetanus status. Do not suture unless cosmetically essential and there is minimal tissue damage—refer if in doubt. Give prophylaxis against infection (e.g. co-amoxiclav or erythromycin).

Human bites Are especially prone to infection. Also consider risk of hepatitis B and HIV. If HIV prophylaxis is indicated, it needs to be started immediately—refer urgently to A&E for local policy implementation.

Snake bites The adder is the only poisonous snake in the UK. Bites are only rarely lethal. Attempt to identify the snake and refer the patient urgently to hospital. Do not apply a tourniquet or cut/suck the wound.

Rabies risk Consider post-exposure prophylaxis for rabies (vaccination ± immunoglobulin) if:
- Any exposure to bat secretions or bat bites in the UK or elsewhere (people who work with bats should be vaccinated prior to exposure)
- Animal bite or exposure to animal secretions elsewhere in the world—risk depends on the location

Further information HPA ℘ www.hpa.org.uk

Insect stings Response depends on the insect involved and the individual's response. Ranges from blisters through papules to urticarial wheals—2° infection is common.

Anaphylaxis Follow algorithm in Figure 29.10, ⊞ p. 1073 and admit to hospital as a blue light emergency.

Immediately after the sting Remove any sting present in the wound; often no further treatment is needed.
- **If severe local reaction occurs** Apply an ice pack; give oral antihistamine (e.g. chlorphenamine 4mg stat); continue antihistamine 4–6 hourly as needed
- **If 2° bacterial infection** Treat with oral or topical antibiotics

Remove sources of insects, e.g. remove fleas from carpets with household flea spray (multiple bites on ankles and lower legs).

Weaver fish sting Common on sandy beaches. The fish lurks under the sand so usually trodden on—presents with severe pain in the foot. Immerse the affected area in uncomfortably hot (but not scalding) water. Give analgesia. Pain resolves after 2–3d.

Jellyfish sting
- Remove the patient from the sea as soon as possible
- Scrape or wash adherent tentacles off
- Alcoholic solutions including suntan lotions should *not* be applied because they may cause further discharge of stinging hairs
- Ice packs ↓ pain and a slurry of baking soda (sodium bicarbonate), but not vinegar, may be useful for treating stings from UK species

Home safety Every year >4,000 people die due to accidents in the home and nearly 3 million seek treatment in A&E departments. Spot the dangers; offer safety advice (e.g. from HV if young children in the house); fit smoke alarms and safety devices (e.g. stair gates for toddlers); ensure adequate supervision of children or elderly confused people; maintain equipment correctly.

Fractures

- **Symptoms** Pain—worse on movement, ↓ function
- **Signs** Swelling; bruising; deformity; local tenderness; impaired function; crepitus; abnormal mobility

⚠ *Action*

- Immobilize the affected part and give analgesia
- If available and the patient is shocked, start an IV infusion
- Refer to A&E for assessment, X-ray, and treatment

Ottawa rules for ankle or foot injury Foot and ankle injuries are common. It can be difficult to distinguish between a sprain and a fracture. The Ottawa rules ↓ need for X-ray by a quarter:

Ankle injury Refer for an ankle X-ray if there is pain in the malleolar area AND:
- Bone tenderness at the posterior tip of the lateral malleolus, or
- Bone tenderness at the posterior tip of the medial malleolus, or
- Unable to weight bear at the time of the injury and when seen

Foot injury Refer for a foot X-ray if there is pain in the mid-foot AND:
- Bone tenderness at the 5th metatarsal base, or
- Bone tenderness at the navicular, or
- Unable to weight bear at the time of injury and when seen

Otherwise diagnose a sprain Treat sprains with rest, ice, compression, elevation, and analgesia (paracetamol ± NSAIDs). If severe (or the patient is an athlete), refer to physiotherapy.

Fractures See Table 29.7.

 Always consider assessment and treatment for osteoporosis in all men and women >50y who have had a Colles' fracture, hip fracture, and/or vertebral collapse.

Head and facial injury 📖 p. 1112

Fracture complications Often occur after the patient has been discharged from hospital and may present as a primary care emergency. Refer back to the fracture clinic or A&E if:
- Persistent pain
- Offensive odour or discharge
- Wound infection that is not settling with oral antibiotics
- External pins/wires become infected
- External pins/wires are catching on clothing or other parts of the body
- Cast edges are abrading the skin
- Cast has deteriorated in structural strength, e.g. from getting wet

- Limb swelling that is not settling

Compartment syndrome Crush injury, fracture, prolonged immobility, or tight splints, dressings, or casts can result in ↑ pressure within muscle compartments and eventually vascular occlusion. Presents with swelling, severe pain—↑ on passive stretch of muscles, distal numbness, redness, mottling, blisters. ❶ Pulses may be present distally. Loosen any restricting bandage/cast. Refer as an emergency to orthopaedics—fasciotomy may be needed to relieve the pressure.

Table 29.7 Common fractures seen in primary care

Fracture	Features and management
Clavicle	Common injury (5% all fractures). Usually results from a fall onto an outstretched arm. 80% fractures are in the middle third; 15% the lateral third; and 5% the medial third
	Refer to A&E for confirmation of diagnosis and fracture clinic follow-up. Treatment is with sling support and analgesia. Most heal well
	Complications Pneumothorax, malunion, and nerve/vessel damage
Colles'	Most commonly due to a fall onto an outstretched hand in an elderly lady. Pain and swelling of the wrist ('dinner fork' deformity)
	Refer any suspected fracture for X-ray and reduction
	Complications Include rupture of the extensor pollicis longus tendon, carpal tunnel syndrome, and reflex sympathetic dystrophy
Scaphoid	Caused by falling onto an outstretched hand. Pain, swelling, and tenderness in the anatomical snuffbox
	Symptoms may be mild and fracture is easily missed—refer suspected cases for scaphoid view X-rays. If X-ray is inconclusive and pain continues, repeat 2wk later–bone scan or MRI can help if still –ve
	Non-union and avascular necrosis of the proximal fragment is a potential complication, which can lead to long-term problems of arthritis and pain
Fingers	Common injuries. Often associated with sport. Refer all suspected fractures for X-ray + reduction
Hip	Common amongst the elderly and carries high morbidity and mortality (~25%). ♀>♂. Usually occurs through the neck of the femur
	Risk factors Maternal hip fracture, osteoporosis; unsteadiness; sedative medication, poor eyesight, and polypharmacy
	There may be a history of a fall but not always. Suspect in any patient who is elderly or has risk factors for osteoporosis who is 'off legs'. Occasionally, patients can still weight bear with difficulty
	Signs External rotation, shortening, and adduction of leg
	Refer urgently to A&E for X-ray
Ankle	History is of a fall over an obstacle or trip down a step. The ankle rapidly becomes swollen and tender—often bilaterally
	Decide whether an X-ray is needed. If so, refer to A&E
Metatarsals	The most common fracture is of the base of the 5th metatarsal in an 'ankle twisting' injury. March or stress fractures occur in people who do a lot of walking or running and affect the neck/shaft of the 2nd metatarsal
	Decide whether an X-ray is needed. If so, refer to A&E. Undisplaced fractures are usually treated with analgesia and support
Toes	Caused by stubbing the toe or dropping a heavy object on it
	Undisplaced suspected fractures Do not X-ray unless diagnosis is in doubt. Support the injured toe by 'buddy' strapping it to the adjacent toe. Give analgesia
	Fracture displacement and/or dislocation Refer for X-ray and reduction

Head and facial injury

Severe head injury
- Perform basic life support (📖 p. 1054)
- Protect the cervical spine (see 📖 p. 1071)
- Transfer to A&E by ambulance

Less severe head injuries

History If possible take the history from a witness as well as the patient. Ask about circumstances of injury, loss of consciousness (LOC), seizures, current symptoms, and behaviour.

Examination Check scalp, head for injury, neurological examination (including fundi), other injuries—accompanying neck injuries are common.

⚠ *Refer to A&E if*[N]
- Glasgow Coma Scale <15 at any time since injury—📖 p. 1068
- Loss of consciousness
- Focal neurological deficit since injury—problems speaking, understanding, reading, writing, ↓ sensation, loss of balance, weakness, visual changes, abnormal reflexes, problems walking, irritability, or altered behaviour especially in young children
- Any suspicion of skull fracture; penetrating head injury; blood or CSF in the nose, ear, or wound; serious scalp laceration or haematoma
- Amnesia for events before or after injury
- Persistent headache
- Vomiting
- Seizure
- Any previous cranial neurosurgical interventions
- High-energy head injury (e.g. pedestrian hit by motor vehicle, fall >1m or >5 stairs)
- History bleeding or clotting disorder or on anticoagulant therapy
- Difficulty in assessing the patient (e.g. very young, elderly, intoxicated or epileptic) or concern about diagnosis
- Suspicion of non-accidental injury
- Inadequate supervision at home

❶ If Glasgow Coma Scale is <15, neck pain/tenderness, focal neurological deficit, paraesthesiae in the extremities or any other clinical suspicion of cervical spine injury, immobilize the neck and refer to A&E.

If examination is normal
- Warn the patient (+ carer) that he/she may suffer mild headaches, tiredness, dizziness, tinnitus, poor concentration, and poor memory for the next few days
- Advise rest and paracetamol (but not codeine-based analgesics) for the headache
- Young children can be difficult to assess—sleepiness is common and not a worrying sign as long as the child is rousable
- Give written head injury information regarding warning signs to trigger reconsultation—drowsiness, severe headache, persistent vomiting, visual disturbance, and/or unusual behaviour

Injury to the face Mostly due to RTAs and violent incidents. Carefully document injuries as your notes may be required for legal proceedings. Look for other injuries, e.g. airway problems, head injury, neck injury. Palpate the face for signs of a fracture—if present refer to maxillofacial surgeons for assessment. Check tetanus status. Post-traumatic stress disorder (📖 p. 998) is common after facial injury.

Specific injuries

- **Facial lacerations** Best sutured by an experienced surgeon. Refer to A&E
- **Fractured mandible** A blow to the jaw can cause unilateral or bilateral fractures. Presents with pain (worse on moving jaw), bruising ± bleeding inside the mouth ± discontinuity of the teeth (displaced fracture) ± numbness of the lower lip (if the inferior dental nerve has been damaged). Refer for X-ray
- **Dislocated jaw** Presents with pain and the mouth is stuck open—refer for X-ray and reduction
- **Fractured zygoma/malar complex** A blow on the cheek may fracture the zygomatic arch in isolation or more usually cause a 'tripod' fracture. *Signs:* bony tenderness, flattening of the malar process— best seen from above (may be masked by swelling), epistaxis, subconjunctival haemorrhage extending posteriorly, and infraorbital numbness ± jaw locked. Refer for X-ray. Advise not to blow nose
- **Middle third facial fractures (Le Fort)** Usually bilateral. *Signs:* epistaxis, CSF rhinorrhoea, crepitus on palpation, swelling, open bite, and risk of airway compromise. Refer for X-ray
- **Haematoma of the pinna** Usually after trauma (e.g. rugby). Must be evacuated urgently (aspirated via large-bore needle or surgically) to prevent necrosis of the cartilage and 'cauliflower' ear—refer
- **Nasal fracture and other nasal injuries** 📖 p. 941
- **'Blow out' fracture of orbit** 📖 p. 959
- **Whiplash** 📖 p. 475
- **Avulsed tooth** 📖 p. 1108
- **Dog bite** 📖 p. 1108

Post-concussion syndrome Seen following even quite minor head injury. Due to neuronal damage. Features include all, or some, of:

- Headache
- Dizziness
- Poor concentration
- Fatigue
- Depression
- Memory problems

Treatment is supportive and symptoms usually resolve with time (although can take months or even years).

Further information

NICE Triage, assessment investigation and early management of head injury in infants, children and adults (2007) ℘ www.nice.org.uk

Scalds and burns

Assess
- Cause, size, and thickness of the burn
- Use the 'rule of nines' to estimate the extent of the burn (see Box 29.1)
- Partial thickness burns are red, painful, and blistered; full thickness burns are painless and white or grey
- Always consider non-accidental injury in children—📖 p. 924

⚠ Action
- Remove clothing from the affected area and place under cold running water for >10min or until pain is relieved
- Do not burst blisters
- Prescribe/give analgesia
- Refer all but the smallest (<5%) partial thickness burns for assessment in A&E
- Refer all electrical burns for assessment in A&E
- Refer all chemical burns for assessment in A&E unless burn area is minimal and pain-free
- Consider referral to A&E for smoke inhalation

If managing the burn in the community
- Check tetanus immunity, and give immunization ± prophylaxis as necessary—📖 p. 1107
- Apply silver sulfadiazine cream (Flamazine®) or paraffin-impregnated gauze and non-adherent dressings and review for healing and infection every 1–2d
- Cover burns on hands in Flamazine® and place in a plastic bag—elevate the hand in a sling and encourage finger movement
- Refer if burns are not healed in 10–12d

Prevention of scalds and burns
- Prevention through public education is important
- Children often sustain burns by pulling on the flex of boiling kettles or irons, pulling on saucepan handles, or climbing onto hot cookers
- Refer any children who have sustained accidental burns to the health visitor for follow-up

Smoke inhalation
- Refer all patients who have potentially inhaled smoke for assessment—a seemingly well patient can deteriorate later
- Smoke can cause thermal injury, carbon monoxide poisoning, and cyanide poisoning
- Airway problems occur due to thermal and chemical damage to the airways causing oedema—suspect if singed nasal hairs, a sore throat, or a hoarse voice
- Carbon monoxide poisoning may result in the classic cherry-red mucosa—but this may be absent
- Cyanide poisoning is commonly due to smouldering plastics and causes dizziness, headaches, and seizures

Box 29.1 'Rule of nines' Ignore areas of erythema only.

Palm	1%
Arm (all over)	9%
Leg (all over)	18% (14% children)
Front	18%
Back	18%
Head (all over)	9% (14% children)
Genitals	1%

 The 'rule of nines' is inaccurate for children <10y. For children and for small burns, estimate the extent of the burn by comparison with the area of the patient's hand. The area of the fingers and palm ~1% total body surface area burn.

Sunburn Susceptibility depends on skin type.
- Tingling is followed 2–12h later by erythema. Redness is maximal at 24h and fades over 2–3d. Desquamation and pigmentation follow
- Severe sunburn may cause blistering, pain, and systemic upset. Treatment is symptomatic with calamine lotion prn (some advocate application of vinegar) and paracetamol for pain
- Rarely, dressings are required for blisters or, in severe cases, hospital admission for fluid management
- Predisposes to skin cancer and photoageing

The sun safety code Take care not to burn in the sun
- Cover up with loose cool clothing, a hat, and sunglasses
- If swimming outdoors or on the beach, dress in a UV protective sunsuit. When out of the water, add a T-shirt, sunglasses, and sun hat
- Seek shade during the hottest part of the day
- Apply sunscreen (≥SPF 25) on sun-exposed parts of the body

Burns in special situations

Chemical burns
- Usually caused by strong acids or alkalis
- Wear gloves to remove contaminated clothing
- Irrigate with cold running water for ≥20min
- Do not attempt to neutralize the chemical—this can exacerbate injury by producing heat
- Refer all burns to A&E, unless the burn area is minimal and pain-free

Electric shock
- Causes thermal tissue injury and direct injury due to the electric current passing through the tissue
- Skin burns may be seen at the entry and exit site of the current
- Muscle damage can be severe with minimal skin injury
- Cardiac damage may occur and rhabdomyolysis can → renal failure
- Refer all patients for specialist management

Poisoning or overdose

On receiving the call for assistance

- Try to establish what has happened—substances involved, ongoing dangers, state of the patient
- Advise the caller to stay with the patient until you arrive
- If the patient is unconscious, immediately arrange for an ambulance to attend, then visit
- Arrange for the patient to be removed from any source of danger, e.g. contaminated clothing or inhaled gases. DO NOT put yourself or anyone else in danger attempting to do this. If necessary call the fire brigade, who have protective clothing and equipment, to help remove a patient from a dangerous environment

Assessment of the unconscious patient

Assess the need for basic life support

- **A**irway patent?
- **B**reathing satisfactory?
- **C**irculation adequate?

Resuscitation (🕮 p. 1116) takes priority over everything else.

Additionally

- If breathing is depressed and opioid overdose is a possibility, give naloxone 0.4–2mg IV every 2–3min to a maximum of 10mg (*child*—10 micrograms/kg and then, if no response, 100 micrograms/kg)
- Check BM—if low, give 50–250mL 10% glucose IV in 50mL aliquots

General examination

- BP
- Pulse
- Temperature
- Level of coma (🕮 p. 1068)
- Pupil responses
- Evidence of IV drug abuse
- Obvious injury

❶ The coma may not be due to poisoning/overdose.

If unconscious, turn into the recovery position 🕮 p. 1071. Check no contraindications first, e.g. spinal injury.

Note down any information about the exposure

- **Product name** As much detail as possible—if unidentified tablets, see if any are left and send them to the hospital in their own container (if there is one) with the patient
- **Time of the incident**
- **Duration of exposure/amount ingested**
- **Route of exposure** Swallowed, inhaled, injected, etc.
- **Whether intentional or accidental**
- **Take a general history from any attendant** Medical history, current medication, substance abuse, alcohol, social circumstances

Assessment of the conscious patient

- Note down any information about the exposure as for the unconscious patient
- Record symptoms the patient is experiencing as a result of exposure

- Examine—pulse, BP, temperature (if necessary), level of consciousness or confusion, evidence of IV drug abuse, any injuries
- If non-accidental exposure assess suicidal intent (📖 p. 1119)
- Take a general history from the patient and/or any attendant—medical history, current medication, substance abuse, alcohol, social circumstances

Consider admission if
- The patient's clinical condition warrants it: unconsciousness, respiratory depression, etc.
- The exposure warrants admission for treatment or observation:
  - **Symptomatic poisoning** Admit to hospital
  - **Agents with delayed action** Aspirin, iron, paracetamol, tricyclic antidepressants, co-phenotrope, paraquat, and modified-release preparations. Admit to hospital even if the patient seems well
  - **Other agents** Consult poisons information
- You judge there is serious suicidal intent (📖 p. 1119) or the patient has another mental health condition which warrants acute admission
- There is a lack of social support

 Overdose and poisoning in children Peak incidence of accidental poisoning is at 2y—mainly household substances, prescribed or OTC drugs, or plants. Teenagers may take deliberate overdoses—especially of OTC medication, e.g. paracetamol.
⚠ Poisoning can be a form of non-accidental injury (📖 p. 924).

Deliberate self-harm (DSH) Deliberate non-fatal act committed in the knowledge that it was potentially harmful and, in the case of drug overdose, that the amount taken was excessive. 90% DSH is due to self-poisoning and it accounts for 20% of admissions to general medical wards—the most frequent reason for admission for young ♀ patients. Paracetamol or aspirin are the most common drugs used. Self-harm is often aimed at changing a situation (e.g. to get a boyfriend back), communication of distress ('cry for help'), a sign of emotional distress, or may be a failed genuine suicide attempt.

Management 📖 p. 1118

❶ People who have self-harmed should be treated with the same care respect and privacy as any other patient.

Poisons information
UK National Poisons Information Service ☎ 0844 892 1111 (Ireland: (01) 809 2566)
TOXBASE poisons database 🖱 www.toxbase.org (registration required)

Suicide and attempted suicide

Calls to patients who have deliberately self-harmed themselves, are threatening suicide or if relatives are worried about suicide risk are common primary care emergencies.

- **Assessment** See Figure 29.20
- **Management** See Figure 29.19

Compulsory admission 📖 p. 1122

Suicide prevention In the UK, 1 in 5,600 ♂ and 1 in 18,000 ♀ commits suicide. Suicide risk can be ↓ by:

- Early recognition, assessment, and treatment of those likely to attempt suicide—many visit their GP just weeks before suicide
- Planning follow-up care for those discharged from psychiatric hospitals
- ↓ availability and lethality of suicide methods, e.g. avoid TCAs and carefully monitor antidepressant repeat prescriptions

```
              ┌─────────────────────────┐
              │   Assess suicide risk   │
              │   (see Figure 29.20)    │
              └─────────────────────────┘
```

High risk of suicide
- Direct statement of intent
- Severe mood change
- Hopelessness
- Alcohol or drug dependence
- Abnormal personality
- Living alone

Lower risk of suicide

Admit as a psychiatric emergency using the Mental Health Act for compulsory admission (📖 p. 1122) if voluntary admission is declined.

Arrange for someone to stay with the patient until follow-up. Remove all potentially harmful drugs. Liaise with the mental health services according to the individual patient about mental health follow-up.

⚠ Mothers of young children who deliberately self-harm/attempt suicide have ↑ risk of child abuse. Assess risks, offer support, arrange for health visitor, or social services to visit.

Figure 29.19 Management of patients who have deliberately self-harmed, threatened or attempted suicide

Further information

NICE Self-harm (2004) 🖰 www.nice.org.uk
DH National Suicide Prevention Strategy for England (2012) 🖰 www.dh.gov.uk

Information and support for patients and relatives:
Self-Injury and Related Issues (SIARI) 🖰 www.siari.co.uk
Samaritans 24h emotional support via telephone ☎ 08457 90 90 90 🖰 www.samaritans.org
Survivors of Bereavement by Suicide ☎ 0844 561 6855 🖰 www.uk-sobs.org.uk

If any self-harm Assess the situation and admit to A&E as needed

Ask about suicidal ideas and plans in a sensitive but probing way. It is a common misconception that asking about suicide can plant the idea into a patient's head and make suicide more likely. Evidence is to the contrary

Ask about present circumstances
What problems are making the patient feel this way?
Does he/she still feel like this?
Would the act of suicide be aimed to hurt someone in particular?
What kind of support does the patient have from friends, relatives, and formal services (e.g. community mental health services)?

Assess suicidal risk Ask patient and any relatives/friends present. *Risk factors:*
• ♂ > ♀
• Social isolation
• Depression
• Personality disorder
• Serious illness (e.g. cancer)
• Divorced > widowed > never married > married
• Certain professions: vets, pharmacists, farmers, doctors
• Admission or recent discharge from psychiatric hospital
• Peak age 35–49y
• History of deliberate self-harm (100x ↑ risk)
• Alcohol or substance abuse
• Schizophrenia
• Contact with the criminal justice system

Assess mental health Features associated with ↑ suicide risk are:
• Depression
• Agitation
• Presence of suicidal ideation
• Hopelessness—good predictor of subsequent and immediate risk
• Early schizophrenia with retained insight—especially young patients who see their ambitions restricted
• Presence of delusions of control, poverty, and/or guilt

Useful questions for assessing suicidal ideas and plans
• Do you feel you have a future?
• Do you feel that life's not worth living?
• Do you ever feel completely hopeless?
• Do you ever feel you'd be better off dead and away from it all?
• Have you ever made any plans to end your life (if drug overdose—have you handled the tablets)?
• Have you ever made an attempt to take your own life? If so, was there a final act, e.g. suicide note?
• What prevents you doing it?
• Have you made any arrangements for your affairs after your death?

Figure 29.20 Assessment of patients who have deliberately self-harmed, threatened or attempted suicide

Disturbed behaviour

⚠ **Look after your own safety**
- If the patient is known to be violent, get back-up from the police before entering the situation
- Tell someone you are going in and when to expect an 'exit' call. Advise them to call for help if that call is not made
- Do not put yourself in a vulnerable situation—sit where there is a clear, unimpeded exit route
- Do not make the patient feel trapped
- Do not try to restrain the patient

Acute hyperventilation/panic attack

Features Fear, terror, and feeling of impending doom accompanied by some or all of the following:
- Palpitations
- Shortness of breath
- Choking sensation
- Dizziness
- Paraesthesiae
- Chest pain/discomfort
- Sweating
- Carpopedal spasm

Differential diagnosis
- Dysrhythmia
- Asthma
- Anaphylaxis
- Thyrotoxicosis
- Temporal lobe epilepsy
- Hypoglycaemia
- Phaeochromocytoma (very rare)

Action

- **Talking down** Explain the nature of the symptoms to the patient:
  - Racing of the heart is due to adrenaline produced by the panic
  - Paraesthesiae/feelings of dizziness are secondary to overbreathing due to panic
  - Count breaths in and out gently slowing breathing rate
- **Rebreathing techniques**
  - Place a paper bag over the patient's mouth, and ask him/her to breathe in and out through the mouth
  - A connected but not switched on O_2 mask or nebulizer mask is an alternative in the surgery
  - This raises the partial pressure of CO_2 in the blood and symptoms due to low CO_2 (e.g. tetany, paraesthesiae, dizziness) resolve and also demonstrates the link between hyperventilation and symptoms
- **Propranolol** 10–20mg stat may be helpful—DO NOT USE for asthmatics or patients with heart failure or on verapamil

Recurrent panic attacks 📖 p. 994

Violent or agitated behaviour When a patient becomes very agitated or violent or starts to behave oddly, the GP is usually called—by the patient, relatives or friends, or police attending the disturbance.

Causes of disturbed behaviour

- **Physical illness causing acute delirium** Infection (e.g. UTI, chest infection); hypoglycaemia; hypoxia; head injury; epilepsy—📖 p. 1010

- **Drugs** Alcohol (or alcohol withdrawal); prescribed drugs (e.g. steroid psychosis); illicit drugs (e.g. amphetamines)
- **Mental health problems** Schizophrenia; mania; anxiety/depression; dementia; personality disorder (e.g. attention-seeking; uncontrolled anger)

Assessment

- Before seeing the patient gather as much information as possible from notes, relatives—even neighbours
- Ask the patient and family for any history of drugs or alcohol excess
- Listen to the patient and talk calmly—choose your words carefully
- Try to look for organic causes—this can be difficult in the heat of the moment—physical examination except from a distance may be impossible. Do not put yourself at risk
- Suspect an organic cause where there are visual hallucinations
- Discuss and explain your suggested management with the patient and any attendants
- If the patient is an immediate danger to himself or others, admission is warranted
- If the cause of the behaviour is unclear, admission for investigation is needed
- Instigate management of treatable causes identified, e.g. admit if acute coronary syndrome or stroke is suspected; treat UTI or chest infection
- Consider sedation to cover the period before admission or to alleviate symptoms if admission is inappropriate

Acute management After assessing the problem, decide if hospitalization is required and whether this can be done on a voluntary or involuntary basis.

Suitable drugs to use for sedation

- **Oral** Diazepam 5–10mg po or lorazepam 1mg po/sublingually; chlorpromazine 25mg po (lower dose if elderly)
- **Intramuscular** Lorazepam 1.5–2.5mg; chlorpromazine 25mg; haloperidol 1–3mg

⚠ Avoid sedating patients with COPD, epilepsy, or if the patient has been taking illicit drugs, barbiturates, or alcohol.

Compulsory admission under the Mental health Act 📖 p. 1122

⚠ **Acute dystonia** Can occur soon after giving phenothiazines or butyophenones. *Signs:*

- Torticollis
- Tongue protrusion
- Grimacing
- Opisthotonus

Dystonia can be relieved with IM procyclidine 5–10mg (repeated prn after 20min to a maximum dose of 20mg).

Compulsory admission and treatment of patients with mental illness

Most requiring inpatient care for mental disorder agree to hospital admission and become 'informal' patients. A minority (~5%) require compulsory admission and detention under the Mental Health Act of 2007* and are termed 'sectioned'—in reference to the Section of the Mental Health Act under which they are detained (see Figure 29.21).

Procedure for 'sectioning' a patient

Applications can be made for
- Admission for assessment under Section 2 (📖 p. 1125)
- Admission for treatment under Section 3 (📖 p. 1125)
- Emergency admission under Section 4 (📖 p. 1125)
- Guardianship under Section 7 (📖 p. 1125)

Applications can be made by
- An approved mental health professional (AMHP)
- The nearest relative of the person concerned. Nearest relative is defined in the Act as the 1st surviving person out of:
  - Spouse (or cohabitee for >6mo)
  - Oldest child (if >18y)
  - Parent
  - Oldest sibling (if >18y)
  - Grandparent
  - Grandchild (>18y)
  - Uncle or aunt (>18y)
  - Nephew or niece (>18y)
  - Non-relative living with patient for ≥5y

The applicant (AMHP or nearest relative) must have seen the patient <2wk (<24h in the case of Section 4) before the date of the application.

❶ The AMHP should be chosen rather than the nearest relative wherever possible, to avoid affecting family relationships.

Applications must be based on
- Two medical recommendations (except Section 4 which only needs one). Clinicians may examine the patient together or separately, but there must be <6d between examinations. Recommendations must be signed on or before the date of application
- Where two medical recommendations are required, the clinicians should not be from the same hospital or practice *and* one of the clinicians must be 'approved' under the Mental Health Act
- One clinician, if practicable, must have prior knowledge of the patient (ideally a GP—but GPs are not obliged to attend outside the practice area). If neither clinician has prior knowledge of the patient, the applicant must state on the application why this was so
- Medical recommendation(s) and application must concur on at least one form of mental disorder

* Applies in England and Wales only. In Northern Ireland, similar provisions apply under the Mental Health (Northern Ireland) Order 1986. Scotland—see 📖 p. 1124.

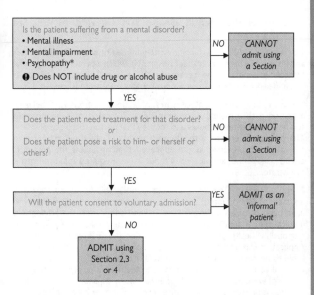

* Personality disorder characterized by inability to make loving relationships, antisocial behavior, and lack of guilt

In practice 'sectioning' means calling in the duty social worker (or other social services approved mental health professional) and duty psychiatrist. It can be a time-consuming and frustrating business. Always try to obtain voluntary admission—it is better for you and the patient.

Keep a supply of forms you might need for sectioning—Forms 3, 7, and 10 (GP recommendation for Section 2, 4, and 3, respectively) and Form 5 (application for Section 4 for a 'nearest relative').

Deputizing doctors should always try to contact the patient's own GP.

Figure 29.21 Deciding whether a 'section' is needed

❶ The Mental Health Act only allows for compulsory assessment and treatment of a patient's mental health problems—the patient may refuse consent for investigation and/or treatment of other health problems whilst 'sectioned'.

Sections of the Mental Health Act relevant to GPs See Table 29.8.

Section 115 Allows an approved mental health professional to enter and inspect any premises (except hospital) in which a person with a mental disorder is living if he/she has reasonable cause to believe that person is not under proper care. Application through a magistrate is needed.

Section 135 Gives right of entry of a police officer who believes a person with a mental disorder is being ill-treated or suffering from self-neglect to enter premises and remove that person to a place of safety. The police officer who attends must be accompanied by an approved mental health professional and approved clinician unless the person is already 'sectioned' and absent without leave. Requires application to a magistrate.

Mental Health Community Act (1995) This Act aims to 'provide a system of supervision of care in the community of certain patients who have been detained in hospital'. In England and Wales, the responsible medical officer applies for 'after care under supervision' (ACUS) to the responsible health authority 6-monthly for the first year then yearly. Application can only be made in respect of a patient (≥16y old) currently liable to be detained in hospital due to a mental disorder where:
- There could be serious risk of harm to the patient or others if the patient were not to receive further care services, *and*
- Supervision would help to ensure receipt of further care services

If patients refuse treatment, they cannot be treated against their will but can be conveyed to a day centre or hospital.

Scotland The Mental Health Act (Care and Treatment) (Scotland) 2003 provides for compulsory admission under Part 5 for 72h. The application is made by a fully registered medical practitioner in consultation with a mental health officer, unless this is impracticable. In hospital Part 6 (lasting 28d) can be applied and then, if necessary, Part 7 (Compulsory Treatment Order) for 6mo.

Further information 🖰 www.scotland.gov.uk

Further information
DH Mental Health Act 2007—overview 🖰 www.dh.gov.uk

Table 29.8 Sections of the Mental Health Act relevant to primary care

Section	Notes	Application
Section 2: *Admission for assessment*	Most commonly used section in the community Admission for 28d for assessment Not renewable after that time Patients may appeal within 2wk of detention via the Mental Health Tribunal	Application must be made by the nearest relative or an AMHP on the recommendation of 2 doctors—one approved and the other who has prior knowledge of the patient If application is made by the AMHP, the nearest relative should be informed before application or as soon as possible afterwards Application is valid for 14d
Section 3: *Admission for treatment*	Admission for treatment for ≤6mo The exact mental disorder must be stated Detention is renewable for a further 6mo. and annually thereafter	Application must be made by the nearest relative or an AMHP on the recommendation of 2 doctors—one approved and the other who has prior knowledge of the patient Application is valid for 14d
Section 4: *Emergency admission for assessment*	Used in situations where admission is urgent and compliance with Section 2 would cause undesirable delay Admission to hospital for 72h only Not renewable Usually converted to a Section 2 on arrival at hospital	Application must be made by the nearest relative or an AMHP If application is made by the AMHP, the nearest relative should be informed before application or as soon as possible afterwards Medical recommendation is from *either* an approved clinician (not necessarily a doctor) *or* a doctor with prior knowledge of the patient Application is only valid for 24h
Section 7: *Guardianship*	A Guardian has power to: • Require a person to live at a particular place • Require a person to go to specific places at specific times for medical treatment, work, education, or training • Require a doctor, AMHP, or other specified person be given access to the person under Guardianship ❶ Guardians can insist a person sees a doctor but cannot force treatment	Application must be made by the nearest relative or an AMHP on the recommendation of 2 clinicians—one approved and the other who has prior knowledge of the patient Application is valid for 14d

Miscellaneous emergencies

Acute limb ischaemia

Causes
- Acute thrombotic occlusion of pre-existing stenotic segment (60%)
- Embolus (30%)
- Trauma, e.g. compartment syndrome or traumatic vessel damage

Presentation
- Pain
- Pallor
- Paraesthesiae
- Pulselessness
- Paralysis
- Perishing cold

Action Admit acutely under the care of a vascular surgeon. Treatment can be surgical (e.g. embolectomy) or medical (e.g. thrombolysis).

Drowning Most common in drunk adults and children poorly supervised around water. Children can drown in a few centimetres of water.

Action
- Call for help
- Start basic life support (Airway, Breathing, Circulation)—📖 p. 1054 (adults); 📖 p. 1060 (children)

⚠ Attempted resuscitation of a seemingly dead child is worthwhile as cooling ↓ metabolic rate and recovery can occur after prolonged immersion.

Prevention Drowning is the third most common cause of accidental death among the under 16s. More than half of those who drown can swim. Most people drown in rivers (25%) or the sea (17%) but for children <4y garden ponds are the most common place of drowning. For adults, alcohol is a contributory factor in 25–50% cases. The best way to ↓ drowning is prevention—spot the dangers; take safety advice; do not go near water alone; learn how to help others.

Hypothermia Defined as a core temperature of <35°C.

Causes
- Not feeling the cold, e.g. neuropathy, confusion, dementia
- Inadequate heat in the home, e.g. poor housing, poverty, and fear of high fuel bill
- Immobility
- Hypothyroidism
- DM
- Alcohol
- ↑ heat loss, e.g. psoriasis, erythroderma
- Inadequate protection from the cold, e.g. unsuitable clothing whilst doing outdoor sports
- Drugs—antipsychotics, antidepressants, barbiturates, tranquillizers—may lower the level of consciousness and ↓ ability to shiver
- Falls—may remain still and cold on the floor until discovered
- Unconsciousness, e.g. overdose, stroke

Presentation Skin pale and cold to touch; puffy face; listlessness, drowsiness, and/or confusion.

When severe ↓ breathing—slow and shallow; ↓ pulse volume—faint and irregular; stiff muscles; loss of consciousness.

Investigation

- Rectal temperature on low-reading thermometer <35°C
- ECG—'J' wave on the end of the QRS complex

Action

- Remove from the cold environment
- Wrap in blankets—including head
- *Do not* use direct heat (e.g. hot water bottles), as this can cause rapid fluid shifts and potentially fatal pulmonary oedema
- Transfer to hospital
- Consider the cause of the incident; liaise with the hospital, primary healthcare team, and social services to prevent recurrence

Heat stroke and heat exhaustion Exercising in excessive heat leads to dehydration, salt depletion, and metabolite accumulation.

Signs Headache, nausea, confusion, incoordination, cramps, weakness, dizziness, malaise.

Treatment Rest, fluid and salt replacement. Admit for IV fluids and supportive measures in severe cases.

Sunburn 📖 p. 1115

Acute altitude sickness Altitude sickness is a potentially fatal complication of rapidly climbing to altitudes >2,500m (8,000 feet). 2 main forms: pulmonary oedema and cerebral oedema. Presents with fatigue, headache, dizziness, nausea/loss of appetite, breathlessness, palpitations, and/or insomnia. Treatment is with oxygen therapy and descent to a lower altitude. Prevent by gradual ascent. Use of prophylactic acetazolamide is controversial.

Wound dehiscence Breakdown of a surgical wound—usually abdominal. May be partial or complete.

- **Partial breakdown** Skin remains intact but muscle layers break down → incisional hernia. Typically the patient feels something 'give' ± sudden ↑ in pain and pink fluid discharge. Refer for urgent reassessment by the operating surgeon
- **Complete dehiscence** Wound breaks down entirely. The patient becomes shocked and distressed. Lie flat; give strong opioid analgesia; cover the wound with a sterile pack soaked in saline; admit as a '999' emergency

Risk factors

- Malnutrition
- Obesity
- ↑ intra-abdominal pressure, e.g. from coughing
- Wound infection
- Haematoma formation
- Ascites draining through a wound

Index

W

waddling gait 545
waist circumference 178, 179
Wales, NHS structure 11
walk-in clinics 99
walking problems 544–5
war pensions scheme 223
warfarin 672, 673
warts, viral 634
  genital 748–9
weaning 872
weaver fish sting 1109
websites 42–3
Wegener's granulomatosis 524
weight loss 175
  maintenance of 179
  respiratory disease 300
Wells' diagnostic algorithm 291
Wernicke's encephalopathy 581
West's syndrome 899
wheelchairs 228
wheeze 298
  in children 886
whiplash injuries 475
Whipple's disease 407
Whipple's procedure 432
white cell count 660, 661

white coat hypertension 246
white patches 592
white reflex asystolic (anoxic) attacks 896
white spots 592
white-coat concordance 142
whitlow, staphylococcal (felon) 633
whole body donation 113
whooping cough 328, 813
widowed parent's allowance 115
Wilms' nephroblastoma 858–9
Wilson–Jungner criteria 170
Wilson's disease 423
Wiskott–Aldrich syndrome 683
Wolff–Parkinson–White syndrome 269
women
  genital tract, congenital abnormalities 720
  sexual problems 774–5
Work Capability Assessment (WCA) 124
work-related upper limb pain 485
working abroad 71
working hours 4

Working Time Regulations (1998) 37
workload 4
Workplace (Health, Safety and Welfare) Regulations (1992) 39
Workplace-Based Assessment 66
wound care 1036, 1037
wounds 1107–8
  dehiscence 1127
  infection 633
wrist/hand problems 484–7
writer's cramp 546
wry neck 475

X

xanthelasma 640
xanthomata 233, 640

Y

yohimbine 777

Z

zanamivir 323
Zollinger–Ellison syndrome 388
zygomatic fracture 1113

Adult basic life support algorithm

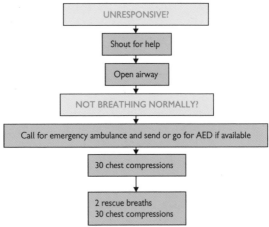

❶ Give 15 chest compressions for every 2 rescue breaths for children

Automated external defibrillator algorithm

Adult advanced life support algorithm: 📖 p. 1059
Paediatric advanced life support algorithm: 📖 p. 1065
Newborn advanced life support algorithm: 📖 p. 1067